Hematological Malignancies
in Children, Adolescents and Young Adults

Hematological Malignancies
in Children, Adolescents and Young Adults

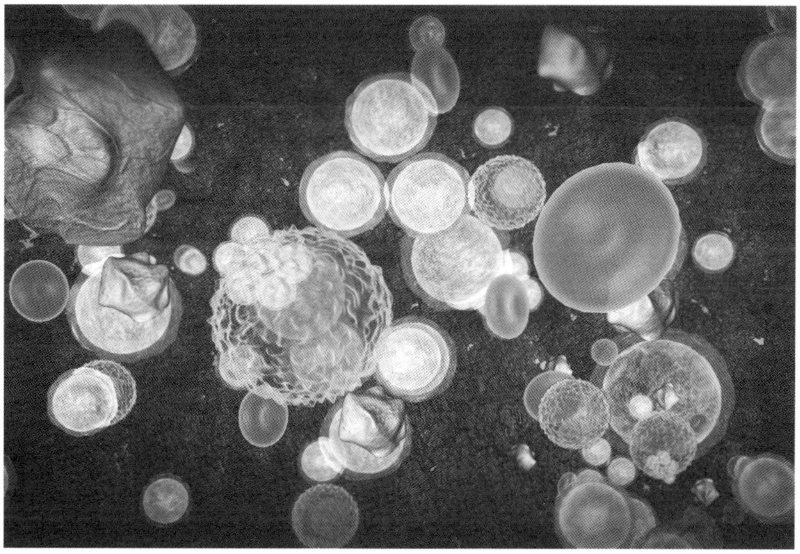

Edited by

Mitchell S Cairo
New York Medical College, USA

Sherrie L Perkins
The University of Utah, USA

World Scientific

NEW JERSEY · LONDON · SINGAPORE · BEIJING · SHANGHAI · HONG KONG · TAIPEI · CHENNAI

Published by

World Scientific Publishing Co. Pte. Ltd.

5 Toh Tuck Link, Singapore 596224

USA office: 27 Warren Street, Suite 401-402, Hackensack, NJ 07601

UK office: 57 Shelton Street, Covent Garden, London WC2H 9HE

British Library Cataloguing-in-Publication Data
A catalogue record for this book is available from the British Library.

HEMATOLOGICAL MALIGNANCIES IN CHILDREN, ADOLESCENTS AND YOUNG ADULTS (With CD-ROM)

ISBN-13 978-981-4299-60-2
ISBN-10 981-4299-60-X

Typeset by Stallion Press
Email: enquiries@stallionpress.com

Printed in Singapore by Mainland Press Pte Ltd.

Contents

Contributing Authors

Chapter 1

Mark B. Geyer, MD
Resident Physician, Department of Medicine
Clinical Fellow in Medicine
Massachusetts General Hospital
Harvard Medical School
Boston, MA

Judith S. Jacobson, DrPH, MBA
Associate Professor of Clinical Epidemiology
Mailman School of Public Health and
Herbert Irving Comprehensive Cancer Center
Columbia University
New York, NY, USA

Chapter 2

Martine Raphaël, MD, PhD
Professor of Hematology
AP-HP, Bicêtre Hospital,
Paris-Sud University
France

Nicole Brousse, MD
Professor of Pathology
Necker-Enfants Malades Hospital, Paris Descartes University
France

Chapter 3

Gregory H. Reaman, M.D.
Associate Director
Office of Hematology and Oncology Products
OND Center for Drug Evaluation and Research
U.S. Food and Drug Administration
Silver Spring, MD, USA

Maura O'Leary, MD
Medical Officer
Center for Biologics Evaluation & Research (CBER)
U.S. Food and Drug Administration
Rockville, MD, USA

Chapter 4

Sherrie L. Perkins, M.D., Ph.D.
Professor of Pathology
Chief of Hematopathology
University of Utah Health Sciences and ARUP Laboratories
Salt Lake City, UT, USA

Russell A. Higgins, M.D.
Assistant Professor of Pathology
University of Texas, San Antonio
San Antonio, TX, USA

Marsha Kinney, M.D.
Professor of Pathology
Chief of Hematopathology
University of Texas, San Antonio
San Antonio, TX, USA

Jerry Hussong, M.D., D.D.S.
Associate Professor of Pathology
Professor of Pathology
University of Utah Health Sciences and ARUP Laboratories
Salt Lake City, UT, USA

Chapter 5

Susana C. Raimondi, Ph.D., FACMG
Director of Cytogenetics Laboratory
St. Jude Children's Research Hospital
Memphis, Tennessee,USA

Nyla A. Heerema, PhD
Professor of Pathology
The Ohio State University
Director of Cytogenetics Laboratory
The Ohio State University Medical Center
Columbus, OH, USA

Chapter 6
Charles G. Mullighan, MBBS(Hons), MSc, MD
Department of Pathology
St. Jude Children's Research Hospital
Memphis, TN, USA

Stephen P. Hunger, MD
Chief of Pediatric Hematology, Oncology and Bone Marrow Transplantation
Professor of Pediatrics
Children's Hospital Colorado
University of Colorado School of Medicine
Aurora, CO, USA

Soheil Meshinchi, MD, PhD
Associate Member
Fred Hutchinson Cancer Center
Associate Professor of Pediatrics
University of Washington
Seattle, WA, USA

Chapter 7
John Swansbury, FRCPath
Section of Haemato-Oncology
Royal Marsden Hospital and Institute of Cancer Research
Sutton, Surrey, UK

Warren G. Sanger, PhD
Munroe Meyer Institute for Genetics and Rehabilitation
University of Nebraska Medical Center
Nebraska Medical Center, Omaha, NE, USA

Chapter 8
Itziar Salaverria, PhD
Alexander von Humboldt Post Doctoral Scientist
Christian-Albrechts University Kiel
University Hospital Schleswig-Holstein Campus Kiel
Kiel, Germany

Reiner Siebert, MD
Professor and Chair Human Genetics
Director of the Institute of Human Genetics
Christian-Albrechts University Kiel
University Hospital Schleswig-Holstein Campus Kiel
Kiel, Germany

Megan S. Lim, MD, PhD
Professor of Pathology
Director of Hematopathology
Department of Pathology
University of Michigan Medical School
Ann Arbor, Michigan, USA

Chapter 9

Monique L. den Boer, MSc, PhD
Erasmus MC-Sophia Children's Hospital
University Medical Center
Dept. of Pediatric Oncology and Hematology
The Netherlands

Rob Pieters, MD, MSc, PhD
Erasmus MC — Sophia Children's Hospital
University Medical Center
Dept. of Pediatric Oncology and Hematology
Rotterdam, The Netherlands

Chapter 10

Lara Mussolin, PhD
Department of Pediatric Hematology-Oncology
University of Padova
Padova, Italy

Dario Campana, MD, PhD
Department of Pediatrics
Yong Loo Lin School of Medicine
National University of Singapore
Singapore

Angelo Rosolen, MD
Professor of Pediatrics
Department of Pediatric Hematology-Oncology
University of Padova
Padova, Italy

Chapter 11

Paul S. Gaynon, MD
Professor of Pediatrics
University of Southern California
Children's Hospital Los Angeles
Division of Hematology/Oncology
Los Angeles, CA, USA

Martin Schrappe, MD
Professor of Pediatrics
Christian-Albrechts University Kiel
University Medical Center Schleswig-Holstein (UKSH), Campus Kiel
Kiel, Germany

Simon Modlich, MD
Childrens Hospital
University Medical Center Schleswig-Holstein, Campus Kiel
Kiel, Germany

Gunnar Cario, MD
Childrens Hospital
University Medical Center Schleswig-Holstein, Campus Kiel
Kiel, Germany

Chapter 12

James Nachman, MD
Professor of Pediatrics
University of Chicago
Director, Leukemia/Lymphoma Program
Comer Children's Hospital
Chicago, IL, USA

Hagop Kantarjian, MD
Professor of Medicine
University of Texas
Chairman, Leukemia Department
MD Anderson Cancer Center
Houston, TX, USA

Chapter 13

Robert J. Arceci, MD, PhD
King Fahd Professor of Pediatric Oncology
Professor of Pediatrics
Oncology and Cellular and Molecular Medicine
Editor-in-Chief, Pediatric Blood & Cancer
Kimmel Comprehensive Cancer Center at Johns Hopkins
The Bunting & Blaustein Cancer Research Building
Baltimore, MD, USA

Soheil Meshinchi, MD, PhD
Associate Member
Fred Hutchinson Cancer Center
Associate Professor of Pediatrics
University of Washington
Seattle, WA, USA

Todd L. Rosenblat, MD
Assistant Member, Leukemia Service
Memorial Sloan-Kettering Cancer Center
Clinical Instructor of Medicine
Weill Cornell Medical College
New York, NY, USA

Joseph G. Jurcic, MD
Associate Member, Leukemia Service
Memorial Sloan-Kettering Cancer Center
Associate Professor of Medicine
Weill Cornell Medical College
New York, NY, USA

Martin S. Tallman, MD
Chief, Leukemia Service, Department of Medicine
Memorial Sloan-Kettering Cancer Center
Professor of Medicine
Weill Cornell Medical College
New York, NY, USA

Chapter 14

Mignon L. Loh, MD
Assistant Professor of Pediatrics
Hematology/Oncology
University of California, San Francisco
San Francisco, CA, USA

Franco Locatelli, MD
Professor Pediatrics
Pediatric Haematology and Oncology
IRCCS Ospedale Bambino Gesù, Rome
University of Pavia, Italy

Chapter 15

Shalini Shenoy, MD
Director, Pediatric Stem Cell Transplant Program,
Division of Pediatric Hematology Oncology
Washington University School of Medicine
St. Louis, MO, USA

Michael Deininger, MD, PhD
Division of Hematology and Hematologic Malignancies
University of Utah
Huntsman Cancer Institute
Salt Lake City, UT, USA

Chapter 16

Ross Pinkerton, MD
Professor of Oncology, University of Queensland
Director of Oncology, Royal Children's Hospital
Brisbane, Queensland, Australia

Mitchell S. Cairo, MD
Chief, Pediatric Hematology, Oncology and Stem Cell Transplantation
Director, Children and Adolescent Cancer and Blood Diseases Center
Medical and Scientific Director, Stem and Cellular Therapy and Engineering Clinical Laboratory
Associate Chairman, Department of Pediatrics
Professor of Pediatrics, Medicine, Pathology, Microbiology & Immunology and Cell Biology & Anatomy
Maria Fareri Children's Hospital at Westchester Medical Center
New York Medical College
Valhalla, NY, USA

Chapter 17

Birgit Burkhardt, MD, PhD
University Hospital Münster
Pediatric Hematology and Oncology
Münster, Germany

Ian Waxman, MD
Medical Officer
Office of Oncology Drug Products
US Food and Drug Administration
Bethesda, MD, USA

Chapter 18

Debra L. Friedman, M.D., M.S.
Associate Professor Pediatrics
E. Bronson Ingram Chair in Pediatric Oncology
Director, Division of Pediatric Hematology/Oncology
Leader Cancer Control and Prevention
Vanderbilt University and Vanderbilt-Ingram Cancer Center
Nashville, TN, USA

Anas Younes, M.D.
Professor of Medicine
Director, Clinical Investigation and Translational Research
Department of Lymphoma/Myeloma
M. D. Anderson Cancer Center
Houston, TX, USA

Chapter 19

Nader Kim El-Mallawany, M.D.
Departments of Pediatric Hematology, Oncology, Blood & Marrow Transplantation
Columbia University
New York, NY, USA

Michael R. Bishop, MD
Section Head, Hematologic Malignancies
Professor of Medicine
Medical College of Wisconsin
Milwaukee, WI, USA

Bruce Shiramizu, M.D.
Professor
Departments of Pediatrics and Medicine
Hawaii Center for AIDS
University of Hawaii
Honolulu, HI, USA

Chapter 20

Mary Eapen, MD, MS
Associate Professor
Center for International Blood and Marrow Transplant Research
Medical College of Wisconsin
Milwaukee, WI, USA

Vanderson Rocha, MD, PhD
Eurocord office — European Blood and Marrow Transplant Group
Hôpital Saint Louis
Paris, France

Chapter 21

Prakash Satwani, MD
Assistant Professor of Pediatrics
Pediatric Blood and Marrow Transplantation
Morgan Stanley Children's Hospital New York-Presbyterian
Columbia University
New York, NY, USA

Alan S. Wayne, MD
Clinical Director
Senior Clinician
Head, Hematologic Diseases Section
Pediatric Oncology Branch
Center for Cancer Research
National Cancer Institute
National Institutes of Health
Bethesda, MD, USA

Chapter 22

Nita L. Seibel, MD
Senior Investigator, Pediatric Section, Cancer Therapy Evaluation Program,
National Cancer Institute, National Institutes of Health, Bethesda, MD, USA
Adjunct Professor of Pediatrics
George Washington University School of Medicine and Health Sciences
Attending Physician
Children's National Medical Center
Washington DC, USA

Malcolm A. Smith, MD, PhD
Associate Branch Chief, Pediatrics
Cancer Therapy Evaluation Program
National Cancer Institute
Bethesda, MD, USA

Chapter 23

Laurence J.N. Cooper, MD, PhD
Professor
University of Texas, MD Anderson Cancer Center
Section Chief, Cell Therapy
Children's Cancer Hospital
Houston, TX, USA

Helen Heslop, MD
Dan L Duncan Chair
Professor of Medicine and Pediatrics
Director Adult Stem Cell Transplant Program
Center for Cell and Gene Therapy
Baylor College of Medicine, The Methodist Hospital and Texas Chiildren's Hospital
Houston, TX, USA

Chapter 24

Paul C. Nathan, M.D. MSc, FRCPC
Director-AfterCare Program, Division of Hematology/Oncology
The Hospital for Sick Children
Associate Professor of Pediatrics and Health Policy, Management & Evaluation
The University of Toronto
Toronto, ON, Canada

Tara Henderson, MD, MPH
Assistant Professor of Pediatrics
Director, Childhood Cancer Survivors Center
University of Chicago Comer Children's Hospital
Chicago, IL, USA

Laura Janzen, PhD, ABPP-CN
Neuropsychologist, The Hospital for Sick Children
Assistant Professor (Status-Only) of Pediatrics
The University of Toronto
Toronto, ON, Canada

Chapter 25

Thomas J. Walsh, MD
Professor of Medicine
Weill Cornell Medical College
Director, Transplantation-Oncology Infectious Diseases Program
New York Presbyterian Hospital
New York, NY, USA

Andreas H. Groll
Infectious Disease Research Program
Center for Bone Marrow Transplantation and
Department of Pediatric Hematology/Oncology
Children's University Hospital
Münster, Germany

Emmanuel Roilides
Laboratory of Infectious Diseases
3rd Department of Pediatrics
Hippokration Hospital
Aristotle University
Thessaloniki, Greece

Chapter 26

Shana S. Jacob, MD
Assistant Professor
George Washington University
Leukemia/ Lymphoma Program
Pediatric Advanced Needs Assessment and Care Team (PANDA)
Center for Cancer and Blood Disorders
Children's National Medical Center
Washington DC, USA

Kara M. Kelly, M.D.
Professor of Clinical Pediatrics
Columbia University Medical Center
Division of Pediatric Oncology
New York, NY, USA

Chapter 27

Rita Secola, RN, PhD, CPHON
Patient Care Services Director, Hematology/Oncology/Bone Marrow Transplantation
Children's Hospital Los Angeles
Los Angeles, CA, USA

Lauren Harrison, RN, MSN
Clinical Research Nurse
New York Medical College
Valhalla, NY, USA

Diane Altounji, RN, MSN, CPHON
Registered Nurse IV
Children's Hospital Los Angeles
Los Angeles, CA, USA

Chapter 28

Stephen A. Sands, Psy.D.
Associate Professor, Departments of Pediatrics and Psychiatry
Director, Valerie Fund Psycho-Social Programs
Columbia University Medical Center
Pediatric Oncology, Herbert Irving Pavilion
New York, NY, USA

Keith P. Pasichow, M.D.
Department of Pediatrics
Cohen Children's Medical Center of New York
New Hyde Park, NY, USA

Chapter 29

Shripad D. Banavali, MD (Med; Bom), BC (Ped; USA), BE (Hem-Onc; USA)
Professor & Head, Dept. of Medical & Pediatric Oncology
Convener, Pediatric Hem-Onc DMG
Co-ordinator, TMC-Rural Outreach Program
Tata Memorial Center
Parel, Mumbai, India

Scott C. Howard, MD, MS
Departments of Oncology and Information Sciences
St. Jude Children's Research Hospital
Memphis, TN, USA

Parth S. Mehta, MD, MPH
Assistant Professor
Chair, International Program at TCCC
Texas Children's Cancer & Hematology Centers Director, Haemophilia & Paediatric Oncology Program of Botswana
Baylor College of Medicine
Houston, TX, USA

Alessandra Sala, MD, PhD
Department of Pediatrics
University of Milano Bicocca
Azienda Ospedaliera S. Gerardo
Monza, Italy

Ronald Barr, MB, ChB, MD
Department of Pediatrics, McMaster University
Hamilton, Ontario, Canada L

Ian Magrath, DSc (Med), FRCP, FRCPath
President, International Network for Cancer Treatment and Research
Brussels, Belgium
Adjunct Professor of Pediatrics
Uniformed Services University of the Health Sciences
Bethesda, MD, USA

Chapter 30

Jessica C. Hochberg, MD
Assistant Professor of Pediatrics
Department of Pediatrics
New York Medical College
Maria Fareri Children's Hospital
Valhalla, NY, USA

Stanton C. Goldman, MD
Department of Pediatric Hematology/Oncology
Medical City Children's Hospital
Dallas, TX, USA

1

Epidemiology of Hematological Malignancies of Children, Adolescents, and Young Adults

Mark B. Geyer and Judith S. Jacobson

Introduction

Cancer is, in general, associated with aging. In the United States, cancer incidence rates per 100,000 persons per year rise almost 100-fold, from 23.4 in the first year of life to 2177.2 in the 85th year and beyond.[1] Among adults, the four most common cancers are solid tumors of the prostate, breast, colon, and lung. Hematologic malignancies, leukemias and lymphomas, are much less common. However, among children, leukemias and lymphomas account for a much larger share of all malignancies (Fig. 1.1). At ages 2–14 years, the hematologic malignancies account for more than 40% of new cancer diagnoses. At ages 15–19 years, they account for 40.1% of malignant diseases among males but only 33.3% among females. At ages 20–39 years, hematologic malignancy incidence rates are slightly lower among females than males, but all-site incidence rates are much higher among females, primarily due to breast, cervical, and thyroid cancer.[2] As a result, by the late 1930s, hematologic malignancies account for 18.6% of newly diagnosed cancers per year among males but only 6.7% among females (Table 1.1).

Leukemia is a set of diseases of the blood or bone marrow (in which blood cells originate), involving an abnormal proliferation of (white) blood cells. The acute leukemias involve the rapid proliferation of immature blood cells, crowding the bone marrow and spreading through the bloodstream into other organs. The chronic leukemias involve a more gradual increase in more mature blood cells. The acute leukemias are the most common hematologic malignancies in children; incidence rates peak among 2–3-year-olds.

Lymphoma is a term used for cancers that originate in lymphocytes, usually within lymph nodes, but, unlike lymphoid leukemias, which involve only circulating blood and bone marrow, lymphomas typically present as solid tumors of the lymph nodes. More than 40 types of lymphoma have been identified,[3] but most can be classified as involving T-cells, B-cells, or NK cells. Lymphomas are very rare among young children; incidence rates are lower than 1/100,000 per year among children younger than 8 years, but are as high as leukemia rates by the early teens and rise considerably higher by the early 1920s (Figs. 1.2A–B).

The Leukemias

Among children aged 0–14 in the United States, leukemias are responsible for 33% of cancers and 30% of cancer deaths.[2] Incidence rates of leukemia are 5.0 per 100,000 per year in that age range, age-specific rates rise from birth to age 2 and then fall; the association

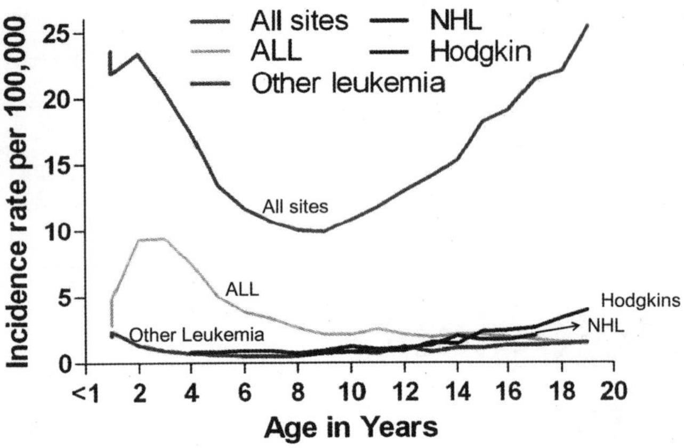

Fig. 1.1. Incidence rates of hematologic malignancies per 100,000, by age.

Table 1.1. Incidence rates (per 100,000) of all sites and hematologic malignancies in children, adolescents, and young adults.

	All sites	Leukemias	Lymphomas	Hematologic as % of all sites
Males				
< 1	25.1	5.3	0.0	21.1
1–4	22.3	10.1	0.7	48.4
5–9	12.2	4.3	1.8	50.0
10–14	13.6	3.5	2.9	47.1
15–19	22.2	3.7	5.2	40.1
20–24	33.4	3.0	7.2	30.5
25–29	46.7	3	8	23.6
30–34	61.3	3.3	9.5	20.9
35–39	86.5	4.2	11.9	18.6
Females				
< 1	21.6	4.3	0.0	19.9
1–4	19.0	8	0.4	44.2
5–9	10.5	3.6	0.8	41.9
10–14	12.8	2.7	1.9	35.9
15–19	20.1	2.4	4.3	33.3
20–24	37.0	2.2	6.4	23.2
25–29	63.2	2.1	7.4	15.0
30–34	105.3	2.8	7.7	10.0
35–39	166.9	3.0	8.1	6.7

with age is driven by acute lymphoblastic leukemia (ALL), the most commonly diagnosed leukemia of children (Fig. 1.1). Untreated acute leukemias are uniformly fatal. However, leukemia was the first cancer in which chemotherapy was successful, and in the past 35 years, combination chemotherapy has achieved dramatic results (Fig. 1.3). Overall 5-year survival among children and adolescents with leukemia has risen from 50% to nearly 80%. Several etiologic factors

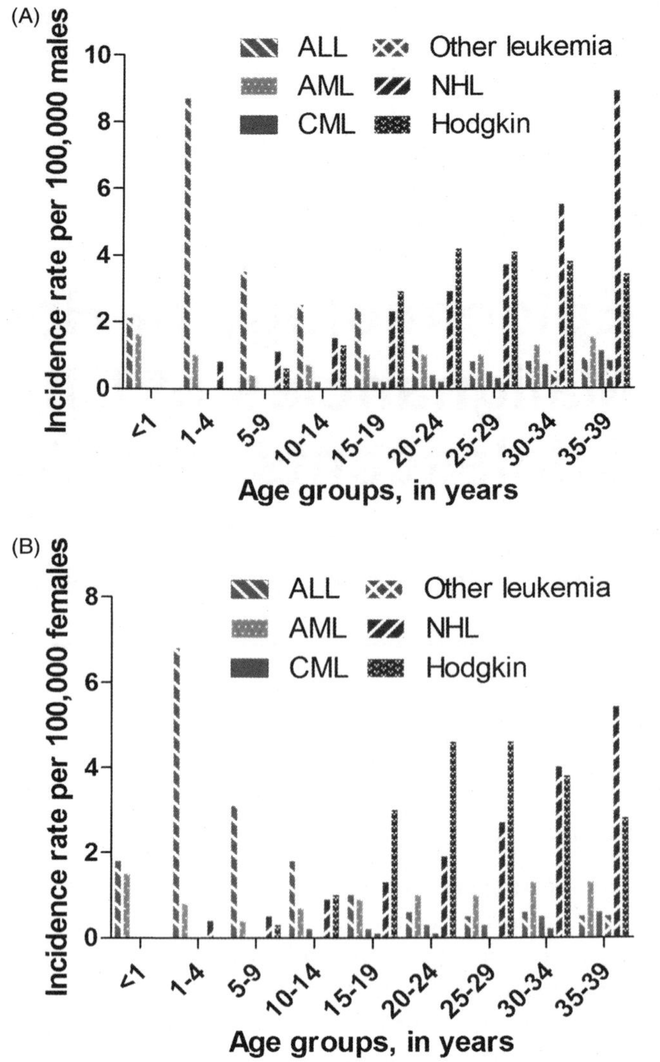

Fig. 1.2. (A) Incidence rates of hematologic malignancies per 100,000 males, by age group. (B) Incidence rates of hematologic malignancies per 100,000 females, by age group.

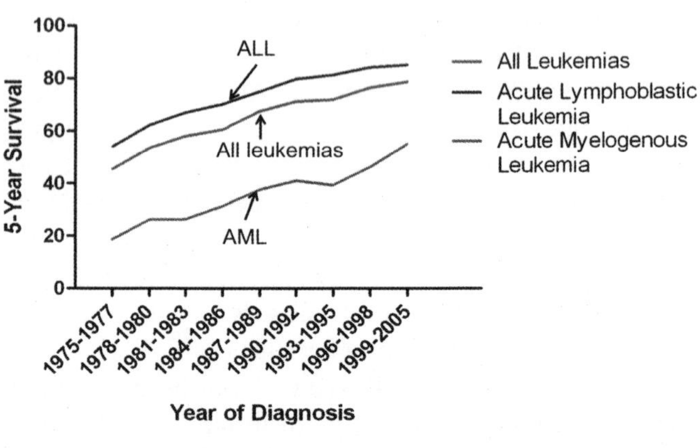

Fig. 1.3. Leukemia in children and adolescents age 0–19: 5-year survival by year of diagnosis (data from Horner, 2009).

Table 1.2. Etiologic factors in leukemia.

Subtype	Factor
ALL	Male gender[2]
	White race (in USA)[2]
	Down Syndrome[4–7]
	Kleinfelter Syndrome?[9]
	Born with TEL-AML1 translocation[62]
	Born with 11q23 rearrangement[22]
	Prior chemoradiotherapy[13]
	Ionizing radiation[16]
	Unidentified infection?[24,25]
	Lack of early daycare attendance[62]
AML	Male gender[2]
	White race (in USA)[2]
	Down Syndrome[4–7]
	Prior chemoradiotherapy[13–15,17,18]
	Ionizing radiation[16]
	Inherited marrow failure syndromes[10–12]
MDS	Inherited marrow failure syndromes[10–12]
	Prior chemoradiotherapy[13–15,17,18]
CML	Male gender[2]
	Ionizing radiation[16]
JMML	Neurofibromatosis type 1[31]

in leukemia in children and young adults are summarized in Table 1.2.

Some childhood leukemias have been linked to certain genetic disorders, including Down syndrome (trisomy 21). Children with Down syndrome (DS) have a 10- to 20-fold increased risk of developing acute leukemia, compared to children without DS.[4] A large case control study from the Children's Cancer Group found significantly increased risk of ALL (odds ratio 4.85) and dramatically increased risk of acute myelogenous leukemia (AML) (odds ratio 76.80) among children with DS.[5] However, children with DS account for only 2% of cases of pediatric ALL, and 15% of cases of pediatric AML).[6] Among children with acute leukemia, children with DS differ substantially from those without DS in leukemia-related cytogenetics and acquired gene mutations. Children with DS also have more than a 400-fold increased risk for acute megakaryoblastic leukemia (AMkL), the most common subtype of DS-associated AML.[7] AMkL is frequently preceded by a preleukemic myelodysplastic syndrome (MDS) in children with DS.[8] Kleinfelter syndrome (XXY) has been inconsistently associated with ALL.[9]

Several inherited marrow failure syndromes, including Fanconi anemia (FA), Schwachman–Diamond Syndrome (SDS), and to a lesser extent Diamond Blackfan anemia (DBA) are associated with increased risk of MDS and AML. FA is a rare, genetic disorder, usually with an autosomal recessive pattern of inheritance, affecting some 1–5 per million. The incidence of FA is considerably higher among Spanish Gypsies, white Afrikaners in South Africa, and Ashkenazi Jews[10] than among other groups, probably due to founder mutations in small, isolated populations. FA is associated with progressive marrow failure, numerous congenital abnormalities, and high incidence of cancer. Among patients with FA, approximately 8% develop AML by age 20, and 22% by age 36.[11] SDS is a rare, autosomal recessive disorder (approximately 1.33 per 100,000 live births) characterized by marrow failure, pancreatic insufficiency, and skeletal abnormalities; some 30% of SDS patients develop MDS or AML.[12] DBA is a rare disorder characterized by macrocytic anemia and erythroblastopenia, associated with several mutations in genes encoding for ribosomal proteins. Familial DBA seems to be autosomal dominant with incomplete penetrance and an incidence rate of approximately 1 in 100,000. DBA is associated with increased risk of hematologic malignancies, particularly MDS and AML, as well as solid tumors. However, the incidence of AML and MDS in children with DBA is considerably lower than in children with FA or SDS.

Children and adolescents who have received chemotherapy or radiation therapy for a prior malignancy are at increased risk for acute leukemia (usually AML) and other myeloproliferative disorders, compared to individuals of similar age who have not been treated for cancer. It is not clear whether genetic factors play a role in this association. Patients treated with mechlorethamine or cyclophosphamide for Hodgkin lymphoma (HL), have a more than 300-fold or 100-fold, respectively, increased risk of acute leukemia compared to that in the general population. Patients receiving mechlorethamine-containing combination chemotherapy (the MOPP regimen) for HL have a cumulative 3.4–9.5% risk of leukemia in the 15 years following treatment.[13] Such cases of AML are often preceded by MDS and tend to occur 5–7 years after the primary diagnosis.[14] Other chemotherapeutic agents used in the treatment of childhood hematologic or solid cancers, such as the epipodophyllotoxins (e.g. etoposide, teniposide) and the anthracyclines (e.g. doxorubicin, daunorubicin), also increase the risk of secondary AML significantly; these cases of AML tend to occur more acutely, without antecedent MDS, at a mean of 2–3 years following the primary diagnosis. The dose of epipodophyllotoxins and the frequency of dosing are positively associated with increased risk of secondary AML.[15]

Children exposed to ionizing radiation also face an increased risk for hematological and other malignancies, including the leukemias. Among more than 86,000 survivors of the 1945 atomic bomb blasts in Hiroshima and Nagasaki, long-term follow-up has suggested that 103 leukemia deaths were attributable to radiation exposure; about 28 of these deaths occurred in children, adolescents and young adults under age 30. A dose-response relationship between radiation dose and excess leukemia risk was observed; individuals who received radiation doses > 2 Gy, 10.4, 14.5, and 59.1 times the risk of ALL, AML, and chronic myelogenous leukemia (CML), respectively, compared to those receiving only background levels of radiation exposure.[16] The therapeutic use of ionizing radiation also predisposes patients to ALL, AML, and CML, with risk greatest 5–9 years following exposure. For example, among 10,000 patients receiving 25 Gy of radiotherapy for testicular cancer, an excess of nine leukemias is predicted over 15 years.[17] Patients treated with combination chemotherapy and total body irradiation (mean: 12.6 Gy) for non-Hodgkin lymphoma (NHL) had a 17% risk of AML in 15 years of follow-up.[18]

Acute lymphoblastic leukemia

Acute lymphoblastic leukemia is an aggressive, malignant neoplasm of B- or T-lymphocyte precursor cells (lymphoblasts) (see Chapters 11 and 12). Unlike other leukemias, ALL is primarily a disease of childhood, with a median age at diagnosis of 13 years. In the United States, ALL is the most common malignancy of children aged 0–14, representing 26% of all cancers and 79% of all leukemias.[2] Among children aged 0–14, the incidence of ALL is 4.0 per 100,000 per year, peaking at 9.4 per 100,000 per year at age 3. In 2002–2006, an estimated 5,760 individuals per year, approximately 3,500 of them under the age of 20, were diagnosed with ALL.

Acute lymphoblastic leukemia incidence rates are higher among males than among females at all ages. Among children aged 0–14, incidence rates are 4.4 per 100,000 in boys and 3.5 per 100,000 in girls. ALL is more common in whites (1.7 per 100,000) than in blacks (0.9 per 100,000) across all age groups. Acute lymphoblastic leukemia incidence is highest among children aged 1–4 in both groups, but is substantially higher in whites (8.5 per 100,000) than blacks (3.3 per 100,000). From 1975 to 2006, the incidence of childhood ALL increased by nearly 50% in children aged 0–14; the average annual increase was 0.8%.

Aneuploidy is the most commonly observed acquired abnormality in ALL, occurring in some form in 92% of cases of childhood ALL.[19] Specific genetic abnormalities have been observed in childhood ALL, including the *TEL-AML1* gene fusion generated by a translocation involving chromosomes 12 and 21 (see Chapters 5 and 6). This fusion gene is present in approximately 25% of cases of ALL; studies by the Children's Oncology Group and others suggest the *TEL-AML1* gene carries positive prognostic significance.[20] However, although approximately 1% of children are born with the TEL-AML1 translocation, only approximately 1 in 8000 of those with the translocation will develop childhood ALL.[21] Translocations involving chromosome 11q23, with resulting arrangement of the *MLL* gene, may occur *in utero* and are found in some infants with ALL; such translocations are also frequently observed in secondary AML following therapy with topoisomerase II inhibitors, including etoposide and doxorubicin.[22] The Philadelphia chromosome, generated by translocation involving chromosomes 9 and 22, is observed in 3–5% of children with ALL and is associated with poor prognosis; in one large retrospective study, only 28% of patients achieved 5-year event-free survival. Matched sibling donor allogeneic stem cell transplantation and good response to initial glucocorticoid therapy were associated with superior outcomes in these patients.[23]

Several investigators have hypothesized an infectious etiology for childhood ALL. Greaves has postulated that two genetic events — one occurring *in utero* and a second following antigenic stimulation — may underlie childhood ALL. He suggests that among infants whose exposure to pathogens is delayed, proliferation may occur in the preleukemic clone.[24] Kinlen believes that exposure to a yet-unidentified viral infection leads to ALL as a rare outcome, particularly when infectious and susceptible populations come into contact. He has identified several studies demonstrating a significantly increased incidence of leukemia in situations where different populations mix, such as urban and rural populations or groups with very different socioeconomic backgrounds.[25] These hypotheses are not wholly inconsistent; abnormal immune responses to infection could be leukemogenic. Although numerous small clusters of childhood ALL have been observed in the United States, no specific environmental etiology has been identified.[26]

However, a recent meta-analysis has demonstrated an association of daycare attendance before age 2 with reduced risk of pediatric ALL[21]; investigators have suggested that the hygiene hypothesis, originally proposed as a risk factor for asthma,[27] may also apply to ALL; early daycare attendance is hypothesized to be a marker of early exposure to pathogens, which may protect against ALL.

Treatment of childhood ALL consists of several phases of combination chemotherapy to induce remission, to eradicate leukemia cells in the central nervous system, and ultimately to suppress leukemic cell growth. Sibling or unrelated donor stem cell transplantation may be employed for children with relapsed or refractory ALL and for those with other poor prognostic features, as will be discussed in subsequent chapters (see Chapters 11, 12 and 20). Five-year survival for ALL has increased substantially in the past 35 years and is currently 89.2% for children aged 0–14 and 85.9% for children and adolescents aged 0–19.[1]

Acute myelogenous leukemia

Acute myelogenous leukemia (AML) is an aggressive cancer of myeloid precursor cells that crowd the bone marrow and interfere with normal hematopoiesis (see Chapter 13). It is estimated that 12,810 individuals, more than 800 of whom were younger than 20 years, were diagnosed with AML in the United States in 2009. AML is primarily a disease of older adults, with a median age at diagnosis of 67 years. AML incidence rates have a J-shaped age distribution. Among children aged 0–14 years, the AML incidence rate is 0.8 per 100,000 per year, but among infants (< 1 year old), the rate is 2.1 per 100,000 per year. In adolescents (15–19 years), the incidence rate is 1.0 per 100,000 per year and continues to rise through middle and older age groups, peaking at 22.9 cases per 100,000 among those aged 80–84. AML is the second most common leukemia in childhood, representing 16% of leukemias in children aged 0–14 and 18% in adolescents aged 15–19.[2]

Although age-adjusted AML incidence rates are higher among males than among females (4.3 per 100,000 in males and 2.9 per 100,000 in females), age-specific rates are similar in males and females younger than 30 years. AML is slightly more common in whites (3.6 per 100,000) than blacks (3.0 per 100,000) overall. Like that of childhood ALL, childhood AML incidence increased significantly between 1975 and 2006 (63.3% in children aged 0–14), with an average annual increase of 1.4%.

Treatment of AML employs combination chemotherapy to induce disease remission. Consolidation therapy for pediatric AML generally consists of high-dose chemotherapy or stem cell transplantation. Treatment regimens will be reviewed in subsequent chapters (see Chapters 13 and 20). Like that of patients with ALL, the survival of patients with AML has increased substantially in the past 35 years; five-year survival is currently 60.2% for children aged 0–14 and 55.0% for children and adolescents aged 0–19. Although pediatric AML carries a less favorable prognosis than ALL, children and adolescents with AML have a far better 5-year survival rate than the general population of AML patients, whose 5-year survival is only 23.8%.[2]

Chronic myelogenous leukemia

Chronic myelogenous leukemia (CML) is a neoplasm of pluripotent stem cells still capable of terminal differentiation (see Chapter 15). It is uniformly associated with the presence of the *BCR-ABL* fusion gene; 95% of patients have a translocation involving chromosomes 9 and 22. Some 5,050 Americans, of whom approximately 120 were aged 0–19 years, were diagnosed with CML in 2009; the median age at diagnosis is 66 years. The incidence of CML approaches 0.1 per 100,000 in children aged 0–14 years and increases to 0.2 per 100,000 among those aged 15–19 years. CML accounts for approximately 3% of leukemias in children and adolescents aged 0–19. Like the acute leukemias, CML has a male predominance; incidence rates are 1.9 per 100,000 among males and 1.1 per 100,000 among females. In children and adolescents, however, CML is similarly rare in both sexes.

Chronic myelogenous leukemia is associated with slow progression from indolent growth in chronic phase, through an acute phase characterized by treatment failure and worsening hematologic derangements, to a blast crisis similar to that in the acute leukemias. Historically, busulfan, hydroxyurea, and interferon-α were used for cytoreduction in chronic phase CML. However, the development and success of tyrosine kinase inhibitors (such as imatinib) that target the *Bcr-abl* fusion protein has changed the treatment of CML. Upfront therapy with imatinib has become the standard care for most patients with pediatric CML. Although tyrosine kinase inhibitors are not curative therapy, they achieve very high rates of cytogenetic response and can extend survival substantially. Allogeneic stem cell transplantation offers the potential for cure, although it entails substantial risks of morbidity and mortality, particularly for unrelated donor transplants. Children with CML undergoing matched sibling donor transplantation in chronic phase have had 60–75% 5-year relapse-free survival, while those undergoing matched unrelated donor transplantation have had less favorable 5-year survival rates, approximately 55% in one recent large study.[28] In some pediatric patients, such as those in whom tyrosine kinase inhibitors fail to control disease, or those in accelerated phase or blast crisis, allogeneic stem cell transplant from related or unrelated donors may clearly be indicated. Subsequent chapters will review the therapeutic approach to childhood and adolescent CML. Significant unresolved questions remain regarding the ideal front-line treatment of CML in this population.[29]

Chronic lymphocytic leukemia

Chronic lymphocytic leukemia (CLL) is a clonal proliferation of B lymphocytes arrested in differentiation. Although CLL is the most common leukemia, with 15,490 new diagnoses among Americans in 2009, it primarily affects older adults; the median age at diagnosis is 72.[2] Cases of CLL in children and adolescents are vanishingly rare. Those described in case reports may be associated with a translocation involving chromosomes 2 and 14.[30]

Myelodysplastic syndromes

The myelodysplastic syndromes (MDS) are a group of disorders characterized by clonal proliferation of pluripotent hematopoietic stem cells, resulting in disordered and ineffective hematopoiesis (see Chapter 15). MDS in the setting of the congenital marrow failure syndromes, severe aplastic anemia, or prior chemotherapy or radiation therapy is known as secondary MDS. MDS/AML observed in the setting of DS is considered to be a separate entity, as previously discussed. Other cases of MDS are considered "primary" or "*de novo*," but may still be associated with genetic predisposition. Monosomy 7 or loss of the long arm of chromosome 7 occurs in approximately 30% of childhood MDS cases and 50% of therapy-related MDS.[31] Abnormalities of chromosome 5 are frequently observed in adult MDS but are very rare in childhood MDS.

Childhood MDS is very rare; in the United Kingdom, which has an MDS registry, the incidence rate of non–DS-related MDS among children under 15 is estimated at 0.81 per million (0.66 per million for de novo MDS). In Denmark and British Columbia, incidence rates are estimated at 2.1 per million and 1.4 per million, respectively.[32]

Myelodysplastic syndrome may progress to AML. Different subtypes of MDS demonstrate differing rates of progression; patients with the subtype of MDS known as refractory anemia with excess blasts (i.e. 5–20% marrow blasts) have approximately 50% risk of developing AML within 5 years; patients with less than 5% marrow blasts have a 20% 5-year risk of progression to AML.[33]

Juvenile myelomonocytic leukemia

Juvenile myelomonocytic leukemia (JMML) is a rare hematopoietic disorder of early childhood characterized by uncontrolled proliferation of monocytes and granulocytes, as well as myelodysplastic features of anemia and thrombocytopenia (see Chapter 14). According to the UK MDS registry, the JMML incidence rate is estimated at 0.69 per million among children under 15. In Denmark and British Columbia, estimates are 1.3 and 1.0 per million, respectively.[32] JMML usually presents in children younger than 6 years; the median age at diagnosis is 2 years. Later presentation of disease is an adverse prognostic indicator.

About 11% of JMML patients have neurofibromatosis type 1, an autosomal dominant disorder found in 1 in 4,000 births and characterized by *café au lait* spots on the skin and predisposition to neurofibromas, and schwannomas. A genetic defect in the *NF1* gene underlies neurofibromatosis type 1; NF1 is a negative regulator of the *Ras* signal transduction pathway.[31] For children born with one defective copy of Ras, a second somatic mutation in NF1 can lead to uncontrolled Ras activation and cell proliferation. Indeed, the pathogenesis of JMML is related to abnormalities in the *Ras* signaling pathway.[34] Similar to MDS, JMML is associated with monosomy 7, which is found in approximately 25% of cases. However, many cases are associated with a normal karyotype.[31]

Standard chemotherapy is generally ineffective in treating JMML and allogeneic stem cell transplantation offers the only potential for cure. Even with stem cell transplantation, the high risk of leukemic relapse lowers 5-year event-free survival to only 50%.[35]

The Lymphomas

The lymphomas are cancers of the lymphatic system, which consists of lymph (interstitial fluid similar to blood plasma, containing white blood cells and other components) and the lymphatic vessels, lymph nodes, and other lymphatic organs (tonsils, spleen, thymus, and Peyer patches on the small intestine) through which the lymph circulates (SEER training). Lymphomas are categorized by cell type as T-cell, representing about 10% of lymphomas, or B-cell, representing the other 90%. Chapter 2 of this volume deals with the 2008 World Health Organization (WHO) classification of lymphomas.

Lymphoma incidence rates rise with age, although patterns of incidence vary by cell type. All the lymphomas diagnosed among children are more common among adults; some types found among adults are virtually unknown among children. These include the chronic/small/prolymphocytic/mantle and B-cell NHLs, which account for more than 15% of adult lymphomas. Malignant lymphoma is the most common cancer affecting adolescents.[36]

Overall, lymphoma incidence has been rising in the past few decades.[1] Although lymphomas have generally been more common among whites than non-whites, the recent increase is greater and the age distribution is younger among blacks than among whites. Lymphomas are overall more common among males than females, although the gender difference is smaller among adults than among children.

Hodgkin lymphoma

Hodgkin lymphoma, first described by the British pathologist Thomas Hodgkin in 1832, is usually distinguished from the many and collectively more common NHLs. Four cell types of HL have been identified: nodular sclerosing (NS), lymphocyte predominant (LP), lymphocyte depletion (LD), and mixed cellularity (MD) (see Chapter 18). Most, but not all, HL involves B cells. Although rare among young children, HL is the most common cancer of young adults and the most common hematologic malignancy among males and females aged 15–30 years (Figs. 1.2A–B) (see Chapter 3). Incidence rates are less than 1.0 per 100,000 per year among children younger than 10 years, 1.0 among those aged 10–14 years, and rise to 4.0 per 100,000 among those aged 15–30 years (The age distribution of HL incidence is bimodal, peaking for the second time among persons aged > 55 years.). Among children < 15 years, HL is at least twice as common in males as in females.[37] In older age groups, the gender difference is not evident (Figs. 1.2A–B). Unlike the incidence rates of the NHLs, those of HL had been relatively stable in the final decades of the 20th century, but they now appear to be rising overall, especially among individuals aged 20–29 years.

Family history is a strong risk factor for HL, especially among relatives of young probands. In a study conducted in the Swedish and Danish cancer registries, linked to other registries, first-degree relatives of cases diagnosed at age < 40 years had a fourfold increased risk compared to relatives of controls; the associations were stronger for siblings than for parents or offspring and for male than for female relatives of probands,[38] although the latter association may reflect the generally higher risk in males than in females.

For more than a decade, the Epstein–Barr virus (EBV) has been understood to play a causal role in HL, especially among young children.[39] EBV has been identified in close to 50% of patients < 15 years and 25% of those aged 15–35 years.[39] In specimens from those patients, the multinucleated Reed–Sternberg cells that confirm the diagnosis of HL contain the EBV genome, and EBV gene products are expressed in those cells. Other viruses have also been associated with HL. An association with human immunodeficiency virus (HIV) is well established, but most HL patients with HIV also appear to have EBV (see Chapter 19).[40] Measles virus has been associated with HL[41] in some, but not all, studies.[42]

In the 0–14 age group, patients diagnosed with HL have more siblings and come from families of lower socioeconomic status (SES) than controls. Incidence rates are higher in developing countries than in industrialized countries[43–44]; they are highest in Western Asia and North Africa. Among adolescents and young adults 15–35 years of age, those associations are generally reversed. The socioeconomic risk factor pattern among young children is consistent with an etiology involving infectious agents (viruses) and underdevelopment of the immune system that may be genetic in origin. The pattern among adolescents and young adults may reflect a relative lack of exposure to infectious agents in childhood among individuals of higher SES, and the expansion of social networks that leads to EBV and infectious mononucleosis among college-age youth and young adults. In a study of EBV and lymphoma among 18,642 organ transplant recipients in Europe, North America, and Australia, 40% of kidney transplant patients aged 0–9 years, 70% of those 10–19 years, 85% of those 20–29 years, and ≥ 90% of older patients were EBV-seropositive prior to transplant.[45] EBV prevalence among transplant recipients may not be representative of EBV prevalence in the general population, but its association with age is unlikely to be very different.

Among young children, the histology of HL, especially EBV-related HL, is most commonly of mixed cellularity; among adolescents and young adults, it is predominantly nodular sclerosis.

Autoimmune disorders, notably rheumatoid arthritis and systemic lupus eythematosus, sarcoidosis, and immune thrombocytopenic purpura have been associated with HL,[46] but their relevance to adolescents and young adults is difficult to establish because of the very small numbers of cases and controls in that age group with a history of such disorders.

Survival among young people with HL is one of the great success stories of hematology and oncology in the latter part of the 20th century and HL treatment has played a key role in the development of the field. In the 1940s, the effects of nitrogen mustard and radiation therapy on the lymphatic system were discovered; the implications of the discoveries for HL were quickly explored in clinical trials. Subsequently, chemotherapy was introduced and steadily improved. Five-year survival among children, adolescents, and young adults is now > 90%. However, the increasing numbers of HL survivors have found themselves at risk for second cancers and other late effects of treatment (see Chapter 24).[47] Many patients who received radiation therapy prior to puberty before standard doses were lowered, have experienced bone or soft tissue hypoplasia. Doxorubicin has been found to have greater cardiotoxicity among children than among adults. Treatment can also have adverse effects on fertility.[48] Second malignant neoplasms associated with prior HL and its treatment include leukemias, sarcomas, and breast, thyroid, gastrointestinal, and lung carcinomas;[49] overall, HL survivors have more than a 10-fold higher risk of those malignancies than the general population. These increased risks may be due in part to the HL or to the exposures that caused it, but they are also clearly related to treatment. Both overall and HL-specific mortality risk have been associated with low SES and non-white race.[50] Improvements in long-term survival and quality of life for patients with HL depend on modifying existing treatments, facilitating access to care, and developing new treatments with fewer side effects.

Non-Hodgkin lymphoma

The past few decades have seen a dramatic rise in the incidence of NHL, *except* in the youngest age groups.[51] In the United States, from the 1970s to the 1990s, rates increased by 3–4% each year, and NHL became the fifth most commonly diagnosed malignancy.[52] However, among children, adolescents, and young adults < 30 years of age, NHL is still less common than HL (Figs. 1.2A–B).

Like HL, NHL is associated with the male gender, family history, infectious agents, autoimmune disorders, immunosuppression,[53] birth order (at least for some cell types)[54] and perhaps some chemical exposures, mainly in the setting of occupational exposures[55] (Table 1.3). An association with white race has also been observed.[56–57] The most common NHLs are diffuse large B-cell lymphoma, lymphoblastic lymphoma, anaplastic large cell lymphoma, and Burkitt lymphoma (see Chapters 16 and 17).

Table 1.3. Etiologic factors in lymphoma.

Subtype	Factor
HL	Male gender[37]
	White race (in USA)[57]
	Epstein-Barr virus[62]
	Family history[38]
	Measles?[41]
	Residing in Western Asia or North Africa[43,44,59]
	Socioeconomic status[37]
	Low for ages 0–14 years
	High for ages 15–30 years
	Transplant recipient status[45]
	Autoimmune disorders?[46]
	Birth order[37]
	Late/last for ages 0–14 years
	Early/first for ages 15–30 years
NHL	Male gender[2]
	White race (in USA)[57]
	Epstein–Barr virus[62]
	Family history[38]
	Birth order[54]
	Socioeconomic status[51]
	Immunosuppression[53]
DLBCL	Primary congenital immunodeficiency[51]
	Ataxia telangiectasia
	Wiskott–Aldrich syndrome
	Epstein–Barr virus[62]
	Birth order (late/last)[54,72]
BL	Male gender[60]
	Epstein–Barr virus[62]
	HIV[62]
LL	Male gender[64]
	HIV[65]
ALCL	Adolescent predominance[66,67]
PMBCL	No male predominance[68]
	Older age distribution[68]

Diffuse large B-cell lymphoma (DLBCL)

Diffuse large B-cell lymphoma (DLBCL) is the most common NHL among adolescents and young adults in industrialized countries, and the second most common, after Burkitt lymphoma, among children.[36] Nearly 40% of new lymphoma cases in adolescents and about 20% in children under 14 years are DLBCL. However, incidence rates are lower than 1 per 100,000 per year for those aged 0–20 years and rises above 1 per 100,000 only for those older than 25 years. Pediatric patients have better outcomes than older patients, possibly because treatment strategies or tumor biology vary by age group.[58] Birth order (having many older siblings) has been associated with DLBCL.[71] Congenital immunodeficiency syndromes, including ataxia telangiectasia and Wiskott–Aldrich syndrome are associated with a 10–15% risk of DLBCL.[51]

Burkitt lymphoma (BL)

Burkitt lymphoma (BL) is the most common childhood cancer in much of tropical Africa[59]; it is much less common in industrialized countries, including the United States; incidence rates hover around 0.6 per 100,000 per year among males and 0.2 per 100,000 among females aged 0–30 years. Among children, it is 3–4 times as common among males as among females. Overall, BL has been found to have a trimodal age-specific incidence pattern, with peaks near ages 10, 40, and 75 years among males; the peak near age 40 years is much less pronounced among females than males.[60] From 1982–1985 to 2002–2005, incidence rates in the US population aged 0–20 years increased from 0.41 to 0.55 per 100,000 or 34%, but the increase in older age groups was much greater. Data from Surveillance Epidemiology and End Results (SEER) for those aged 0–29 years illustrate the increase and the peak around age 10 years.[61] In Africa, BL also has almost the same geographical distribution as *Plasmodium falciparum* malaria; mosquito eradication programs and sickle cell trait are associated with reduced risk of BL.[62] Most adult-onset BL also appears to be AIDS-related. Both DLBCL and BL are also associated with EBV.[63]

Lymphoblastic lymphoma

Lymphoblastic lymphoma is a T-cell lymphoma that overlaps in many respects with T-cell lymphoblastic leukemia.[64] It is the second most common NHL among patients younger than 15 years, but is less common in older adolescents and young adults.[36] Incidence rates are 0.4 per 100,000 among children younger than 5 years but close to 0.1 per 100,000 in older age groups. It is similar to pediatric T-cell acute lymphoblastic leukemia in gender and age, but generally does not present with bone marrow involvement. In Africa, LL has been associated with HIV.[65]

Anaplastic large cell lymphoma (ALCL)

Anaplastic large cell lymphoma (ALCL) is a relatively rare NHL, with incidence rates of about 0.2 per 100,000 per year overall. About 13% of NHL among children, and somewhat more among adolescents, but much less among adults is ALCL.[66,67]

Primary mediastinal B-cell lymphoma (PMBCL)

Primary mediastinal B-cell lymphoma (PMBCL) is another rare NHL that has been classified by WHO as a subtype of DLBCL but appears to be a distinct entity that also has some features of classical HL.[36,68]

Although the varying descriptive features of the various cell types suggest differences in etiology, their rarity makes it difficult to study them, and their commonalities also appear to be informative.

For example, an important clue to the etiology of the NHLs among children is the occurrence of post-transplant lymphoproliferative (usually B-cell) disease,[69] a relatively common complication of organ transplantation, probably due to the immunosuppression that transplantation requires. Risk is greatest among children who are EBV- or CMV-negative prior to receiving a transplant from an EBV- or CMV-positive donor. A similar risk factor is atopic dermatitis treated with topical steroids. Immunosuppression favors infectious agents, perhaps in the presence of a genetic factor or factors that also facilitate malignant transformation.

Other environmental factors that may play a role in pediatric lymphomas as well as other cancers are agricultural chemicals and occupational exposures of parents. Future studies with larger samples may make it possible to home in on these exposures and to develop effective interventions to improve outcomes for children, adolescents, and young adults at risk.

As Figs. 1.4A–B shows, survival continues to improve for most lymphoma subtypes, but is better for children and adolescents than for young adults.[70] Tai *et al.* suggest that lack of health insurance leading to late

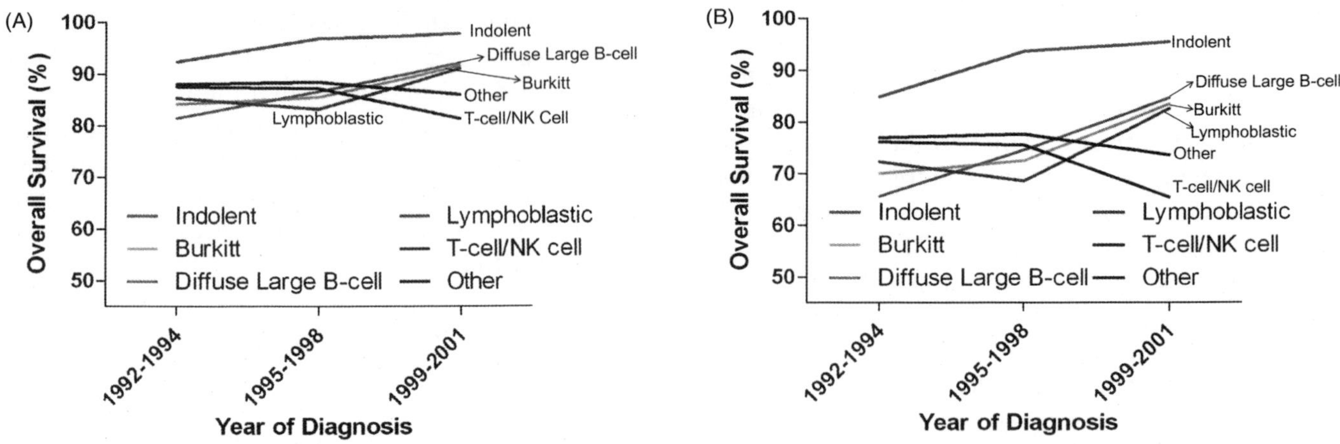

Fig. 1.4. (A) Changes in survival for patients with NHL subtypes, ages 0–19 years, 1992–2001. (B) Changes in survival for patients with NHL subtypes, ages 20–29 years, 1992–2001.

diagnosis contributes to the inferior survival of young adult patients.

Conclusions

If childhood cancers were as common as adult cancers, their etiology would be much better understood. The example of lung cancer and smoking illustrates the contrast. The rise in smoking prevalence preceded the identification of the causal role of smoking in lung cancer by about 20 years; without that increase, lung cancer would still be rare and the association might still be controversial. Childhood cancers, by definition, take less than 20 years from initial exposure to diagnosis, but because cancers in the young are, fortunately, rare it has generally been difficult to identify and recruit enough cases for well-designed epidemiologic studies. Even to the extent that etiologic agents are known, the rarity of childhood cancer is a deterrent to effective prevention. For example, EBV is now implicated in HL as well as several NHL, but EBV infection is almost ubiquitous. The pathway by which it increases the risk of lymphoma, the co-factors in that pathway, and their relationship to specific lymphoma subtypes need to be much better understood. Other infectious agents, genetic factors, and other environmental factors, such as nutrition, are likely to affect individual risk and specific disease outcome. Age at exposure may also play a role, as it does in the hygiene hypothesis invoked to explain the rise of asthma.[71] However, childhood ALL rates have not risen in parallel with asthma rates. The crossover association between socioeconomic status and HL is also suggestive of a similar pattern.

The acquired immune deficiency (AIDS) epidemic and the related rising rates of lymphoma among children and young adults, especially in the third world, are tragic. However, they give us the opportunity to observe whether AIDS treatment increases risk by prolonging life or reduces risk by addressing the immunocompromised state; and the role of concomitant tuberculosis and other co-infections and their treatment may also be instructive. Studying these patterns may help us to improve outcomes for all children and young adults with hematologic malignancies. The dramatic successes in treating patients with these diseases have not depended on knowledge of etiology, but they have come at a cost in long-term morbidity and risk of second malignancies. Epidemiologic studies now in progress are identifying etiologic factors, teasing out interactions between infectious agents, and other associations that may provide a basis for more targeted treatments. Such treatments may lead to further improvement in outcomes for young patients and those at risk for hematologic malignancies.

References

1. Altekruse SF KC, Krapcho M, Neyman N, Aminou R, Waldron W, Ruhl J, Howlader N, Tatalovich Z, Cho H, Mariotto A, Eisner MP, Lewis DR, Cronin K, Chen HS, Feuer EJ, Stinchcomb DG, Edwards BK (eds). (2010) *SEER Cancer Statistics Review, 1975–2007.* National Cancer Institute. Bethesda, MD.
2. Horner MJ RL, Krapcho M, Neyman N, Aminou R, Howlader N, Altekruse SF, Feuer EJ, Huang L, Mariotto A,

Miller BA, Lewis DR, Eisner MP, Stinchcomb DG, Edwards BK (eds). (2009) *SEER Cancer Statistics Review*, 1975–2006. National Cancer Institute. Bethesda, MD.

3. Jaffe ES. (2009) The 2008 WHO classification of lymphomas: Implications for clinical practice and translational research. *Hematology Am Soc Hematol Educ Program* 523–531.
4. Fong CT, Brodeur GM. (1987) Down's syndrome and leukemia: Epidemiology, genetics, cytogenetics and mechanisms of leukemogenesis. *Cancer Genet Cytogenet* **28**: 55–76.
5. Mertens AC, Wen W, Davies SM, Steinbuch M, Buckley JD, Potter JD, Robison LL. (1998) Congenital abnormalities in children with acute leukemia: A report from the Children's Cancer Group. *J Pediatr* **133**: 617–623.
7. Lange BJ, Kobrinsky N, Barnard DR, Arthur DC, Buckley JD, Howells WB, Gold S, Sanders J, Neudorf S, Smith FO, Woods WG. (1998) Distinctive demography, biology, and outcome of acute myeloid leukemia and myelodysplastic syndrome in children with Down syndrome: Children's Cancer Group Studies 2861 and 2891. *Blood* **91**: 608–615.
10. Callen E, Casado JA, Tischkowitz MD, Bueren JA, Creus A, Marcos R, Dasi A, Estella JM, Munoz A, Ortega JJ, de Winter J, Joenje H, Schindler D, Hanenberg H, Hodgson SV, Mathew CG, Surralles J. (2005) A common founder mutation in FANCA underlies the world's highest prevalence of Fanconi anemia in Gypsy families from Spain. *Blood* **105**: 1946–1949.
11. Rosenberg PS, Alter BP, Ebell W. (2008) Cancer risks in Fanconi anemia: Findings from the German Fanconi Anemia Registry. *Haematologica* **93**: 511–517.
12. Dror Y. (2005) Shwachman-Diamond syndrome. *Pediatr Blood Cancer* **45**: 892–901.
13. Travis LB. (2006) The epidemiology of second primary cancers. *Cancer Epidemiol Biomarkers Prev* **15**: 2020–2026.
15. le Deley MC, Leblanc T, Shamsaldin A, Raquin MA, Lacour B, Sommelet D, Chompret A, Cayuela JM, Bayle C, Bernheim A, de Vathaire F, Vassal G, Hill C. (2003) Risk of secondary leukemia after a solid tumor in childhood according to the dose of epipodophyllotoxins and anthracyclines: A case-control study by the Societe Francaise d'Oncologie Pediatrique. *J Clin Oncol* **21**: 1074–1081.
16. Richardson D, Sugiyama H, Nishi N, Sakata R, Shimizu Y, Grant EJ, Soda M, Hsu WL, Suyama A, Kodama K, Kasagi F. (2009) Ionizing radiation and leukemia mortality among Japanese Atomic Bomb Survivors, 1950–2000. *Radiat Res* **172**: 368–382.
17. Travis LB, Andersson M, Gospodarowicz M, van Leeuwen FE, Bergfeldt K, Lynch CF, Curtis RE, Kohler BA, Wiklund T, Storm H, Holowaty E, Hall P, Pukkala E, Sleijfer DT, Clarke EA, Boice JD, Jr., Stovall M, Gilbert E. (2000) Treatment-associated leukemia following testicular cancer. *J Natl Cancer Inst* **92**: 1165–1171.
18. Travis LB, Weeks J, Curtis RE, Chaffey JT, Stovall M, Banks PM, Boice JD, Jr. (1996) Leukemia following low-dose total body irradiation and chemotherapy for non-Hodgkin's lymphoma. *J Clin Oncol* **14**: 565–571.
19. Wartenberg D GF, Adelman AS. (2008) Acute lymphoblastic leukemia: Epidemiology and etiology. In: EH Estey SF, HM Kantarjian. NY: Springer, ed. *Acute Leukemias.*
20. Rubnitz JE, Wichlan D, Devidas M, Shuster J, Linda SB, Kurtzberg J, Bell B, Hunger SP, Chauvenet A, Pui CH, Camitta B, Pullen J. (2008) Prospective analysis of TEL gene rearrangements in childhood acute lymphoblastic leukemia: A Children's Oncology Group study. *J Clin Oncol* **26**: 2186–2191.
22. Eguchi M, Eguchi-Ishimae M, Greaves M. (2003) The role of the MLL gene in infant leukemia. *Int J Hematol* **78**: 390–401.
23. Arico M, Valsecchi MG, Camitta B, Schrappe M, Chessells J, Baruchel A, Gaynon P, Silverman L, Janka-Schaub G, Kamps W, Pui CH, Masera G. (2000) Outcome of treatment in children with Philadelphia chromosome-positive acute lymphoblastic leukemia. *N Engl J Med* **342**: 998–1006.
24. Greaves MF. (1997) Aetiology of acute leukaemia. *Lancet* **349**: 344–349.
25. Kinlen LJ. (1995) Epidemiological evidence for an infective basis in childhood leukaemia. *Br J Cancer* **71**: 1–5.
27. Strachan DP. (1989) Hay fever, hygiene, and household size. *BMJ* **299**: 1259–1260.
28. Muramatsu H, Kojima S, Yoshimi A, Atsuta Y, Kato K, Nagatoshi Y, Inoue M, Koike K, Kawase T, Ito M, Kurosawa H, Tanizawa A, Tono C, Hamamoto K, Hotta N, Watanabe A, Morishima Y, Kawa K, Shimada H. Outcome of 125 children with chronic myelogenous leukemia who received transplants from unrelated donors: The Japan Marrow Donor Program. *Biol Blood Marrow Transplant* **16**: 231–238.
31. Niemeyer CM, Kratz CP. (2008) Paediatric myelodysplastic syndromes and juvenile myelomonocytic leukaemia: Molecular classification and treatment options. *Br J Haematol* **140**: 610–624.
32. Passmore SJ, Chessells JM, Kempski H, Hann IM, Brownbill PA, Stiller CA. (2003) Paediatric myelodysplastic syndromes and juvenile myelomonocytic leukaemia

in the UK: A population-based study of incidence and survival. *Br J Haematol* **121**: 758–767.

33. Germing U, Aul C, Niemeyer CM, Haas R, Bennett JM. (2008) Epidemiology, classification and prognosis of adults and children with myelodysplastic syndromes. *Ann Hematol* **87**: 691–699.
35. Chan RJ, Cooper T, Kratz CP, Weiss B, Loh ML. (2009) Juvenile myelomonocytic leukemia: A report from the 2nd International JMML Symposium. *Leuk Res* **33**: 355–362.
36. Hochberg J, Waxman IM, Kelly KM, Morris E, Cairo MS. (2009) Adolescent non-Hodgkin lymphoma and Hodgkin lymphoma: State of the science. *Br J Haematol* **144**: 24–40.
37. Punnett A, Tsang RW, Hodgson DC. (2010) Hodgkin lymphoma across the age spectrum: Epidemiology, therapy, and late effects. *Semin Radiat Oncol* **20**: 30–44.
38. Goldin LR, Bjorkholm M, Kristinsson SY, Turesson I, Landgren O. (2009) Highly increased familial risks for specific lymphoma subtypes. *Br J Haematol* **146**: 91–94.
39. Jarrett RF. (2002) Viruses and Hodgkin's lymphoma. *Ann Oncol* **13** Suppl 1: 23–29.
42. Wilson KS, Freeland JM, Gallagher A, Cosby SL, Earle JA, Alexander FE, Taylor GM, Jarrett RF. (2007) Measles virus and classical Hodgkin lymphoma: No evidence for a direct association. *Int J Cancer* **121**: 442–447.
43. Glaser SL, Lin RJ, Stewart SL, Ambinder RF, Jarrett RF, Brousset P, Pallesen G, Gulley ML, Khan G, O'Grady J, Hummel M, Preciado MV, Knecht H, Chan JK, Claviez A. (1997) Epstein-Barr virus-associated Hodgkin's disease: Epidemiologic characteristics in international data. *Int J Cancer* **70**: 375–382.
45. Opelz G, Daniel V, Naujokat C, Dohler B. (2009) Epidemiology of pretransplant EBV and CMV serostatus in relation to posttransplant non-Hodgkin lymphoma. *Transplantation* **88**: 962–967.
46. Landgren O, Engels EA, Pfeiffer RM, Gridley G, Mellemkjaer L, Olsen JH, Kerstann KF, Wheeler W, Hemminki K, Linet MS, Goldin LR. (2006) Autoimmunity and susceptibility to Hodgkin lymphoma: A population-based case-control study in Scandinavia. *J Natl Cancer Inst* **98**: 1321–1330.
49. O'Brien MM, Donaldson SS, Balise RR, Whittemore AS, Link MP. (2010) Second malignant neoplasms in survivors of pediatric Hodgkin's lymphoma treated with low-dose radiation and chemotherapy. *J Clin Oncol* **28**: 1232–1239.
50. Keegan TH, Clarke CA, Chang ET, Shema SJ, Glaser SL. (2009) Disparities in survival after Hodgkin lymphoma: A population-based study. *Cancer Causes Control.*
51. Fisher SG, Fisher RI. (2004) The epidemiology of non-Hodgkin's lymphoma. *Oncogene* **23**: 6524–6534.
53. Kinlen LJ. (1992) Immunosuppression and cancer. *IARC Sci Publ*: 237–253.
54. Grulich AE, Vajdic CM, Falster MO, Kane E, Smedby KE, Bracci PM, de Sanjose S, Becker N, Turner J, Martinez-Maza O, Melbye M, Engels EA, Vineis P, Costantini AS, Holly EA, Spinelli JJ, La Vecchia C, Zheng T, Chiu BC, Franceschi S, Cocco P, Maynadie M, Foretova L, Staines A, Brennan P, Davis S, Severson RK, Cerhan JR, Breen EC, Birmann B, Cozen W. (2010) Birth order and risk of non-Hodgkin lymphoma — true association or bias? *Am J Epidemiol* **172**: 621–630.
55. Carozza SE, Li B, Wang Q, Horel S, Cooper S. (2009) Agricultural pesticides and risk of childhood cancers. *Int J Hyg Environ Health* **212**: 186–195.
56. Morton LM, Wang SS, Devesa SS, Hartge P, Weisenburger DD, Linet MS. (2006) Lymphoma incidence patterns by WHO subtype in the United States, 1992–2001. *Blood* **107**: 265–276.
57. Li J, Thompson TD, Miller JW, Pollack LA, Stewart SL. (2008) Cancer incidence among children and adolescents in the United States, 2001–2003. *Pediatrics* **121**: e1470–e1477.
58. Oschlies I, Klapper W, Zimmermann M, Krams M, Wacker HH, Burkhardt B, Harder L, Siebert R, Reiter A, Parwaresch R. (2006) Diffuse large B-cell lymphoma in pediatric patients belongs predominantly to the germinal-center type B-cell lymphomas: A clinicopathologic analysis of cases included in the German BFM (Berlin-Frankfurt-Munster) Multicenter Trial. *Blood* **107**: 4047–4052.
59. Stiller CA. (2004) Epidemiology and genetics of childhood cancer. *Oncogene* **23**: 6429–6444.
61. Surveillance E, and End Results (SEER) Program (www.seer.cancer.gov) SEER*Stat Database: Incidence — SEER 9 Regs Research Data, Nov 2009 Sub (1973–2007) <Katrina/Rita Population Adjustment> — Linked To County Attributes — Total U.S., 1969–2007 Counties, National Cancer Institute, DCCPS, Surveillance Research Program, Cancer Statistics Branch, released April 2010, based on the November 2009 submission.
62. Crawford DH. (2001) Biology and disease associations of Epstein-Barr virus. *Philos Trans R Soc Lond B Biol Sci* **356**: 461–473.
64. Burkhardt B. (2010) Paediatric lymphoblastic T-cell leukaemia and lymphoma: One or two diseases? *Br J Haematol* **149**: 653–668.
65. Bolarinwa RA, Ndakotsu MA, Oyekunle AA, Salawu L, Akinola NO, Durosinmi MA. (2009) AIDS-related lymphomas in Nigeria. *Braz J Infect Dis* **13**: 359–361.

66. Jaglowski SM, Linden E, Termuhlen AM, Flynn JM. (2009) Lymphoma in adolescents and young adults. *Semin Oncol* **36**: 381–418.
67. Patte C, Ribrag V, Brugieres L. (2007) Non Hodgkin's lymphoma in adolescents. *Bull Cancer* **94**: 339–348.
68. Attias D, Hodgson D, Weitzman S. (2009) Primary mediastinal B-cell lymphoma in the pediatric patient: Can a rational approach to therapy be based on adult studies? *Pediatr Blood Cancer* **52**: 566–570.
69. Katz BZ, Pahl E, Crawford SE, Kostyk MC, Rodgers S, Seshadri R, Proytcheva M, Pophal S. (2007) Case-control study of risk factors for the development of post-transplant lymphoproliferative disease in a pediatric heart transplant cohort. *Pediatr Transplant* **11**: 58–65.
70. Tai E, Pollack LA, Townsend J, Li J, Steele CB, Richardson LC. (2010) Differences in non-Hodgkin lymphoma survival between young adults and children. *Arch Pediatr Adolesc Med* **164**: 218–224.
71. Ma X, Urayama K, Chang J, Wiemels JL, Buffler PA. (2009) Infection and pediatric acute lymphoblastic leukemia. *Blood Cells Mol Dis* **42**: 117–120.
72. Morton LM, Wang SS, Cozen W, Linet MS, Chatterjee N, Davis S, Severson RK, Colt JS, Vasef MA, Rothman N, Blair A, Bernstein L, Cross AJ, de Roos AJ, Engels EA, Hein DW, Hill DA, Kelemen LE, Lim U, Lynch CF, Schenk M, Wacholder S, Ward MH, Hoar Zahm S, Chanock SJ, Cerhan JR, Hartge P. (2008) Etiologic heterogeneity among non-Hodgkin lymphoma subtypes. *Blood* **112**: 5150–5160.

2

The WHO Classification of Hematological Malignancies (2008)

Martine Raphaël and Nicole Brousse

Introduction

Historic aspects, REAL classification and the 3rd edition of WHO classification

The recent fourth edition of the World Health Organization (WHO) handbook for the classification of hematopoietic and lymphoid tissues published in 2008[1] is a revision and update of the third edition of the WHO in 2001,[2] and the first true worldwide consensus classification of hematologic malignancies that was based on a large experience under the joint auspices of the European Association for Hematopathology (EAHP) and the Society for Hematopathology (SH) with the input of clinical advisory committee and experts. At that time, 10 committees for T- and B-cell lymphomas and leukemias and myeloid and histiocytic tumors were created to propose a list of diseases with relevant criteria[2] for the WHO handbook. This proposal became the standard accepted as the standard classification of hematological malignancies. The advances of techniques in genetics, cytogenetics, and molecular biology led to a revolution in the ability to diagnose and classify hematological malignancies by a combination of morphologic, immunophenotypic, and genetic criteria in addition to clinical features defining each disease entity (see Chapters 4–8).

The clinical advisory committee appointed by the steering committee ensured that the classification meets clinical questions in term of diagnoses and therapeutic strategies. Clinical issues related to the classification were discussed at a meeting gathering the Clinical Advisory Committee and the representatives of the different committees of pathologists (Airlie). This meeting, organized around a series of controversial clinical questions, was able to reach a consensus on most of questions concerning lymphoid, myeloid, and histiocytic neoplasms.[3]

The principles of the WHO classification were based on those of the Revised European–American Classification of lymphoid neoplasms (REAL) which identified entities associated with distinctive clinical presentations and natural history such as age, nodal vs. extranodal presentation, specific anatomic site, history of cytotoxic, and other therapies. This classification published by the International Lymphoma Study Group in 1994[4] was based on the updated Kiel Classification developed by K. Lennert on the principle of a related normal counterpart of malignant lymphoid proliferation[5] and the similar concept proposed by Lukes and Collins.[6]

To characterize these neoplasms, morphology is the first step of analysis of the tumor and is always important independent of the category of hematological malignancy. Immunophenotype, which is specific in some neoplasms, must complete both the morphological and cytogenetic analyses, showing specific genetic abnormalities that can have prognostic significance.[7]

A postulated normal counterpart of the neoplastic cells should be proposed when possible. This postulated cell of origin represents the stage of differentiation of the tumor but not the notion of the cell where the initial transforming event occurs. For lymphoid neoplasms, besides the identification of the lineage B, T and natural killer (NK), they are further divided into precursor neoplasms and mature neoplasms. For the latter, the clinical manifestations were subdivided into disseminated/leukemic, extranodal, and nodal malignancies. In contrast to previous classifications,[5,8] the lymphoid neoplasms were grouped neither according to their histological grade nor according to their clinical aggressiveness. The importance of clinical factors with the International Prognostic Index (IPI) is now used to determine clinical outcome and response to therapy within disease entities.[9]

The reproducibility of the REAL classification was tested by the review of more than 1000 cases of non-Hodgkin lymphoma at centers around the world by a team of five experts in hematopathology. The results of this study demonstrated the relevance of this classification: more than 95% of cases with adequate material could be classified into one or another of the categories with a much better reproducibility than the previous classifications.[7,10] These results emphasized the principles of the WHO, which was based on this classification.

The principles of these disease definitions were extended to the myeloid, mast cells, and histiocytic/dendritic neoplasms. However, in myeloid tumors, whatever the stage of cell differentiation at clinical presentation, the stem cell is involved in most of the neoplasms. Thus, the hematological malignancies are stratified according to lineage: lymphoid neoplasms, myeloid neoplasms, mast cell disorders and histiocytic/dendritic neoplasms. Within each category, distinct diseases are defined according to an integrated approach by the combination of morphology, immunophenotype, genetic feature, and clinical syndrome. The relative importance of each of these criteria differs among these neoplasms. In the third edition, four major groups of myeloid diseases were identified: (1) chronic myeloproliferative diseases (CMPD) arising from clonal hematopoietic stem cell disorders, (2) myelodysplastic/myeloproliferative diseases (MDS/MPD) showing overlapping features between MDS and CMPD, MDS, (3) clonal stem cell disorders characterized by ineffective hematopoiesis, and (4) acute myeloid leukemia (AML) *de novo* or arising from myelodysplasia or therapy related. In AML, numerous genetic lesions that predict clinical outcome were incorporated into the classification. In this field of hematological malignancies, many progresses from basic science are arising, leading to the incorporation of the new molecular features which underlined the relationships between those entities.

Thus, the rapid acquisition of knowledge in the different fields of the WHO classification concerning lymphoid and myeloid malignancies as well as mast cell disorders justified the upgrading of the third edition to incorporate new information in a collaborative project of the EAHP and the SH.

The 4th edition of the WHO classification

As any classification must be periodically reviewed and upgraded, the classification of tumors of hematopoietic and lymphoid tissues will continue to be reviewed under the auspices of the two societies, EAHP and SH. These societies have initiated cooperation and communication between pathologists, hematologists, oncologists as well as researchers for exchanging continued progress not only from basic science to pathology and clinics but also from the microscope to basic science laboratory for new discovery.[11] The fourth edition of the WHO classification exemplifies these progresses in lymphoid and myeloid neoplasms.

The update of the fourth edition of the WHO classification began in 2006. It is a worldwide consensus coming from the same organization as the third edition: two clinical advisory committees; myeloid neoplasms and other acute leukemias and lymphoid neoplasms were created and, in addition, more than 100 authors and experts in hematopathology participated. Meetings around a series of questions were set up and a consensus final meeting was held in Lyon at the headquarters of International Agency for Research on Cancer (IARC) to finalize the decisions on the incorporation of new information in the different chapters.[1]

From this methodology, new information would have emerged from basic and clinical investigations in the interval since publication of the third edition in 2001, due to an increased number of entities being described in the new 2008 WHO classification. In fact, some heterogeneous or ambiguous subcategories are better defined with new basic insights. On the contrary, some changes allowed the identification of certain provisional borderline categories in order to analyze and study the so-called "grey zone" neoplasms. Among these new entities, pediatric lymphomas are identified; they are represented by the frequency of some categories of lymphomas such as: precursor lymphoid neoplasms, aggressive mature B-cell lymphoma and they are also listed as new variants of different subtypes of non-Hodgkin lymphoma, usually described in the adult population, such as follicular lymphomas (FL) or nodal marginal zone lymphomas (NMZL). In myeloid neoplasms, they may have more specific clinical presentation such as in mastocytosis. These differences emphasized the need to describe more specifically hematological malignancies occurring in children, adolescents, and young adults.

In the WHO classification, the defined diseases are clinically distinctive facilitating the interpretation of clinical and translational studies as well as more precise pathogenic approaches, such as in infection-associated lymphoma.[12] A scheme of pathogenic insights based on a disease-oriented approach to lymphoma classification identified six different predominant pathogenic mechanisms of lymphoma: (1) lymphomas associated with infectious agents, (2) lymphomas with deregulation of apoptosis with survival pathways, (3) lymphomas with deregulation of the cell cycle, (4) lymphoma with deregulation with cell signaling or transcriptional regulation, (5) lymphoma associated with susceptibility factors, congenital or acquired.[11] Furthermore, besides these pathogenic mechanisms, more complexity begins to be identified such as the ability of lineage plasticity in hematopoietic cells and their neoplasms. This phenomenon may complicate the interpretation of some biological markers used to identify the lineage of a neoplasm.

Moreover, epidemiologic studies will take benefice from such reproducible, well-defined entity classifications. For example, previous epidemiologic observations[13] were confirmed by the review of lymphoid neoplasms using the REAL[10] and then the WHO classification.[2] This approach allows better epidemiologic research[14] for which the reproducibility of classification is a key factor.[15,16]

Today and in the near future, the development of targeted therapies and the recognition of additional markers of clinical behavior will lead to additional modifications. This evolution illustrates the need of a continuum from basic science to clinical features, for accurate and precise classification of disease entities, which is the clue and the first step for discovering new genetic basis of hematological neoplasms.

Classification of Lymphoid Neoplasms

Tumors developed from the immune system comprise B- and T/NK-cell neoplasms. Almost all lymphoid proliferations can be related to normal counterparts sharing the same immunophenotype and functional property, however, at that time, the normal counterpart of the neoplastic cell cannot be the unique basis of the classification. Three major categories are described: B-cell neoplasms, T/NK-cell neoplasms and Hodgkin lymphomas. The WHO classification contains many groups, which are subclassified using different criteria: either morphological, immunohistochemical, clinical, or genetic.[1]

This chapter will not describe all the lymphomas but recalls the categories of lymphomas and will emphasize the new subtypes in the classical types of lymphomas, the provisional and borderline categories, and finally the new entities devoted to children.

Precursor lymphoid neoplasms

These neoplasms include B lymphoblastic leukemia/lymphoma (B-LBL/ALL) and T lymphoblastic leukemia/lymphoma (T-LBL/ALL), most of them (about 75%) occur in children with male predominance, whatever B or T cell lineage. The term "lymphoma" is confined to clinical presentation with predominant mass, with no or minimal peripheral blood or bone marrow infiltration. B-LBL represents about 15% of cases of precursor B neoplasms. The term "leukemia" is arbitrarily dedicated when the percentage of blasts in the bone marrow is higher than 20%. The subcategories according to the genetic abnormalities introduced in the third revision are confirmed in the fourth revision of the WHO classification,[1] identifying B-LBL/ALL with or without recurrent genetic abnormalities (Table 2.1).

B-LBL/ALL, arising from either a hematopoietic stem cell or B-cell progenitor, is primarily a disease of children. The involvement of bone marrow and frequent

Table 2.1. WHO classification of precursor lymphoid neoplasms (2008).

- B lymphoblastic leukemia/lymphoma
- B lymphoblastic leukemia/lymphoma, not otherwise specified
- B lymphoblastic leukemia/lymphoma with recurrent genetic abnormalities
    - With t(9;22)(q34;q11.2); *BCR-ABL1*
    - With t(v;11q23); *MLL* rearranged
    - With t(12;21)(p13;q22); *TEL-AML1 (ETV-RUNX1)*
    - With hyperdiploidy
    - With hypodiploidy
    - With t(5;14)(q31;q32); *IL3-IGH*
    - With t(1;19)(q23;p13.3); *E2A-PBX1 (TCF3-PBX1)*
- T lymphoblastic leukemia/lymphoma

infiltration of central nervous system (CNS), lymph node, spleen, and testis are the hallmark of B-ALL while skin, soft tissue, bone, and lymph nodes are involved in B-LBL.[17] B-LBL/ALL not otherwise specified (NOS) are associated with genetic lesions such as del6q, del9p del12p.[1] Seven subtypes with recurrent genetic abnormalities: t(9;22)(q34;q11.2); *BCR-ABL1*, t(v;11q23); *MLL* rearranged, t(12;21)(p13;q22); *TEL-AML1 (ETV6-RUNX1)*, with hyperploidy, with hypoploidy, t(5;14)(q31;q32); *IL3-IGH*, t(1;19)(q23;p13.3); *E2A-PBX1 (TCF3-PBX1)* are now described and their prognoses differ according to those genetic abnormalities.[1]

Cases of T-LBL/ALL arising from T cell progenitors (T-ALL) or thymic lymphocytes (T-LBL) are mostly presented by the primary involvement of thymus associated (or not) with other extranodal sites. Leukemia represents about 15% of cases. Their diagnosis is also based on morphology, immunophenotype, and cytogenetics. Chromosomes abnormalities are found in 50–70% of cases. The most frequent anomaly is represented by the translocation involving the alpha and delta loci at 14q11.2, the beta locus at 7q35 and the gamma locus at 7p14-15, with different partner genes. The genes of transcription factors *HOX11L2 (TLX3)* and *HOX11* (*TLX1*) are involved either in adult or children with different frequency;[18] deletions and mutations implicating mostly NOTCH1 are also described with significant prognosis for the latter.[19]

Mature B-cell lymphoma

The long list of mature B-cell neoplasms comprises at least 20 different categories, which can be identified as chronic lymphoproliferative neoplasms, that are very rare if not described in children, while aggressive mature B-cell neoplasms are the most frequent mature lymphoid neoplasms in children and adolescents. Among these neoplasms, diffuse large B-cell lymphoma (DLBCL) is a large group where new subtypes were introduced in the last revised version as listed on Table 2.2.[1]

The recent development of molecular analysis has helped to identify, in DLBCL, gene expression signatures associated with good or poor responses to therapy, according to germinal center or activated phenotype, independent from the IPI.[20]

The group of DLBCL NOS is a large group of heterogeneous lymphomas, with different subtypes, according to the morphologic variants, the immunophenotype, the genetics, the postulated cell of origin (of either germinal center or post-germinal center origin) and the predictive factors (based on the IPI). Thus, morphological variants comprise mostly common morphologic variants: centroblastic, immunoblastic, and anaplastic. The molecular subgroups are composed of germinal center B cell-like (GCB) and activated B cell-like (ABC) while the immunohistochemical subgroups include: CD5+ DLBCL, GCB and non-GCB DLBCL.[21] The stratification according to gene expression profiles GCB vs. ABC

Table 2.2. WHO classification of the mature B-cell neoplasms (2008).

- Chronic lymphocytic leukemia/small lymphocytic lymphoma
- B-cell prolymphocytic leukemia
- Splenic B-cell marginal zone lymphoma
- Hairy cell leukemia
  - Splenic lymphoma/leukemia unclassifiable*
    - Splenic diffuse red pulp small B-cell lymphoma*
    - Hairy cell leukemia-variant*
- Lymphoplasmacytic lymphoma
  - Waldenström macroglobulinemia
- Heavy chain disease
  - Alpha heavy chain disease
  - Gamma heavy chain disease
  - Mu heavy chain disease
- Plasma cell myeloma
- Solitary plasmacytoma of bone
- Extraosseous plasmacytoma
- Extranodal marginal zone lymphoma of mucosa-associated lymphoid tissue (MALT lymphoma)
- Nodal marginal zone lymphoma
  - Pediatric nodal marginal zone lymphoma*
- Follicular lymphoma
  - Pediatric follicular lymphoma*
- Primary cutaneous follicle center lymphoma
- Mantle cell lymphoma
- Diffuse large B-cell lymphoma (DLBCL), not otherwise specified (NOS)
  - T-cell/histiocyte rich large B-cell lymphoma
  - Primary DLBCL of the Central Nervous System (CNS)
  - Primary cutaneous DLBCL, leg type
  - EBV+ DLBCL of the elderly*
- DLBCL associated with chronic inflammation
- Lymphomatoid granulomatosis
- Primary mediastinal (thymic) large B-cell lymphoma
- Intravascular large B-cell lymphoma
- ALK+ large B-cell lymphoma
- Plasmablastic lymphoma
- Large B-cell lymphoma arising in HHV8-associated multicentric Castleman disease
- Primary effusion lymphoma
- Burkitt lymphoma
- B-cell lymphoma, unclassifiable with features intermediate between diffuse large cell lymphoma and Burkitt lymphoma
- B-cell lymphoma, unclassifiable with features intermediate between large B-cell lymphoma and classical Hodgkin lymphoma

*Provisional entities

types as having prognostic value, but as yet does not direct therapy.[20]

DLBCL have been also separated into their specificity representing different entities according to their morphologic aspect, localization, and clinical presentation with the identification of subtypes as listed in Table 2.2: T cell/histiocyte-rich large B-cell lymphoma at morphologic level. The identification of diseases characterized by the involvement of specific anatomic sites is recognized as entities such as: primary mediastinal (thymic) large B-cell lymphoma, primary DLBCL of the CNS including intracerebral and intraocular lymphomas, cutaneous DLBCL leg type, and intravascular large B-cell lymphoma. Specific clinical features with decreased immune surveillance are associated with other DLBCLs like Epstein–Barr virus (EBV), positive DLBCL of the elderly, DLBCL associated with chronic inflammation often associated with EBV, lymphomatoid granulomatosis, plasmablastic lymphoma, large B-cell lymphoma arising in HHV8-associated multicentric Castleman disease and primary effusion lymphoma, the subcategory of ALK-positive large B-cell lymphoma has been also listed.[1]

Burkitt lymphoma

Among the mature B-cell lymphoma, Burkitt lymphoma (BL), which is one of the most frequent lymphomas in childhood and adolescents, is defined by a very short doubling time tumor and the involvement of the *MYC* gene, which is highly characteristic but not specific, justifying a combination between morphology, immunophenotype and genetic analysis for diagnosis.[22] Three clinical variants are described, namely: endemic BL, sporadic BL, and immunodeficiency-associated BL. The frequency of EBV varies according to those clinical variants as well as the clinical presentation.[1,2,23]

Borderline categories

These two subcategories of DLBCL with features intermediate between DLBCL and BL are identified in the revised edition of the 2008 WHO classification in order to recognize this group more clearly which is not considered as a distinct entity. It is more frequent in adults than in children and young adults but needs to be individualized at the light of new molecular and genetic approach.[1,24] The same goals justify the identification of the subgroup of B-cell lymphoma, unclassifiable with features intermediate between DLBCL and classical Hodgkin lymphoma. These lymphomas most commonly associated with mediastinal mass are mostly present in young adults.[1,25]

Mature T and NK-cell lymphoma

These lymphomas are relatively uncommon, representing less than 15% of all lymphomas.[10] These neoplasms that comprise numerous categories summarized in Table 2.3 are rare in children, except anaplastic large cell lymphoma (ALCL), which represents the third most common lymphoma in children and adolescents (Table 2.3).[26]

The incidence of T- and NK-cell lymphomas shows significant differences according to geographical regions and racial populations. These lymphomas display the immunophenotype of post-thymic T lymphocytes or NK cells. The predominant clinical features of these neoplasms can be leukemic or disseminated, extranodal including cutaneous primary localizations and nodal.

In cutaneous primary lymphomas, the different nosological entities defined by the previous WHO/European Organisation for Research and Treatment of

Table 2.3. WHO classification of mature and NK-cell neoplasms (2008).

- T-cell prolymphocytic leukemia
- T-cell large granular lymphocyte leukemia
- Chronic lymphoproliferative disorders of NK cells*
- Aggressive NK cell leukemia
- Systemic EBV positive T-cell lymphoproliferative disease of childhood
- Hydroa vacciniforme-like lymphoma
- Adult T-cell leukemia/lymphoma
- Extranodal NK/T-cell lymphoma, nasal type
- Enteropathy-associated T-cell lymphoma
- Hepatosplenic T-cell lymphoma
- Subcutaneous panniculitis-like T-cell lymphoma
- Mycosis fongoïde
- Sezary syndrome
- Primary cutaneous CD30+ T-cell lymphoproliferative disorders
  - o Lymphomatoid papulosis
  - o Primary cutaneous anaplastic large cell lymphoma
- Primary cutaneous gamma-delta T-cell lymphoma
  - o Primary cutaneous CD8+ aggressive epidermotropic cytotoxic T-cell lymphoma*
  - o Primary cutaneous CD4+ small/medium-cell lymphoma*
- Peripheral T-cell lymphoma NOS
- Angioimmunoblastic T-cell lymphoma
- Anaplastic large cell lymphoma, ALK+
  - o Anaplastic large cell lymphoma, ALK–*

*Provisional entities

Cancer (EORTC) classification[27] are incorporated, underlining the final diagnosis that implies clinicopathological correlation as the clinical manifestation, an essential element in the diagnostic approach to primary cutaneous lymphomas.[28] In addition to the previous categories of cutaneous lymphomas which were listed in the third edition of the WHO classification, primary cutaneous peripheral T-cell lymphomas rare subtypes (namely primary gamma-delta T-cell lymphoma, primary cutaneous $CD8^+$ aggressive epidermotropic cytotoxic T-cell lymphoma, primary cutaneous $CD4^+$ small/medium T-cell lymphoma) have been added.[1] Among the recent changes in the terminology, in the T-cell system, primary cutaneous $CD30^+$ T-cell lymphoproliferative disorders have been listed.[2,28] These disorders include primary cutaneous ALCL (C-ALCL),[29] lymphomatoid papulosis (LyP)[30,31] and borderline cases. C-ALCL must be distinguished from systemic ALCL with cutaneous involvement, which is a separate disease. Primary C-ALCL sporadically affects children, contrary to LyP, a clonal T-cell proliferation that also has limited malignant potential. Thus, it is not considered a malignant disorder, even with the presence of monoclonality in many cases; it is a recurrent, chronic, self-healing disease.[30,31]

Among the other T-cell lymphomas, peripheral T-cell lymphoma NOS has been already described in children but it is very rare.[32]

In situ or early lesions in lymphomas

These lesions must be mentioned since they are identified in the fourth revision of the WHO classification. *In situ* or early lesions have been recognized for both FL and mantle cell lymphoma, and to early gastric MALT lymphomas. The risk for progression is unknown. They are often incidental findings. The recognition of small clonal lymphoid populations such as clonal expansions of B cells, or less often T cells, appears to have limited potential for histologic or clinical progression. For example, although up to 70% of healthy adults have circulating clonal memory B cells with the t(14;18)(q32;q21), these cells presumably lack other genetic alterations necessary for development of malignant behavior. A total of 3% to 5% of healthy adults have circulating monoclonal B cells with the immunophenotype of chronic lymphocytic leukemia (monoclonal B lymphocytosis). They rarely progress to overt, progressive leukemia.[33]

The 2008 WHO classification relevance to pediatric non-Hodgkin lymphomas

Non-Hodgkin lymphomas in children and adolescents frequently observed in children, adolescents and young adults or identified as new variants of different subtypes of lymphomas described in adults, such as FL or nodal marginal zone lymphomas (NMZL) are summarized in Table 2.4.

Lymphomas account for about 10% of childhood malignancies in the US and Europe. Pediatric lymphomas are usually extranodal, have a rapid growth and are rarely follicular. Some categories are not described or very rare such as lymphocytic lymphoma, or mantle cell lymphoma.

The most frequent lymphomas in children and adolescents are T-cell LBL and BL which are the two most common lymphomas. DLBCL accounts for less than 20% and ALCL anaplastic lymphoma receptor tyrosine kinase (ALK)-positive represents the third most frequent type of lymphoma in children (around 20%). All these lymphomas have the characteristics of the equivalent ones in the adult population and will not be described in detail in this chapter. However, while they are morphologically and immunophenotypically similar to lymphomas occurring in adults, pediatric lymphomas may differ in pathogenesis from their equivalent in adults.[34]

The new variants of different subtypes of lymphomas described in children in the 2008 WHO classification comprise pediatric FL and pediatric NMZL.

Pediatric FL, a variant of FL described in the 2008 WHO classification, is a very rare disease. It often involves

Table 2.4. WHO classification of pediatric variants of lymphomas (2008).

- T-cell lymphoblastic lymphoma
- B-cell lymphoblastic lymphoma
- Burkitt lymphoma
- Anaplastic large cell lymphoma
- Diffuse large B-cell lymphoma

- Specific variants of other lymphomas:
  - Pediatric nodal marginal zone lymphoma
  - Pediatric follicular lymphoma
  - Pediatric follicular hyperplasia with monoclonal B cells
  - EBV-positive T-cell lymphoproliferative (LPD) disorders of childhood
    - Systemic EBV-positive T-cell LPD
    - Hydroa vacciniform-like lymphoma
  - Lymphoproliferative disorders (LPD) associated with primary immune disease (PID)

cervical lymph nodes, other peripheral lymph nodes, Waldeyer ring or testis.[35] Children with FL typically have early-stage disease. They have many features resembling adult FL, but an increased proportion is localized, lacks BCL2 protein expression and t(14;18) and is grade 3. The diagnosis is said to be made with the morphological features of malignancy.[36] The prognosis is good. The 2008 WHO classification asks the question of the nature of pediatric follicular hyperplasia with monoclonal B cells; in fact, cases of follicular hyperplasia in children have been reported that contain clonal populations of CD10 GCB cells.[36] Are they an early involvement by a neoplasm, a precursor lesion or an inconsequential finding? Yet, they do not progress to overt lymphoma.

Pediatric NMZL, a clinical variant of NMZL has distinctive clinical and morphological characteristics.[37] NZML is mostly described in males, with asymptomatic and localized disease, mainly in the head and neck lymph nodes. The histology and immunophenotype are similar to adult NMZL. The differential diagnosis with atypical marginal zone hyperplasia with monotypic Ig expression may be difficult and necessitates studies for clonal IgH rearrangement.[38] The prognosis is excellent.

EBV-positive T-cell lymphoproliferative disorders of childhood (LPD)

These disorders include two types: systemic EBV-positive T-cell LPD and Hydroa vacciniform-like lymphoma. The systemic EBV-positive T-cell LPD is a clonal proliferation of EBV-infected T-cells with an activated cytotoxic phenotype. It has a rapid progression with multiple organ failure.[39] Hydroa vacciniform-like lymphoma is an EBV-positive cutaneous T-cell lymphoma occurring in children and associated with sun sensitivity affecting the sun-exposed skin, particularly the face. The cells have a cytotoxic T-cell phenotype, less often a NK cell phenotype (see Chapter 19).[40]

Primary immune disease (PID) might be associated with LPD

The pathology and pathogenesis of the more than the 60 PIDs are heterogeneous, such as the manifestations and clinical aspects. The most frequent PIDs associated with LPD are: ataxia telangiectasia, Wiskott–Aldrich syndrome, common variable immune deficiency, severe combined immune deficiency, X-linked LPD, Nijmegen breakage syndrome and autoimmune lymphoproliferative syndrome (ALPS) (see Chapter 19).[1,2]

With the exception of common variable immune deficiency (CVID), these diseases present primarily in the pediatric age group. Because of the genetic abnormalities, most often X-linked, they are more common in males. The cause and mechanisms (defective T-cell immune surveillance to EBV, defects in function of T cells, B cells, mutations in the gene for CD40 or CD40-ligand, mutations in the *FAS* or *FASL* gene, abnormal DNA repair mechanism etc.) of the LPD are related to the underlying primary immune deficiency.[41] Type, frequency and presentation are dependent of the underlying disease, often in extranodal sites, most commonly the gastrointestinal tract, lung and CNS. At the morphologic level, they include reactive hyperplasia, polymorphous lymphoid infiltrates and frank lymphomas involving EBV in the majority of cases. Lymphomatoid granulomatosis is a rare variant of DLBCL observed in that clinical context. It is an EBV-driven lymphoproliferative B cell disease involving extranodal sites, especially pulmonary with angiocentricity and angiodestruction.[42]

Hodgkin lymphoma

Since the third edition of WHO classification, the term Hodgkin lymphoma is now preferred over Hodgkin's disease, as the origin of the Reed–Sternberg cell is known to be a lymphoid cell, most often of the B-cell type at the germinal center stage of differentiation.

Hodgkin lymphoma comprises two diseases entities:[43] nodular lymphocyte predominant Hodgkin lymphoma, which rarely occurs during childhood, contrary to classical Hodgkin lymphoma showing a bimodal age curve with a first peak at 15–35 years of age (Table 2.5). These two entities differ in their clinical features and behavior, as well as in the composition of their cellular background and, most important for diagnosis, in the morphology, immunophenotype and preservation or extinction of B-cell gene expression program.[1]

The four different subtypes of the classical Hodgkin lymphoma (nodular sclerosis, mixed cellularity, lymphocyte-rich and lymphocyte-depleted subtype) (Table 2.5) differ in their sites of involvement, clinical features, growth pattern, presence of fibrosis, composition of cellular background, number and/or degree of atypia

Table 2.5. WHO classification of Hodgkin lymphoma (2008).

- Nodular lymphocytic-predominant Hodgkin lymphoma
- Classical Hodgkin lymphoma
  - Nodular sclerosis classical Hodgkin lymphoma
  - Lymphocyte-rich classical Hodgkin lymphoma
  - Mixed cellularity classical Hodgkin lymphoma
  - Lymphocyte-depleted classical Hodgkin lymphoma

of the tumor cells and frequency of EBV infection, but not in the immunophenotype of the tumor cells, which is the same in all four variants ($CD30^+$, $CD15^+$, variable CD20 expression only in a minority of the neoplastic cells).[1]

Conclusion and pitfalls in the diagnosis of pediatric lymphoma

Despite the development of new techniques, particularly at the molecular and genetic levels, and the better understanding of the immune system and its tumor counterpart, the diagnosis of lymphomas is still difficult in some cases, especially in children. One should first have all the clinical signs, ask for infections, vaccination, drugs etc. The specimen must be sent to a pathologist with special expertise in lymph node pathology and also with a special experience in pediatric pathology. A descriptive report outlining the diagnostic dilemma may be the wisest option in difficult cases. Pathologists must also keep in mind that a lymphoproliferative disorder may reveal an immune deficiency and also that infections and benign reactions are much more common than lymphomas.[44]

Although these are important progresses in the knowledge of the immune system and in the technical approach to characterize lymphoid neoplasms, there are still unresolved issues including defining pathologic predictors of prognosis, outcome and response to treatment, in common diseases such as FL, DLBCL and peripheral T-cell lymphomas. The host immune response, the so-called microenvironment, may have a strong impact on the clinical outcome after chemotherapy.

Classification of the Myeloid Neoplasms

The third edition of the WHO classification for myeloid neoplasms introduced genetic information into diagnostic approach for the described entities. This approach which emphasized the role of molecular and genetic abnormalities in the definition and clinical relevance of myeloid neoplasms was confirmed by the discovery of new molecular insights that became part of the diagnosis in chronic myeloproliferative neoplasms and AML.

So, in the fourth edition, defined myeloid entities are based on a combination of morphologic, immunophenotype, and genetic features (Table 2.5). The first example is chronic myelogenous leukemia, in which the well-known genetic abnormality *BCR-ABL1* is useful for diagnosis and therapy targeting. The last revision individualizes a subgroup of myeloid neoplasms associated with eosinophilia that have genetic abnormalities involving the platelet-derived growth factor, which respond to anti-tyrosine kinase therapy.[45] The major revolution was the discovery of *JAK2* mutations which is now included in the diagnosis algorithm of myeloproliferative neoplasm;[46,47] however *JAK2* mutations are not specific since they are also reported in some myelodysplastic syndrome or myelodysplastic/myeloproliferative neoplasms and AML, underlining the need of a combination of features: cytology, histology, immunophenotype, and genetics to characterize myeloid entities. The blast percentage remains one of the gold standards to categorize these neoplasms and to follow their evolution. Examination of peripheral blood smears, bone marrow aspirate, and trephine biopsy constitute the morphologic approach for evaluation of bone marrow cellularity, percentage of blasts, maturation, morphology, and hematopoiesis. Morphology must be completed by cytochemistry and other special stains such as myeloperoxidase, Sudan black, nonspecific and specific esterases, and immunophenotype, mostly with multiparameters flow cytometry which is essential for the characterization using a combination of monoclonal antibodies. Genetics study using classical karyotypes should be performed at the initial diagnosis. Molecular techniques including RT-PCR, FISH and gene sequencing are important to finalize the characterization according to the criteria of the 2008 WHO classification.

Myeloproliferative neoplasms

For this category of myeloid neoplasms, (Table 2.6) several changes are done such as the nomenclature: neoplasms instead of diseases, the chronic eosinophilic leukemia with genetic abnormalities of *PDGFRA, PDGFRB or FGFR1* are now categorized as myeloid or lymphoid neoplasms since cases associated with *PDGFRA* rearrangements can have presentation according to AML or T cell lymphoblastic neoplasms,[48]

Table 2.6. WHO classification of myeloproliferative neoplasms myeloid and lymphoid neoplasms with éosinophilia and abnormalities of PDGFRA, PDGFRB, FGFR1 (2008).

- Chronic myelogenous leukemia
  - BCR-ABL1 positive
- Chronic neutrophilic leukemia
- Polycythaemia vera
- Primary myelofibrosis
- Essential thrombocythaemia
- Chronic eosinophilic leukemia, NOS
- Mastocytosis
  - Cutaneous mastocytosis
  - Systemic mastocytosis
  - Mast cell leukemia
  - Mast cell sarcoma
  - Extracutaneous mastocytoma
- Myeloproliferative neoplasm, unclassifiable
- Myeloid and lymphoid neoplasms with *PDGFRA* rearrangement
- Myeloid neoplasms with *PDGFRB* rearrangement
- Myeloid and lymphoid neoplasm with *FGFR1* rearrangement

the mastocytosis are included in this category of hematopoietic neoplasms, the discovery of *JAK2* mutations has changed the criteria of diagnosis of these myeloproliferative neoplasms, the threshold of platelets count for essential thrombocythemia has been lowered and finally, the criteria to evaluate accelerated phase for chronic myeloid leukemia must be reviewed with the era of anti-tyrosine kinase. Among these neoplasms which occurred mostly in adults in the fourth to seventh decade, some subtypes such as chronic myeloid leukemia,[49] chronic neutrophilic leukemia[50] and essential thrombocytemia[51] are reported in childhood and adolescence. Polycythemia vera[52] and primary myelofibrosis[53] are only very rarely reported.

Mastocytosis may occur at any age; in childhood, cutaneous mastocytosis is more frequent and may be present at birth or the children who present with this proliferation developed the skin lesions within the first 6 months of age.[54,55] Diffuse cutaneous variants are also reported in childhood.[56]

Myelodysplastic/myeloproliferative neoplasms and myelodysplastic syndromes

Among these two categories of hematopoietic neoplasms (Table 2.7), while the atypical chronic myeloid leukemia *BCR-ABL1* negative, categorized as borderline type between myelodysplastic and myeloproliferative neoplasms have been described in only few cases of adolescents,[57] two neoplasms occurred specifically in

Table 2.7. WHO classification of myelodysplastic/myeloproliferative and myelodysplastic neoplasms (2008).

- Chronic myelomonocytic leukemia
- Atypical chronic myeloid leukemia
  - BCR-ABL1 negative
- Juvenile myelomonocytic leukemia
- Myelodysplastic/myeloproliferative neoplasm unclassifiable
  - Refractory anemia with ring sideroblasts associated with marked thrombocytosis*
- Refractory cytopenia with unilineage dysplasia
  - Refractory anemia
  - Refractory neutropenia
  - Refractory thrombocytopenia
- Refractory anemia with ring sideroblasts
- Refractory cytopenia with multilineage dysplasia
- Refractory anemia with excess of blasts
- Myelodysplastic syndrome, unclassifiable
- Childhood myelodysplastic syndrome
  - Refractory cytopenia of childhood

*Provisional entities

childhood and adolescents: the juvenile myelomonocytic leukemia and the childhood myelodysplastic syndrome. The former, a clonal hematopoietic disorder described in childhood, occur between 0–14 years of age but 75% of cases occur in children less than 3 years of age with a male predominance. Several criteria must be reached to confirm the diagnosis, one of the most remarkable is the increased synthesis of hemoglobin F.[58,59] The diagnosis of this disorder is based on a combination of arguments, namely morphology, cytochemistry, immunophenotype, and genetics showing abnormalities in 35% of cases without any fusion gene *BCR-ABL1*. While the majority of myelodysplastic syndromes occur in older adults with a median age of 70 years, the childhood myelodysplastic syndrome neoplasm, which shares morphologic, immunophenotypic and genetic features observed in adults, is also described as well as those with some specificity observed in childhood like the predominance of neutropenia, thrombocytopenia and hypocellular bone marrow. A provisional entity, refractory cytopenia of childhood, is introduced in the fourth edition of the WHO classification[60] which represent about 50% of cases.

Acute myeloid leukemia

Since the third edition of the WHO classification, AMLs are first classified according to their cytogenetics patterns, namely with recurrent genetic abnormalities

Table 2.8. WHO classification of acute myeloid leukemia (AML) and related precursor neoplasms (2008).

- AML with recurrent genetic abnormalities
  - AML with t(8;21)(q22;q22); *RUNX1-RUNX1T1*
  - AML with inv(16)(p13.1q22) or t(16;16)(p13.1q22); *CBF-MYH11*
  - Acute promyelocytic leukemia with t(15;17)(q22;q12); *PML-RARA*
  - AML with t(9;11)(p22;q23); *MLLT3-MLL*
  - AML with t(6;9)(p23;q34); *DEK-NUP214*
  - AML with inv(3)(q21q26.2) or t(3;3)(q21;q26.2); *RPN-EVI1*
  - AML (megakaryoblastic) with t(1;22)(p13;q13); *RBM15-MKL1*
  - AML with mutated *NPM1**
  - AML with mutated *CEBPA**
- AML with myelodysplasia-related changes
- Therapy-related myeloid neoplasms
- Acute myeloid leukemia NOS
  - AML with minimal differentiation
  - AML without maturation
  - AML with maturation
  - Acute myelomonocytic leukemia
  - Acute monoblastic and monocytic leukemia
  - Acute erythroid leukemia
  - Acute megakaryoblastic leukemia
  - Acute basophilic leukemia
  - Acute panmyelosis with myelofibrosis
- Myeloid sarcoma
- Myeloid proliferation related to Down syndrome
- Transient abnormal myelopoiesis
- Myeloid leukemia associated with Down syndrome
- Blastic plasmacytoid dendritic cell neoplasm

*Provisional entities

or NOS or myeloid sarcoma (Table 2.8).[2] Other categories identified as AML with myelodysplasia, therapy-related myeloid neoplasms, and blastic plasmacytoid dendritic cell neoplasm are rare in children and young adults. Myeloid proliferations related to Down syndrome are clearly identified in the fourth edition since their clinical behavior differs from that in non-affected children.[1]

Among the acute leukemias with recurrent genetic abnormalities[1] which can occur in all age groups, the t(9;22)(p22;q23), *MLLT3-MLL* from a hematopoietic stem cell with multilineage potential as a postulated normal counterpart, usually associated with monocytic features, the t(8;21)(q22;q22), *RUNX1-RUNX1T1*, arising from myeloid stem cell with predominant neutrophilic differentiation, the inv(16)(p13.1q22) or t(16;16)(p13.1;q22), *CBFB-MYH11* from hematopoietic stem cells with potential to differentiate into granulocytic or monocytic lineage, occur predominantly in younger patients. The t(6;9)(p23;q34); *DEK-NUP214* from a hematopoietic stem cell with multilineage potential occurring in both children and adults, has a median age of 13 years in childhood.[61] Among rare subtypes of AML, acute megakaryoblastic leukemia with t(1;22)(p13;q13), *RBM5-MKL1* representing less than 1% in AML, most often occur in children without Down syndrome almost in the first 6 months of life. In AML with *NPM1* mutations in about 5% of cases occur in childhood.[1]

Table 2.9. WHO classification of acute leukemia with ambiguous lineage (2008).

- Acute undifferentiated leukemia
- Mixed phenotype acute leukemia with t(9;22)(q34;q11.2); *BCR-ABL1*
- Mixed phenotype acute leukemia with t(v;11q23); *MLL* rearranged
- Mixed phenotype acute leukemia B/myeloid NOS
- Mixed phenotype acute leukemia T/myeloid NOS
  - Natural killer (NK) cell lymphoblastic leukemia/lymphoma*

*Provisional entities

Mostly, all subcategories of AML NOS, such as with minimal differentiation, with maturation, monoblastic and monocytic lineage, erythroid leukemia, and acute megakaryoblastic leukemia, are described in childhood and adolescence.[1] In children with Down syndrome, the myeloid proliferations have been individualized in the 2008 WHO classification with two presentations: the transient abnormal myelopoiesis occurring in about 10% of newborn with Down syndrome, and acute megakaryoblastic leukemia in 50% of cases of AML in children with Down syndrome.[62]

Rare acute leukemias of ambiguous lineage occurring in both children and adults comprise several subcategories according to the degree of differentiation, the type of mixed phenotype (B/myeloid, T/myeloid) and the characteristics of cytogenetic abnormalities (Table 2.9).

Histiocytic and Dendritic Cell Neoplasms

These tumors are very rare, representing less than 1% of tumors from lymphoid and soft tissues. These proliferations occur from myeloid-derived macrophages, myeloid-derived dendritic cells and stromal-derived dendritic cells.[63] Tumors from this system are developed in a wide age range occurring from infancy to elderly. These tumors comprise histiocytic sarcoma, interdigitating dendritic cell sarcoma, and follicular dendritic cell sarcoma (Table 2.10).[1] Some of these tumors are preferentially observed during childhood, such as

Table 2.10. WHO classification of histiocytic and dendritic cell neoplasms (2008).

- Histiocytic sarcoma
- Langerhans cell histiocytosis
- Langerhans cell sarcoma
- Follicular dendritic cell sarcoma
- Fibroblastic reticular cell tumor
- Disseminated juvenile xanthogranuloma

Langerhans cell histiocytosis and disseminated juvenile xanthogranuloma.[1] The former presents with multiple or sequential destructive bone lesions associated with tissues masses with preferential skull, mandibular and pulmonary involvement.[64] The latter occurring in infancy is mostly characterized by a solitary dermal localization or visceral and disseminated presentation. The association with neurofibromatosis type 1 is known, as well as the increased risk of juvenile myelomonocytic leukemia.[65]

Among the list of hematopoietic and lymphoid neoplasms identified as entities from a combination of morphologic, immunophenotypic and genetic features as well as clinical findings, variants identified from children and young adults were mentioned in the last edition of WHO classification. However, more accurate diagnoses, especially applied in these categories of individuals will lead to a better understanding of the pathogenesis of these tumors and to improve the outcome of these neoplasms in children, adolescents and young adults.

References

1. Swerdlow SH, Campo E, Harris NL, Jaffe ES, Pileri SA, Stein H, Thiele J, Vardiman JW (eds.) (2008) *WHO Classification of Tumors of Hematopoietic and Lymphoid Tissues* (4th ed). Lyon: IARC Press.
2. Jaffe ES, Harris NL, Stein H, Vardiman JW (eds.) (2001) *WHO Classification of Tumors of Hematopoietic and Lymphoid Tissues* (3rd ed). Lyon: IARC Press.
3. Harris NL, Jaffe ES, Diebold J, Flandrin G, Muller-Hermelink HK, Vardiman J, Lister TA, Bloomfield CD. (2000) The World Health Organization classification of neoplasms of the hematopoietic and lymphoid tissues: Report of the Clinical Advisory Committee meeting — Airlie House, Virginia, November 1997. *Hematol J* **1**: 53–66.
4. Harris NL, Jaffe ES, Stein H, Banks PM, Chan JK, Cleary ML, Delsol G, de Wolf-Peeters C, Falini B, Gatter KC, *et al.* (1994) A revised European-American classification of lymphoid neoplasms: A proposal from the International Lymphoma Study Group. *Blood* **84**: 1361–1392.
9. A predictive model for aggressive non-Hodgkin's lymphoma. (1993) The International Non-Hodgkin's Lymphoma Prognostic Factors Project. *N Engl J Med* **329**: 987–994.
10. A clinical evaluation of the International Lymphoma Study Group classification of non-Hodgkin's lymphoma. (1997) The Non-Hodgkin's Lymphoma Classification Project. *Blood* **89**: 3909–3918.
11. Jaffe ES, Harris NL, Stein H, Isaacson PG. (2008) Classification of lymphoid neoplasms: The microscope as a tool for disease discovery. *Blood* **112**: 4384–4399.
12. Suarez F, Lortholary O, Hermine O, Lecuit M. (2006) Infection-associated lymphomas derived from marginal zone B cells: A model of antigen-driven lymphoproliferation. *Blood* **107**: 3034–3044.
14. Morton LM, Wang SS, Devesa SS, Hartge P, Weisenburger DD, Linet MS. (2006) Lymphoma incidence patterns by WHO subtype in the United States, 1992–2001. *Blood* **107**: 265–276.
16. Sant M, Allemani C, de Angelis R, Carbone A, de Sanjose S, Gianni AM, Giraldo P, Marchesi F, Marcos-Gragera R, Martos-Jimenez C, Maynadie M, Raphael M, Berrino F. (2008) Influence of morphology on survival for non-Hodgkin lymphoma in Europe and the United States. *Eur J Cancer* **44**: 579–587.
17. Lin P, Jones D, Dorfman DM, Medeiros LJ. (2000) Precursor B-cell lymphoblastic lymphoma: A predominantly extranodal tumor with low propensity for leukemic involvement. *Am J Surg Pathol* **24**: 1480–1490.
18. Graux C, Cools J, Michaux L, Vandenberghe P, Hagemeijer A. (2006) Cytogenetics and molecular genetics of T-cell acute lymphoblastic leukemia: From thymocyte to lymphoblast. *Leukemia* **20**: 1496–1510.
19. Malyukova A, Dohda T, von der Lehr N, Akhoondi S, Corcoran M, Heyman M, Spruck C, Grander D, Lendahl U, Sangfelt O. (2007) The tumor suppressor gene hCDC4 is frequently mutated in human T-cell acute lymphoblastic leukemia with functional consequences for Notch signaling. *Cancer Res* **67**: 5611–5616.
20. Alizadeh AA, Eisen MB, Davis RE, Ma C, Lossos IS, Rosenwald A, Boldrick JC, Sabet H, Tran T, Yu X, Powell JI, Yang L, Marti GE, Moore T, Hudson J, Jr., Lu L, Lewis DB, Tibshirani R, Sherlock G, Chan WC, Greiner TC, Weisenburger DD, Armitage JO, Warnke R, Levy R, Wilson W, Grever MR, Byrd JC, Botstein D, Brown PO, Staudt LM. (2000) Distinct types of diffuse large B-cell lymphoma identified by gene expression profiling. *Nature* **403**: 503–511.

21. Hans CP, Weisenburger DD, Greiner TC, Gascoyne RD, Delabie J, Ott G, Muller-Hermelink HK, Campo E, Braziel RM, Jaffe ES, Pan Z, Farinha P, Smith LM, Falini B, Banham AH, Rosenwald A, Staudt LM, Connors JM, Armitage JO, Chan WC. (2004) Confirmation of the molecular classification of diffuse large B-cell lymphoma by immunohistochemistry using a tissue microarray. *Blood* **103**: 275–282.
22. Magrath I. (1990) The pathogenesis of Burkitt's lymphoma. *Adv Cancer Res* **55**: 133–270.
24. Hummel M, Bentink S, Berger H, Klapper W, Wessendorf S, Barth TF, Bernd HW, Cogliatti SB, Dierlamm J, Feller AC, Hansmann ML, Haralambieva E, Harder L, Hasenclever D, Kuhn M, Lenze D, Lichter P, Martin-Subero JI, Moller P, Muller-Hermelink HK, Ott G, Parwaresch RM, Pott C, Rosenwald A, Rosolowski M, Schwaenen C, Sturzenhofecker B, Szczepanowski M, Trautmann H, Wacker HH, Spang R, Loeffler M, Trumper L, Stein H, Siebert R. (2006) A biologic definition of Burkitt's lymphoma from transcriptional and genomic profiling. *N Engl J Med* **354**: 2419–2430.
25. Savage KJ, Monti S, Kutok JL, Cattoretti G, Neuberg D, De Leval L, Kurtin P, Dal Cin P, Ladd C, Feuerhake F, Aguiar RC, Li S, Salles G, Berger F, Jing W, Pinkus GS, Habermann T, Dalla-Favera R, Harris NL, Aster JC, Golub TR, Shipp MA. (2003) The molecular signature of mediastinal large B-cell lymphoma differs from that of other diffuse large B-cell lymphomas and shares features with classical Hodgkin lymphoma. *Blood* **102**: 3871–3879.
26. Stein H, Foss HD, Durkop H, Marafioti T, Delsol G, Pulford K, Pileri S, Falini B. (2000) CD30(+) anaplastic large cell lymphoma: A review of its histopathologic, genetic, and clinical features. *Blood* **96**: 3681–3695.
28. Kempf W, Sander CA. (2010) Classification of cutaneous lymphomas — an update. *Histopathology* **56**: 57–70.
29. Bekkenk MW, Geelen FA, van Voorst Vader PC, Heule F, Geerts ML, van Vloten WA, Meijer CJ, Willemze R. (2000) Primary and secondary cutaneous CD30(+) lymphoproliferative disorders: A report from the Dutch Cutaneous Lymphoma Group on the long-term follow-up data of 219 patients and guidelines for diagnosis and treatment. *Blood* **95**: 3653–3661.
30. El Shabrawi-Caelen L, Kerl H, Cerroni L. (2004) Lymphomatoid papulosis: Reappraisal of clinicopathologic presentation and classification into subtypes A, B, and C. *Arch Dermatol* **140**: 441–447.
32. Rizvi MA, Evens AM, Tallman MS, Nelson BP, Rosen ST. (2006) T-cell non-Hodgkin lymphoma. *Blood* **107**: 1255–1264.
33. Kussick SJ, Kalnoski M, Braziel RM, Wood BL. (2004) Prominent clonal B-cell populations identified by flow cytometry in histologically reactive lymphoid proliferations. *Am J Clin Pathol* **121**: 464–472.
34. Miles RR, Raphael M, McCarthy K, Wotherspoon A, Lones MA, Terrier-Lacombe MJ, Patte C, Gerrard M, Auperin A, Sposto R, Davenport V, Cairo MS, Perkins SL. (2008) Pediatric diffuse large B-cell lymphoma demonstrates a high proliferation index, frequent c-Myc protein expression, and a high incidence of germinal center subtype: Report of the French-American-British (FAB) international study group. *Pediatr Blood Cancer* **51**: 369–374.
36. Lorsbach RB, Shay-Seymore D, Moore J, Banks PM, Hasserjian RP, Sandlund JT, Behm FG. (2002) Clinicopathologic analysis of follicular lymphoma occurring in children. *Blood* **99**: 1959–1964.
37. Taddesse-Heath L, Pittaluga S, Sorbara L, Bussey M, Raffeld M, Jaffe ES. (2003) Marginal zone B-cell lymphoma in children and young adults. *Am J Surg Pathol* **27**: 522–531.
38. Swerdlow SH. (2004) Pediatric follicular lymphomas, marginal zone lymphomas, and marginal zone hyperplasia. *Am J Clin Pathol* **122 Suppl**: S98–S109.
39. Kimura H, Hoshino Y, Kanegane H, Tsuge I, Okamura T, Kawa K, Morishima T. (2001) Clinical and virologic characteristics of chronic active Epstein-Barr virus infection. *Blood* **98**: 280–286.
41. Anagnostopoulos I, Hansmann ML, Franssila K, Harris M, Harris NL, Jaffe ES, Han J, van Krieken JM, Poppema S, Marafioti T, Franklin J, Sextro M, Diehl V, Stein H. (2000) European Task Force on Lymphoma project on lymphocyte predominance Hodgkin disease: Histologic and immunohistologic analysis of submitted cases reveals 2 types of Hodgkin disease with a nodular growth pattern and abundant lymphocytes. *Blood* **96**: 1889–1899.
43. Haque AK, Myers JL, Hudnall SD, Gelman BB, Lloyd RV, Payne D, Borucki M. (1998) Pulmonary lymphomatoid granulomatosis in acquired immunodeficiency syndrome: Lesions with Epstein-Barr virus infection. *Mod Pathol* **11**: 347–356.
44. Isaacson PG. (2007) Haematopathology practice: The commonest problems encountered in a consultation practice. *Histopathology* **50**: 821–834.
45. Bain BJ, Fletcher SH. (2007) Chronic eosinophilic leukemias and the myeloproliferative variant of the hypereosinophilic syndrome. *Immunol Allergy Clin North Am* **27**: 377–388.
47. James C, Ugo V, le Couedic JP, Staerk J, Delhommeau F, Lacout C, Garcon L, Raslova H, Berger R, Bennaceur-Griscelli A, Villeval JL, Constantinescu SN, Casadevall N,

Vainchenker W. (2005) A unique clonal JAK2 mutation leading to constitutive signalling causes polycythaemia vera. *Nature* **434**: 1144–1148.
48. Metzgeroth G, Walz C, Score J, Siebert R, Schnittger S, Haferlach C, Popp H, Haferlach T, Erben P, Mix J, Muller MC, Beneke H, Muller L, del Valle F, Aulitzky WE, Wittkowsky G, Schmitz N, Schulte C, Muller-Hermelink K, Hodges E, Whittaker SJ, Diecker F, Dohner H, Schuld P, Hehlmann R, Hochhaus A, Cross NC, Reiter A. (2007) Recurrent finding of the FIP1L1-PDGFRA fusion gene in eosinophilia-associated acute myeloid leukemia and lymphoblastic T-cell lymphoma. *Leukemia* **21**: 1183–1188.
49. Redaelli A, Bell C, Casagrande J, Stephens J, Botteman M, Laskin B, Pashos C. (2004) Clinical and epidemiologic burden of chronic myelogenous leukemia. *Expert Rev Anticancer Ther* **4**: 85–96.
50. Hasle H, Olesen G, Kerndrup G, Philip P, Jacobsen N. (1996) Chronic neutrophil leukaemia in adolescence and young adulthood. *Br J Haematol* **94**: 628–630.
51. Randi ML, Putti MC, Fabris F, Sainati L, Zanesco L, Girolami A. (2000) Features of essential thrombocythaemia in childhood: A study of five children. *Br J Haematol* **108**: 86–89.
52. Passamonti F, Malabarba L, Orlandi E, Barate C, Canevari A, Brusamolino E, Bonfichi M, Arcaini L, Caberlon S, Pascutto C, Lazzarino M. (2003) Polycythemia vera in young patients: A study on the long-term risk of thrombosis, myelofibrosis and leukemia. *Haematologica* **88**: 13–18.
53. Cervantes F, Barosi G, Demory JL, Reilly J, Guarnone R, Dupriez B, Pereira A, Montserrat E. (1998) Myelofibrosis with myeloid metaplasia in young individuals: Disease characteristics, prognostic factors and identification of risk groups. *Br J Haematol* **102**: 684–690.
55. Bodemer C, Hermine O, Palmerini F, Yang Y, Grandpeix-Guyodo C, Leventhal PS, Hadj-Rabia S, Nasca L, Georgin-Lavialle S, Cohen-Akenine A, Launay JM, Barete S, Feger F, Arock M, Catteau B, Sans B, Stalder JF, Skowron F, Thomas L, Lorette G, Plantin P, Bordigoni P, Lortholary O, de Prost Y, Moussy A, Sobol H, Dubreuil P. (2010) Pediatric mastocytosis is a clonal disease associated with D816V and other activating c-KIT mutations. *J Invest Dermatol* **130**: 804–815.
56. Heide R, Zuidema E, Beishuizen A, den Hollander JC, van Gysel D, Seyger MM, Pasmans SG, Kakourou T, Oranje AP. (2009) Clinical aspects of diffuse cutaneous mastocytosis in children: Two variants. *Dermatology* **219**: 309–315.
57. Niemeyer CM, Arico M, Basso G, Biondi A, Cantu Rajnoldi A, Creutzig U, Haas O, Harbott J, Hasle H, Kerndrup G, Locatelli F, Mann G, Stollmann-Gibbels B, van't Veer-Korthof ET, van Wering E, Zimmermann M. (1997) Chronic myelomonocytic leukemia in childhood: A retrospective analysis of 110 cases. European Working Group on Myelodysplastic Syndromes in Childhood (EWOG-MDS). *Blood* **89**: 3534–3543.
58. Breccia M, Biondo F, Latagliata R, Carmosino I, Mandelli F, Alimena G. (2006) Identification of risk factors in atypical chronic myeloid leukemia. *Haematologica* **91**: 1566–1568.
60. Passmore SJ, Chessells JM, Kempski H, Hann IM, Brownbill PA, Stiller CA. (2003) Paediatric myelodysplastic syndromes and juvenile myelomonocytic leukaemia in the UK: A population-based study of incidence and survival. *Br J Haematol* **121**: 758–767.
61. Byrd JC, Mrozek K, Dodge RK, Carroll AJ, Edwards CG, Arthur DC, Pettenati MJ, Patil SR, Rao KW, Watson MS, Koduru PR, Moore JO, Stone RM, Mayer RJ, Feldman EJ, Davey FR, Schiffer CA, Larson RA, Bloomfield CD. (2002) Pretreatment cytogenetic abnormalities are predictive of induction success, cumulative incidence of relapse, and overall survival in adult patients with de novo acute myeloid leukemia: Results from Cancer and Leukemia Group B (CALGB 8461). *Blood* **100**: 4325–4336.
62. Dixon N, Kishnani PS, Zimmerman S. (2006) Clinical manifestations of hematologic and oncologic disorders in patients with Down syndrome. *Am J Med Genet C Semin Med Genet* **142C**: 149–157.
64. Pileri SA, Grogan TM, Harris NL, Banks P, Campo E, Chan JK, Favera RD, Delsol G, de Wolf-Peeters C, Falini B, Gascoyne RD, Gaulard P, Gatter KC, Isaacson PG, Jaffe ES, Kluin P, Knowles DM, Mason DY, Mori S, Muller-Hermelink HK, Piris MA, Ralfkiaer E, Stein H, Su IJ, Warnke RA, Weiss LM. (2002) Tumours of histiocytes and accessory dendritic cells: An immunohistochemical approach to classification from the International Lymphoma Study Group based on 61 cases. *Histopathology* **41**: 1–29.
65. Dehner LP. (2003) Juvenile xanthogranulomas in the first two decades of life: A clinicopathologic study of 174 cases with cutaneous and extracutaneous manifestations. *Am J Surg Pathol* **27**: 579–593.

3

Special Considerations in Infants and Adolescents with Hematological Malignancies

Gregory Reaman and Maura O'Leary

Introduction

The diagnosis and management of hematological malignancies at the extreme age groups of the pediatric population propose significant and sometimes unique challenges for clinicians and clinical investigators. Lymphoid malignancies in infants less than 1 year of age are almost exclusively attributed to acute lymphoblastic leukemia (ALL).[1] The disease presents with a unique constellation of clinical and biological features. The distinct biological characteristic of the disease in infants has enormous impact on treatment considerations and response to therapy.[2] In the adolescent and young adult (AYA) age group, ALL, non-Hodgkin lymphoma (NHL), myeloid leukemias (acute and chronic), and Hodgkin lymphoma (HL) present a unique set of challenges by virtue of specific differences in distribution frequency of diseases in this age group as well as management issues related to psychosocial, behavioral and developmental domains typical of this particular age group which require sensitivity and consideration during diagnosis and therapy. Even within the AYA spectrum of ages (15–29 years), the incidence of these malignancies changes significantly.[3] Between the ages of 15 and 19 years, lymphoma, followed by leukemia are the most common malignancies. In the 20–29-year-old group, lymphoma remains the most common diagnoses but the incidence of leukemia falls in proportion to other diagnoses, such as melanoma and thyroid cancer. An important challenge also relates to the diminished access to clinical trials and the relative infrequency of participation in such by the adolescent and young adult age group, which has direct impact on their inferior outcomes when compared to younger children.

This chapter will review distinct epidemiologic differences and provide some guidelines and special recommendations for professionals faced with the challenge of treating these unique patient populations as well as strategies to assure that AYAs gain access to appropriate multidisciplinary care and approved participation in clinical trials. The diagnosis and management of specific hematological malignancies will be described in detail in the relevant chapters of this text.

Acute Lymphoid Leukemia in Infancy

ALL represents 3–4% of childhood ALL with an annual incidence of 20 per million infants at risk, with a slight female predominance (see Chapter 11). The incidence of ALL is nearly twice that of acute non-lymphoid leukemia during the first year of life.[4] ALL in infancy differs significantly from the disease in older children, not only in presentation but also in specific clinical and biological factors which impact response to therapy and ultimately outcome. While the 5-year event-free survival (EFS) overall for ALL approaches 90%, the current 5-year EFS for infants is less than half of that.[2,5] Although most infants with ALL achieve complete remission (CR), early treatment failure and an increased incidence of central nervous system (CNS) and other extramedullary relapse account for the extremely poor outcome of this group. Historically, toxic death related to chemotherapy accounted for a significant number of deaths, but improvements in supportive care and accepted modifications in chemotherapy dose have significantly altered this natural history. ALL in infants is characterized by hyperleukocytosis and extreme organomegaly and patients are therefore at increased risk for hyperuricemia and subsequent renal compromise.[2,5,6] Historically, prognostic factors associated with ALL in infants have included evidence of *MLL* gene rearrangement, absence of CD10 antigen expression, coexpression of myeloid antigens and hyperleukocytosis, especially at ages less than 3 to 6 months. These clinical and biological factors appear significantly interrelated since more than 80% of infants have evidence of *MLL* gene rearrangement, which is nearly always associated with CD10 negativity. Virtually, all infants less than 3 months of age have evidence of *MLL* rearrangement.[7]

ALL in infants is characterized by a high incidence of nonrandom structural chromosomal abnormalities (see Chapter 5), notably translocations affecting 11q23, the region of the *MLL* gene, resulting in rearrangements that can be detected using molecular analysis in nearly 80% of patients. The most prevalent translocation is the t(4;11), which accounts for 70% of these abnormalities. The other translocations, t(11;19) and t(9;11), are much less common and there is evidence to suggest that leukemogenesis in response to therapy in infants with such *MLL* gene rearrangements may differ depending on the specific fusion partner.[8] More than 40 partner genes have been identified in these *MLL* translocations and such fusion proteins demonstrate structural motifs of nuclear transcription factors or other nuclear proteins, which may be involved in transcriptional regulation and are thought to play a role in leukemogenesis. The more commonly associated cytogenetic abnormalities seen in children older than 1 year of age with ALL are almost never seen in infants less than 1 year of age, again giving support to the likely role of the *MLL* gene in leukemogenesis in general and specifically in this population.

Specific immunophenotypic patterns are also observed in infants with ALL which vary considerably from those typical patterns seen in older children with this disease (see Chapter 6). Although most infants have diseases of B-cell precursor origin, CD10 is not expressed in the overwhelming majority and the incidence of coexpression of myeloid-associated antigens is more common in this population than in older children.[2] Other important prognostic factors in this population of patients includes the rapidity of response to induction therapy as determined by response to prednisone prophase in the Berlin-Franfurt-Munster (BFM) trials and by assessment of remission status by bone marrow aspiration on day 14 of induction therapy. Both day 14 marrow status of M1 as well as clinical response to prednisone prophase are highly significant predictors of outcome in infants with ALL, including those with *MLL* gene rearrangements.

Treatment approaches to ALL in infants

Several historical reports confirm the poor prognosis of this population of patients with small stepwise improvements made in subsequent studies by a number of cooperative groups. Even the larger clinical trial experiences have resorted to single arm studies using historical controls; randomized trials being impossible because of small sample size. The intensity of therapy provided for infants with ALL has evolved over time resulting in improved EFS rates that still do not exceed 50%. Even in the most recently reported series, age less than 3 months, *MLL* gene rearrangement, and early response to therapy, remain significantly predictive of outcome.

Two concurrent and parallel studies in North America shared an identical 3-week induction followed by post-induction intensification phases of therapy designed to address the typical pattern of early relapse seen in this population, which included high-dose methotrexate (HD MTX), cyclophosphamide, and cytarabine. Dosages were based on body surface area rather than body weight, resulting in increases in dose of individual chemotherapeutic agents delivered. Further intensification was attempted with allogeneic stem cell transplantation in first remission, given the typical early relapse pattern.[9] Analysis of the studies taken together confirmed the importance of age (less than 3 months), hyperleukocytosis, and *MLL* gene rearrangement. However, the impact of *MLL* gene rearrangement on outcome was less; a prolonged EFS rate of 56% was observed, which improved when compared to earlier trials as a result of the intensive therapy. The prognostic significance of *MLL* rearrangement in this age group was confirmed in a large European collaborative study, Interfant 99. Intensification of therapy was associated with a significantly increased incidence of infectious complications associated with treatment-related myelotoxicity and necessitated reduction in dose of anthracyclines during induction as well as reduction in dose and disruption of administration of corticosteroids and the change from dexamethasone to prednisone due to significant increases in fungal infections in this population of patients. Of note in these parallel North American studies, CNS preventive therapy was provided with intensified systemic chemotherapy plus combination intrathecal therapy, which both reduced the incidence of CNS relapse and decreased the incidence and severity of neurocognitive defects in this patient population when compared to historical controls.

The recent analysis of the role of allogeneic stem cell transplantation, both unrelated cord blood transplants as well as matched sibling transplants, has not demonstrated an improvement in outcome when compared, albeit in a small number of patients. Despite questionable randomization compliance, a beneficial effect of stem cell transplantation on prolonging EFS was not observed. A significant impediment to successful transplantation attempts in infants with ALL is the lack of suitable family donors, resulting in the identification of alternative donor sources including cord blood. Even in the subpopulation of infants at highest risk for treatment failure (those with *MLL* gene rearrangements) wherein the most recent historical controls demonstrated 5-year EFS of 30–40%; the prospective assessment of the impact of transplantation in a series of 53 infants with *MLL*-rearranged ALL demonstrated 5-year EFS of 48.8% compared to a 5-year EFS of 48.7% in patients treated with chemotherapy alone.[10] No differences in transplant-outcome related to either preparatory regimen nor donor source were observed. There appears to be no compelling clinical evidence to support a role for allogeneic stem cell transplantation in first remission in infants with ALL including those with *MLL*-rearranged leukemia.

Epidemiology of ALL in infants

Increasing molecular epidemiologic evidence suggests that perhaps all ALL in infants arises *in utero* (see Chapter 1). As two mutational events are believed necessary for the development of leukemia, at least one of these events likely takes place *in utero*. Genetic evidence for mutational events *in utero* includes the fact that ALL in infants exhibit fetal type DJ joining sequences in the immunoglobulin gene; cases diagnosed within the first few days of life typically have 11q23 chromosomal rearrangements. In addition, molecular studies of leukemic identical twins with *MLL*-rearranged genes support the suggestion that such rearrangements are acquired *in utero* and likely spread through the monochorionic placenta from one twin to the other. In children with ALL diagnosed from age 5 months to 2 years, *MLL* genomic fusion patterns and the same genotypic patterns seen in leukemia are found upon examination of the patients' neonatal blood spots, again suggesting that at least one mutagenic event occurs *in utero*, while additional genetic or post-natal events may be required. As exposure to topoisomerase II inhibitors, such as the epipodophyllotoxins, has been associated with the development of secondary leukemias characterized by *MLL* gene rearrangements, it is postulated that given the high incidence of *MLL* rearrangements in infants with ALL, exposure to topoisomerase II inhibitors such as flavonoids, soybeans, quinolone antibiotics, catechins (tea and wine), podophyllin resin, benzene metabolites, and estrogens in pregnant woman may play a role in leukemogenesis in infants.[11,12] In addition, the risk of potential dietary intake of soy-based infant formula is also under investigation. The potential role of parental genetic susceptibility factors related to modulating parental exposure to carcinogens and subsequent leukemogenesis in infants is suggested by the observation of increased frequency of single and double glutathione S-transferase (GST) gene deletions and GST gene polymorphisms in parents of infants with acute leukemia when compared to the general population. Although always thought to be an important consideration, the effect of parental exposure to radiation therapy on leukemogenesis *in utero* remains controversial since neither a large Germany study nor the European childhood leukemia lymphoma incidence study demonstrated an increase in childhood and infant ALL specifically following the Chernobyl accident.

Acute myeloid leukemia

The relative incidence of acute myeloid leukemia (AML) in the infant population nearly equals that of

ALL (see Chapter 13). No specific epidemiologic risk factors have been identified to differentiate potential causal relationships in infants as compared to older children. There does appear to be a slight excess of myelomonocytic and monoblastic subtypes in the infant population.[13] Infants are observed to have a higher incidence of hyperleukocytosis, CNS leukemia at diagnosis, skin infiltration, and 11q23 cytogenetic abnormalities than older children. No special therapeutic strategies have been developed for infants with this disease and no differences in outcome, including both overall survival and EFS, are noted in infants when compared to older children.

Late effects of successful leukemia therapy in infants

Although it is expected that infants cured of their ALL should experience a normal lifespan, this particular survivor population presents unique challenges with respect to evaluation of those factors contributing to quality of life and quality of survivorship (see Chapter 24). Obviously, survivors of ALL diagnosed during infancy must be followed closely for delayed effects of therapy as well as for those immediate effects connected to successful anti-leukemia therapy. Inherent in this is the challenge to design therapies that are effective yet which avoid exposure to known toxicities and to those modalities which are known to present significant risk including excessive anthracycline exposure and radiation therapy. Although the EFS rate remains suboptimal over the past 10–15 years, improvement has been demonstrated, resulting in a reasonable cohort for long-term longitudinal evaluation. Previously, the study of late effects was hampered by the historically poor EFS and compounded by the relative scarcity of the disease in this population. It is highly probable that the use of radiation therapy, both as prophylaxis and treatment for CNS leukemia and as part of the preparative regimen for patients undergoing stem cell transplantation, represents the greatest hazard with respect to late effects, notably neurocognitive damage and endocrine dysfunction. Historical series of patients who survived the disease and its therapy and who had received cranial radiation as CNS preventive therapy demonstrated profound neurotoxicity. Other frequently observed late effects in a relatively small series of survivors included growth retardation, hypothyroidism, delayed onset of puberty, cataracts, cardiac abnormalities and hearing loss. In at least one small longitudinal study of infant survivors who were treated with HD systemic MTX in place of cranial radiation, no neurologic toxicity was demonstrated, confirming the present approach for alternative modes of CNS preventive therapy.[14] As allogeneic stem cell transplantation represents the treatment of choice for many patients with AML, including infants, at high risk of treatment failure defined by specific genetic alterations, continued longitudinal follow-up of survivors transplanted in infancy with current preparative approaches is warranted.

Future direction for infants with ALL

Continued progress in increased EFS for infants with ALL is highly dependent on the use of existing therapies; however, the maximum tolerability of current therapy intensification has likely been demonstrated with intensive therapy approaches. Future success will likely depend on the identification of specific molecular targets in ALL in this population and exploiting these molecular legions therapeutically (see Chapter 22). The recent demonstration of overexpression of FMS-like tyrosine kinase 3 (Flt-3) in a subclass of infants with ALL has led to *in vitro* evaluation of specific Flt-3 inhibitors since its increased expression is likely key to the etiology of the disease. The *in vitro* activity of the specific Flt-3 inhibitor, CEP-701, in ALL cell lines and diagnostic marrow samples from infants with ALL, specifically those with *MLL* rearrangements, demonstrated compelling activity and has resulted in the clinical evaluation of this agent in newly diagnosed infants with ALL with *MLL* rearrangement.[15] As continued molecular genetic discoveries are made, further evaluation of targeted therapy strategies may be possible. In addition, the presence of slow early response and the presence of minimal residual disease at the time of completion of induction therapy have been utilized to intensify therapy in older children with high risk ALL. Similar therapeutic approaches may prove feasible for infants with this disease.

Leukemia in Adolescents and Young Adults

In the AYA population, leukemia represents about 6% of the malignancies diagnosed based on SEER data from 1975–2000 as described in the SEER monograph on Cancer in Adolescents and Young Adults (see Chapters 12 and 13).[16] Recently updated statistics for 2003–2007 continue to affirm this finding.[17] The AYA age group is actually a nadir period for the diagnosis of leukemia if all age groups in the SEER data base are considered. Furthermore, for ALL within the interval 15–29 years, the incidence decreases while the incidence of AML increases. For ALL in 2003–2007, the incidence in the 15–19-year-old group is 1.8 per 100,000, 20–24-year-old group is 1.0 per 100,000 and for 25–29-year-old group is 0.7 per 100,000.[17] For the same groups for AML, 15–19 years is 0.8 per 100,000, 20–24 years is 0.9 per 100,000 and 25–29 years is 1.0 per 100,000 — this is the group where the shift to AML predominance occurs. When gender is considered, there is a definite male predominance in ALL in the AYA population but in AML there is no gender trend except in the 25–29-year-old group. If one looks at incidence in terms of race and ethnicity, Hispanics experience the highest rates of leukemia and this is particularly noted if ALL is analyzed separately. Furthermore, Asians or Pacific Islanders had a slightly higher incidence AML in the AYA group. Chronic myeloid leukemia (CML) is rarely seen in pediatric patients; the AYA age group is when it becomes significant. In children less than 15 years, the incidence of CML is 1.7 per million, while in the 25–29-year-old group it increases to 5.2 per million and is more common than ALL.[16]

Overall, the mortality rate for all leukemias is higher in males than females in all age groups. Hispanics have the highest mortality in those under the age of 25 while African Americans had a higher mortality in those above the age of 25. If this is broken down further into 15–19, 20–24 and 25–29-year-old age groups, Hispanics have the highest mortality in the first two groups and in the 25–29 group; the change to African American predominance is first noted.[18] Survival figures for CML in the period before 2000 for all age groups are lower than the post-imatinib era of treatment. Looking at survival in the under 45 age group in the SEER Statistics review,[17] CML survivors have almost doubled.

Treatment approaches to ALL in AYA

ALL in the AYA population represents a different spectrum of the disease. In this group, a higher incidence of Ph+ disease, T-cell disease, and a decrease in favorable cytogenetic categories such as trisomy of 4, 10, 17, and ETV6-RUNX1 are observed. There has been an ongoing discussion of the treatment of this group since they are not all seen in a pediatric center and the historical approach to the disease tends to be less aggressive. Numerous articles have been published looking at similar populations treated with either a pediatric or adult approach. While overall survival is often better with the pediatric approach, the average age of the patients treated on the pediatric protocols is usually 2 years younger than those on the adult protocols.[18] If one looks at data from the pediatric cooperative group studies over the last 30 years, age and white blood count at diagnosis remain the most important predictors of outcome. All patients are initially staged with those criteria and patients over the age of 10 are treated more aggressively (even within the pediatric community) because successive studies have established this as necessary to improve outcome.

The overall survival rate of 60–70% in these AYA patients treated on pediatric protocols does not approach the overall survival rate of 90% in patients between the ages of 1 and 10. Recent advancements in the treatment of Ph+ ALL in pediatric patients, with the use of an aggressive backbone of chemotherapy augmented with imatinib, has produced an overall 3-year EFS of 80.5% with no advantage for bone marrow transplantation in those who received sibling donor transplant.[19] The median age of this population was 10 with a range of 1.3 to 21 years. Looking at the adult experience within the age range of 15–84 and an average of 45, the disease-free survival range is from 48% to 62% — a summary of data from 9 studies. The long-term impact here is difficult to assess since the patients were able to achieve CR at a higher rate and often went on to stem cell transplantation in CR1, which in the pediatric study was less common due to the restriction of sibling-matched donors.[18]

The Children's Oncology Group (COG) has also published an analysis of the AYA patients on the recently competed protocol CCG-1961.[20] The original analysis[21] detailed the benefits of intensified post-induction therapy, regardless of the duration of therapy in patients with a rapid early response to induction therapy. EFS in all rapid early responers (RER) was 81% for the augmented therapy vs. 72% for the standard treatment. In this second report, the AYA patients (16–21 years of age) are analyzed separately and those who were RER and received the augmented post-induction therapy had an EFS of 82% vs. 67% for those who received standard therapy.[20] Two hundred and sixty-two patients were included in this analysis. Increased duration of therapy (one vs. two interim maintenance and delayed intensification) again had no effect, as per the original cohort. In a recently completed collaborative study (MRC UKALL XII/ECOG E2993) of adults (ages 15–55) with ALL, the overall survival rate was 53% for

ALL PH– patients with a suitable allogeneic donor vs. 45% for those without a donor and treated with chemotherapy or autologous transplant.[22] Both figures are below what was achieved in the adolescent population on 1961. Further analysis of this international cohort[22] of the 234 Ph– patients under 20 years of age detailed a survival rate of 43%.

AYAs with T-cell ALL are treated separately in COG protocols from B precursor leukemia patients. This is based on reports of studies from the Children's Cancer Group, the Pediatric Oncology Group, and the Dana Farber Cancer Institute.(G. Reaman, personal communication).[23,24] The incidence of T-cell ALL is about 15–20% in adults and children — there is a male predominance. Treatment includes a focus on extramedullary disease, in particular the CNS, due to the propensity of the disease to extend here. The current outcome for pediatric patients is 70–75%. There is questionable benefit to HD MTX regimens vs. augmented post-induction therapy in separately reported trials.[23,25,26] The current COG protocol is utilizing nelarabine for high-risk patients in addition to the augmented backbone therapy of 1961 with a randomized question of HD MTX vs. Capizzi I therapy for all patients. In the adult setting, T-cell patients are often treated on the same regimens as the pre-B cell ALL patients, making it difficult to compare treatments.

Treatment approaches to AML/CML in AYA

AML in the AYA patients is a complex disease. The COG dictates treatment by risk group and subtype. Patients with acute promyelocytic leukemia (APML) are treated separately on a backbone of treatment with anthracyclines and cytosine arabinoside with the addition of All-transretinoic acid and arsenic. The overall survival for APML over the age of 15 on the last protocol was 86% for the arm that included arsenic and the EFS was 77%.[27]

All other patients with AML are treated with an aggressive chemotherapy protocol for 6 months and/or stem cell transplantation if indicated by risk group. For AML, the last published study for the COG was CCG 2961. The study had an overall survival rate of 52% and EFS of 42%. The overall remission rate was 88%. The age range for this study was 0–21 with a median of 9.5. Patients in the age range 16–21 had an inferior overall survival rate and EFS which was attributed to increased induction mortality.[28] Patients on 2961 that received bone marrow transplants because they had a suitable donors had a disease-free survival rate of 60% at 5 years, significantly better than those without donors treated with chemotherapy intensification. Overall survival was comparable and not statistically significantly different: 67% for bone marrow transplant vs. 62% for chemotherapy. In Medical Research Council trials, it was also noted that older AYAs (16–39-year-olds) had a decreased survival but improved over older adults.[29] Currently, low-risk patients even with a donor are treated with chemotherapy alone. Risk categories are determined primarily by criteria including the presence of Flt3-ITD, cytogenetics, response to initial therapy and other molecular criteria. Patients with such cytogenetics or molecular abnormalities such as t(8, 21) or inv (16), NPM1 mutant, CEBPA mutant, Flt3-ITD, are considered favorable. Patients with Flt3-ITD, MLL-PTD, monosomy 7, other unfavorable cytogenetics and complex patterns with greater than 3 abnormalities, fall into the unfavorable group. All others are considered intermediate.[30] These categories are reviewed frequently as new treatments emerge. Most protocols recommend stem cell transplantation for patients with intermediate adverse criteria. Patient with Flt3-ITD are also considered for unrelated donor transplants if a suitable donor can be found.

CML has a peak incidence in the fourth and fifth decades.[31] In the 25–29-year-olds, the incidence exceeds that of ALL and AML (see Chapter 15). The established treatment for chronic phase CML is the use of the tyrosine kinase inhibitor, imatinib, but recent publications indicate that a new generation of these inhibitors is even more effective in front-line treatment.[32,33] Nilotinib was evaluated at two dose levels in comparison to imatinib. With a primary endpoint of molecular response, patients receiving either dose of nilotinib had a better response than those receiving imatinib. Adverse events for nilotinib were comparable and uncommon in both groups. Cardiac toxicity was also not significant. Dose reductions were also comparable in all groups.[33] In the dasatinib vs. imatinib study,[32] the dasatinib had a faster response with respect to cytogenetics and major molecular response. With a *p*-value of 0.007, the dasatinib group achieved a cytogenetic response compared to the imatinib group. For molecular response, it was 52% vs. 34% for any time period in the study. Adverse events such as fluid retention and superficial edema were more common in the dasatinib group and pleural effusions were more common in the dasatinib group. Both drugs had comparable cardiac profiles.[32]

Epidemiology of leukemia in AYA

The etiology of acute leukemias is not known (see Chapter 1). In ALL, ionizing radiation and chemical mutagens have been implicated. Certain genetic syndromes such as Down syndrome, ataxia telangiectasia, Nijmegen breakage syndrome, and Bloom Syndrome have an increased risk of lymphoid malignancy. In patients with ataxia telangiectasia, it is more likely to be a T-cell malignancy.[34] Patients with immunodeficiency syndromes such as Wiskott–Aldrich and congenital hypogammaglobulinemia, also have an increased risk of ALL. There is felt to be clonal pathogenesis with a specific event occurring that affects the committed lymphoid precursor. The regulatory process that controls the lymphoid cell's life cycle can be influenced[34] by molecular alterations in the lymphoid cell lines genetic makeup.

In AML, there are ethnic and racial differences, as previously described. Environmental predisposition includes ionizing irradiation as in post-atomic bomb reports from Nagasaki and Hiroshima, Japan. Benzene and pesticides have been linked to the development of AML. Down syndrome, dyskaratosis congenita, Bloom syndrome, congenital agranulocytosis, neurofibromatosis and Noonan's syndrome are also known risk factors. The development of monosomy 7 has also been linked to subsequent diagnosis of AML.[35] In CML, ionizing radiation had been implicated as a risk factor.[31]

Future direction for AYA with leukemia

Further definition of the biology of leukemia in this group of patients will enable oncologists to adapt the therapy to the biology and molecular characteristics of the disease. In CML, we have seen the effect of tyrosine kinase inhibitors on the overall treatment and prognosis of the disease. In ALL, we have identified new prognostic indicators for successful treatment such as early response and increased intensity for post-induction treatment to improve survival.[20] Using new molecular techniques including gene expression classifiers, we are attempting to refine our prognostic information. Through these studies, new mutations and potential targets such as IKZF1 and JAK have been identified.[36,37]

Similar work is being done in AML and with the emergence of Flt3-ITD as a poor prognostic indicator, Flt3 inhibition utilizing a variety of targeted small molecule tyrosine kinase inhibitors is under investigation in the treatment of AML.[38] As discussed for CML, the newer generation of tyrosine kinase inhibitors have increased efficacy without an increase in toxicity.

The future of treatment for the AYA patient will likely include more targeted biological agents, and hopefully, will allow the intensity of the current chemotherapy regimens to be modified to decrease overall morbidity and mortality while improving overall survival.

Lymphoma in the AYA Population

Overall, lymphomas are the most common hematologic malignancy and the 15–29-year-old age group represent 19% of all cancers from 1975–1999,[39] as compared to 5% of all new malignancies diagnosed in the United States (see Chapters 17 and 18). Within the AYA age group, the younger patients have a higher incidence (26%) while the older 5-year bracket of 25–29 is 15.8%. Overall males have a higher incidence in this AYA age group except for the 15–19-year-olds with HL where female gender has a higher incidence. Twelve percent of the lymphomas are HL and the remaining 7% is NHL.[39]

The white non-Hispanic population has the highest incidence of HL in the AYA population. The incidence is bimodal with a peak at 20–25 years and later at 75–80 years.[40] NHL is highest in white non-Hispanic for the younger portion of the AYA cohort[15–19] but in the 20–29-year-old group, African Americans have the highest incidence.[39]

Mortality for all lymphomas is higher in males. African Americans have higher mortality in those older than 20 for the AYA group. The overall survival rate in the 15–29-year-old population has remained steady while the survival for younger patients has improved significantly; the 5-year survival rate is similar for all racial/ethnic groups.[39]

NHL has multiple histologic types and the emergence of follicular lymphoma in the AYA population is noteworthy since it is not found in patients less than 15 years of age. Other subtypes increase; and that includes mantle cell lymphoma and diffuse small-cell lymphoma.[39] Decreases are noted in the incidence of lymphoblastic lymphoma (12% to 4%) and Burkitt lymphoma (10% to 4%) in the 15–19 to the 25–29 year age groups.[39] Also noted in the SEER monograph is the more detailed assessment of histologic subtype in the more recent era of 1996–2002 as applied to the diagnosis of Burkitt lymphoma, cutaneous lymphomas, diffuse anaplastic large-cell lymphoma, and diffuse marginal zone lymphoma.[39]

Overall, the SEER registry from 1975 to 1999 noted a statistically significant increase in lymphomas for all age groups over 19 years. Some of this can be associated with the known risk factor of human immunodeficiency virus (HIV).

Epidemiology of lymphoma in AYA

HL is associated with an improved standard of living and Epstein–Barr virus (EBV) infections in adolescence.[41–43] Family histories of malignancy or blood disorder, immunodeficiency and Jewish ethnicity are also risk factors for HL. HIV has been associated with both HL and NHL. Other factors that contribute to the development of NHL include EBV infection, autoimmune disorders, *Helicobacter pylori* infection, genetic history, male gender, smoking, and chemical exposure (see Chapters 1 and 19).[44–51]

Treatment approaches to lymphoma in AYA

The AYA population with HL has experienced two different approaches to therapy. For patients seen in the pediatric oncology clinic, the focus is dose intensive and response-based with its chemotherapeutic approach and radiation utilized at lower doses concentrated on the involved areas of disease, than a therapeutic approach that uses radiation alone in lower stages of disease. For advanced stage HL, the chemotherapy has been modified even more than the adult model to modify the late effects to this younger population. COG studies of HL include mostly adolescents with a trend to the 10–14-year-olds and 15–19-year-olds of the AYA group. They have shown a benefit to response-based therapies in COG's initial pilot studies. In a disease with good response and survival to multiple approaches, this focus has to be considered to avoid long-term issues such as infertility, congestive heart failure, and second malignancies.[52–54]

Therapy in this group should also be response-based. The COG has recently completed a study on intermediate risk patients with HL and the results are pending. In this study, the patients with an early response were randomized to either receive involved field radiation or not. This was based on the previous study that indicated radiation still had a role post-chemotherapy but the randomization was not tied to the initial response.[54] Current response evaluations of FDG-PET scan to initial cycles of therapy[55] will dictate subsequent type and amount of chemotherapy as well as radiation.

The approach to therapy for NHL depends on the type of disease treated. Burkitt lymphoma treatment has improved significantly in the last 20 years. Children with the disease have a 75% 5-year survival. The therapy involves a period of tumor reduction followed by aggressive chemotherapy over 6–9 months with alkylating agents (cyclophosphamide), antimetabolites (MTX), anthracyclines, and aggressive intrathecal therapy.[56–59] Other subsets of NHL that are increased in this age groups — follicular lymphoma and mantle cell lymphoma — have shown responses to combination-targeted therapy with anti-CD20 antibody and aggressive chemotherapy with cyclophosphamide, adriamycin, vincristine, and prednisone.[60–62]

Late effects of successful leukemia and lymphoma therapy in AYA

The Children's Oncology Group has published guidelines for the follow-up of patients treated for malignancy based on available evidence for current and past therapies. (see Chapter 24).[63,64]

For ALL, AML, and lymphoma, aggressive and augmented regimens are used to treat the AYA patients. These are patients in their early reproductive years. For the most part, their growth has been completed or near complete. As survival has improved in this group, the best approach to their successful follow-up should include their transition as survivors to a program that will accommodate their life-long follow-up to allow surveillance and, when necessary, interventions for possible clinical, social, and behavioral sequelae which will permit them to succeed in life.

Most of the leukemia regimens for ALL, AML and lymphoma include significant doses of anthracyclines. Therefore, routine cardiac evaluations, based on their dose exposure, are warranted.[64] Fertility should also be monitored and recommendations based on doses of alkylating agents particularly in ALL protocols. Patients with AML who have undergone stem cell transplantation will require specific follow-ups tailored to their preparative regimen and exposure to total body irradiation as well as their conventional chemotherapy prior to transplant. If followed in a comprehensive center, these resources are available.

Perhaps the most significant new and developing issue for AYA survivors of ALL and in some histologic types of lymphoma is the development of osteonecrosis. Osteonecrosis is now reported in up to 20% of ALL survivors. It is not uncommon for it to affect multiple sites, particularly the hip joints, and require replacement surgery in relatively young individuals. Patients with lymphoblastic lymphoma and HL also receive significant amounts of corticosteroids and should also be monitored for this complication. There is not a known effective intervention to prevent osteonecrosis. Alteration of steroid regimens in the delayed intensification portion of ALL therapy from continuous to intermittent dexamethasone, as well as avoidance of dexamethasone in induction, is noted to have a lower incidence of osteonecrosis (G. Reaman, personal communication). Surgical intervention early in the course is controversial which leaves joint replacement as the only viable therapy is severe cases. While the AYA population is usually through their major skeletal growth phase, this is a life-long commitment to multiple surgeries as artificial joints wear out. This complication is more common in females than males.[58,65–67]

Future direction for AYA with lymphoma

Treatment for HL has, over the last 20 years, evolved into a number of choices. Multiple combination chemotherapy approaches have produced durable and sustained responses. Radiation therapy either alone or in combination with chemotherapy is a known benefit to therapy but its appropriate use is still being defined. In a population that is young and planning to be assimilated with their peers, we must evaluate therapies not only for efficacy but for sequelae. We need to focus on approaches that target the disease not the host. Pediatric centers have started this with dose intensive, response-based therapy. Biologic agents should also be evaluated and added to frontline regimens (see Chapter 22).[67] Due to the excellent prognosis for HL, new drug development is stagnant. Unfortunately, for those who fail initial and second line therapy which includes stem cell transplantation, the subsequent survival is less than 3 years (see Chapter 20). The most encouraging responses seen in relapsed patients is to the compound SGN-35, a conjugate of anti-CD30 antibody and a synthetic anti-microtubule agent (monomethyl auristatin E) (see Chapter 21).[68,69]

NHL treatment strategies in the future will also include targeted biologic agents to augment. The COG has completed a pilot protocol for frontline Burkitt patients with COPAD therapy and rituximab[69] and the combination was well tolerated. Overall results are not yet available. Other subtypes of NHL have also benefited from the addition of anti-CD20 antibody and other targeted approaches are also under evaluation such as proteosome inhibitors in mantle cell lymphoma (see Chapters 21 and 22).[70]

References

1. Gurney JG, Severson RK, Davis S, Robison LL. (1995) Incidence of cancer in children in the United States. Sex-, race-, and 1-year age-specific rates by histologic type. *Cancer* **75**: 2186–2195.
3. Bleyer A. (2007) Young adult oncology: The patients and their survival challenges. *CA Cancer J Clin* **57**: 242–255.
5. Reaman GH, Sposto R, Sensel MG, Lange BJ, Feusner JH, Heerema NA, Leonard M, Holmes EJ, Sather HN, Pendergrass TW, Johnstone HS, O'Brien RT, Steinherz PG, Zeltzer PM, Gaynon PS, Trigg ME, Uckun FM. (1999) Treatment outcome and prognostic factors for infants with acute lymphoblastic leukemia treated on two consecutive trials of the Children's Cancer Group. *J Clin Oncol* **17**: 445–455.
6. Biondi A, Cimino G, Pieters R, Pui CH. (2000) Biological and therapeutic aspects of infant leukemia. *Blood* **96**: 24–33.
7. Pui CH, Gaynon PS, Boyett JM, Chessells JM, Baruchel A, Kamps W, Silverman LB, Biondi A, Harms DO, Vilmer E, Schrappe M, Camitta B. (2002) Outcome of treatment in childhood acute lymphoblastic leukaemia with rearrangements of the 11q23 chromosomal region. *Lancet* **359**: 1909–1915.
8. Raffini LJ, Slater DJ, Rappaport EF, lo Nigro L, Cheung NK, Biegel JA, Nowell PC, Lange BJ, Felix CA. (2002) Panhandle and reverse-panhandle PCR enable cloning of der(11) and der(other) genomic breakpoint junctions of MLL translocations and identify complex translocation of MLL, AF-4, and CDK6. *Proc Natl Acad Sci USA* **99**: 4568–4573.
10. Dreyer ZE, Dinndorf PA, Camitta B, Sather H, La MK, Devidas M, Hilden JM, Heerema NA, Sanders JE, McGlennen R, Willman CL, Carroll AJ, Behm F, Smith FO, Woods WG, Godder K, Reaman GH. (2011) Analysis of the role of hematopoietic stem-cell transplantation in infants with acute lymphoblastic leukemia in first remission and MLL gene rearrangements: A report from the Children's Oncology Group. *J Clin Oncol* **29**: 214–222.
11. Ross JA, Potter JD, Reaman GH, Pendergrass TW, Robison LL. (1996) Maternal exposure to potential inhibitors of DNA topoisomerase II and infant leukemia (United States): A report from the Children's Cancer Group. *Cancer Causes Control* **7**: 581–590.

12. Spector LG, Xie Y, Robison LL, Heerema NA, Hilden JM, Lange B, Felix CA, Davies SM, Slavin J, Potter JD, Blair CK, Reaman GH, Ross JA. (2005) Maternal diet and infant leukemia: The DNA topoisomerase II inhibitor hypothesis: A report from the children's oncology group. *Cancer Epidemiol Biomarkers Prev* **14**: 651–655.
14. Kaleita TA, Reaman GH, MacLean WE, Sather HN, Whitt JK. (1999) Neurodevelopmental outcome of infants with acute lymphoblastic leukemia: A Children's Cancer Group report. *Cancer* **85**: 1859–1865.
15. Brown P, Levis M, Shurtleff S, Campana D, Downing J, Small D. (2005) FLT3 inhibition selectively kills childhood acute lymphoblastic leukemia cells with high levels of FLT3 expression. *Blood* **105**: 812–820.
16. Bleyer A, O'Leary M, Barr R, Ries LAG (eds). (2006) *Cancer Epidemiology in Older Adolescents and Young Adults 15 to 29 Years of Age, Including SEER Incidence and Survival: 1975–2000* (ed NIH Pub No 06–5767). Bethesda: National Cancer Institute.
17. Altekruse SF, Kosary CL, Krapcho M, Neyman N, Aminou R, Waldron W, Ruhl J, Howlader N, Tatalovich Z, Cho H, Mariotto A, Eisner MP, Lewis DR, Cronin K, Chen HS, Feuer EJ, Stinchcomb DG, Edwards BK (eds). (2009) *SEER Cancer Statistics Review 1975–2007*. Bethesda: National Cancer Institute.
19. Schultz KR, Bowman WP, Aledo A, Slayton WB, Sather H, Devidas M, Wang C, Davies SM, Gaynon PS, Trigg M, Rutledge R, Burden L, Jorstad D, Carroll A, Heerema NA, Winick N, Borowitz MJ, Hunger SP, Carroll WL, Camitta B. (2009) Improved early event-free survival with imatinib in Philadelphia chromosome-positive acute lymphoblastic leukemia: A children's oncology group study. *J Clin Oncol* **27**: 5175–5181.
20. Nachman JB, La MK, Hunger SP, Heerema NA, Gaynon PS, Hastings C, Mattano LA, Jr., Sather H, Devidas M, Freyer DR, Steinherz PG, Seibel NL. (2009) Young adults with acute lymphoblastic leukemia have an excellent outcome with chemotherapy alone and benefit from intensive postinduction treatment: A report from the children's oncology group. *J Clin Oncol* **27**: 5189–5194.
21. Seibel NL, Steinherz PG, Sather HN, Nachman JB, Delaat C, Ettinger LJ, Freyer DR, Mattano LA, Jr., Hastings CA, Rubin CM, Bertolone K, Franklin JL, Heerema NA, Mitchell TL, Pyesmany AF, La MK, Edens C, Gaynon PS. (2008) Early postinduction intensification therapy improves survival for children and adolescents with high-risk acute lymphoblastic leukemia: A report from the Children's Oncology Group. *Blood* **111**: 2548–2555.
23. Silverman LB, Stevenson KE, O'Brien JE, Asselin BL, Barr RD, Clavell L, Cole PD, Kelly KM, Laverdiere C, Michon B, Schorin MA, Schwartz CL, O'Holleran EW, Neuberg DS, Cohen HJ, Sallan SE. (2010) Long-term results of Dana-Farber Cancer Institute ALL Consortium protocols for children with newly diagnosed acute lymphoblastic leukemia (1985–2000). *Leukemia* **24**: 320–334.
25. Gaynon PS, Angiolillo AL, Carroll WL, Nachman JB, Trigg ME, Sather HN, Hunger SP, Devidas M. (2010) Long-term results of the children's cancer group studies for childhood acute lymphoblastic leukemia 1983–2002: A Children's Oncology Group Report. *Leukemia* **24**: 285–297.
26. Salzer WL, Devidas M, Carroll WL, Winick N, Pullen J, Hunger SP, Camitta BA. (2010) Long-term results of the pediatric oncology group studies for childhood acute lymphoblastic leukemia 1984–2001: A report from the children's oncology group. *Leukemia* **24**: 355–370.
28. Lange BJ, Smith FO, Feusner J, Barnard DR, Dinndorf P, Feig S, Heerema NA, Arndt C, Arceci RJ, Seibel N, Weiman M, Dusenbery K, Shannon K, Luna-Fineman S, Gerbing RB, Alonzo TA. (2008) Outcomes in CCG-2961, a children's oncology group phase 3 trial for untreated pediatric acute myeloid leukemia: A report from the children's oncology group. *Blood* **111**: 1044–1053.
32. Kantarjian H, Shah NP, Hochhaus A, Cortes J, Shah S, Ayala M, Moiraghi B, Shen Z, Mayer J, Pasquini R, Nakamae H, Huguet F, Boque C, Chuah C, Bleickardt E, Bradley-Garelik MB, Zhu C, Szatrowski T, Shapiro D, Baccarani M. (2010) Dasatinib versus imatinib in newly diagnosed chronic-phase chronic myeloid leukemia. *N Engl J Med* **362**: 2260–2270.
33. Saglio G, Kim DW, Issaragrisil S, le Coutre P, Etienne G, Lobo C, Pasquini R, Clark RE, Hochhaus A, Hughes TP, Gallagher N, Hoenekopp A, Dong M, Haque A, Larson RA, Kantarjian HM. (2010) Nilotinib versus imatinib for newly diagnosed chronic myeloid leukemia. *N Engl J Med* **362**: 2251–2259.
36. Kang H, Chen IM, Wilson CS, Bedrick EJ, Harvey RC, Atlas SR, Devidas M, Mullighan CG, Wang X, Murphy M, Ar K, Wharton W, Borowitz MJ, Bowman WP, Bhojwani D, Carroll WL, Camitta BM, Reaman GH, Smith MA, Downing JR, Hunger SP, Willman CL. (2010) Gene expression classifiers for relapse-free survival and minimal residual disease improve risk classification and outcome prediction in pediatric B-precursor acute lymphoblastic leukemia. *Blood* **115**: 1394–1405.
37. Mullighan CG, Su X, Zhang J, Radtke I, Phillips LA, Miller CB, Ma J, Liu W, Cheng C, Schulman BA, Harvey RC, Chen IM, Clifford RJ, Carroll WL, Reaman G, Bowman WP, Devidas M, Gerhard DS, Yang W, Relling

MV, Shurtleff SA, Campana D, Borowitz MJ, Pui CH, Smith M, Hunger SP, Willman CL, Downing JR. (2009) Deletion of IKZF1 and prognosis in acute lymphoblastic leukemia. *N Engl J Med* **360**: 470–480.

38. Meshinchi S, Alonzo TA, Stirewalt DL, Zwaan M, Zimmerman M, Reinhardt D, Kaspers GJ, Heerema NA, Gerbing R, Lange BJ, Radich JP. (2006) Clinical implications of FLT3 mutations in pediatric AML. *Blood* **108**: 3654–3661.
39. O'Leary M, Sheaffer J, Keller F, Shu X-O, Cheson B. (2006) Lymphomas and reticuloendothelial neoplasms. In: A Bleyer, M O'Leary, R Barr, LAG Ries (eds.), *Cancer Epidemiology in Older Adolescents and Young Adults 15 to 29 Years of Age, Including SEER Incidence and Survival: 1975–2000*. pp. 25–38. Bethesda: National Cancer Institute.
42. Jarrett RF. (2003) Risk factors for Hodgkin's lymphoma by EBV status and significance of detection of EBV genomes in serum of patients with EBV-associated Hodgkin's lymphoma. *Leuk Lymphoma* **44 Suppl 3**: S27–S32.
43. Sleckman BG, Mauch PM, Ambinder RF, Mann R, Pinkus GS, Kadin ME, Sherburne B, Perez-Atayde A, Thior I, Mueller N. (1998) Epstein-Barr virus in Hodgkin's disease: Correlation of risk factors and disease characteristics with molecular evidence of viral infection. *Cancer Epidemiol Biomarkers Prev* **7**: 1117–1121.
46. Cote TR, Biggar RJ, Rosenberg PS, Devesa SS, Percy C, Yellin FJ, Lemp G, Hardy C, Geodert JJ, Blattner WA. (1997) Non-Hodgkin's lymphoma among people with AIDS: Incidence, presentation and public health burden. AIDS/Cancer Study Group. *Int J Cancer* **73**: 645–650.
47. Fritschi L, Johnson KC, Kliewer EV, Fry R. (2002) Animal-related occupations and the risk of leukemia, myeloma, and non-Hodgkin's lymphoma in Canada. *Cancer Causes Control* **13**: 563–571.
49. Morton LM, Hartge P, Holford TR, Holly EA, Chiu BC, Vineis P, Stagnaro E, Willett EV, Franceschi S, la Vecchia C, Hughes AM, Cozen W, Davis S, Severson RK, Bernstein L, Mayne ST, Dee FR, Cerhan JR, Zheng T. (2005) Cigarette smoking and risk of non-Hodgkin lymphoma: A pooled analysis from the International Lymphoma Epidemiology Consortium (interlymph). *Cancer Epidemiol Biomarkers Prev* **14**: 925–933.
50. Muller AM, Ihorst G, Mertelsmann R, Engelhardt M. (2005) Epidemiology of non-Hodgkin's lymphoma (NHL): Trends, geographic distribution, and etiology. *Ann Hematol* **84**: 1–12.
51. Westergaard T, Melbye M, Pedersen JB, Frisch M, Olsen JH, Andersen PK. (1997) Birth order, sibship size and risk of Hodgkin's disease in children and young adults: A population-based study of 31 million person-years. *Int J Cancer* **72**: 977–981.
52. Hodgson DC, Hudson MM, Constine LS. (2007) Pediatric Hodgkin lymphoma: Maximizing efficacy and minimizing toxicity. *Semin Radiat Oncol* **17**: 230–242.
53. Kelly KM, Sposto R, Hutchinson R, Massey V, McCarten K, Perkins S, Lones M, Villaluna D, Weiner M. (2011) BEACOPP chemotherapy is a highly effective regimen in children and adolescents with high-risk Hodgkin lymphoma: A report from the Children's Oncology Group. *Blood* **117**: 2596–2603.
54. Nachman JB, Sposto R, Herzog P, Gilchrist GS, Wolden SL, Thomson J, Kadin ME, Pattengale P, Davis PC, Hutchinson RJ, White K. (2002) Randomized comparison of low-dose involved-field radiotherapy and no radiotherapy for children with Hodgkin's disease who achieve a complete response to chemotherapy. *J Clin Oncol* **20**: 3765–3771.
55. Friedberg JW, Fischman A, Neuberg D, Kim H, Takvorian T, Ng AK, Mauch PM, Canellos GP, van den Abbeele AD. (2004) FDG-PET is superior to gallium scintigraphy in staging and more sensitive in the follow-up of patients with *de novo* Hodgkin lymphoma: A blinded comparison. *Leuk Lymphoma* **45**: 85–92.
56. Cairo MS, Gerrard M, Sposto R, Auperin A, Pinkerton CR, Michon J, Weston C, Perkins SL, Raphael M, McCarthy K, Patte C. (2007) Results of a randomized international study of high-risk central nervous system B non-Hodgkin lymphoma and B acute lymphoblastic leukemia in children and adolescents. *Blood* **109**: 2736–2743.
57. Gerrard M, Cairo MS, Weston C, Auperin A, Pinkerton R, Lambilliote A, Sposto R, McCarthy K, Lacombe MJ, Perkins SL, Patte C. (2008) Excellent survival following two courses of COPAD chemotherapy in children and adolescents with resected localized B-cell non-Hodgkin's lymphoma: Results of the FAB/LMB 96 international study. *Br J Haematol* **141**: 840–847.
58. Marchese VG, Connolly BH, Able C, Booten AR, Bowen P, Porter BM, Rai SN, Hancock ML, Pui CH, Howard S, Neel MD, Kaste SC. (2008) Relationships among severity of osteonecrosis, pain, range of motion, and functional mobility in children, adolescents, and young adults with acute lymphoblastic leukemia. *Phys Ther* **88**: 341–350.
59. Patte C, Auperin A, Gerrard M, Michon J, Pinkerton R, Sposto R, Weston C, Raphael M, Perkins SL, McCarthy K, Cairo MS. (2007) Results of the randomized international FAB/LMB96 trial for intermediate risk B-cell non-Hodgkin lymphoma in children and adolescents: It is

possible to reduce treatment for the early responding patients. *Blood* **109**: 2773–2780.

60. Hiddemann W, Kneba M, Dreyling M, Schmitz N, Lengfelder E, Schmits R, Reiser M, Metzner B, Harder H, Hegewisch-Becker S, Fischer T, Kropff M, Reis HE, Freund M, Wormann B, Fuchs R, Planker M, Schimke J, Eimermacher H, Trumper L, Aldaoud A, Parwaresch R, Unterhalt M. (2005) Frontline therapy with rituximab added to the combination of cyclophosphamide, doxorubicin, vincristine, and prednisone (CHOP) significantly improves the outcome for patients with advanced-stage follicular lymphoma compared with therapy with CHOP alone: Results of a prospective randomized study of the German Low-Grade Lymphoma Study Group. *Blood* **106**: 3725–3732.
61. Romaguera JE, Fayad L, Rodriguez MA, Broglio KR, Hagemeister FB, Pro B, McLaughlin P, Younes A, Samaniego F, Goy A, Sarris AH, Dang NH, Wang M, Beasley V, Medeiros LJ, Katz RL, Gagneja H, Samuels BI, Smith TL, Cabanillas FF. (2005) High rate of durable remissions after treatment of newly diagnosed aggressive mantle-cell lymphoma with rituximab plus hyper-CVAD alternating with rituximab plus high-dose methotrexate and cytarabine. *J Clin Oncol* **23**: 7013–7023.
62. Vose JM, Link BK, Grossbard ML, Czuczman M, Grillo-Lopez A, Fisher RI. (2005) Long-term update of a phase II study of rituximab in combination with CHOP chemotherapy in patients with previously untreated, aggressive non-Hodgkin's lymphoma. *Leuk Lymphoma* **46**: 1569–1573.
64. Landier W, Bhatia S, Eshelman DA, Forte KJ, Sweeney T, Hester AL, Darling J, Armstrong FD, Blatt J, Constine LS, Freeman CR, Friedman DL, Green DM, Marina N, Meadows AT, Neglia JP, Oeffinger KC, Robison LL, Ruccione KS, Sklar CA, Hudson MM. (2004) Development of risk-based guidelines for pediatric cancer survivors: The Children's Oncology Group Long-Term Follow-Up Guidelines from the Children's Oncology Group Late Effects Committee and Nursing Discipline. *J Clin Oncol* **22**: 4979–4990.
65. Karimova EJ, Rai SN, Howard SC, Neel M, Britton L, Pui CH, Kaste SC. (2007) Femoral head osteonecrosis in pediatric and young adult patients with leukemia or lymphoma. *J Clin Oncol* **25**: 1525–1531.
66. Niinimaki RA, Harila-Saari AH, Jartti AE, Seuri RM, Riikonen PV, Paakko EL, Mottonen MI, Lanning M. (2007) High body mass index increases the risk for osteonecrosis in children with acute lymphoblastic leukemia. *J Clin Oncol* **25**: 1498–1504.
67. Younes A. (2009) Novel treatment strategies for patients with relapsed classical Hodgkin lymphoma. *Hematology Am Soc Hematol Educ Program*: 507–519.
69. Goldman S, Lynch J, Harrison L, Gross T, Shiramizu B, Sanger W, Perkins SL, Cairo MS. (2009 (abstract)) Preliminary results of the addition of rasburicase to the reduction cycle and rituximab to the induction and consolidation cycles of FAB group C chemotherapy in children and adolescents with advanced stage (bone marrow ±CNS) mature B-cell non-Hodgkin lymphoma (B-NHL): A Children's Oncology Group Report. *Blood* **114**: 104.
70. Goy A, Bernstein SH, Kahl BS, Djulbegovic B, Robertson MJ, de Vos S, Epner E, Krishnan A, Leonard JP, Lonial S, Nasta S, O'Connor OA, Shi H, Boral AL, Fisher RI. (2009) Bortezomib in patients with relapsed or refractory mantle cell lymphoma: Updated time-to-event analyses of the multicenter phase 2 PINNACLE study. *Ann Oncol* **20**: 520–525.

4

Pathologic Diagnosis of Hematologic Malignancies in Children, Adolescents and Young Adults

Sherrie L. Perkins, Russell A. Higgins, Marsha C. Kinney and Jerry Hussong

Pathologic Diagnosis of Hematologic Malignancies in CAYA

Diagnosis of pediatric hematologic neoplasms using the 2008 WHO Classification (see Chapter 3) often requires extensive workup to ensure proper diagnosis as well as to obtain important prognostic information.[1] Because of similar morphologic appearances of many pediatric tumors, diagnosis often requires additional studies such as immunophenotyping by flow cytometry or immunohistochemistry, cytogenetic and molecular analysis. In addition, many prognostic factors have been identified by immunophenotyping or molecular/cytogenetic studies. Important roles for the pathologist in the workup of a suspected pediatric hematologic tumor include collecting appropriate samples for ancillary testing (Table 4.1).

Morphology provides the keystone for most pathologic diagnoses and requires adequate, properly fixed tissue. Most diagnoses will require tissue sampling either by biopsy or needle core biopsy or analysis of blood and marrow. A few diagnoses may be able to be made on the basis of cytologic analysis using fine needle aspiration of tumors, however this may not be definitive and often requires subsequent tissue biopsy. The pathologist and the personnel performing the biopsy must work together to ensure adequate tissue is collected for both ancillary testing and diagnosis. While blood samples are often easily obtainable, bone marrow and tissue biopsies may have sample limitations requiring knowledge about the requirements and utility of additional testing modalities to allow optimal collection of data. The pathologist is responsible for allocation tissue, based on the size of the specimen, desired additional testing and the suspected diagnosis.

For diagnostic morphology, proper tissue fixation and slide preparation are essential. Most tissues should be fixed in formalin, allowing for good morphology as well as optimal immunophenotypic analysis by immunohistochemistry. Zinc formalin fixatives may provide better preservation of nuclear and cytoplasmic morphologic features but may interfere with some immunophenotyping and molecular analyses. Other fixatives, including Bowen fixative, Zenker's fixative and alcohol-based fixatives, provide no advantages in the analysis of hematologic malignancies and should not be

Table 4.1. Approaches to work-up of pediatric and young adult hematopoietic neoplasms.

Approach	**Utility**	**Tissue requirement**
Morphology	Required for diagnosis	Fixed
Immunophenotypic analysis	Very helpful, usually required	Fixed (immunoperoxidase staining) Fresh (flow cytometry)
Cytogenetics	May provide diagnostic or prognostic information. May not be required for diagnosis.	Fresh
Molecular analysis	May provide diagnostic or prognostic information. May not be required for diagnosis.	Fresh, Fixed
FISH for specific translocation	May provide diagnostic or prognostic information	Fresh, Fixed
Immunoglobulin gene arrangements	May help in diagnosis, often not required for diagnosis.	Fresh, Frozen, Fixed

routinely used. Most fixatives penetrate tissue at a rate of 1–2 mm per hour and fixation of large pieces of tissue for short times will have a negative impact upon morphology. If rapid processing is required, a small, thinly cut portion of the tissue may be fixed and processed, while other materials are allowed to fix for a longer period. Rapid processing of small biopsies may be performed using microwaves, however, this may impact morphologic quality.

Characterization of pediatric hematologic malignancies usually requires immunophenotypic analysis by either immunohistochemical (IHC) staining in fixed tissues or flow cytometric analysis (FCA) on fresh cell preparations. Each tumor type will have specific antigens expressed by the tumor that may be more or less specific for that type of tumor (see Table 4.2 and below). Use of antibody panels usually provides a diagnosis in conjunction with morphology. The choice of antibodies to be used will be influenced by morphologic and clinical features. Diagnoses should not be made on the basis of a single antibody, but require the integration of positive and negative staining results using antibody panels.

In frozen sections, or in paraffin-embedded fixed tissues, immunophenotyping is usually done by cell cytospins immunohistochemical staining. An antibody that recognizes a specific protein epitope in cells is linked to a colorimetric detection molecule, such as alkaline phosphatase or dramino (DAB). This allows for visualization of the antigen/antibody binding and allows for characterization of the tissue or cellular antigen expression patterns. These are a wide variety of nuclear-, cytoplasmic- and membrane-specific antibodies available for use in IHC staining that allows most tumors to be fully characterized. IHC provides the advantage of allowing morphologic features to be evaluated at the same time as antigen detection. Knowledge of staining patterns for each tumor is essential for correct interpretation of IHC.

Immunophenotyping on fresh tissues using FCA is most useful in hematologic neoplasms with non-adherent cells, such as leukemias, allowing for a cell suspension to be easily obtained. FCA allows for the measurement of numerous cell properties including cell size, complexity and antigenic expression. Using this approach, a specific fluorescently labeled antibody will bind to the cell if a specific antigen epitope is present. Cells will be analyzed by a laser light source to generate data on cell size and cell complexity (granularity) as well as antigen expression profiles. Analysis of up to 4 to 10 different fluorochrome stains simultaneously allows for integration of multiple antigenic signals expressed by a cell.

Many pediatric hematologic neoplasms also have specific cytogenetic and molecular features that impart additional diagnostic as well as prognostic information (discussed below and further in Chapters 5–8). Karyotypic analysis requires fresh samples that contain malignant cells. Extensive necrosis, or normal (non-neoplastic) tissue, may affect the ability to do adequate cytogenetic analysis. Samples should be processed rapidly to ensure optimal cell viability. Molecular testing using fluorescent *in situ* hybridization (FISH) is another cytogenetic approach that is often utilized in pediatric hematologic neoplasms. FISH technology uses specific, fluorescent-labeled probes to identify specific chromosomal abnormalities. This approach is

Table 4.2. Antigens useful in work-up of hemalogic malignancies.

Antigen	Expression distribution	Technology
CD2	T-cells, some T-ALLs, some T-cell lymphomas	IHC, FCA
CD3	T-cells, some T-ALLs, some T-cell lymphomas	IHC, FCA
CD4	T-helper cells, some T-ALLs, some T-cell lymphomas, monocytes	IHC, FCA
CD5	T-cells, some T-ALLs, some T-cell lymphomas	IHC, FCA
CD7	T-cells, some T-ALLs, some T-cell lymphomas	IHC, FCA
CD8	T-suppressor cells, some T-ALLs, some T-cell lymphomas	IHC, FCA
CD10	B-ALL, pediatric follicular lymphoma, granulocytes	IHC, FCA
CD15	Hodgkin lymphoma, granulocytes	IHC, FCA
CD19	B-cells, B-ALLs, B-cell lymphomas	FCA
CD20	B-cells, some B-ALLs, some B-cell lymphomas	IHC, FCA
CD30	Hodgkin lymphoma, ALCL, some other B and T-cell lymphomas	IHC
CD34	Immature lymphoid and myeloid cells, some leukemias/lymphomas, hematogones	IHC, FCA
CD99	Immature lymphoid cells, some leukemias/lymphomas, hematogones	IHC
Tdt	Immature lymphoid and myeloid cells, some leukemias/lymphomas, hematogones	IHC, FCA
PAX-5	B-cells, some B-ALLs, some B-cell lymphomas	IHC
ALK-1	ALCL	IHC

ALL: acute lymphoblastic leukemia; ALCL: anaplastic large cell lymphoma; FCA: flow cytometric analysis; IHC: immunohistochemistry.

useful because it is much more rapid, requiring only 24–48 hours compared to 5–10 days for conventional cytogenetics. However, FISH technology will identify only those abnormalities for which the specific probe is created and is unable to identify additional cytogenetic abnormalities. However, when a specific diagnosis is suspected, such as acute promyelocytic leukemia (APL) where cytogenetic analysis is essential for directing therapy, FISH technology provides a rapid means to identify the abnormality. FISH technology is also useful in following minimal residual disease when a specific abnormality is known to be present in a tumor. In some cases, FISH approaches are more sensitive than conventional cytogenetics, e.g. identification of the translocations inv(16) or t(8;21), where conventional cytogenetics often fails to identify a cryptic cytogenetic abnormality.

Molecular testing for specific molecular and cytogenetic abnormalities may be required for diagnosis and prognosis in some pediatric hematologic malignancies using either Southern Blot analysis (requiring fresh or frozen tissue) or real-time polymerase chain reaction (RT-PCR) (which can use fresh, frozen or fixed tissue). The sensitivity of molecular testing is very high and it has the ability to detect very small numbers of cells harboring a specific defect, making it particularly useful in monitoring minimal residual disease (see Chapter 10). Formalin fixation is considered optimal for subsequent PCR testing as it provides the best preservation of nucleic acids.

Other molecular testing modalities, including microarray and competitive genomic hybridization (CGH) analysis, may become important in the future as specific molecular profiles are identified that affect the diagnosis and therapy of specific tumors. When sufficient tissue to allow for appropriate morphologic review and ancillary testing for diagnosis and prognosis is present and additional tissue is left over, tissue banking should be considered. Tissue banking will provide samples of specific tumor types to allow for additional biological studies to be performed in the future. Use of banked tissue materials have led to many of the advances in understanding the biology as well as therapeutic and prognostic approaches to diagnosis of pediatric tumors.

Myelodysplastic and Myeloproliferative Neoplasms

Non-acute myeloid leukemia (AML) myeloid neoplasms are rare in children. In order of decreasing incidence in children from 0–14 years of age, these myeloid neoplasms include pediatric myelodysplastic syndrome (MDS), myeloid leukemia of Down syndrome (DS), juvenile myelomonocytic leukemia (JMML), chronic myeloid leukemia (CML), and polycythemia vera/essential thrombocytosis (PV/ET) (Table 4.3).[2] Because of their rarity, the diagnostic criteria for most myeloid neoplasms are based on adult experience. Notable exceptions

Table 4.3. Relative incidence of myeloproliferative, myelodysplastic/myeloproliferative and mastocytosis in children, adolescents and young adults (CAYA).

Diagnosis	Relative incidence in age groups
TAM	Children only (Down syndrome infants)
JMML	Children only
CML	Adults >> Young adults > Adolescents > Children
PV/ET/PMF	Adults >> CAYA
CEL	Adults >> CAYA
PDGFR-related disorders	Adults >> CAYA
Atypical CML	Adults >> Adolescents
CNL	Adults
Cutaneous mastocytosis	CAYA > Adults
Systemic mastocytosis	Adults > CAYA

CEL: chronic eosinophilic leukemia; CML: chronic myelogenesis leukemia; ET: essential thrombocythemia; JMML: juvenile myelomonocytic leukemia; PV: polycythemia vera; PDGFR: platelet-derived growth factor receptor; PMF: primary myelofibrosis; TAM: transient abnormal myeloporesis.

are JMML, transient abnormal myelopoiesis, and more recently, pediatric MDS.

MDS is associated with ineffective hematopoiesis, characterized by abnormal dysplastic hematopoietic cells and peripheral blood cytopenias. In contrast, the myeloproliferative neoplasms (MPN) have somewhat effective hematopoiesis, characterized by the proliferation of one or more hematopoietic lineages, resulting in elevated peripheral blood cell counts, at least early in the disease; dysplasia is not a prominent feature of these neoplasms. MDS/MPN are neoplasms with combined features of both categories.

CML, PV, ET, and primary myelofibrosis (PMF) are the classic myeloproliferative neoplasms. CML, defined by the presence of the Philadelphia chromosome, resulting in the *BCR-ABL1* fusion gene is the most common of these neoplasms in the pediatric population. Other *BCR-ABL1* negative myeloproliferative neoplasms include chronic eosinophilic leukemia, myeloid neoplasms with eosinophilia and abnormalities of platelet-devolved growth factor receptor A (*PDGFRA*), *PDGFRB*, and fibroblast growth factor receptor 1 (*FGFR1*), and mastocytosis.

JMML is by far the most frequent pediatric MDS/MPN. Chronic myelomonocytic leukemia (CMML) occurs in older adults and is considered a separate entity from JMML. Atypical CML, lacking *BCR-ABL* and displaying severe dysgranulopoiesis, is a neoplasm of elderly adults that may very rarely occur in teenagers.

Myeloid proliferations related to Down syndrome

Clinical

Although DS is associated with an increased risk of both acute lymphoblastic leukemia (ALL) and AML, acute megakaryoblastic leukemia (AML-MK) occurring in young DS children (usually less than 5 years of age) has unique clinicopathologic and molecular features, which qualify its recognition by the World Health Organization (WHO) as a separate entity.[1] Ten percent of DS newborns develop a transient abnormal myelopoiesis (TAM) characterized by peripheral blood findings indistinguishable from AML-MK. Cases of TAM resolve spontaneously, but 10–20% of DS children with TAM develop AML, most commonly in the following 1 to 3 years. Unlike TAM, AML arising in this setting does not resolve spontaneously thus requiring therapy. Almost all AML associated with DS is preceded by a relatively short MDS phase, so AML and MDS are considered a single entity — myeloid leukemia associated with DS (MDS/AML-DS). Seventy percent of the AML that develops in young children with DS is AML-MK, an otherwise very uncommon subtype in non-DS children; furthermore, AML-MK in this setting responds well to chemotherapy. These clinicopathologic features and the presence of *GATA1* mutations in almost all TAM and DS-associated AML-MK form the basis for the WHO designation.[1,3,4]

Morphology

TAM presents with leukocytosis and circulating blasts (Fig. 4.1A). Cytopenias are variable but usually mild. Blasts often have megakaryoblastic features with basophilic cytoplasm, basophilic granules, and cytoplasmic blebbing in addition to the usual dispersed chromatin and prominent nucleoli. Blast percentages vary and may represent up to 50% of leukocytes, while blasts may be fewer in the bone marrow (Fig. 4.1C). Dysplasia of the megakaryocytic and erythroid lineages may be seen. Megakaryocytes may be uni- or hypolobated or may have abnormal nuclei with separate lobes (Fig. 4.1B). Erythroid dysplasia is characterized by megaloblastic change, binucleation, and/or nuclear fragmentation.

AML-DS is preceded by a preleukemic phase of MDS consisting of thrombocytopenia, macrocytic anemia, dyspoiesis, and less than 20% blasts in the peripheral blood and bone marrow. The leukemic phase of DS children with AML-MK is morphologically similar to TAM, but

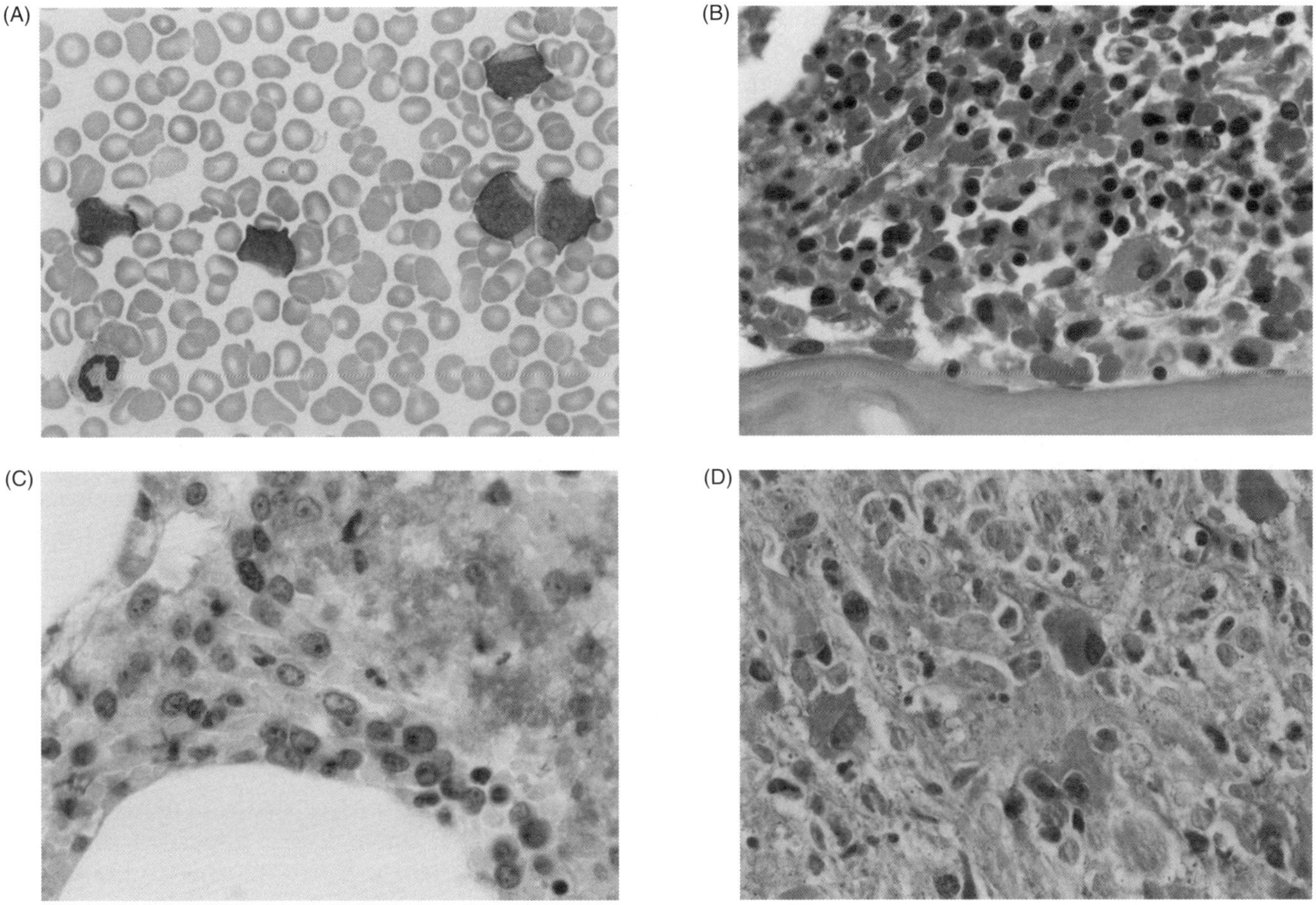

Fig. 4.1. (A–C) Transient abnormal myelopoiesis (TAM) in an infant with Down syndrome. (A) A Wight stained peripheral blood smear (1000× magnification) shows numerous circulating blasts (>50%) in an infant with TAM. (B) A bone marrow biopsy (600× magnification) shows decreased normal hematopoietic elements and a proliferation of small megakaryocytic cells. (C) A PAS-stained section of bone marrow clot shows increased blasts (600× magnification). The TAM resolved spontaneously. (D) An H&E-stained section of a bone marrow core biopsy involved by acute megakaryoblastic leukemia (400× magnification). There are numerous atypical megakaryocytes and a background of immature cells.

anisopoikilocytosis and thrombocytopenia are more pronounced. Blasts exceed 20% in the peripheral blood or bone marrow and often have characteristics of megakaryoblasts, as described above (Fig. 4.1D). The bone marrow is typically hypercellular with a background of erythroid and megakaryocytic dysplasia but granulocytic dysplasia may also be seen. Reticulin fibrosis, which may be prominent, along with a variety of dysplastic megakaryocytes sometimes impart a menacing sarcomatous-like appearance. Extramedullary sites of involvement, especially liver and spleen, are frequent and consist of immature-appearing blasts and dyplastic megakaryocytes.

Immunophenotype

Blasts of TAM and DS-associated AML-MK commonly display a degree of megakaryocytic differentiation and share a similar immunophenotype. The blasts express immature markers (CD34 and CD117), myeloid associated markers (CD13 and CD33), megakaryocytic markers (CD41, CD42, and CD61) and aberrantly express CD4, CD7, and CD56. The blasts lack myeloperoxidase, CD15, and CD14. HLA-DR is positive in 30% of cases. There is a less frequent expression of CD34 (50%), CD61, and CD56 in AML-MK compared to TAM. Non-megakaryocytic AML-DS express a variety of other myeloid and monocytic lineage differentiation patterns.

Genetics

GATA1 mutation analysis is helpful to support the diagnosis of TAM or MDS/AML-DS, but available assays are not sufficiently sensitive to follow response or to identify early relapse. *GATA1* mutations are identified in most TAM and DS-associated AML-MK.[5,6] Rare cases of DS-related minimally differentiated AML have been reported to have *GATA1* mutation,[7,8] but other DS-related AML, DS-related ALL, and non-DS AML (including non-DS AML-MK) are negative for *GATA1* mutations.[6] Finding *GATA1* mutations in monozygotic twins (with acquired trisomy 21) with AML-MK has been reported as evidence supporting the prenatal acquisition of *GATA1* mutations.[7] Trisomy 21 is thought to create an increased dosage of a yet unidentified gene, possibly *RUNX1*, resulting in increased proliferation; in the setting of increased proliferation, an acquired mutation of *GATA1*, which is important in megakaryocytic and erythroid differentiation, produces the clinical syndrome of TAM. Several examples of identical *GATA1* mutations in TAM and subsequent AML-MK in DS children support the current model that *GATA1* mutations are necessary, but are not the inciting events that cause progression to AML.[5,7] Instead, acquisition of additional genetic abnormalities may allow progression of TAM to AML-MK. This is supported by increased numbers of cytogenetic abnormalities in DS-related AML-MK compared to TAM. A large study of 404 AML of DS found +21, +8, and dup(1q) to be the three most common secondary abnormalities identified by conventional cytogenetic techniques.[9] The t(1;22) rearrangement, which is associated with AML-MK in non-DS children, is not seen in AML-MK of DS children.

Diagnostic issues

Although a very specific relationship of DS, TAM, and AML-MK has been delineated above, it is important to remember that other subtypes of AML, as well as ALL, occur in DS children. The importance of identifying the DS-related AML with *GATA1* mutations lies in the predicted good response to reduced intensity therapy in this entity. AML in DS children > 5 years of age are less likely to have *GATA1* mutations and may not respond as well to chemotherapy; the WHO recommends that AML without *GATA1* mutations in these older children should be considered to be "conventional" AML similar to that of non-DS children.[3] In DS children ≥ 4 years of age, recurrent rearrangements of AML such as t(8;21), t(15;17), and 11q23 occur at a rate similar to that seen in "conventional" AML; moreover, the relapse rate in the older age group is greater than that of most DS AML-MK.[8] It is important to note, however, that there is no absolute age cutoff, as rare cases of DS-related AML in children > 4 years of age may carry a *GATA1* mutation.[8]

Pediatric myelodysplastic syndrome

Clinical

Pediatric myelodysplastic syndrome (PMDS) is a newly appreciated WHO category. As with adult MDS, this is a stem cell defect that produces cytopenias and ineffective hematopoiesis. MDS associated with bone marrow failure syndromes, therapy-related MDS, and DS-related TAM have been excluded from the PMDS designation, making PMDS a rare entity with an incidence of 1.8 per million population per year.[2] The WHO recognizes PMDS apart from the general classification of adult MDS based on a number of clinicopathologic differences including the following: (1) presentation with thrombocytopenia and neutropenia along with macrocytic anemia is common in children, as opposed to frequent isolated anemia in adults; (2) hypocellular bone marrow is common (up to 75%) in children, whereas the typical adult MDS is associated with marrow hypercellularity; and (3) stable disease associated with blast counts between 20% and 30% has been observed in some pediatric cases. In children, the latter are better regarded as refractory anemia with excess blasts in transformation (RAEB-t) rather than AML. The subtype distribution differs in children and adults; refractory anemia with ringed sideroblasts and isolated del(5q) subtypes are rare in children. The most common subtype of PMDS, provisionally called refractory cytopenia of childhood (RCC), presents with cytopenias (thrombocytopenia > anemia > neutropenia) in various combinations with < 2% blasts in peripheral blood and < 5% blasts in bone marrow and evidence of dysplasia in the blood and marrow (Table 4.4).[10]

Morphology

Dysplastic changes are requisite for a diagnosis of PMDS (Table 4.4). The peripheral blood usually shows macrocytic anemia and thrombocytopenia with giant platelets. Peripheral blood is helpful to identify dyspoietic granulocytes with hypolobulated or binucleated (pseudo-Pelger-Huet) forms and/or hypogranulation. Bone marrow aspirate smears demonstrate dyspoiesis of the erythroid, granulocytic, and/or megakaryocytic lineages. Dyserythropoiesis is characterized by multinucleation,

Table 4.4. Morphologic features of pediatric MDS.

	Bone marrow biopsy	Bone marrow aspirate cytology
Erythropoiesis	Patchy distribution	Nuclear lobulation
	Left shift	Multinuclearity
	Increased mitoses	Megaloblastoid changes
Granulopoiesis	Marked decrease	Pseudo-Pelger-Huët anomaly
	Left shift	Agranulation of cytoplasm
		Hypogranulation of cytoplasm
		Nuclear-cytoplasmic maturation defects
Megakaryopoiesis	Marked platelet decrease	Micromegakaryocytes
	Dysplastic changes	Multiple separated nuclei
	Micromegakaryocytes (in blood)	Small round nuclei
Lymphocytes	May be increased focally or dispersed	May be increased
CD34+ cells	No increase	

nuclear budding, nuclear bridges, nuclear fragmentation, karyorrhexis, and nuclear cytoplasmic dyssyncrony (megaloblastoid change). Dysgranulopoiesis is characterized by hypolobulation, hypogranulation, giant bands, and nuclear–cytoplasmic dyssyncrony. In order for a lineage to be considered dysplastic, >10% of the lineage must be dysplastic. Micromegakaryocytes are a very helpful indication of dyspoiesis of the megakaryocytic lineage. In addition, megakaryocytes may have hypolobulated nuclei or forms with separated nuclei. The erythroid to myeloid ratio may be slightly increased.

The bone marrow trephine biopsy is vital for assessing PMDS morphology. Age-matched hypocellarity is seen in 75% of cases but normocellularity or hypercellularity may be seen. Megakaryocyte dysplasia may be assessed on biopsy sections as well and may be adequate, decreased, or increased in number. When the marrow is hypocellular, small scattered collections of erythroid precursors are present with scant granulopoiesis and few megakaryocytes — findings helpful in the distinction from aplastic anemia.

Immunophenotype

Immunophenotypic analysis by flow cytometry may be helpful to quantify CD34/CD117 positive blasts, which should be <5% in the bone marrow. PMDS more commonly demonstrates aberrant CD7 (50%) on myeloblasts than AML. Myeloid maturational asynchrony is most commonly encountered as early acquisition of CD11a and CD11b (usually acquired at the promyelocyte stage) on myeloblasts (CD34+/CD117+) without other myeloid markers CD64, CD65, and CD15.[11] Immunohistochemistry on paraffin sections may be helpful to establish the number and topography of CD34 or CD117 positive blasts. CD34 positive blasts are usually rare and scattered, so clusters of immature appearing cells expressing CD34 or CD117 raise suspicion for AML. Megakaryocytic markers (CD61, CD41, or von Willebrand factor) help to identify megakaryoctyes and micromegakaryocytes, which may be more numerous than appreciated on hematoxalin- and eosin-stained sections.

Genetics

Identifying a clonal abnormality that is associated with MDS, in the appropriate clinicopathologic setting, allows for a more definitive diagnosis of PMDS. Monosomy 7 (49%), trisomy 8 (8–9%), and partial loss of 7q are the most common clonal chromosomal abnormalities identified in PMDS by routine chromosome banding techniques;[12,13] however, numerous other chromosomal abnormalities including complex abnormalities and abnormalities associated with adult MDS have been reported in PMDS. Due to the limited resolution of conventional cytogenetic techniques (~5MB), small abnormalities may not be detected, while clonal abnormalities are detected in only approximately 50% of PMDS,[12] so other techniques such as FISH and CGH may be helpful to target common MDS abnormalities in the face of a normal karyotype. Clonal evolution may be seen in patients with existing abnormalities as well as a previously normal karyotype, so genetic studies at periodic intervals may be helpful.

Diagnostic issues

The diagnosis of PMDS truly requires clinicopathologic correlation. Morphologic evidence of dysplasia in the bone marrow is necessary but is not diagnostic of PMDS in isolation. Features of dyspoiesis may be caused by stress erythropoiesis (e.g. hemolytic anemia, aplastic anemia, paroxysmal nocturnal hemoglobinuria), metabolic disease, rheumatic disease, vitamin deficiencies, mineral deficiencies, drugs, toxins, and infections. Moreover, the inherited bone marrow failure disorders (e.g. Fanconi anemia, dyskeratosis congeniti, Shwachman–Diamond syndrome) may cause secondary MDS or AML and need to be excluded by physical examination, clinical history, and appropriate laboratory studies.

The presence of dyspoiesis and clonal cytogenetic abnormalities are not specific for PMDS. For example, monosomy 7 and dyspoiesis may be seen in evolving congenital bone marrow failure syndromes due to chromosomal instability. A clinical history of congenital anomalies and/or a prior cytogenetic study revealing a normal karyotype would suggest a congenital bone marrow failure syndrome. Monosomy 7 is also found in JMML and CMML; however, monocytosis and other clinicopathologic findings easily resolve this difference. Likewise, trisomy 8 is associated with PMDS, but is also the most commonly acquired cytogenetic abnormality in DS-AML. These findings highlight the need to correlate pathologic findings with the clinical history to arrive at a PMDS diagnosis.

The definition of AML based on blast count is no longer uniform throughout the WHO classification. Because PMDS can exhibit stable disease with relatively high blast counts and the adult AML blast count of ≥ 20% has not been verified in the pediatric population, the WHO has arbitrarily assigned the cutoff for AML arising from PMDS at ≥ 30% blasts in the bone marrow or peripheral blood. PMDS with blast counts of 2–19% in peripheral blood or 5–19% in the bone marrow should be classified as refractory anemia with excess blasts, as in adult MDS. PMDS with blast counts from 20% up to 30% should be classified as RAEB-t. However, it is important to note that blasts counts of ≥ 20% are consistent with transformation to AML when arising from other MPN or MDS/MPN in pediatric patients.

Juvenile myelomonocytic leukemia

Clinical

JMML is classified as a MDS/MPN disorder presenting with granulocytic and monocytic proliferation and variable (usually slight) myelodysplastic changes. JMML is a disorder of pediatric population with an annual incidence of 1.3 per million children aged 0–14 years, accounting for approximately 20–30% of non-AML myeloid disorders.[2] JMML presents rarely at birth.[14] JMML presents with leukocytosis and splenomegaly secondary to leukemic infiltrate. Infiltrates of lymph nodes, tonsils, and lungs make the distinction from an infectious process difficult; viral infections including Epstein–Barr virus (EBV), cytomegalovirus, and human herpes virus-6 closely mimic JMML. A diagnosis of JMML requires core criteria of monocytosis (1×10^9/L), less than 20% blasts, and absence of *BCR-ABL1* translocation. The WHO also requires two of the following: elevated hemoglobin F for age, immature granulocytes in peripheral blood, white blood count of greater than 10×10^9/L, clonal chromosomal abnormality, and *in vitro* hypersensitivity of myeloid progenitors to granulocyte-macrophage colony-stimulating factor (GM-CSF) (Table 4.5).[15] Newer recommendations from the International JMML Symposium state that evidence of somatic mutations in one of several GM-CSF signaling pathway-related genes (see “Genetics” below), a clinical diagnosis of neurofibromatosis, or monosomy 7 supports a diagnosis of JMML along with the core criteria.[16] Although transformation to AML is uncommon, JMML is an aggressive disease with frequent mortality in untreated children due to leukemic infiltrates. Hematopoietic stem cell transplant is the mainstay of treatment.

Table 4.5. Diagnostic criteria of juvenile myelomonocytic leukemia.

1. Peripheral blood monocytosis $>1 \times 10^3/\text{mm}^3$ ($>1 \times 10^9$/L)
2. Blasts (including promonocytes)[a] are > 20% of the leukocytes in the blood and of the nucleated bone marrow cells
3. Plus 2 or more of the following:
   - Hemoglobin F increased for age
   - Immature granulocytes in the peripheral blood
   - WBC count $>10 \times 10^3/\text{mm}^3$ ($>10 \times 10^9$/L)
   - Clonal chromosomal abnormality (may be monosomy 7)
   - GM-CSF hypersensitivity of myeloid progenitors *in vitro*

[a] In this classification, promonocytes are equivalent to blasts.

Morphology

The peripheral blood demonstrates increased leukocytes comprised of granulocytes with left shifted forms, nucleated red blood cells, and monocytes (Fig. 4.2). Promonocytes, which display more dispersed chromatin and basophilic cytoplasm, may be present and are considered blast equivalents. Hypolobulated and hypogranulated neutrophils may be seen as evidence of granulocytic dysplasia. Nucleated red blood cells are common along with normocytic, macrocytic, or rarely microcytic anemia. Thrombocytopenia is common. Circulating blasts (plus promonocytes) are usually < 5% but are < 20% by definition.

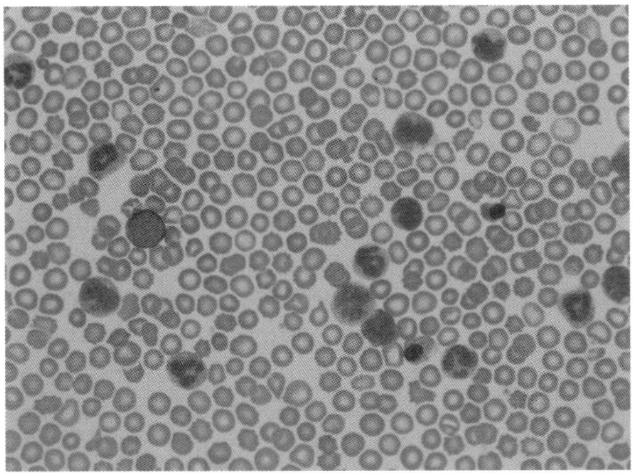

Fig. 4.2. Juvenile myelomonocytic leukemia in an infant. Peripheral blood (600× magnification) shows an elevated white blood cell count, neutrophilia with a left shift, monocytosis, nucleated red blood cells, and blasts (< 5%). An extensive workup for an infectious process was negative, and karyotypic analysis demonstrated monosomy 7. A bone marrow sample at autopsy showed a hypercellular marrow with granulocytic hyperplasia.

Bone marrow aspirate sections demonstrate hypercellularity due to granulocytic hyperplasia. Dysgranulopoiesis, as well as possible dyplasia of the erythroid or megakaryocytic lineages, may be appreciated. Despite significant peripheral blood monocytosis, monocytic cells may be subtle in bone marrow aspirates and core biospies. This is a well-known paradox based on pure morphology; however, cytochemical stains on aspirate material or immunohistochemical stains on paraffin embedded tissue may help to identify the increased monocytic population. In patients with CMML, a morphologically similar disease of adults, the same paradox exists and may be due to increased promonocytes, which are difficult to distinguish from maturing granulocytic cells in bone marrow samples.

Bone marrow trephine biopsies show hypercellularity due to granulocytic hyperplasia. Again, the monocytic component is difficult to appreciate on hematoxalin- and eosin-stained sections. Megakaryocytes are decreased in many cases and do not usually display prominent dysplasia. Acute monocytic leukemia should be considered if sheet-like proliferations of immature monocytic cells are seen.

Immunophenotype

The immunophenotype of monocytes and other lineages is normal. The utility of immunophenotyping studies is primarily to exclude AML with monocytic or myelomonocytic differentiation, which may be included in the differential diagnosis.

The number and distribution of monocytes and granulocytes may be demonstrated on paraffin embedded sections with CD68 or myeloperoxidase (MPO) staining.

Genetics

In vitro GM-CSF hypersensitivity of myeloid progenitors is a unifying feature of the molecular defects underlying JMML.[15,17] In the last few decades, defective GM-CSF signaling pathway-related genes have been identified as the mediators of this hypersensitivity. Increased activation of the RAS signaling pathway is now recognized as the core pathologic pathway resulting in JMML (see Chapter 14). The first clues came from JMML's association with neurofibromatosis type 1 and its known germline mutation in *NF1*. This was followed by the recognition of *PTPN11* germline mutations in Noonan syndrome, which is associated with a JMML-like disorder. Somatic mutations resulting in RAS activation are now clearly implicated in JMML. Mutations of *PTPN11* (35%), *NF1* (~15%), *NRAS*, *KRAS* (*NRAS* + *KRAS* = 25%), or *c-CBL* (17%) are found in the majority of JMML.[16,18] Identifying these mutations is diagnostically helpful.

Most cases of JMML (65%) demonstrate a normal karyotype by conventional banding techniques. Monosomy 7 (25%) is the most common karyotypic abnormality and is helpful in supporting the diagnosis of JMML. Other non-recurrent abnormalities are found in approximately 10% of cases.[19]

Diagnostic issues

Some of the characteristic features discussed above for JMML are not specific and must be considered with the entire clinicopathologic context of the patient. Monosomy 7 and, to a lesser extent, increased hemoglobin F are associated with PMDS but should be easily excluded on the basis of leukocytosis or monocytosis.

Other causes of monocytosis need to be excluded. Another myeloproliferative disorder with monocytosis is CML with the p190 isoform, which is rare in children. Causes of reactive monocytosis including infection, drugs, and other neoplasms should be considered. Leukemic infiltrates of the lungs may be misinterpreted as evidence of infection. Therapeutic drugs such as cytotoxic drugs, growth factor therapy, or immunomodulatory drugs may produce dysplastic morphologic features. Various other clinical scenarios are described to be associated with JMML or a JMML-like disorder including leukocyte adhesion deficiency type 1, infantile malignant osteopetrosis, and infective endocarditis.[20] In difficult cases, molecular studies to identify mutations in the GM-CSF signaling pathway, as described above, may be particularly helpful.

Eosinophilia is not a characteristic finding, but 8% of JMML cases have peripheral blood eosinophilia greater than 5%.[19] Genomic alterations involving oncogenic tyrosine kinases seem to be very rare (or unrecognized) in children; nonetheless, JMML with significant eosinophilia may incite the differential diagnosis of *PDGFRA*, *PDGFRB*, or *FGFR1*-related disease. Thus far, only one case report in an 18-month-old male with JMML and eosinophilia has documented a t(5;17)(q33;p11.2), which resulted in a chimeric fusion of *HCMOGT-1* and *PDGFRB*. The importance of identifying these cases lays in the potential responsiveness to tyrosine kinase inhibitors.

Chronic myeloid leukemia

Clinical

CML is generally a myeloproliferative neoplasm of adults, but CML is seen rarely in children age 0 to 14 years with an annual incidence of 0.6 per million.[2] The incidence increases with age, and the majority of cases (~60%) occur in children > 10 years of age.[21] The *BCR-ABL1* fusion gene is necessary for the diagnosis of CML. Like adults, the disease progresses from a chronic phase to a blast phase.[22] Pediatric CML in chronic phase presents with a higher white blood cell count (median = 242×10^9/L) than adult CML.[21] A high white count may contribute to leukostasis presenting with symptoms such as headache, dizziness, hearing or visual changes, or priapism in pediatric CML.[21–23] Otherwise, many of the clinical features are similar to adult patients. The most common symptoms are asthenia, splenic discomfort, bleeding, and weight loss. Splenomegaly (70%) is by far the most common physical finding. Like adult CML, incidental discovery of pediatric CML is frequent (23%).[21] The survival of childhood and adult CML has dramatically improved during the last decade, likely due to the use of small molecule tyrosine kinase inhibitors.[24]

Morphology

The morphology of the peripheral blood and bone marrow is similar to that of adults. There is a neutrophilic leukocytosis and a left shift, consisting primarily of myelocytes and metamyelocytes with lesser numbers of promyelocytes and blasts (Fig. 4.3A). Blasts are usually less than 5% and are always < 10% in chronic phase; blast percentages from 10–19% indicate accelerated phase of CML. Notably, dysgranulopoiesis is absent or minimal, affecting < 10% of granulocytes. Approximately one third of children have moderate anemia (< 8 g/dL).[22] Basophilia is present, and eosinophilia is common. Platelets are most often increased (60% of pediatric CML) but may be decreased or normal.[21]

(A)

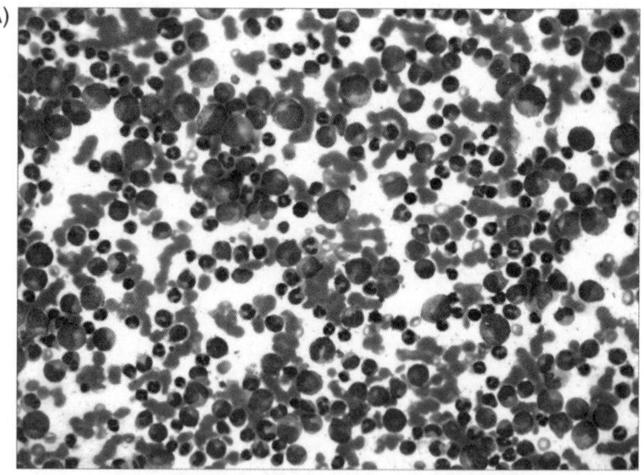

(B)

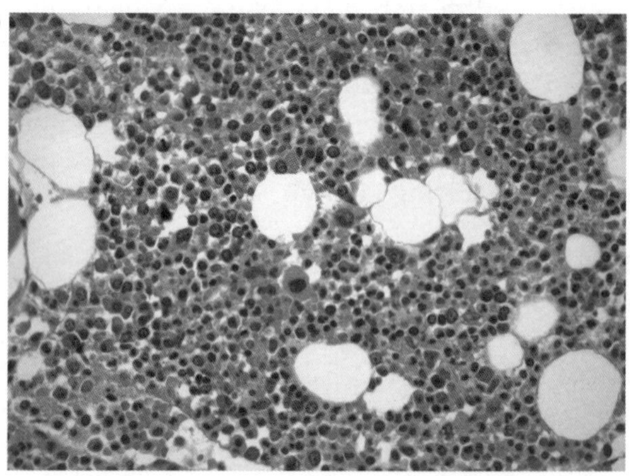

Fig. 4.3. Chronic myelogenous leukemia in a 16-year-old child. (A) Peripheral blood (1000× magnification) shows leukocytosis due to increased numbers of left-shifted myeloid cells with occasional myeloblasts and increased eosinophils and basophils. (B) A bone marrow biopsy (400× magnification) shows a hypercellular marrow with increased granulocytic precursors and numerous mononuclear and hypolobated megakaryocytes.

The bone marrow is hypercellular with granulocytic hyperplasia, creating a markedly elevated myeloid to erythroid ratio. Granulocytes show orderly maturation to the neutrophil stage without significant dysplasia. Megakaryocytes may be increased and are often small, in the form of micromegakaryocytes, and may be loosely clustered (Fig. 4.3B). Pseudo-Gaucher cells, seen on Wright-stained aspirate smears as histiocytes with abundant blue foamy cytoplasm, may be present as a reflection of the increased cell turnover.

Genetics

The t(9;22)(q34;q11.2), also known as the Philadelphia chromosome, results in *BCR-ABL1* gene fusion that is required for the diagnosis of CML.[25] Quantitative reverse transcriptase polymerase chain reaction (QRT-PCR) is used to follow CML responsiveness to tyrosine kinase inhibitors. A major molecular response is a 3-log reduction from the initial diagnosis.[26] Failure to achieve a major molecular response may require a change in management such as changing to another tyrosine kinase inhibitor.

Depending on the breakpoint the BCR gene, one of three BCR-ABL1 fusion protein isoforms are generated: p210, p190, and p230. The p210 isoform is most common in adult and pediatric CML. The p190 isoform is associated with monocytosis, which is not a characteristic feature of the more common p210 CML.[27] The p230 isoform is associated with mature neutrophilia without the usual prominent left shift. Due to alternative splicing, those with p210 protein also produce a small amount of p190 protein. This small amount of p190 should not be misinterpreted as a p190 CML.

Karyotypic analysis to identify the t(9;22)(q34;q11.2) is helpful to determine cytogenetic response to therapy. These conventional cytogenetic studies are particularly important when patients are not achieving a major molecular response in order to globally assess the genome for addition abnormalities. Cytogenetic evolution, commonly including duplication of t(9;22), +8, +19, inv(17q), are indicators of accelerated or blast phase of CML.

Diagnostic issues

Neutrophilic leukocytosis without a detectable *BCR-ABL1* fusion requires additional workup and diagnostic considerations. Philadelphia chromosome negative myeloid neoplasms with granulocytic proliferation include JMML or extremely rare cases of atypical CML, chronic neutrophilic leukemia, and primary myelofibrosis. Atypical CML (aCML) is a Ph– MDS/MPN that can best be distinguished from CML by the presence of severe dysgranulopoiesis.[25,28] Chronic neutrophilic leukemia (CNL) is associated with a proliferation of mature neutrophils without the left shift of usual CML. As mentioned briefly above, the rare p230 isoform of *BCR-ABL1* presents with mature neutrophilia but should be labeled CML. A diagnosis of true CNL requires careful exclusion of reactive neutrophilia and may be difficult when cytogenetic studies demonstrate a normal karyotype.

Monocytic proliferations may be seen in CML with the p190 isoform of BCR-ABL, thus it is important that laboratories evaluate both p210 and p190 isoforms. If *BCR-ABL1* fusion is not detectable and monocytes are prominent, then aCML, JMML, or AML with monocytic differentiation are included in the differential diagnosis. When aCML is associated with a very high white blood cell count, the absolute monocyte count may exceed 1×10^9/L; however, the percentage of monocytes is usually less than 10%. Cytogenetic or molecular studies are helpful in evaluating abnormalities associated with JMML or acute monocytic leukemia.

While eosinophilia can be characteristic of CML, it is not a characteristic feature of JMML, aCML or CNL; therefore, Ph– MDS/MPN with significant eosinophilia should raise the possibility of *PDGFRA*, *PDGFRB*, or *FGFR1*-related neoplasms.

BCR-ABL1 negative myeloproliferative neoplasms

Clinical

PV, ET, and PMF are extremely uncommon myeloproliferative neoplasms in children and young adults. The most common of these uncommon neoplasms is ET, which is a proliferation of megakaryocytes with a peripheral thrombocytosis. The hematologic parameters of ET, PV, and PMF are similar to their adult counterparts. PV/ET has an annual incidence of 0.1 per million children aged 0–14 years.[2] PMF is extremely rare.

Morphology

Since *BCR-ABL1* negative myeloproliferative neoplasms are extremely rare in children and young adults, the diagnostic criteria and morphologic features are based on the adult counterparts.

PV is characterized by an early prepolycythemic phase, an overt polycythemic phase and a late postpolycythemia myelofibrotic phase. The polycythemia phase is characterized by erythrocytosis, variable neutrophilia, and variable thrombocytosis. The bone marrow shows hypercellularity due to proliferation of myeloid, erythroid, and megakaryocytic lineages (panmyelosis). The megakaryocytes often display hyperlobated nuclei, but erythroid and myeloid maturation is orderly without dysplasia. The prepolycythemia phase resembles the bone marrow of ET, thus identification of panmyelosis is important. The postpolycythemic phase can resemble primary myelofibrosis.

ET presents with thrombocytosis in the peripheral blood and proliferation of megakaryocytes in the bone marrow. The bone marrow is normocellular or hypercellular. Megakaryocytes are large to giant (in size) and display hyperlobated nuclei and abundant cytoplasm. Loose clustering of megakaryocytes is seen while Panmyelosis is not observed.

Primary myelofibrosis presents with an early prefibrotic phase and a late fibrotic phase. The prefibrotic phase presents with thrombocytosis and variable leukocytosis. The bone marrow demonstrates hypercellularity due to megakaryocytic and granulocytic hyperplasia. Megakaryocytic proliferation consists of abnormally small and large megakaryocytes with very atypical nuclear lobulation. Reticulin may be minimal in the early phase and increases as cases progress to the fibrotic phase, as the majority of cases will do. The fibrotic phase presents with leukoerythroblastosis and anemia with tear drop-shaped red blood cells in the peripheral blood. Thrombocytopenia is uncommon in pediatric PMF.[29] The bone marrow is hypocellular except for very atypical megakaryocytes within a fibrotic background. Extramedullary hematopoiesis in the spleen and liver is common. A mass of immature myeloid cells at extramedullary sites should incite a differential diagnosis of myeloid sarcoma.

Genetics

An acquired mutation in exon 10 of Janus 2 kinase (*JAK2*), V617F, has been identified in > 90% of adult PV and about 50% of adult ET and adult PMF. *JAK2* V617F was found in only 3 out of 8 pediatric PV cases compared to 24 out of 26 adult PV. Studies have found a variable percentage of *JAK2* V617F mutation in pediatric ET ranging from 0–38%.[30–32] The *BCR-ABL1* fusion gene is absent.

Clonal karyotypic abnormalities may be present in a minority of cases and are helpful to support the diagnosis of a neoplastic process in the present of typical morphologic features. Disease progression or development of MDS or AML increases the likelihood of a clonal abnormality.

Diagnostic issues

Hereditary thrombocytosis and/or erythrocytosis may be identified more readily in the pediatric setting, as siblings may be affected. Mutations in the gene for erythropoietin (*EPO*), thrombopoietin (*TPO*), or the thrombopoietin receptor (*MPL*) are identified in a proportion of these familial cases.[32][31] Mutations in *MPL* are also rarely identified in ET (1%) and PMF (5%) in adults.[33]

The *JAK2* V617F mutation is not specific for these disorders, and the mutation has even been found in healthy individuals. Therefore, complete clinical and morphologic assessments are necessary to correlate with this finding. The full diagnostic criteria for PV, ET, and PMF are available elsewhere.[34–36]

Myeloid disorders with eosinophilia

Clinical

Chronic eosinophilic leukemia (CEL) and related disorders have a median age of presentation in the fourth or fifth decade. However, rare, well-documented reports of CEL occur in the pediatric population.[37] CEL, as defined by the current WHO, is a myeloproliferative disorder with eosinophilia $\geq 1.5 \times 10^9/\mu l$ and either evidence of clonality or increased myeloblasts in the peripheral blood or bone marrow. When one of the latter two criteria is not met, and there is evidence of organ damage due to eosinophilia, then a diagnosis of idiopathic hypereosinophilic syndrome (HES) is made.[38] A diagnosis of CEL must exclude cases with *BCR-ABL1* (CML) and rearrangements of platelet-derived growth factor receptor alpha (*PDGFRA*), platelet-derived growth factor receptor beta (*PDGFRB*), and fibroblast growth factor receptor (*FGFR1*) that result in constitutive tyrosine kinase activity.[39]

The WHO recognizes myeloid disorders with eosinophilia and recurrent rearrangements *PDGFRA*, *PDGFRB*, or *FGFR1* as a separate category because of specific clinicopathologic features, but these disorders are discussed together with CEL here for comparison.

PDGFRA and *PDGFRB*-related myeloid neoplasms are rare in children and young adults; however, identification of these abnormalities has potential impact on outcome, since these neoplasms often respond to tyrosine kinase inhibitors (e.g. imatinib mesylate).[40,41] *FGFR1*-related myeloid disease is not responsive tyrosine kinase inhibitors.

Morphology

Abnormal eosinophils with irregularly distributed granules, abnormal basophilic granules, or hypersegmented nuclei may be seen but do not separate neoplastic from reactive eosinophilia. Eosinophils may infiltrate any tissue. Bone marrow is generally hypercellular with increased eosinophils and sometimes Charcot–Leyden crystals.

Genetics

Many cases of HES may be CEL, but clonality often is difficult to prove. Cytogenetic studies revealing abnormalities associated with myeloid neoplasms support a diagnosis of CEL. Rarely, X-linked polymorphism analysis has been used to document clonality in females when cytogenetic studies revealed a normal karyotype.[37,38]

The *PDGFRA-FIP1L1* fusion, resulting from the cryptic interstitial deletion of *CHIC2* at 4q12, is a common molecular genetic abnormality in patients with CEL-like picture and mast cell proliferation.[40] Occasionally the presentation may be AML or T-LBL, and some cases may progress to AML, indicated by a blast count ≥20% in peripheral blood or bone marrow. The most common *PDGFRB*-related abnormality is t(5;12)(q31~33;p12). These cases usually presents with a CMML-like picture, but the clinicopathologic setting of *PDGFRB*-related disorders varies and includes CEL, aCML, or even JMML.[15] Abnormalities of the *FGFR1* locus at 8p11, previously referred to as 8p11 stem cell leukemia/lymphoma syndrome, are associated with CEL, AML, and T- or B-lymphoblastic leukemia/lymphoma.[39]

Immunophenotype

Eosinophil immunophenotyping is not diagnostically helpful. Mast cells may aberrantly coexpress CD2 and/or CD25. Immunophenotyping may be helpful to enumerate blasts or to subtype acute leukemias.[39]

Diagnostic issues

The presentation of hematopoietic neoplasms with eosinophilia and abnormalities of *PDGFRA*, *PDGFRB*, and *FGFR1* are heterogeneous, and thus require exclusion in any myeloid neoplasm with eosinophilia. Cases presenting as CMML, JMML, atypical chronic myelogenous leukemia, or even acute leukemia, with coexisting eosinophilia require molecular genetic studies of oncogenic tyrosine kinases.

An extensive workup to exclude reactive eosinophilia such as allergic, drug, infection, neoplasms, and autoimmune disorders is necessary before considering HES, CEL, or *PDGFRA*, *PDGRFRB*, or *FGFR1*-related disease. Solid tumors or hematopoietic neoplasms (myeloid neoplasms or lymphomas) can have a reactive secondary eosinophilia due to increased secretion of cytokines such as IL-5 or GM-CSF. Other rare reactive causes of eosinophilia like Kimura disease, hyper-IgE syndrome, or autoimmune lymphoproliferative disorder may be considered in the differential diagnosis in children.

Mastocytosis

Clinical

Mast cells, which are derived from bone marrow stem cells, reside in many organs (e.g. skin) where they mediate inflammatory reactions through the release of their granular contents. Mastocytosis is a neoplastic proliferation of mast cells classified as myeloproliferative neoplasms by the WHO.[42] Mastocytosis comprises two main groups of disease based on distribution of disease: cutaneous mastocytosis (CM) limited to the skin and systemic mastocytosis (SM) involving multiple organs. Symptoms of CM include pruritis and flushing, whereas systemic symptoms include flushing, diarrhea, abdominal pain, and muscle aches. Children are primarily affected by CM, most commonly appearing within the first year of life, and frequently show spontaneous regression by puberty. Uzzaman Ashraf *et al.* studied a series of pediatric CM who had bone marrow biopsies at the time of diagnosis and showed complete or major regression in 87% upon follow up after 20 years; moreover, a rare systemic mastocytosis displayed stable disease in the bone marrow.[43] In contrast, adults are primarily affected by systemic mastocytosis and have persistent disease. Altogether, these clinical features affect the diagnostic approach in children, who do not routinely require bone marrow biopsies unless there is evidence of systemic disease (e.g. organomegaly or high serum tryptase level). Common forms of CM are uticaria pigmentosa (UP) presenting as macules and papules, diffuse cutaneous mastocytosis (DCM) presenting with diffuse thickening without individual lesions, and mastocytoma presenting as a solitary lesion. All types of CM characteristically demonstrate Darier's sign, in which a wheal and flare reaction develops after physical irritation.

Morphology

Childhood UP, DCM, and mastocytoma are all characterized by multifocal aggregates (> 15 mast cells) or diffuse proliferations of mast cells in the skin, requiring clinical correlation to correctly classify them into these clinicopathohistologic entities. There is usually increased intraepidermal melanin, which gives the lesions their pigmented appearance clinically. Mast cells proliferation in UP involve the papillary dermis and extends into the reticular dermis along adnexal and vascular structures (Fig. 4.4A). DCM is similar except the mast cell proliferation is limited to a band-like distribution in the papillary dermis and upper reticular dermis. Mast cells often show an abnormal morphology, most frequently characterized by spindled forms in UP and DCM (Fig. 4.4B). On the other hand, mastocytoma comprises sheets of mast cells (Fig. 4.4C) without cytologic atypia (Fig. 4.4D).[42]

Bone marrow involvement is seen as masses of mast cell, usually in the peritrabecular or perivascular pattern. In cases where large masses of mast cells are absent, multifocal aggregates consisting of >15 mast cells each, are supportive of mastocytosis. Abnormal morphology, typically spindled mast cells, in >25% of cells are an indicator of mastocytosis.

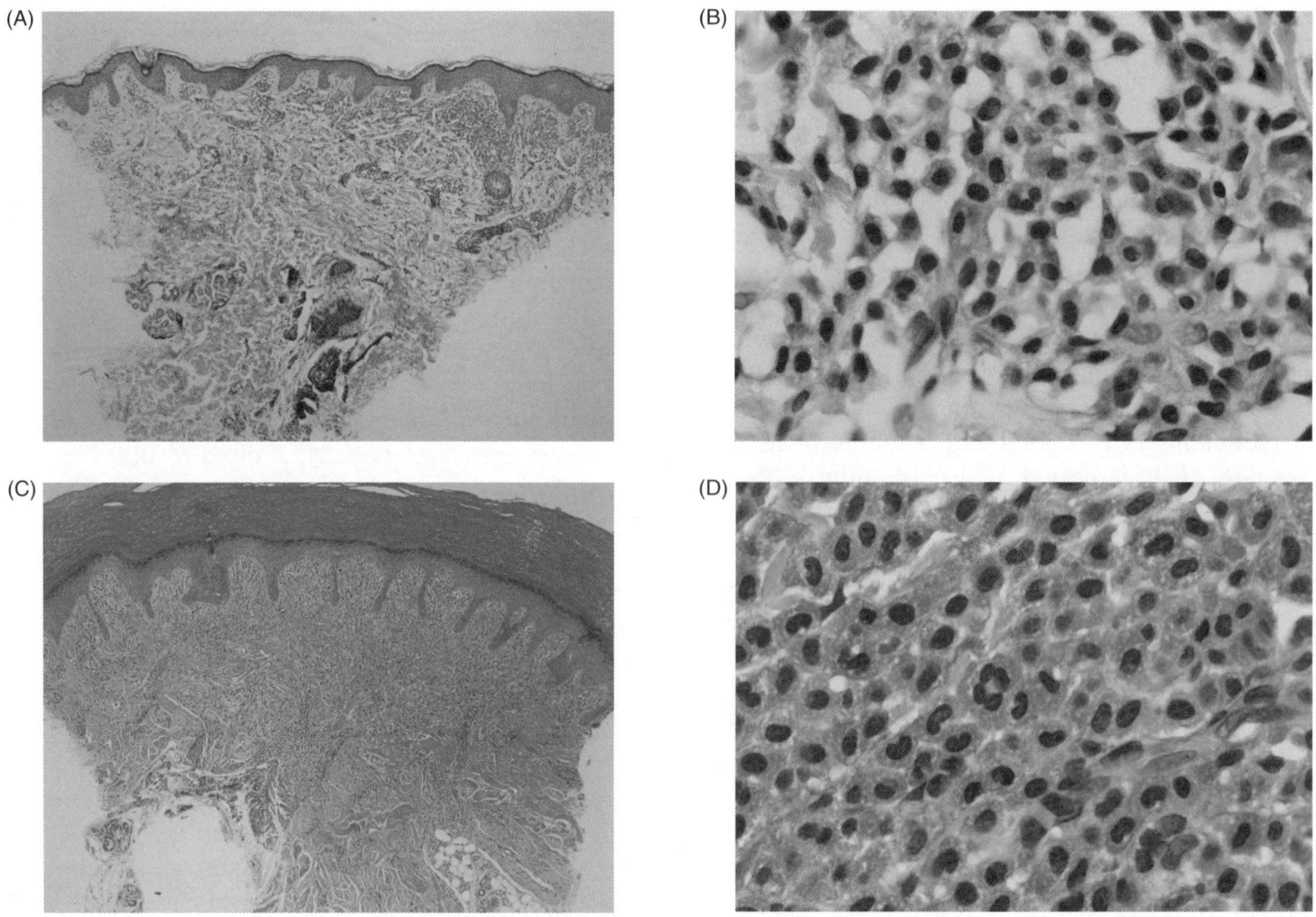

Fig. 4.4. Cutaneous mastocytosis. Uticaria pigmentosa (UP) at (A) low power (2× magnification), and (B) high power (600× magnification) showing collections of mast cells with spindled morphology. (C) Mastocytoma at low power (2× magnification) showing a large mass of mast cells extending to subcutaneous adipose tissue. (D) Mastocytoma at high power (600× magnification). The mast cells of mastocytoma are slightly more round and regular than those of UP.

Immunophenotype

Immunohistochemistry for mast cell tryptase or CD117 is useful to clearly confirm the identity of mast cells or to identify rare aggregates that are difficult to see, as in hypercellular bone marrow cores. CD25 and/or CD2 expression on aggregates of mast cells is abnormal. The demonstration of these aberrant markers is not necessary for a diagnosis of CM but is supportive of SM when multifocal aggregates of mast cells are present in an extracutaneous organ (e.g. bone marrow).

Genetics

A D816V mutation in *KIT*, the gene coding for a receptor tyrosine kinase for stem cell factor, causes unregulated activation of the tyrosine kinase. The D816V mutation is identified in most cases of adult mastocytosis. In children, the 816 mutation has been found in about one third of CM.[1,42] Bodemer *et al.* reported the D816V mutation in 42% of pediatric CM; however, sequencing of the entire *KIT* gene revealed a variety of other *KIT* mutations, which were mutually exclusive of the D816V mutation.[44] Therefore, a total of 86% of pediatric CM cases carried *KIT* mutations, and, interestingly, all of the *KIT* mutations resulted in receptor-independent tyrosine kinase activity.

Diagnostic issues

In reactive mast cell hyperplasia, mast cells are diffusely increased as scattered cells without clustering or formation of sheets. In some instances, the distinction may be difficult, so immunohistochemistry or molecular studies for *KIT* may be helpful. However, molecular studies may be somewhat limited because the D816V *KIT* mutation is less frequent in children, and sequencing the gene to look for the variety of other mutations that occurring in children is not feasible for most laboratories.

The diagnosis of CM requires the exclusion of SM, thus correlation with clinical history, physical exam, and laboratory data are needed. Mastocytosis of extracutaneous organs is considered to be supportive of SM. The detailed diagnostic criteria are available elsewhere.[42]

Acute Myeloid Leukemia

AML accounts for only 15–20% of all acute leukemias in children and adolescents[45] as the majority of the acute leukemias in this age group are ALL. The peak incidence of AML is at 2 years of age. Most patients present with *de novo* AML but there has been an increase in the number of secondary AMLs seen in patients treated with radiation or chemotherapeutic agents. Using the WHO Classification,[1] AML is subclassified based on cytogenetic, clinical and immunophenotypic features (Table 4.6), as discussed below. Typically, a diagnosis of AML requires a demonstration of ≥20% blood or bone marrow blasts, with exceptions as noted below.

Acute myeloid leukemia with recurrent genetic abnormalities

This group of acute leukemias is unique in that they are defined not only by the origin of the blast population (i.e. myeloid) but more precisely by specific cytogenetic abnormalities.[1,46] Many of the AML in this category have unique morphologic and immunophenotypic features, but are defined by cytogenetic findings.[47] Most often they are associated with balanced translocations, such as t(15;17)(q22;q12), and require appropriate

Table 4.6. WHO 2008 classification of acute myeloid leukemia.

Acute myeloid leukemia with recurrent genetic abnormalities

- AML with t(8;21)(q22;q22); (*RUNX1-RUNX1T1*)
- AML with inv(16)(p13.1q22) or t(16;16)(p13.1;q22); (*CBFB-MYH11*)
- APL with t(15;17)(q22;q12); (*PML-RARA*)
- AML with t(9;11)(p22:q23); (*MLLT3-MLL*)
- AML with t(6;9)(p23;q34); (*DEK-NUP214*)
- AML with inv(3)(q21q26.2) or t(3;3)(q21;q26.2); (*TPN1-EVI1*)
- AML (megakaryoblastic) with t(1;22)(p13;q13); (*RBM15-MLK1*)
- Provisional entity: AML with mutated *NPM1*
- Provisional entity: AML with mutated *CEBPA*

Acute myeloid leukemia with myelodysplasia-related changes
Therapy-related myeloid neoplasms
Acute myeloid leukemia, not otherwise specified

- AML with minimal differentiation
- AML without maturation
- AML with maturation
- Acute myelomonocytic leukemia
- Acute monoblastic/monocytic leukemia
- Acute erythroid leukemias
    - Pure erythroid leukemia
    - Erythroleukemia, erythroid/myeloid
- Acute megakaryoblastic leukemia
- Acute basophilic leukemia
- Acute panmyelosis with myelofibrosis

Myeloid sarcoma
Myeloid proliferations related to Down syndrome

- Transient abnormal myelopoiesis
- Acute myeloid leukemia associated with Down syndrome

specimen handling so that all of cytogenetic information can be obtained prior to the start of therapy. The categories of AML with t(15;17)(q22;q12), t(8;21)(q22;q22), inv(16)(p13.1q22) and t(16;16)(p13.1q22) are considered acute leukemias regardless of blast count.[1] The following are the recognized *de novo* AMLs with recurrent genetic abnormalities.

AML with t(8;21)(q22;q22); RUNX1-RUNX1T1

Clinical

This entity represents approximately 5% of AMLs. Patients tend to be of younger age and thus are not uncommon in the pediatric/young adult population. Myeloid sarcoma may be seen at presentation and may represent the first manifestation.

Morphologic features

Blasts are typically large in size with abundant basophilic cytoplasm and often contain azurophilic granules. Perinuclear clearing or hofs, may be seen. Thin Auer rods are common and may even be present in mature neutrophils. Some of the granulocytes may exhibit dysplasia, but it is not a prominent feature and is usually limited to the myeloid series.

Immunophenotype

Most cases express CD13, CD33, CD34, myeloperoxidase and HLA-DR. CD15 and TdT (weak) expression can be seen. Aberrant expression of the lymphoid markers CD19, PAX-5 or CD79a is not uncommon. If CD56 is expressed, it may indicate a poorer overall prognosis.

Genetics

By definition, this acute leukemia exhibits a t(8;21)(q22;q22). Approximately three quarters of the patients have additional abnormalities such as del 9q or loss of sex chromosomes. FISH studies may also used to identify this translocation and are often quicker than conventional karyotyping (Fig. 4.5).

Diagnostic issues

This AML is typically not a diagnostic challenge. Often the blasts contain thin Auer rods. Initially, before the cytogenetic findings are known, some cases with less than 20% blasts in the blood or bone marrow may raise a differential diagnosis of myelodysplasia. Once the translocation is identified, these cases are classified as AML regardless of the peripheral blood or bone marrow blast count.

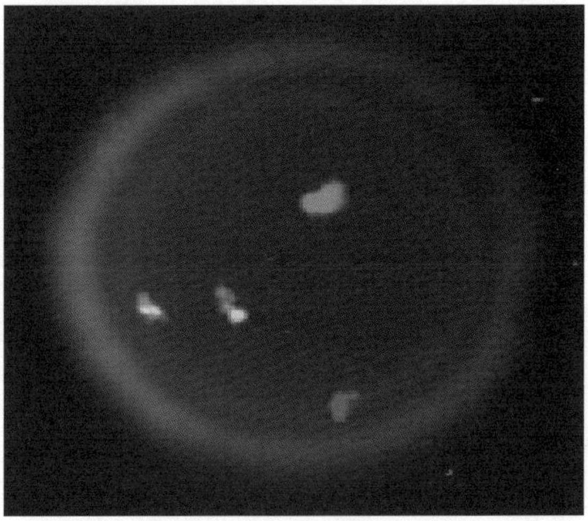

Fig. 4.5. Fluorescence *in situ* hybrization (FISH) showing a yellow fusion signal resulting from a translocation involving RUNX1 (green) and RUNX1T1 (red) seen in acute myeloid leukemia with t(8;21)(q22;q22);RUNX1-RUNX1T1 (1500× magnification).

Acute promyelocytic leukemia (APL) with t(15;17)(q22;q12); PML-RARA

Clinical

APL is an acute leukemia that truly requires emergent diagnosis and treatment. Due to the marked association with disseminated intravascular coagulopathy (DIC), these patients have a marked propensity for life-threatening bleeding. APL occurs at any age, but is seen more commonly in adults. It accounts for 5–10% of de novo AMLs in children.[48]

Morphologic features

Morphologically, there are two variants including the "classic" (hypergranular) type and the microgranular type. In the classic type, the promyelocytes vary in size and shape but often resemble normal promyelocytes. Prominent granules fill and commonly distend the cytoplasm, and single to multiple Auer rods are often seen (Fig. 4.6A). The latter cells are referred to as "faggot cells." The cytoplasmic granules are strongly positive for myeloperoxidase; often there are few circulating

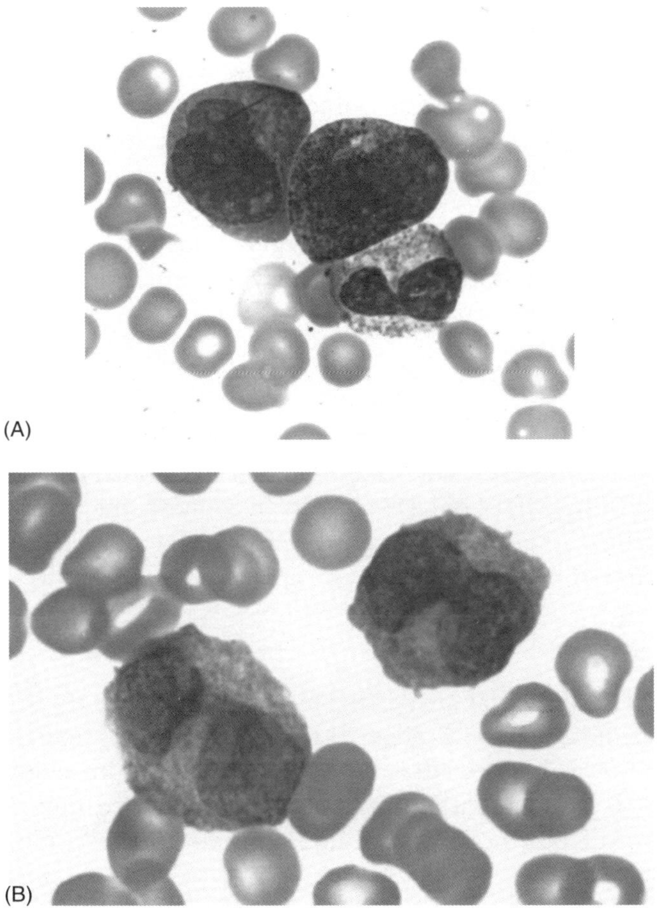

Fig. 4.6. Acute promyelocytic leukemia with t(15;17)(q22;q12). (A) Classical morphology of acute promyelocytic leukemia including prominent granulation and auer rods. (B) Hypogranular variant showing a classic bi-lobed morphology without easily distinguishable granules in the cytoplasm. Both subtypes would be strongly positive with myeloperoxidase and have similar propensity for association with disseminated intravascular coagulation (1000× magnification).

blasts. Within the hypogranular variant, the cytoplasmic granules are much smaller, making it difficult to identify them with light microscopy. The granules show strong positivity with myeloperoxidase staining. The nuclei in the hypogranular variant are almost always bilobed in appearance (Fig. 4.6B). The hypogranular variant commonly presents with a markedly elevated circulating blast count.

Immunophenotype

As the neoplastic cells or blast equivalents are promyelocytes, they typically express CD13, CD33, myeloperoxidase but not HLA-DR or CD34. CD64 may be expressed and aberrant CD2 expression is seen a subset of cases.

Genetics

The cytogenetic abnormality that defines this entity is the t(15;17)(q22;q12). It involves the retinoic acid receptor alpha gene on chromosome 17 which fuses with the PML nuclear regulatory factor gene on chromosome 15. This results in a PML-RARA fusion gene. Additional abnormalities are seen in up to 40% of cases. Variant translocations with the RARA gene on chromosome 17 are well described.

Diagnostic issues

APL is initially treated with all-*trans* retinoic acid (ATRA) for which it is very sensitive and decreases bleeding complications by enhancing cellular differentiation of the tumor cells. The differential diagnosis may include growth factor therapy and myelodysplasia.

AML with inv(16)(p13.1q22) or t(16;16)(p13.1;q22): CBFβ-MYH11

Clinical

This subtype comprises approximately 5–8% of all AMLs. Not uncommonly, myeloid sarcoma may be present at the time of initial diagnosis or may be seen during relapse.

Morphologic features

This AML is somewhat unique in that in addition to the blast population, there is characteristically an abnormal eosinophil population including immature forms. The cytoplasmic granules within the eosinophils are commonly large and blue-purple in color resembling basophilic granules. In addition, there is often both granulocytic and monocytic blast differentiation. Mature neutrophils are decreased. The blast population is often in the range of 15–25%. Cases in which the blast population is > 20% but exhibit a inv(16)(p13.1q22) or t(16;16)(13.1;q22) should still be considered as AML.

Immunophenotype

The blast population typically expresses CD34 and HLA-DR. Evidence of both myeloid differentiation (expression of CD13, CD33, CD15 and myeloperoxidase) as well as monocytic differentiation (expression of CD14, CD4, CD11c, CD64 and lysozyme) is often seen. CD2 may be aberrantly expressed.

Genetics

Inv(16)(p13.1q22) is seen in the majority of cases. A smaller subset of cases exhibit t(16;16)(p13.1;q22). Additional changes including +8, +21, +22 or del 7q may be present in up to 40% of cases. Conventional karyotyping may not pick up all cases of inv(16)(p13.1q22) or t(16;16)(p13.1;q22) and thus FISH and/or RT-PCR may need to be utilized.

Diagnostic issues

The presence of prominent eosinophils within a background of AML should always raise the differential diagnosis of this leukemia. Some cases may not have prominent eosinophilia or may have striking monocytosis. In addition, not all cases will have 20% blasts in the bone marrow or blood, however, if either of these translocations are present, they should be classified as AML.

AML with t(9;11)(p22;q23); MLLT3-MLL

Clinical

This acute leukemia often presents with myeloid sarcoma and prominent monocytic differentiation. A subset of patients has accompanying DIC at diagnosis.

Morphologic features

In many cases, the blasts exhibit monocytic differentiation similar to acute myelomonocytic leukemia or acute monoblastic leukemia. Often the blast population is represented by a combination of promonocytes and monoblasts. The neoplastic cells have abundant pale blue cytoplasm, round to irregular nuclear contours and fine azurophilic granules. Cytoplasmic vacuolization may be seen.

Immunophenotype

In children, the blasts typically express CD4, CD33, CD65 and HLA-DR. Only minimal to dim expression of CD13, CD14 or CD34 is seen. In addition, the monocytic blast population is positive for nonspecific esterase but not myeloperoxidase.

Genetics

These leukemias are defined by the presence of a t(9;11)(p22;q23) (Fig. 4.7). The MLL gene on chromosome 11, however, has been described in translocations involving > 50 partner genes.[49] Some of them are more common in ALL but the t(9;11)(p22;q23) results are most common in AML.

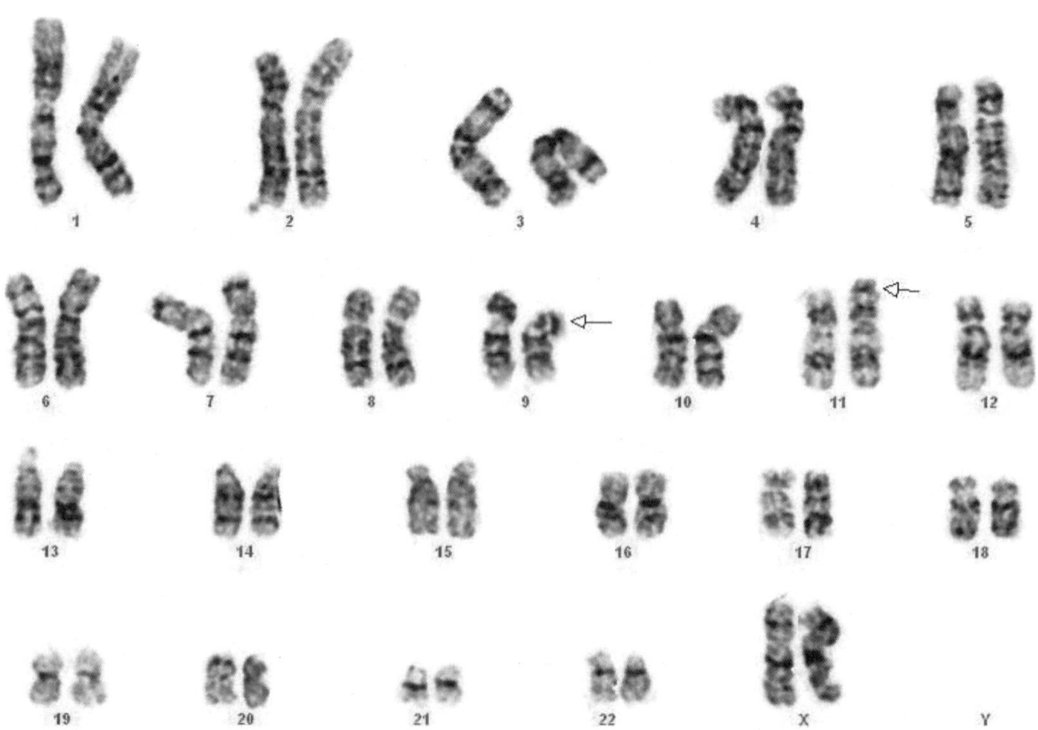

Fig. 4.7. Karyotype from patient with acute myeloid leukemia with t(9;11)(p22;q23);MLLT3-MLL. This patient presented with disseminated intravascular coagulopathy.

Diagnostic issues

This leukemia is defined by its cytogenetic abnormality and thus requires identification of t(9;11)(p22;q23). As it commonly exhibits monocytic differentiation, it must be distinguished from acute myelomonocytic leukemia (not otherwise specified [NOS]), acute monoblastic leukemia (NOS), CMML and JMML.

AML with t(6;9)(p23;q34); DEK-NUP214

Clinical

This leukemia typically presents with cytopenias and often with pancytopenia. Not uncommonly, there is a normal to only slightly elevated white blood cell counts in contrast to many of other AMLs which present with markedly elevated blast counts. This leukemia represents approximately 1–2% of all AMLs. In children, it presents at a median age of 13 years.

Morphologic features

The blast population may exhibit monocytic differentiation but can present with morphologic features of any AML, NOS except APL and AML-MK. There is frequently an associated basophilia and multilineage dysplasia. Ring sideroblasts may be seen. The blast population contains Auer rods in a minor subset of cases.

Immunophenotype

The blasts do not exhibit any unique expression pattern and often express CD13, CD33, CD15, CD117, CD34, HLA-DR and myeloperoxidase. Some cases may express CD64 and TdT.

Genetics

The t(6;9)(p23;q34) is the defining cytogenetic abnormality of this AML and often the only clonal abnormality identified by karyotyping (Fig. 4.8). Many patients with this translocation will also have *FLT3-ITD* mutations.[46,50]

Diagnostic issues

This acute leukemia can be confused with other AML with monocytic differentiation. It tends to have an overall worse prognosis than AML without cytogenetic abnormalities.

AML with inv(3)(q21q26.2) or t(3;3) (q21;q26.2); RPN1-EVI1

Clinical

The AMLs with inv(3)(q21q26.2) or t(3;3)(q21;q26.2) are more common in adults than in children. This leukemia is rare and accounts for 1–2% of all AMLs. Patients typically present with anemia and normal to elevated platelet counts. Organomegaly may be present.

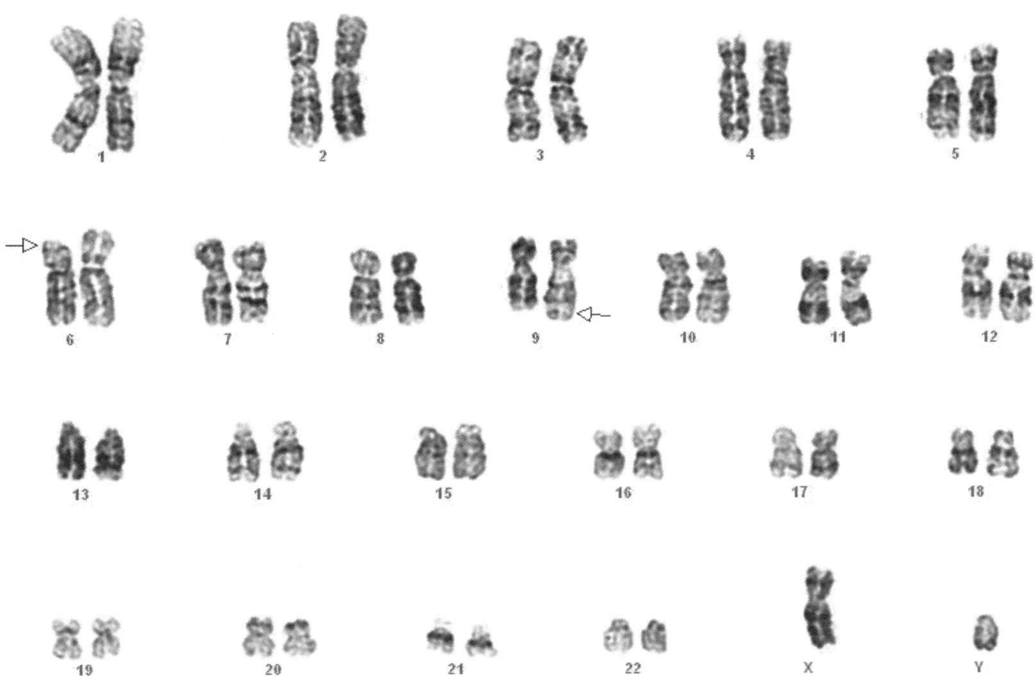

Fig. 4.8. Karyotype from patient with acute myeloid leukemia with t(6;9)(p23;q34);DEK-NUP214.

These leukemias may present *de novo* or arise out of a previously known MDS.

Morphologic features

Within the peripheral blood as well as the bone marrow, there are typically dysplastic features including pseudo-Pelger-Huet neutrophils and hypogranular platelets. The bone marrow will contain numerous atypical megakaryocytes, some of which may be monolobated. The remaining marrow elements often exhibit some degree of dysplasia. The blast population will be nondescript in appearance and in some cases will represent less than 20% of the marrow elements which does not preclude a diagnosis of acute leukemia if an inv(3)(q21q26.2) or t(3;3)(q21;q26.2) is identified.

Immunophenotype

The blast population typically expresses CD13, CD33, HLA-DR, and CD34. Expression of the megakaryocytic markers CD41 and CD61 may be seen. Aberrant expression of CD7 is not uncommon.

Genetics

In addition to the inv(3)(q21q26.2) or t(3;3)(q21;q26.2) identified in these AMLs, many also have additional karyotypic abnormalities including del 5q or del 7. Some patients with chronic myelogeous leukemia may acquire an inv(3)(q21q26.2) or t(3;3)(q21;q26.2), which typically indicates progression of disease into accelerated or blast phase.

Diagnostic issues

This leukemia is aggressive with an overall shorter survival than that seen in many patients with other subtypes of AML. It can morphologically be confused with AML with myelodysplastic-related changes and occasionally with AML-MK. Identification of the defining cytogenetic abnormality is imperative.

AML (Megakaryoblastic) with t(1;22)(p13;q13); RBM15-MKL1

Clinical

This leukemia occurs almost exclusively in infants and young children, most often within the first 6 months of life. Typically, patients have a leukocytosis, anemia and thrombocytopenia. There is also frequent hepatosplenomegaly. Overall, this acute leukemia is rare, accounting for < 1% of all acute myeloid leukemias. It is more common in females and is seen more often in infants without DS.

Morphologic features

The morphologic features are similar to AML-MK, NOS including undifferentiated blasts admixed with megakaryoblasts. The megakaryoblasts can vary in size from medium to large and often have abundant pale blue to basophilic agranular cytoplasm. Cytoplasmic blebs are common. Occasional dysplastic megakaryocytes may be seen. There is frequently prominent reticulin fibrosis.

Immunophenotype

The megakaryoblasts commonly express CD41, CD61, CD36, CD13, CD33 and CD34. CD42 may be expressed. CD45, HLA-DR and myeloperoxidase are typically negative.

Genetics

By definition, this acute leukemia must have the t(1;22)(p13;q13) karyotypic translocation.

Diagnostic issues

This leukemia is most easily confused with AML-MK, NOS or in young children with DS with the *GATA1*-related MK-AML.

In addition to the specific entities described above, other gene mutations may be seen in patients with AML. These can be seen in patients who have identifiable translocations or deletions as well as in patients with normal karyotypes. In patients with a normal karyotype, mutations of *FLT3*, *NPM1* or *CEBPA* have been shown to have some prognostic significance. *FLT3* (fms-related tyrosine kinase 3) mutations can be of two types. The first involves internal tandem duplications (*FLT3-ITD*) and accounts for 75–80% of *FLT3* mutations and is associated an overall worse prognosis in patients with a normal karyotype.[46,50] The second involves mutations affecting the second tyrosine kinase domain (*FLT3-TKD*) and are not specifically related with a worse prognosis. *NPM1* (nucleophosmin) mutations occur in one third of all AMLs in adults and 2–8%

in children. *NPM1* mutations are heterogenous and can involve various exons. AMLs with a *NPM1* mutation and no *FLT3-ITD* mutations are associated with a favorable prognosis. *CEBPA* (CCAAT/enhancer-binding protein-alpha) mutations that are seen in acute myeloid leukemia, which have a normal karyotype and are negative for the *FLT3-ITD* mutation, are associated with a favorable overall prognosis.

Acute myeloid leukemia, not otherwise specified

The AML, NOS represents those leukemias which do not exhibit the criteria to fall into another category based on specific cytogenetic abnormalities, associated myelodysplasia or a history of prior radiation or chemotherapy. Generally, they resemble the AMLs that were recognized within the previous French-American-British (FAB) classification and require identification of 20% blasts or blast equivalents within the peripheral blood or bone marrow.[1]

AML with minimal differentiation

Clinical

Patients typically present with cytopenias secondary to marrow failure. There may be a leukocytosis with numerous circulating blasts. Within the pediatric population, this leukemia is more commonly seen in infants. It accounts for 5% of all AML cases.

Morphologic features

The blast population is characterized by medium to large size, finely dispersed chromatin, round to irregular nuclear contours and one or more prominent nucleoli. The cytoplasm is scant to moderately prominent and agranular. Auer rods are not seen (Fig. 4.9).

Immunophenotype

The blasts typically express CD13, CD33, CD117, CD34, CD38 and HLA-DR. More mature myeloid markers, as well as most lymphoid markers, are negative. Myeloperoxidase expression may be seen by flow cytometry but is usually negative by cytochemical staining. CD7 and/or TdT expression can be seen in up to 50% of cases.

Genetics

There are no specific or recurrent cytogenetic abnormalities identified.

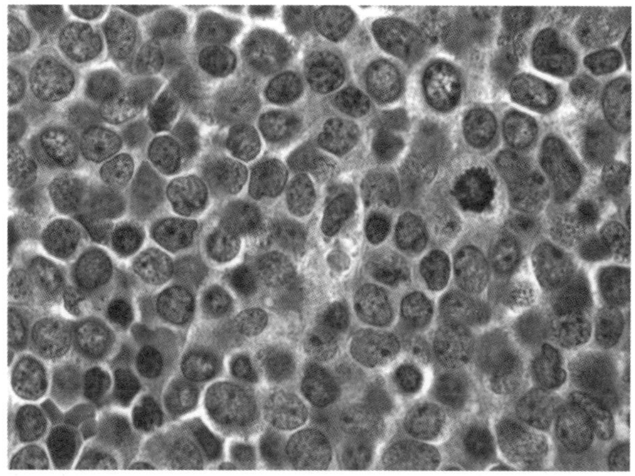

Fig. 4.9. H&E section from a bone marrow biopsy with acute myeloid leukemia with minimal differentiation. Note the finely dispersed chromatin and occasional nucleoli. Auer rods were not seen in this case (800× magnification).

Diagnostic issues

As the blasts may appear undifferentiated and contain few granules, they can readily be confused with ALL morphologically.

AML without maturation

Clinical

Patients present with cytopenias. There may be a leukocytosis with numerous circulating blasts. This leukemia may occur at any age and accounts for 5–10% of all AML.

Morphologic features

The blast population can vary from apparent undifferentiated blasts to easily recognized myeloblasts with

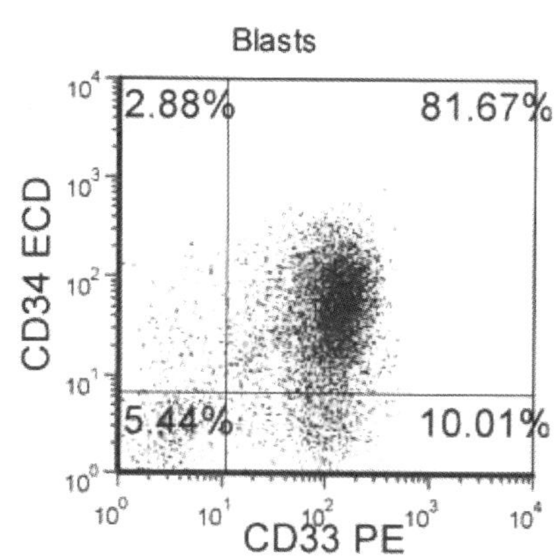

Fig. 4.10. Flow cytometry histogram showing expression of CD33 and CD34 by the blast population in this child with acute myeloid leukemia without maturation.

abundant cytoplasm, azurophilic granules and Auer rods. Within the bone marrow, the blast population must constitute > 90% of the non-erythroid cells, as significant maturation should not be present. In the blood, there may be a leukocytosis secondary to circulating blasts and cytopenias, including anemia and/or thrombocytopenia.

Immunophenotype

CD13, CD33, CD34, CD117, myeloperoxidase, and HLA-DR are commonly expressed by the blasts (Fig. 4.5). Monocytic markers CD14 and CD64 are negative. CD7, CD2, CD4, CD19 and/or CD56 can be expressed by a subset of cases.

Genetics

There are no specific or recurrent cytogenetic abnormalities identified.

Diagnostic issues

Due to the fact that the blast population can look undifferentiated, the differential diagnosis morphologically may include ALL as well as AML with minimal differentiation.

AML with maturation

Clinical

This subtype represents 10% of all cases of AML and can be seen at any age. Patients often present with cytopenias, including anemia and/or thrombocytopenia. The blood leukocyte count may be elevated due to circulating blasts.

Morphologic features

By definition, AML with maturation requires 20% blasts within the peripheral blood or bone marrow and there must be evidence of maturation (> 10% of the myeloid cells must be maturing, i.e. not blasts) and < 20% of the marrow elements should be of monocytic lineage.

Immunophenotype

The blast population typically expresses CD13, CD15, CD33, CD117, CD34, HLA-DR and myeloperoxidase. A minor subset of cases may express CD7. The monocytic markers CD14 and CD64 are usually absent.

Genetics

There are no specific or recurrent cytogenetic abnormalities identified.

Diagnostic issues

Depending on the blast count, the differential diagnosis would include MDSs such as refractory anemia with excess blasts.

Acute myelomonocytic leukemia

Clinical

This acute leukemia can occur at any age but is more common in adults. It accounts for 5–10% of all AML. Patients often present with a leukocytosis (comprised of myeloblasts, monoblasts and promonocytes) as well as anemia and/or thrombocytopenia.

Morphologic features

These leukemias often contain more than one population of blasts. By definition, there must be at least 20% blasts or blast equivalents (including promonocytes); greater than 20% and less than 80% of the blasts should be of monocytic origin. There are often numerous mature and immature monocytic cells within the peripheral blood.

Immunophenotype

The myeloid blast population often expresses CD13, CD33, CD34 and HLA-DR. Another of the blast populations exhibits monocytic differentiation with expression of CD4, CD13, CD14, CD33, CD64 and HLA-DR. An immature population of blasts only expressing CD117 and CD34 may also be identified.

Genetics

There are no specific or recurrent cytogenetic abnormalities identified. In many cases, a +8 can be identified.

Diagnostic issues

The differential diagnosis includes CMML as well as acute monocytic leukemia. The blast count and type can help distinguish between these cases. Cases with at least 20% blasts with >80% of the blasts exhibiting monocytic differentiation should be classified as acute monoblastic or acute monocytic leukemia.

Acute monoblastic and acute monocytic leukemia

Clinical

This group of leukemias represent <5% of all AMLs. They can occur at any age but are most common in children and young adults. They are slightly more common in males than females. Extramedullary proliferations involving the skin, mucous membranes, and gingiva are common. Central nervous system (CNS) involvement can also be seen. Spontaneous bleeding is not uncommon.

Morphologic features

More than 80% of the blasts should be of monocytic origin (monoblasts or promonoblasts). If the blasts predominantly comprises monoblasts, these cases are classified as acute monoblastic leukemia. If the blasts or blast equivalents predominantly comprises promono cytes, they are classified as acute monocytic leukemia. Monoblasts are characterized by increased size, abundant basophilic cytoplasm, and round nuclei. The chromatin is fine and they often have prominent nucleoli. Promonocytes also have abundant cytoplasm but is often paler in appearance. The nuclei are folded to convoluted. Cytoplasmic vacuoles or granules may be seen.

Immunophenotype

The blasts typically express ≥2 monocytic markers such as CD4, CD14, CD11b, CD64, CD68 or lysozyme. CD13, CD33, and HLA-DR are often expressed. CD34 and myeloperoxidase are expressed in a minor subset of cases.

Genetics

Most cases will have cytogenetic abnormalities but they are typically nonspecific. The t(8;16)(p11.2;p13.3) can be seen in cases of acute monocytic or acute myelomonocytic leukemia and are often associated with hemophagocytosis by the leukemic cells.

Diagnostic issues

The differential diagnosis includes acute myelomonocytic leukemia as well as CMML. Acute monoblastic leukemia can be confused with AML with minimal differentiation or AML without maturation.

Acute erythroid leukemia

Clinical

These patients often present with cytopenias including marked anemia. It is extremely rare in children and young adults. This leukemia accounts for <5% of all AMLs.

Morphologic features

By definition, at least 50% of the bone marrow elements must be erythroid precursors. One subtype requires that at least 50% of the marrow elements represent erythroid precursors and of the remaining non-erythroid marrow elements, at least 20% must be myeloblasts. The second subtype, referred to as pure erythroid leukemia, comprises neoplastic erythroid precursors representing at least 80% of the marrow elements and 20% erythroblasts. Occasional circulating erythroblasts can be seen in the blood.

Immunophenotype

The erythroblasts will express hemoglobin A and glycophorin; some may express CD71. They are commonly negative for CD34 and myeloperoxidase. In cases with an associated myeloblast population, the markers typically expressed by the myeloblasts include CD13, CD33, HLA-DR, CD34, and myeloperoxidase.

Genetics

There are no specific or recurrent cytogenetic abnormalities identified. Complex karyotypes are common.

Diagnostic issues

These cases can easily be confused with high-grade MDSs such as refractory anemia with excess blasts. In addition, erythropoietin therapy as well as folate and B12 deficiency can lead to changes within the marrow that can resemble acute erythroid leukemia. Knowing the clinical history and B12 or folate levels is extremely important.

Acute megakaryoblastic leukemia

Clinical

Similar to many other AMLs, patients often present with cytopenias including thrombocytopenia. Some may present with a thrombocytosis. This leukemia is seen in both adults and children and accounts for < 5% of all AMLs. There may be an association between this leukemia and mediastinal germ cell tumors in young adult males. The overall prognosis of this leukemia is poor.

Morphologic features

By definition, this AML requires at least 20% blasts within the peripheral blood or bone marrow and at least 50% of the blasts must be of megakaryocytic lineage. The megakaryoblasts are medium to large in size with round to irregular nuclear contours, dispersed chromatin, occasional nucleoli and variably abundant cytoplasm.

Immunophenotype

The megakaryoblasts commonly express CD36, CD41, CD61 and/or CD42. CD13 and CD33 may be expressed but HLA-DR and CD34 are typically negative. CD7 may be aberrantly expressed.

Genetics

There are no specific or recurrent cytogenetic abnormalities identified. Complex karyotypes are common.

Diagnostic issues

The differential diagnosis includes AML with myelodysplasia-related changes as well as AML with inv(3)(q21q26.2), t(3;3)(q21;q26.2), or t(1;22)(p13;q13). The latter cytogenetic translocation will allow placing the leukemia into that specific category. In young children, AML with t(1;22)(p13;q13) and AML associated with DS should be excluded.

Acute panmyelosis with myelofibrosis

Clinical

This leukemia occurs predominantly in adults but rarely has been reported in children and young adults. Most patients present acutely with fever, lethargy, weakness and bone pain. There is nearly always pancytopenia at presentation. Significant organomegaly is not typically seen.

Morphologic features

The peripheral blood often exhibits dyspoiesis and features consistent with marrow fibrosis including circulating nucleated red blood cells, teardrop cells and occasional fragments. There are frequently circulating immature myeloid precursors including blasts. The bone marrow is hypercellular with extensive fibrosis often precluding successful aspiration. There is panmyelosis with dysplastic megakaryocytes and increased blasts. The blast count, however, can vary considerably.

Immunophenotype

Often a dry tap precludes flow cytometry of the bone marrow. The blasts within the peripheral blood are typically myeloid in origin. A CD34 stain by immunohistochemistry will allow for quantitation of the immature cells and identification of 20% blasts.

Genetics

If cytogenetic studies are successful, there is usually an abnormal karyotype. No consistent abnormalities are seen.

Diagnostic issues

The differential diagnosis often includes chronic myeloproliferative neoplasms such as primary myelofibrosis as well as AML-MK.

Therapy-related acute myeloid leukemia

Therapy-related AML occurs as a late sequelae of radiation therapy and/or cytotoxic chemotherapy. Some patients may present first with a therapy-related MDS or MDS/MPN. In one study in children, therapy-related AMLs and MDSs were seen most commonly in patients treated for osteosarcoma, Hodgkin lymphoma (HL) and B-cell acute lymphoblastic leukemia/lymphoma.[45,51]

Clinical

The incidence varies depending on the course of therapy as well as the duration. Alkylating agents and topoisomerase II inhibitors are among the chemotherapeutic agents most often associated with this acute leukemia. The incidence increases with age for patients who received alkylating agents or radiation therapy. Some patients treated with intensified chemotherapy and autologous bone marrow transplant also develop therapy-related AML.

Patients treated with alkylating agents generally develop therapy-related myelodysplasia prior to developing frank acute leukemia. It typically occurs 5–10 years following the initial chemotherapy. Patients treated with topoisomerase II inhibitors generally proceed outright to acute leukemia without first developing a MDS. This occurs more quickly after initial therapy with a latency period of 1–5 years. Often patients may have received both drugs.

Morphologic features

Those cases associated with prior alkylating and/or radiation therapy often will present with cytopenias with associated dyspoiesis which can be seen in one or more cell lines (Fig. 4.11). The bone marrow may be hypercellular, normocellular, or hypocellular. Often there is marrow fibrosis. Ring sideroblasts are common. Those cases associated with topoisomerase II inhibitors most often present as frank acute leukemia. These acute leukemias are morphologically similar to other subtypes of AML.

Immunophenotype

There is no one unique immunophenotype seen with this group of acute leukemias. The blasts commonly express CD34 as well as the myeloid markers CD13 and CD33. Aberrant expression of CD7 and CD56 can be seen.

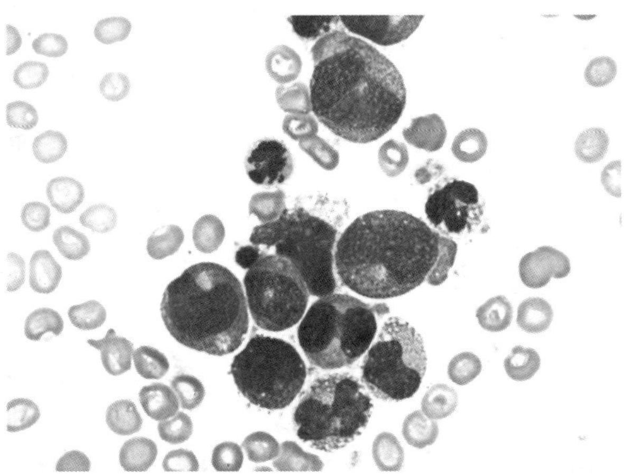

Fig. 4.11. Bone marrow aspirate in a young adult patient previously treated with alkylating agents fort-lymphoblastic non-Hodgkin lymphoma. There were approximately 25% blasts (arrow) in the bone marrow aspirate, myeloid dysplasia and the karyotype identified a 12p deletion (1000× magnification).

Genetics

Nearly all cases of therapy-related AML will have cytogenetic abnormalities.[1] Those leukemias associated with alkylating and/or radiation therapy often exhibit unbalanced translocations or deletions frequently involving chromosome 5 or 7. Other deletions and/or additions, such as −13q, −20q, −21, or +8, are not uncommon. The acute leukemias seen in patients treated with prior topisomerase II inhibitors often exhibit balanced chromosomal translocations involving 11q23, inv (16)(p13q22), t(15;17)(q22q12) as well as 21q22 as is seen in t(8;21)(q22q22).

Diagnostic issues

A history of prior therapy with alkylating agents, radiation therapy and/or topoisomerase II inhibitors, is crucial for this diagnosis. Morphologically and cytogenetically, this group of leukemias can resemble their counterpart AMLs which are not associated with prior therapy. It is important to recognize this group of acute leukemias because they have an overall worse prognosis. A subset of those cases associated with balanced translocations tends to do better than those with unbalanced translocations or deletions. Those with a t(15:17), t(16;16) and inv(16) do poorer than their counterparts that arise as *de novo* disease.

Acute leukemias of ambiguous lineage

This group of acute leukemias includes those that lack clear differentiation into a single lineage. They encompass those that show no differentiation (acute undifferentiated leukemia) as well as those showing differentiation along more than one lineage (mixed phenotype acute leukemia). The latter leukemias present as two or more separate blasts populations, each expressing single lineage antigens or a single blast population exhibiting multiple lineage antigen expression.[45] Overall, acute leukemias of ambiguous leukemias (ALAL) are rare and account for less than 5% of all acute leukemias. By definition, ALAL excludes cases that can be classified into another category of acute leukemia by clinical or genetic features. The most recognized categories of ALAL are summarized in Table 4.7.

Table 4.7. Acute leukemias of ambiguous lineage.

Acute undifferentiated leukemia
Mixed phenotype acute leukesmia with t(9;22)(q34;q11.2); *BCR-ABL1*
Mixed phenotype acute leukemia with t(v;11q23); *MLL* rearranged
Mixed phenotype acute leukemia, B/myeloid, NOS
Mixed phenotype acute leukemia, T/myeloid, NOS

Clinical

There are no specific nor unique clinical features of this group of leukemias that reliably distinguish them from more classic AML or ALL. The mixed phenotype acute leukemia with t(9;22)(q34;q11.2); *BCR-ABL1* may be associated with high white counts at presentation.

Morphologic features

Depending on the category of the ALAL, the morphologic features of the blast population may be indistinguishable from other acute leukemias. The mixed phenotypic subsets, often have a dimorphic blast population, one resembling lymphoblasts and one resembling myeloblasts.

Immunophenotype

The identification of this group of leukemias requires immunophenotyping which is best achieved by flow cytometry. Considerable confusion has arisen regarding the terms undifferentiated and mixed phenotype acute leukemia. Acute undifferentiated leukemia lacks expression of lineage specific myeloid, lymphoid, plasmablastic dendritic cell or megakaryocytic antigens. They often only express HLA-DR, CD34 and TdT. Mixed phenotype acute leukemia presents with either two or more separate lineage-specific blast populations or a single blast population which expresses more than one lineage specific antigens.

Genetics

A subset of the mixed phenotype acute leukemias have either a t(9;22)(q34;q11.2) or t(v;11q23) translocation and are classified as such (see Table 4.7). The remainder of the leukemias in this group frequently have cytogenetic abnormalities but do not show specificity.

Diagnostic issues

These leukemias can be difficult to diagnose either because they lack specific antigen expression or because they express antigens of different lineage. The distinction between this group of leukemias and other leukemias which exhibit aberrant antigen expression can, in some cases, be problematic, if not impossible. These entities should only be considered in the differential diagnosis if all other categories of acute leukemia have been excluded.

Blastic plasmacytoid dendritic cell neoplasm

Clinical

Blastic plasmacytoid dendritic cell neoplasm (BPDCN) is an aggressive neoplasm presenting with asymptomatic skin lesions which can be solitary or multiple.[52] Some patients may also have lymphadenopathy. Initially, bone marrow involvement is minimal or absent but occurs with progression of disease. Cytopenias may be present at diagnosis. While most commonly seen in the elderly, BPDCN can occur at any age including in children. Most patients show initial response the chemotherapy but relapse or progress in nearly all cases. Ten to twenty percent develop AML which may have monocytic differentiation. The median survival is 12–14 months despite therapy, but long-term survival is reported in patients who received an allogeneic stem cell transplant following acute leukemia type induction chemotherapy.

Morphologic features

Skin biopsies in BPDCN reveal a diffuse infiltrate of medium-sized monomorphic cells with scant cytoplasm, irregular nuclear contours and fine, dispersed chromatin (Figs. 4.12A–B). Occasional mitosis can be seen. The neoplastic cells fill the dermis and spare the overlying epidermis. Involvement of lymph nodes is commonly seen in an interfollicular or medullary pattern. Bone marrow involvement may be interstitial or replace the majority of the marrow elements. In peripheral blood or aspirate smears, the neoplastic cells can exhibit cytoplasmic vacuolization.

Immunophenotype

The neoplastic cells typically express CD4, CD43, CD45RA, CD56, CD123, TCL1, and CLA (Fig. 4.12C). CD68 is expressed in approximately half of the cases with dot-like cytoplasmic positivity and TdT is expressed in one third of cases. Other myeloid and lymphoid markers can be expressed including CD7, CD33 and less commonly CD2 and CD38. These neoplasms are typically

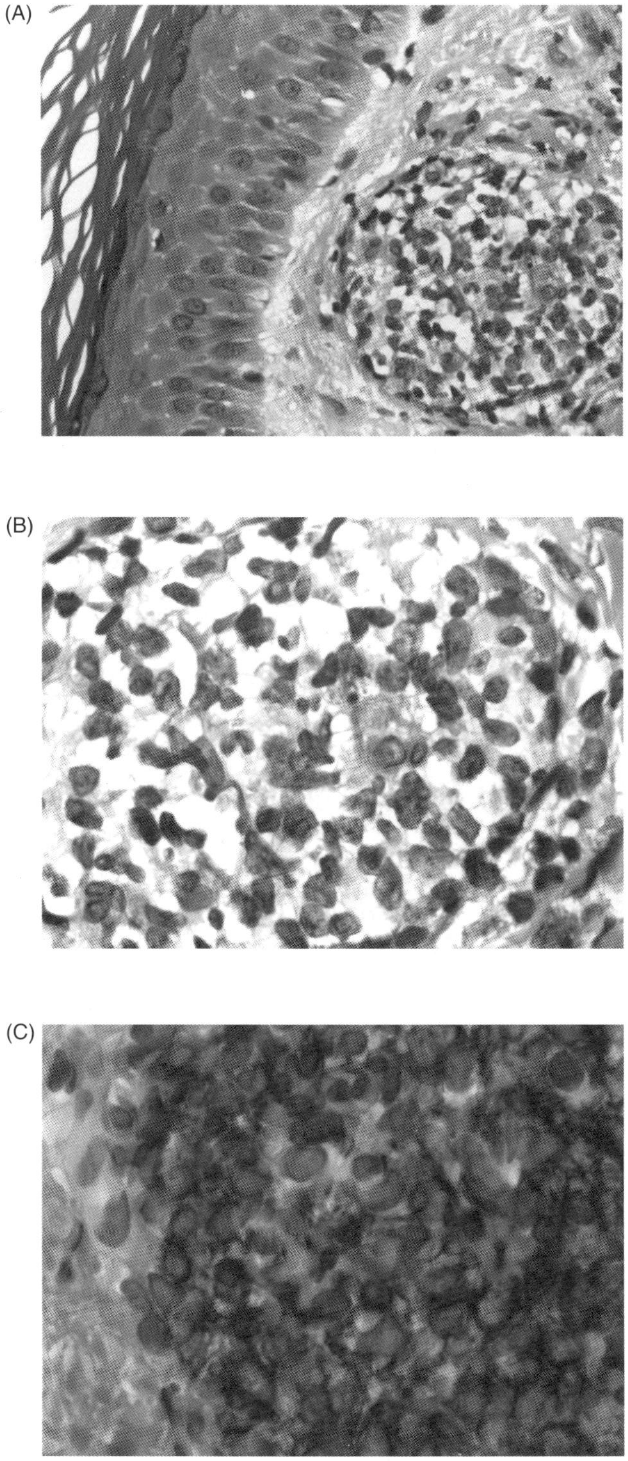

Fig. 4.12. Skin biopsy from an 8-year-old male with a subcutaneous mass of the thigh. (A) Within the superficial and deep dermis, there was a mononuclear infiltrate that formed occasional nodules of tumor cells (200× magnification). (B) Higher magnification shows the blastic morphology of tumor cells with fine chromatin and inconspicuous nucleoli (1000× magnification). (C) Positive CD56 immunohistochemical stain from the skin biopsy. The blast cells also expressed CD45, staining was also negative (1000× magnification).

negative for CD3, CD5, CD13, CD19, CD20, CD34, CD79a, CD117, myeloperoxidase, and EBV.

Genetics

The majority of cases will exhibit an abnormal karyotype, often complex, but no specific findings are seen. More commonly seen abnormalities include those associated with 5q21 or 5q34, 12p13, 13q13-21, 6q23-qter, 15q and del 9. B and T-cell gene rearrangements are negative.

Diagnostic issues

The differential diagnosis may initially be broad including non-Hodgkin lymphoma (NHL), myeloid sarcoma and non-hematopoietic neoplasms. The immunophenotypic profile, however, is relatively specific and quite helpful in the diagnosis. Correlation with peripheral blood and bone marrow involvement is necessary to rule out progression to acute myeloid leukemia.

Precursor Lymphoid Neoplasms

Precursor lymphoid neoplasms include three specific subcategories in the current WHO classification: B-lymphoblastic leukemia/lymphoma (B-ALL/LBL) (NOS), (B-ALL/LBL) with recurrent genetic abnormalities and T-lymphoblastic leukemia/lymphoma (Table 4.8).[1] These neoplasms are seen with relatively high frequency in pediatric populations, with over 75% cases occurring in children under the age of 6 years. Lymphoblastic neoplasms have the capacity to present as either leukemic or lymphomatous processes involving nodal or extranodal sites. The process is usually classified by its predominant presentation, but there is significant overlap. By convention, the terminology of lymphoma

Table 4.8. WHO classification of acute lymphoblastic leukemia/lymphoma.

Precursor lymphoid neoplasms
B lymphoblastic leukemia/lymphoma, NOS
B lymphoblastic leukemia/ lymphoma with recurrent genetic abnormalities
• t(9;22)(q34;q11.2);*BCR-ABL1*
• t(v;11q23); *MLL* rearranged
• t(12;21)(p13;q22); *TEL-AML1 (ETV6-RUNX1)*
• Hyperdiploidy
• Hypodiploidy (hypodiploid ALL)
• t(5;14)(q31;q32); *IL3-IGH*
• t(1;19)(q23;p13.3); *E2A-PBX1 (TCF3-PBX1)*
T lymphoblastic leukemia/lymphoma

is used to refer to disease presenting as a mass with no or minimal bone marrow involvement, and a cutoff of > 25% marrow blasts is used to distinguish leukemia from lymphoma in most pediatric trials.[53,54] B-lymphoblastic disease is more likely to present as ALL and over 80% of ALL is B-cell phenotype. In contrast, T-lymphoblastic disease is more likely to present as a lymphoma, with 85–90% of LBL being of T-cell phenotype.[55]

B-Lymphoblastic leukemia/lymphoma (NOS)

Clinical

B-ALL/LBL (NOS) is primarily a disease of childhood with most of the cases occurring in young children. Patients with B-ALL often present with cytopenias and the leukocyte count may be decreased, normal or increased. Marrow involvement is usually extensive. Extramedullary involvement of the CNS, nodes, spleen, liver and testis is also frequently seen.[53] Patients presenting with B-LBL frequently show involvement of skin, nodes and bone. Nodal presentations frequently involve the head and neck and are associated with limited stage disease.[55] There may be minimal marrow involvement, but B-LBL is defined by < 25% marrow blasts.[1]

Morphologic features

B-lymphoblasts vary in size and may be small with minimal cytoplasm, condensed chromatin and indistinct chromocenters or intermediate in sized with moderate amounts of pale cytoplasm (Fig. 4.13). The chromatin is variably dispersed and nuclear contours range from round to convoluted. Larger blasts may have variably prominent nucleoli. Usually the marrow shows near complete effacement by a relatively uniform blast population. B-LBL typically shows a diffuse infiltrate of blast-like cells. The cells may infiltrate in single file through soft tissues. Mitotic activity is usually high and there may be a "starry sky" pattern seen focally.[1]

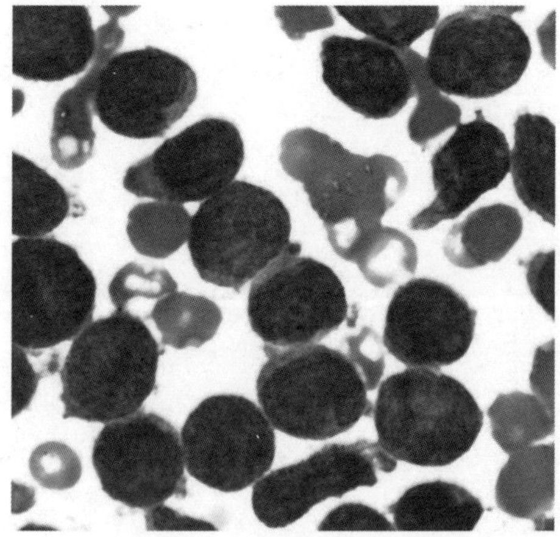

Fig. 4.13. Blood smear from a patient with precursor B-ALL showing characteristic lymphoblastic morphology. The blasts are intermediate in size with fine chromatin. Nucleoli are not prominent. There is minimal amounts of cytoplasm noted (1000× magnification).

Immunophenotype

B-ALL/LBL demonstrates evidence of B-cell lineage and usually will express CD19, CD22 and CD79a. Most cases will also express CD10, PAX-5, TdT, and BCL-2. Usually CD45 is low to absent. There is variable expression of CD34 and CD20 and usually cell surface immunoglobulin expression is absent or diminished. There may be aberrant expression of myeloid markers, particularly CD13 and CD33.[56,57] Many times the immunophenotype of the B-lymphoblasts will recapitulate that of normal B-cell maturation (Table 4.9), although the majority of ALL cases are precursor B-phenotype and CD10+ (Table 4.10).

Genetics

Genetic abnormalities are an important prognostic feature of B-ALL (Table 4.11), although several recurrent abnormalities have been identified as specific diagnostic entities (see below and Table 4.9).[1] B-ALL/LBL (NOS) frequently has cytogenetic abnormalities, but

Table 4.9. Common antigen expression patterns of B-acute lymphoblastic leukemia/lymphoblastic lymphoma.

	CD19	CD20	CD22	CD24	CD10	CD34	Tdt	HLA-DR	SIg
Pre precursor B-ALL	+	−/+	−	+	+/−	+	+	+	−
Precursor B-ALL	+	+/−	−/+	+	+	+	+/−	+	−

Table 4.10. Distribution of immunophenotypic subtypes in acute lymphoblastic leukemia.

Immunophenotype	Patients (%)
Early precursor B, CD10–	5%
Precursor B, CD10+	66%
Late precursor B	17%
Pre-T	12%

Table 4.11. Cytogenetics and prognosis.

Prognosis	Cytogenetic findings
Favorable	Hyperdiploidy >50 chromosomes
	t(12;21)
Intermediate	Hyperdiploidy 47–50 chromosomes
	Normal (diploidy)
	del(6q)
	t(1;19)
Unfavorable	Hypodiploidy-near haploidy
	Near tetraploidy
	del(17p)
	t(9;22)
	t(v;11q23) e.g. t(4;11)
	9p abnormalities
	t(17;19)
	t(5;14)

these may not include the recurrent abnormalities. Normal cytogenetics may be seen in up to 10–20% of pediatric and young adult patients. Nearly all patients will have clonal rearrangements of the immunoglobulin heavy chain and up to 70% may also have rearrangements at the T-cell receptor locus.[58]

Diagnostic issues

Because of the marked impact on prognosis, cytogenetics is considered an essential part of the work-up of ALL. Immunophenotypic abnormalities, including expression of CD13 and CD33 may provide useful markers for the monitoring of minimal residual disease by flow cytometric analysis. Little information identifying cytogenetic or immunophenotypic differences between B-ALL and B-LBL is available and this distinction is made purely on clinical findings.

B-Lymphoblastic leukemia/lymphoma with recurrent genetic abnormalities

Clinical

This diagnostic grouping of B-ALL/LBL are characterized by recurrent genetic abnormalities that impact on prognosis and are primarily described in B-ALL.[1] Clinical features are similar to those described above except for the prognostic implications of each specific abnormality, as discussed below.[59,60]

B-ALL/LBL with t(9;22)(q34;q11)

This B-ALL is more common in adults but makes up about 2–4% of cases in children, and typically is seen in older children. Often patients have higher WBC counts. Lymphomatous presentations are very rare. The blasts are usually express CD10, CD19 and TdT and there is frequent aberrant myeloid antigen expression by CD13 and CD33.[57,61] Expression of CD25 is common. Genetically, t(9;22) leads to the formation of a BCR-ABL1 fusion protein. In children, this is usually the p190kd fusion protein that varies from the p210kd protein seen in cases of CML.[62] This genetic abnormality is associated with a very poor outcome.

B-ALL/LBL with t(v;11q23)

Translocations of the 11q23 locus may occur with a wide variety of fusion partners.[63] This translocation is the most common genetic alteration seen in children <1 year of age (infantile ALL) but is relatively infrequent in older children with B-ALL. Patients typically present with very high WBC counts and there is a high incidence of CNS involvement. Presentation as LBL is rare.[64] The most common cytogenetic abnormality seen in infantile ALL is the t(4;11) which has a CD19+, CD10–, CD24– phenotype and usually coexpresses CD15.[61,64] The 11q23 gene encodes the MLL (mixed lineage leukemia) locus and is also seen in AML.[1] Patients with the t(4;11) have a poor prognosis, particularly those under the age of 6 months.[64] It is unclear whether other 11q23 fusion partners also impart such a poor prognosis.[1,63]

B-ALL/LBL with t(12;21)(p13;q22)

This is a common type of B-ALL seen in children, comprising about 25% of cases, but is rare in infants and older children.[1] The blasts display a CD19+, CD10+ and CD34+ phenotype with frequent expression of myeloid antigens, such as CD13.[61] The t(12;21) creates an ETV6-RUNX1 (TEL-AML1) fusion protein that impacts on normal transcription.[65] This genetic abnormality is associated with a favorable prognosis.[1]

B-ALL/LBL with hyperdiploidy

This entity includes patients whose blasts contain >50 chromosomes, usually without other structural abnormalities. This is commonly seen in children, where it comprises about 25% of of B-ALL. It is infrequent in infants and older children.[1] Blasts are usually CD19, CD10 and CD34 positive.[61] Cytogenetic analysis shows increased numbers of chromosomes, most commonly chromosomes 21, X, 14 and 4. This subtype of B-ALL may be detected either by karyotyping, DNA ploidy analysis or FISH analysis. It is associated with a good prognosis, particularly when trisomies of chromosome 4, 10 and 17 are identified. Patients with near tetraploidy may have a poorer prognosis.[1,66]

B-ALL/LBL with hypodiploidy

This subtype of B-ALL contains < 46 chromosomes and accounts for about 5% of B-ALL, although those cases with < 45 chromosomes make up about 1% of cases. Children may have a near haploid ALL (23–29 chromosomes).[1] The blasts are usually a precursor B phenotype (CD19, CD10+).[61] Genetically there may be other structural abnormalities, although these are rare in the near haploid cases. Endoreduplication may make cytogenetic analysis difficult, but hypodiploidy is usually be identified by FISH or DNA ploidy studies.[66,67] Hypodiploidy is associated with a poor prognosis, especially those patients with near haploidy.[1,68]

B-ALL/LBL with t(5;14)(q31;q32)

This subtype of B-ALL is associated with a reactive eosinophilia. It is rare (<1% of cases). The blasts have a CD19, CD10+ phenotype. The translocation leads to fusion of the IgH gene with the IL-3 gene, leading to IL-3 overexpression and this may be a cause of the reactive increase in benign eosinophils. These cases are thought to have an intermediate prognosis.[1]

B-ALL/LBL with t(1;19)(q23;p13)

This genetic subtype of B-ALL makes up about 6% of cases in children.[1,66] The blasts will have a CD19, CD10 cytoplasmic heavy chain positive phenotype but often lack CD34.[61] This translocation leads to the formation of an E2A-PBX1 fusion protein that is thought to act as a transcriptional activator.[62] With current pediatric ALL therapy, this is associated with an intermediate prognosis.[1]

T-Lymphoblastic leukemia/lymphoma (T-ALL/LBL)

Clinical

T-lymphoblastic leukemia/lymphoma may also present as either ALL or LBL, but lymphomatous presentations are more common. Common sites of presentation include the mediastinum (thymus), lymph nodes as well as extranodal sites.[55] T-ALL makes up about 15% of pediatric ALL. It is more common in older children or adolescents and males. Presentation is often with a high peripheral blast counts. Patient may also have lymphomatous masses, particularly in the mediastinum.[69] T-LBL makes up >85% of all LBL and is most commonly seen in adolescent males. A rapid proliferation rate may lead to presentation as respiratory compromise.[54,55]

Morphologic features

T-lymphoblasts may be indistinguishable from B-lymphoblasts and are usually intermediate in size with fine chromatin. Variable amounts of cytoplasm, nuclear convolutions and number of nucleoli may be seen. Lymphomatous presentations show a diffuse effacement of architecture or a cortical infiltration pattern with sparing of the germinal centers. The neoplastic cells have fine chromatin and scanty cytoplasm (Fig. 4.14). Mitotic figures may be prominent and a starry sky pattern may be present.[1]

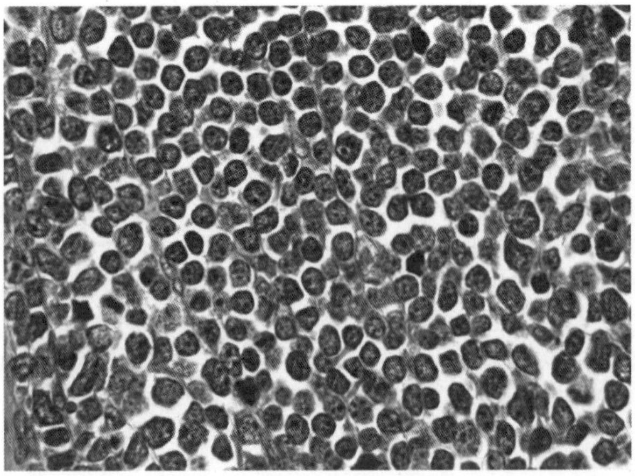

Fig. 4.14. T-lymphoblastic lymphoma. Sections are from a mediastinal mass in a 14-year-old boy. The neoplastic cells show fine chromatin without prominent nucleoli. There is minimal cytoplasm. Immunophenotypic analysis showed a cortical phenotype with coexpression of CD4 and CD8 with no cell surface CD3. Cytoplasmic CD3 and CD1a were positive, as was TdT (1000× magnification).

Table 4.12. Immunophenotypes of precursor T-cell lymphoblastic leukemia/lymphoma.

Antigen	Prethymocyte	Prothymocyte	Common thymocyte	Mature thymocyte	
				T-H	T-S
CD1a	–	–	+	–	–
CD2	±	±	±	+	+
cCD3	±	+	±	–	–
sCD3	–	–	–/+	+	+
CD5	–/+	+	+	+	+
CD7	+	+	+	+	+
CD4	–	–	+	+	–
CD8	–	–	+	–	+
HLA-DR	±	–	–	–	–
CD34	±	–	–	–	–
TdT	+	+	+	+	+

cCD3: cytoplasmic CD3; sCD3: surface CD3, T-H: T-helper (CD4+); T-S: T-suppressor (CD8+).

Immunophenotype

The blasts variably express T-cell antigens including CD2, CD4, CD5, CD7 and CD8. Of these, CD2, CD5 and/or CD7 are seen in most cases (Table 4.12). Usually CD3 is expressed in the cytoplasm, but may not be seen on the cell surface except in later stages of differentiation. Most cases will express markers of immaturity, including CD1a, CD34 and TdT. CD10 is seen in about half of cases.[1,57] T-cell antigen expression will roughly correlate with normal stages of T-cell maturation (Table 4.12). The pro- and pre-thymocyte stage will lack expression of both CD4 and CD8, cortical thymocyte stage will have coexpression of CD4 and CD8 and the medullary thymocyte stage will express either CD4 or CD8.[1]

Genetics

T-ALL/LBL often shows clonal T-cell receptor rearrangements and about 20% of cases may also show IgH rearrangements.[61] An abnormal karyotype is seen in about 50–70% of T-ALL and often involves the T-cell receptor loci at 14q11, 7q35 and 7p14–15. Other commonly involved loci include *HOX11* (10q24), *HOX11L2* (5q35), *TAL-1* (1p32), *MYC* (8q24), *LMO1* (11p15), *LMO2* (11p13) and *LYL1* (19p13).[70,71] Often these are cryptic by standard karyotyping and require molecular analysis to detect. Activating mutations of *NOTCH1* also appear to be common.[58]

Diagnostic issues

Little is known about the cytogenetic, molecular and immunophenotypic patterns in T-LBL and whether there is significant variation from T-ALL.[1,71] Microarray studies suggest that there are distinct gene expression profile differences between T-ALL and T-LBL but it is uncertain if these are relevant to diagnosis and therapy.[72] There is no clear correlation between cytogenetics or molecular findings and prognosis, as is seen in B-ALL/LBL.[1]

Mature B-cell non-Hodgkin lymphomas

The WHO Classification recognizes a large spectrum of mature B-cell NHL with a variety of clinical presentations, including nodal disease and those that are primarily leukemic in presentation.[1] The distribution of diseases described in the WHO Classification differs between pediatric and adult populations, with a much more limited subset of mature B NHL subtypes seen in children, adolescents and young adults (see Table 4.13). The most common subtype of mature B-cell NHL is Burkitt lymphoma (BL). Also commonly seen in older children,

Table 4.13. Mature B-cell lymphomas seen in children and young adults.

Type of lymphoma	Incidence
Burkitt lymphoma	Common
Diffuse large B-cell lymphoma	Less common
Primary mediastinal (thymic) large B-cell lymphoma	Uncommon
Follicular lymphoma	Rare
Nodal and extranodal marginal zone lymphomas	Rare
Lymphomatoid granulomatosis	Very rare
Mantle cell lymphoma	Extremely rare

adolescents and young adults is diffuse large B-cell lymphoma (DLBCL). It has been increasingly recognized that children may have a low incidence of mature B-cell neoplasms that are more characteristically seen in adults, such as follicular lymphoma and marginal zone lymphoma; however the new WHO Classification recognizes that there are pathologically and clinically distinct pediatric follicular and nodal marginal zone lymphomas. Other low-grade B-cell lymphoproliferative disorders that are predominantly seen in adults, such as chronic lymphocytic leukemia/small lymphocytic lymphoma or the more aggressive mantle cell lymphoma, are extremely rare in children and limited to a few case reports.[55]

One feature of the majority of pediatric mature B-cell NHL is the relatively high proportion of lymphomas that are derived from follicular center cells.[1,73,74] This may reflect the developing immune system and predominance of primary responses to antigens in the pediatric and young adult age groups as compared to older adults. Many of the pediatric mature B-cell NHL have a high proliferation rate and may have overexpression of pro-proliferative proteins, such as cMYC, which suggest the mechanism of lymphomagenesis in these patients is more closely linked to abnormal regulation of proliferation than the mechanism of defective apoptosis seen in many adult B-cell lymphomas.[74–76]

Burkitt lymphoma

Clinical

Burkitt lymphoma (BL) is the most common subtype of NHL diagnosed in pediatric populations.[77] Present ations in extranodal sites, including the gastrointestinal track and ovaries are common in non-endemic areas (US and Europe) whereas presentation as a jaw mass or extranodal sites is seen in endemic areas (equatorial Africa and Papua, New Guinea). BL may also be seen in some immunodeficiency states, in particular in HIV infection and post-transplant. A leukemic form is also described and CNS involvement is seen. The tumor is rapidly proliferating and is often manifested as bulky disease.[55]

Morphologic features

BL is a diffuse lymphoma composed of medium-sized cells with a typically relatively monomorphic appearance. The nuclei are round and have finely clumped to dispersed chromatin with 3–5 peripherally placed inconspicuous nucleoli (Fig. 4.15A). The cytoplasm is typically moderate in amount, basophilic and contains lipid vacuoles that may be best appreciated in cytologic preparations (Fig. 4.15B). The tumor cells may appear to grow in a syncitial pattern and may preferentially invade reactive germinal centers. Due to the high proliferation rate, numerous macrophages ingesting apoptotic debris are often admixed with the tumors cells, giving rise to a characteristic "starry sky" appearance (Fig. 4.15C).[78] In the past, cases with slightly irregular nuclear contours or single prominent central nucleoli were called Burkitt-like lymphoma or atypical BL; however these cases appear, at least in children, to be identical to more classical forms of BL by immunophenotypic analysis and gene expression profiling and are currently included within the acceptable morphologic spectrum of BL.[1]

Immunophenotype

The classic phenotype is that of a mature B-cell with expressions of CD19, CD20, CD22, CD38 and monoclonal cell surface immunoglobulin. The cells will express markers of germinal center derivation and will be positive for CD10 and bcl-6.[1] The tumor is negative for BCL-2 (although up to 20% of cases may have weak positivity), and those cases with strong expression of BCL-2 may be considered grey zone lymphomas (described below).[79] TdT is negative. The tumor is highly proliferative and will have MIB-1 staining in nearly 100% of neoplastic cells. The tumor cells will also express cMYC protein.[75] The EBV genome is integrated into the neoplastic cells in all endemic cases and up to 30% of non-endemic cases.[80]

Genetics

Translocations involving the *cMYC* locus with immunoglobulin heavy or light chain genes are characteristic and seen in >90% of cases.[81] Many cases will have secondary abnormalities, such as deletion 1q, that may affect prognosis. All cases will have clonal immunoglobulin gene rearrangements.[82]

Diagnostic issues

Diagnosis of BL requires integration of morphologic, immunophenotypic, and genetic features. In cases with a classic clinical presentation, morphology and

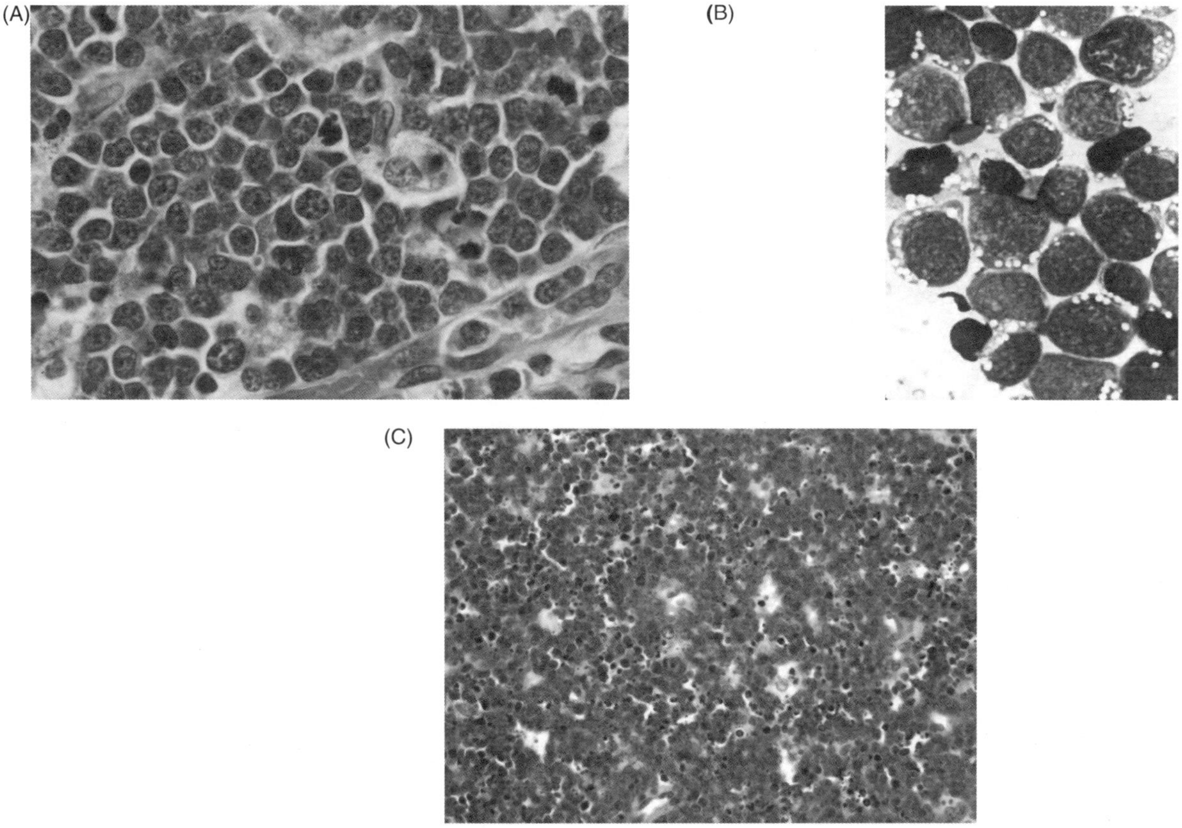

Fig. 4.15. Burkitt lymphoma. (A) High power of Burkitt lymphoma shows the relatively monotonous neoplastic infiltrate of intermediate-sized cells with modest amounts of cytoplasm. There is some degree of nuclear molding. Mitotic figures are seen and there is a tangible body macrophage present that is ingesting apoptotic debris (1000X magnification). (B) Cytologic preparation of Burkitt lymphoma showing characteristic Burkitt cells with condensed chromatin, modest amounts of basophilic cytoplasm with prominent cytoplasmic vaculation (1000× magnification). (C) Burkitt lymphoma showing the characteristic starry sky pattern due to multiple interspersed tangible body macrophages that are ingesting phagocytic debris. There is also focal necrosis. The neoplastic cells form a uniform sheet that show evidence of extensive apoptosis (200× magnification).

immunophenotype without additional genetic studies to demonstrate a *cMYC* translocation are sufficient for diagnosis.[1] Molecular profiling studies have demonstrated a specific molecular signature for BL and have suggested that this is more reliable than morphologic and immunophenotypic characterization, particularly in adult cases or cases associated with immunodeficiency.[83–85] It should be noted that *cMYC* translocations are seen in up to 30% of pediatric DLBCL and should thus not be used as a single criterion for the diagnosis of BL.[82]

Diffuse large B-cell lymphoma (NOS)

Clinical

DLBCL comprises 15–20% of pediatric NHL and has a heterogeneous clinical presentation including nodal disease, abdominal masses, GI tract tumors, as well as primary bone lymphomas.[55] Both nodal and extranodal disease are seen although nodal disease is more common. Involvement of bone marrow and CNS is uncommon. In immunocompromised individuals, extranodal DLBCL may be more common.[86]

Morphologic features

DLBCL has diffuse nodal infiltration by large cells that may have of a variety of morphologic appearances including centroblastic, immunoblastic, anaplastic, and T-cell/histiocyte-rich subtypes. The large neoplastic cells have a nucleus that is at least the size of a tissue histiocyte or twice the size of a small reactive lymphocyte. Cytoplasm is variable in appearance, ranging from pale to plasmacytoid or granular. Cytoplasm is variable in volume but is more abundant than in Burkitt lymphoma (Fig. 4.16).[1]

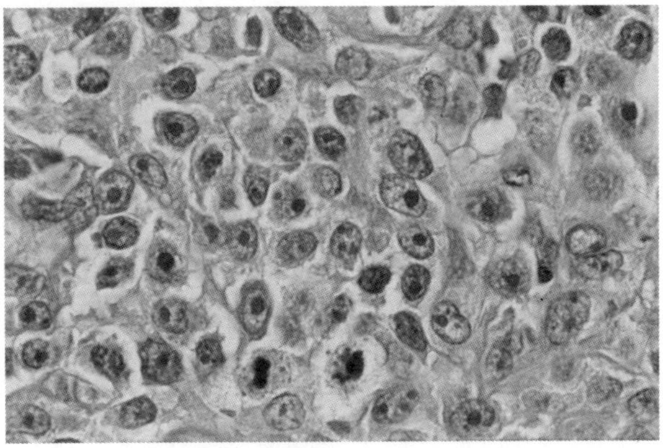

Fig. 4.16. Diffuse large B-cell lymphoma. There is diffuse effacement by an infiltrate of large neoplastic cells, many of which have prominent central eosinophilic nucleoli, consistent with an immunoblastic cytology. Mitotic figures are present (1000× magnification).

Immunophenotype

DLBCL demonstrates a mature B-cell phenotype with expression of cell surface immunoglobulin and B-specific antigens including CD19, CD20, CD22, CD79a and PAX5. CD30 expression may be seen in some cases of DLBCL, representing nonspecific activation.[1] Mitotic activity, as determined by Ki-67 or MIB1 staining is usually high in pediatric cases but less than that seen in BL (<90%). Pediatric DLBCL is more likely to have overexpression of cMYC protein compared to adults (84% vs. 10%) but will have decreased levels of BCL2 (28% vs. 40–50%).[74,73] The majority (>80%) of pediatric DLBCL will demonstrate immunophenotypic evidence of germinal center derivation including expression of BCL6 and CD10.[74] CD5 coexpression is uncommon.

Genetics

There are no specific or recurrent cytogenetic abnormalities associated with DLBCL in children and adolescents. Most cases show cytogenetic complexity with three or more abnormalities. *BCL2* translocations are extremely rare. Translocations involving the *cMYC* locus are more common in children than in adults and have been reported in 30–40% of cases.[82,87]

Diagnostic issues

Because of *cMYC* translocations and overexpression of cMYC protein, there may be differential diagnostic difficulties with BL. Molecular profiling studies demonstrating a specific DLBCL profile that differs from the BL gene expression profile have shown that morphology may not be reliable for the diagnosis of DLBCL.[83,84] Molecular profiling has also confirmed a high incidence of germinal center-derived tumors with increased expression of proliferation signatures. As noted with BL, diagnosis often requires correlation of clinical, immunophenotypic, morphologic and genetic features.[1]

Primary mediastinal (thymic) large B-cell lymphoma

Clinical

Primary mediastinal large B-cell lymphoma (PMBL) in the current WHO has been identified as a unique subtype that differs from DLBCL (NOS). PMBL is thought to arise from thymic B-cells and patients present with a localized superior mediastinal mass that may invade into adjacent structures such as lung, pleura or pericardium. Spread to supraclavicular or cervical lymph nodes may occur, but the absence of other lymph node or bone marrow involvement is a prerequisite that helps to exclude a diagnosis of DLBCL (NOS).[1] Patients may present with a superior vena cava syndrome. Dissemination to extranodal sites including kidney, adrenal, liver or CNS may occur, but bone marrow involvement is rare.[88] Response to therapy in children appears to be inferior to that of DLBCL.[88,89]

Morphologic features

The morphology of PMBL is diverse but is commonly associated with compartmentalizing sclerosis. Tumor cells are medium to large with abundant pale cytoplasm and typically regular, round or ovoid nuclei (Fig. 4.17). Occasional pleomorphic or multi-lobated cells may be seen. Nucleoli are typically inconspicuous but may occasionally be more prominent. Some cases may have features which overlap with that of HL, the so-called grey-zone or borderline lymphomas.[1]

Immunophenotype

The tumor cells of PMBL express B-cell antigens including CD19, CD20, CD22, and CD79a but most often lack cell surface expression of immunoglobulin. CD30 is often expressed (>80% of cases) but is often weak and patchy in distribution. CD15 is usually negative but may occasionally be focally positive.[1] Tumor cells are frequently positive for IRF4/MUM1 and CD23.

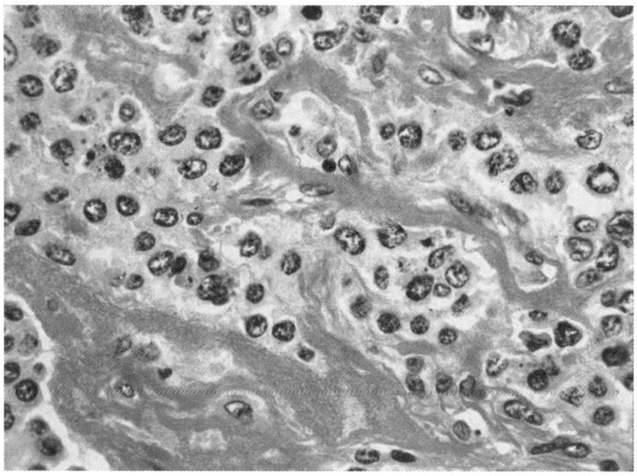

Fig. 4.17. Primary mediastinal B-cell lymphoma. Sections show a neoplastic infiltrate of large cells with clear cytoplasm. There is prominent compartmentalizing sclerosis that is characteristic of this neoplasm (400× magnification).

BCL6 and CD10 expression is less common and BCL2 is frequently expressed.[1,74] In addition, the tumor cells are positive for MAL antigen, and coexpress TRAF1 and nuclear REL.[1]

Genetics

PMBL shows clonally rearranged immunoglobulin genes. Comparative genomic hybridization often demonstrates gains in chromosome 9p24 and 2p15. Rearrangements of *BCL2*, *BCL6* and *MYC* genes are absent or rare.[90]

Diagnostic issues

Molecular profiling of PMBL shows a genetic signature that shares features with classical HL. This signature also shows evidence of constitutively activated *NFκB* and *JAK-STAT* signaling pathways.[90–92] Some cases may show morphologic overlap with DLBCL (NOS) or classical HL and may be better classified as a grey zone lymphoma requiring extensive immunophenotypic and molecular analysis for definitive diagnosis.[1] (See discussion below.)

Pediatric follicular lymphoma

Clinical

Pediatric follicular lymphoma (FL) is a rare neoplasm of children, comprising <5% of pediatric NHL. The tumor often involves cervical lymph nodes, Waldeyer ring and extranodal sites. In males, there is frequent involvement of the testes. Pediatric FL typically has limited stage disease with localized tumor.[93,94]

Morphologic features

Pediatric FL are nodular neoplasms that usually contain large expansile follicles (Fig. 4.18A). There is often more variation in size and shape than seen in adult-type FL. Mantle zones may be preserved or absent. The majority of pediatric FL are grade 3 (follicular large cell lymphoma) (Fig. 4.18B) but other lower grade disease, including follicular mixed small cleaved and large-cell tumors, are also well described.[1,94]

(A)

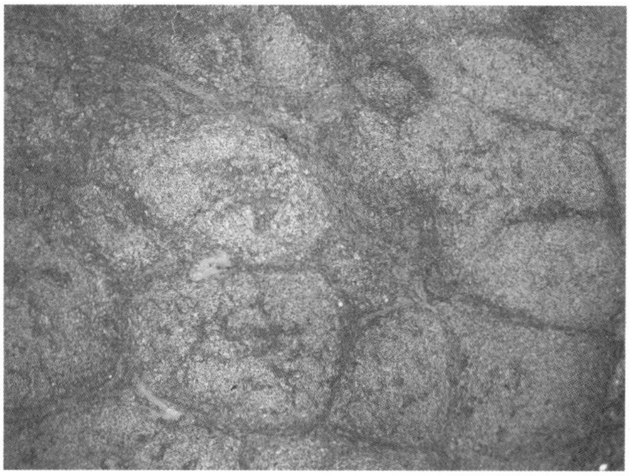

(B)

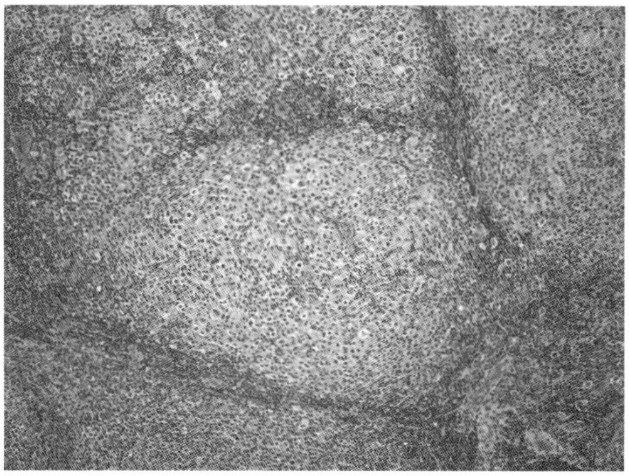

Fig. 4.18 Pediatric follicular lymphoma. (A) Low power view showing the back-to-back follicular structures present in a cervical lymph node of a 16-year-old boy with pediatric follicular lymphoma. There is a lack of follicle polarization and the neoplastic follicles lack intact mantle zones (100× magnification). (B) Higher magnification showing the neoplastic follicle that is comprised predominantly of large cells (follicular grade 3 morphology). Scattered mitotic figures and tangible body macrophages are present within the neoplastic follicle (400× magnification).

Immunophenotype

Immunophenotypic features of pediatric FL include expression of mature B-cell markers including CD19, CD20, CD22 and PAX5. The tumor cells will also express antigens associated with follicular center cell derivation including CD10 and BCL6. Proliferation, particularly in grade 3 lesions, may be high. In contrast to adult FL, pediatric FL is typically negative for BCL2 expression. In pediatric patients who have FL with BCL2 expression, the tumor tends to act more like adult-type FL with disseminated disease.[1,93–95]

Genetics

Pediatric FL is unlikely to have *BCL2* gene rearrangements or evidence of t(14;18)(q32;q21) rearrangements.[96] Alternative mechanisms of lymphomagenesis may involve mutations of the *BCL6* gene as well as isochromosome 17q.[97,98]

Diagnostic issues

Pediatric FL may be considered in a differential with florid follicular hyperplasia.[99] Rare cases of florid follicular hyperplasia in young males may demonstrate clonality of CD10+ B-cells by flow cytometry and molecular analyses.[100,101] A diagnosis of pediatric FL requires correlation of morphologic features of malignancy, and demonstration of monoclonality.[1]

Pediatric nodal marginal zone lymphoma

Clinical

Pediatric nodal marginal zone lymphoma (NMZL) has unique clinical and morphologic features and is recognized as a provisional diagnostic entity in the WHO classification.[1] It is a rare disorder (< 5% of pediatric NHL). There is a strong male predominance (M:F ratio of 20:1) in the pediatric population.[102,103] Over 90% of the disease presents with localized adenopathy and is often clinically stage 1. Patients are usually asymptomatic.[102]

Morphologic features

The morphologic features of pediatric NMZL are similar to that seen in adults with morphologic diversity of neoplastic cells including small to medium lymphocytes, centrocyte-like cells with irregular nuclear contours, large centroblasts, monocytoid B-cells with abundant cytoplasm and plasma cells (Fig. 4.19A).

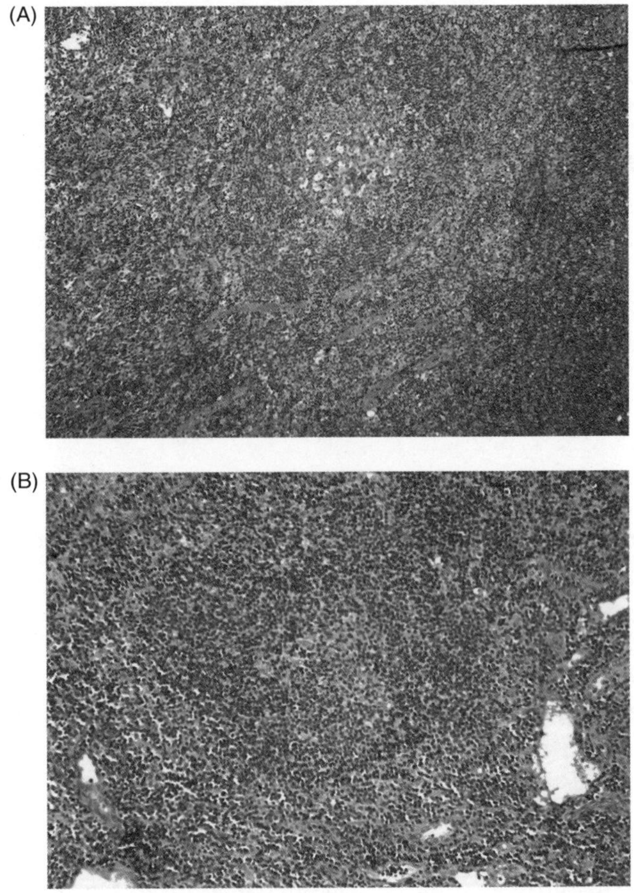

Fig. 4.19. Pediatric nodal marginal zone lymphoma. Sections from a 14-year-old boy with cervical adenopathy. (A) Sections show the polymorphous neoplastic infiltrate with infiltration into a germinal center. There is a mixture of monocytoid B cells, small lymphocytes and large cells in the neoplastic infiltrate (200× magnification). (B) Evidence of progressive transformation of germinal centers associated with a pediatric nodal marginal zone lymphoma. Progressive transformation of germinal centers is unique to the pediatric subtype and is characterized by infiltration of follicles by small, dark-colored mantle cell lymphocytes (200× magnification).

Often times there are numerous reactive components including reactive germinal centers and polyclonal plasma cells. These often infiltrate in a diffuse pattern and there may be infiltration of reactive germinal centers by the tumor cells.[1] In contrast to adult NMZL, pediatric cases often have an increase in follicles with progressively transformed germinal centers with disruption of the outer borders of the follicle by neoplastic cells (Fig. 4.19B).[1,102]

Immunophenotype

Pediatric NMZL is a mature B-cell neoplasm that expresses pan-B-cell markers such as CD19, CD20,

CD22, CD79a and PAX5. There is often coexpression of CD43. The tumor will be monoclonal by flow cytometry. The plasma cell component may be monoclonal or polytypic.[104]

Genetics

Pediatric NMZL will show clonal rearrangement of the immunoglobulin heavy chain; this is essential to be distinguished from reactive marginal zone hyperplasia. There are no clear cut cytogenetic abnormalities associated with pediatric NMZL.[103]

Diagnostic issues

There are reports of atypical marginal-zone hyperplasia in children, particularly in tonsils that have monotypic immunoglobulin expression by immunoperoxidase. These may be confused with a pediatric NMZL but may be distinguished by lacking evidence for clonal rearrangements by molecular testing.[1]

Other mature B-cell lymphomas in children

Other types of pediatric mature B-cell MHL are extremely rare and appear primarily as individual case reports or small series. Cases of lymphomatoid granulomatosis,[105] mantle cell lymphoma[106] and extranodal marginal zone lymphoma (MALT lymphoma)[102,103] have been described. There is also increased recognition that there may be a population of patients with tumors that have features intermediate between DLBCL and classical HL, the/so-called "grey-zone lymphomas".[1,107–109] These typically present in the mediastinum and have morphologic and immunophenotypic features that are intermediate between PMBL and classical HL including prominence of pleomorphic large cells or Reed-Sternberg (RS)-like cells, variable amounts of fibrotic stroma or necrosis, and a sparse amount of reactive inflammatory cells. Immunopheotypically, the neoplastic cells express CD45 and have strong expressions of CD30 and CD15 or lack of uniform expression of pan-B-cell markers such as CD79a or CD20.[1,110] It is uncertain what the clinical ramifications of this diagnosis are at this time, but it has been suggested that they are more clinically aggressive than either PMBL or classical HL.[108,109]

Peripheral T-cell lymphoma

Although T-cell lymphoma represents approximately 25–50% of pediatric lymphoma (compared to 10% of adult lymphoma), more than half of these are immature tumors arising in the thymus (T lymphoblastic lymphoma).[77] Peripheral (mature) T-cell lymphomas (PTCL) in children and adolescents represent approximately 20% of childhood NHL and are primarily anaplastic large cell lymphoma (ALCL) with other types being rare (Table 4.14).[111] In recent reports from the United States Children's Oncology Group (COG), the United Kingdom, and Japan, the most frequent non-anaplastic PTCL was PTCL, NOS (43–68%) followed by extranodal natural killer (NK)/T-cell lymphoma nasal type (12–48%), angioimmunoblastic T-cell lymphoma (AITL) (5–12%), subcutaneous panniculitis-like T-cell lymphoma (SPTCL) (5–8%), and EATL (5%).[112–114]

Table 4.14. Mature T and NK cell neoplasms seen in children and young adults.

Lymphoproliferative disorder	Frequency
Systemic anaplastic large cell lymphoma, ALK positive	Common
Peripheral T-cell lymphoma, not otherwise specified	Less common
Angioimmunoblastic T-cell lymphoma	Uncommon
Primary cutaneous anaplastic large cell lymphoma	Uncommon
Systemic EBV-positive T-cell lymphoproliferative disease of childhood	Uncommon
Mycosis fungoides/Sézary syndrome	Uncommon
Subcutaneous panniculitis-like T-cell lymphoma	Uncommon
Hydroa vacciniforme-like lymphoma	Rare
Hepatosplenic T-cell lymphoma	Very rare
Enteropathy-type T-cell lymphoma	Very rare
T-cell granular lymphocytic leukemia	Very rare
Adult T-cell lymphoma/leukemia (HTLV 1+)	Very rare

EBV: Epstein–Barr virus; HTLV: human T-cell leukemia virus.

Anaplastic large cell lymphoma, ALK-positive

ALCL, a CD4+, CD30+ pleomorphic large T-cell lymphoma is the most common peripheral T-cell lymphoma in children. ALCL represents approximately 10–15% of pediatric/adolescent NHL as compared to 2% of adult NHL.[115] ALCL is subdivided into two groups based on dysregulation of the *ALK* (anaplastic lymphoma kinase) gene on chromosome 2p23, primarily detected by immunohistochemical staining with the ALK-1 antibody.[1] More than 90% of pediatric ALCL are ALK+.[116,117]

Clinical

ALK+ ALCL patients are predominantly male with a bimodal age distribution, with most cases occurring in children, adolescents and young adults (pediatric median age 10.2–11.0 years).[118] Approximately 70% of patients have advanced stage III/IV disease due to peripheral, mediastinal and abdominal lymphadenopathy. Extranodal disease is frequent (approximately 40%) with skin, bone, lung, and soft tissue being the most common sites.[119] Bone marrow involvement occurs in approximately 10–30% based on morphology and immunohistochemistry and up to 61% by molecular studies,[120,121] and is most common in the small cell variant. CNS disease is rare. Clinical features associated with a worse prognosis and higher relapse rate include bone marrow and blood involvement (at the morphologic and molecular level),[119–121] B-symptoms, visceral organ involvement, mediastinal mass, skin lesions, and advanced stage.[118,120,122] Circulating antibodies against the NPM-ALK fusion protein have been detected in approximately 91% of pediatric ALCL and appear to be inversely correlated with relapse and stage.[123,124]

Morphologic features

ALCL classically presents as a cohesive appearing, pleomorphic large cell infiltrate in the paracortical and subcapsular areas of the lymph node (Figs. 4.20A–B).[1] The tumor cells have abundant, eosinophilic cytoplasm and vary from large cells with large indented, horseshoe, kidney-shaped or embryoid nuclei (hallmark cells) to multinucleated wreath-like or RS-like cells. ALCL has a morphologic spectrum,[125] which includes a monomorphic variant that resembles diffuse large cell lymphoma. The most difficult variants to recognize are the small cell (approximately 5–10% of cases) (Fig. 4.20C) and the lymphohistiocytic variants (approximately 10–15% of cases). The small cell variant is composed predominantly of small, irregular lymphocytes with fewer large cells that have a tendency to surround blood vessels.[126] The lymphohistiocytic variant has numerous admixed histiocytes including those with plasmacytoid features.[127] There is overlap in morphology between the small cell variant and the lymphohistiocytic variant. Simultaneous small cell variant and classical histology may be present in the same tissue.[117] A Hodgkin-like pattern is seen in less than 5% of cases and mimics nodular sclerosing HL.[128]

Based on morphology, bone marrow involvement is infrequent (less than 20%), except in the small cell variant which tends to have disseminated disease including peripheral blood involvement.[126] Marrow involvement is usually subtle with only scattered or small clusters of tumor cells rather than mass lesions; immunohistochemistry with ALK-1 and CD30 is recommended.[129] On Wright stain, the large tumor cells have a characteristic appearance with large nuclei and abundant, dark blue cytoplasm containing small vacuoles.

Immunophenotype

Virtually all large cells express the activation antigen CD30 and by definition ALK (Figs. 4.20D–E). In the small cell variant, the large cells and a subset of small cells are CD30+ ALK+ (Fig. 4.20F). The tumor cells are predominantly CD4+ cytotoxic (TIA-1, granzyme B, perforin and granulysin positive) T-cells that often have weak expression or loss of CD3 and the alpha-beta T-cell receptor protein.[1] Most ALK+ ALCL are EMA+ and CD25+. CD56 is expressed in a small number of cases (approximately 15%, with a broad range reported in various studies).[117,130] EBV is negative. Virtually all cases are EBV negative, and there is no evidence of involvement by HTLV-1.

Genetics

Approximately 90% of ALCL have a detectable clonal *TCR* gene rearrangement.[131] More than 90% of pediatric ALCL have dysregulation of ALK on 2p23 detectable by immunohistochemical staining.[116,117] The ALK fusion protein contains oligomerization domains that lead to the activation of the ALK tyrosine kinase signaling pathway. The most common fusion partner in adult and pediatric patients with ALK+ ALCL is NPM, occurring in approximately 80–95%.[117] At least 10 other partners have been

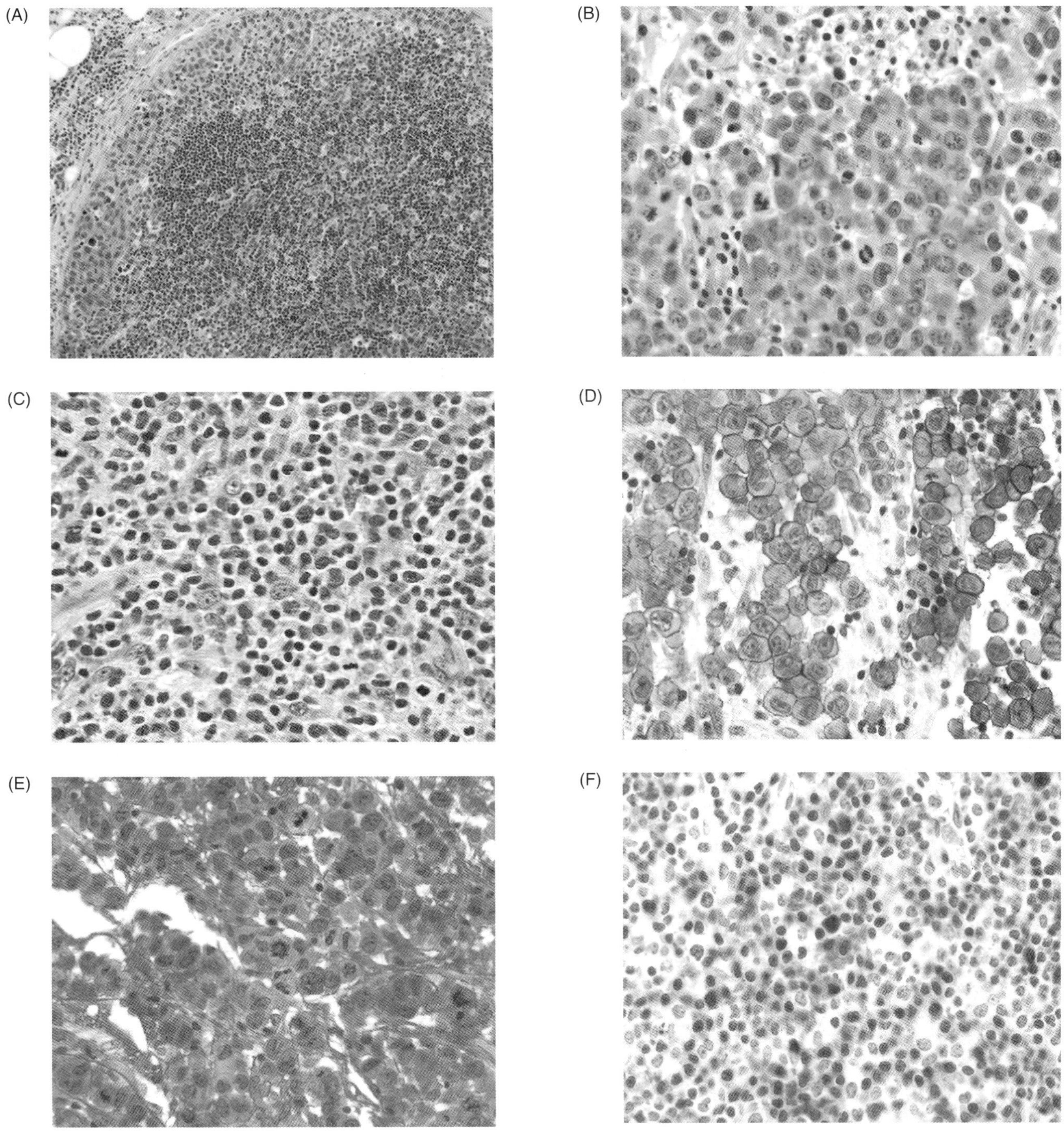

Fig. 4.20. This figure illustrates the morphologic spectrum of systemic anaplastic large cell lymphoma (ALCL). (A) In classical ALK+ ALCL, pleomorphic large cells infiltrate the lymph node in the subcapsular sinus and paracortical region (100× magnification). (B) Tumor cells have large, folded, and indented nuclei with abundant pink cytoplasm (hallmark cells) (600× magnification). (C) In contrast to classical ALCL, the tumors cells in the small cell variant are predominantly small with irregular, hyperchromatic nuclei, and indistinct to clear cytoplasm, and only rare large cells with indented large nuclei are present (600× magnification). (D) Tumor cells have strong membrane and golgi expression of CD30 in virtually every cell (1000× magnification). (E) ALK protein is present in the nucleus and cytoplasm of the tumor cells. (F) ALK protein is expressed in the small and large cells; large cells tend to be more prominent near blood vessels (600× magnification). (G) In ALK–ALCL, the tumor cells show identical morphologic features to ALK+ ALCL and (H) have strong expression of CD30 in every cell (600× magnification).

(G)

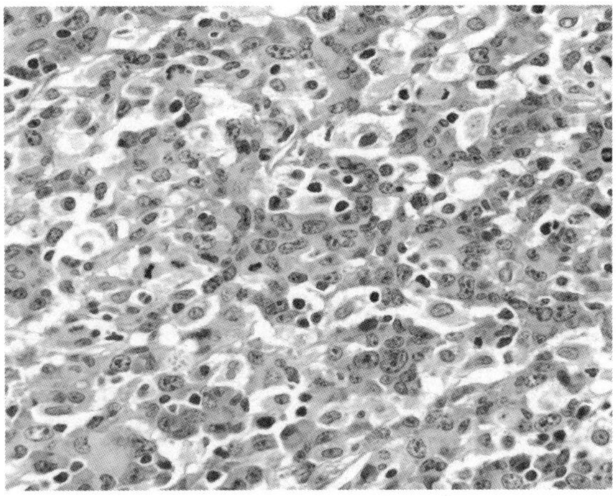

(H)

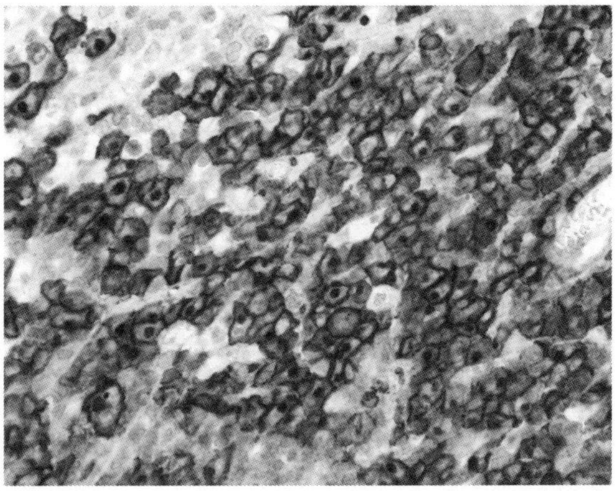

Fig. 4.20. (*Continued*)

described.[1] The NPM-ALK fusion is associated with a nuclear, nucleolar, and cytoplasmic staining pattern, whereas the other variants predominantly show diffuse cytoplasmic staining except for the granular staining seen in t(2;17)(p23;q23) associated with the clathrin gene, *CLTC* (predominantly seen in ALK+ B-cell lymphoma)[132] and the t(2;X) with the moesin gene (Xq11-12) that produces membrane staining. Other cytogenetic abnormalities that occur in ALK+ ALCL include losses of chromosome 4, 11q, and 13q and gains of 7, 17p, and 17q.[133]

Diagnostic issues

ALCL with variant histology, particularly the small cell and the lymphohistiocytic variants may be confused with reactive processes or other peripheral T-cell lymphomas due to the small number of large tumor cells, numerous admixed reactive cells, and in some cases preservation of lymph node architecture.[134]

Anaplastic large cell lymphoma, ALK-negative

ALK-negative anaplastic large cell lymphoma, (ALK– ALCL) is a provisional entity in the 2008 WHO classification defined by strong expression of membrane and Golgi-associated CD30 in virtually every tumor cell.[1] ALK– ALCL shares morphologic features with classical ALCL. ALK– ALCL is a systemic disease and separated from primary cutaneous ALCL. Less than 10% of pediatric ALCL lack ALK, therefore the clinicopathologic features in this age group are not well defined.[116]

Clinical

ALK– ALCL in the pediatric age group is limited to single case reports or small numbers of patients in larger series. Involvement of extranodal sites appears less frequent than seen in ALK+ ALCL. Most patients have advanced state III/IV disease and systemic symptoms.

Morphology

The morphology of ALK– ALCL is similar to ALK+ ALCL with a paracortical, sinus, or diffuse infiltrate of cohesive appearing pleomorphic or anaplastic large cells which may be more pleomorphic than in ALK+ ALCL (Fig. 4.20G). Hallmark cells and multinucleated, very large, RS-like cells may be present. Small cell and lymphohistiocytic variants have not been recognized in this group.

Immunophenotype

Virtually every tumor cell should uniformly, strongly express CD30 in a membrane and Golgi-associated pattern (Fig. 4.20H). Expression of T-cell antigens appears similar to ALK+ ALCL with a predominance of a CD4+ phenotype and variable expression of other T-cell antigens. CD3 and T-cell receptor protein expression is decreased.[135] CD43 is usually strongly expressed. Expression of cytotoxic granule proteins and EMA is decreased compared to ALK+ ALCL. Expression of CD15 is rarely present, and HL must be excluded.

Genetics

The majority of cases have a clonal T-cell receptor gene rearrangement, even in the absence of T-cell antigen expression.[136] No recurrent cytogenetic abnormalities have been described.

Diagnostic issues

The differential diagnosis of ALK– ALCL primarily includes PTCL, NOS and HL. PTCL, NOS has less expression of CD30 and more abnormal small- to medium-sized cells than typically seen in the homogeneous large cell population found in ALCL. Also, sinus involvement is much more typical of ALCL. If sclerosis, prominent eosinophils or expression of CD15 are present, HL must be excluded. Immunostaining for PAX-5, weakly present in RS-cells and absence in ALCL may be useful. Expression of EBV would also be more supportive of HL. The demonstration of a T-cell receptor gene rearrangement would be keeping with ALK– ALCL.

Primary cutaneous anaplastic large cell lymphoma

CD30+ lymphoproliferative disorders are the second most common clonal T-cell proliferations in the skin and include lymphomatoid papulosis (LyP) and primary cutaneous ALCL (C-ALCL) LyP and ALCL form a clinicopathologic spectrum with overlapping features. Integration of clinical and pathologic features is essential in making a diagnosis.

Clinical

C-ALCL is usually a disorder of adults with most patients over the age 50 years. C-ALCL is rare in children and young adults.[137] C-ALCL is usually a solitary tumor or nodule that is often ulcerated and present on the extremities, face, or (less frequently) the trunk. Multifocal lesions are present in approximately 20% of cases and, more frequently, have extracutaneous spread (approximately 10% of patients). Spontaneous regression occurs in approximately 25%. Systemic disease must be ruled out with careful staging as skin lesions in systemic ALCL are associated with an aggressive course. Long-term follow-up of C-ALCL patients is necessary due to the high relapse rate and the rare occurrence of evolution to systemic disease.

Morphologic features

Tumor cells spread diffusely throughout the dermis into the subcutaneous tissue, often showing a perivascular distribution with some infiltration and expansion, but not destruction, of the vessel wall (Fig. 4.21A). Reactive lymphocytes may be prominent particularly at the periphery of the infiltrate, and acute inflammatory cells are often admixed with ulcerated lesions. The cytologic appearance of C-ALCL is similar to that seen in ALK+ ALCL with cohesive large anaplastic cells with indented to slightly irregular nuclei and abundant pink cytoplasm (Fig. 4.21B).

Immunophenotype

Tumor cells in C-ALCL have strong Golgi and membrane expression of CD30 in virtually every cell (Fig. 4.21C). Most tumors are CD4+ with variable loss of pan T-cell antigens and expression of cytotoxic proteins (TIA-1, granzyme B and perforin). Approximately 20–30% of C-ALCL express EMA,[138] but it is more focal and weak than seen in ALK+ ALCL. Most C-ALCL are ALK negative (Fig. 4.21D). ALK expression is highly associated with systemic disease. Clusterin expression is seen in 41–100% of cases.[139] CD56 expression is present in a subset of cases but is not associated with a worse prognosis.[140]

Genetics

Most cases have a clonal T-cell receptor gene rearrangement. Recurrent cytogenetic abnormalities have not been identified and ALK gene translocations are very rare.[141]

Diagnostic issues

The principal diagnostic issue is confirming that the C-ALCL is limited to the skin and not part of the systemic disease. Differentiating C-ALCL and LyP may be difficult and is principally based on clinical features (number and size of the lesions and time course)[142] and morphology, including the number and distribution of CD30+ large cells and the depth of invasion of the infiltrate. The infiltrate of LyP is perivascular and wedge-shaped and usually does not involve the subcutaneous tissue (Fig. 4.22A). In LyP, the CD30+ large cells are scattered or in small clusters of 5–10 cells (Fig. 4.22B). LyP occurs very rarely in children.[143]

Mycosis fungoides

Mycosis fungoides (MF) is the most common cutaneous T-cell lymphoma in adults and children, representing

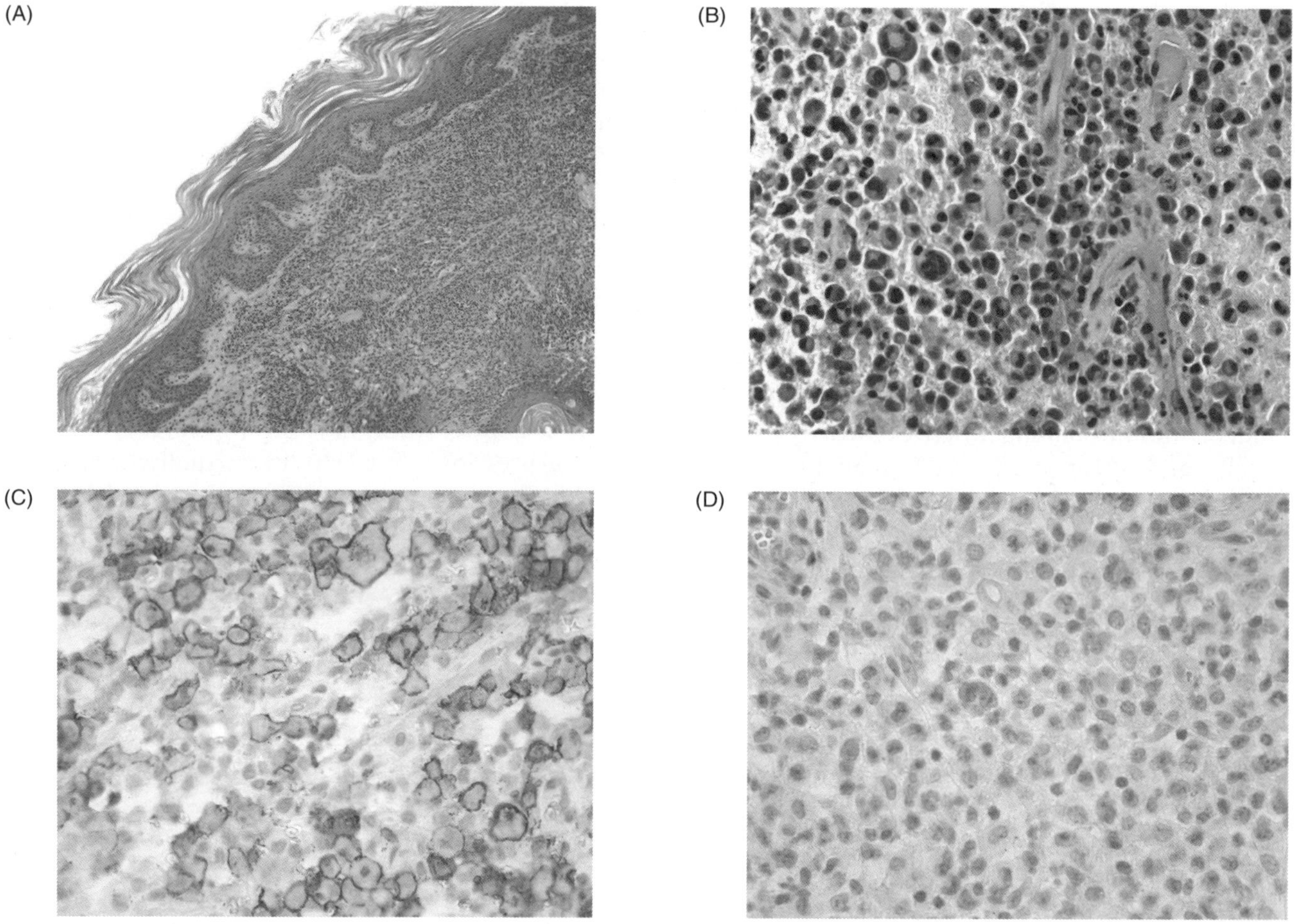

Fig. 4.21. Cutaneous anaplastic large cell lymphoma. (A) Sheets of large dysplastic cells diffusely infiltrate the dermis (15× magnification). (B) Rare large cells are multinucleated and have the appearance of Reed-Sternberg cells (400X magnification). (C) The tumor cells strongly express CD30 and (D) lack ALK expression (400× magnification).

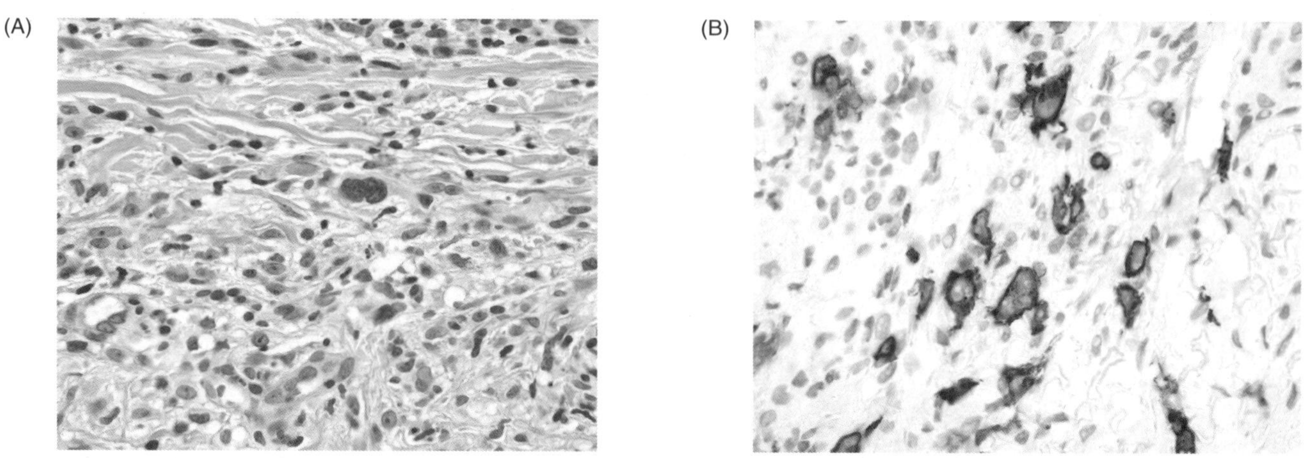

Fig. 4.22. Lymphomatoid papulosis, type A. (A) The skin is involved by a moderately dense, perivascular and interstitial lymphocytic infiltrate with numerous small lymphocytes and rare, large dysplastic cells, some having Reed-Sternberg-like morphology (400× magnification). (B) The abnormal large cells are CD30+ (400× magnification) and lack ALK (not shown).

approximately 40% of primary cutaneous lymphoma in childhood.[1] Approximately 4–5% of MF occur in patients younger than 20 years of age and there is increasing recognition of this entity in the pediatric population.[144]

Clinical

In the pediatric population, MF can occur at any age, with a median of 10–14 years of age in most series.[145] The lesions may be hypo- or hyperpigmented, hyperkeratotic, ichthyosiform, vesicular, pustular, granulomatous, verrucous, lichenoid, and pityriasis lichenoides-like.[144] Hypopigmented and poikilodermatous variants (reticulate dyspigmentation, follicular atrophy, and telangiectasia) are more common in pediatric populations.[146] Approximately 20% of the pagetoid reticulosis variant occurs in patients less than 20 years of age.[147]

Most pediatric patients have early stage disease with patches or plaques, and up to 85% are misdiagnosed as reactive skin conditions such as eczema, psoriasis, tinea corporis, or vitiligo resulting in a delayed diagnosis for 5 years or more.[145] A useful distinguishing feature is the persistent nature of MF despite treatment. Most pediatric patients do not have progression of their disease to large cell lymphoma, Sézary syndrome, or systemic disease.

Morphologic features

Lymphocytes with atypical, hyperchromatic, cerebriform nuclei are present in the upper dermis in a perivascular, band-like distribution (Fig. 4.23A). The cerebriform lymphocytes infiltrate the epidermis with little associated spongiosis, line-up along the basal layer surrounded by halos (clear spaces), and in a smaller percentage of cases form intraepidermal clusters called Pautrier microabscesses (Fig. 4.23B). The epidermal lymphocytes tend to be larger and more hyperchromatic and dysplastic than the dermal lymphocytes.[148] The pagetoid reticulosis variant has marked invasion of the epidermis, and the dermal lymphocytes are predominantly reactive.

Immunophenotype

Two thirds of pediatric MF cases have a CD4+ T-cell phenotype with approximately one third being CD8+. Hypopigmented MF and pagetoid reticulosis, in particular, have more frequent CD8 expression. Loss of pan T-cell antigens such as CD2, CD5, or CD7 is a useful diagnostic feature, however, decreased expression of CD7 can be seen in reactive processes as well. Only a small number of CD30+ large cells are present.

(A)

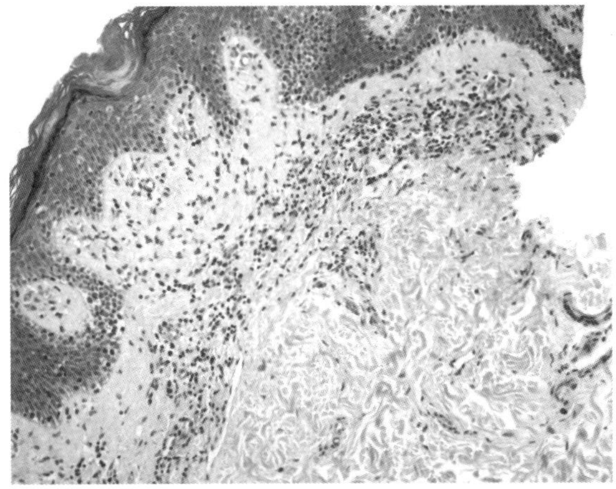

(B)

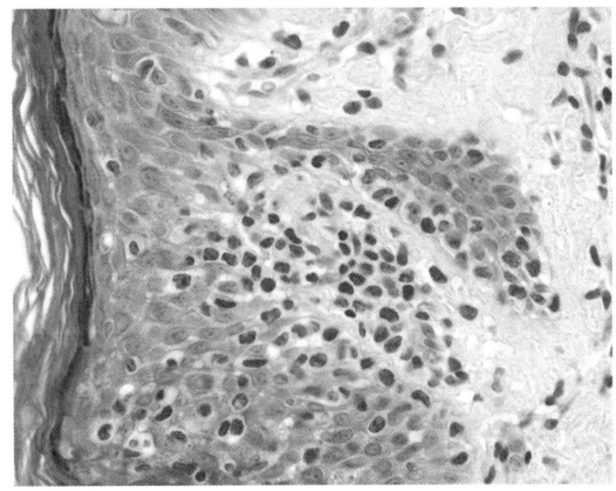

Fig. 4.23. Skin biopsy from a patient with hypopigmented skin lesions of mycosis fungoides. (A) A perivascular and interstitial band-like lymphocytic infiltrate is present in the superficial dermis (40× magnification). (B) The lymphocytes have hyperchromatic, irregular cerebriform nuclei and infiltrate the epidermis with virtually no associated spongiosis. Although tumor cells in most types of mycosis fungoides are CD4+, the hypopigmented variant is often CD8+ (400× magnification).

Genetics

Numerous random and non-random structural chromosome abnormalities have been reported in up to 70% of MF particularly in later stage disease. The most frequent abnormalities involve chromosomes 1, 8, 9, 10, 11, 12, and 17, and include loss of chromosome material at 1p22 and 1p36, and 9p21, 10q and 17p.[149]

Diagnostic issues

Early MF may be extremely difficult to diagnose and relies on the demonstration of distinct cytologic atypia in the cerebriform lymphocytes, loss of pan T-cell antigens (particularly CD2 or CD5), or the demonstration of a clonal T-cell population. The latter also can be nonspecific, as reactive conditions (particularly pityriasis lichenoides)[150] can have a T-cell clone. The hypopigmented form of MF may be initially misdiagnosed as vitiligo, lichen sclerosis et atrophicus, or pityriasis alba.[151]

Angioimmunoblastic T-cell lymphoma

AITL is predominantly a node based, disseminated, peripheral T-cell lymphoma.[1] The tumor arises from a CD4+ follicular helper T-cell and is characterized by expanded follicular dendritic meshwork, vascular proliferation with prominent high endothelial venules, and a minor population of EBV+ B-cells.

Clinical

AITL typically occurs in middle-aged to elderly males or females. Patients have systemic symptoms, polyclonal hypergammaglobulinemia, generalized lymphadenopathy, and hepatosplenomegaly; skin rash and pruritus may be present. Immune dysregulation is manifest by circulating immune complexes, autoimmune hemolytic anemia, cold agglutinins, rheumatoid factor, and anti-smooth muscle antibodies. AITL occurs infrequently in pediatric patients (5–12% of PTCL). The clinical course in AITL is aggressive with median survivals of less than 3 years. Progression to large B-cell lymphoma, which may or may not be EBV+, may rarely occur.

Morphology

Nodal architecture is effaced by a paracortical or interfollicular polymorphous infiltrate composed predominantly of small- to medium-sized lymphocytes with atypical folded nuclei and clear to pale cytoplasm and small numbers of large lymphocytes (Figs. 4.24A–B). Variable numbers of histiocytes, plasma cells, and eosinophils are admixed. There is marked proliferation of arborizing blood vessels with prominent high endothelial venules often surrounded by clusters of tumor cells. The B-cell follicles may be burned out or hyperplastic with ill-defined borders (early lesions).[152] Prominent proliferation of follicular dendritic meshwork is present, and it extends beyond the follicle and wraps around high endothelial venules (Fig. 4.24C).

(A) (B) (C)

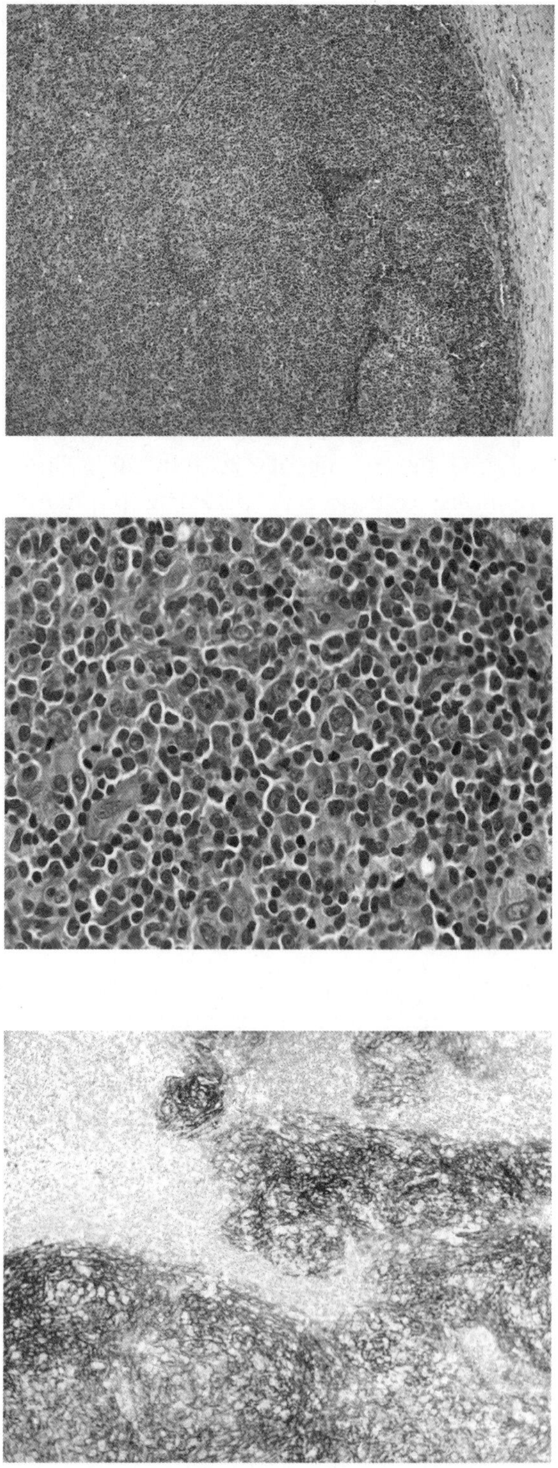

Fig. 4.24. Angioimmunoblastic T-cell lymphoma. (A) Lymph node architecture is effaced by a predominantly diffuse infiltrate (100× magnification) of (B) small- to medium-sized lymphocytes with irregular, folded nuclei and pale to clear cytoplasm (400× magnification). (C) Expanded follicular dendritic cell meshwork extends beyond germinal center as demonstrated by CD21 expression (15× magnification).

EBV+ large B-cells with immunoblastic features are present in most cases and may cause confusion with HL if they are large and atypical.[153]

Immunophenotype

AITL has a phenotype of a follicular helper T-cell (CD4+, CD10+/–, BCL6+/–, CXCL13+, PD-1+). There is little loss of pan T-cell antigens CD2, CD5, and CD7. Numerous reactive CD8+ T-cells may be present. EBV+ B-immunoblasts and plasma cells are polytypic. Immunostaining for follicular dendritic cell markers (CD21, CD23, CD35, and CNA.42) is useful (Fig. 4.24C). The EBV+ B-cells are often CD30+.

Genetics

Clonal T-cell receptor rearrangements are detected in 75–90% of cases and clonal IgH rearrangements in 25–30% (EBV+ B-cells).[1] Cytogenetic abnormalities include trisomy 3 and 5 and an additional copy of the X chromosome.[154,155] Compared to PTCL-NOS and ALCL, AITL has fewer structural abnormalities and lacks polyploidy or gains of chromosome 7.

Diagnostic issues

The differential diagnosis of AITL includes reactive and neoplastic processes that expand the lymph node paracortex. Due to its polymorphous appearance and lack of T-cell antigen loss in most cases, AITL can be misdiagnosed as a reactive process such as a drug reaction or abnormal immune reactions, e.g. autoimmune lymphoproliferative syndrome (ALPS). The presence of EBV+ cells and CD30+ large cells could be confused with HL.

Peripheral T-cell lymphoma, not otherwise specified

PTCL, NOS is a poorly defined, heterogeneous category of mature T-cell lymphomas that do not fit precisely into other diagnostic categories.[1] PTCL, NOS represents approximately 30% of peripheral T-cell lymphomas in adults and is rare in children.[114] These tumors predominantly arise in lymph nodes.

Clinical

Patients present with systemic symptoms and lymphadenopathy with generalized disease involving the bone marrow, liver, and spleen. The skin and the gastrointestinal tract are the most frequent extranodal sites.

(A)

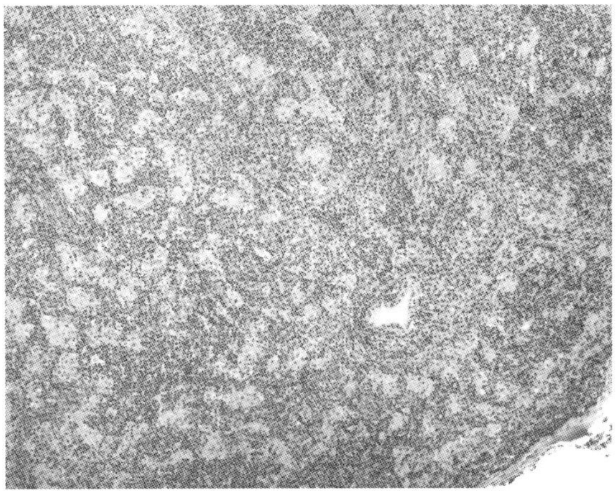

(B)

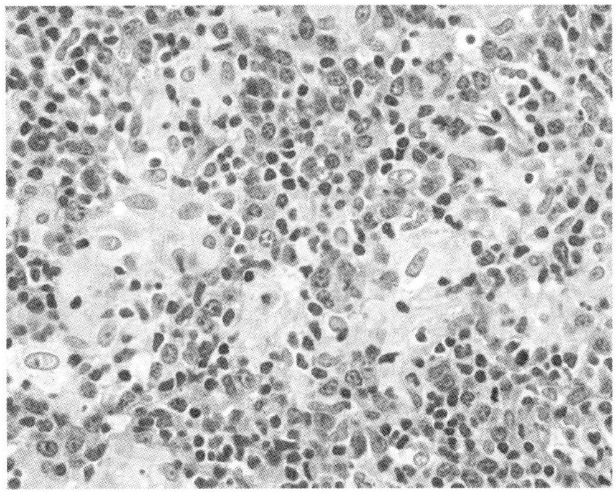

Fig. 4.25. Peripheral T-cell lymphoma, not otherwise specified. (A) Lymph node architecture is diffusely effaced by an infiltrate of lymphocytes and histiocytes (40× magnification). (B) The lymphocytes are predominantly small to medium-sized with atypical, folded nuclei; in this case numerous epithelioid histiocytes are present (400× magnification).

Morphology

Lymph node architecture is effaced in a paracortical or diffuse or, less frequently, a T-zone pattern (perifollicular) pattern (Fig. 4.25A). Tumor cells have cytologic atypia and vary from small to medium to large. Numerous small lymphocytes, plasma cells, eosinophils, and histiocytes may be admixed with prominent endothelial venules, giving the infiltrate a reactive appearance (Fig. 4.25B).

Immunophenotype

Most PTCL, NOS arise from CD4+ T-cells, however, CD8+ or rarely CD4– CD8– or CD4+ CD8+ phenotypes are described. The phenotype is often aberrant with loss of CD7 or CD5. Variable expression of CD30 is reported, and ALK is negative. Most cases are EBV negative. Rare cases express CD15 or CD20.

Genetics

PTCL-NOS is usually associated with a complex karyotype with recurrent numerical abnormalities including gains of chromosomes 1q, 3p, 7q (7q22–q31), 5p, 8q (8q24qter), 17q and 22q and losses in 4q, 5q, 6q (6q22q24), 9p, 10q, 10p13pter, 12q, and 13 q.[1,156]

Diagnostic issues

Autoimmune lymphoproliferative syndrome (ALPS) may be confused with PTCL, NOS[157] as patients present with lymphadenopathy and splenomegaly. In ALPS, an abnormal α-β T-cell population lacking both CD4 and CD8 is present, and the T-cells are polyclonal. PTCL-NOS is distinguished from ALK– ALCL by a more polymorphic mixed cell appearance, lack of a sinus growth pattern, and variable rather the strong CD30 seen in virtually every cell in ALCL.

Hepatosplenic T-cell lymphoma

Hepatosplenic T-cell lymphoma (HSTL) is an extranodal, systemic, cytotoxic T-cell lymphoma commonly typically presenting as hepatosplenomegaly in male adolescents and young adults.[1] The tumor has a characteristic sinusoidal pattern of infiltration of the liver, spleen, and bone marrow.

Clinical

Most patients have hepatosplenomegaly without peripheral adenopathy, and the bone marrow is involved at presentation in most patients. Approximately 80–85% of patients have thrombocytopenia and anemia with leukopenia in approximately 45%. Circulating tumor cells are present in 25–50% of patients during the course of disease. Up to 20% of HSTL arise in an abnormal immune background, either immunodeficiency, immunosuppressive therapy, or antitumor necrosis factor (TNF) therapy (infliximab and less frequently adalimumab).[158] Adolescents with Crohn's disease treated with TNF-α blockade, particularly in combination with other immunosuppressive agents, appear to be at increased risk.[159]

Morphology

Tumor cells infiltrate sinuses of the liver, spleen, and bone marrow and are composed of homogeneous populations of medium-sized lymphocytes with partially dispersed chromatin and somewhat indistinct nucleoli (Fig. 4.26). There is little cytologic atypia. On Wright stain, the tumor cells have partially condensed chromatin and pale cytoplasm with a variable presence of granules. Hemophagocytosis by macrophages or tumor cells is rarely reported.[160]

Immunophenotype

HSTL is the prototypic γ-δ T-cell tumor, however, an α-β T-cell phenotype is seen in a minority of cases.[161] Most tumor cells are CD4– CD8– with approximately 15% expressing CD8. The tumor cells express CD2 and CD3 but lack CD5. Virtually all tumor cells express the cytolytic granule protein TIA-1 but most lack granzyme B or perforin, indicating a non-activated cytotoxic phenotype. CD56 is expressed in >60%. EBV is generally negative.

Genetics

TCR γ genes are rearranged. TCR β genes are rearranged in the α-β cases, however, nonproductive rearrangement of the TCR β genes may be present in some cases with a γ-δ phenotype.[162] Isochromosome 7q is a recurrent cytogenetic abnormality.

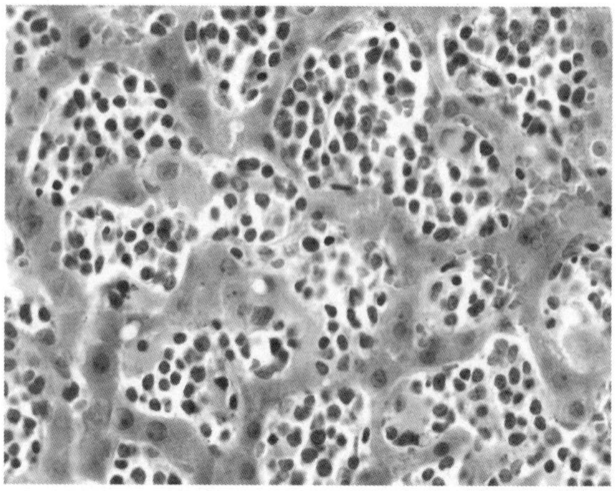

Fig. 4.26. Hepatosplenic lymphoma (1000× magnification). The liver sinuses are distended by relatively monomorphic small- to medium-sized lymphocytes with partially dispersed chromatin.

Diagnostic issues

The main differential diagnostic consideration for HSTL is aggressive NK-cell leukemia, as discussed below.

Epstein–Barr virus (EBV)-positive T-cell lymphoproliferative disorders of childhood

EBV+ T-cell lymphoproliferative disorders (LPD) of childhood are very rare and include systemic EBV+ LPD of childhood, an aggressive process with a fulminant course and Hydroa vacciniforme-like lymphoma, an initially indolent cutaneous lymphoma with progression over time.

Systemic EBV+ LPD of childhood

Systemic EBV+ LPD of childhood includes previously described fulminant EBV+ T-cell LPD of childhood, sporadic fatal infectious mononucleosis (FIM); fulminant haemophagocytic syndrome in children in Taiwan,[163] fatal EBV-associated haemophagocytic syndrome in Japan,[164] and severe chronic active EBV infection (CAEBV).[165]

Clinical

Although rare, EBV+ T-cell LPD is a disease of children and young adults who are predominantly Asians, Native Americans from Central and South America, and Mexicans. EBV+ T-cell LPD may arise *de novo* as a primary EBV infection or in a very small subset of patients with CAEBV, an infectious mononucleosis-like condition persisting for at least 3–6 months.[165] Patients presenting with a primary, *de novo* acute EBV infection have abnormal EBV serology with low or absent anti-VCA IgM antibodies. Patients with CAEBV have high titers of EBV-capsid antigen (VCA-IgG) and early antigen (EA-IgG)[166] and a prodrome with expansion of polyclonal or oligoclonal EBV+ T-cells. Patients with EBV+ T-cell LPD present with chronic intermittent or acute onset of fever and malaise and develop hepatosplenomegaly within weeks to months and fulminant multiorgan failure, systemic hemophagocytosis, sepsis and death in days to weeks. There is little adenopathy. The clinical features suggest a genetic defect in patient's immune response to EBV infection. A severe form of CAEBV has been reported in Japan characterized by high fever, hepatosplenomegaly, extensive lymphadenopathy and pancytopenia. These patients have very high peripheral blood EBV viral loads due to infected NK- and T-cells and frequently have monoclonal T-cell populations. As most of these Japanese patients progress to frank lymphoma, this should be considered part of the spectrum of EBV+ T-cell LPD.[167]

Morphologic features

The lymphocytes are usually small with normal morphology and infiltrate the sinuses of the liver and spleen. Splenic white pulp is depleted, and periportal areas of the liver are also involved. Lymph node architecture is preserved and tumor cells are present in the paracortical areas. Erythrophagocytosis is often present throughout the reticuloendothelial system. Cases with pleomorphic medium to large tumor cells have been described.[167]

Immunophenotype

The T-cells are EBV+, express CD2, CD3, and TIA-1, and lack CD56. T-cell subset expression varies with the clinical presentation. A mixture of T-cell subsets has been reported; cases secondary to acute primary EBV infection are CD8+ whereas those arising in CAEBV are more often CD4+.[168]

Genetics

TCR genes are clonally rearranged. EBV is clonal and Type A either with wild type or the 30 bp deleted product of the *LMP1* gene.[167] No recurrent chromosomal abnormalities have been described.

Diagnostic issues

The clinical presentation of EBV+ LPD of childhood is similar to aggressive NK-cell leukemia, which would show a true NK-cell phenotype. In addition, patients with hemophagocytic lymphohistiocytosis (either of familial origin or infection associated) could have similar features, and differentiation would require T-cell receptor gene rearrangement studies, and in familial cases, demonstration of a perforin (*PRF*), MUNC13-14 (*UNC13D*, chromosome 17q25), or syntaxin (*STX11*, chromosome 6q24) mutations.[169]

Hydroa vacciniforme-like lymphoma

Clinical

Hydroa vacciniforme is a photosensitivity disorder of childhood with the development of vesiculopapular lesions on sun-exposed skin that usually resolves by young adulthood. Hydroa vacciniforme-like T-cell lymphoma is an EBV+ clonal T-cell proliferation associated with a history of hypersensitivity to sun and (often) insect bites. Rare patients, particularly of Asian, Native American, or Mexican descent, develop persistent or more aggressive disease with facial swelling, lesions on non-sun-exposed skin and high grade fever and liver damage.[170,171] Patients present with papulovesicular lesions that progress to ulcerated, crusted lesions with scarring. Patients have systemic symptoms and may have lymphadenopathy and hepatosplenomegaly, particularly late in the disease course. The clinical course is variable and recurrent lesions may occur over 10–15 years. When the disease spreads to non-cutaneous sites the course is usually aggressive.

Morphologic features

The neoplastic infiltrate is angiocentric and angioinvasive with necrosis, extends from the papillary dermis to the deep dermis, and may involve the subcutaneous tissue (Figs. 4.27A–B). The cells are small- to medium-sized without significant atypia.

Immunophenotype

The T-cells have a cytotoxic (TIA-1+, granzyme B+, perforin+) phenotype with variable expression of CD56;[172] rarely the tumor cells have a NK-cell origin. Both CD4+ and CD8+ phenotypes have been reported. The tumor cells are EBV+ (Fig. 4.27C).

Genetics

Most cases have clonal TCR rearrangements with a small number being of true NK-cell origin. EBV is clonal without expression of LMP. No recurrent cytogenetic abnormalities have been reported.

Diagnostic issues

Extranodal NK/T-cell lymphoma, nasal type may show similar lesions in the skin. Both tumors have a similar EBV+ phenotype, however the expression of CD56 is more common in extranodal NK/T-cell lymphoma, nasal

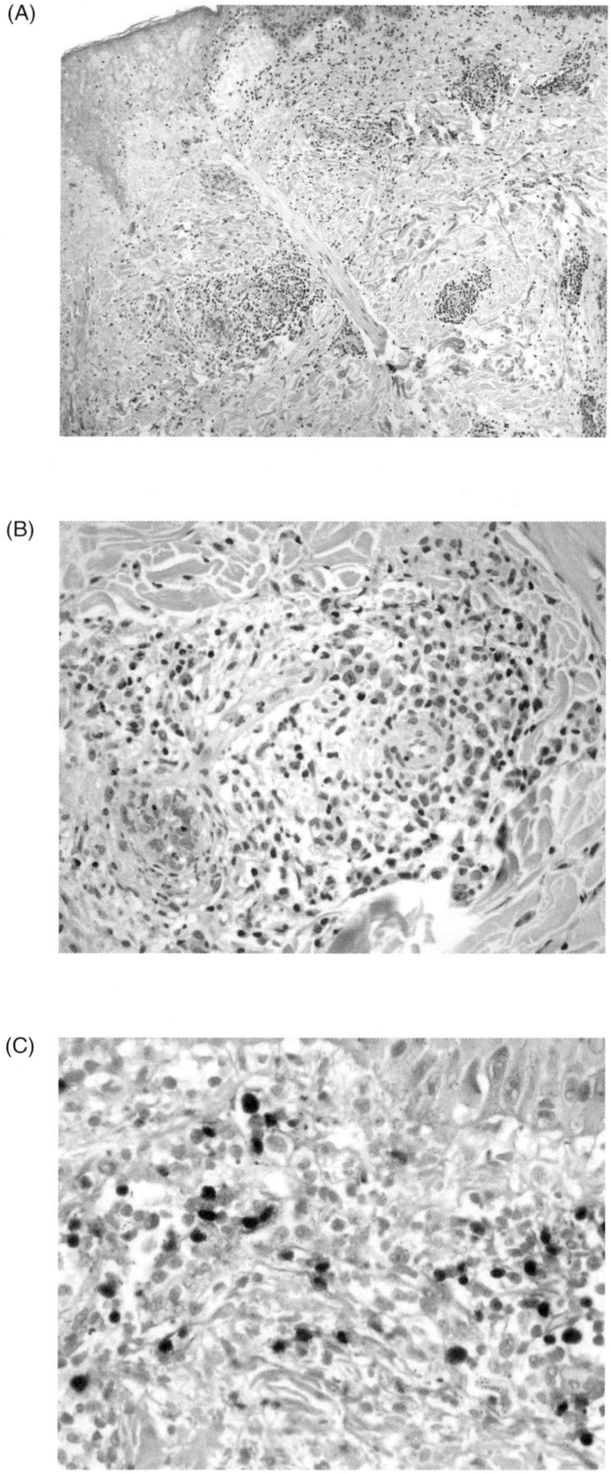

Fig. 4.27. Hydroa vacciniforme-like lymphoma. (A) The skin has an ulcerated epidermis with a predominantly perivascular lymphoid infiltrate (15× magnification). (B) The lymphocytes have large, folded, pleomorphic nuclei with dispersed chromatin and prominent nucleoli and invade and disrupt the vessel wall (400× magnification). (C) The large tumor cells are EBV+ (EBV encoded RNA, EBER) (600× magnification) and phenotyped as CD8+ cytotoxic T cells (not shown).

type. The clinical association with hypersensitivity to sunlight or insect bites and distribution of sun-exposed skin would be more common in Hydroa vacciniforme-like lymphoma. In addition, the expression of CD4, as seen in a subset of cases of Hydroa vacciniforme-like lymphoma, would be very unusual in extranodal NK/T-cell lymphoma, which is usually CD4–, CD8– or CD4–, CD8+.

Subcutaneous panniculitis-like T-cell lymphoma

Subcutaneous panniculitis-like T-cell lymphoma (SPTCL) is a rare (< 1% of all NHL) extranodal cytotoxic T-cell lymphoma that preferentially involves the subcutaneous tissue.[1] Cutaneous γ-δ T-cell lymphomas involving the subcutaneous tissue are now recognized as a separate entity with a more aggressive course.[1,173]

Clinical

Patients with SPTCL are typically young (median age approximately 35 years) but any age can be affected. Pediatric and young adult patients have been described and include infants, toddlers, children, and teenagers. Up to 20% of patients have autoimmune disease, most frequently systemic lupus erythematosus. Patients present with multiple subcutaneous nodules, and 50% have systemic symptoms including fever and weight loss. The course may be protracted, but the overall survival is favorable with a greater than 80% 5 year survival. Approximately 20% of the patients have an associated hemophagocytic syndrome which may lead to decreased survival.[173]

Morphologic features

SPTCL is limited to the subcutaneous fat and infiltrates the fat lobules in a delicate lace-like pattern rimming the fat spaces (Fig. 4.28A). The lymphocytes are variable in size but most are small- to medium-sized with hyperchromatic nuclei (Fig. 4.28B). Lymphocytes infiltrate small vessels but do not destroy the vessels (Fig. 4.28C). Fat necrosis with apoptotic debris is present. Histiocytes with lipid-laden cytoplasm, and in some cases phagocytosis of red blood cells and other cellular debris, are present. Plasma cells are absent or scarce.

Immunophenotype

The tumor cells are CD3+, CD8+, cytotoxic (TIA-1+, granzyme B+, perforin+) α-β T-cells that lack CD30, CD56, and EBV (Figs. 4.28D–E).

Genetics

No recurrent cytogenetic abnormalities have been reported. Frequent copy number changes particularly gains of 5q and 13q and losses of 1p, 2p, 10q, 11q, 12q, 16, 19, 20 and 22 have been described.[174]

Diagnostic issues

Other reactive and neoplastic causes of panniculitis have to be excluded[175] including cutaneous γ-δ T-cell lymphomas,[1,173] lupus profundus, erythema nodosum, and cytophagic histiocytic panniculitis.

Extranodal NK/T-cell lymphoma, nasal type

Extranodal NK/T-cell lymphoma, nasal type is an EBV+ extranodal lymphoma with a cytotoxic phenotype and a characteristic angiocentric and angiodestructive growth pattern with prominent necrosis.[1]

Clinical

Extranodal NK/T-cell lymphoma, nasal type is a rare tumor occurring more often in Asians and Native American populations in Mexico, Central America, and South America with a median age of approximately 45–50 years with a wide range. Extranodal NK/T-cell lymphoma, nasal type is particularly rare in childhood.

The classic presentation of extranodal NK/T-cell lymphoma, nasal type is a localized nasal mass with nasal obstruction, epistaxis, or midfacial destructive lesions and local extension. The tumor may also initially occur or later relapse at other extranasal sites including skin, gastrointestinal tract or testis.[176] Compared to adults, many pediatric patients have more disseminated disease (bone marrow, liver involvement) suggesting overlap with aggressive NK-cell leukemia.[177,178] Approximately 10–20% of cases are complicated by the development of a systemic hemophagocytic syndrome.[179]

Morphology

The most characteristic feature is the presence of an angiocentric, angioinvasive and angiodestructive infiltrate producing zonal, coagulative necrosis. The tumor cells may be small, medium-sized, or large with variable degrees of cytologic atypia and chromatin dispersal (Fig. 4.29A).

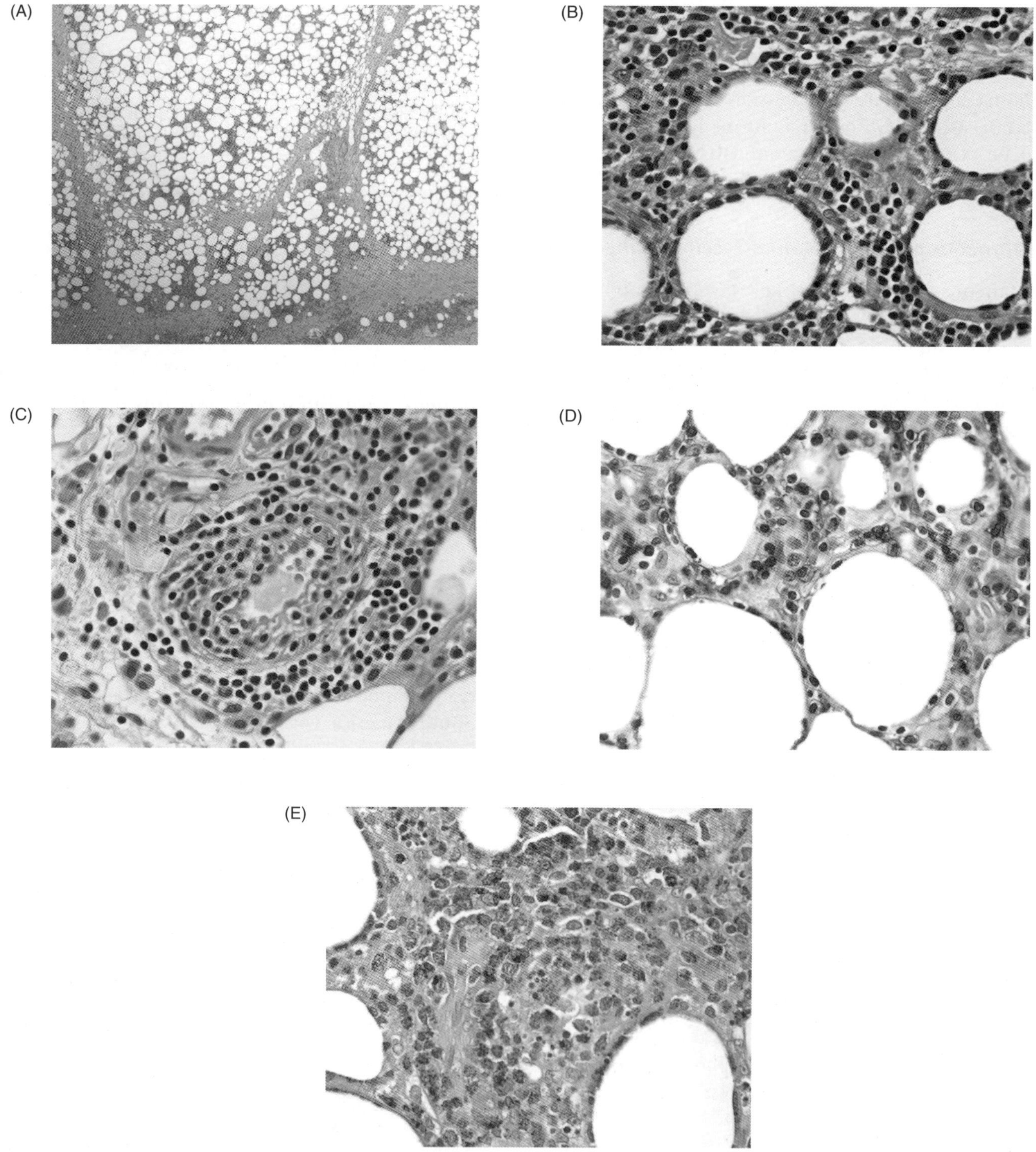

Fig. 4.28. Subcutaneous panniculitis-like T-cell lymphoma. (A) Subcutaneous tissue with a predominantly lobular lymphoid infiltrate (40× magnification). (B) Subcutaneous tissue composed of predominantly small atypical lymphocytes that rim fat spaces; focal fat necrosis is present (600× magnification). (C) Lymphocytes infiltrate but do not destroy small vessels (600× magnification). (D) Tumor cells are alpha-beta T cells as shown by staining with the antibody Beta-F1 (600× magnification) and (E) express cytotoxic granule protein TIA-1 (600× magnification).

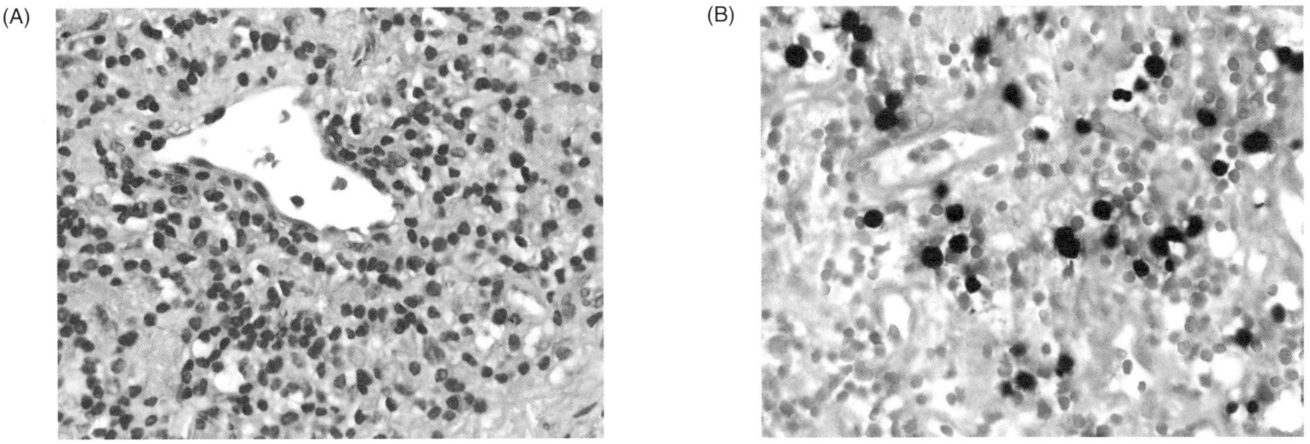

Fig. 4.29. Extranodal NK/T-cell lymphoma, nasal type. (A) Tumor cells are medium to large pleomorphic cells that infiltrate vessels (400× magnification). (B) EBV+ (EBER *in situ* hybridization) (600× magnification).

Immunophenotype

Most tumors have a true NK-cell origin (CD2+, CD7+, surface CD3–, cytoplasmic CD3+, CD4–, CD8–/+, CD5–). Tumors with a T-cell phenotype also express CD3 and CD5 and are CD4– with variable expression of CD8 and often lack the T-cell α-β receptor protein (as detected by the antibody Beta-F1), compatible with a γ-δ T-cell phenotype. The tumor cells express CD56 and cytotoxic granule proteins TIA-1, granzyme B, and perforin. Most cases express EBV (EBV encoded RNA, EBER+) (Fig. 4.29B).

Genetics

There is a suggestion from the literature that pediatric extranodal NK/T-cell lymphoma may more often have a T-cell phenotype/genotype[177] than in adults. Many cytogenetic abnormalities have been reported,[180] the most frequent being del(6)(q21q25) or i(6)p10.

Diagnostic issues

With skin involvement, extranodal NK/T-cell lymphoma must be distinguished from Hydroa vacciniforme-like T-cell lymphoma.

Aggressive NK-cell leukemia

Aggressive NK-cell leukemia is a very rare EBV+ systemic proliferation of mature NK-cells associated with a fulminant course.[1] The tumor was previously classified as aggressive NK-cell leukemia/lymphoma due to its disseminated nature and relatively minor component of tumor cells in the bone marrow and blood as compared to other leukemias.

Clinical

Aggressive NK-cell leukemia is rare, occurring predominantly in young to middle-aged Asians with a median age of approximately 42 years. It is uncommon in pediatric patients. Patients are generally very ill with fever and constitutional symptoms, and involvement of the peripheral blood, bone marrow, liver, and spleen; lymphadenopathy is present in some. Virtually any site can be affected; however, skin lesions are uncommon. The number of circulating tumor cells is variable, but most patients have neutropenia, anemia, and thrombocytopenia. As there can be overlap with extranodal NK/T-cell lymphoma, nasal type, it is unclear at present if aggressive NK-cell leukemia is a distinct entity.[181]

Morphologic features

Circulating tumor cells may vary from small to large with differing degrees of nuclear atypia (Fig. 4.30A). Cytoplasm is abundant and pale with fine to coarse azurophilic granules. In tissue sections, the infiltrate can be dense or patchy, and the tumor cells can also range from small to large with more pleomorphism. Necrosis is common; angioinvasion is variable. Liver and splenic involvement may be sinusoidal resembling hepatosplenic lymphoma (Fig. 4.30B).

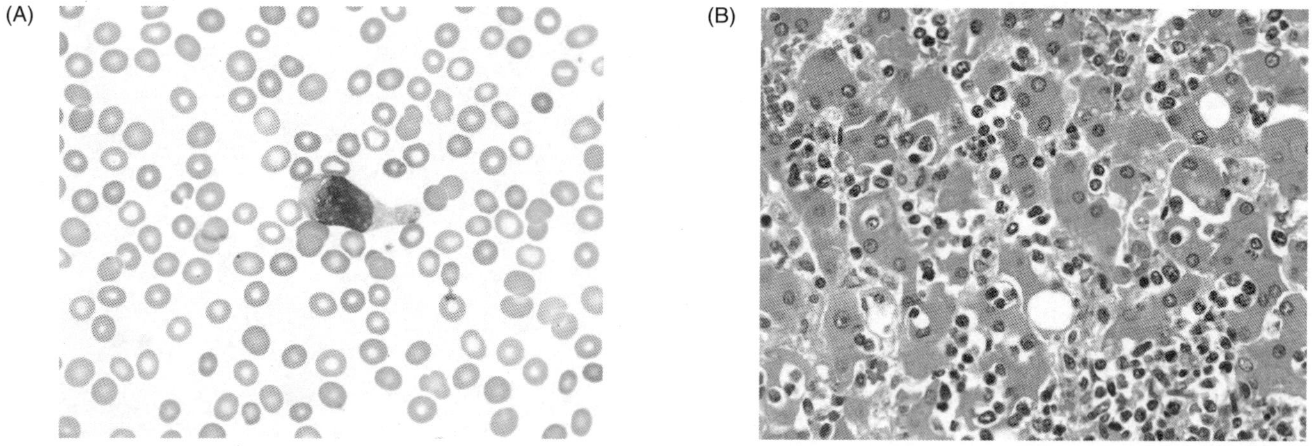

Fig. 4.30. Aggressive NK cell leukemia. (A) Large atypical lymphocytes in the peripheral blood have dysplastic, irregular nuclei with prominent nucleoli and cytoplasm containing fine, azurophilic granules (1000× magnification). (B) Tumor cells infiltrate liver sinuses and resemble hepatosplenic lymphoma but have more irregular, pleomorphic nuclei and vary more from cell to cell (600× magnification).

Immunophenotype

The tumor cells have an NK-cell phenotype with expression of CD2, CD3 epsilon chain and CD7 with lack of CD5, surface CD3, and T-cell receptor proteins.[182] CD56 is positive as well as CD16, while CD57 is usually negative. More than 90% of cases are EBER+.

Genetics

By definition, T-cell receptor genes are not rearranged. Cytogenetic abnormalities, evidence of X-chromosome inactivation in females, or clonal EBV by terminal repeat analysis are the only available clonal markers. The most frequent cytogenetic abnormalities include del(6)(q21q25) and 11q deletion.[183]

Diagnostic issues

The clinical presentation may resemble hepatosplenic T-cell lymphoma, however, there is generally more lymphadenopathy in aggressive NK-cell leukemia, and the phenotype is that of a true NK-cell rather than a cytotoxic, γ-δ T-cell. EBV is also absent in hepatosplenic γ-δ T-cell lymphoma in most cases.

Classical Hodgkin Lymphoma

Clinical

There are two categories of HL. Classical HL (95% of HL) will be discussed here, and nodular lymphocyte predominant HL will be discussed below. HL comprises 30% of lymphomas and is the most common cancer in the pediatric population. Classical HL has two age-related peaks in incidence: a peak in adolescents/young adults and a second peak in the elderly (> 50 years old). Classical HL is uncommon in younger children but becomes more frequent in adolescents.

Based on distinct clinicopathologic differences such as sites of involvement, median age of presentation, and histopathologic patterns, classical HL can be further subclassified into nodular sclerosis, mixed cellularity, lymphocyte rich, and lymphocyte-depleted HL. Nodular sclerosis HL is by far the most common subtype in children, adolescents, and adults. There is a nearly uniform response to current radiation and chemotherapy strategies among all of the subtypes.

Classical HL is predominantly a disease of lymph nodes, and extranodal involvement is rare (14% of cases).[184] Cervical, mediastinal, and axillary lymph nodes are common sites of involvement. Notably, the nodular sclerosis subtype of classical HL involves the mediastinum in 80% of cases. Splenic and bone marrow involvement may occur in 20% and 5% of cases, respectively.[185] B symptoms occur in about 40% of cases.[184]

Morphologic features

Classical HL may have a nodular or diffuse pattern of lymph node involvement. HL is an unusual neoplasm because the neoplastic cells are generally the cell of minority in a background of reactive inflammatory cells. Reactive background cells include lymphocytes (mostly T cells), eosinophils, neutrophils, and plasma cells. Large neoplastic Hodgkin cells are present in all HLs; however, the appearance of Hodgkin cells on hematoxylin and eosin-stained sections varies. The most characteristic of classical HL is the RS cells, a binucleate cell with central inclusion-like eosinophilic nucleoli and perinuclear clearing (Fig. 4.31A). The majority of large neoplastic cells often consist of mononuclear Hodgkin cells with prominent eosinophilic nuclei. Various other morphologic variants of Hodgkin cell have been described including the mummified Hodgkin cell characterized by its smudged chromatin and the lacunar Hodgkin cell characterized by its shrunken appearance and location within lacunar spaces (Fig. 4.31B). Lacunar Hodgkin cells are a formalin fixation artifact whereby the nuclei of Hodgkin cells shrink away from the surrounding tissue, giving the appearance of cells sitting in lacunae.

Each subtype of Classical HL has a characteristic morphology. Nodular sclerosis HL is a nodular tumor created by broad bands of fibroblast poor collagen (Fig. 4.31C). Within nodules are RS cells, mononuclear Hodgkin cells, and characteristically lacunar Hodgkin cells all in a background of lymphocytes, histiocytes, eosinophils, and neutrophils. Lymphocyte-rich HL is composed of nodules composed of B cells (mantle cells) within which are RS and Hodgkin cell variants. In contrast to other classical HL, lymphocyte-rich HL lacks the mixed background of eosinophils and neutrophils. Mixed cellularity HL is diffuse or nodular lymphoma and contains scattered RS cells and Hodgkin cells in a background of eosinophils and neutrophils.

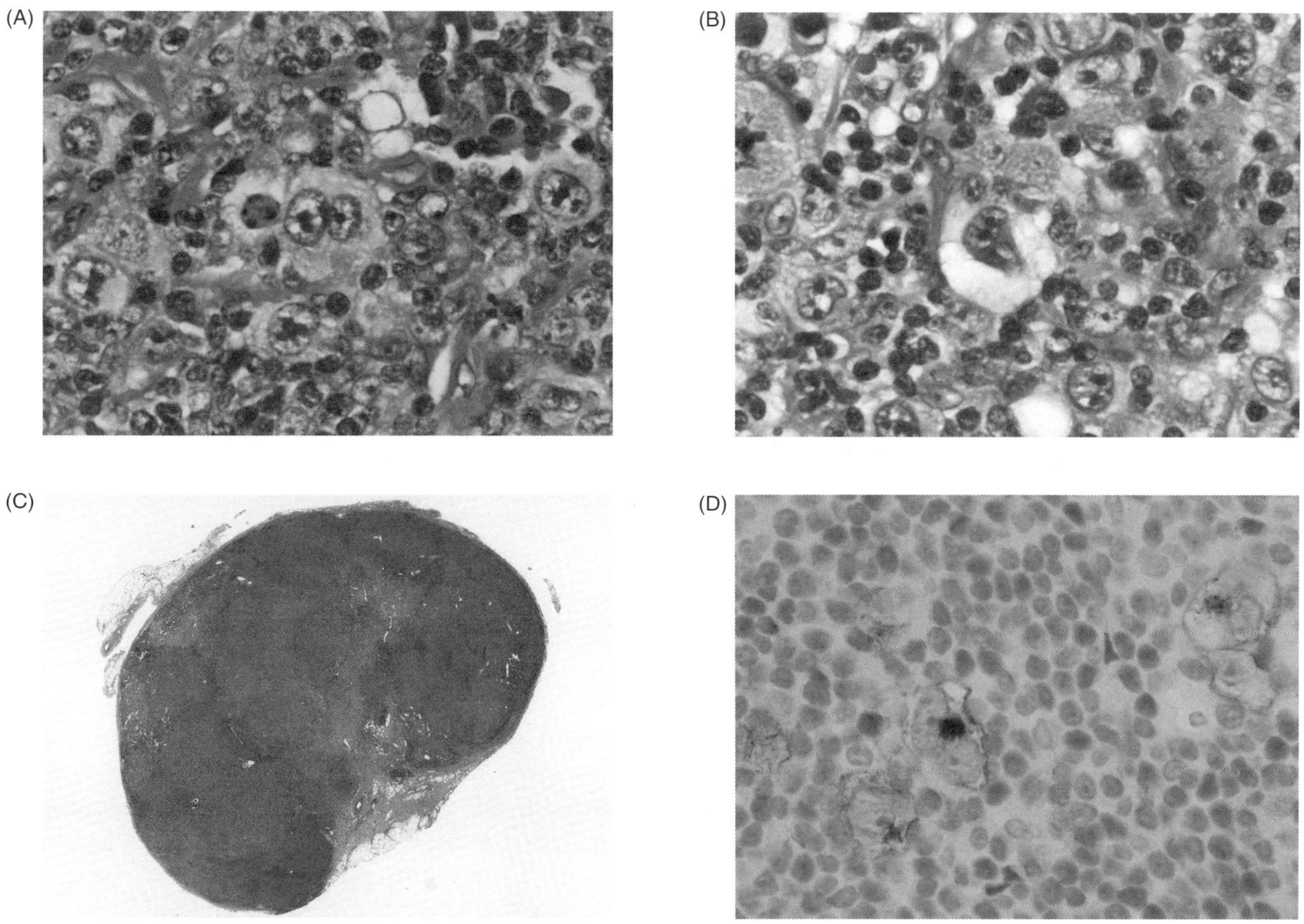

Fig. 4.31. Nodular sclerosing Hodgkin lymphoma. (A) High power (600× magnification) H&E stain showing a classic Reed-Sternberg cell, a background of small lymphocytes, and scattered large mononuclear forms of Hodgkin cells. (B) Low-power (15× magnification) hematoxylin and eosin-stained lymph node showing effacement of the lymph node by nodules. Some nodules are surrounded by bands of fibrous tissue. (C) Lacunar Hodgkin cells (600× magnification). (D) Classical Hodgkin cells show membrane and golgi positivity for CD30 (1000× magnification).

Lymphocyte-depleted HL is usually a diffuse lymphoma, in which Hodgkin cells are the predominant cell or the background lymphocytes are diminished. Two main patterns are seen. In the first pattern, sheets of Hodgkin cells in a scant background of reactive cells result in a likeness to sarcoma. In the second pattern, there is a background of fibrous tissue with variable numbers of Hodgkin cells.

Immunophenotype

Hodgkin/RS cells of classical HL have a relatively consistent core immunophenotype: CD45 is negative; CD30 (almost 100%) is positive (Fig. 4.31D); and CD15 (75–85%) is positive. A significant proportion of classical HL are EBV driven, varying by subtype (mixed cellularity > lymphocyte-rich > nodular sclerosis).[185] In these cases, the presence of EBV can be demonstrated in Hodgkin cells by *in situ* hybridization for EBER or by a immunohistochemical stain for LMP1. Zhou *et al.* tabulated published data from 39 countries and found EBER and/or immunohistochemical evidence of EBV in Hodgkin cells in 83% and 42% of HL in children ≤ 10 and > 10 years old, respectively.[186] The rate of EBV-related HL in the United States and United Kingdom is lower (~ 60%) in children ≤ 10 years old, suggesting an effect of earlier EBV exposure in developing countries.[186] EBV is found in 100% of HIV-associated HL.

Classical HL has been described as a B-cell lymphoma with an incomplete B-cell program. Hence, B-cell markers are commonly demonstrated, but some B-cell markers are incomplete or absent. PAX-5 is almost always positive (95%). CD20 is present in approximately 30% of cases but shows a variable expression with negative, weak, and moderate intensity. CD79a is less frequent. Transcription factors OCT-2 and BOB.1 are coexpressed in normal B cells but are rarely coexpressed in classical HL.

Genetics

Classical HL is a B-cell lymphoma with somatic mutation in the immunoglobulin heavy chain gene, indicating a germinal center cell origin. Genetic and molecular tests are not usually helpful for diagnosis or prognosis. Immunoglobulin heavy chain clonality studies usually do not detect a B-cell clone in whole tissue because of the paucity of Hodgkin cells. Cytogenetics typically show complex changes.

Diagnostic issues

Several close diagnostic differentials of classical HL exist. Cases in which the Hodgkin cells are numerous are often troublesome. A variant of nodular sclerosis HL, known as syncytial variant, and some lymphocyte depleted HLs contain sheets of Hodgkin cells that may be confused with anaplastic appearing tumors. In these scenarios, ALCL, which strongly expresses CD30, may be a diagnostic consideration. ALK positive cases are easily identified as ALCL, but rare cases of pediatric ALK– ALCL may be problematic. Expression of CD20 or PAX-5, a B cell-associated antigen, would confirm a diagnosis of HL.

PMBL (or DLBCL) may also be difficult to distinguish from classical HL. Indeed, composite lymphomas consisting of PMBL and classical HL, as well as, unusual lymphomas with intermediate morphologic and immunophenotypic characteristics of these two lymphomas have been well described.[107] These cases emphasize a spectrum of disease that cannot always be classified neatly. A new diagnostic category recognizes these conundrums as B-cell lymphoma, unclassifiable, with features intermediate between DLBCL and classical HL, or "grey zone lymphoma",[1] as discussed previously.

Infectious mononucleosis (EBV) or infection mononucleosis-like (e.g. cytomegalovirus) lymphadenopathy may be especially problematic, as large CD30 positive RS-like cells may be present. Preservation of architecture is helpful on morphologic grounds. Correlation with clinical presentation and EBV serologic studies is imperative.

Nodular lymphocyte predominant Hodgkin lymphoma

Clinical

Nodular lymphocyte predominant Hodgkin lymphoma (NLPHL) presents at a median age of 37 years old. NLPHL is rare in adults, comprising only 5% of HL and is even rarer in children. NLPHL is predominantly a disease of lymph nodes. Rare (6%) extranodal involvement does occur in a variety of anatomic sites.[184] Compared with classical HL, lymphocyte predominant HL is more common in males, is less frequently associated with B-symptoms, presents at an earlier stage, and has a more favorable treatment outcome.[184]

Morphologic features

NLPHL usually demonstrates nodular effacement of lymph nodes (Fig. 4.32A), but nodular and diffuse

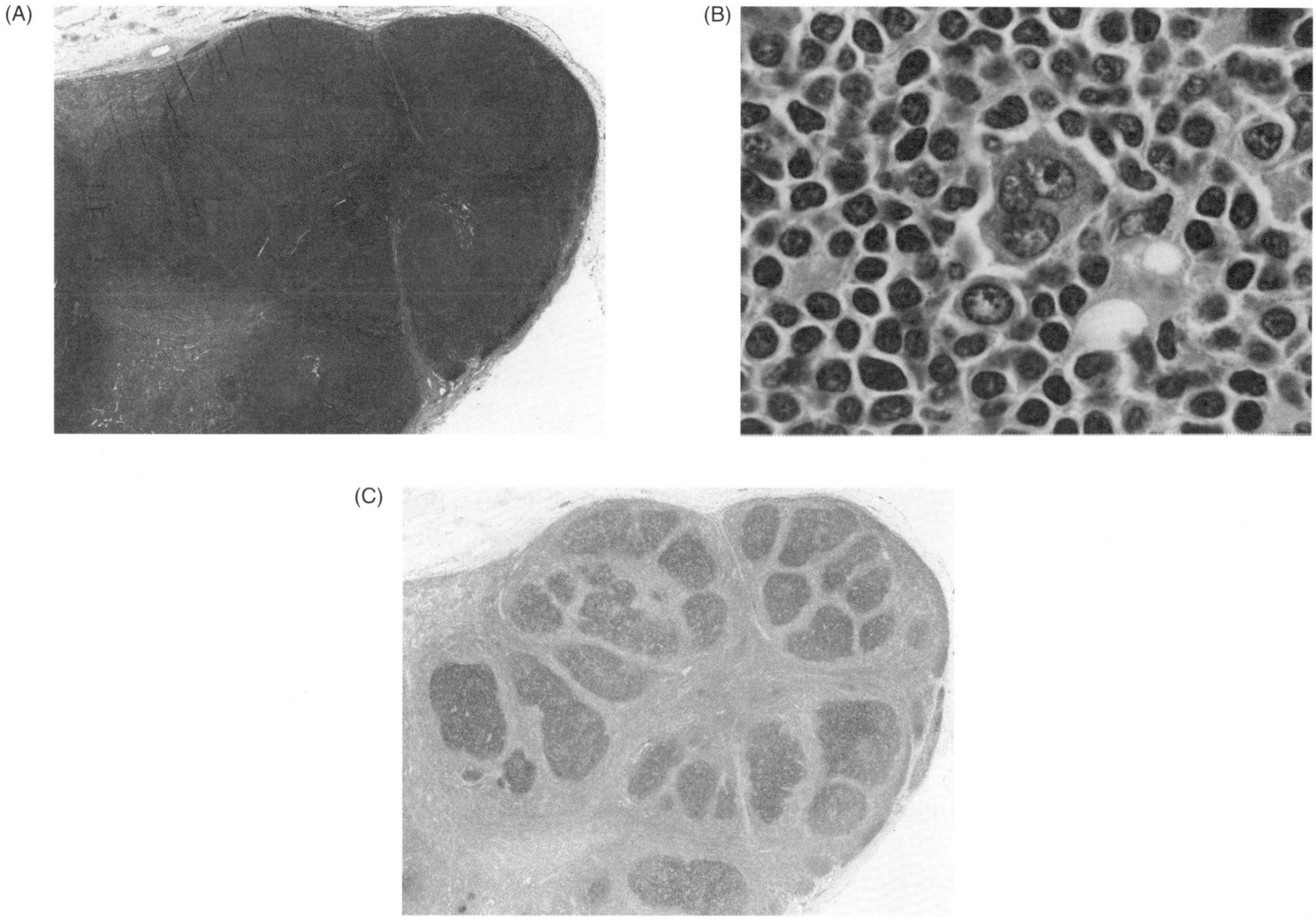

Fig. 4.32. Nodular lymphocyte predominant Hodgkin lymphoma showing. (A) Nodular effacement of a lymph node (15× magnification). (B) Scattered neoplastic LP are present within the nodules (1000× magnification). (C) A CD20 immunohistochemical stain (15× magnification) highlights nodules composed of numerous small B-lymphocytes.

patterns are described. Like all HL, NLPHL comprises of numerous reactive cells with a minority of scattered large neoplastic cells. The neoplastic lymphocyte predominant (LP) cells, also called popcorn cells, are large and highly lobated with scant cytoplasm (Fig. 4.32B). Characteristic nodules consist predominantly of smallB cells with scattered T cells and popcorn cells (Fig. 4.32C). The predominance of small B cells in the back-ground contrasts with the background of T cells in classical HL.

Immunophenotype

NLPHL has an intact B-cell program. LP cells are negative for CD30 and CD15 and are positive for CD45 and B-cell markers: PAX-5, CD20, and CD79a. BCL-6 is positive reflecting the cell of origin, the germinal center B cell. LP cells are positive for EMA in > 50% of cases. Follicular dendritic cell markers such as CD21 and CD23 are useful to demonstrate the expanded residual follicular dendritic meshwork within the nodular areas. T cells are present in the nodules, particularly CD4 positive/CD57 positive T cells, which may form rosettes around LP cells. PD-1, a marker of germinal center T cells, may also be helpful to highlight T cell rosettes around LP cells.

Genetics

NLPHL are B-cell lymphomas with somatic mutation in the immunoglobulin heavy chain gene indicating a germinal center cell origin. Genetic and molecular tests are not usually helpful for diagnosis or prognosis. *BCL6* rearrangements, including *IGH-BCL6* rearrangements are frequent but are not specific for NLPHL.

Diagnostic issues

A common diagnostic differential of nodular lymphocyte predominant HL is T-cell rich large B-cell lymphoma. This only becomes a problem when there is a purely diffuse pattern but warrants different therapies.

NLPHL should also be distinguished from progressive transformation of germinal centers (PTGC), a reactive process, that may occur in isolation or be associated with NLPHL in a variety of temporal relationships. PTGC occurs in a background of normal appearing reactive follicles with germinal centers and likely represents a progression from follicular hyperplasia to follicular lysis and PTGC.[187]

Langerhans cell histiocytosis

Clinical

Langerhans cell histiocytosis (LCH) is rare, occurring in about 5 per million person;[188] however, the incidence in children is much higher. The cell of origin is the Langerhans cell, which is a dendritic cell specialized in antigen presentation. LCH may be grouped into three general categories based on disease distribution: unifocal unisystem, multifocal unisystem, and disseminated LCH. Unifocal disease primarily occurs in older children/young adults. Unifocal disease is usually identified clinically as a lytic bone lesion, but isolated lymph node, skin, and lung lesions can rarely be seen. Isolated lung lesions in young adult smokers are likely a reactive process rather than an neoplasm of Langerhans cells. Multifocal disease occurs in younger children and primarily affects bone. Extension into adjacent tissue is not uncommon; most notably, diabetes insipidus may be seen when lesion involving cranial bones extend into pituitary or hypothalamic regions. Disseminated LCH occurs in infants and may involve skin, bone, liver, spleen, and bone marrow. Prognosis is related to disease burden/distribution with excellent survival in unifocal LCH. Rarely skin lesions without visceral involvement are present at birth or appear early in infancy. Roughly one third of these regress spontaneously and are referred to as self-regressing cutaneous LCH.[189]

Morphology

Tumors are composed of numerous Langerhans cells and background inflammatory cells including variably numerous eosinophils, histiocytes, and lymphocytes. The oval nuclei of neoplastic Langerhans cells are deeply folded and grooved, giving the characteristic coffee bean appearance when cut longitudinally. Pink cytoplasm is abundant. Eosinophils are often a clue for the diagnosis on initial microscopic examination (Fig. 4.33A).

Electron microscopy can be used to identify characteristic Birbeck granules of Langerhans cells. Birbeck granules are pentalaminar structures that sometimes have swelling at one end and have been likened to tennis racquets.

Immunophenotype

Immunophenotypic studies are used to confirm the identity of Langerhans cells. The tumor cells are positive for S100, CD1a (Fig. 4.33B), and langerin. Langerin

(A)

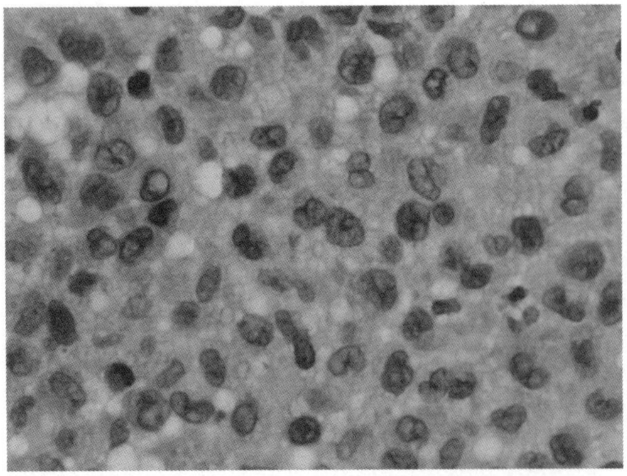

(B)

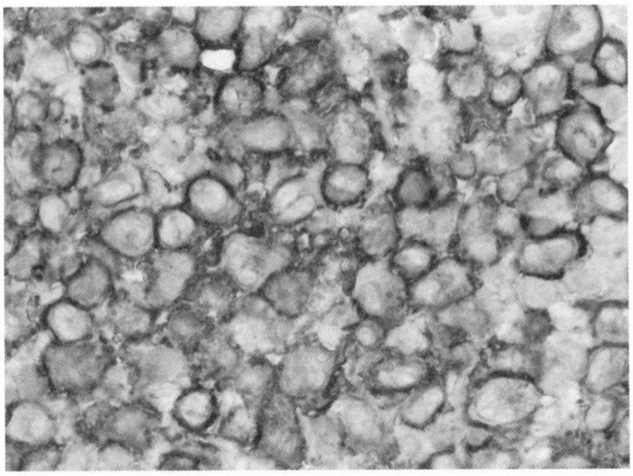

Fig. 4.33. Langerhans cell histiocytosis presenting. (A) High power (600× magnification) image of an H&E stained section showing Langerhans cells and scattered eosinophils. The Langerhans cells have deeply folded nuclei and occasional demonstrate classic longitudinal grooves (600× magnification). (B) Immunohistochemical staining for CD1a confirm the identity of the histocytic cells as Langerhans cells (600× magnification).

targets the Birbeck granules and provides an alternative to electronmicroscopy.

Genetics

Routine molecular and genetic studies are not useful for diagnosis. Clonality of LCH has been demonstrated by X-linked androgen receptor gene assay.

Diagnostic issues

Other S-100 positive histiocytic neoplasms may cause a diagnostic dilemma. Interdigitating dendritic cell sarcoma, a rare tumor usually involving lymph nodes, is S-100 positive. Solitary or disseminated juvenile xanthogranuloma may resemble LCH morphologically, especially when Touton-giant cells are sparse or absent. Juvenile xanthogranulomas can rarely express S-100 in a variable pattern. Both of these entities are negative for CD1a, and Birbeck granules are absent.

References

1. WHO. (2008) *WHO Classification of Tumours of Haematopoietic and Lymphoid Tissues*. Lyon, France: IARC.
2. Hasle H, Niemeyer CM, Chessells JM, Baumann I, Bennett JM, Kerndrup G, Head DR. (2003) A pediatric approach to the WHO classification of myelodysplastic and myeloproliferative diseases. *Leukemia* **17**: 277–282.
5. Hitzler JK, Cheung J, Li Y, Scherer SW, Zipursky A. (2003) GATA1 mutations in transient leukemia and acute megakaryoblastic leukemia of Down syndrome. *Blood* **101**: 4301–4304.
9. Forestier E, Izraeli S, Beverloo B, Haas O, Pession A, Michalova K, Stark B, Harrison CJ, Teigler-Schlegel A, Johansson B. (2008) Cytogenetic features of acute lymphoblastic and myeloid leukemias in pediatric patients with Down syndrome: An iBFM-SG study. *Blood* **111**: 1575–1583.
14. Foucar K. (2009) Myelodysplastic/myeloproliferative neoplasms. *Am J Clin Pathol* **132**: 281–289.
16. Chan RJ, Cooper T, Kratz CP, Weiss B, Loh ML. (2009) Juvenile myelomonocytic leukemia: A report from the 2nd International JMML Symposium. *Leuk Res* **33**: 355–362.
18. de Vries AC, Zwaan CM, van den Heuvel-Eibrink MM. Molecular basis of juvenile myelomonocytic leukemia. *Haematologica* **95**: 179–182.
21. Millot F, Traore P, Guilhot J, Nelken B, Leblanc T, Leverger G, Plantaz D, Bertrand Y, Bordigoni P, Guilhot F. (2005) Clinical and biological features at diagnosis in 40 children with chronic myeloid leukemia. *Pediatrics* **116**: 140–143.
26. Hughes T, Deininger M, Hochhaus A, Branford S, Radich J, Kaeda J, Baccarani M, Cortes J, Cross NC, Druker BJ, Gabert J, Grimwade D, Hehlmann R, Kamel-Reid S, Lipton JH, Longtine J, Martinelli G, Saglio G, Soverini S, Stock W, Goldman JM. (2006) Monitoring CML patients responding to treatment with tyrosine kinase inhibitors: Review and recommendations for harmonizing current methodology for detecting BCR-ABL transcripts and kinase domain mutations and for expressing results. *Blood* **108**: 28–37.
32. Teofili L, Giona F, Martini M, Cenci T, Guidi F, Torti L, Palumbo G, Amendola A, Foa R, Larocca LM. (2007) Markers of myeloproliferative diseases in childhood polycythemia vera and essential thrombocythemia. *J Clin Oncol* **25**: 1048–1053.
37. Thiele J. (2009) Philadelphia chromosome-negative chronic myeloproliferative disease. *Am J Clin Pathol* **132**: 261–280.
43. Uzzaman A, Maric I, Noel P, Kettelhut BV, Metcalfe DD, Carter MC. (2009) Pediatric-onset mastocytosis: A long term clinical follow-up and correlation with bone marrow histopathology. *Pediatr Blood Cancer* **53**: 629–634.
44. Bodemer C, Hermine O, Palmerini F, Yang Y, Grandpeix-Guyodo C, Leventhal PS, Hadj-Rabia S, Nasca L, Georgin-Lavialle S, Cohen-Akenine A, Launay JM, Barete S, Feger F, Arock M, Catteau B, Sans B, Stalder JF, Skowron F, Thomas L, Lorette G, Plantin P, Bordigoni P, Lortholary O, de Prost Y, Moussy A, Sobol H, Dubreuil P. (2010) Pediatric mastocytosis is a clonal disease associated with D816V and other activating c-KIT mutations. *J Invest Dermatol* **130**: 804–815.
45. Rubnitz JE, Gibson B, Smith FO. (2008) Acute myeloid leukemia. *Pediatr Clin North Am* **55**: 21–51, ix.
46. Manola KN. (2009) Cytogenetics of pediatric acute myeloid leukemia. *Eur J Haematol* **83**: 391–405.
50. Advani AS, Hunger SP, Burnett AK. (2009) Acute leukemia in adolescents and young adults. *Semin Oncol* **36**: 213–226.
51. Aguilera DG, Vaklavas C, Tsimberidou AM, Wen S, Medeiros LJ, Corey SJ. (2009) Pediatric therapy-related myelodysplastic syndrome/acute myeloid leukemia: The MD Anderson Cancer Center experience. *J Pediatr Hematol Oncol* **31**: 803–811.
52. Cota C, Vale E, Viana I, Requena L, Ferrara G, Anemona L, Metze D, Fink-Puches R, Wiesner T, Cerroni L. (2010) Cutaneous manifestations of blastic plasmacytoid dendritic cell neoplasm-morphologic and

phenotypic variability in a series of 33 patients. *Am J Surg Pathol* **34**: 75–87.

53. Pieters R, Carroll WL. (2010) Biology and treatment of acute lymphoblastic leukemia. *Hematol Oncol Clin North Am* **24**: 1–18.
54. Ribera JM, Oriol A. (2009) Acute lymphoblastic leukemia in adolescents and young adults. *Hematol Oncol Clin North Am* **23**: 1033–1042, vi.
55. Gross TG, Termuhlen AM. (2007) Pediatric non-Hodgkin's lymphoma. *Curr Oncol Rep* **9**: 459–465.
61. Basso G, Case C, Dell'Orto MC. (2007) Diagnosis and genetic subtypes of leukemia combining gene expression and flow cytometry. *Blood Cells Mol Dis* **39**: 164–168.
67. Haferlach T, Bacher U, Kern W, Schnittger S, Haferlach C. (2007) Diagnostic pathways in acute leukemias: A proposal for a multimodal approach. *Ann Hematol* **86**: 311–327.
73. Oschlies I, Klapper W, Zimmermann M, Krams M, Wacker HH, Burkhardt B, Harder L, Siebert R, Reiter A, Parwaresch R. (2006) Diffuse large B-cell lymphoma in pediatric patients belongs predominantly to the germinal-center type B-cell lymphomas: A clinicopathologic analysis of cases included in the German BFM (Berlin-Frankfurt-Munster) Multicenter Trial. *Blood* **107**: 4047–4052.
78. de Leval L, Hasserjian RP. (2009) Diffuse large B-cell lymphomas and burkitt lymphoma. *Hematol Oncol Clin North Am* **23**: 791–827.
82. Poirel HA, Cairo MS, Heerema NA, Swansbury J, Auperin A, Launay E, Sanger WG, Talley P, Perkins SL, Raphael M, McCarthy K, Sposto R, Gerrard M, Bernheim A, Patte C. (2009) Specific cytogenetic abnormalities are associated with a significantly inferior outcome in children and adolescents with mature B-cell non-Hodgkin's lymphoma: Results of the FAB/LMB 96 international study. *Leukemia* **23**: 323–331.
83. Klapper W, Szczepanowski M, Burkhardt B, Berger H, Rosolowski M, Bentink S, Schwaenen C, Wessendorf S, Spang R, Moller P, Hansmann ML, Bernd HW, Ott G, Hummel M, Stein H, Loeffler M, Trumper L, Zimmermann M, Reiter A, Siebert R. (2008) Molecular profiling of pediatric mature B-cell lymphoma treated in population-based prospective clinical trials. *Blood* **112**: 1374–1381.
87. Gualco G, Weiss LM, Harrington WJ Jr., Bacchi CE. (2009) Nodal diffuse large B-cell lymphomas in children and adolescents: Immunohistochemical expression patterns and c-MYC translocation in relation to clinical outcome. *Am J Surg Pathol* **33**: 1815–1822.
92. Calvo KR, Traverse-Glehen A, Pittaluga S, Jaffe ES. (2004) Molecular profiling provides evidence of primary mediastinal large B-cell lymphoma as a distinct entity related to classic Hodgkin lymphoma: Implications for mediastinal gray zone lymphomas as an intermediate form of B-cell lymphoma. *Adv Anat Pathol* **11**: 227–238.
96. Oschlies I, Salaverria I, Mahn F, Meinhardt A, Zimmermann M, Woessmann W, Burkhardt B, Gesk S, Krams M, Reiter A, Siebert R, Klapper W. (2010) Pediatric follicular lymphoma — a clinico-pathological study of a population-based series of patients treated within the Non-Hodgkin's Lymphoma — Berlin-Frankfurt-Munster (NHL-BFM) multicenter trials. *Haematologica* **95**: 253–259.
101. Kussick SJ, Kalnoski M, Braziel RM, Wood BL. (2004) Prominent clonal B-cell populations identified by flow cytometry in histologically reactive lymphoid proliferations. *Am J Clin Pathol* **121**: 464–472.
102. Taddesse-Heath L, Pittaluga S, Sorbara L, Bussey M, Raffeld M, Jaffe ES. (2003) Marginal zone B-cell lymphoma in children and young adults. *Am J Surg Pathol* **27**: 522–531.
103. Rizzo KA, Streubel B, Pittaluga S, Chott A, Xi L, Raffeld M, Jaffe ES. (2010) Marginal zone lymphomas in children and the young adult population; characterization of genetic aberrations by FISH and RT-PCR. *Mod Pathol* **23**: 866–873.
107. Traverse-Glehen A, Pittaluga S, Gaulard P, Sorbara L, Alonso MA, Raffeld M, Jaffe ES. (2005) Mediastinal gray zone lymphoma: The missing link between classic Hodgkin's lymphoma and mediastinal large B-cell lymphoma. *Am J Surg Pathol* **29**: 1411–1421.
112. Hutchison RE, Laver JH, Chang M, Muzzafar T, Desai S, Murphy S, Schwenn M, Shuster J, Link MP. (2008) Non-anaplastic peripheral T-cell lymphoma in childhood and adolescence: A Children's Oncology Group study. *Pediatr Blood Cancer* **51**: 29–33.
116. Perkins SL, Pickering D, Lowe EJ, Zwick D, Abromowitch M, Davenport G, Cairo MS, Sanger WG. (2005) Childhood anaplastic large cell lymphoma has a high incidence of ALK gene rearrangement as determined by immunohistochemical staining and fluorescent in situ hybridisation: A genetic and pathological correlation. *Br J Haematol* **131**: 624–627.
117. d'Amore ES, Menin A, Bonoldi E, Bevilacqua P, Cazzavillan S, Donofrio V, Gambini C, Forni M, Gentile A, Magro G, Boldrini R, Pillon M, Rosolen A, Alaggio R. (2007) Anaplastic large cell lymphomas: A study of 75 pediatric patients. *Pediatr Dev Pathol* **10**: 181–191.

120. Mussolin L, Pillon M, d'Amore ES, Santoro N, Lombardi A, Fagioli F, Zanesco L, Rosolen A. (2005) Prevalence and clinical implications of bone marrow involvement in pediatric anaplastic large cell lymphoma. *Leukemia* **19**: 1643–1647.
121. Damm-Welk C, Busch K, Burkhardt B, Schieferstein J, Viehmann S, Oschlies I, Klapper W, Zimmermann M, Harbott J, Reiter A, Woessmann W. (2007) Prognostic significance of circulating tumor cells in bone marrow or peripheral blood as detected by qualitative and quantitative PCR in pediatric NPM-ALK-positive anaplastic large-cell lymphoma. *Blood* **110**: 670–677.
125. Falini B, Bigerna B, Fizzotti M, Pulford K, Pileri SA, Delsol G, Carbone A, Paulli M, Magrini U, Menestrina F, Giardini R, Pilotti S, Mezzelani A, Ugolini B, Billi M, Pucciarini A, Pacini R, Pelicci PG, Flenghi L. (1998) ALK expression defines a distinct group of T/null lymphomas ("ALK lymphomas") with a wide morphological spectrum. *Am J Pathol* **153**: 875–886.
138. Vergier B, Beylot-Barry M, Pulford K, Michel P, Bosq J, de Muret A, Beylot C, Delaunay MM, Avril MF, Dalac S, Bodemer C, Joly P, Groppi A, de Mascarel A, Bagot M, Mason DY, Wechsler J, Merlio JP. (1998) Statistical evaluation of diagnostic and prognostic features of CD30+ cutaneous lymphoproliferative disorders: A clinicopathologic study of 65 cases. *Am J Surg Pathol* **22**: 1192–1202.
143. Nijsten T, Curiel-Lewandrowski C, Kadin ME. (2004) Lymphomatoid papulosis in children: A retrospective cohort study of 35 cases. *Arch Dermatol* **140**: 306–312.
151. Fink-Puches R, Chott A, Ardigo M, Simonitsch I, Ferrara G, Kerl H, Cerroni L. (2004) The spectrum of cutaneous lymphomas in patients less than 20 years of age. *Pediatr Dermatol* **21**: 525–533.
152. Ree HJ, Kadin ME, Kikuchi M, Ko YH, Go JH, Suzumiya J, Kim DS. (1998) Angioimmunoblastic lymphoma (AILD-type T-cell lymphoma) with hyperplastic germinal centers. *Am J Surg Pathol* **22**: 643–655.
159. Mackey AC, Green L, Leptak C, Avigan M. (2009) Hepatosplenic T-cell lymphoma associated with infliximab use in young patients treated for inflammatory bowel disease: Update. *J Pediatr Gastroenterol Nutr* **48**: 386–388.
168. Park S, Kim K, Kim WS, Yoo KH, Koo HH, Ko YH. (2008) Systemic EBV+ T-cell lymphoma in elderly patients: Comparison with children and young adult patients. *Virchows Arch* **453**: 155–163.
171. Feng S, Jin P, Zeng X. (2008) Hydroa vacciniforme-like primary cutaneous CD8-positive T-cell lymphoma. *Eur J Dermatol* **18**: 364–365.
175. Parveen Z, Thompson K. (2009) Subcutaneous panniculitis-like T-cell lymphoma: Redefinition of diagnostic criteria in the recent World Health Organization-European Organization for Research and Treatment of Cancer classification for cutaneous lymphomas. *Arch Pathol Lab Med* **133**: 303–308.
181. Falcao RP, Rizzatti EG, Saggioro FP, Garcia AB, Marinato AF, Rego EM. (2007) Flow cytometry characterization of leukemic phase of nasal NK/T-cell lymphoma in tumor biopsies and peripheral blood. *Haematologica* **92**: e24–e25.
184. Nogova L, Reineke T, Brillant C, Sieniawski M, Rudiger T, Josting A, Bredenfeld H, Skripnitchenko R, Muller RP, Muller-Hermelink HK, Diehl V, Engert A. (2008) Lymphocyte-predominant and classical Hodgkin's lymphoma: A comprehensive analysis from the German Hodgkin Study Group. *J Clin Oncol* **26**: 434–439.

5

Cytogenetics in Children, Adolescents and Young Adults with ALL and AML

Susana C. Raimondi and Nyla A. Heerema

Introduction

Cytogenetics is the study of chromosomes, the carriers of DNA in the cell nucleus. The chromosomes are frequently abnormal in malignant cells, and these abnormalities may be diagnostic and prognostic and may predict response to specific treatments. They reflect the genetic abnormalities that contribute to the malignant phenotype, and they may be used for treatment assignment. The abnormalities are acquired and are found only in the malignant cells; therefore, it is important that disease cells be used for analysis. In acute lymphoblastic leukemia (ALL), approximately 80% of cases have abnormalities that can be detected by metaphase analysis at diagnosis, and in acute myeloid leukemias (AML), the abnormality detection rate is approximately 80% in children and 60% in adults.

Cytogenetic analyses have become part of the standard diagnostic approach to pediatric and adult patients suspected of having acute leukemia, allowing the distinction, at the microscopic level, of specific subtypes of disease with different prognoses. However, an accurate cytogenetic diagnosis depends on the presence of dividing cells from the abnormal cell population, chromosome morphology, and banding resolution. Fluorescence *in situ* hybridization (FISH) is a complementary method that evaluates a known or suspected chromosomal aberration in leukemic cells. For clinical purposes, several methods are currently being used to detect chromosomal rearrangements, including conventional cytogenetics, FISH, and reverse transcriptase polymerase chain reaction (RT-PCR). There is correlation among these methods; however, in some instances, FISH and RT-PCR are more sensitive than G-banding due to the presence of subtle or cryptic rearrangements that cannot be detected microscopically. Of note, a disadvantage of RT-PCR is that the primers used must cover all the variant breakpoints generated by each particular translocation.

The tissue of choice for cytogenetic analysis of acute leukemias is the bone marrow, either part of the first draw or from a repositioned needle. This is because blood may dilute subsequent samples, and an accurate analysis may not be possible. A peripheral blood sample may be used if there are ≥ 15% blasts in the periphery; however, a normal result in the periphery may not reflect normal bone marrow, because the dividing cells may be reactive rather than malignant. Cytogenetic laboratories typically culture direct or 24-hour unstimulated cultures, fix and band the cells with standard procedures, completely analyze 20 cells, and prepare karyograms of the abnormal clones (Figs. 5.1A–B).

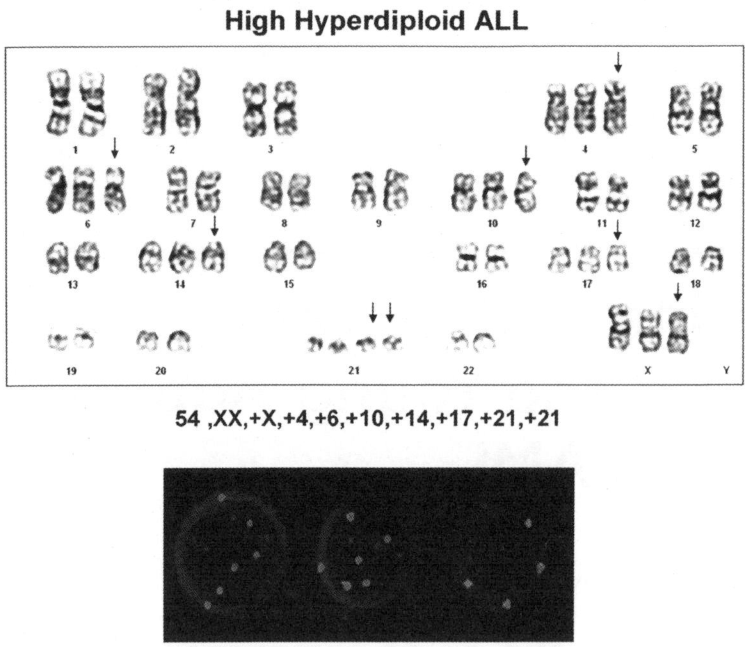

Fig. 5.1. (A) Upper: Karyogram of high hyperdiploid acute lymphoblastic leukemic cell. Lower: FISH showing triple trisomy (left and center cells) using centromere probes (Abbott Molecular) for chromosomes 4 (red), 10 (green) and 17 (aqua). The cell on the right is normal.

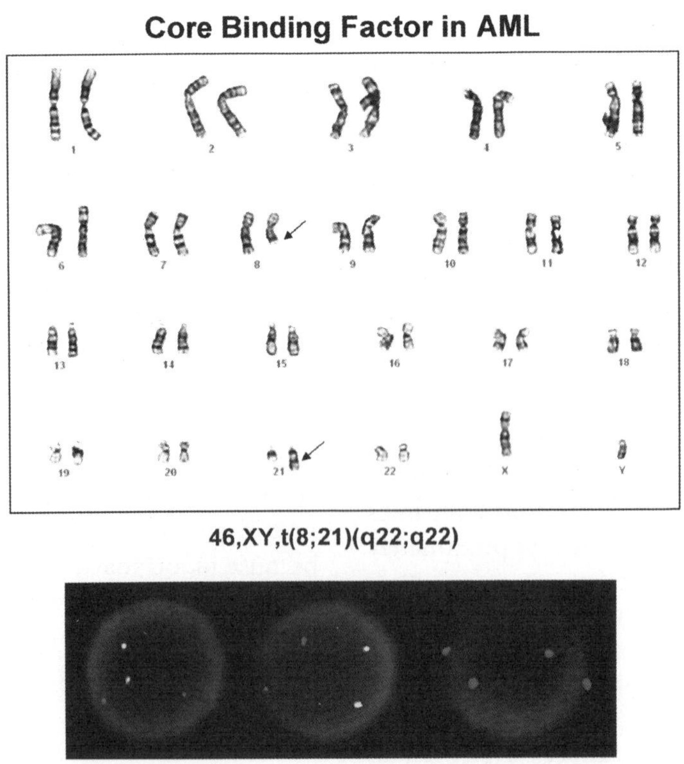

Fig. 5.1. (B) Upper: Karyogram of t(8;21) core binding factor acute myeloid leukemia cell. Lower: FISH with dual fusion *ETO-AML1* probes (Abbott Molecular) showing dual fusion (left and center cells). The cell on the right is normal.

Many genetic lesions are frequently required for a cell to become overtly malignant. These changes occur primarily in pathways controlling cell cycle regulation, cell differentiation and cell death, and cytogenetic aberrations often alter genes in such pathways. Other genetic lesions are cryptic (not visible) cytogenetically, usually because they are below the limit of cytogenetic resolution (~2 Mb).

This chapter will highlight the conventional and molecular cytogenetic findings that may alter clinical outcome, but the discussion of genetic lesions will be limited unless there is a strong association with a specific cytogenetic subgroup.

Cytogenetics of Acute Lymphoblastic Leukemia

For more than 30 years, cytogenetic abnormalities in ALL have been recognized to have prognostic significance and are still being used to direct patients' therapies. Pediatric ALL has an excellent prognosis, with more than 80% of children predicted to be cured of their disease.[1,2] Adult ALL does not share this good prognosis, and less than 45% are expected to be cured.[1,3] Adolescents and young adult (AYA, defined herein as 15–30 years old) ALL have a prognosis that falls between those of pediatric and adult patients.[4] This difference probably results from several factors, such as treatment, sociological factors, and the genetics of the disease. More than 50% of pediatric patients have relatively good genetic prognostic features, whereas very few adults have these features. Conversely, a large proportion of adults have poor genetic prognostic features. The cytogenetic features of AYA with ALL have not been uniquely described.

For this chapter, to investigate whether the cytogenetics of ALL in AYA contribute to their worse outcome, the incidence of various cytogenetic abnormalities in children 1–14 years old with ALL was compared with those of AYA with ALL in the Children's Oncology Group (COG) cytogenetic database. Infants younger than 12 months were not included because their cytogenetics differ from those of children 1–14 years old and AYA. The database was divided into B-cell precursor (BCP) cases and T-cell (T-ALL) cases because the cytogenetics of these lineages differ. There were 7975 cases, 7365 BCP and 610 T-ALL. Of the BCP patients, 6642 (90.2%) were 1–14 years old, and 723 (9.8%) were AYA. Of the T-lineage patients, 500 (82.0%) were 1–14 years old, and 110 (18.0%) were AYA. Cytogenetic results were accepted in 6435 (87.3%) BCP patients; of those, 5849 (90.7%) were 1–14 years old, and 586 (9.3%) were AYA. In the T-ALL patients, 486 (79.7%) had accepted cytogenetics; of those, 394 (82.0%) were 1–14 years old, and 92 (18.0%) were AYA. Thus, AYA were represented more frequently in T-ALL than in BCP ALL (18.9% vs 9.3%).

The cytogenetic features of ALL that contribute to its biology, prognosis, and treatment risk assignment include both numerical and structural aberrations. Prognostic implications of both the numerical and structural aberrations have long been recognized, and many have maintained their significance. What are these genetic features, and how do the genetics of AYA compare with those of pediatric and adult patients?

B-cell precursor ALL

The significance of normal chromosomes in ALL is not known, and these cases probably have cryptic abnormalities not detectable by cytogenetics or only normal cells were analyzed. Only normal chromosomes were found in 9.0% of BCP ALL: 8.2% of 1- to 14-year-olds and 17.7% of AYA.

Numerical abnormalities

Numerical aberrations are defined by the modal number, which, for these analyses, was defined as the number of chromosomes in the simplest abnormal clone (See Fig. 5.2A for comparisons of modal numbers in BCP ALL between 1- to 14-year-olds and AYA). Hyperdiploidy with more than 50 chromosomes (Fig. 5.1A, Table 5.1), specifically 51–67 chromosomes, called high hyperdiploidy (HH), has long been recognized as indicative of a good prognosis.[5] Interestingly, the extra chromosomes present in HH ALL are not random, with chromosomes X, 4, 6, 10, 14, 17, 18, and 21 found in extra copy numbers most often.[6] Several groups have defined specific extra chromosomes as having prognostic significance. The COG showed that trisomies of chromosomes 4, 10, and 17 (triple trisomy [TT]) were the significant indicators of a good prognosis.[6] The Medical Research Council (MRC) of the United Kingdom described trisomies of chromosomes 10 and 18 as having a significant effect on prognosis.[7] The frequency of HH in adults is much lower, only 2–11%,[8] and the frequencies and prognostic significance of specific extra chromosomes in adults have not been studied (Fig. 5.3A). We compared the frequencies of HH and of TT in COG patients 1–14 years old with

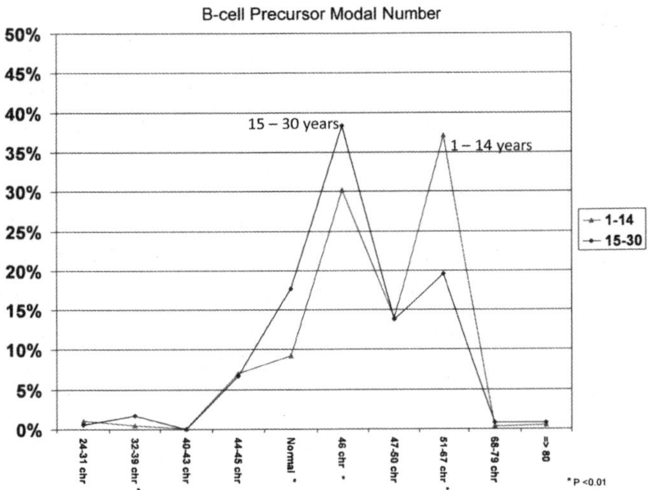

Fig. 5.2. (A) Comparisons of frequencies of modal numbers in Children's Oncology Group B-cell precursor acute lymphoblastic leukemia patients age 1–14 years old and AYA. Asterisks (*) indicate differences that are significant at $p < 0.01$.

those in AYA. HH was found in 37.1% of children 1–14 years old, and 16.6% had TT. In contrast, 19.6% of AYA had HH, and 8.5% had TT (Fig. 5.2A, Table 5.1). This has been reported in other series as well.[9] Thus, the frequency of HH, a good prognostic feature, in AYA falls between those of children and adults. Furthermore, the frequency of TT is much lower in AYA than in children 1–14 years old. Approximately 50% of HH cases have structural abnormalities; the most common is a duplication of chromosome arm 1q, which does not have prognostic significance. Few of the cases have other recurring structural abnormalities, with the exception of a der(19)t(1;19)(q23;p13.3).

Low hyperdiploidy (LH), defined as 47–50 chromosomes, occurs in similar frequencies in children 1–14 years old and AYA (14.0% and 13.8%, respectively, Fig. 5.2A, Table 5.1). A similar frequency (10–15%) has been reported for adult patients with ALL.[8] Children with LH frequently also have a structural abnormality, and their prognosis is correlated with the structural abnormality. Patients with LH who do not have a recurring structural abnormality have an intermediate prognosis.[10]

Near-triploidy (68–79 chromosomes) and near-tetraploidy (≥80 chromosomes) are found in less than 1% of pediatric cases, but in approximately 5% of adult ALL.[8] The outcome for these patients is not well defined, probably because they are diverse and few in number. In the COG study, only 0.3% of cases were near-triploid and 0.5% near-tetraploid. Near-triploidy was found in 0.3% of patients 1–14 years old and in 0.8% of AYA. Near-tetraploidy was found in 0.5% of patients 1–14 years old and in 0.8% of AYA (Fig. 5.2A, Table 5.1).

Hypodiploidy is defined as fewer than 46 chromosomes. It can be further differentiated by modal numbers. Pediatric cases with 44 or 45 chromosomes have an intermediate prognosis.[11] However, children with 43 or fewer chromosomes have a very poor outcome.[11] Cases with 39 and fewer chromosomes, particularly those with fewer than 30 chromosomes, frequently have a doubled hypodiploid clone. This can be difficult to recognize because the cytogenetics appear to be hyperdiploid. However, the chromosomes generally will be present in

Table 5.1. Frequencies of numerical abnormalities in B-cell precursor acute lymphoblastic leukemia patients 1–14 years old compared with adolescents and young adults.[a]

			Frequency %	
		Modal number	**1–14 years old**	**15–30 years old**
Hypodiploidy	Near haploidy	24–31 chr	1.1	0.6
	Low hypodiploidy	32–39 chr	0.5	1.7
		40–43 chr	0.1	0.0
		44–45 chr	7.0	6.7
Normal		Normal	9.2	17.7
Pseudodiploidy		46 chr	30.2	38.3
Hyperdiploidy	Low hyperdiploidy	47–50 chr	14.0	13.8
	High hyperdiploidy	51–67 chr	37.1	19.6
	Near triploidy	68–79 chr	0.3	0.8
	Near tetraploidy	=> 80 chr	0.5	0.8
	Hyperdiploid karyotypes with +4, + 10, +17		16.6	8.5

[a] Data from the Children's Oncology Group Database

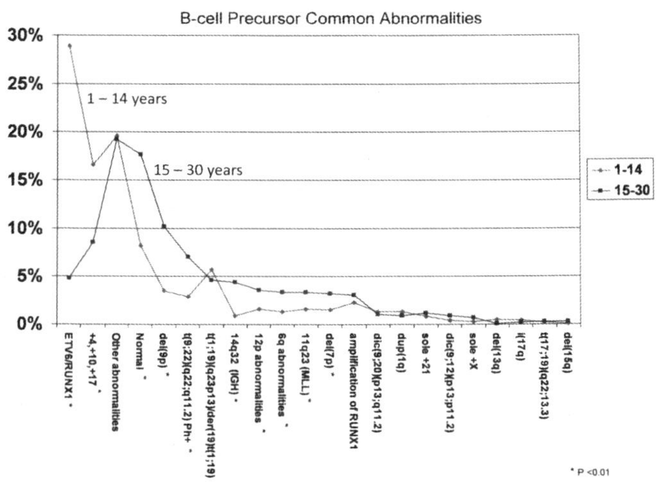

Fig. 5.2. (B) Comparisons of frequencies of common abnormalities in Children's Oncology Group B-cell precursor acute lymphoblastic leukemia patients age 1–14 years old and AYA. Asterisks (*) indicate differences that are significant at $p < 0.01$.

two and four copies, as opposed to the usual three copies present in HH. DNA analysis for microsatellite differences between alleles may be necessary to confirm a hypodiploid clone.[12] Only numerical aberrations are found in approximately 40% of these cases.[11] Conversely, most cases with 40–43 chromosomes do not have doubling of the hypodiploid clone, but they do have structural abnormalities in approximately 90% of cases. Although prognostically significant, hypodiploidy with < 44 chromosomes is rare, occurring in only 1.7% of the current COG studies, 1.7% of patients 1–14 years old and 2.3% of AYA (Fig. 5.2A, Table 5.1).

Pseudodiploidy is defined as 46 chromosomes, but with an abnormality that is usually, although not always, a structural abnormality. The prognostic significance of many of these structural abnormalities has been defined. The same abnormalities may occur in cases with other modal numbers, particularly LH, in which case the prognosis is associated with the structural abnormality.

Structural abnormalities (See Table 5.2 for a summary of BCP ALL structural abnormalities)

A specific structural genetic abnormality associated with a good prognosis in pediatric BCP ALL is t(12;21)(p13;q22), which is cryptic cytogenetically and must be detected by FISH or other molecular techniques such as RT-PCR. The aberration results in an *ETV6-RUNX1* (formerly *TEL-AML1*) fusion gene. It

Table 5.2. Frequencies of structural abnormalities in B-cell precursor acute lymphoblastic leukemia patients 1–14 years old compared with adolescents and young adults.[a]

	Frequency %	
Abnormality	**1–14 years old**	**15–30 years old**
amplification of *RUNX1*	2.3	3.1
ETV6-RUNX1	28.9	4.8
11q23 (*MLL*)	1.6	3.4
t(9;22)(q22;q11.2) Ph+	2.9	7.0
t(1;19)(q23p13)/der(19)t(1;19)	5.7	4.6
del(9p)[2]	3.5	10.2
dic(9;20)(p13;q11.2)[2]	1.3	1.0
14q32 (*IGH*)	0.9	4.4
12p abnormalities	1.6	3.6
6q abnormalities	1.3	3.4
del(7p)	1.5	3.2
dup(1q)	1.3	0.9
sole +21	0.8	1.2
dic(9;12)(p13;p11.2)[b]	0.4	0.9
sole +X	0.3	0.7
del(13q)	0.5	0.1
i(17q)	0.4	0.2
t(17;19)(q22;13.3)	0.2	0.3
del(15q)	0.1	0.3

[a] Data from the Children's Oncology Group Database
[b] All result in loss of 9p

was found in 26.7% of COG cases with BCP ALL (Figs. 5.2B and 5.3A, Table 5.2), but it occurs rarely in adults (< 1%) and then only in young adults (< 30 years old).[13] In the present evaluation of the COG database, children 1–14 years old had a 28.9% incidence of an *ETV6-RUNX1* rearrangement, whereas AYA had only a 4.8% frequency of this aberration (Figs. 5.2B and 5.3A). A very low frequency of *ETV6-RUNX1* cases are near-tetraploid with doubling of the aberration. The *ETV6-RUNX1* fusion occurs prenatally and is thought to be an "initiating mutation"; it initiates but is insufficient in itself to cause leukemia, and additional mutations are required for overt leukemia.[1] Loss of *ETV6* is a frequent secondary abnormality and is often, although not always, cytogenetically visible.

Amplification of a region of chromosome 21 that includes the *RUNX1* gene has been described in patients with ALL. In pediatric ALL, it has been associated with older age, a low white blood cell count, and a poor outcome.[14] Amplification of *RUNX1* does not appear to occur in adult ALL.[15] This aberration can be reliably detected by FISH with *ETV6-RUNX1* probes. It is usually present as a homogeneously staining region on an abnormal chromosome 21. By definition, three extra copies of *RUNX1* on a single chromosome are required to confirm this abnormality.[14] In the COG database, amp(*RUNX1*) was present in 2.3% of patients 1–14 years old and 3.1% of AYA (Fig. 5.2B, Table 5.2); with an average age of 9, confirming that it is more frequent in older children. Although the region invariably contains *RUNX1*, it is not known if this is the significant gene, because it has not been shown to be overexpressed in these cases.[14]

Rearrangements of chromosome band 11q23 are recurrent in ALL. They usually, although not always, involve the *MLL* gene. *MLL* rearranges with many partners and rearranges in both ALL and AML. Some partners occur in both ALL and AML, some are specific to AML, and some to ALL. A t(4;11)(q21;q23) is specific to ALL and is especially frequent in infants younger than 1 year at diagnosis. The t(11;19)(q23;p13.3) and t(9;11)(p22;q23) aberrations occur in both ALL and AML. *MLL* rearrangements are indicative of a poor outcome in ALL, although there may be a difference in outcome depending on the patient's age. Infants do very poorly, with children over 1 year old doing somewhat better but still with a poor outcome, especially for those with t(4;11) or t(9;11).[16] In the BCP COG patients, 1.7% of patients 1–14 years old and 3.4% of AYA had an *MLL* rearrangement at diagnosis (Figs. 5.2B and 5.3A, Table 5.2). *MLL* rearrangements also occur in 10% of adults with ALL, a somewhat higher frequency, where they also are associated with a poor outcome.[1]

Interestingly, it has been shown that *MLL* rearrangements occur *in utero*, at least for cases that occur in infants and young children.[1] Whether these rearrangements in ALL in AYA also occur prenatally is unknown, although some patients with confirmed prenatal origin have been older than 10 years. Additionally, some *MLL* rearrangements in AML, which typically presents in young adults (20–40 years), have been shown to occur prenatally.[10] Since these and other abnormalities occur prenatally, yet leukemia usually occurs much later, most if not all of the primary (initiating) abnormalities found in ALL are insufficient to cause disease, and additional mutations are required for overt leukemia.[1]

The Philadelphia chromosome (Ph) is the abnormal chromosome 22 that results from a t(9;22)(q34;q11.2). It encodes a chimeric oncogene, *BCR-ABL1*, and the resulting protein is necessary for leukemogenesis. The cytogenetic abnormality is identical to the abnormality present in chronic myeloid leukemia (CML). However, at the molecular level, the rearrangement results in a 190-kD protein in children with ALL (frequency, 5%) and in half of adults with ALL (frequency, 25%), whereas in most patients with CML and some adult ALL, a 210-kD protein is produced. Nevertheless, no clinical differences have been observed in adults with ALL with the two different rearrangements.[17] The molecular rearrangement in AYA has not been described.

Until recently, the presence of a Ph was a very poor prognostic indicator in ALL.[18] The incorporation of kinase inhibitors as a part of treatment for Ph+ ALL has favorably changed outcome for these patients. In COG Ph+ ALL patients ages 1.3 to 21 years (median, 10 years), there was no significant difference in 3-year event-free survival (EFS) between patients with continuous treatment with chemotherapy plus imatinib mesylate (a tyrosine kinase inhibitor) and those who had a matched sibling bone marrow transplant, and outcome was significantly better than that of Ph+ historical controls.[19] In the COG database, a Ph chromosome occurred in 2.9% of patients 1–14 years old and 7.0% of AYA (Figs. 5.2B and 5.3A, Table 5.2).

A t(1;19)(q23;p13.3) is a recurring aberration in BCP ALL with a pre-B phenotype. It results in a chimeric oncogene, *TCF3(E2A)-PBX1*, which is a potent transcriptional activator.[20] The aberration occurs both as a balanced rearrangement and an unbalanced der(19)t(1;19).

Some cases with a der(19)t(1;19) are also hyperdiploid and have a *TCF3-PBX1* rearrangement, while other hyperdiploid der(19)t(1;19) cases do not, thus molecular studies are required to establish the molecular basis of the aberration. Early reports indicated a poor outcome for these cases, but recent studies show an intermediate outcome with current intensive therapies. The t(1;19) is found in 2–3% of adult ALL.[8] The frequencies of t(1;19) in the COG database for patients age 1–14 years old and AYA are 5.7% and 4.6%, respectively (Fig. 5.2B, Table 5.2).

Another frequent aberration in ALL is a deletion of 9p, although its frequency is difficult to establish because it is often cryptic. It results in loss of the *INK4a-ARF* locus, which encodes p16INK4A, p14ARF, and p15INK4B. It is seen in both BCP ALL and T-ALL. The frequencies of cases with a karyotypic deletion or loss of 9p in the COG database for patients age 1–14 and AYA are 5.2% and 12.1%, respectively (Fig. 5.2B, Table 5.2). The prognostic significance of del(9p) in BCP ALL has been controversial.[21]

Cytogenetically, many different structural aberrations occur involving 9p (Fig. 5.2B, Table 5.2). Dicentric chromosomes are common in ALL and most frequently involve chromosome 9. The most common are dic(9;12) and dic(9;20). Although dic(9;V) all result in loss of 9p, their clinical significance may be related to the formation of chimeric oncogenes rather than to the loss of genes. Approximately half of dic(9;12) cases result in a *PAX5-ETV6* fusion gene;[22] others have an *EVT6-RUNX1* fusion.[23] In these cases, the genes, if any, involved in the dic(9;12) are not known.[23] The frequencies of cases with a dic(9;12) in the COG database for patients age 1–14 years old and AYA are 0.4% and 0.9%, respectively (Fig. 5.2B, Table 5.2). It is very rare in adult ALL.

The dic(9;20) has a peak incidence at approximately 3 years, and it has a female predominance. The dic(9;20) occurs in approximately 0.5% of adult ALL. The frequencies of cases with a dic(9;20) in the COG database for patients age 1–14 years old and AYA are 1.3% and 1.0%, respectively (Fig. 5.2B, Table 5.2). The molecular breakpoints of both partners of the dic(9;20) are heterogeneous, with some 9p11–13 breakpoints in the repetitive region near the centromere and some involving *PAX5* on 9p; *ASXL1* on 20q is disrupted frequently in this rearrangement.[24]

Rearrangements in 14q32, usually involving the *IGH* gene, are also recurrent in ALL. The t(8;14)(q22;q32) and its variants t(2;8)(p12;q22) and t(8;22)(q22;q11.2) occur in B-cell ALL, namely Burkitt leukemia. Children with this aberration are not considered BCP ALL patients in the COG but are classified as having Burkitt leukemia.

Other 14q32 rearrangements occur in BCP ALL. The frequencies of cases with 14q32 rearrangements other than a Burkitt rearrangement in the COG database for patients age 1–14 years old and AYA are 0.9% and 4.4%, respectively (Fig. 5.2B, Table 5.2). These findings confirm that *IGH* rearrangements are more common in older pediatric patients.[14] A recurrent *IGH* aberration is t(8;14)(q11.2;q34). It is especially frequent in children with Down syndrome (DS) and ALL, who have an excellent prognosis.[25] It was present in 0.2% of 1- to 14-year-olds and 1.4% of AYA. A t(14;19)(q32;q13) is an additional recurrent *IGH* rearrangement in ALL. It involves the *CEBPA* gene, which is overexpressed as a result of the translocation; other *CEBP* gene family members also rearrange with *IGH* and are overexpressed in some BCP ALL. A cryptic t(X or Y;14)(pter;q32) or del(X or Y)(pter) has been described recently. The X or Y gene is *CRLF2*, which is on the pseudoautosomal region of X and Y. The gene is overexpressed either as a result of its juxtaposition to *IGH* or resulting from the deletion, which juxtaposes its coding region with *P2RY8*. The deletion is particularly common in children with DS.[26]

In summary, the frequencies of "good risk" cytogenetics BCP ALL (HH and *ETV6-RUNX1* rearrangements) in the COG database for patients age 1–14 and AYA are 66.0% and 24.4%, respectively. Conversely, the frequencies of "poor risk" cytogenetics in BCP ALL (Ph+, *MLL* rearrangements, and <44 chromosomes) for patients age 1–14 years old and AYA are 6.2% and 12.7%, respectively (Fig. 5.3A). These results indicate that one factor contributing to the poorer outcome of BCP ALL in AYA than in patients 1–14 years old is the genetics of the disease.

T-cell ALL

T-ALL is distinct from BCP ALL. It accounts for approximately 15% of pediatric ALL and 25% of adult ALL.[27] Outcome and treatment differ for children with T-ALL compared with BCP ALL. The overall survival for pediatric T-ALL is 80–85%, while for adults it is less than 50%. Cytogenetically, some of the same aberrations occur in BCP and T-ALL, but some are unique to each subgroup. Cytogenetic aberrations are not known to contribute significantly to outcome in pediatric T-ALL. As the T-ALL COG study started much later than the BCP ALL COG studies, their relative frequencies within the database have not yet been determined.

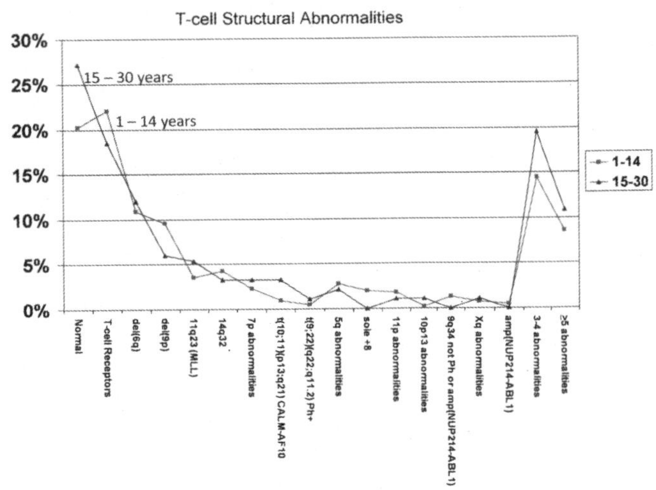

Fig. 5.2. (C) Comparisons of frequencies of cytogenetic abnormalities in Children's Oncology Group T-cell acute lymphoblastic leukemia patients age 1–14 years old and AYA. None of the differences was significant.

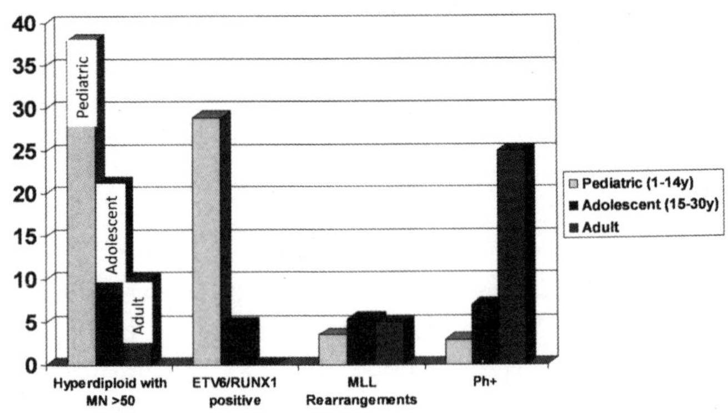

Fig. 5.3. (A) Comparisons of frequencies of prognostically significant aberrations among patients 1–14 years old, AYA, and adults with B-cell precursor acute lymphoblastic leukemia. Fewer adults and more children have favorable cytogenetic abnormalities (hyperdiploidy and *ETV6-RUNX1* rearrangements) and fewer children and more adults have the unfavorable Philadelphia chromosome abnormality. Frequencies of adolescents with these abnormalities are between children and adults. The frequencies of *MLL* rearrangements do not appear to differ in the different age groups.

The COG database for T-ALL is much smaller than that for BCP ALL. The frequency of normal analyses in T-ALL is much higher than in BCP ALL. Of the 486 accepted COG T-ALL cases, 105 (20.3%) had normal analyses, accounting for 20.3% of patients 1–14 years old and 27.2% of AYA. (See Figs. 5.2C, 5.3B and Table 5.3 for comparisons of frequencies of cytogenetic aberrations in

Table 5.3. Frequencies of abnormalities in T-cell acute lymphoblastic leukemia patients 1–14 years old compared with adolescents and young adults.[a]

	Frequency %	
	1–14 years old	**15–30 years old**
Unknown prognosis		
24–31chr	0.0	0.0
32–39 chr	0.0	0.0
40–43 chr	0.0	0.0
44–45 chr	1.0	2.2
46 chr	6.9	5.4
47–50 chr	4.8	4.4
51–67 chr	1.0	2.2
68–79 chr	0.0	0.0
≥ 80	0.5	0.0
Normal	20.3	27.2
7p other	2.3	3.3
t(9;12)(p24;p13)	0.0	0.0
t(9;12)(q34;p13)	0.0	0.0
9q34 other	1.3	0.0
10p13 other	1.5	0.0
11p abnormalities	1.8	1.1
t(9;14)(q34;q32)	0.0	0.0
14q32 other	2.3	2.2
10q23.31 abnormalities	0.0	0.0
Xq abnormalities	0.8	1.1
5q abnormalities	2.8	2.2
del(9)(p13-p22)	9.6	6.5
+8 sole abnormality	2.0	0.0
6q-	10.9	12.0
Total	**69.8**	**69.8**
Not prognostically significant		
t(14;21)(q11.2;q22)	0.3	0.0
t(1;7)(p34;q34)	0.0	1.1
t(7;9)(q34;q32)	0.2	0.0
t(7;9)(q34;q34)	0.0	0.0
t(7;12)(q34;p13)	0.0	0.0
t(7;19)(q34;p13)	0.0	0.0
7p15	1.5	2.2
7q34 other	3.0	5.4
inv(14)	0.5	1.1
14q11.2 other	3.5	1.1
t(6;7)(q23;q34)	0.8	0.0
inv(7)(p15q34)	1.3	0.0
t(11;14)(p13;q11.2)	6.9	2.2
t(11;14)(p15;q11.2)	0.8	0.0
Total	**18.8**	**13.1**
Poor prognosis		
t(9;22)(q34;q11.2)	0.5	1.1
amp(NUP214/ABL1)	0.5	0.0
t(10;11)(p12;q14)	0.5	1.1
t(10;11)(p13;q21)	1.0	3.3

(*Continued*)

Table 5.3. (***Continued***)

	Frequency %	
	1–14 years old	**15–30 years old**
t(6;11)(q27;q23)	1.5	2.2
t(X;11)(q13;q23)	0.0	1.1
11q23 other	0.3	0.0
t(5;14)(q35;q32)	2.0	1.1
Total	**6.3**	**9.9**
Good prognosis		
t(1;14)(p32;q11.2)	2.0	2.2
t(10;14)(q24;q11.2)	1.3	3.3
t(11;19)(q23;p13.3)	1.8	2.2
Total	**5.1**	**7.7**

[a] Data from the Children's Oncology Group Database

T-ALL patients age 1–14 years old and AYA. Many of these aberrations are not discussed, as their frequencies are low and their prognostic significance unknown.) This may result from many cryptic cytogenetic aberrations in T-ALL that requires FISH or another molecular method for detection. Ploidy is not a significant factor in T-ALL, with few HH cases (6 in the COG database) and very few cases with < 44 chromosomes (none in the COG database).

The most frequent aberrations in T-ALL are rearrangements with breakpoints at the T-cell receptor (TCR) loci, 14q11.2 (*TCRA/D*), 7q34 (*TCRB*), and 7p15 (*TCRG*). Rearrangements with any of these TCRs result in an oncogene fused to the TCR; the oncogene is overexpressed as it comes under the promoter and enhancer elements of the TCR.[14] Aberrations involving the TCR in the COG T-ALL patients 1–14 years old and AYA T-ALL occurred in 22.3% and 18.6%, respectively (Fig. 5.2C, Table 5.3).

One TCR rearrangement of note, t(1;14)(p32;q11.2), results in the juxtaposition of *TAL1* and *TCRD*. A t(1;14) was found in 2.0% of COG patients 1–14 years old and 2.2% of AYA; it has been reported in 3% of adult T-ALL. However, a cryptic deletion of chromosome 1 resulting in a *TAL1-SIL* fusion is common and has been reported in 15–25% of T-ALL.[28] This deletion can be detected using FISH. *TAL1* is overexpressed, both in cases with a *TAL1-TCRD* rearrangement and in those with *TAL1-SIL* fusion.

A second *TCR* rearrangement that occurs fairly frequently in T-ALL is t(11;14)(p13;q11.2). The gene on chromosome 11p13 is *LMO2*. This aberration was found in 6.9% of COG patients 1–14 years old and 2.2% of AYA. It results in the overexpression of *LMO2*. Overexpression of *LMO2* also results from a cryptic deletion of 11p.[14]

TLX (formerly *HOX*) genes are frequently deregulated in T-ALL, often by rearrangement. They are homeobox genes and are involved in both organismal and hematopoietic differentiation. The rearrangements (10;14)(q24;q11.2) and t(7;10)(q34;q24) result in overexpression of *TLX1*(*HOX11*) and are associated with a good prognosis. However, many T-ALL cases have overexpression of *TLX1* without one of these translocations,[29] and they also have a good prognosis (Table 5.3). *TLX3*(*HOX11A2*) also may be overexpressed in T-ALL, typically as a result of the cryptic translocation t(5;14)(q35;q32) (Table 5.3). The 14q32 gene in this rearrangement is *BCL11B*. Interestingly, although the t(5;14) is cryptic, most of these cases have cytogenetically detectable 5q aberrations.[14]

Deletions of 9p are also very frequent cytogenetic abnormalities in T-ALL (cytogenetically detected in 9.4% of T-ALL COG cases, Fig. 5.2C, Table 5.3) and in some series are the most frequent abnormality reported. They are found in approximately 10% of adult T-ALL when studied cytogenetically. However, deletions of 9p are frequently cytogenetically cryptic and are detected at a much higher frequency when studied by FISH or other molecular techniques, as discussed above in BCP ALL. Recent reports indicate that del(9p) is not of prognostic significance in adult T-ALL.[3]

Another cryptic abnormality in T-ALL is the amplification of the chimeric oncogene, *ABL-NUP214*. *NUP214* is slightly distal to *ABL1* on chromosome 9. The rearrangement is on an episome but can be detected by FISH using an *ABL1* probe.[30] It is very rare in pediatric T-ALL (0.5% of COG patients 1–14 years old and no AYA, Fig. 5.2C, Table 5.3), but may be present in approximately 5% of adult T-ALL. *NUP214* also rearranges with *SET*, (*SET-NUP214*) resulting from a cryptic deletion of 9q34 found in approximately 4% of adult and pediatric T-ALL. Patients with this abnormality have a poor response to induction therapy.[31]

The oncogene *MYB* (6q23) can be translocated with *TCRB* (7q34) as a partner or it may be cryptically amplified.[14] It is overexpressed as a result of either of these aberrations. Visible deletions of 6q also are frequent in T-ALL and were present in 10.9% of COG patients 1–14 years old and 12.0% of AYA (Fig. 5.2C, Table 5.3). Del(6q) also occurs in BCP ALL but less frequently, being found in only 1.3% of children 1–14 years old and 3.4% of AYA (Fig. 5.2B). Deletions of 6q do not appear to have prognostic significance.

MLL rearrangements also occur in T-ALL, where they are a distinct subtype with early thymocyte differentiation.[32] They were found in 3.6% of patients 1–14 years old and 5.4% of AYA among the COG cases (Fig. 5.2C, Table 5.3). In T-ALL, *MLL-ENL* fusion, resulting from t(11;19)(q23;p13.3), is associated with a good outcome, in contrast to its poor prognosis in BCP ALL.[2]

In pediatric ALL, complexity has not been shown to influence prognosis; however, in adult T-ALL, complexity, defined as at least five unrelated abnormalities, has been associated with an inferior outcome.[3] In the COG T-ALL cases, 8.6% of children 1–14 years old and 10.9% of AYA had complexity of 5 or greater (Fig. 5.2C). It is not yet known whether complexity in pediatric T-ALL is associated with prognosis.

In summary, in T-ALL, cytogenetic abnormalities did not appear to differ between patients 1–14 years old and AYA. The frequencies of modal number, the presence of specific abnormalities, and complexity ≥ 5 were not significantly different in the two age groups (Fig. 5.2C). Thus, cytogenetic aberrations do not appear to contribute to differences in outcome between AYA and patients 1–14 years old with T-ALL (Fig. 5.3B).

Cytogenetics of Acute Myeloid Leukemia

AML increases exponentially with age, accounting for 15–20% of all childhood leukemias, about 33% in adolescence, and about 50% in adulthood. AML is the most common acute leukemia in adults. Cytogenetic alterations are important predictors of outcome (Table 5.4). Risk classifications based on cytogenetics typically include favorable-risk mutations: t(8;21)(q22;q22), inv(16)(p13.1q22), or t(16;16)(p13.1;q22), called core binding factor (CBF) leukemia, and t(15;17), which is excluded from current myeloid treatments; unfavorable-risk mutations: monosomy 5 (−5), deletion of the q arm of chromosome 5 [del(5q)], monosomy 7 (−7), t(6;9)(p23;q34), 3q abnormalities, t(8;16)(p11;q13), and complex karyotypes, defined as ≥ 3 aberrations; intermediate-risk mutations: normal and other karyotypes excluding favorable and unfavorable abnormalities. The fourth edition of the World Health Organization (WHO 2008) classification of tumors of hematopoietic tissues recommends a multidisciplinary approach to diagnosing and classifying myeloid disease.[33]

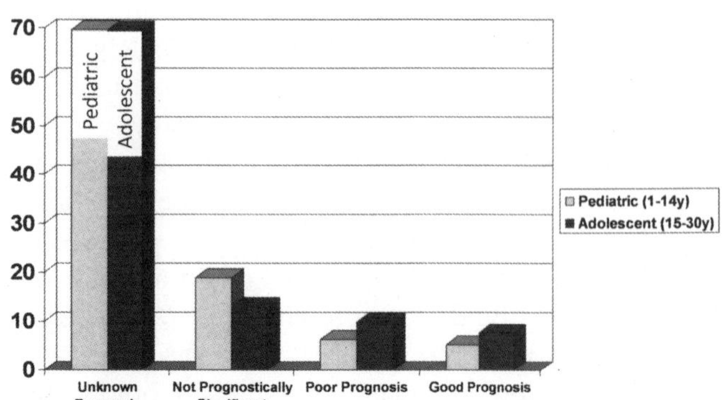

Fig. 5.3. (B) Comparisons of frequencies of prognostic groups between patients 1–14 years old and AYA with T-cell acute lymphoblastic leukemia. The aberrations included in each group are indicated in Table 5.3.

Table 5.4. Frequencies of common chromosomal abnormalities in children and adults with acute myeloid leukemia.

Chromosome abnormality	Children (%)	Adults (%)
Normal	20	40
t(8;21)(q22;q22)	12	6
inv(16)/t(16;16)(p13.1;q22)	6	5
t(15;17)(q22;q21)	9 (rare in infants)	7 (~15% <45 y/o; rare after 45 y/o)
t(9;11)(p22;q23)	7	2
11q23/*MLL* rearranged -other than t(9;11)	15 (50% of infant AML)	3
Monosomy 7	3	5 (increase >60 y/o)
Monosomy 5/del(5q)	1	7 (increase >60 y/o)
t(6;9)(p23;q34)	1	<1
inv(3)/t(3;3)(q21;q26)	<1 (>12 y/o)	2
t(1;22)(p13;q13)	1 (mostly M7 infants)	rare

Translocations involving core binding factors

t(8;21)(q22;q22)/AML1(RUNX1, CBFA2)-ETO(RUNX1T1, MTG8)

The t(8;21) translocation (Fig. 5.1B) is one of the most frequently associated with AML, 12% in children and 6% in adults, accounting for about 40–50% of the French-American-British (FAB) M2 subtype and, in rare cases, M0, M1, and M4, subtypes. Patients with t(8;21) have a more favorable outcome. Three-way variants or other complex t(8;21) translocations are found in about 4% of the cases. By FISH, a cryptic/submicroscopic chromosomal aberration has been described in 8.5% of patients with t(8;21), this being a small hidden insertion resulting in an *AML1-ETO* fusion; others have shown a large deletion of the 5′*ETO* region in 4.3–9% of the cases. These cryptic deletions do not appear to have any prognostic significance. The most frequent additional cytogenetic abnormalities include loss of a Y chromosome in males and loss of an X in females; del(9q), +8, +4, and +21.[34,35] The translocation juxtaposes *AML1* to *ETO*, resulting in *AML1-ETO* fusion, which has transcriptional activity. The generated oncoprotein functions mainly as a dominant-negative repressor of the *AML1* gene, which normally controls several hematopoietic genes by binding to the core enhancer sequence.

inv(16)(p13.1q22) or t(16;16)(p13.1;q22)/MYH11 (SMMHC)-CBFB

The inv(16)/t(16;16), henceforth abbreviated as inv(16), is mostly associated with AML subtype M4 with eosinophilia, which accounts for 6% of AML in children and 5% in adults. The inv(16) fuses the *CBFB* gene with the *MYH11* gene to produce a chimeric protein. Patients have a more favorable clinical course with this than with any of the other AML cytogenetic subgroups. The most frequent additional cytogenetic abnormalities include +22, +8, and +21.[35] When the chromosome banding is suboptimal, it is difficult to detect inv(16), and in some instances, the abnormality may be submicroscopic; also in rare instances, a microinsertion of *MYH11* into 16q22 creates a masked *CBFB-MYH11* fusion gene. Thus, FISH or PCR should be performed to test for this subtle chromosomal aberration because is important for risk assignment. In general, inv(16) is rarely involved in complex rearrangements, but the application of locus-specific probes can detect deletions of 16p (*MYH11*) in as many as 30% of cases with an inv(16); the deletion of 16q (*CBFB*) has been observed in fewer cases.[36]

Patients with CBF AML have a more favorable outcome with regimens including high-dose cytarabine than patients with other cytogenetic subgroups. Creutzig *et al.*[37] compared biological features in AML patients younger than 30 years and found that favorable CBF karyotypes were rarely seen in infants (4.5%) as compared to older patients; they were most frequent in the 2- to < 13-year-olds (32%) and less frequent in adolescents (25%) and young adults (22%).

Translocations involving the retinoic acid receptor alpha: Acute promyelocytic leukemia

Acute promyelocytic leukemia (APL) accounts for 9% of pediatric AML and 15% in adult patients younger than 45 years; it is infrequent in patients older than 45 years. APL in children often presents with hyperleukocytosis (defined as a leukocyte count greater than 10×10^9/L), affecting 40% vs. only 20–25% in adults. As it is frequently associated with disseminated intravascular coagulopathy, a prompt diagnosis is critical for APL.[38] Chromosomal abnormalities in addition to t(15;17) are found in about 30% of APL patients; the most frequent are: +8, isoderivative -ider(17)t(15;17), or isochromosome -i(17)(q). APL has the t(15;17)(q22;q21), resulting in the fusion of the promyelocytic leukemia (*PML*) and retinoic acid receptor alpha (*RARA*) genes. The fusion product (*PML-RARA*) homodimerizes, binds to DNA, and works as a transcriptional repressor together with corepressors, including histone deacetylase. A combination regimen to treat patients with APL including all-*trans* retinoic acid (ATRA), arsenic trioxide, and anthracycline-based therapy achieves complete remission rates of up to 95% in adult patients with APL. Such regimens currently are being investigated for children with APL but long-term follow-up is not yet available.[38]

Variant chromosomal rearrangements or cryptic insertions can be detected in about 9% of APL patients, who respond to ATRA combination regimens much the same as APL patients with the typical t(15;17). Three-way or more complex translocations represent 3% of APL. Cryptic/submicroscopic rearrangements due to insertions have been described in about 6% of all APL, with the same proportion of insertions of *PML* to *RARA* or vice versa, and are detectable only by FISH. Approximately 1% of all APL cases have variant translocations involving only *RARA*. The most frequent is t(11;17)(q23;q21)/*PLZF-RARA* that is partially resistant to ATRA.

Translocations involving chromatin remodeling proteins: MLL

11q23/MLL(MLL1, ALL1, TRX, HTRX1)

Rearrangements of the *MLL* gene located at 11q23 are associated with aggressive ALL and AML, leukemia in infants, and therapy-related leukemia. A variety of chimeric oncoproteins are generated, which include the amino terminal region of *MLL*, implicated in protein–protein interactions and transcriptional repression, with the carboxy terminal portion of a variety of mostly unrelated fusion partners. To date, about 100 different 11q23 chromosomal abnormalities have been reported and more than 60 *MLL* fusion partner genes have been cloned.[39]

The frequency of 11q23 abnormalities is higher in children with AML (>18%) than in adult patients (about 5%), with a peak incidence of about 50% in infants with AML; however, it is rarely observed in patients older than 60 years.[37] However, such frequencies are underestimated, because an additional 5% of cryptic and subtle *MLL* rearrangements are not always detected by conventional cytogenetics. In most cases, *MLL* is broken in an 8.3-kb breakpoint cluster region and fused in-frame with its corresponding partners, generating an aberrant fusion protein responsible for leukemogenesis. In some instances, *MLL* or the partner gene must change orientation to form the fusion protein, and FISH using an *MLL* probe may produce an atypical signal pattern. In clinical practice, FISH using the *MLL* probe in conjunction with cytogenetics is the best method to evaluate rearrangements of this promiscuous gene. However, FISH alone in interphase nuclei (without metaphases) cannot precisely identify the involved partner gene or *MLL* partial tandem duplication (PTD; described below). Most important, it should be noted that FISH occasionally shows a concurrent deletion of 3′*MLL*, and rarely of 5′*MLL*, because these translocations may involve the gain or loss of genetic material at the genomic breakpoint junctions without affecting the production of the fusion transcript. Molecular studies to evaluate *MLL* rearrangements or the numerous generating fusions include standard or multiplex RT-PCR with specific primers to identify most common *MLL* fusion transcripts. Furthermore, cDNA panhandle PCR or long-distance inverse PCR allows identification of infrequent or novel *MLL* partner genes. Sequencing and bioinformatics analysis also may be used, but these methods have not been validated for routine clinical use. In pediatric AML, the main translocations are t(9;11)(p22;q23), t(10;11)(p12;q23), t(11;19)(q23;p13.3), t(6;11)(q27;q23), and t(10;11)(p11.2;q23), accounting for 15–20% of cases.[35]

In a recent collaborative group study of 756 children with an 11q23/*MLL* rearrangement, the overall 5-year EFS rate was 44%. The outcome of the subgroups varied greatly; for example, patients with a t(1;11)(q21;q23) had a 5-year EFS of 92%, whereas those with a t(6;11)(q27;q23) had the worst outcome (5-year EFS, 11%). The subgroups t(10;11)(p12;q23), t(4;11)(q21;q23), and t(10;11)(p11.2;q23) had a 5-year EFS of 31%, 29%, and 17%, respectively.[40]

The **t(9;11)(p22;q23)/*MLL-AF9*(*MLLT3*)** aberration is the most frequent 11q23 abnormality in children and adults with AML and is also occasionally found in patients with ALL. Some pediatric AML clinical trials have reported that patients with t(9;11) fared better than patients with variable 11q23, whereas other studies found no differences. In a study by Balgobind *et al.*,[40] the favorable prognosis of t(9;11) was not confirmed but rather revealed heterogeneity in this subgroup since FAB-M5 was an independent favorable prognostic indicator. These discrepancies probably reflect the different protocols used and the distinct biologic heterogeneity of 11q23, generating numerous variants and rare genetic events. WHO-2008 classifies t(9;11) as an entity and recommends that partners in the variant *MLL* translocations be specified.[33] The **t(10;11)(p12;q23)/*MLL-AF10*(*MLLT10*)** aberration is a frequent 11q23 abnormality, but because the orientation of the genes is in the opposite direction, most cases have concurrent inversions, insertions, or multiple breaks to juxtapose the genes in the proper orientation to generate a functional fusion gene.[39] In such cases, FISH using the subtelomeric probes for 10p and 11q are helpful to clarify the nature of the abnormality. Other cryptic rearrangements of *MLL* in which the genes have opposite orientation include Xq24 (*SEPT6*), 5q31 (*AF5Q31*/*AFF4*), and many other cases reported in the literature.[39] Infrequently, some cases with t(10;11)(p12;q21) lack *MLL* involvement because they generate the *CALM-AF10* gene fusion. The patients with t(10;11)(p12;q21) are characterized by young age, AML or T-ALL with a mixed-lineage phenotype and coexpression of T-cell and myeloid antigens, frequent occurrence of a mediastinal mass, and poor clinical outcome. It is difficult to distinguish the two subtypes of t(10;11) by conventional cytogenetics, but FISH and RT-PCR can aid in differentiating these genetic lesions with accuracy. The **t(6;11)(q27;q23)/*MLL-AF6*(*MLLT4*)** is a very subtle abnormality that can be easily missed by conventional cytogenetics. Although the incidence is low, it is important to accurately detect the t(6;11), because patients with that aberration have a dismal outcome and should be placed in the high-risk arm of protocols.[40] The **t(11;19)(q23;p13)** juxtaposes *MLL* with several partners at 19p. The two most frequently observed distinct breakpoints are at 19p13.3 and 19p13.1, where the *ENL*(*MLLT1*) and *ELL* genes are mapped, respectively. The t(11;19)(q23;p13.1) is found only in association with AML, but the t(11;19)(q23;p13.3) is seen in both myeloid and lymphoid (B- and T-lineage) leukemias. At the cytogenetic G-banded level of resolution, it is not always possible to differentiate between these two 19p breakpoints. Laboratory-developed FISH probes or RT-PCR can aid in an accurate molecular classification. Balgobind *et al.*[40] found no statistical differences between patients with t(11;19), irrespective of the breakpoint assignment. Of note, there are other infrequent t(11;19)(q23;p13) abnormalities with *MLL* rearranged with genes other than those described above, such as *EEN*, *MYO1F*, *ACER1(ASAH3)*, and *VAV1*. Although RT-PCR is the most sensitive method for studying these fusions, it is not performed in routine studies, so we rely on FISH testing using an *MLL* probe on sequentially G-banded FISH metaphases. Thus, it should be noted that due to the complexity of *MLL* with genes at 19p, the accuracy of the detection of the specific genetic lesion may be limited in such rare cases.

Abnormalities associated with infants in AML

t(1;22)(p13;q13)/RBM15(OTO)-MKL1(MAL)

The t(1;22) abnormality is strongly associated with acute megakaryoblastic leukemia (AMkL, AML-M7) and is seen in 3–5% of all AML cases; it is incorporated in the WHO-2008 classification. This translocation has been found mostly in infants and young children but has also been seen in a few adults. The karyotype in AMkL is usually complex and has many abnormalities in addition to the t(1;22), which is seen in half of the cases as a derivative form, der(22)t(1;22)(q13;p13). The diagnosis of this translocation may be hampered by a fibrotic bone marrow, often resulting in a dry tap during sampling. Thus, RT-PCR is a good method to evaluate samples with AMkL to assess the *RBM15-MKL1* fusion transcript. The prognosis of this translocation is contentious; earlier, it was associated with a poor prognosis, but in later reports, it was shown that these patients respond well to intensive chemotherapy.

t(7;12)(q36;p13)/TEL(ETV6)-HLXB9(MNX1) (plus unknown genes)

The t(7;12) aberration has been identified by several cooperative groups in one third of infants with AML, and it has an undifferentiated FAB morphology subtype and a poor clinical outcome.[41] The translocation is strongly associated with 7q or 12p abnormalities with a +8 or +19; the +19 is rarely observed in other cytogenetic subgroups of AML except for AMkL. The translocation can be subtle and difficult to observe by conventional cytogenetics. The juxtaposition of *TEL* (*ETV6*, 12p13) with *HLXB9* (7q36) generates the *TEL-HLXB9* chimeric fusion that has been detected by RT-PCR in several, but not all, reported cases of t(7;12) because the 7q breakpoints are molecularly heterogeneous; these cases overexpress *HLXB9*. Of importance, t(7;12) appears to be the second most frequent rearrangement after 11q23 in infants with AML and has a worse outcome than the cases with 11q23.[41]

Cytogenetically normal AML

Cytogenetically normal AML (CN-AML) is found in 20% of children and 40% of adults with AML and is considered an intermediate risk. Submicroscopic gene mutation evaluations have identified many genetic alterations in patients with AML; some are associated with a normal karyotype that does not delineate a specific leukemic subtype but contributes as a prognostic indicator. *NPM1* (5q31) mutations in adults with AML are found in 24–35% of all cases and in 50–60% of patients with a CN-AML; in children, they are found in 8% of all cases and in 22% of those with CN-AML. The mutations are age dependent, found in children with a median age of 10.9 years and not seen in children younger than 3 years. Most AML patients with *NMP1* mutations and either a normal or abnormal karyotype respond well to chemotherapy and have a favorable prognosis (in the absence of a concomitant *FLT3*-ITD mutation, which is seen in as many as 30% of patients with CN-AML).[42] *CEBPA* (19q13.1) mutations are found in about 5% of older children with AML, most having CN-AML (accounting for 17% of the cohort with a normal karyotype), and are associated with a good prognosis in the absence of *FLT3* mutations. In some instances, these genetic alterations are not mutually exclusive, and the survival rate may be altered. To incorporate recent findings, WHO recommended two "provisional entities" for two mutated genes in AML: *NPM1* and *CEBPA*.[33]

Most frequent deletions in AML

Monosomy 5/del(5q)

AML with isolated −5/del(5q) is associated with a poor prognosis and places children in the unfavorable risk group. The −5/del(5q) can be found in very complex karyotypes, and the interpretation of −5/del(5q) is sometimes equivocal. Contrary to its frequency of 7% in adult AML, −5/del(5q) is very rare in childhood AML. The region-specific FISH probes generally used to evaluate del(5q) include *EGR1* (5q31) and *CSF1R* (5q33–34).

Monosomy 7 (–7) and deletion 7q (7q–)

In children with AML, –7 is found in 3% of the population, but it increases exponentially in adults with myelodysplastic syndrome (MDS) or AML. These patients have an adverse prognosis and are treated in high-risk protocols. A –7 is the most common acquired abnormality in children with MDS, accounting for 40% of cases.[35] Deletion of 7q is a consistent finding in AML, MDS, and therapy-related disease (both AML and MDS). In the past, children with a del(7q) were also considered to be at high risk for treatment failure. However, Hasle *et al.* [43] showed that the outcome for children with a del(7q), but not monosomy 7, are comparable to that for other patients with AML. The presence of a del(7q) does not abrogate the prognostic significance of favorable cytogenetic subgroups like inv(16), t(8;21). There is high heterogeneity in 7q– and complexity of 7q rearrangements, and it is suggested there may be multiple genes involved in their pathogenesis.

del(9q)

The deletion of the q arm of chromosome 9 is seen in about 2% of AML cases, with 9q21–22 being the most commonly deleted region. Most del(9q) cases are associated with t(8;21) or other chromosomal abnormalities; a sole del(9q) is seen less frequently. Recently, it was shown that AML with del(9q) as the sole abnormality or in combination with a single abnormality other than t(8;21) is strongly associated with *CEBPA* (19q13.1) loss-of-function mutations. Thus, the loss of critical genes at 9q and the disruption of *CEBPA* possibly cooperate in the pathogenesis of this leukemia.

Most frequent trisomies in AML

Trisomy 4 (+4): A +4 as the sole abnormality in myeloid disease is rare (<1%). Some of these cases have a mixed-lineage phenotype. **Trisomy 8 (+8)**: A trisomy of chromosome 8 as a sole abnormality is seen in AML and is among the most frequent secondary numerical abnormalities with usually complex karyotypes. When the additional abnormalities are associated with either a favorable or unfavorable outcome, the +8 does not affect the prognosis. Some reports have associated +8 with a poor prognosis, but the outcome for these patients is controversial, and most protocols include such patients in the intermediate-risk group.[44] **Trisomy 11 (+11)**: A +11 as a sole abnormality is rare in children. In adults with AML or MDS, a +11 is most often found with other chromosomal aberrations as part of a complex karyotype and confers a poor prognosis. As mentioned below, patients with +11 have a nonrandom association with *MLL*-PTD. The incidence of *MLL*-PTD in +11 cases ranges from 20% to 73%.[45] **Trisomy 21 (+21)**: An isolated trisomy or tetrasomy 21 is uncommon in non-DS children with AML. Tetrasomy 21 is common in DS patients with AMkL. Of note, *GATA1* (localized to Xp11.23) mutations are present in most DS children with either transient myeloproliferative disorders or AMkL. *GATA1* mutation is not observed in non-DS children with AMkL or in DS with other types of leukemia. In WHO-2008, there is a new category for myeloid proliferations related to DS that incorporates transient abnormal myelopoiesis, as well as MDS and AML, that is DS related.[33] **Trisomy 22 (+22)**: A +22 has been reported as a recurring secondary abnormality in AML, particularly in association with inv(16). As a sole abnormality, +22 is a rare event.

Infrequent recurrent chromosomal abnormalities in children with AML

t(6;9)(p23;q34)/DEK-CAN(NUP214)

The t(6;9) is a rare recurrent abnormality that is found in 1% of patients with AML or MDS and generates a *DEK-CAN* chimeric fusion. The patients are young at diagnosis; the bone marrow has signs of multilineage dysplasia, frequently with basophilia, a high incidence of *FLT3* mutations, and a dismal prognosis. Another rare translocation involves 9q34 generating a *CAN-SET* oncogenic fusion in AML.

t(7;11)(p15;p15.5)/NUP98-HOXA9 or t(5;11)(q35;p15.5)/NUP98-NSD1

The t(7;11)(p15;p15.5) is rare and subtle in childhood AML but is recurrent and associated with a poor prognosis. The translocation generates the *NUP98-HOXA9* chimeric fusion, facilitating detection by RT-PCR. It also can be detected by FISH with split *NUP98* probes.[46] Of interest, another recurrent *NUP98* translocation is the cryptic t(5;11)(q35;p15.5)/*NUP98-NSD* with a frequency of 5%; these patients have a poor response to treatment and a short survival. However, in clinical practice, the t(7;11)(p15;p15.5) and (5;11)(q35;p15.5) are often missed because FISH and PCR methods are not routinely performed to evaluate these genetic lesions. The *NUP98* gene encodes a nucleoporin protein, which contains nuclear pore complexes that facilitate mRNA export from the nucleus. Approximately 20 translocations (many cryptic) involving *NUP98* are found in AML, MDS, and T-ALL.

t(8;16)(p11.1;p13.3)/MOZ(MYST3, KAT6A)-CBP (CREBBP)

The 8p11.1 region is involved in rare translocations including: inv(8)(p11.1q13)/*MOZ-NCOA2*(*TIF2*), t(8;16)(p11.1;p13)/*MOZ-CBP*(*CREBBP*), t(8;22)(p11;q13)/*MOZ-P300*(*EP300*), and t(8;20)(p11.1;q12)/*MOZ-NCOA3*. It has been proposed that aberrant acetylation by these fusion proteins might participate in the process of leukemogenesis through aberrant chromatin remodeling. Among these 8p11.1 translocations, t(8;16)(p11.1;p13.3) is the most frequently observed with an incidence of less than 1%. Most have a monocytic morphology subtype and confer a dismal outcome. The *CBP* gene is also involved in other translocations in AML, t(10;16)(q22;p13)/*MORF*(*MYST4*)-*CBP*, and t(11;16)(q23;p13), which results in *MLL-CBP* fusion and is strongly associated with treatment-related hematologic malignancies.

3q26 (EVI1, EAP, MDS1)

Abnormalities of the q arm of chromosome 3 are seen rarely in children with AML. The breakpoints involved are most often 3q21 and 3q26, with the deregulation of *EVI1* or flanking *EAP* and *MDS1* genes. The abnormalities at 3q26 are described in 5% of adult patients with *de novo* AML or treatment related-AML, blast crisis of CML, and MDS evolving into leukemia. WHO-2008 defines all patients with inv(3)/t(3;3) as having AML.[47] Monosomy 7 or 7q abnormalities are among the most frequent additional abnormalities observed in such cases. The most common translocations involving 3q26 are: t(3;3)(q21;q26) or inv(3)(q21q26)/*RPN1-EVI1*, t(3;12)(q26;p13)/*TEL-EVI1*, and t(3;21)(q26;q22)/*AML1-EVI1*. Other rare 3q26 aberrations include: t(2;3)(p15–22;q26)/*EVI1-BCL11*/*EVI1-THADA*, t(3;6)(q26;q25), t(3;7)(q26;q21), t(3;8)(q26;q24), t(3;13)(q26;q13–14), and t(3;17)(q26;q22)/*MSI2-EVI1*.[48] Because of the molecular heterogeneity in the region and because 3q abnormalities are often subtle and difficult to identify by conventional cytogenetics, FISH probes can be helpful in identifying the chromosome breakpoints affecting the *EVI1* locus in these patients.

Complex karyotypes

The classification of complex karyotypes in AML has differed in the past but currently is best defined as three or more aberrations, excluding the chromosomal abnormalities described as entities in WHO-2008. The comprehensive evaluation of complex karyotypes is limited by G-banding techniques; other multicolor FISH methods are needed to analyze the origin of marker chromosomes, reveal subtle rearrangements, and determine the structure of complex derivative chromosomes. Most data regarding complex karyotypes have been derived from studies of adult patients with AML, which account for only 10–15% of the cases and have high-risk chromosome abnormalities and a worse outcome. Among the recurrent abnormalities included in complex karyotypes are losses of 5q, 7q, and 17p, and gains of 8q, 11q, and 21q. In children, complex karyotypes are less common and are most often seen in association with AMkL; the risk assignment of complex karyotypes is controversial and needs to be re-evaluated in future prospective studies.

Mutations and genetic lesions in the pathogenesis of AML

In numerous studies, submicroscopic gene mutations are increasingly being recognized as important diagnostic and prognostic markers in myeloid neoplasia. These include mutations of *NPM1*, *CEBPA*, *FLT3*, *RUNX1*, *KIT*, *NRAS*, *WT1*, and *MLL*-PTD. For example, *GATA1* indicates myeloid proliferations associated with DS. A few genetic lesions were incorporated within the cytogenetics entities because of their importance and frequencies, which vary among cytogenetic groups.[42] These mutations are important for the development of molecules that target these specific mutations directly or that act downstream in their disrupted signal transduction pathways

In summary, it is recommended that FISH methods be used as an adjunct to increase the yield of useful cytogenetic results. To detect the most significant abnormalities in AML, it is important to incorporate FISH with probe sets for t(8;21), 11q23/*MLL*, inv(16)/t(16;16), −5/5q-, and −7 for cases with normal or unknown cytogenetics; for APL, the identification of t(15;17) is critical for treatment decisions. Subtle translocations that could be missed in AML include inv(3)(q21q26), t(6;9)(p23;q34), t(6;11)(q27;q23), t(7;12)(q36;p13), t(10;11)(p12;q23), t(11;19) (q23;p13.1), and t(11;19)(q23;p13.3). Known molecular genetic mutations and others that will emerge may be used as genetic markers with clinical value, underscoring patient variability and disease heterogeneity. These genetic events alter cellular pathways and functions that may affect the clinical phenotype of the disease and treatment response, which will require individual-targeted therapy.

Conclusion

The use of conventional and molecular cytogenetics has led to many gene discoveries in cancer biology over the past 3 decades. The cloning of chromosome translocation breakpoints, like the t(8;21), inv(16), 11q23, t(12;21), t(9;22) and many others, has helped identify the genes involved in these translocations and allowed the development of DNA probes for FISH and RT-PCR that are used to diagnose and monitor minimal residual disease. Many of the genetic lesions are currently used as tools for the diagnosis, classification, and management of patients with acute leukemia.

The advent of new DNA array and sequencing technologies has enabled the simultaneous detection of mutations, deletions, amplifications, and epigenetic changes; RNA arrays have allowed the evaluation of associated biochemical pathways (see Chapter 6). Thus, the detection of additional tumor markers via innovative genetic technologies will help pinpoint the genes that act cooperatively in a particular malignant cell type, complementing the current WHO-2008 assignment of genetic lesions used in acute leukemias.

The most successful examples of targeted therapy currently used have benefited patients with chromosomal abnormalities like Ph+ and t(15;17) leukemias (see Chapter 22). In Ph+ leukemias, imatinib (and other novel tyrosine kinase inhibitors) specifically targets an abnormal, constitutively active BCR-ABL1 tyrosine kinase found in most patients with CML and Ph+ ALL. In APL, the patients are treated with ATRA in combination with chemotherapy to achieve a successful outcome.

The recent application of genome-wide microarray and high-throughput sequencing technologies has identified new high-risk subgroups in ALL, such as the genetic alteration of IKZF1 and JAK whose patients have a high-risk of relapse (see Chapter 6). The outcome for such patients will undoubtedly improve with innovative treatments which require the identification of target molecules for new therapies.

Currently known molecular genetic mutations as well as novel ones that remain to be identified are potential genetic markers that have clinical significance, underscoring the patient variability in and heterogeneity of acute leukemias. These genetic events alter cellular pathways and functions, which may in turn affect the clinical phenotype of the disease and treatment response, thereby necessitating individualized targeted therapy.

Acknowledgments

We regret that the original work of numerous investigators could not be acknowledged because of limited space only the latest references in various topics have been included in this chapter. Special thanks to the COG cytogeneticists who contributed cytogenetic results used in this text. Thanks also to COG investigators for their tireless efforts on behalf of children and adolescents with acute leukemia. A special thanks to Heather Breidenbach, who helped with data compilation and with the manuscript and to Aaron Hunt for statistical analyses. We also thank David Galloway for expert scientific editing.

References

1. Pui CH, Relling MV, Downing JR. (2004) Acute lymphoblastic leukemia. *N Engl J Med* **350**: 1535–1548.
2. Pui CH, Schrappe M, Ribeiro RC, Niemeyer CM. (2004) Childhood and adolescent lymphoid and myeloid leukemia. *Hematology Am Soc Hematol Educ Program* 118–145.
3. Marks DI, Paietta EM, Moorman AV, Richards SM, Buck G, de Wald G, Ferrando A, Fielding AK, Goldstone AH, Ketterling RP, Litzow MR, Luger SM, McMillan AK, Mansour MR, Rowe JM, Tallman MS, Lazarus HM. (2009) T-cell acute lymphoblastic leukemia in adults: Clinical features, immunophenotype, cytogenetics, and outcome from the large randomized prospective trial (UKALL XII/ECOG 2993). *Blood* **114**: 5136–5145.
4. Stock W, La M, Sanford B, Bloomfield CD, Vardiman JW, Gaynon P, Larson RA, Nachman J. (2008) What determines the outcomes for adolescents and young adults with acute lymphoblastic leukemia treated on cooperative group protocols? A comparison of Children's Cancer Group and Cancer and Leukemia Group B studies. *Blood* **112**: 1646–1654.

5. (1981) Third International Workshop on Chromosomes in Leukemia, 1980 Clinical significance of chromosomal abnormalities in acute lymphoblasic leukemia. *Cancer Genet Cytogenet* **4**: 111–137.
6. Sutcliffe MJ, Shuster JJ, Sather HN, Camitta BM, Pullen J, Schultz KR, Borowitz MJ, Gaynon PS, Carroll AJ, Heerema NA. (2005) High concordance from independent studies by the Children's Cancer Group (CCG) and Pediatric Oncology Group (POG) associating favorable prognosis with combined trisomies 4, 10, and 17 in children with NCI Standard-Risk B-precursor Acute Lymphoblastic Leukemia: A Children's Oncology Group (COG) initiative. *Leukemia* **19**: 734–740.
7. Moorman AV, Richards SM, Martineau M, Cheung KL, Robinson HM, Jalali GR, Broadfield ZJ, Harris RL, Taylor KE, Gibson BE, Hann IM, Hill FG, Kinsey SE, Eden TO, Mitchell CD, Harrison CJ. (2003) Outcome heterogeneity in childhood high-hyperdiploid acute lymphoblastic leukemia. *Blood* **102**: 2756–2762.
8. Mrozek K, Heerema NA, Bloomfield CD. (2004) Cytogenetics in acute leukemia. *Blood Rev* **18**: 115–136.
9. Usvasalo A, Raty R, Knuutila S, Vettenranta K, Harila-Saari A, Jantunen E, Kauppila M, Koistinen P, Parto K, Riikonen P, Salmi TT, Silvennoinen R, Elonen E, Saarinen-Pihkala UM. (2008) Acute lymphoblastic leukemia in adolescents and young adults in Finland. *Haematologica* **93**: 1161–1168.
10. Heerema N, Sather H, Reaman G, Hutchinson R, Lange B, Nachman J, Stinherz P, Uckun F, Gaynon P, Trigg M, Arthur D. (1998) Cytogenetic studies of acute lymphoblastic leukemia: Clinical correlations results form the children's cancer group. *Journal of Association of Genetic Technologists* **24**: 206–212.
11. Nachman JB, Heerema NA, Sather H, Camitta B, Forestier E, Harrison CJ, Dastugue N, Schrappe M, Pui CH, Basso G, Silverman LB, Janka-Schaub GE. (2007) Outcome of treatment in children with hypodiploid acute lymphoblastic leukemia. *Blood* **110**: 1112–1115.
12. Carroll AJ, Heerema NA, Gastier-Foster JM, Astbury C, Pyatt R, Reshmi SC, Borowitz MJ, Devidas M, Linda S, Loh ML, Raetz EA, Wood B, Winick NJ, Hunger SP, Carroll WL. (2009) Masked hypodiploidy: Hypodiploid acute lymphoblastic leukemia (ALL) in children mimicking hyperdiploid ALL: A report from the children's oncology group (COG) AALL03B1 study. *Blood (ASH Annual Meeting Abstracts)* **114**: 1580.
13. Douet-Guilbert N, Morel F, le Bris MJ, Herry A, le Calvez G, Marion V, Abgrall JF, Berthou C, de Braekeleer M. (2003) A fluorescence *in situ* hybridization study of TEL-AML1 fusion gene in B-cell acute lymphoblastic leukemia (1984–2001). *Cancer Genet Cytogenet* **144**: 143–147.
14. Harrison CJ. (2009) Cytogenetics of paediatric and adolescent acute lymphoblastic leukaemia. *Br J Haematol* **144**: 147–156.
15. Penther D, Preudhomme C, Talmant P, Roumier C, Godon A, Mechinaud F, Milpied N, Bataille R, Avet-Loiseau H. (2002) Amplification of AML1 gene is present in childhood acute lymphoblastic leukemia but not in adult, and is not associated with AML1 gene mutation. *Leukemia* **16**: 1131–1134.
16. Pui CH, Gaynon PS, Boyett JM, Chessells JM, Baruchel A, Kamps W, Silverman LB, Biondi A, Harms DO, Vilmer E, Schrappe M, Camitta B. (2002) Outcome of treatment in childhood acute lymphoblastic leukaemia with rearrangements of the 11q23 chromosomal region. *Lancet* **359**: 1909–1915.
17. Melo JV. (1996) The molecular biology of chronic myeloid leukaemia. *Leukemia* **10**: 751–756.
18. Arico MVM, Camitta B, Scrappe M, Chessells J, Baruchel A, Gaynon P, Silverman L, Janka-Schaub G, Kamps W, Pui C-H, Masera G, Conter V, Riehm H, Heerema N, Sallan S, Auclerc M-F, Pullen J, Shuster J, Carroll A, Raimondi S, Richards S. (2000) Outcome of treatment in children with Philadelphia chromosome-positive acute lymphoblastic leukemia. *N Engl J Med* **342**: 998–1006.
19. Schultz KR, Bowman WP, Aledo A, Slayton WB, Sather H, Devidas M, Wang C, Davies SM, Gaynon PS, Trigg M, Rutledge R, Burden L, Jorstad D, Carroll A, Heerema NA, Winick N, Borowitz MJ, Hunger SP, Carroll WL, Camitta B. (2009) Improved early event-free survival with imatinib in Philadelphia chromosome-positive acute lymphoblastic leukemia: A children's oncology group study. *J Clin Oncol* **27**: 5175–5181.
20. Devaraj PE, Foroni L, Secker-Walker LM. (1995) The detection of E2A rearrangement or E2A-PBX1 fusion transcript in t(1;19) leukemia. *Genes Chromosomes Cancer* **12**: 157–158.
21. van Zutven LJ, van Drunen E, de Bont JM, Wattel MM, den Boer ML, Pieters R, Hagemeijer A, Slater RM, Beverloo HB. (2005) CDKN2 deletions have no prognostic value in childhood precursor-B acute lymphoblastic leukaemia. *Leukemia* **19**: 1281–1284.
22. Strehl S, Konig M, Dworzak MN, Kalwak K, Haas OA. (2003) PAX5/ETV6 fusion defines cytogenetic entity dic(9;12)(p13;p13). *Leukemia* **17**: 1121–1123.
23. Gastier-Foster JM, Carroll AJ, Ell D, Harvey R, Chen I-M, Ketterling R, Meloni-Ehrig A, Opheim KE, Patil S, Pettenati M, Rao K, Wu S, Heerema NA. (2007) Two

distinct subsets of dic(9;12)(p12;p11.2) among children with B-cell precursor acute lymphoblastic leukemia (ALL): PAX5-ETV6 and ETV6-RUNX1 rearrangements: A report from the children's oncology group. *ASH Annual Meeting Abstracts* **110**: 1439.

24. An Q, Wright SL, Moorman AV, Parker H, Griffiths M, Ross FM, Davies T, Harrison CJ, Strefford JC. (2009) Heterogeneous breakpoints in patients with acute lymphoblastic leukemia and the dic(9;20)(p11–13;q11) show recurrent involvement of genes at 20q11.21. *Haematologica* **94**: 1164–1169.
25. Messinger YH, Higgins R, Devidas M, Hunger SP, Carroll AJ, Heerema NA. (2008) Acute lymphoblastic leukemia (ALL) with t(8;14)(q11.2;q32): B-lineage disease with high proportion of down syndrome. A Children's Oncology Group (COG) Study. *Blood (ASH Annual Meeting Abstracts)* **112**: 1477.
26. Mullighan CG, Collins-Underwood JR, Phillips LA, Loudin MG, Liu W, Zhang J, Ma J, Coustan-Smith E, Harvey RC, Willman CL, Mikhail FM, Meyer J, Carroll AJ, Williams RT, Cheng J, Heerema NA, Basso G, Pession A, Pui CH, Raimondi SC, Hunger SP, Downing JR, Carroll WL, Rabin KR. (2009) Rearrangement of CRLF2 in B-progenitor- and Down syndrome-associated acute lymphoblastic leukemia. *Nat Genet* **41**: 1243–1246.
27. Asnafi V, Beldjord K, Libura M, Villarese P, Millien C, Ballerini P, Kuhlein E, Lafage-Pochitaloff M, Delabesse E, Bernard O, Macintyre E. (2004) Age-related phenotypic and oncogenic differences in T-cell acute lymphoblastic leukemias may reflect thymic atrophy. *Blood* **104**: 4173–4180.
28. Janssen JW, Ludwig WD, Sterry W, Bartram CR. (1993) SIL-TAL1 deletion in T-cell acute lymphoblastic leukemia. *Leukemia* **7**: 1204–1210.
29. Kees UR, Heerema NA, Kumar R, Watt PM, Baker DL, La MK, Uckun FM, Sather HN. (2003) Expression of HOX11 in childhood T-lineage acute lymphoblastic leukaemia can occur in the absence of cytogenetic aberration at 10q24: A study from the Children's Cancer Group (CCG). *Leukemia* **17**: 887–893.
30. Graux C, Cools J, Melotte C, Quentmeier H, Ferrando A, Levine R, Vermeesch JR, Stul M, Dutta B, Boeckx N, Bosly A, Heimann P, Uyttebroeck A, Mentens N, Somers R, MacLeod RA, Drexler HG, Look AT, Gilliland DG, Michaux L, Vandenberghe P, Wlodarska I, Marynen P, Hagemeijer A. (2004) Fusion of NUP214 to ABL1 on amplified episomes in T-cell acute lymphoblastic leukemia. *Nat Genet* **36**: 1084–1089.
31. Gorello P, la Starza R, Varasano E, Chiaretti S, Elia L, Pierini V, Barba G, Brandimarte L, Crescenzi B, Vitale A, Messina M, Grammatico S, Mancini M, Matteucci C, Bardi A, Guarini A, Martelli MF, Foa R, Mecucci C. (2010) Combined interphase fluorescence *in situ* hybridization elucidates the genetic heterogeneity of T-cell acute lymphoblastic leukemia in adults. *Haematologica* **95**: 79–86.
32. Ferrando AA, Armstrong SA, Neuberg DS, Sallan SE, Silverman LB, Korsmeyer SJ, Look AT. (2003) Gene expression signatures in MLL-rearranged T-lineage and B-precursor acute leukemias: Dominance of HOX dysregulation. *Blood* **102**: 262–268.
33. Swerdlow S, Campo E, Harris N, Jaffe E, Pileri S, Stein H, Thiele J, Vardiman J (eds.). (2008) *World Health Organization Classification of Tumours of Haematopoietic and Lymphoid Tissues* (4th ed). Lyon: IARC Press.
34. Mrozek K, Marcucci G, Paschka P, Bloomfield CD. (2008) Advances in molecular genetics and treatment of core-binding factor acute myeloid leukemia. *Curr Opin Oncol* **20**: 711–718.
35. Raimondi SC, Chang MN, Ravindranath Y, Behm FG, Gresik MV, Steuber CP, Weinstein HJ, Carroll AJ. (1999) Chromosomal abnormalities in 478 children with acute myeloid leukemia: Clinical characteristics and treatment outcome in a cooperative pediatric oncology group study-POG 8821. *Blood* **94**: 3707–3716.
36. Kolomietz E, Al-Maghrabi J, Brennan S, Karaskova J, Minkin S, Lipton J, Squire JA. (2001) Primary chromosomal rearrangements of leukemia are frequently accompanied by extensive submicroscopic deletions and may lead to altered prognosis. *Blood* **97**: 3581–3588.
37. Creutzig U, Buchner T, Sauerland MC, Zimmermann M, Reinhardt D, Dohner H, Schlenk RF. (2008) Significance of age in acute myeloid leukemia patients younger than 30 years: A common analysis of the pediatric trials AML-BFM 93/98 and the adult trials AMLCG 92/99 and AMLSG HD93/98A. *Cancer* **112**: 562–571.
38. Sanz MA, Grimwade D, Tallman MS, Lowenberg B, Fenaux P, Estey EH, Naoe T, Lengfelder E, Buchner T, Dohner H, Burnett AK, Lo-Coco F. (2009) Management of acute promyelocytic leukemia: Recommendations from an expert panel on behalf of the European LeukemiaNet. *Blood* **113**: 1875–1891.
39. Meyer C, Kowarz E, Hofmann J, Renneville A, Zuna J, Trka J, Ben Abdelali R, Macintyre E, De Braekeleer E, de Braekeleer M, Delabesse E, de Oliveira MP, Cave H, Clappier E, van Dongen JJ, Balgobind BV, van den Heuvel-Eibrink MM, Beverloo HB, Panzer-Grumayer R, Teigler-Schlegel A, Harbott J, Kjeldsen E, Schnittger S, Koehl U, Gruhn B, Heidenreich O, Chan LC, Yip SF, Krzywinski M, Eckert C, Moricke A, Schrappe M,

Alonso CN, Schafer BW, Krauter J, Lee DA, Zur Stadt U, Te Kronnie G, Sutton R, Izraeli S, Trakhtenbrot L, lo Nigro L, Tsaur G, Fechina L, Szczepanski T, Strehl S, Ilencikova D, Molkentin M, Burmeister T, Dingermann T, Klingebiel T, Marschalek R. (2009) New insights to the MLL recombinome of acute leukemias. *Leukemia* **23**: 1490–1499.

40. Balgobind BV, Raimondi SC, Harbott J, Zimmermann M, Alonzo TA, Auvrignon A, Beverloo HB, Chang M, Creutzig U, Dworzak MN, Forestier E, Gibson B, Hasle H, Harrison CJ, Heerema NA, Kaspers GJ, Leszl A, Litvinko N, Nigro LL, Morimoto A, Perot C, Pieters R, Reinhardt D, Rubnitz JE, Smith FO, Stary J, Stasevich I, Strehl S, Taga T, Tomizawa D, Webb D, Zemanova Z, Zwaan CM, van den Heuvel-Eibrink MM. (2009) Novel prognostic subgroups in childhood 11q23/MLL-rearranged acute myeloid leukemia: Results of an international retrospective study. *Blood* **114**: 2489–2496.
41. von Bergh AR, van Drunen E, van Wering ER, van Zutven LJ, Hainmann I, Lonnerholm G, Meijerink JP, Pieters R, Beverloo HB. (2006) High incidence of t(7;12)(q36;p13) in infant AML but not in infant ALL, with a dismal outcome and ectopic expression of HLXB9. *Genes Chromosomes Cancer* **45**: 731–739.
42. Dohner K, Dohner H. (2008) Molecular characterization of acute myeloid leukemia. *Haematologica* **93**: 976–982.
43. Hasle H, Alonzo TA, Auvrignon A, Behar C, Chang M, Creutzig U, Fischer A, Forestier E, Fynn A, Haas OA, Harbott J, Harrison CJ, Heerema NA, van den Heuvel-Eibrink MM, Kaspers GJ, Locatelli F, Noellke P, Polychronopoulou S, Ravindranath Y, Razzouk B, Reinhardt D, Savva NN, Stark B, Suciu S, Tsukimoto I, Webb DK, Wojcik D, Woods WG, Zimmermann M, Niemeyer CM, Raimondi SC. (2007) Monosomy 7 and deletion 7q in children and adolescents with acute myeloid leukemia: An international retrospective study. *Blood* **109**: 4641–4647.
44. Schaich M, Schlenk RF, Al-Ali HK, Dohner H, Ganser A, Heil G, Illmer T, Krahl R, Krauter J, Sauerland C, Buchner T, Ehninger G. (2007) Prognosis of acute myeloid leukemia patients up to 60 years of age exhibiting trisomy 8 within a non-complex karyotype: Individual patient data-based meta-analysis of the German Acute Myeloid Leukemia Intergroup. *Haematologica* **92**: 763–770.
45. Rege-Cambrin G, Giugliano E, Michaux L, Stul M, Scaravaglio P, Serra A, Saglio G, Hagemeijer A. (2005) Trisomy 11 in myeloid malignancies is associated with internal tandem duplication of both MLL and FLT3 genes. *Haematologica* **90**: 262–264.
46. Romana SP, Radford-Weiss I, Ben Abdelali R, Schluth C, Petit A, Dastugue N, Talmant P, Bilhou-Nabera C, Mugneret F, Lafage-Pochitaloff M, Mozziconacci MJ, Andrieu J, Lai JL, Terre C, Rack K, Cornillet-Lefebvre P, Luquet I, Nadal N, Nguyen-Khac F, Perot C, van den Akker J, Fert-Ferrer S, Cabrol C, Charrin C, Tigaud I, Poirel H, Vekemans M, Bernard OA, Berger R. (2006) NUP98 rearrangements in hematopoietic malignancies: A study of the Groupe Francophone de Cytogenetique Hematologique. *Leukemia* **20**: 696–706.
47. Swerdlow SH, Wright SA. (1986) The spectrum of Leu-M1 staining in lymphoid and hematopoietic proliferations. *Am J Clin Pathol* **85**: 283–288.
48. Poppe B, Dastugue N, Vandesompele J, Cauwelier B, de Smet B, Yigit N, de Paepe A, Cervera J, Recher C, de Mas V, Hagemeijer A, Speleman F. (2006) EVI1 is consistently expressed as principal transcript in common and rare recurrent 3q26 rearrangements. *Genes Chromosomes Cancer* **45**: 349–356.

6

Molecular Genetics in Children, Adolescents and Young Adults with Acute Lymphoblastic Leukemia and Acute Myeloid Leukemia

Charles G. Mullighan, Stephen P. Hunger and Soheil Meshinchi

Introduction

Over the past several decades, genomic analyses of acute lymphoblastic and acute myeloid leukemia (ALL and AML) have led to major insights into the mechanisms of leukemogenesis. Studies of ALL, AML and other tumors have demonstrated that cancer develops through a process of successive mutations, the most critical of which are "driver" mutations that are fundamental to the process of oncogenesis and often are critical in specifying the clinical phenotype of disease. Mutations affect both oncogenes and tumor suppressor genes (TSGs). Chromosome translocations are considered to be early and perhaps initiating events in many cases of acute leukemia. Specific sentinel chromosome translocations are often associated with distinct molecular and clinical subtypes of disease and can have important prognostic implications; the protein products of these translocations may serve as critical targets for therapeutic intervention. More recently, large-scale genomic studies have begun to uncover the complexity of genetic changes that occur in the acute leukemias of children, adolescents, and young adults (CAYA) and have shown that mutations affecting key regulators of normal lymphoid and myeloid differentiation occur in many, if not most, cases of ALL and AML.

Molecular genetics of cancer

Mathematical models predict that cancers have acquired at least 6–8 different mutations at the time they become clinically evident,[1] with fewer mutations likely required for childhood acute leukemias as compared to epithelial cancers that are common in adults. While germline mutations are linked with predisposition to some cancers, the prototype being hereditary *RB1* gene mutations in retinoblastoma,[2] almost all mutations that occur in ALL/AML of CAYA are acquired in somatic cells rather than being present in the germline. The causes of these somatic mutations remain largely unknown, particularly in childhood cancers, for which environmental or host lifestyle factors issues seem to have little influence.

Fundamentally different types of mutations occur in oncogenes and TSGs, with very different functional consequences. Oncogenes are targeted by gain-of-function mutations that are genetically and functionally dominant, because they can be transforming even when a wild type protein from the unaffected normal allele is still expressed. In contrast, mutations that affect TSGs are most often genetically and functionally recessive because they typically inactivate the TSG protein product. In most cases, the normal protein produced by the intact wild type allele can carry out necessary cellular functions. Thus, inactivating mutations of both alleles of a TSG are generally required during leukemogenesis. It is quite common that the two alleles are inactivated by different mechanisms; for example, point mutation of one allele and deletion of the other. There are some instances in which TSG mutations can be dominant and have important consequences even if only one allele is mutated. For example, mutant proteins can function in a "dominant-negative" manner and have phenotypic consequences even in the presence of an intact wild type protein, or there can be gene dosage effects if the amount of protein produced from one allele is suboptimal when compared to that produced from two alleles.

Mechanisms of oncogene activation and TSG inactivation in acute leukemias of CAYA

Chromosomal translocations are the most common mechanism of oncogene activation in ALL and AML and are generally believed to either initiate the cascade of genetic alterations that culminate in leukemia, or at least occur very early in this process (see Chapter 5). As discussed in more detail below, chromosome translocations frequently occur *in utero* and have years of latency before acute leukemia is detected clinically.[3]

There are two major types of chromosome translocations that occur in leukemia. In the first type, which also occurs commonly in mesenchymal sarcomas of CAYA, two genes from different chromosomes are joined to create a fusion gene that encodes a chimeric protein with novel structural and functional properties not present in the parental wild type proteins. A prototypic example of this type of translocation is the t(9;22)(q34;q11), or "Philadelphia chromosome" (Ph), that occurs in almost all cases of chronic myeloid leukemia (CML) and a subset of ALL cases (Ph+ ALL).[4] An inversion of a single chromosome can have the same consequences, as exemplified by the inv(16)(p13;q22) that occurs in AML subtype M4Eo.[5] Fusion genes and their mRNA products are extremely useful for molecular diagnosis, while the novel proteins they encode can provide excellent targets for therapeutic intervention.[4]

Chromosome translocations in leukemia can also activate proto-oncogenes by moving them into the vicinity of active regulatory elements of other genes, most commonly one of the immunoglobulin (Ig) or T-cell receptor (TCR) genes, leading to dysregulated expression of a structurally intact protein. Such translocations in B-lineage ALL involve the Ig heavy chain gene (*IGH@*, or IgH) at 14q32, the kappa light chain gene (*IGK@*, IgK) at 2q12, or the lambda light chain gene (*IGL@*, Igλ) at 22q11, while T-cell ALLs have translocations that target T-cell antigen receptor genes *TRB@* (TCRβ) at 7q35, *TCRG* (TCRγ) at 7q35 and TRD@ (TCRδ) at 14q11.[6] The *c-MYC* gene is frequently involved in translocations of this type with almost all cases of Burkitt's leukemia or lymphoma having a translocation that joins *c-MYC* with one of the three Ig loci; similar translocations involve *c-MYC* and T-cell antigen receptor genes in T-ALL.[7] These translocations lead to high-level and inappropriately timed expression of the Myc transcription factor, which activates expression of target genes and leads to entry into S phase, decreased growth factor requirements, and escape from normal regulation of cell cycle progression.[8]

Focal interstitial deletions can have similar functional consequences and place a proto-oncogene under control of an active promoter. The *SCL/TAL-1* gene, which was first discovered by virtue of its involvement in the rare t(1;14)(p32;q11) translocation, is more commonly activated in T-ALL by a focal interstitial deletion of chromosome 1 that places *SCL/TAL-1* under the control of the adjacent *SIL* promoter.[9] The result of both types of rearrangements is the inappropriate expression of SCL/TAL-1 protein, which is now known to be a transcription factor that plays critical roles in specifying the fate of hematopoietic stem and/or progenitor cells and maturation of erythroid cells.[10] As discussed in more detail later in this chapter, an analogous interstitial deletion of the pseudoautosomal region of chromosome Xp/Y brings the lymphoid cytokine receptor gene *CRLF2* under control of the *P2RY8* promoter, leading to the overexpression of an intact CRLF2 protein.[11,12]

Not all modes of oncogene activation involve cytogenetically visible chromosome alterations. Point mutations that alter a single nucleotide at the DNA level can, by changing a single amino acid in a gene's protein product (missense mutations), activate a proto-oncogene. The most common known target of oncogenic point mutations in acute leukemia are the Ras genes *KRAS* and *NRAS*, which are mutated in many cases of both AML and ALL.[13]

Tumor suppressor genes can also be inactivated by a variety of different genetic mechanisms. Missense point mutations can inactivate TSGs by interfering with key functions of the encoded protein. For example, missense *TP53* mutations produce mutant p53 proteins that are impaired in important transcriptional and cell cycle–regulatory functions.[14] The most common mechanism of

TSG inactivation in leukemia is gene deletion, which occurs through large cytogenetically evident deletions involving millions of base pairs, or small targeted deletions that can only be identified by targeted assays or those that interrogate the entire genome at high resolution (reviewed in Ref. 15). The *CDKN2A* and *CDKN2B* genes, that are located within about 25 kb of one another on chromosome 9, are common targets of deletion in ALL, particularly T-ALL.[16,17] These genes encode proteins of approximately 16 ($p16^{INK4a}$) and 15 ($p15^{INK4b}$) kD that function as cyclin-dependent kinase inhibitors, and negatively regulate cell cycle progression by inhibiting specific cyclin-dependent protein kinase/cyclin complexes. The *CDKN2A* locus encodes a second key protein known as ARF (Alternate Reading Frame, p14 in humans and p19 in mice) that activates p53 via inhibition of the negative regulator MDM2. Other genetic mechanisms of TSG inactivation include nonsense and frameshift mutations. Nonsense mutations are point mutations that introduce a stop codon leading to the of a truncated and frequently unstable protein product that is functionally inactive. Frameshift mutations result when a small number (not divisible by three) of nucleotides are deleted or introduced in the coding region of a gene, thereby altering the reading frame of the gene and generating a protein that has extraneous amino acids (and often stop codons) downstream of the insertion/deletion site.

Specific sentinel chromosome translocations are associated with distinct subtypes of leukemia, define clinical phenotypes and can serve as therapeutic targets

Many chromosome translocations that occur in leukemia are closely linked to specific clinical characteristics (see Chapters 11–13). Gene expression profiling studies show that leukemias sharing specific recurrent sentinel chromosome translocations cluster together with one another in unsupervised analyses, indicating that the oncogenic proteins produced by these translocations are largely responsible for specifying the clinical phenotype (Fig. 6.1).[18,19]

The presence or absence of specific translocations can be associated with a better or worse treatment outcome, and the proteins produced by the translocation can serve as therapeutic targets. Perhaps the best examples of this genotype/phenotype association in leukemia are the t(15;17)(q22;q21) and *PML-RARA*

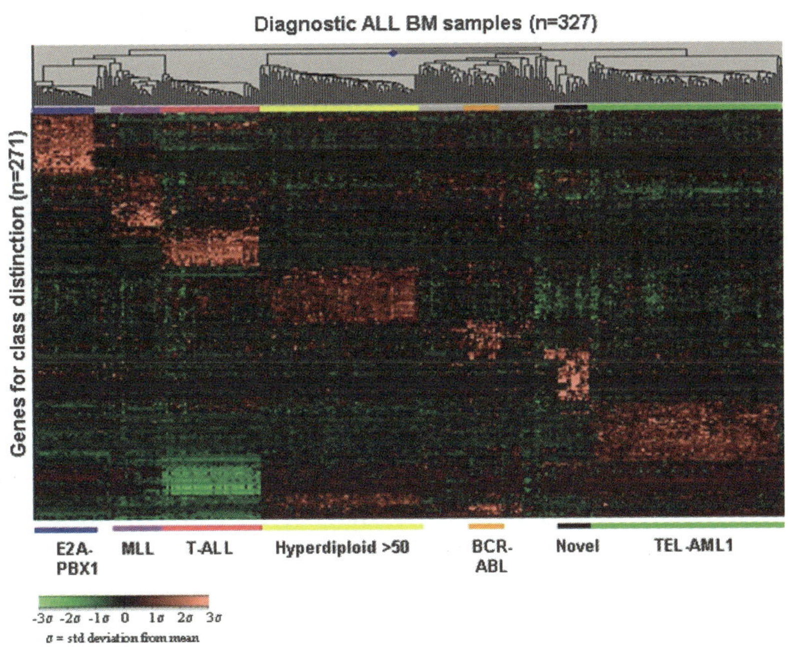

Fig. 6.1. Hierarchical clustering of Affymetrix U95 microarray gene expression profiling of 327 diagnostic ALL samples (columns) vs.271 genes (rows). The genes shown represent the top 40 genes most highly correlated with each ALL subtype. Red representing high expression and green representing low expression, with the scale shown at the lower left. Reprinted from *Cancer Cell*, Vol. 1, Yeoh EJ, Ross ME, Shurtleff SA, Williams WK, Patel D, Mahfouz R, Behm FG, Raimondi SC, Relling MV, Patel A, Cheng C, Campana D, Wilkins D, Zhou X, Li J, Liu H, Pui CH, Evans WE, Naeve C, Wong L, Downing JR, Classification, subtype discovery, and prediction of outcome in pediatric acute lymphoblastic leukemia by gene expression profiling, © (2002), with permission from Elsevier.[18]

fusion that occurs almost universally in acute promyelocytic leukemia (APML)[20] and *BCR-ABL1* fusion in CML and Ph+ ALL.[4]

These sentinel translocations can identify patients with identical clinical characteristics that have very different risks of relapse, and therefore often play a key role in risk stratification schemes used to allocate patients to different treatments.[21] For example, children with ALL that have similar clinical features (age, initial white blood cell count [WBC]) may have very different risks of relapse, requiring different therapies if one has a cryptic t(12;21) and *ETV6-RUNX1* fusion while the other has Ph+ ALL. The former child has a 90% or better expected cure rate with relatively modest intensity treatment.[22] The child with Ph+ ALL has a low chance of cure with conventional therapy, but outcome is improved markedly if treatment includes intensive chemotherapy and the tyrosine kinase inhibitor imatinib.[23,24]

The concept of "oncogene addiction" is critical for the development of therapies targeted at specific recurrent molecular lesions ("molecularly targeted therapy").[25,26] Leukemic cells commonly contain mutations in multiple genes, some of which are integral to the process of leukemogenesis ("driver mutations"), while others may have limited or no importance in pathogenesis or treatment response ("passenger mutations").[27] Molecularly targeted therapy is likely to be most effective when an agent inhibits a specific protein produced by a driver mutation that is critical to leukemia growth and/or survival and retained over time, particularly a sentinel lesion that is an initiating or very early step in leukemogenesis. Oncogene addiction predicts that the more dependent a tumor is on a particular genetic lesion, the more effective an inhibitor of this abnormality will be.

Sentinel chromosome translocations can develop years before acute leukemia occurs

Transgenic and knock-in mouse models show that forced overexpression of human leukemia oncogenes often leads to tumor development, but penetrance and latency are variable and tumors that arise are clonal.[28] These observations are consistent with human studies and show that a series of mutations are required to cause overt leukemia. Elegant studies of childhood leukemia have confirmed this model. The first clues derived from studies of monozygotic twins, in which concordance for leukemia approaches 100% if leukemia is diagnosed in the first year of life but then decreases markedly with increasing age of the index case. These and other observations suggested that leukemia might arise in one twin and be transferred to the other twin via shared placental circulation. Definitive proof of this was provided in 1993 when Ford and colleagues reported three sets of monozygotic twins concordant for infant leukemia in which the leukemia of each twin showed identical somatic *MLL* gene rearrangements.[29] Subsequent studies by these and other investigators showed a number of twins with leukemia in which each twin had identical (at the genomic level) non-germline sentinel chromosome translocations.[30] Storage of neonatal blood spots on "Guthrie cards" provided the opportunity to "backtrack" the timing of sentinel chromosome translocations and other somatic lesions. When blood obtained and stored at birth is analyzed retrospectively from children who later developed leukemia in the first 3–5 years of life, most, but not all, have evidence of cells harboring the chromosome translocation at birth.[31] The need for multiple mutations is underscored by the fact that approximately 1% of cord blood samples from healthy children contain cells with *ETV6-RUNX1* fusion, a rate that is about 100 times larger than the number that will eventually develop *ETV6-RUNX1*+ ALL,[32] and recent evidence showing that in the majority of *ETV6-RUNX1* ALL cases, leukemic cells harbor multiple deletions and gains of DNA, many of which target genes controlling lymphoid differentiation, tumor suppression and cell cycle regulation (see below).[17,33–35] Recent evidence suggests that the majority of these mutations, particularly the drivers, occur postnatally.[36]

Genome-wide profiling of genetic alterations in ALL

Although structural chromosomal rearrangements are important events in leukemogenesis and strongly influence therapeutic outcome, several observations indicate that these alterations do not fully explain the biology and clinical behavior of ALL. As described above, many children harbor chromosomal alterations such as *ETV6-RUNX1*, but may not develop leukemia for many years, if at all. Also, these chromosomal alterations frequently fail to induce leukemia in experimental models, suggesting that additional genetic alterations are required. Moreover, a substantial minority of children lack a structural chromosomal alteration identifiable on cytogenetic analysis. The proportion of ALL cases lacking a known chromosomal alteration increases through adolescence and into adulthood, with a corresponding decline in prognosis. While the frequency of Ph+ ALL rises with increasing age, this is insufficient to explain the generally poor outcome of ALL in the CAYA and adult population.[37]

The completion of the human genome project has enabled the development of genome-wide approaches to identify genomic alterations in large cohorts of cancer samples at high resolution conveniently and at low cost. Microarray-based studies of transcriptional profiling and structural genetic alterations have been performed in large childhood ALL cohorts, including B-progenitor and T-lineage cases with known chromosomal rearrangements, and cases lacking known genetic rearrangements. Importantly, these studies have integrated transcriptional profiling, DNA copy number alteration, and sequence mutation data in well-annotated cohorts of ALL patients, and have identified multiple genetic alterations contributing to the pathogenesis of ALL previously unsuspected from cytogenetic analyses.

Gene expression profiling studies, in which microarrays are used to quantitate the levels of expression of thousands of coding RNA transcripts in leukemic cells, have shown that sentinel chromosomal alterations are associated with distinct gene expression profiles (Fig. 6.1).[18,19,38] These studies have provided important insights into the cellular pathways perturbed in leukemogenesis, but do not readily identify driver mutation(s) influencing gene expression. Microarrays may also be used to identify structural genetic alterations in ALL. In this approach, microarrays comprising thousands to millions of probes are generated from bacterial artificial chromosomes (BACs) or oligonucleotides. ligonucleotide arrays are now more widely used as they can use millions of probes to identify genetic alterations at extremely high resolution. Multiple platforms are available, but common to all is the principle that the strength of probe hybridization to target DNA (as reflected by signal intensity on array scanning) is proportional to DNA content in the test sample. Oligonucleotide arrays from (e.g.) Agilent (Santa Clara, CA) and NimbleGen (Madison, WI) are two-channel designs, in which DNA from a tumor sample and a reference sample (ideally matched normal DNA from the same individual) are labeled with different fluorochromes and cohybridized to the same array, and identify gains and losses in DNA acquired by the tumor. Single nucleotide polymorphism (SNP) arrays are a type of oligonucleotide array in which probes interrogate DNA sequences flanking SNPs, and use different probes specific for each allele at individual SNP loci. SNP arrays were initially developed for genome-wide SNP genotyping studies, such as genome-wide association studies (GWAS). However, by providing both SNP genotype and DNA copy number data, SNP arrays are a powerful tool to: (i) interrogate cancer genomes, (ii) identify tumor-acquired gains and losses in DNA, (iii) identify regions of DNA copy "neutral" loss-of-heterozygosity (CN-LOH; also known as somatic-acquired uniparental disomy, aUPD), (iv) identify inherited DNA copy number variants, or polymorphisms (CNPs), (v) perform genome-wide analysis of associations between SNP genotype and cancer susceptibility.[39,40] The ability of SNP arrays to identify CN-LOH in addition to DNA copy number alterations is particularly desirable in genome-wide studies of cancer genomes, as regions of CN-LOH may indicate the presence of a mutated or epigenetically silenced tumor suppressor gene that has been reduplicated. Currently available SNP arrays (e.g. Illumina San Diego, CA, Affymetrix, Santa Clara, CA) examine up to two million genetic features, with sub-kilobase resolution. A detailed description of the methodologic aspects of SNP array aspects of cancer can be found elsewhere.[41,42]

Several groups have used Affymetrix SNP arrays and oligonucleotide array-CGH to characterize DNA copy number alterations and loss of heterozygosity in large cohorts of childhood ALL cases.[17,33–35,43–48] These studies have examined both B-progenitor and T-lineage cases with known recurring chromosomal rearrangements, including t(12;21) *ETV6-RUNX1*, t(9;22) *BCR-ABL1*, rearrangement of *MLL* at 11q23 and t(1;19) *TCF3-PBX1*, rearrangements involving the T-cell receptor genes in T-lineage ALL, and cases with aneuploidy (high hyperdiploidy and hypodiploidy), as well as cases lacking recurring chromosomal rearrangements. These studies have been highly informative in identifying novel targets of genetic alteration in ALL, in defining the nature of lesions that occur in conjunction with known cytogenetic abnormalities, and in identifying new ALL subtypes with distinct complements of genetic alterations.

In contrast to many solid tumors, which commonly harbor a high number of large genomic alterations suggestive of genomic instability,[49] the average number of DNA copy number alterations in ALL is relatively low at 6–8 lesions per case, many of which are the whole chromosomal gains characteristic of ALL with high hyperdiploidy.[17] However, detailed studies have identified over

50 recurring regions of deletion or gain in ALL, many of which are focal (arbitrarily defined as less than 1 Mb in size) and involve a single or few genes. Focal deletions are more common than gains, with high level DNA amplification a rare phenomenon in ALL. Many of the regions of deletion or gain involve genes that encode proteins with known roles in lymphoid development or tumorigenesis, including transcriptional regulators of lymphoid development (*PAX5, EBF1, IKZF1*, and *LEF1*), tumor suppressors and cell cycle regulators (*PTEN, RB1, CDKN2A, CDKN2B*), putative mediators of apoptosis (*BTG1*), lymphoid signaling genes (e.g. *BTLA* and *CD200*) drug response genes (e.g. the glucocorticoid receptor gene *NR3C1*), microRNA genes (mir-15a and mir-16), as well as a number of genes that currently lack a known role in lymphoid leukemogenesis. The number of genetic alterations is associated with ALL subtype. For example, *MLL*-rearranged leukemias harbor an average of less than one alteration per case, suggesting that few cooperating genetic alterations are required to induce leukemia.[17,50] In contrast, *ETV6-RUNX1* and *BCR-ABL1* rearranged leukemias harbor over eight lesions per case, suggesting that these lesions cooperate in leukemogenesis. One of the most striking findings from these studies has been the observation that the majority of B-progenitor ALL cases harbor genetic alterations targeting the transcriptional control of lymphoid development, most commonly deletions, sequence mutations or translocations involving *PAX5* (over 40% of B-progenitor ALL cases) and less commonly, deletions or point mutations of *IKZF1* (IKAROS), and deletions of *IKZF2* (HELIOS), *IKZF3* (AIOLOS) and *EBF1* (early B-cell factor). Notably, the deletion of *IKZF1* is a hallmark of Ph+ lymphoid leukemia, is observed in over 80% of *de novo* Ph+ ALL cases and CML in lymphoid blast crisis,[43,51] and is associated with poor outcome in both Ph+ and Ph– ALL (Fig. 6.2).[52–54] Furthermore, these genetic alterations commonly involve only a single copy of the gene. As coordinated expression of these genes is required for normal lymphoid development,[55,56] these findings suggest that genetic disruption of this pathway contributes to the block in lymphoid maturation characteristic of B-progenitor ALL. Formal demonstration of a role of these genetic alterations in lymphoid leukemogenesis is an area of active study, but existing data from murine models of leukemia, including retroviral bone marrow transplant models of Ph+ ALL and approaches using chemical or retroviral mutagenesis, indicates that haploinsufficiency for transcriptional regulators such as *Pax5* and *Ikzf1* does increase the penetrance and reduce the latency of leukemia.[57–59] Moreover, genomic profiling of the tumors generated by these mouse models commonly identifies additional genetic lesions involving the murine orthologs of genes involved by structural genetic alterations in human ALL, providing additional support for a role of these genes in leukemogenesis.

Genomic profiling of high risk ALL

Relapse of leukemia occurs in up to one quarter of childhood ALL cases, is associated with a poor outcome, and is a leading cause of childhood and young adult cancer-related deaths (Chapters 11 and 12). The biologic determinants of disease relapse are poorly understood, and recent studies have performed integrated genomic profiling of high-risk childhood ALL in order to identify genetic basis of treatment failure, and to identify new potential therapeutic targets.

A study of over 200 high-risk B-progenitor ALL cases (the Children's Oncology Group (COG) P9906 cohort) performed microarray profiling of DNA copy number alterations, gene expression, and candidate gene sequencing, and identified genetic alterations disrupting lymphoid development in over two thirds of cases.[53] Remarkably, deletion or sequence mutation of the early lymphoid transcription factor *IKZF1* (IKAROS) was present in one third of cases, most of which lacked a known cytogenetic alteration, and was associated with a tripling of the risk of treatment failure to over 75% (Fig. 6.1).[53] Importantly, this cohort lacked Ph+ ALL cases, a subtype of leukemia which commonly has a poor outcome and in which *IKZF1* is also common, suggesting that perturbation of *IKZF1* activity is a key determinant of pathogenesis and resistance to therapy in multiple subtypes of ALL. A role for *IKZF1* in ALL pathogenesis is further supported by recent results of genome-wide association studies of ALL, in which inherited SNP alleles at the *IKZF1* locus are associated with increased risk of ALL.[39,40,60] Moreover, the high-risk *IKZF1*-mutated cases had a gene expression profile similar to that of Ph+ ALL, suggesting the presence of previously unidentified mutations resulting in kinase signaling in these Ph– cases.[53] This "BCR-ABL1-like" subtype of ALL has also been identified by gene expression profiling analysis of other cohorts.[61] Candidate gene sequencing of over 100 genes, including multiple receptor and non-receptor tyrosine kinases[62] identified activating Janus kinase mutations in 10% of these high-risk ALL cases (Fig. 6.3).[63] JAK mutations are associated with a Ph-like gene expression

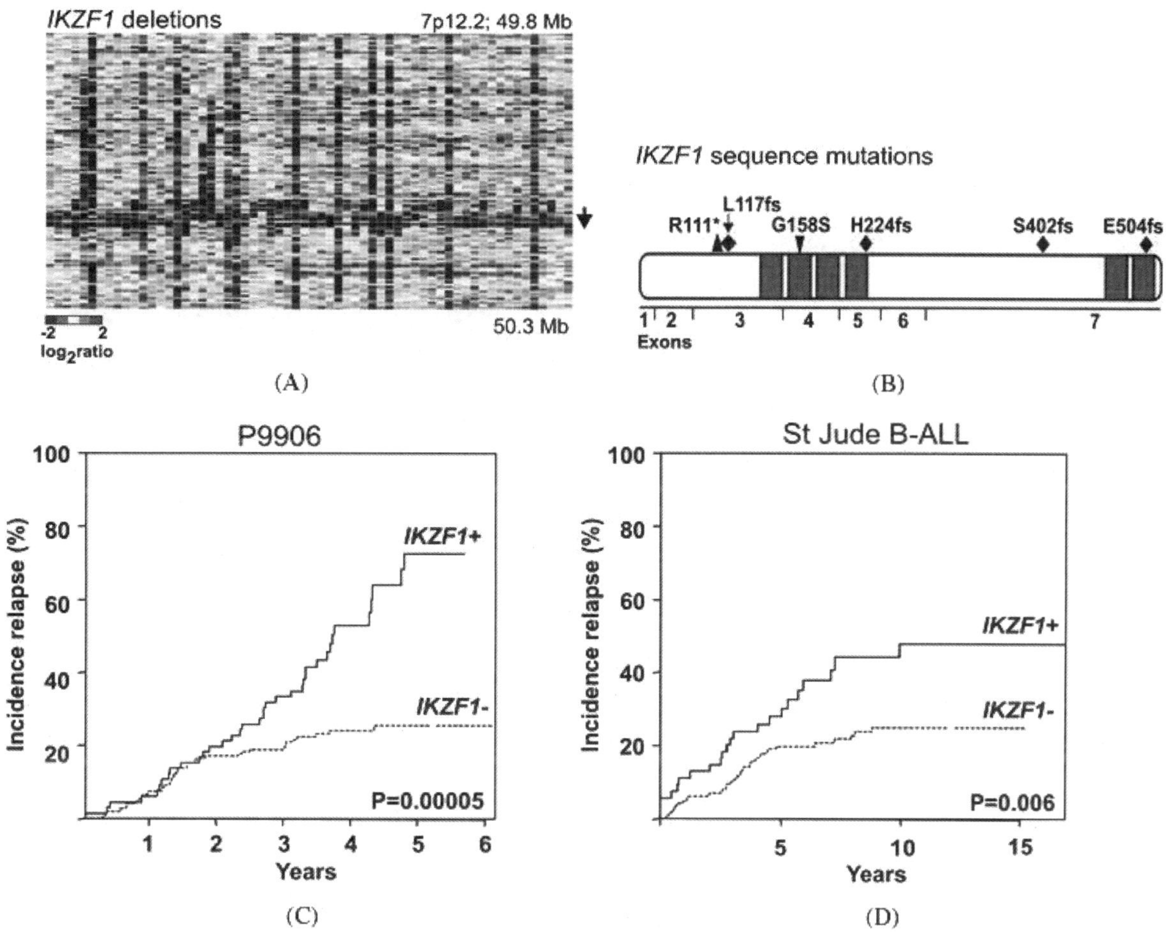

Fig. 6.2. *IKZF1* (IKAROS) alterations in ALL. (A) dChip DNA copy number heatmap showing focal and broad *IKZF1* deletions in ALL. Deletions are shown as blue. (B) Sequence mutations of *IKZF1*, and alignment with IKZF1 domains. IKAROS has four N-terminal zinc fingers that mediate DNA binding, and two C-terminal zinc fingers that mediate dimerization (green). The dominant negative isoform IK6 lacks the N-terminal zinc fingers, and the ability to bind DNA. (C) association between *IKZF1* alteration and poor outcome in two cohorts of childhood ALL. B-A, BCR-ABL1 positive; hypodiploid; H50, hyperdiploidy with greater than 50 chromosomes; E-R, ETV6-RUNX1; T-P, TCF3-PBX1. Adapted and used with permission from Mullighan CG, Su X, Zhang J, Radtke I, Phillips LA, Miller CB, Ma J, Liu W, Cheng C, Schulman BA, Harvey RC, Chen IM, Clifford RJ, Carroll WL, Reaman G, Bowman WP, Devidas M, Gerhard DS, Yang W, Relling MV, Shurtleff SA, Campana D, Borowitz MJ, Pui CH, Smith M, Hunger SP, Willman CL, Downing JR. (2009) Deletion of IKZF1 and Prognosis in Acute Lymphoblastic Leukemia. *N Engl J Med* **360**: 470–480; © Massachusetts Medical Society.[53]

profile, *IKZF1* mutations and poor outcome (Fig. 6.4). The mutations involved the pseudokinase domains of JAK1 and JAK2, and the kinase domain on JAK2, most commonly at or near R683 in the pseudokinase domain of JAK2, a previously reported site of mutation in ALL associated with Down syndrome.[64–66] JAK2 is also commonly mutated in myeloproliferative diseases (MPD) such as polycythemia vera and essential myelofibrosis,[67] but the JAK2 V617F mutation commonly observed in MPD has not been observed in ALL. An additional important finding from this study was that expression of the JAK mutations observed in ALL transformed the pro-B cell Ba/F3-EpoR cell line to cytokine-independent growth and induced constitutive Jak-Stat pathway activation. This transformation was abrogated by pharmacologic JAK1/2 inhibitors, suggesting these drugs may represent a useful therapeutic option in patients harboring these mutations.[63]

An unanswered question from these studies was why two different hematologic neoplasms — ALL and myeloproliferative diseases — were associated with different types of JAK mutations. As the most common sites of JAK2 mutation in MPD (V617) and ALL (R683) involve different faces of the JAK2 pseudokinase domain, it was tempting to speculate the mutants selectively interacted with different cytokine receptors or signaling pathways in

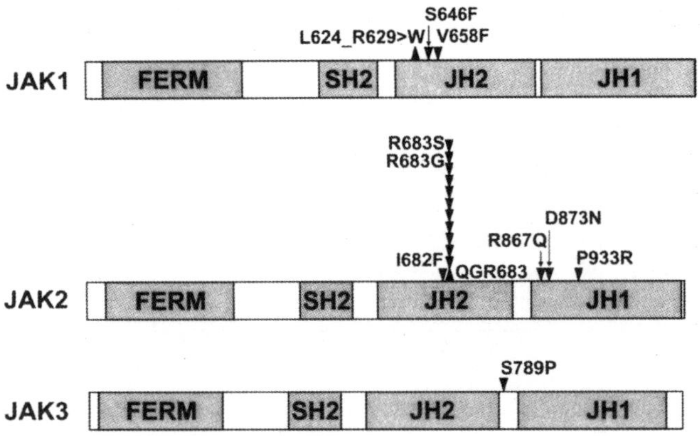

Fig. 6.3. Janus kinase mutations in ALL. Primary structure of JAK1, JAK2, and JAK3, showing the location of missense (▼) and insertion/deletion (▲) mutations. FERM, band 4.1 ezrin, radixin and moesin domain; SH2, src-homology domain; JH2, pseudokinase domain; JH1, kinase domain. The mutations involve the kinase (JH1) and pseudokinase (JH2) domains of JAK1 and JAK2. The V617F mutation observed in myeloproliferative disease is not identified in ALL. From Mullighan CG, Zhang J, Harvey RC, Collins-Underwood JR, Schulman BA, Phillips LA, Tasian SK, Loh ML, Su X, Liu W, Devidas M, Atlas SR, Chen IM, Clifford RJ, Gerhard DS, Carroll WL, Reaman GH, Smith M, Downing JR, Hunger SP, Willman CL. (2009) JAK mutations in high-risk childhood acute lymphoblastic leukemia. *Proc Natl Acad Sci U S A* **106**: 9414–9418.[63]

each disease.[63,64] Detailed analysis of SNP array and gene expression data in this P9906 cohort identified focal DNA copy number alterations adjacent to the *CRLF2* gene (encoding cytokine receptor-like factor 2, also known as the thymic stromal lymphopoietin receptor, TSLPR), and overexpression of CRLF2 in JAK-mutated ALL cases (Fig. 6.3).[11] *CRLF2* was recently identified as a target of rearrangement in B-ALL by rearrangement into the immunoglobulin heavy chain (*IGHa*) locus.[12] Subsequent work demonstrated *CRLF2* rearrangement in 5–7% of childhood ALL cases, and a significant association of *CRLF2* rearrangement and activating JAK mutations.[11,68,69] The rearrangement is most commonly a focal deletion upstream of *CRLF2* at the pseudoautosomal region 1 (PAR1) of Xp/Yp that results in fusion of the first, non-coding exon of the purinergic receptor gene *P2RY8* to the full coding region of *CRLF2* (Fig. 6.3).[11] The *P2RY8-CRLF2* fusion and *IGH@-CRLF2* rearrangement result in overexpression of CRLF2 at the cell surface of leukemic cells, which may be readily detected via flow cytometry (Fig. 6.5). *CRLF2* rearrangement, most commonly as *P2RY8-CRLF2* is particularly common in DS-ALL, being present in over 50% of cases.[11,12,69] Less commonly, activating sequence mutations in *CRLF2* have also been identified.[70,71] In both DS- and non-DS-ALL, *CRLF2* rearrangement is strongly associated with JAK mutations.[11,12,69] Over half of the cases with *CRLF2* rearrangement have activating JAK mutations, and almost all JAK-mutated cases have *CRLF2* rearrangement. The nature of the "JAK-like" mutations in other *CRLF2*-rearranged cases is at present unknown. Together, these data suggest that *IKZF1* alteration, *CRLF2* rearrangement and JAK mutations cooperate in leukemogenesis. Studies testing this hypothesis are ongoing, but existing data have shown that expression of CRLF2 in murine hematopoietic cells results in increased colony replating *in vitro*,[12,71] and coexpression of *P2RY8-CRLF2* and mutated Jak in Ba/F3 cells expression IL7 receptor alpha (the heterodimeric partner of CRLF2) is transforming (Fig. 6.3).[11] Moreover, the presence of these three alterations — *IKZF1* mutation, *CRLF2* rearrangement, and JAK mutation — is associated with poor outcome in high-risk ALL cohorts,[68] adding further impetus to clinical studies exploring JAK inhibitor therapy in these patients.

Genomic Alterations in AML

Disease-associated genomic alterations in AML can be grouped into several broad categories. Large structural alterations of the chromosomes identified in leukemic cells including duplications, deletions and translocations are identified by standard cytogenetic analyses in the majority of children with AML (Fig. 6.6). Karyotypic abnormalities remain the most significant tools for diagnosis as well as for defining prognosis in AML. More recently, mutations of genes regulating hematopoietic development have been identified; these mutations may contribute to AML pathogenesis. Such mutations have come to define AML biology, provide prognostic information and act as potential targets for directed therapy. Additional areas are emerging as major contributors to the pathogenesis of AML, including regulation of translation by non-coding RNA (miRNA) as well as epigenetic alterations due to aberrant DNA dysregulation methylation and altered histone modifications.

Cytogenetic alterations

Nonrandom numerical and structural chromosome aberrations are identified in approximately 80% of children with AML and are considered to be major contributors in an early stage of disease development. Karyotypic

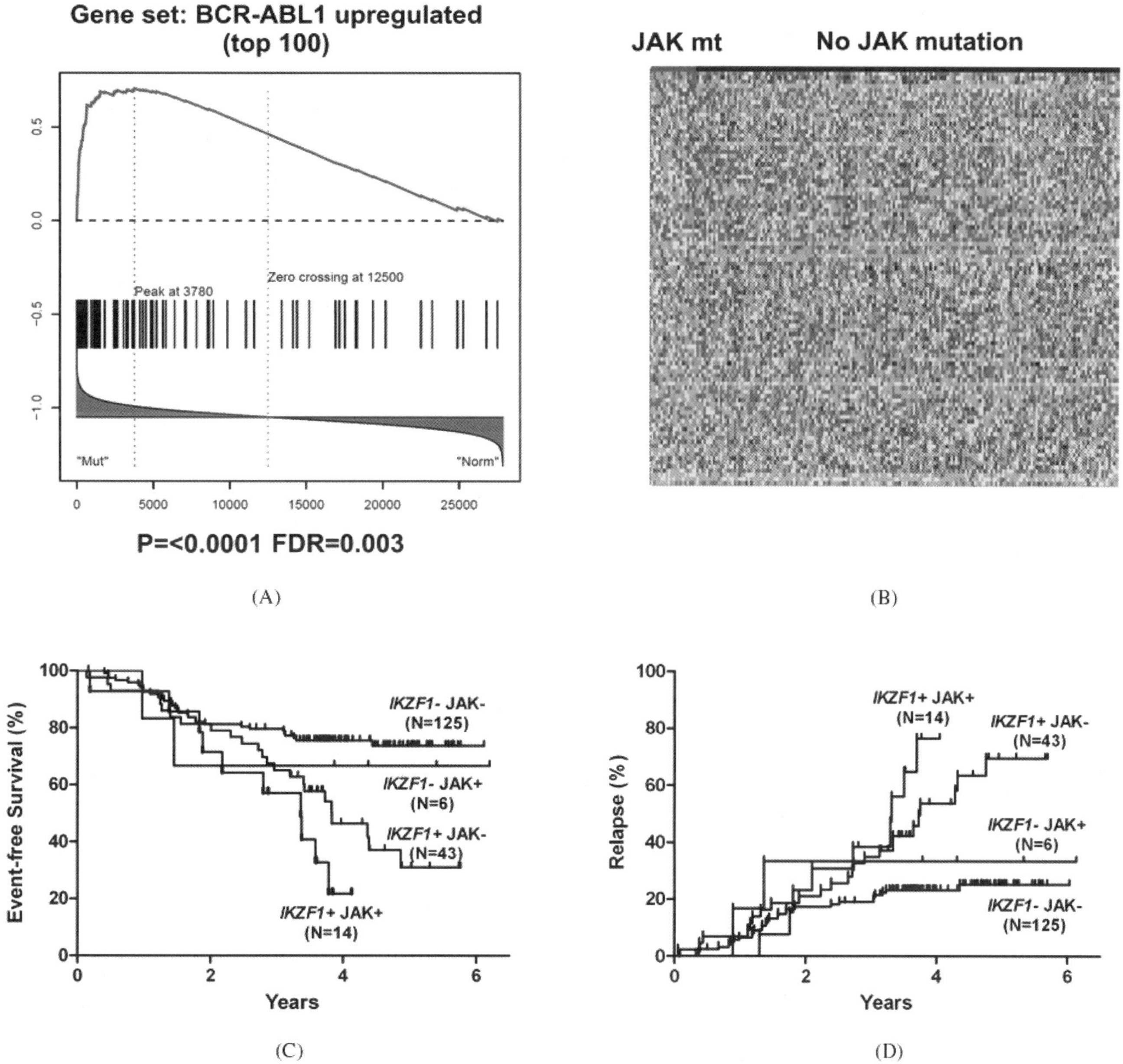

Fig. 6.4. Gene expression profiling and outcome of JAK-mutated high-risk B-progenitor ALL. (A) Gene set enrichment analysis demonstrates significant enrichment of the BCR-ABL1 gene expression signature in JAK-mutated ALL. (B) Heatmap of the enriched *BCR-ABL1* upregulated gene set in the P9906 cohort, showing overexpression of *BCR-ABL1* upregulated genes in JAK-mutated ALL. Notably, several cases lacking JAK mutations also have a *BCR-ABL1* signature, suggesting the presence of additional kinase mutations in these cases. (C–D) JAK mutation and *IKZF1* alteration are associated with a high incidence of (C) events and (D) relapse. From Mullighan CG, Zhang J, Harvey RC, Collins-Underwood JR, Schulman BA, Phillips LA, Tasian SK, Loh ML, Su X, Liu W, Devidas M, Atlas SR, Chen IM, Clifford RJ, Gerhard DS, Carroll WL, Reaman GH, Smith M, Downing JR, Hunger SP, Willman CL. (2009) JAK mutations in high-risk childhood acute lymphoblastic leukemia. *Proc Natl Acad Sci U S A* **106**: 9414–9418.[63]

alterations of leukemic cells are one of the most significant biological markers that define AML biology and the presence of specific chromosomal abnormalities have significant prognostic implications (see Chapter 5). The new WHO classification of AML has recognized this association of cytogenetic alterations with diagnosis and prognosis in AML by including the cytogenetic alterations as part of the classification schema of AML (see Chapter 3). Nearly 80% of children with AML carry at least one and frequently multiple cytogenetic abnormalities.[72,73] Core

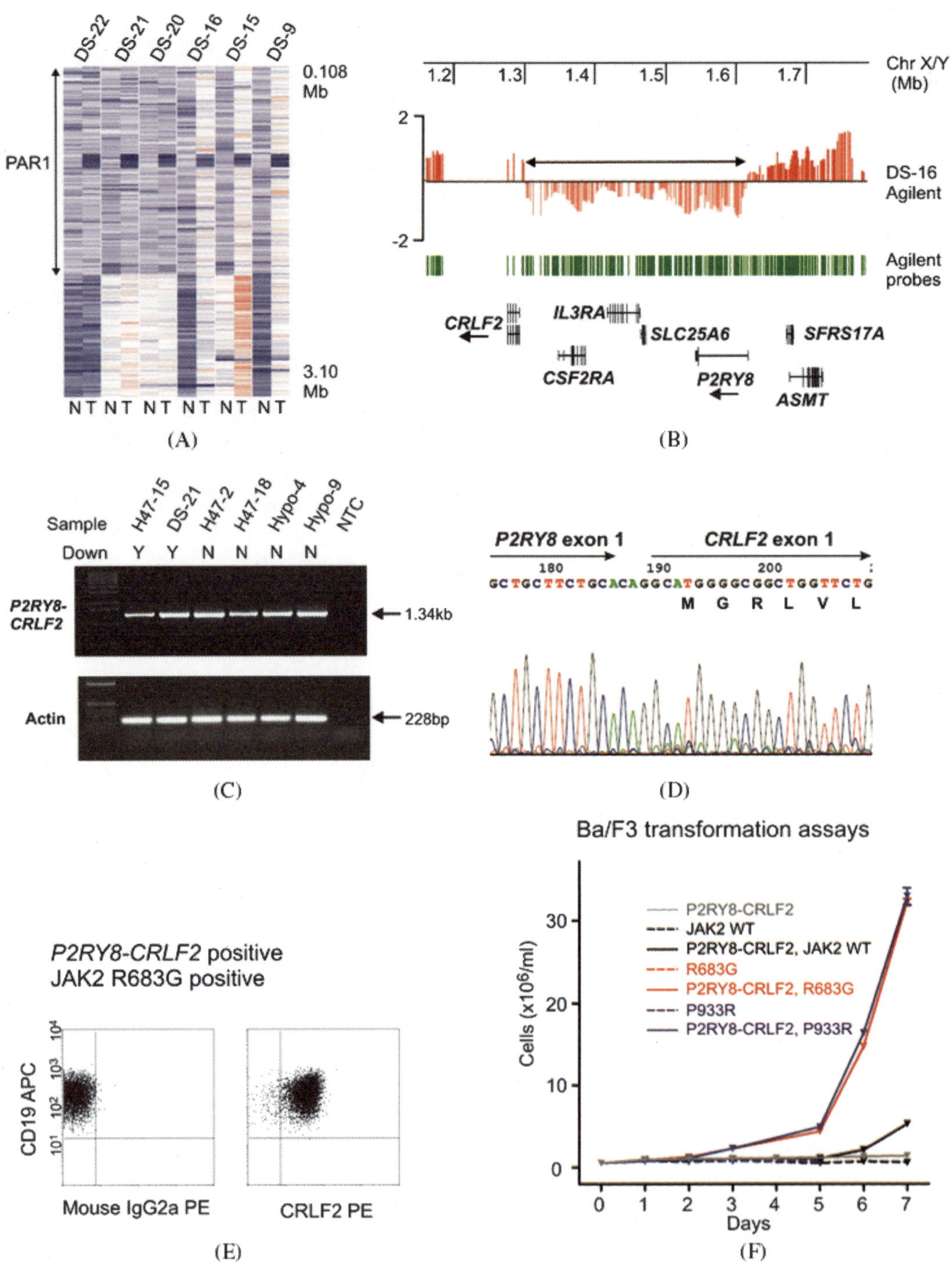

Fig. 6.5. *CRLF2* and JAK alterations in ALL. (A) Focal deletions in the pseudoautosomal 1 region of Xp/Yp in ALL. (B) Mapping of the PAR1 deletion (probe level data is shown as vertical red lines) to between intron 1 of *P2RY8* and upstream of CRLF2. (C–E) The PAR1 deletion results in *P2RY8-CRLF2* fusion that may be detected by RT-PCR (C–D), and by immunophenotyping of leukemic cells (E). (F) Expression of JAK2 mutations and *P2RY8-CRLF2* results in transformation of Ba/F3-IL7R cells to cytokine independent growth. Two examples of JAK2 mutant alleles are shown: the R683G mutation in the JAK2 pseudokinase domain, and the P933R mutation in the kinase domain. B7, Ba/F3-IL7R; DS, Down syndrome; H47, low hyperdiploid (ALL); hypo, hypodiploid; P2C, P2RY8-CRLF2; WT, wild type. From Mullighan CG, Collins-Underwood JR, Phillips LA, Loudin MG, Liu W, Zhang J, Ma J, Coustan-Smith E, Harvey RC, Willman CL, Mikhail FM, Meyer J, Carroll AJ, Williams RT, Cheng J, Heerema NA, Basso G, Pession A, Pui CH, Raimondi SC, Hunger SP, Downing JR, Carroll WL, Rabin KR. (2009) Rearrangement of CRLF2 in B-progenitor- and Down syndrome-associated acute lymphoblastic leukemia. *Nat Genet* **41**: 1243–1246.[11]

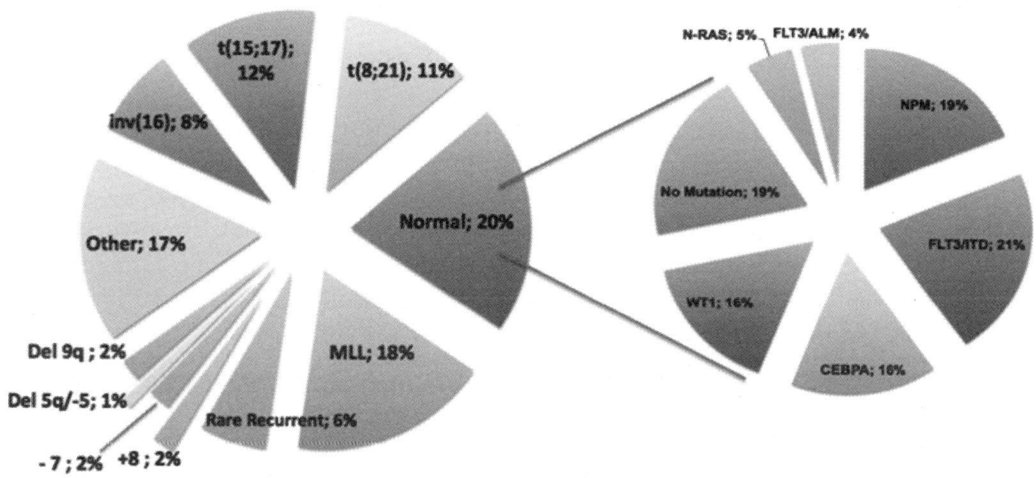

Fig. 6.6. Genomic alterations in childhood AML. The left panel demonstrates the most common cytogenetic alterations in childhood AML. Eighty percent of all children with AML have disease-associated genomic structural karyotypic alterations. The mutation profile in those without cytogenetic abnormalities (normal karyotype) is shown in the right panel, where 81% of those in the normal karyotype population have one of the known mutations.

From Childhood Leukemias, ed. Gregory Reaman and Frank Smith, Springer, 2010.

binding factor AML (CBF AML) that includes t(8;21) and inv(16) are present in 25% of childhood AML, *MLL* rearrangements in 20% and t(15;17) in 12%. In addition to karyotypic alterations, disease-associated mutations are identified in AML, with the highest prevalence in those with normal karyotype, where nearly 90% of those with normal karyotype have at least one disease-associated mutation.

t(15;17) translocations

Acute promyelocytic leukemia (APL), which is due to the abnormal accumulation of promyelocytes, is defined by a chromosomal translocation involving the retinoic acid receptor alpha (*RARα* or *RARA*) gene and is unique from other forms of AML in its biology as well as responsiveness to targeted therapy with retinoids.[74] The t(15;17) translocation juxtaposes the PML and RARA gene and leads to the expression of a novel fusion product, which is a potent recruiter of transcriptional repressors that are resistant to derepression by physiologic concentrations of retinoic acid (RA). Leukemic cells with t(15;17) are arrested in the immature, promyelocytic stage of differentiation. Identification of underlying molecular biology of APL allowed for the utility of pharmacologic doses of retinoic acid (RA) to overcome the transcription repression induced by the PML/RARA fusion product, allowing for continued differentiation of the leukemic cells down the granulocytic pathway. Such findings led to APL being the first disease to be treated by a molecularly targeted therapy. With the incorporation of all-*trans* retinoic acid (ATRA) into the therapeutic regimen, patients with APL have an excellent outcome with an overall survival of approximately 75–85% at 3 years; thus, patients with APL are currently treated differently from those having other types of AML. Understanding the biological basis of APL allowed for the development of a rational targeted therapy for this AML subtype. The resultant fusion transcript is also used for monitoring response to therapy and predicting relapse, where emergence of the fusion transcript can be detected in advance of morphologic relapse, allowing for initiation of treatment at the time of minimal disease, thus improving the survival for those with impending relapse.

Core-binding factor (CBF) AML

Recurrent chromosome translocations, inversions, and deletions result in structural genomic rearrangements often involving genes that encode transcription factors.[75,76] CBF is an α/β heterodimeric transcription factor complex involved in the transcriptional regulation of several genes important in hematopoiesis. They are characterized by a DNA binding (CBF-α) and a non-DNA binding (CBF-β) subunit. Disruption of the CBF subunit α and β genes are observed in t(8;21)(q22;q22) and inv(16)(p13q22), respectively.[77,78] The CBF α subunit binds directly to the enhancer core DNA sequence of target genes, whereas the β subunit increases the affinity and stabilizes the binding of the α subunit to the DNA. Data from *in vitro* studies and transgenic animal models suggest a dominant negative role for the fusion genes created by these rearrangements leading to the expression of a leukemic phenotype through a possible common pathway.

The balanced translocation between chromosomes 8 and 21 juxtaposes the *RUNX1* (*AML1*) gene on chromosome 21 to the *RUNX1T1* (*ETO*) gene on chromosome 8, resulting in a novel fusion transcript. The N-terminus of RUNX1 contains the DNA binding domain, and the C-terminus has the transcriptional activation function.[77] The *RUNX1T1* gene on chromosome 8 encodes a protein that functions as a transcription factor. This functional domain of the protein includes two zinc finger domains as well as a proline-rich region.[79] The chimeric *RUNX1-RUNX1T1* (*AML1-ETO*) fusion gene created as a result of t(8;21) translocation contains virtually the entire *RUNX1T1*-coding region fused to the DNA-binding domain of the *RUNX1* gene minus the activation domain. Overexpression of this chimeric protein, which retains the DNA-binding function of the AML1 gene without its activation function, acts as a dominant negative regulator of AML1 function, thus preventing transactivation of CBF targets contributing to leukemic transformation.

Two distinct translocations, inv(16)(p13q22) and t(16;16)(p13;q22), collectively referred to as inv(16), result in the fusion of the *CBFB* gene from chromosome 16q22 with the *MYH11* gene from chromosome 16p13. The *MYH11* gene encodes a myosin heavy chain.[80] A number of variants of the *CBFB-MYH11* fusion transcripts have been identified in those with inv(16) AML, with the most common variant detected in approximately 85% of patients inv(16). It is not known whether the different fusion transcripts have any clinical or biological significance.

The exact mechanism whereby the *CBFB-MYH11* fusion gene contributes to malignant transformation is unclear; however, data from murine models suggest *CBFB-MYH11* interferes with normal hematopoiesis in a dominant-negative manner, resulting from the N-terminal portion of the CBFB fusing to the C-terminal domain of the MYH11. Such an interaction directly represses the AML1-mediated transcriptional activation by sequestering AML1 into a functionally inactive complex, resulting in a similar leukemogenic paradigm as in t(8;21).

Cumulatively, CBF AML (inv(16) and t(8;21)) account for nearly a quarter of all childhood AML cases, and the prevalence of these translocations declines with age; in contrast, where the prevalence is 10–15% in adults and < 5% in AML patients older than 60 years. The presence of t(8;21) or inv(16) are associated with clinical outcome, where those with either of these translocations have a more rapid response to chemotherapy, and improved survival.[81] Although the exact mechanism of response in this subtype is not clear, there are data supporting the conclusion that patients with CBF AML benefit from intensification of cytarabine arabinoside as part of their consolidation therapy.

Acute megakaryoblastic leukemia (AMKL)

AMKL occurs almost always in childhood, and represents up to 15% of AML cases,[82] and occurs in three main contexts: AMKL associated with Down syndrome (DS-AMKL),[83] AMKL associated with translocations t(1;22), or less commonly, t(1;3),[84] and AMKL not associated with DS or these translocations. DS is associated with an up to 20-fold risk of developing acute leukemia, most commonly AMKL but also ALL.[85] DS-AMKL commonly arises after prior transient myeloproliferative disorder, a clonal myeloid disorder characterized by megakaryocytic proliferation and mutation of the transcription factor *GATA1*. *GATA1* mutations are associated with the expression of a truncated form of GATA1, and are uniquely observed in DS but not sporadic AMKL. The nature of the secondary genetic alterations cooperating with *GATA1* mutations in DS-AMKL are unknown. AMKL with t(1;22)(p13;q13) occurs in infants and young children, and is associated with bone marrow fibrosis and very poor outcome. The translocation results in rearrangement of *RBM15* (*OTT*) at 1p13 to *MKL1* (*MAL*) at 22q13.

AML with MLL rearrangement

MLL is a large protein with multiple functional domains ubiquitously expressed in hematopoietic cells and is involved in the regulation of hematopoietic differentiation and proliferation. The *MLL* gene is located on chromosome 11, band 23 (11q23) and encodes a methyltransferase involved in the regulation of *HOX* gene expression and methylation of histone residue H3K4. *In vitro* data have demonstrated that MLL fusion proteins can transform hematopoietic precursors to leukemia-initiating cells, implicating this gene in stem cell maintenance and hematopoietic regulation.[86] Structural alterations involving the mixed-lineage leukemia gene (MLL) are common in AML and appear to have an age-dependent prevalence, with a prevalence of nearly 30% in those less than 2 years of age. There is a high prevalence of *MLL* rearrangements in AML patients less than 2 years of age, and less than 10% of patients 10 years or older.[87] The prevalence of *MLL* rearrangements in adults with AML is less than 5%.[88,89] *MLL* rearrangements result in the juxtaposition of the N terminus of MLL to the C terminus of over 50 different partners, resulting in the loss of the methyltransferase domain. Some MLL fusion partners appear to positively regulate transcription by methylation of specific histone lysine residues. Studies using gene expression profiling in patients with *MLL*-rearranged AML, ALL or biphenotypic leukemia have demonstrated that those with *MLL* translocations have a unique gene expression profile regardless of the morphologic diagnosis of their disease, suggesting a common set of regulated pathways that could be therapeutically exploited.[90]

In addition to the above translocations present in nearly 70% of all childhood AML, less common structural alterations are described that are associated with worse outcome. Patients with monosomy 7 (−7), monosomy 5 and deletion 5q, which are present in less than 5% of childhood AML, have a higher rate of induction failure and extremely poor survival.[91]

Sub-karyotypic (cryptic) chromosomal abnormalities in AML

Gross cytogenetic abnormalities involving large chromosomal regions can be detected by conventional cytogenetics, and the frequency and implication of these changes have been described above. Karyotypic analysis in AML is limited by the ability to grow leukemic cells *in vitro* prior to analysis as well as the size of the region involved. Small structural alterations, including deletions or duplications, can escape detection by conventional cytogenetics and may require more specialized techniques such as fluorescence *in situ* hybridization (FISH). Loss of heterozygosity (LOH) which is generally associated with deletions, may lead to haploinsufficiency and may contribute to malignant transformation. SNP microarrays have identified regions of CN-LOH in AML.[92–94] CN-LOH may arise from homologous recombination, in which a homozygous state is achieved subsequent to an initial acquisition of a heterozygous mutation. Such an event leading to acquisition of LOH can alter the gene dosage of a particular mutation and may have significant clinical implications. CN-LOH has been described in specific populations of AML including *FLT3*/ITD and *CEBPA* mutations with varying prevalence in different studies.[95,96]

Disease-associated mutations in signal transduction pathways in AML

Cytogenetic alterations are thought to be the initiating events in leukemic transformation in AML pathogenesis. However, such events are not sufficient for acquisition of the full leukemic phenotype. In a multistep model of leukemic evolution, it is thought that additional "hits" are required to provide proliferative signal to a clone with differentiation arrest caused by the initial transforming event (translocation). Mutations of the receptor tyrosine kinases and their downstream signal transduction mediators (RAS, STAT) are implicated in AML pathogenesis and are thought to be another piece of the regulatory puzzle in AML pathogenesis. Mutations of the kinase-mediated RAS/MAP signal transduction pathways lead to constitutive activation of the signal transduction pathway. Activation of the specific membrane-bound receptors either by a ligand or by an intrinsic mutation leads to the activation of their intracellular kinase moieties. The activated receptor recruits and activates a number of proteins in the cytoplasm to form a complex of protein–protein interactions in the intracellular domain, resulting in a cascade of phosphorylation reactions that culminates in the activation of a number of secondary mediators, including MAP kinase, STAT, and AKT/PI3 kinase signal transduction pathways.[97–100] These activated mediators trigger a series of events, culminating in the regulation of cell differentiation, proliferation, apoptosis, and cell survival. Mutations in the signaling cascades are common in AML and their prevalence and biologic significance is described below (Fig. 6.7).

FLT3 mutations

FMS-like tyrosine kinase 3 (*FLT3*), a receptor tyrosine kinase (RTK), is a membrane-bound receptor with an intrinsic tyrosine kinase activity that is highly expressed in hematopoietic stem/progenitor cells and regulates hematopoietic differentiation and proliferation. Mutations in the *FLT3* gene are common in AML and lead to constitutive activation of the receptor kinase. Two distinct mutations of *FLT3* gene have been identified with similar biological but different clinical consequence. Internal tandem duplication of the juxtamembrane domain coding sequence in *FLT3* (*FLT3*/ITD) was initially identified in a high proportion of patients with AML.[100] Additional studies identified missense mutations in the activation loop domain of

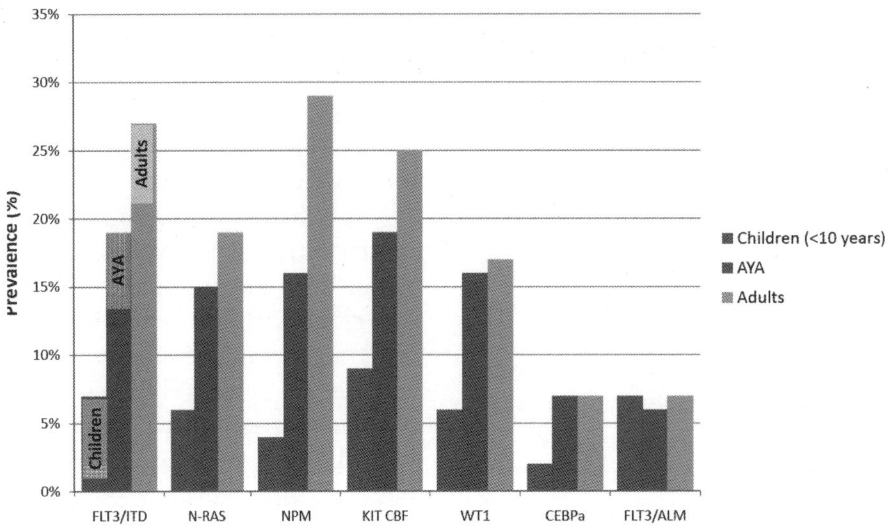

Fig. 6.7. Prevalence of mutations in AML by age category. The prevalence of the most common disease associated mutations in AML is shown for young children, AYA and adults. For the majority of mutations, prevalence increases by increasing age.

the tyrosine kinase moiety of the *FLT3* receptor (*FLT3* activation loop mutation, *FLT3*/ALM).[101]

FLT3 internal tandem duplications (FLT3/ITD)

These mutations are the result of a segmental duplication of a fragment of the juxtamembrane domain-coding region (encoded by exons 14 and 15) of FLT3 and are highly prevalent in myeloid malignancies, occurring in CML (5–10%), myelodysplasia (MDS; 5–10%), and AML (15–35%) patients.[100,102–105] The prevalence of *FLT3*/ITD is age dependent, where it is rare in infant AML, and the prevalence increases in a stepwise manner to 5–10% in age 5–10, 20% in young adults and over 35% in AML patients older than 55 years.[102] There is also considerable variability in the size of the duplicated segment (ranging from 3– > 400 bp) and this variability may have biologic and clinical significance.[100,102,103] *FLT3*/ITDs lead to constitutive activation of the *FLT3* receptor and promote cellular proliferation via the activation of multiple signaling pathways including RAS/MAPK, STAT and the AKT/PI3 kinase pathways. Studies have demonstrated that cytokine-independent cellular proliferation of *FLT3*/ITD-transduced cells was mediated by RAS and STAT5 pathways.[106] Demonstration of STAT5 activation in *FLT3*/ITD highlighted that some of the effects of *FLT3*/ITDs are unique to the mutated receptor, in contrast to *FLT3*/ITD, in which ligand-induced *FLT3*-WT activation does not lead to STAT5 activation and no STAT5 DNA binding.[106] Other studies have demonstrated that in addition to RAS and STAT pathways, *FLT3*/ITDs constitutively phosphorylate and activate AKT, and that ligand-independent growth requires this aberrant AKT activation by *FLT3*/ITDs, such that the ligand-independent growth is reversed if AKT activation is blocked. The presence of *FLT3*/ITD is associated with laboratory and clinical characteristics and outcome. Patients with *FLT3*/ITD have higher diagnostic white blood count, higher marrow blast percentage and more likely to have normal karyotypes. Furthermore, presence of *FLT3*/ITD is highly associated with clinical outcome, whereas those with *FLT3*/ITD have a higher relapse rate and poor outcome. Large studies have demonstrated the prognostic significance of *FLT3*/ITD in adult and pediatric AML trials. In these studies, survival of patients with *FLT3*/ITD was 20–30% compared to 50% for those without *FLT3*/ITD. In addition, it was demonstrated that the mutant to wild type allelic ratio observed in patients with *FLT3*/ITD appeared to influence outcome.[102,107] Evaluation of various thresholds of *FLT3*/ITD allelic ratio (ITD-AR) established an allelic ratio threshold that demarcates patients with *FLT3*/ITD at high risk of relapse from those expected to have a more favorable outcome, demonstrating it is not merely the presence of *FLT3*/ITD, but the level of mutant allele that determines clinical outcome.[102] Additional reports have demonstrated similar differences in clinical outcome for patients with AML having different mutant to wild type allelic ratios.[108] Currently, AML trials conducted by the COG utilize a *FLT3*/ITD allelic ratio of ≥0.4 to identify *FLT3*/ITD positive patients who are at high risk of relapse; these patients are referred for stem cell transplantation using the most suitable, available donor.

FLT3 activation loop mutation (FLT3/ALM) are missense point mutations within the activation loop of the *FLT3* kinase domain that promote autonomous and constitutive activation of the receptor kinase, similar to that of *FLT3*/ITD.[101,107] However, there are significant biological differences between the two types of *FLT3* mutations[109–112] as *FLT3*/ITDs and *FLT3*/ALMs appear to promote the activation of different downstream effectors[109] and different biological responses. Animal studies have demonstrated that mice harboring *FLT3*/ITDs primarily develop an oligoclonal myeloproliferative disorder, while mice harboring *FLT3*/ALM are more likely to develop oligoclonal lymphoid disorders.[110] In addition, despite their biological similarity, patients who harbor the two different mutations appear to have drastically different clinical outcomes as those with *FLT3*/ALM differ from those with *FLT3*/ITD as their outcome is not different than those without *FLT3* mutations. Prevalence of *FLT3*/ALM is 6–8%, regardless of age, and the presence of *FLT3*/ALM and *FLT3*/ITD appears to be mutually exclusive.[102] These studies further demonstrated that the presence of *FLT3*/ALM is not associated with leukocytosis, and in contrast to *FLT3*/ITD, those patients with *FLT3*/ALM AML do not have adverse outcomes.

c-KIT mutations

c-KIT is a proto-oncogene located on chromosome band 4q11–12 and a member of the type III receptor tyrosine kinase family.[113–114] Ligand stimulation of the c-KIT receptor leads to receptor dimerization and activation of the downstream signaling pathways.[109] Preferential activation of alternative pathways leading to cytokine-independent growth and increased drug resistance have been linked to specific c-KIT mutations.[115–117] Mutations of *c-KIT* mutations are infrequent in adult AML (2–8%) and tend to cluster within the activation loop (exon 17) and a region of the extracellular domain integral to receptor dimerization (exon 8).[114] Their prevalence is higher, however, in CBF AML patients (6–48%) and may be associated with worse clinical outcome in adults.[113,118–121] Although adult data suggested that the presence of KIT mutations are associated with worse clinical outcome, a study conducted in pediatric cooperative trials demonstrated a prevalence of nearly 20% but lack of clinical significance in pediatric CBF AML with *c-KIT* mutations.[122]

Other frequent mutations in AML

RAS mutations

Mutations in *N-RAS* gene occur in approximately 10–30% of adult AML cases,[103,123] and 10% of pediatric AML.[124] Point mutations frequently occur in codons 12, 13, and 61,[125] and prevent the hydrolysis of RAS-GTP, keeping RAS in the "on" or activated state. The coincident occurrence of both a *FLT3* and *RAS* mutation in the same cases is very rare, as might be expected, since there may be no *a priori* selective advantage to two mutations affecting the same pathway. However unlike *FLT3*-ITD mutations, *RAS* mutations are not prognostically important.[124] With both *FLT3* and *RAS* mutations, there may be discordance between diagnostic and relapse specimens. Thus, a patient with either a *RAS* or *FLT3* mutation at diagnosis may relapse without the mutation (or vice versa). This suggests that these mutations may not be primary oncogenic events.

Nucleophosmin (NPM1) mutations

NPM1 encodes a ubiquitously expressed and highly conserved phosphoprotein that is primarily localized to the nucleolus, but shuttles rapidly between the nucleus and cytoplasm in its role as a molecular chaperone. The NPM1 protein has been shown to contribute to many basic cellular processes, including biosynthesis of ribosomes, prevention of protein aggregation in the nucleolus, and regulation of centrosome duplication through cyclin E/cyclin-dependent kinsase 2 phosphorylation. Abnormalities in *NPM1* have been implicated in the pathogenesis of various hematopoietic malignancies, including anaplastic large cell lymphoma with t(2;5) translocation, resulting in expression of the NPM1-ALK fusion protein. Mutations in *NPM1* are common in AML, with a prevalence of 30% in adult and 8–10% in pediatric AML.[104,126–129] *NPM1* mutations appear to be more prevalent in AML with normal karyotype, with a prevalence of nearly 40–50% in adults and 20% in pediatric AML. Disease-associated mutations, characterized by four base insertions in exon 12 of the *NPM1* gene lead to impaired nuclear localization of the nucleophosmin protein. Presence of *NPM1* mutations portends favorable outcome with reduced relapse risk and improved survival, where those with *NPM1* mutations have a similar outcome as those with CBF AML (Fig. 6.8). There is significant overlap between *NPM1* mutations and *FLT3*/ITD, where nearly one third of

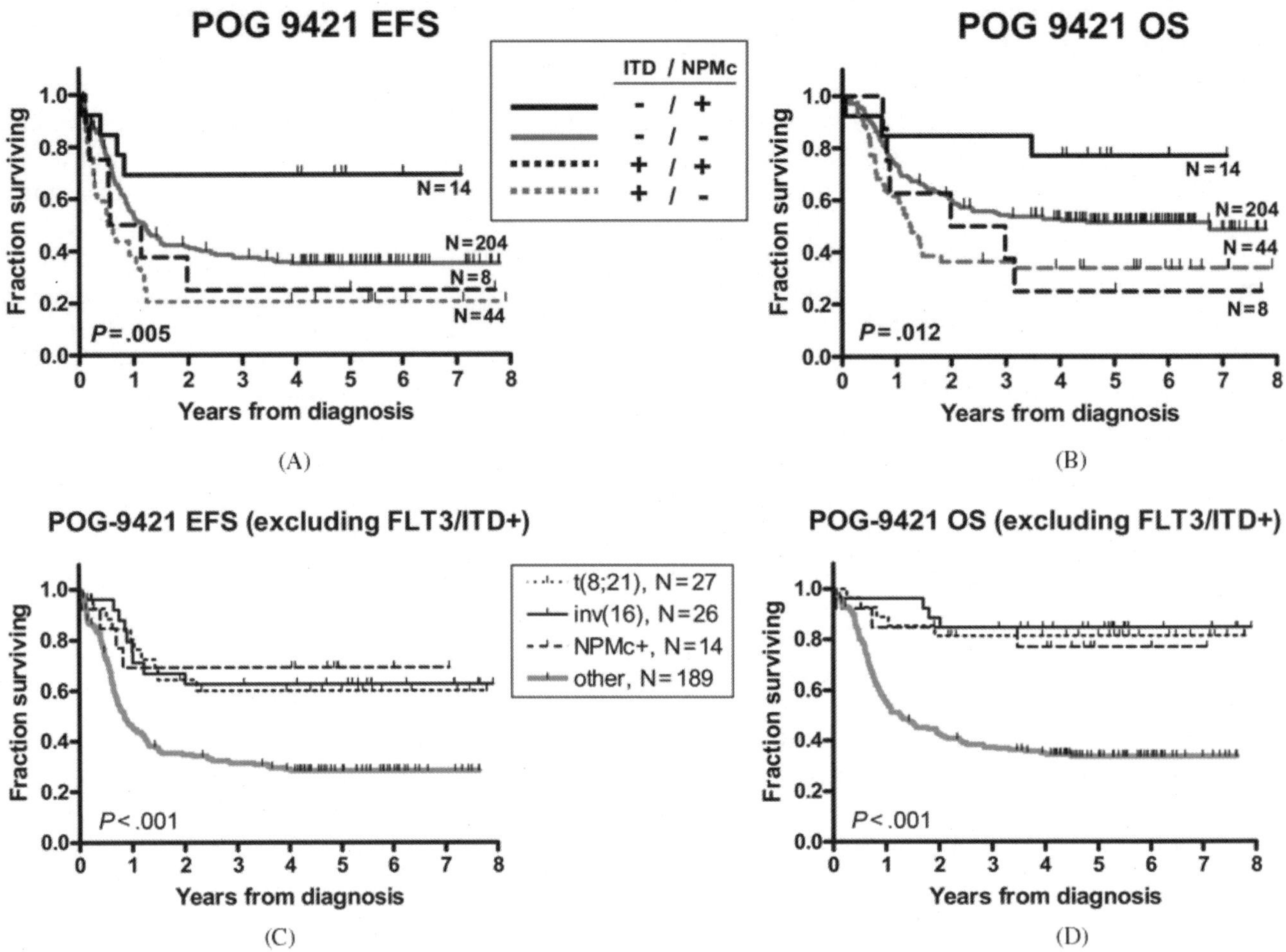

Fig. 6.8. Prognostic impact of *NPM1* mutations in childhood AML. (A–B) *NPM1* mutations (NPMc+) have prognostic value only in FLT3 ITD negative patients. Kaplan–Meier estimates of event-free survival (EFS) and overall survival (OS) according to combination of NPMc+ and FLT3-ITD in the Pediatric Oncology Group (POG) study 9421. (C–D) The prognostic effect of *NPM1* mutations is similar to t(8;21) and inv(16) in predicting favorable outcome in *FLT3* ITD negative patients. This research was originally published in *Blood*. Brown P, McIntyre E, Rau R, Meshinchi S, Lacayo N, Dahl G, Alonzo TA, Chang M, Arceci RJ, Small D. The incidence and clinical significance of nucleophosmin mutations in childhood AML. *Blood* 2007;110:979–985. © The American Society of Hematology.

those with *NPM1* mutations also have *FLT3*/ITD. In adult AML, it has been shown that *FLT3*/ITD retains its high-risk status in the presence of *NPM1* mutations. In pediatric AML, the presence of *NPM1* mutations in the presence of *FLT3*/ITD has been reported to partially ameliorate the poor prognosis conferred by *FLT3*/ITD alone.[127]

CEBPA mutations

CCAAT/enhancer binding protein-α (C/EBPa) is encoded by the *CEBPA* gene is a transcription factor that regulates proliferation and terminal granulocytic differentiation. It is a member of the basic region leucine zipper class of transcription factors, and is expressed in a variety of tissues, including adipocytes, hepatocytes, and Type II alveolar cells. In the hematopoietic system, C/EBPa is expressed in cells of myelomonocytic origin and regulates the expression of genes that regulate granulocyte differentiation. C/EBPa has been shown to inhibit E2F pathways, downregulate *C-MYC* and thus allow myeloid differentiation. CEBPA mutations occur in 4% of childhood AML cases and the overwhelming majority of cases with these mutations occur in a bi-allelic manner, where two distinct mutations occur, one in the N-terminal domain (NTD) and the second in the opposite allele affecting the bZip domain.[130] NTD mutations results in an early termination codon, which truncates the p42 protein, allowing intact translation of only the p30 protein. In a bi-allelic model, the bZip mutation in the opposite allele disrupts the bZip domains of its protein products, resulting in loss of function. Such a bi-allelic mutation would result in the expression of p30 as the only functional protein. Kirstetter *et al.* demonstrated that sole expression of p30 may be sufficient for the development of AML. In this mouse model, expression of the p30 isoform in the absence of p42 resulted in a fully penetrant AML phenotype.[131] This model would argue that both types of mutations are required for AML pathogenesis. COG studies have demonstrated that CEBPA mutations tend to occur in patients with normal cytogenetics and are associated with decreased relapse risk as well as improved survival compared to patients without a mutation (Fig. 6.9).[130]

Wilms tumor (WT1) expression and mutation

The *WT1* gene, located on chromosome 11p13, encodes a zinc-finger protein that exists in multiple isoforms and functions as a transcription factor. *WT1* is expressed in CD34+ hematopoietic progenitors, and is overexpressed in a subset of acute leukemias, including AML, ALL, and CML in blast crisis.[132] Somatic mutations of *WT1* have been reported to have variable prognostic significance.[133] Initial studies in adults suggested that the presence of *WT1* mutations was an independent prognostic factor for poor outcome. However, recent studies, including a comprehensive evaluation of pediatric AML, has identified WT mutations in 8–10% of patients; further, it was demonstrated that a strong association between *WT1* mutations and *FLT3*/ITD existed. In this study, although the presence of *WT1* mutation was associated with a worse outcome, it was shown that the prognostic significance of *WT1* mutation

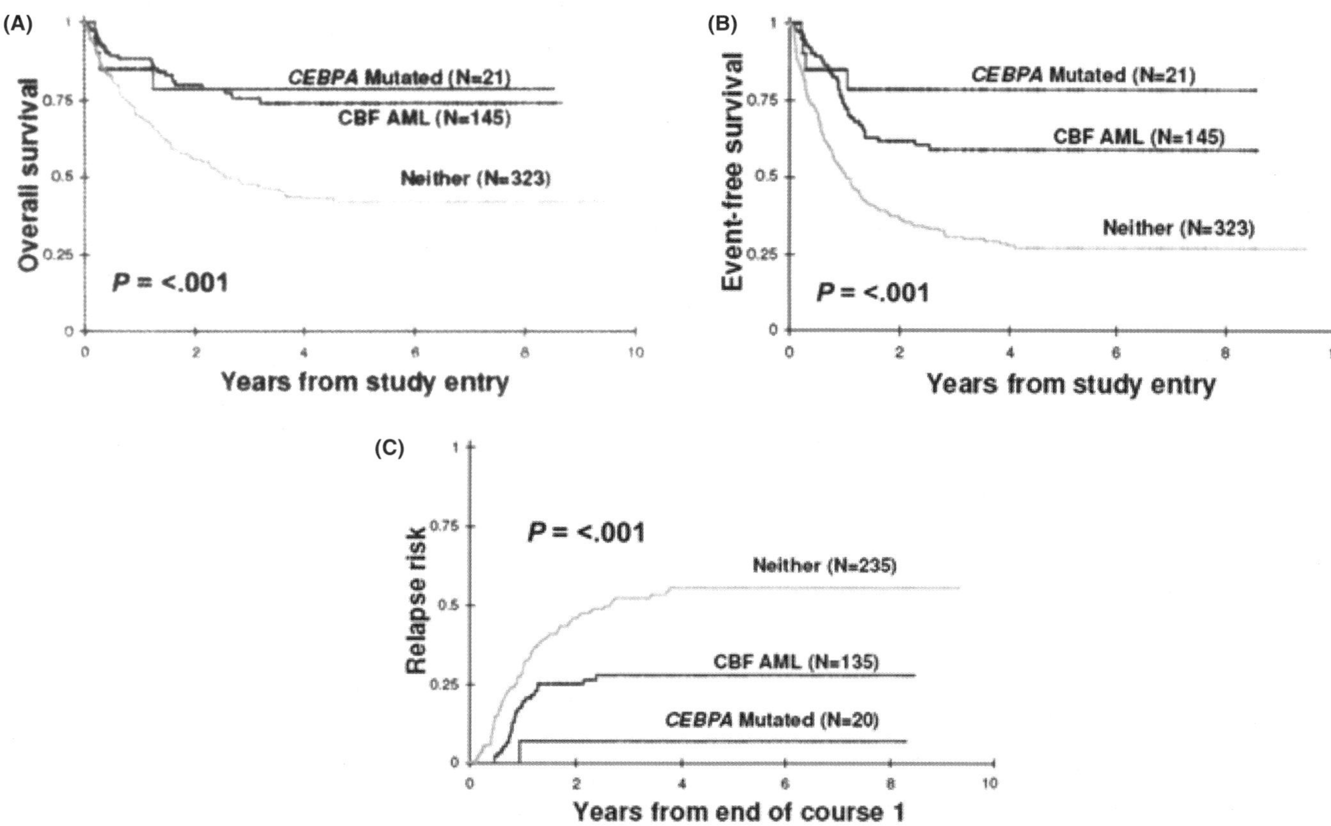

Fig. 6.9. Prognostic impact of CEBPA mutations and core binding factor gene (CBF) rearrangement status in pediatric AML. (A) Overall survival and (B) event-free survival from study entry, and (C) relapse risk from first CR for patients with and without CEBPA mutations compared with those with CBF AML. Data represents 847 pediatric AML patients on the CCG-2941, CCG-2961 and COG-AAML03P1 studies. This research was originally published in *Blood*. Ho PA, Alonzo TA, Gerbing RB, Pollard J, Stirewalt DL, Hurwitz C, Heerema NA, Hirsch B, Raimondi SC, Lange B, Franklin JL, Radich JP, Meshinchi S. Prevalence and prognostic implications of CEBPA mutations in pediatric acute myeloid leukemia (AML): A report from the Children's Oncology Group. *Blood* 2009;113:6558–6566. © The American Society of Hematology.[130]

was due to *FLT3*/ITD*;* however, in patients without *FLT3*/ITD, the presence of a *WT1* mutation did not portend poor outcome.[134]

TET2 mutations

Disease-associated genomic alterations *in TET2* gene (4q24) has recently been demonstrated in myeloid malignancies in adults. The prevalence of these mutations appears to be 20% in MDS, 10–20% in myeloproliferative disease and 12% in adult AML.[135,136] Although the prevalence of *TET2* mutations are not well defined in childhood AML, early data from COG suggest that these mutations are uncommon with a prevalence of 3% with unclear prognostic significance.

Recent advances in whole genome sequencing have enabled interrogation of the entire leukemic genome for identification of novel disease-associated mutations. Initial evaluation of a patient with AML identified numerous previously un-described mutations; however, the screening of an additional 200 patients failed to demonstrate any of these mutations in a larger cohort.[137] This study highlights the need to separate the mutations that promote the leukemic process from "passenger" mutations that do not contribute to AML initiation or progression. Whole exome sequencing and whole transcriptome sequencing allow sequencing of the entire exonic and the transcribed sequences, respectively, allowing additional means of evaluating disease profile. Application of these new technologies to AML will enable identification of genomic alterations that would be impractical to identify on a gene-by-gene basis.

Future Directions in Genomic Analysis of Acute Leukemias

Integrated analysis of DNA copy number alterations, gene expression profiling and candidate gene sequencing analysis has been highly informative in ALL and AML, but the full spectrum of somatic genetic alterations in leukemia remains to be defined, and some clinically problematic subtypes remain poorly studied. For example, there are relatively few data specifically examining ALL in adolescents, young adults and older adults. While several reports have performed genomic profiling of older children and adults,[138,139] and have identified similar genetic alterations to those seen in younger children, these studies have often lacked the resolution to detect lesions now known to be prognostically important (e.g. *IKZF1* deletions) or have lacked sufficient sample size to perform rigorous, genome-wide multivariable analyses of genetic alterations, clinical variables, and outcome. Moreover, several ALL subtypes, including ALL with low hypodiploidy,[140–143] standard risk ALL cases that fail therapy, and cases with "BCR-ABL1-like" or "kinase-like" genomic features lacking recently identified genomic rearrangements warrant further study.

Despite the prevalence of mutations identified in AML, with the exception of few mutations, significance of individual mutations in the context of other genomic alterations is yet to be defined. This molecular heterogeneity divides the AML population into small cohorts with significant genomic overlaps and different outcomes, making clinical decisions based on a single genomic marker challenging.

Additional modalities of genetic interrogation are likely to be valuable and identify new mechanisms of leukemogenesis in leukemias. Extensive candidate gene sequencing studies in ALL have identified new mutations in B-progenitor ALL,[62] indicating that genome-wide sequencing is required to identify the full complement of genetic alterations in this disease. This is now feasible with next-generation, massively parallel sequencing of tumor nucleic acids (either DNA or RNA),[144] and this has identified new targets of mutation in AML,[137,145] T-lineage ALL,[146] and lymphoma,[147] and has identified new targets of rearrangement in B-lineage ALL.[148] It is likely that as the time and cost requirements of these methods declines, sequencing-based approaches will assume greater importance in interrogating cancer genomes, and may supplant array-based methodologies.

This review has not discussed epigenetic alterations in leukemias, but there is compelling data from candidate gene studies[149,150] and genome-wide studies of AML[151] and small ALL patient cohorts[152,153] that epigenetic alterations, including cytosine methylation and histone modifications, are likely to be important initiating or downstream events in the pathogenesis of leukemias.

Acknowledgments

Work described in this review has been supported by the National Cancer Institute TARGET (Therapeutically Applicable Research to Generate Effective Treatments) initiative and the American Lebanese Syrian Associated Charities of St Jude Children's Research Hospital. C.G.M. is a Pew Scholar in the Biomedical Sciences. S.P.H. is the Ergen Family Chair in Pediatric Cancer.

References

1. Renan MJ. (1993) How many mutations are required for tumorigenesis? Implications from human cancer data. *Mol Carcinog* **7**: 139–146.
3. Wiemels J, Kang M, Greaves M. (2009) Backtracking of leukemic clones to birth. *Methods Mol Biol* **538**: 7–27.
6. Harrison CJ. (2009) Cytogenetics of paediatric and adolescent acute lymphoblastic leukaemia. *Br J Haematol* **144**: 147–156.
11. Mullighan CG, Collins-Underwood JR, Phillips LA, Loudin MG, Liu W, Zhang J, Ma J, Coustan-Smith E, Harvey RC, Willman CL, Mikhail FM, Meyer J, Carroll AJ, Williams RT, Cheng J, Heerema NA, Basso G, Pession A, Pui CH, Raimondi SC, Hunger SP, Downing JR, Carroll WL, Rabin KR. (2009) Rearrangement of CRLF2 in B-progenitor- and Down syndrome-associated acute lymphoblastic leukemia. *Nat Genet* **41**: 1243–1246.
12. Russell LJ, Capasso M, Vater I, Akasaka T, Bernard OA, Calasanz MJ, Chandrasekaran T, Chapiro E, Gesk S, Griffiths M, Guttery DS, Haferlach C, Harder L, Heidenreich O, Irving J, Kearney L, Nguyen-Khac F, Machado L, Minto L, Majid A, Moorman AV, Morrison H, Rand V, Strefford JC, Schwab C, Tonnies H, Dyer MJ, Siebert R, Harrison CJ. (2009) Deregulated expression of cytokine receptor gene, CRLF2, is involved in lymphoid transformation in B-cell precursor acute lymphoblastic leukemia. *Blood* **114**: 2688–2698.
17. Mullighan CG, Goorha S, Radtke I, Miller CB, Coustan-Smith E, Dalton JD, Girtman K, Mathew S, Ma J, Pounds SB, Su X, Pui CH, Relling MV, Evans WE, Shurtleff SA, Downing JR. (2007) Genome-wide analysis of genetic alterations in acute lymphoblastic leukaemia. *Nature* **446**: 758–764.
18. Yeoh EJ, Ross ME, Shurtleff SA, Williams WK, Patel D, Mahfouz R, Behm FG, Raimondi SC, Relling MV, Patel A, Cheng C, Campana D, Wilkins D, Zhou X, Li J, Liu H, Pui CH, Evans WE, Naeve C, Wong L, Downing JR. (2002) Classification, subtype discovery, and prediction of outcome in pediatric acute lymphoblastic leukemia by gene expression profiling. *Cancer Cell* **1**: 133–143.
21. Schultz KR, Pullen DJ, Sather HN, Shuster JJ, Devidas M, Borowitz MJ, Carroll AJ, Heerema NA, Rubnitz JE, Loh ML, Raetz EA, Winick NJ, Hunger SP, Carroll WL, Gaynon PS, Camitta BM. (2007) Risk- and response-based classification of childhood B-precursor acute lymphoblastic leukemia: A combined analysis of prognostic markers from the Pediatric Oncology Group (POG) and Children's Cancer Group (CCG). *Blood* **109**: 926–935.
22. Rubnitz JE, Wichlan D, Devidas M, Shuster J, Linda SB, Kurtzberg J, Bell B, Hunger SP, Chauvenet A, Pui CH, Camitta B, Pullen J. (2008) Prospective analysis of TEL gene rearrangements in childhood acute lymphoblastic leukemia: A Children's Oncology Group study. *J Clin Oncol* **26**: 2186–2191.
23. Arico M, Valsecchi MG, Camitta B, Schrappe M, Chessells J, Baruchel A, Gaynon P, Silverman L, Janka-Schaub G, Kamps W, Pui CH, Masera G. (2000) Outcome of treatment in children with Philadelphia chromosome-positive acute lymphoblastic leukemia. *N Engl J Med* **342**: 998–1006.
24. Schultz KR, Bowman WP, Aledo A, Slayton WB, Sather H, Devidas M, Wang C, Davies SM, Gaynon PS, Trigg M, Rutledge R, Burden L, Jorstad D, Carroll A, Heerema NA, Winick N, Borowitz MJ, Hunger SP, Carroll WL, Camitta B. (2009) Improved early event-free survival with imatinib in Philadelphia chromosome-positive acute lymphoblastic leukemia: A children's oncology group study. *J Clin Oncol* **27**: 5175–5181.
26. Weinstein IB, Joe A. (2008) Oncogene addiction. *Cancer Res* **68**: 3077–3080; discussion 3080.
27. Jones S, Zhang X, Parsons DW, Lin JC, Leary RJ, Angenendt P, Mankoo P, Carter H, Kamiyama H, Jimeno A, Hong SM, Fu B, Lin MT, Calhoun ES, Kamiyama M, Walter K, Nikolskaya T, Nikolsky Y, Hartigan J, Smith DR, Hidalgo M, Leach SD, Klein AP, Jaffee EM, Goggins M, Maitra A, Iacobuzio-Donahue C, Eshleman JR, Kern SE, Hruban RH, Karchin R, Papadopoulos N, Parmigiani G, Vogelstein B, Velculescu VE, Kinzler KW. (2008) Core signaling pathways in human pancreatic cancers revealed by global genomic analyses. *Science* **321**: 1801–1806.
29. Ford AM, Ridge SA, Cabrera ME, Mahmoud H, Steel CM, Chan LC, Greaves M. (1993) In utero rearrangements in the trithorax-related oncogene in infant leukaemias. *Nature* **363**: 358–360.
31. Greaves MF, Wiemels J. (2003) Origins of chromosome translocations in childhood leukaemia. *Nat Rev Cancer* **3**: 639–649.
32. Mori H, Colman SM, Xiao Z, Ford AM, Healy LE, Donaldson C, Hows JM, Navarrete C, Greaves M. (2002) Chromosome translocations and covert leukemic clones are generated during normal fetal development. *Proc Natl Acad Sci U S A* **99**: 8242–8247.
33. Kuiper RP, Schoenmakers EF, van Reijmersdal SV, Hehir-Kwa JY, van Kessel AG, van Leeuwen FN, Hoogerbrugge PM. (2007) High-resolution genomic profiling of childhood ALL reveals novel recurrent genetic lesions affecting pathways involved in lymphocyte differentiation and cell cycle progression. *Leukemia* **21**: 1258–1266.

34. Kawamata N, Ogawa S, Zimmermann M, Kato M, Sanada M, Hemminki K, Yamatomo G, Nannya Y, Koehler R, Flohr T, Miller CW, Harbott J, Ludwig WD, Stanulla M, Schrappe M, Bartram CR, Koeffler HP. (2008) Molecular allelokaryotyping of pediatric acute lymphoblastic leukemias by high-resolution single nucleotide polymorphism oligonucleotide genomic microarray. *Blood* **111**: 776–784.
35. Parker H, An Q, Barber K, Case M, Davies T, Konn Z, Stewart A, Wright S, Griffiths M, Ross FM, Moorman AV, Hall AG, Irving JA, Harrison CJ, Strefford JC. (2008) The complex genomic profile of ETV6-RUNX1 positive acute lymphoblastic leukemia highlights a recurrent deletion of TBL1XR1. *Genes Chromosomes Cancer* **47**: 1118–1125.
36. Bateman CM, Colman SM, Chaplin T, Young BD, Eden TO, Bhakta M, Gratias EJ, van Wering ER, Cazzaniga G, Harrison CJ, Hain R, Ancliff P, Ford AM, Kearney L, Greaves M. (2010) Acquisition of genome-wide copy number alterations in monozygotic twins with acute lymphoblastic leukemia. *Blood* **115**: 3553–3558.
39. Trevino LR, Yang W, French D, Hunger SP, Carroll WL, Devidas M, Willman C, Neale G, Downing J, Raimondi SC, Pui CH, Evans WE, Relling MV. (2009) Germline genomic variants associated with childhood acute lymphoblastic leukemia. *Nat Genet* **41**: 1001–1005.
40. Papaemmanuil E, Hosking FJ, Vijayakrishnan J, Price A, Olver B, Sheridan E, Kinsey SE, Lightfoot T, Roman E, Irving JA, Allan JM, Tomlinson IP, Taylor M, Greaves M, Houlston RS. (2009) Loci on 7p12.2, 10q21.2 and 14q11.2 are associated with risk of childhood acute lymphoblastic leukemia. *Nat Genet* **41**: 1006–1010.
43. Mullighan CG, Miller CB, Radtke I, Phillips LA, Dalton J, Ma J, White D, Hughes TP, Le Beau MM, Pui CH, Relling MV, Shurtleff SA, Downing JR. (2008) BCR-ABL1 lymphoblastic leukaemia is characterized by the deletion of Ikaros. *Nature* **453**: 110–114.
45. van Vlierberghe P, van Grotel M, Beverloo HB, Lee C, Helgason T, Buijs-Gladdines J, Passier M, van Wering ER, Veerman AJ, Kamps WA, Meijerink JP, Pieters R. (2006) The cryptic chromosomal deletion del(11)(p12p13) as a new activation mechanism of LMO2 in pediatric T-cell acute lymphoblastic leukemia. *Blood* **108**: 3520–3529.
47. Gutierrez A, Sanda T, Grebliunaite R, Carracedo A, Salmena L, Ahn Y, Dahlberg S, Neuberg D, Moreau LA, Winter SS, Larson R, Zhang J, Protopopov A, Chin L, Pandolfi PP, Silverman LB, Hunger SP, Sallan SE, Look AT. (2009) High frequency of PTEN, PI3K, and AKT abnormalities in T-cell acute lymphoblastic leukemia. *Blood* **114**: 647–650.
48. Mullighan CG, Phillips LA, Su X, Ma J, Miller CB, Shurtleff SA, Downing JR. (2008) Genomic analysis of the clonal origins of relapsed acute lymphoblastic leukemia. *Science* **322**: 1377–1380.
52. Martinelli G, Iacobucci I, Storlazzi CT, Vignetti M, Paoloni F, Cilloni D, Soverini S, Vitale A, Chiaretti S, Cimino G, Papayannidis C, Paolini S, Elia L, Fazi P, Meloni G, Amadori S, Saglio G, Pane F, Baccarani M, Foa R. (2009) IKZF1 (Ikaros) deletions in BCR-ABL1-positive acute lymphoblastic leukemia are associated with short disease-free survival and high rate of cumulative incidence of relapse: A GIMEMA AL WP report. *J Clin Oncol* **27**: 5202–5207.
53. Mullighan CG, Su X, Zhang J, Radtke I, Phillips LA, Miller CB, Ma J, Liu W, Cheng C, Schulman BA, Harvey RC, Chen IM, Clifford RJ, Carroll WL, Reaman G, Bowman WP, Devidas M, Gerhard DS, Yang W, Relling MV, Shurtleff SA, Campana D, Borowitz MJ, Pui CH, Smith M, Hunger SP, Willman CL, Downing JR. (2009) Deletion of IKZF1 and Prognosis in Acute Lymphoblastic Leukemia. *N Engl J Med* **360**: 470–480.
56. Nutt SL, Kee BL. (2007) The transcriptional regulation of B cell lineage commitment. *Immunity* **26**: 715–725.
61. den Boer ML, van Slegtenhorst M, de Menezes RX, Cheok MH, Buijs-Gladdines JG, Peters ST, van Zutven LJ, Beverloo HB, van der Spek PJ, Escherich G, Horstmann MA, Janka-Schaub GE, Kamps WA, Evans WE, Pieters R. (2009) A subtype of childhood acute lymphoblastic leukaemia with poor treatment outcome: A genome-wide classification study. *Lancet Oncol* **10**: 125–134.
63. Mullighan CG, Zhang J, Harvey RC, Collins-Underwood JR, Schulman BA, Phillips LA, Tasian SK, Loh ML, Su X, Liu W, Devidas M, Atlas SR, Chen IM, Clifford RJ, Gerhard DS, Carroll WL, Reaman GH, Smith M, Downing JR, Hunger SP, Willman CL. (2009) JAK mutations in high-risk childhood acute lymphoblastic leukemia. *Proc Natl Acad Sci U S A* **106**: 9414–9418.
64. Bercovich D, Ganmore I, Scott LM, Wainreb G, Birger Y, Elimelech A, Shochat C, Cazzaniga G, Biondi A, Basso G, Cario G, Schrappe M, Stanulla M, Strehl S, Haas OA, Mann G, Binder V, Borkhardt A, Kempski H, Trka J, Bielorei B, Avigad S, Stark B, Smith O, Dastugue N, Bourquin JP, Tal NB, Green AR, Izraeli S. (2008) Mutations of JAK2 in acute lymphoblastic leukaemias associated with Down's syndrome. *Lancet* **372**: 1484–1492.
67. Levine RL, Pardanani A, Tefferi A, Gilliland DG. (2007) Role of JAK2 in the pathogenesis and therapy of myeloproliferative disorders. *Nat Rev Cancer* **7**: 673–683.

68. Harvey RC, Mullighan CG, Chen IM, Wharton W, Mikhail FM, Carroll AJ, Kang H, Liu W, Dobbin KK, Smith MA, Carroll WL, Devidas M, Bowman WP, Camitta BM, Reaman GH, Hunger SP, Downing JR, Willman CL. (2010) Rearrangement of CRLF2 is associated with mutation of JAK kinases, alteration of IKZF1, Hispanic/Latino ethnicity, and a poor outcome in pediatric B-progenitor acute lymphoblastic leukemia. *Blood* **115**: 5312–5321.

72. Raimondi SC, Chang MN, Ravindranath Y, Behm FG, Gresik MV, Steuber CP, Weinstein HJ, Carroll AJ. (1999) Chromosomal abnormalities in 478 children with acute myeloid leukemia: Clinical characteristics and treatment outcome in a cooperative pediatric oncology group study-POG 8821. *Blood* **94**: 3707–3716.

74. Lo-Coco F, Ammatuna E. (2006) The biology of acute promyelocytic leukemia and its impact on diagnosis and treatment. *Hematology Am Soc Hematol Educ Program*: 156–161, 514.

79. Miyoshi H, Kozu T, Shimizu K, Enomoto K, Maseki N, Kaneko Y, Kamada N, Ohki M. (1993) The t(8;21) translocation in acute myeloid leukemia results in production of an AML1-MTG8 fusion transcript. *EMBO J* **12**: 2715–2721.

80. van der Reijden BA, Dauwerse JG, Wessels JW, Beverstock GC, Hagemeijer A, van Ommen GJ, Breuning MH. (1993) A gene for a myosin peptide is disrupted by the inv(16)(p13q22) in acute nonlymphocytic leukemia M4Eo. *Blood* **82**: 2948–2952.

83. Roy A, Roberts I, Norton A, Vyas P. (2009) Acute megakaryoblastic leukaemia (AMKL) and transient myeloproliferative disorder (TMD) in Down syndrome: A multi-step model of myeloid leukaemogenesis. *Br J Haematol* **147**: 3–12.

89. Balgobind BV, Raimondi SC, Harbott J, Zimmermann M, Alonzo TA, Auvrignon A, Beverloo HB, Chang M, Creutzig U, Dworzak MN, Forestier E, Gibson B, Hasle H, Harrison CJ, Heerema NA, Kaspers GJ, Leszl A, Litvinko N, Nigro LL, Morimoto A, Perot C, Pieters R, Reinhardt D, Rubnitz JE, Smith FO, Stary J, Stasevich I, Strehl S, Taga T, Tomizawa D, Webb D, Zemanova Z, Zwaan CM, van den Heuvel-Eibrink MM. (2009) Novel prognostic subgroups in childhood 11q23/MLL-rearranged acute myeloid leukemia: Results of an international retrospective study. *Blood* **114**: 2489–2496.

90. Armstrong SA, Staunton JE, Silverman LB, Pieters R, den Boer ML, Minden MD, Sallan SE, Lander ES, Golub TR, Korsmeyer SJ. (2002) MLL translocations specify a distinct gene expression profile that distinguishes a unique leukemia. *Nat Genet* **30**: 41–47.

96. Radtke I, Mullighan CG, Ishii M, Su X, Cheng J, Ma J, Ganti R, Cai Z, Goorha S, Pounds SB, Cao X, Obert C, Armstrong J, Zhang J, Song G, Ribeiro RC, Rubnitz JE, Raimondi SC, Shurtleff SA, Downing JR. (2009) Genomic analysis reveals few genetic alterations in pediatric acute myeloid leukemia. *Proc Natl Acad Sci U S A* **106**: 12944–12949.

100. Nakao M, Yokota S, Iwai T, Kaneko H, Horiike S, Kashima K, Sonoda Y, Fujimoto T, Misawa S. (1996) Internal tandem duplication of the flt3 gene found in acute myeloid leukemia. *Leukemia* **10**: 1911–1918.

102. Meshinchi S, Alonzo TA, Stirewalt DL, Zwaan M, Zimmerman M, Reinhardt D, Kaspers GJ, Heerema NA, Gerbing R, Lange BJ, Radich JP. (2006) Clinical implications of FLT3 mutations in pediatric AML. *Blood* **108**: 3654–3661.

114. Renneville A, Roumier C, Biggio V, Nibourel O, Boissel N, Fenaux P, Preudhomme C. (2008) Cooperating gene mutations in acute myeloid leukemia: A review of the literature. *Leukemia* **22**: 915–931.

122. Pollard JA, Alonzo TA, Gerbing RB, Ho PA, Zeng R, Ravindranath Y, Dahl G, Lacayo NJ, Becton D, Chang M, Weinstein HJ, Hirsch B, Raimondi SC, Heerema NA, Woods WG, Lange BJ, Hurwitz C, Arceci RJ, Radich JP, Bernstein ID, Heinrich MC, Meshinchi S. (2010) Prevalence and prognostic significance of KIT mutations in pediatric patients with core binding factor AML enrolled on serial pediatric cooperative trials for *de novo* AML. *Blood* **115**: 2372–2379.

124. Berman JN, Gerbing RB, Sung L, Miller K, Pollard JA, Ho P, Stirewalt D, Radich J, Hurwitz CA, Heerema NA, Hirsch B, Raimondi SC, Lange B, Gamis AS, Franklin JL, Alonzo TA, Meshinchi S. (2009) Prevalence and clinical implications of N-RAS mutations in childhood AML: A report from the Children's Oncology Group. *Blood (ASH Annual Meeting Abstracts)* **114**: 3115.

128. Brown P, McIntyre E, Rau R, Meshinchi S, Lacayo N, Dahl G, Alonzo TA, Chang M, Arceci RJ, Small D. (2007) The incidence and clinical significance of nucleophosmin mutations in childhood AML. *Blood* **110**: 979–985.

130. Ho PA, Alonzo TA, Gerbing RB, Pollard J, Stirewalt DL, Hurwitz C, Heerema NA, Hirsch B, Raimondi SC, Lange B, Franklin JL, Radich JP, Meshinchi S. (2009) Prevalence and prognostic implications of CEBPA mutations in pediatric acute myeloid leukemia (AML): A report from the Children's Oncology Group. *Blood* **113**: 6558–6566.

137. Ley TJ, Mardis ER, Ding L, Fulton B, McLellan MD, Chen K, Dooling D, Dunford-Shore BH, McGrath S,

Hickenbotham M, Cook L, Abbott R, Larson DE, Koboldt DC, Pohl C, Smith S, Hawkins A, Abbott S, Locke D, Hillier LW, Miner T, Fulton L, Magrini V, Wylie T, Glasscock J, Conyers J, Sander N, Shi X, Osborne JR, Minx P, Gordon D, Chinwalla A, Zhao Y, Ries RE, Payton JE, Westervelt P, Tomasson MH, Watson M, Baty J, Ivanovich J, Heath S, Shannon WD, Nagarajan R, Walter MJ, Link DC, Graubert TA, DiPersio JF, Wilson RK. (2008) DNA sequencing of a cytogenetically normal acute myeloid leukaemia genome. *Nature* **456**: 66–72.

7

Cytogenetics of Lymphoma in Children and Young Adults

John Swansbury and Warren Sanger

Introduction

The volume of published cytogenetic data from children and young adults (CAYA) with lymphoma is small. Although lymphoma is a relatively common type of cancer in this age group, in absolute terms it is still an uncommon disease, so there are relatively few cases available for study. Also, easily accessible tissues such as blood and bone marrow are infrequently infiltrated, thus not all cases are adequately studied; some clones have very complex karyotypes and cannot be fully defined. Also, few modern journals will accept routine cytogenetic results for publication. A substantial proportion of the cases in the literature were published well over a decade ago, when the diseases were less well defined diagnostically, sometimes without the benefit of immunophenotyping and using differing classifications. For all these reasons, cytogenetic data in pediatric lymphomas have not had as much clinical impact as they have had in pediatric leukemia.

Despite these limitations, there is now a sufficient understanding of the available cytogenetic data useful to the clinician in giving an indication of likely differential responses to treatment. Many types of childhood lymphoma respond well to intensive treatment, but such therapies can have potentially harmful sequelae in children, and so it is important to minimize these whenever possible. More data are needed, and it is likely that the newer technologies such as microarray and gene expression arrays will contribute (see Chapter 8). Some information from these sources is already available. Hummel *et al.*,[1] for example, have reported the use of transcriptional and genomic profiling to define Burkitt lymphoma (BL). Because it is too early to assess the practical implications of these new types of data, this chapter will focus on the main lessons from classic cytogenetics and fluorescence *in situ* hybridization (FISH) studies.

Cytogenetics and Disease Types Vary with Age

Although it may be arbitrary to define an age that separates adults from CAYA, it is clear that there are differences in the types of lymphoma prevalent at each end of the age spectrum. Some types of non-Hodgkin lymphoma (NHL) that have well-characterized cytogenetic features in adults are almost unknown in CAYA; others occur far more frequently in CAYA than in adults. In addition, there is increasing evidence that there are age-related biological differences in the same types of lymphoma. Poirel *et al.*[2] describe differences between children and adults in the incidence of both primary and secondary cytogenetic abnormalities. This might suggest that genetics could be a more useful guide to the choice of treatment than mere age. However, a more fruitful approach might be to regard age and cytogenetic data as being complementary: For example, Kim *et al.*[3]

have reported that in acute lymphoblastic leukemia (ALL), homozygous deletions of the *CDKN2A* and *CDKN2B* genes are associated with a poor prognosis in adults but not in children; similar associations may yet be discovered in lymphomas.

Cytogenetic Abnormalities Associated with Disease Types

The proportion of different lymphoma types with available cytogenetic information does not accurately reflect the true pattern since some types are more amenable to cytogenetic study than others. For example, BL and DLBCL are more likely to infiltrate bone marrow than ALCL, in which more than 90% of cases do not have BM involvement. It is a source of frustration to many cytogeneticists that a secondary tissue such as BM (instead of nodal material) is often sent for study, since it proves not to be infiltrated in many cases. If a diagnostic study is required, nodal tissue should be supplied. Cytogenetic studies are not suitable for assessing involvement of bone marrow, which can be done far more accurately by immunophenotyping.

A few cytogenetic abnormalities occur, often as secondary changes, in almost all kinds of lymphoma, and these include translocations involving chromosome 1, and deletion of part of the long arms of chromosome 6 (especially involving bands q21, q23, and q27). Others have a degree of diagnostic specificity, and some of these are described below.

Burkitt lymphoma/leukemia (BL)

Most cytogenetics studies have been of the sporadic form of BL, which accounts for 30–50% of NHL in CAYA.[4] There have been few reports comparing the genetics of the endemic and sporadic forms.[5]

Cytogenetically, BL is indistinguishable from the L3 FAB type of ALL. The great majority of cases have a primary cytogenetic abnormality that involves the *MYC* gene region at 8q24, in the form of one of three translocations:[5,6] the t(8;14)(q24;q32), with a *MYC-IGH@* fusion (70–80%); the t(2;8)(p12;q24), with a *MYC-IGK* fusion (5–10%); and the t(8;22)(q24;q11), with a *MYC-IGL* fusion (5–10%).

In 5–15% of well-studied cases, no *MYC* translocation is detected.[1,2,7–9] There is no evidence so far that the prognosis for the relatively few *MYC*-negative cases is significantly different from that of *MYC*-positive cases of BL.[2]

In 10–40% of cases of BL, the clone has just the primary cytogenetic abnormality.[2,7,10,11] This contrasts with other types of childhood lymphoma, in which a *MYC* translocation, if present, is rarely the sole abnormality.

The most common secondary abnormalities are gains of 1q, 7q and 12q, and losses of 6q, 13q, and 17p.[2,5,8,10–12] A gain of 1q, which is the most common (and often the only) secondary abnormality, appears to have no effect on outcome; it occurs in many types of tumors, thus it clearly has a major role in tumorigenesis or tumor progression that has yet to be identified. Gain of 7q and loss of 13q, particularly the 13q14 region, have been shown to have an adverse effect on prognosis, not only in BL[9] but also in DLBCL.[2] It is important to note that deletion of 13q is often not chromosomally visible, but it is more readily detected by FISH.[9] It has been suggested that these could be secondary abnormalities associated with tumor progression in most or all types of childhood B-NHL.[2] Some other recurrent abnormalities have been reported in too few cases to have a detectable effect on prognosis. However, increasing the use of FISH studies of primary tissue, such as paraffin-embedded lymph nodes, rather than depending on finding chromosome abnormalities in metaphase studies, should help to increase the amount of data available on the incidence of secondary abnormalities.

A complex clone, defined as having at least three abnormalities, has been associated with a poorer prognosis,[2] though this is due, at least in part, to the frequent inclusion of 7q gain and 13q loss in complex karyotypes.

In a small proportion of children, their disease is high grade and is described as being Burkitt-like or atypical BL. Cytogenetically, these are similar to BL in having a high incidence of MYC rearrangements, but in almost all cases, they are part of a complex clone.[2,8,13]

Diffuse large cell lymphoma (DLBCL)

This is the most common class of NHL in adults, constituting 85% of intermediate-grade lymphomas; it includes a variety of disease subtypes. However, it is uncommon in younger adults and rare in children. In adults, the most common cytogenetic abnormalities are translocations involving the *BCL6* gene at 3q27 or the *IGH@* gene at 14q32, and abnormalities of 1q21. *BCL2* at 18q21 is a common *IGH@* partner. In children, however, *BCL6* (3q27) and *BCL2* (18q21) are far less commonly involved; in the large series reported by Poirel *et al.*,[2] these genes were involved in less than 7%

of cases; Dave *et al.*[14] did not find any cases with abnormal *BCL6* and Oschlies *et al.*[15] found no cases with t(14;18)(q32;q21) in their FISH studies of 63 cases of pediatric DLBCL. Conversely, translocations involving *MYC* are rare in adults with DLBCL, and the incidence in children is much higher, being 33% in the series reported by Poirel *et al.*[2] In 93% of their cases, the clone had further abnormalities, and it was suggested that the *MYC* translocation might often be a secondary event. The outcome for these cases was significantly worse than for other children with DLBCL. The contrasting cytogenetic data strongly suggest that DLBCL, in most pediatric cases, is a different disease from that found in adults.

Some cytogenetic abnormalities occur significantly more frequently in DLBCL than in BL. These include deletions of 6q, translocations involving 11q, and trisomy for chromosome 12 (Table 7.1).[2,14]

T-cell lymphomas

Cytogenetically, T-cell ALL and T-cell lymphoblastic lymphoma (LBL) appear to be very similar diseases, with the same chromosome abnormalities occurring in both.[16] The majority of these are translocations that involve the *TCR* genes, *TCR-* and *TCR-δ* at 14q11, *TCR-β* at 7q34–36, and *TCR-γ* at 7p15. There is some evidence that particular partner genes, such as *TAL1, MYC, LMO2*, or *NOTCH1*, may be associated with an inferior prognosis.[17]

Table 7.1. Comparison of cytogenetic abnormalities occurring in BL, Burkitt-like lymphoma, and DLBCL.

	BL	BLL	DLBCL
Number of cases	182	18	30
Translocations involving MYC at 8q24	93%	83%	33%
8q24 with other abnormalities	64%	93%	100%
Gain of 1q	29%	39%	13%
Gain of 7q	14%	11%	27%
Loss of 17p	6%	11%	23%
Rearrangements involving 11q	4%	17%	27%
Gain of 12q	3%	11%	23%
Loss of 6q	10%	11%	43%
Loss of 13q	14%	17%	10%
Aneuploidy	27%	44%	80%
Complexity[a]	27%	50%	80%

[a] Complexity was defined as > 3 abnormalities.

BL: Burkitt lymphoma, BLL: Burkitt-like lymphoma, DLBCL: diffuse large B-cell lymphoma.

Data from the FAB LMB96 Trial shown in graphical form, from Poirel HA *et al. Leukemia* (2009) 23, 323–331.

Burkhardt *et al.*[18] found a greater incidence of 6q deletions (measured by loss of heterozygosity) in T-LBL (21/108 = 19%) than in T-ALL (16/127 = 12.5%); the same study found that deletion of 6q was associated with an increased incidence of relapse in T-LBL but not in T-ALL.

Unlike the claims for B-NHL in CAYA, there has been little suggestion that T-NHL/T-ALL in adults and CAYA are different diseases. Although the data in CAYA are not numerous, and most reported cases are in small series, some larger series have found similar results in patients of all ages.[19,20]

Anaplastic large cell lymphoma (ALCL)

About 10–15% of NHL in CAYA are of ALCL type, mainly systemic or cutaneous. A recurrent abnormality in systemic ALCL is the t(2;5)(p23;q35), resulting in the fusion of the *ALK* (anaplastic lymphoma kinase) and *NPM* (nucleophosmin) genes. Using FISH and molecular methods, involvement of *ALK* has been detected in up to 100% of cases in some series.[21] Aberrant expression of a gene can occur without detectable translocations, and this is true for the *ALK* gene as for other genes. Perkins *et al.*[21] described 43 cases of ALCL, of which 83% had an abnormal *ALK* signal by FISH study, and 97% had *ALK* overexpression by immunohistochemistry. The t(2;5) is less often found in extranodal ALCL.[22] Ten to twenty percent of cases have *ALK* rearrangements with partners other than chromosome 5[23] and these include t(1;2)(q25;p23) [*TPM3-ALK*], t(2;3)(p23;q21) [*TFG-ALK*], inv(2)(p23q35), [*ATIC-ALK*], t(2;17)(p23;q11) [*CLTCL-ALK*], t(2;19)(p23;p13) [*TPM4-ALK*], t(X;2)(q11–12;p23) [*MSN-ALK*], and ins(8;2)(q22;p23). The biological or clinical differences between these have yet to be established. All the variant translocations can be detected in the same way, using a FISH probe that spans the *ALK* gene and breaks apart when there is a rearrangement, whatever the translocation partner (Fig. 7.1).

Karyotypes can be complex[24,25] and complexity has been associated with an inferior prognosis. Recurrent secondary abnormalities include extra copies of all or part of chromosome 11,[26] and breakpoints involving 1p36, 6p25, and 8q24.[22]

The association between ALCL and abnormalities of *ALK* may not be absolute: there are some reports of *ALK* negative cases, and of finding the t(2;5)(p23;q35) in other kinds of lymphoma.[27] However, it has been stated that translocation defines the disease more precisely than morphologic or immunologic methods.[28]

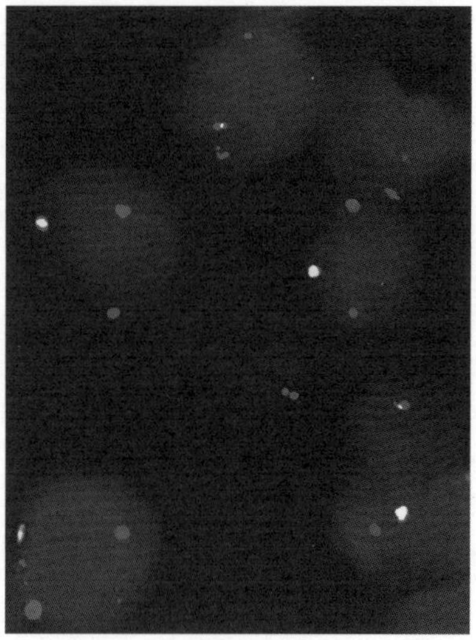

Fig. 7.1. Nuclei from a paraffin-embedded 2-μ section of anaplastic large cell lymphoma, hybridized with a break-apart probe that spans the *ALK* gene at 2p23. The normal gene has a red and green signal. Any translocation involving the gene results in the red and green parts being separated, as shown in several of the nuclei. (Illustration kindly provided by Dr Toon Min, Institute of Cancer Research, UK).

Hodgkin lymphoma (HL)

HL constitutes approximately one third of malignant lymphomas, and occurs most frequently in young male patients. The finding of chromosomally abnormal clones in HL helped to establish that it is not merely a reactive disorder, and the detection in some cases of *IGH@* and *TCR* gene rearrangements has been taken to indicate that it is a type of lymphoma. However, cytogenetics has so far had little impact on the clinical management of the disease. Most cytogenetic studies of HL have had a low success rate and clone detection rate. This is likely because of the limited number of Reed–Sternberg cells present in samples, and their low mitotic index. Also, the karyotype in HL is often very complex (Fig. 7.2) with both numerical and structural abnormalities; no specific recurrent abnormalities have been found. Compared to other types of lymphoma (in patients of all ages), there are very few published cases, probably due to the lack of recurrent abnormalities: it is difficult to interest journal editors in publishing unremarkable

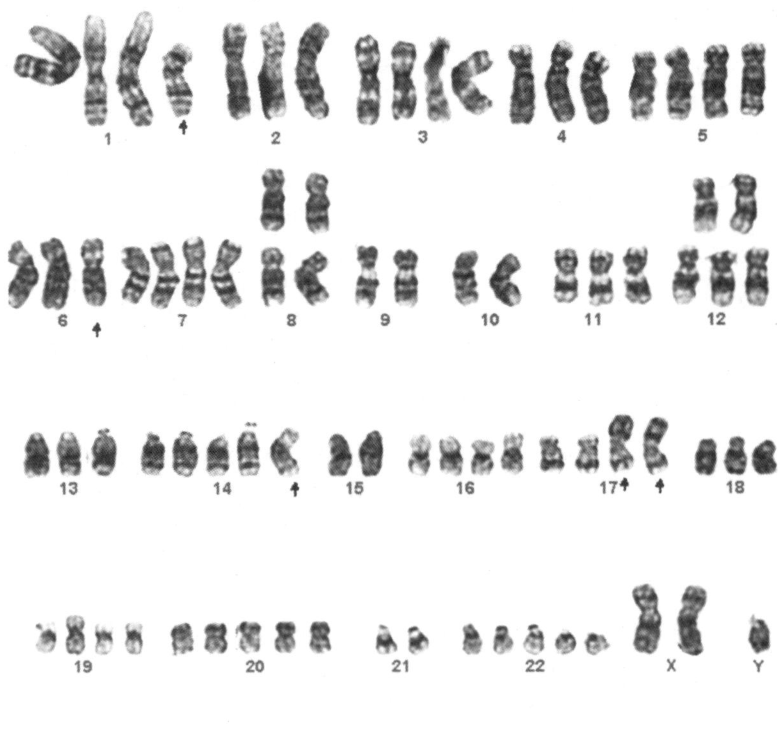

Fig. 7.2. Complex, near-tetraploid karyotype obtained from a 17-year-old male with Hodgkin lymphoma: 81<4n>,XXY,-Y,del(1)(p22p35), −2, −4, −6,del(6)(q23q24) −9, −10, −10, −11, +12, −13, + add(14)(p12), −15, −15, der(17)t(17;18)(p12;q11.2)×2, −18, +20, −21, −21, +22, 2dmin. (Illustration kindly provided by Dr Marilu Nelson, University of Nebraska Medical Center.)

data. A review of nearly 200 published abnormal karyotypes in HL[29] remarked on the paucity of cases available for study, confirmed that no specific cytogenetic–pathologic associations could be identified among the many abnormalities present, but observed that karyotypes with more than 10 abnormalities were more often found in patients with advanced disease. The genetic heterogeneity is thought to arise from an intrinsic genomic instability, and this is supported by the finding of so-called jumping translocations in some cases, i.e. multiple translocation partners to the same breakpoint within the same case.[29] Breakpoint hotspots reported include 12p11–13, 13p11–13, 3q26–28, 6q15–16, and 7q31–35,[30] 1p11–1p13, 1p36, 4q35, 14q11, and 15p11.[31] The smallest overlapping deletion segments have included bands 4q25–4q27 and 6q21–6q23.[31] However, most of the abnormalities in the complex karyotypes of HL are of unknown significance, and it has not yet been possible to distinguish between what are significant and what may be secondary "noise".

Some of the abnormalities that occur in NHL are also found in HL; these include abnormalities of chromosome 1, translocations to 14q32, deletions of 6q, and abnormalities involving 7q and 12p.[32] The *BCL6* gene at 3q27 is involved in nodular lymphocyte predominance HL, but is not recurrent in other kinds of HL.[33] There is also other genetic evidence to suggest that this kind of HL is a distinct disorder.[34] Involvement of the long arms of a chromosome 4 in deletions and translocations has been observed in several cases of HL;[31,32] abnormalities of this region are unusual in other types of lymphoma. Unusually high levels of involvement of the short arms of acrocentric chromosomes (especially 13, 14, 15) have also been found in HL.

The newer technologies may reveal specific associations that have so far been hidden to karyotype analysis. Studies using FISH and comparative genomic hybridization (CGH) have confirmed the unusually high level of complexity in HL. The profuse genetic heterogeneity of HL is further illustrated by the differing results obtained in different series: gains of 17q and 20q were found in 70% and 40% of samples in one[34] and in 20% and 54% in another.[35] However, some significant abnormalities are emerging: parts of the short arms of chromosome 2 and chromosome 9 are frequently found to be gained, and this corresponds to the presence of genes (*REL* and *JAK2*) that are involved in the JAK/STAT signaling pathway. For a more comprehensive review of the applications of these technologies to the study of HL, see Joos and Siebert.[36]

Other cytogenetic abnormalities

Several translocations that are recurrent in adult NHL have been very rarely reported in CAYA, or not at all. It remains to be established whether this is sometimes due to the small number of reported studies, or because there is a biological reason for their absence in younger patients. These abnormalities include the following:

t(9;14)(p13;q32) occurs in a variety of adult NHL, but especially in small lymphocytic plasmacytoid type lymphoma. Only one reported case,[37] was in a 4-year-old boy with post transplant lymphoproliferative disorder.

t(14;18)(q32;q21) This translocation, which fuses the *IGH@* and *BCL2* genes, occurs in a variety of lymphomas, but is most commonly associated with follicular lymphoma (FL). FL is rare in children,[38] and there are only seven reported cases of FL in CAYA with this translocation. There have been no published cases of CAYA with either of the variant forms: the t(2;18)(p12;q21) fusing the *IGK@* and *BCL2* genes, or the t(18;22)(q21;q11), fusing the *BCL2* and *IGL@* genes. FISH studies confirmed the absence of t(14;18)(q32;q21) in a series of 25 pediatric cases of FL,[39] despite BLC2 being expressed in 55% of these cases.

The *t(14;18)(q32;q21)* is considered to be an early event in the pathogenesis of FL. Low levels of this translocation have been detected in normal people, with an incidence that increases with age. Schüler *et al.*[40] found no positivity in 36 cord blood samples or in 48 blood samples from children aged less than 10 years, and only low levels in older CAYA. If the presence of circulating cells with the translocation predisposes to the development of FL, their rarity in CAYA would correlate with the rarity of overt FL.

t(11;14)(q13;q32) This translocation, which fuses the *IGH@* and *CCND1* genes, occurs in a variety of lymphomas (particularly mantle cell lymphoma) and in myeloma. However, there are only three published cases of CAYA with this translocation, all in ALL,[41,42] one without the expression of the *CCND1* gene.[43]

t(8;13)(p11;q13) This translocation is usually associated with chronic myeloproliferative disorders. However, it has been reported in six CAYA cases of lymphoma that proved to be bilineal with T-lymphoma and myeloblasts.[44]

Other cytogenetic abnormalities have been reported too infrequently in lymphoma in CAYA for clinical associations to be established, and have therefore not been included in this review. All published cases for any chromosome abnormality found in oncology are listed in the Mitelman Catalog that is available online at http://cgap.nci.nih.gov/Chromosomes/CytSearchForm.

The Future

In many cases of leukemia, cytogenetic studies are useful in establishing a diagnosis, indicating a broad prognosis, and identifying a target for assessment of response to treatment (usually by a more sensitive technique, such as quantitative PCR). More generally, cytogenetic studies have led to the identification of gene locations for research. However, children and young adults with lymphoma are currently deprived of some of the extensive clinical benefit that diagnostic cytogenetics provides in, for example, the acute leukemias, due to the lack of well-described, published data. The publication of more karyotype and FISH data will make an important contribution to determining the clinical implications of the abnormalities that are found in lymphoma.

New types of genetic data are being generated by techniques such as array CGH and gene expression profiling. Their potential is just beginning to be explored, but there is already promise in what is known.[1] For example, Dave *et al.*[45] have described profiles that distinguish between BL and DLBCL, and have also identified some cases that do not fit the regular patterns; and Schraders *et al.*[46] report the use of high-resolution genomic profiling to detect subtle differences between LBL and ALLs.

The new generation of agents, such as ALK inhibitors, effective in targeted therapy, has enormous potential for controlling cancer without many of the unwanted side effects of systemic chemotherapy (see Chapter 22). These generally require prior identification in the patient of gene rearrangements or gene products; they are wasted and can be harmful in patients without the relevant genetic abnormalities. Therefore, laboratory genetic studies have a new role in oncology; more than establishing a diagnosis, indicating a broad prognosis, or identifying a target for assessment of MRD (see Chapter 10), they are now becoming essential for deciding what therapeutic agent to use.

Acknowledgments

The authors gratefully acknowledge the many informal contributions to this chapter made by colleagues.

References

1. Hummel M, Bentink S, Berger H, Klapper W, Wessendorf S, Barth TF, Bernd HW, Cogliatti SB, Dierlamm J, Feller AC, Hansmann ML, Haralambieva E, Harder L, Hasenclever D, Kuhn M, Lenze D, Lichter P, Martin-Subero JI, Moller P, Muller-Hermelink HK, Ott G, Parwaresch RM, Pott C, Rosenwald A, Rosolowski M, Schwaenen C, Sturzenhofecker B, Szczepanowski M, Trautmann H, Wacker HH, Spang R, Loeffler M, Trumper L, Stein H, Siebert R. (2006) A biologic definition of Burkitt's lymphoma from transcriptional and genomic profiling. *N Engl J Med* **354**: 2419–2430.
2. Poirel HA, Cairo MS, Heerema NA, Swansbury J, Auperin A, Launay E, Sanger WG, Talley P, Perkins SL, Raphael M, McCarthy K, Sposto R, Gerrard M, Bernheim A, Patte C. (2009) Specific cytogenetic abnormalities are associated with a significantly inferior outcome in children and adolescents with mature B-cell non-Hodgkin's lymphoma: Results of the FAB/LMB 96 international study. *Leukemia* **23**: 323–331.
3. Kim M, Yim SH, Cho NS, Kang SH, Ko DH, Oh B, Kim TY, Min HJ, She CJ, Kang HJ, Shin HY, Ahn HS, Yoon SS, Kim BK, Shin HR, Han KS, Cho HI, Lee DS. (2009) Homozygous deletion of CDKN2A (p16, p14) and CDKN2B (p15) genes is a poor prognostic factor in adult but not in childhood B-lineage acute lymphoblastic leukemia: A comparative deletion and hypermethylation study. *Cancer Genet Cytogenet* **195**: 59–65.
4. Sandlund JT, Downing JR, Crist WM. (1996) Non-Hodgkin's lymphoma in childhood. *N Engl J Med* **334**: 1238–1248.
5. Barth TF, Muller S, Pawlita M, Siebert R, Rother JU, Mechtersheimer G, Kitinya J, Bentz M, Moller P. (2004) Homogeneous immunophenotype and paucity of secondary genomic aberrations are distinctive features of endemic but not of sporadic Burkitt's lymphoma and diffuse large B-cell lymphoma with MYC rearrangement. *J Pathol* **203**: 940–945.
6. Kaiser-McCaw B, Epstein AL, Kaplan HS, Hecht F. (1977) Chromosome 14 translocation in African and North American Burkitt's lymphoma. *Int J Cancer* **19**: 482–486.
7. Haralambieva E, Schuuring E, Rosati S, van Noesel C, Jansen P, Appel I, Guikema J, Wabinga H, Bleggi-Torres LF,

Lam K, van den Berg E, Mellink C, van Zelderen-Bhola S, Kluin P. (2004) Interphase fluorescence *in situ* hybridization for detection of 8q24/MYC breakpoints on routine histologic sections: Validation in Burkitt lymphomas from three geographic regions. *Genes Chromosomes Cancer* **40**: 10–18.
8. Lones MA, Sanger WG, Le Beau MM, Heerema NA, Sposto R, Perkins SL, Buckley J, Kadin ME, Kjeldsberg CR, Meadows A, Siegel S, Finlay J, Bergeron S, Cairo MS. (2004) Chromosome abnormalities may correlate with prognosis in Burkitt/Burkitt-like lymphomas of children and adolescents: A report from Children's Cancer Group Study CCG-E08. *J Pediatr Hematol Oncol* **26**: 169–178.
9. Nelson M, Perkins SL, Dave BJ, Coccia PF, Bridge JA, Lyden ER, Heerema NA, Lones MA, Harrison L, Cairo MS, Sanger WG. (2010) An increased frequency of 13q deletions detected by fluorescence *in situ* hybridization and its impact on survival in children and adolescents with Burkitt lymphoma: Results from the Children's Oncology Group study CCG-5961. *Br J Haematol* **148**: 600–610.
10. Lai JL, Fenaux P, Zandecki M, Nelken B, Huart JJ, Deminatti M. (1989) Cytogenetic studies in 30 patients with Burkitt's lymphoma or L3 acute lymphoblastic leukemia with special reference to additional chromosome abnormalities. *Ann Genet* **32**: 26–32.
11. Onciu M, Schlette E, Zhou Y, Raimondi SC, Giles FJ, Kantarjian HM, Medeiros LJ, Ribeiro RC, Pui CH, Sandlund JT. (2006) Secondary chromosomal abnormalities predict outcome in pediatric and adult high-stage Burkitt lymphoma. *Cancer* **107**: 1084–1092.
12. Kornblau SM, Goodacre A, Cabanillas F. (1991) Chromosomal abnormalities in adult non-endemic Burkitt's lymphoma and leukemia: 22 new reports and a review of 148 cases from the literature. *Hematol Oncol* **9**: 63–78.
13. Pezzolo A, Cinti R, Negri F, Parodi F, Garaventa A, Gambini C, Pistoia V. (2006) Chromosomal imbalances in pediatric Burkitt-like lymphoma and review of the literature in relation to other germinal center derived B-cell tumors. *Leuk Lymphoma* **47**: 2359–2364.
14. Dave BJ, Weisenburger DD, Higgins CM, Pickering DL, Hess MM, Chan WC, Sanger WG. (2004) Cytogenetics and fluorescence *in situ* hybridization studies of diffuse large B-cell lymphoma in children and young adults. *Cancer Genet Cytogenet* **153**: 115–121.
15. Oschlies I, Klapper W, Zimmermann M, Krams M, Wacker HH, Burkhardt B, Harder L, Siebert R, Reiter A, Parwaresch R. (2006) Diffuse large B-cell lymphoma in pediatric patients belongs predominantly to the germinal-center type B-cell lymphomas: A clinicopathologic analysis of cases included in the German BFM (Berlin-Frankfurt-Munster) Multicenter Trial. *Blood* **107**: 4047–4052.
16. Uyttebroeck A, Vanhentenrijk V, Hagemeijer A, Boeckx N, Renard M, Wlodarska I, Vandenberghe P, Depaepe P, de Wolf-Peeters C. (2007) Is there a difference in childhood T-cell acute lymphoblastic leukaemia and T-cell lymphoblastic lymphoma? *Leuk Lymphoma* **48**: 1745–1754.
17. Lones MA, Heerema NA, le Beau MM, Sposto R, Perkins SL, Kadin ME, Kjeldsberg CR, Meadows A, Siegel S, Buckley J, Abromowitch M, Kersey J, Bergeron S, Cairo MS, Sanger WG. (2007) Chromosome abnormalities in advanced stage lymphoblastic lymphoma of children and adolescents: A report from CCG-E08. *Cancer Genet Cytogenet* **172**: 1–11.
18. Burkhardt B, Moericke A, Klapper W, Greene F, Salzburg J, Damm-Welk C, Zimmermann M, Strauch K, Ludwig WD, Schrappe M, Reiter A. (2008) Pediatric precursor T lymphoblastic leukemia and lymphoblastic lymphoma: Differences in the common regions with loss of heterozygosity at chromosome 6q and their prognostic impact. *Leuk Lymphoma* **49**: 451–461.
19. Cauwelier B, Dastugue N, Cools J, Poppe B, Herens C, de Paepe A, Hagemeijer A, Speleman F. (2006) Molecular cytogenetic study of 126 unselected T-ALL cases reveals high incidence of TCRbeta locus rearrangements and putative new T-cell oncogenes. *Leukemia* **20**: 1238–1244.
20. Kahl C, Gesk S, Harder L, Harbott J, French L, Deloukas P, Grote W, Schlegelberger B, Siebert R. (2001) Detection of translocations involving the HOX11/TCL3-locus in 10q24 by interphase fluorescence *in situ* hybridization. *Cancer Genet Cytogenet* **129**: 80–84.
21. Perkins SL, Pickering D, Lowe EJ, Zwick D, Abromowitch M, Davenport G, Cairo MS, Sanger WG. (2005) Childhood anaplastic large cell lymphoma has a high incidence of ALK gene rearrangement as determined by immunohistochemical staining and fluorescent *in situ* hybridisation: A genetic and pathological correlation. *Br J Haematol* **131**: 624–627.
22. Ott G, Katzenberger T, Siebert R, DeCoteau JF, Fletcher JA, Knoll JH, Kalla J, Rosenwald A, Ott MM, Weber-Matthiesen K, Kadin ME, Muller-Hermelink HK. (1998) Chromosomal abnormalities in nodal and extranodal CD30+ anaplastic large cell lymphomas: Infrequent detection of the t(2;5) in extranodal lymphomas. *Genes Chromosomes Cancer* **22**: 114–121.
23. Liang X, Meech SJ, Odom LF, Bitter MA, Ryder JW, Hunger SP, Lovell MA, Meltesen L, Wei Q, Williams SA,

Hutchinson RN, McGavran L. (2004) Assessment of t(2;5)(p23;q35) translocation and variants in pediatric ALK+ anaplastic large cell lymphoma. *Am J Clin Pathol* **121**: 496–506.

24. Lones MA, Heerema NA, le Beau MM, Perkins SL, Kadin ME, Kjeldsberg CR, Sposto R, Meadows A, Siegel S, Buckley J, Finlay J, Abromowitch M, Cairo MS, Sanger WG. (2006) Complex secondary chromosome abnormalities in advanced stage anaplastic large cell lymphoma of children and adolescents: A report from CCG-E08. *Cancer Genet Cytogenet* **171**: 89–96.
25. Nelson M, Horsman DE, Weisenburger DD, Gascoyne RD, Dave BJ, Loberiza FR, Ludkovski O, Savage KJ, Armitage JO, Sanger WG. (2008) Cytogenetic abnormalities and clinical correlations in peripheral T-cell lymphoma. *Br J Haematol* **141**: 461–469.
26. Bobos M, Kotoula V, Kaloutsi V, Karayannopoulou G, Papadimitriou CS, Kostopoulos I. (2009) Aberrant CCND1 copies and cyclin D1 mRNA expression do not result in the production of functional cyclin D1 protein in anaplastic large cell lymphoma. *Histol Histopathol* **24**: 1035–1048.
27. Weisenburger DD, Gordon BG, Vose JM, Bast MA, Chan WC, Greiner TC, Anderson JR, Sanger WG. (1996) Occurrence of the t(2;5)(p23;q35) in non-Hodgkin's lymphoma. *Blood* **87**: 3860–3868.
28. Jaffe ES. (2001) Anaplastic large cell lymphoma: The shifting sands of diagnostic hematopathology. *Mod Pathol* **14**: 219–228.
29. Falzetti D, Crescenzi B, Matteuci C, Falini B, Martelli MF, van Den Berghe H, Mecucci C. (1999) Genomic instability and recurrent breakpoints are main cytogenetic findings in Hodgkin's disease. *Haematologica* **84**: 298–305.
30. Tilly H, Bastard C, Delastre T, Duval C, Bizet M, Lenormand B, Dauce JP, Monconduit M, Piguet H. (1991) Cytogenetic studies in untreated Hodgkin's disease. *Blood* **77**: 1298–1304.
31. Dohner H, Bloomfield CD, Frizzera G, Frestedt J, Arthur DC. (1992) Recurring chromosome abnormalities in Hodgkin's disease. *Genes Chromosomes Cancer* **5**: 392–398.
32. Stamatoullas A, Picquenot JM, Dumesnil C, Ruminy P, Penther D, Bertrand P, Courel MN, Maisonneuve C, Francois A, Gaulard P, Tilly H, Bastard C. (2007) Conventional cytogenetics of nodular lymphocyte-predominant Hodgkin's lymphoma. *Leukemia* **21**: 2064–2067.
33. Wlodarska I, Nooyen P, Maes B, Martin-Subero JI, Siebert R, Pauwels P, De Wolf-Peeters C, Hagemeijer A. (2003) Frequent occurrence of BCL6 rearrangements in nodular lymphocyte predominance Hodgkin lymphoma but not in classical Hodgkin lymphoma. *Blood* **101**: 706–710.
34. Chui DT, Hammond D, Baird M, Shield L, Jackson R, Jarrett RF. (2003) Classical Hodgkin lymphoma is associated with frequent gains of 17q. *Genes Chromosomes Cancer* **38**: 126–136.
35. Joos S, Menz CK, Wrobel G, Siebert R, Gesk S, Ohl S, Mechtersheimer G, Trumper L, Moller P, Lichter P, Barth TF. (2002) Classical Hodgkin lymphoma is characterized by recurrent copy number gains of the short arm of chromosome 2. *Blood* **99**: 1381–1387.
36. Joos S, Siebert R. (2007) Cytogenetics of Classical Hodgkin Lymphoma. In: R Hoppe, P Mauch, JO Armitage, V Diehl, L Weiss (eds.), *Hodgkin Lymphoma*. Philadelphia: Lippincott, Williams & Wilkins, pp. 109–120.
37. Djokic M, le Beau MM, Swinnen LJ, Smith SM, Rubin CM, Anastasi J, Carlson KM. (2006) Post-transplant lymphoproliferative disorder subtypes correlate with different recurring chromosomal abnormalities. *Genes Chromosomes Cancer* **45**: 313–318.
38. Lorsbach RB, Shay-Seymore D, Moore J, Banks PM, Hasserjian RP, Sandlund JT, Behm FG. (2002) Clinicopathologic analysis of follicular lymphoma occurring in children. *Blood* **99**: 1959–1964.
39. Oschlies I, Salaverria I, Mahn F, Meinhardt A, Zimmermann M, Woessmann W, Burkhardt B, Gesk S, Krams M, Reiter A, Siebert R, Klapper W. (2010) Pediatric follicular lymphoma — a clinico-pathological study of a population-based series of patients treated within the Non-Hodgkin's Lymphoma-Berlin-Frankfurt-Munster (NHL-BFM) multicenter trials. *Haematologica* **95**: 253–259.
40. Schúler F, Dolken L, Hirt C, Kiefer T, Berg T, Fusch G, Weitmann K, Hoffmann W, Fusch C, Janz S, Rabkin CS, Dolken G. (2009) Prevalence and frequency of circulating t(14;18)-MBR translocation carrying cells in healthy individuals. *Int J Cancer* **124**: 958–963.
41. Kim IS, Kim HJ, Yoo KH, Sung KW, Kim SH. (2006) A boy with acute lymphoblastic leukemia acquired clonal and nonclonal cytogenetic abnormalities including del(7q) and del(20q) without clinical evidence of disease after sex-mismatched cord blood transplantation. *J Pediatr Hematol Oncol* **28**: 540–543.
42. Soszynska K, Mucha B, Debski R, Skonieczka K, Duszenko E, Koltan A, Wysocki M, Haus O. (2008) The application of conventional cytogenetics, FISH, and RT-PCR to detect genetic changes in 70 children with ALL. *Ann Hematol* **87**: 991–1002.

43. Raynaud SD, Gratecos N, Simon MP, Chischportich M, Grosgeorge J, Gaudray P, Ayraud N. (1993) Fluorescent *in situ* hybridization analysis of an atypical t(11;14)(q13;q32) without expression of the cyclin D1 gene. *Leukemia* 7: 1924–1927.
44. Vega F, Medeiros LJ, Davuluri R, Cromwell CC, Alkan S, Abruzzo LV. (2008) t(8;13)-positive bilineal lymphomas: Report of 6 cases. *Am J Surg Pathol* **32**: 14–20.
45. Dave SS, Fu K, Wright GW, Lam LT, Kluin P, Boerma EJ, Greiner TC, Weisenburger DD, Rosenwald A, Ott G, Muller-Hermelink HK, Gascoyne RD, Delabie J, Rimsza LM, Braziel RM, Grogan TM, Campo E, Jaffe ES, Dave BJ, Sanger W, Bast M, Vose JM, Armitage JO, Connors JM, Smeland EB, Kvaloy S, Holte H, Fisher RI, Miller TP, Montserrat E, Wilson WH, Bahl M, Zhao H, Yang L, Powell J, Simon R, Chan WC, Staudt LM. (2006) Molecular diagnosis of Burkitt's lymphoma. *N Engl J Med* **354**: 2431–2442.
46. Schraders M, van Reijmersdal SV, Kamping EJ, van Krieken JH, van Kessel AG, Groenen PJ, Hoogerbrugge PM, Kuiper RP. (2009) High-resolution genomic profiling of pediatric lymphoblastic lymphomas reveals subtle differences with pediatric acute lymphoblastic leukemias in the B-lineage. *Cancer Genet Cytogenet* **191**: 27–33.

8

Molecular Genetics of Lymphomas in Children and Young Adults

Itziar Salaverria, Reiner Siebert and Megan S. Lim

Introduction

This chapter will provide a description of the molecular alterations in lymphomas other than Hodgkin lymphoma (HL) (i.e. previously non-Hodgkin lymphoma [NHL]), occurring in children and young adults (CAYA). It includes a compilation of data regarding molecular genetics of recurrent translocations, gene mutations, gene expression profiling (GEP), methylation profiling and proteomic analyses in these lymphoid malignancies.

Because overall the data on the molecular genetics of most lymphoma in CAYA are rare, the chapter first summarizes the features of these included entities independent of age and then provides specific details on CAYA.

All cancers arise as a result of acquisition of a series of fixed DNA sequence abnormalities, called mutations, many of which ultimately confer a growth advantage. In lymphomas, mutations of specific oncogenes or tumor suppressor genes have been observed to have a role in lymphomagenesis.

As it is well established, for the majority of mature B-cell and T-cell neoplasms, characteristic genetic abnormalities are important in determining their biological features and can be useful in the diagnostic workup of these cases. The most recurrent phenomenon in B-cell malignancies are translocations involving the immunoglobulin heavy chain locus (*IGH*) on 14q32 in which a cellular proto-oncogene comes under the influence of the *IGH* promoter. Translocations involving genes encoding the variant IG light chains, *IGK* and *IGL* have also been described. Moreover, other rearrangements have been demonstrated to have a role in lymphomagenesis. The same has been observed in T-cell–derived malignancies, in which chromosomal rearrangements result in oncogenes becoming juxtaposed to the promoter and enhancer elements of the T-cell receptor genes (*TCR*), leading to their aberrant expression. Consequently, molecular characterization of all these chromosomal translocations and other aberrations is beginning to provide specific markers that may prove useful in the diagnosis and classification of the lymphoid neoplasms, as well as in monitoring the response to therapy (e.g. detecting minimal residual disease in patients in remission).

Recombination of the three genetic components of the heavy chain to create the V-D-J transcriptional unit is a unique feature of B cells. Subsequent events of recombination, somatic mutation, isotype switching, and antigen selection all leave evidence in the variable-gene sequences of the stage of differentiation reached by the B cell of origin. Therefore, specifically, analysis of the rearranged *IGH* variable-gene sequences is a commonly used method to gain insight into the clonality of the cell of origin of B-cell lymphomas showing the differentiation stage of the B lymphocyte that gives rise to the neoplastic clone.

This increasing interest in the molecular origins and consequences of mature lymphoid neoplasms has led to the development of multiple molecular techniques such as GEP and methylation studies, which in the last decades have contributed to a better understanding of the molecular pathogenesis of these tumors. Since, functional state, phenotype, and response to environmental variables of tumoral cells are largely determined by its expression signature, GEP studies using whole genome microarrays are a powerful tool to understand the complex molecular networks in malignant lymphomas. GEP microarrays can interrogate the expression of thousands of genes at the RNA level, helping to elucidate pathways of activation and transformation. It has been shown that GEP can be used for the subclassification of specific categories of lymphomas, adding important information to the WHO classification criteria,[1] which are based on morphology, immunophenotype, and genetics.[2–4]

Aberrant DNA methylation, which is a hallmark of cancer, includes global DNA hypomethylation and hypermethylation of CpG-islands with a pattern that is tumor specific and can be used to identify genes involved in the genesis and progression of different tumor types.

The study of global protein expression is a key area of research that can enhance our understanding of the pathogenesis and phenotypic diversity of lymphoid neoplasms. Many lines of evidence suggest that only a fraction of mRNA is reflected in the protein content. In addition, proteomic methods enable the study of post-translational modifications of gene products. In this sense, different proteomic techniques have been performed in lymphomas.[5–8]

Nevertheless, these recent studies that apply innovative genome-wide technologies suffer from the weaknesses that with very few exceptions they have been performed in a series of adult patients. No age-related host aspects have been considerably taken into account and some studies performed in pediatric cases include also young adult specimens. The following chapter, although the data are scarce, aims to summarize key molecular differences between lymphomas that occur in the adult population from those of children.

B-Cell Lymphomas

Burkitt lymphoma

Burkitt Lymphoma (BL) is an aggressive B-cell lymphoma characterized by typical morphological, immunophenotypic and molecular features (see Chapter 4). Three variants of BL are recognized, each manifesting differences in clinical presentation, morphology and biology, endemic BL, sporadic BL, and immunodeficiency-associated BL. The t(8;14)(q24;q32) translocation or its variants, which juxtapose the locus of the *MYC* oncogene and one of the three immunoglobulin (*IG*) loci, are present in almost all BL.[1]

In endemic BL, most *MYC/IG* breakpoints affect the VDJ region, whereas in sporadic cases, the translocations are mediated by immunoglobulin class switch recombination of the *IGH* locus at 14q32.[9] These differences in *MYC* breakpoint may well be accounted by the different stages of maturation of the cell of origin of Epstein–Barr virus (EBV)-positive (mainly endemic) and EBV-negative (mainly sporadic) BL.[10] Furthermore, mutations in *MYC* may enhance its tumorigenicity; some of these mutations may lead to decreased expression of BIM which binds and inactivates BCL2.[11] Furthermore, the *MYC* translocation is not the only genetic lesion found in BL. *MYC*-transformed cells are usually characterized by the loss of expression of several genes; cooperating alterations of cell cycle-associated genes have been demonstrated to contribute to the pathogenesis of BL. These genetic alterations involve *CDKN2A*, *TP53*, *p73*, *BAX*, *p130/RB2* and *BCL6* genes and may promote cell growth and/or inhibit apoptosis.[1]

Using the GEP approach, several groups have been able to recognize a consistent gene expression signature for BL. The cases that carry this signature cases are described as "molecular BL" (mBL) and can be clearly differentiated from non-mBL, a group mainly composed of DLBCL.[3,4]

Specifically in pediatric B-cell lymphoma entities, a molecular characterization by GEP in patients up to 18 years old has been recently performed.[12] GEP was also able to differentiate between mBL and non-mBL lymphomas in this group of pediatric patients (Fig. 8.1). Interestingly, morphologic BL/Atypical BL, as well as mBL, defined by GEP were more frequent in children than adults among the aggressive lymphoma series. This study based on gene expression data and including also copy number studies,[13] evidenced that genetic and expression differences did not exist between pediatric and adult BL and the attempt to establish a gene

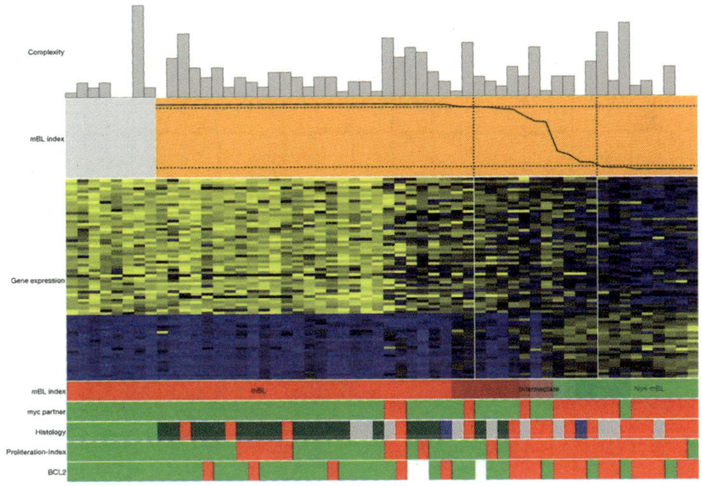

Fig. 8.1. Molecular features of pediatric malignant B-NHL classified by gene expression profiling using the mBL index. Genomic complexity of the cases is shown as bar plots on top of the panels, with complexity increasing with height. Below, the plot with the orange background shows the mBL-index on the y-axes indicating the similarity to the core-BLs[4] (gray box on the left to the mBL-index plot). The vertical lines delineate the 3 groups of lymphomas (mBL on the left, intermediate in the middle, and non-mBL on the right) and the dashed horizontal lines indicate the index-score cutoffs defining the mBL group (0.95) and the non-mBL group (0.05) according to the mBL-index.[4] Below, the heat map shows the gene-expression levels of the 58 mBL-signature genes, with 1 gene shown per row. Bright blue indicates a low level of expression (3 SD below the average of all cases), bright yellow indicates a high level of expression (3 SD above the average), and black the average level of expression across all samples. The cases are ordered from left to right on the basis of decreasing mBL-signature index score, given again below the heat map. Green represents a high index score (mBL), and red a low index score (non-mBL). The color gradient of the intermediate cases highlights the continuous transition of the index score between the mBL and non-mBL cases. The *MYC* translocation partners are shown according *MYC* break (bright green) and *MYC*-breakpoint absent (red). The histological diagnosis is shown in the panel below. Bright green indicates core-Burkitt lymphoma; dark green, Burkitt lymphoma; red, diffuse large-B-cell lymphoma; blue, follicular lymphoma and gray, unclassifiable mature aggressive B-cell lymphoma. The proliferation-index is coded with green for Ki-67 greater than 95% and red for Ki-67 less than 95%. Finally, BCL2 protein expression is indicated in green for negativity and red for positivity. White bars indicate not assessable. This research was originally published in Klapper W, Szczepanowski M, Burkhardt B, Berger H, Rosolowski M, Bentink S, Schwaenen C, Wessendorf S, Spang R, Möller P, Hansmann ML, Bernd HW, Ott G, Hummel M, Stein H, Loeffler M, Trümper L, Zimmermann M, Reiter A, Siebert R; Molecular profiling of pediatric mature B-cell lymphoma treated in population-based prospective clinical trials. *Blood.* 2008;112:1374–1381 © The American Society of Hematology.

expression-based predictor of pediatric and adult BL failed. This finding was somewhat unexpected considering, e.g. the marked male predominance of BL in children but not in adults (Fig. 8.2).

Regarding methylation studies, not only genetics but also epigenetic alterations of different genes such as *CDKN2A* and *TP53*, involving a selective growth advantage even in the presence of constitutively active *MYC*, have been demonstrated in BL.[14] Recent data on combined transcriptional, epigenetic and genetic profiling in a large series of aggressive B-cell lymphomas have shown that DNA methylation of the genes under study does not distinguish between these aggressive lymphoma subtypes with regards to morphology, immunophenotype, genetic aberrations or gene expression signatures. These studies also demonstrate that genes that are *de novo* methylated across different lymphoma subtypes are highly enriched for targets of Polycomb repressor complex in stem cells.[15]

Many lines of evidence suggest that *MYC*-negative BL exist. Some studies pointed that it should be considered that few cases of sporadic BL lack an identifiable *MYC* rearrangement.[4] Also, another study in endemic BL evaluated, using both *MYC* break apart and *MYC/IGH* fusion probes, described several cases that were negative for *MYC* translocation. However, no FISH assay can ultimately rule out an *IG-MYC* fusion due to cryptic insertions.[16] A microRNA (mir) expression study has showed that hsa-mir-34b is downregulated only in BL cases negative for the *MYC* translocation, suggesting that different pathogenetic mechanisms, other than *MYC* translocation, could be involved in the transformation of these cases.[17] Nevertheless, it should not be ignored that for

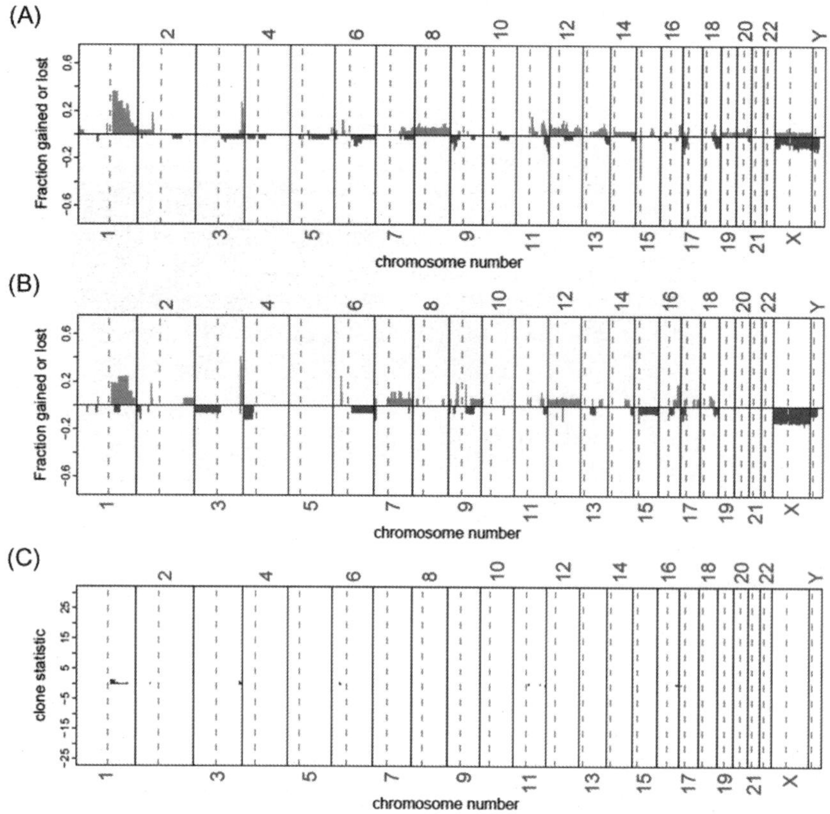

Fig. 8.2. Comparison of chromosomal imbalances detected by matrix-CGH in pediatric (≤14 years, n = 33) and adult (>18 years, n = 17) mBL. Every vertical bar on the plots represents a CGH clone in its genomic position. The green and red bars show relative frequencies of gains and losses, respectively. The heights of the red bars are given a negative value for clarity. Panel A shows the relative frequency of genomic imbalances in pediatric mBL (≤14 years). Panel B refers to the population of adult mBL (>18 years). Panel C illustrates the discrepancies in the frequency of genomic aberrations between the patient groups from Panel A and B with the corresponding chi-square statistics. The chi-square statistics for losses are shown with a negative sign. Clones with more than 10% missing values or having 5 or fewer aberrations overall are not shown. This research was originally published in Klapper W, Szczepanowski M, Burkhardt B, Berger H, Rosolowski M, Bentink S, Schwaenen C, Wessendorf S, Spang R, Möller P, Hansmann ML, Bernd HW, Ott G, Hummel M, Stein H, Loeffler M, Trümper L, Zimmermann M, Reiter A, Siebert R; Molecular profiling of pediatric mature B-cell lymphoma treated in population-based prospective clinical trials. *Blood.* 2008;112:1374–1381 © The American Society of Hematology.

discarding the rearrangement, appropriate probe sets, with a locus-specific *MYC* probe spanning at least 500 kb centromeric and 1 Mb telomeric of the *MYC* gene sequence, should be used and that the probes used in these studies could not cover the whole region of break.[18]

Diffuse large B-cell lymphoma

According to the WHO classification,[1] DLBCL are defined as diffuse proliferations of large neoplasic mature B cells (see Chapter 4). It is, however, recognized that this definition comprises a group of morphologically, immunohistochemically, and clinically heterogeneous tumors rather than one single entity. In this sense, biological subgroups of DLBCL with favorable prognosis, germinal center B-cell–like (GCB), and with poor prognosis, activated B-cell–like (ABC) have been defined by gene expression and genetic profiling and can be distinguished by immunohistochemistry.[2]

Regarding the genetic characteristics of these cases, chromosomal translocation affecting the 3q27 band, where the *BCL6* gene is localized, is one of the most common genetic abnormalities in these lymphomas (30% of the cases). Translocation occurs within the major translocation cluster (MTC) of *BCL6*; as a result of translocation, either one of the three *IG* genes or a variable non-*IG* gene is juxtaposed to the coding regions of *BCL6*. Moreover, translocation of the *BCL2* gene, a hallmark of FL, occurs in 20–30% of the cases. Also, the presence of *MYC* break has been observed in up to 10% of the cases and is linked to complex karyotypes and a very unfavorable outcome.[4] Approximately 20% of the cases with *MYC* break have a concurrent *IGH-BCL2* translocation and/or *BCL6* break or both.[4,19] Also, *TP53* mutations have been associated with poor survival in some series of DLBCL and in one study, mutations in the DNA binding domain proved to be the most important outcome predictor.[20]

The two gene expression profiling subgroups carry specific genetic alterations. Most ABC lymphomas present amplification and overexpression of *BCL2*, present deletions of *INK4* and present alterations, whereas genetic lesions of GCB-DLBCL are the t(14;18) translocation, deletion of the tumor suppressor *PTEN*, and *TP53* mutations. Moreover ABC-DLBCL present a characteristic activation of NF-κB pathway, in close similarity to primary mediastinal B-cell lymphoma (Table 8.1).

By mutating multiple genes, and possibly by favoring chromosomal translocations, aberrant hypermutation may represent the major contributor to the lymphomagenesis of these lymphomas.[21] Somatic hypermutations of *BCL6* are present in DLBCL. The mutations are clustered within a region of the MTC, suggesting that a common molecular mechanism is operating for the two genetic lesions of *BCL6*. Aberrant somatic hypermutations targeting multiple genes, including *PIM1*, *MYC*, *RhoH/TTF* and *PAX5* are also encountered in more than 50% of DLBCL cases. Intriguingly, several of the hypermutable genes are susceptible to chromosomal translocations in the same region, consistent with a role for hypermutation in generating translocations by DNA double-strand breaks.

Immunohistochemical studies have shown that pediatric DLBCL were predominantly lymphomas of the GCB subtype, which, in contrast to their adult counterpart, are virtually devoid of the translocation t(14;18).[22] Nevertheless, in a gene expression study performed by the same group,[23] the classification into ABC and GCB subtypes in pediatric cases showed only a moderate predominance of the GCB over the ABC type compared with adults. Moreover, the group of morphologically defined DLBCL seemed to contain a higher rate of "contamination" with lymphomas with an mBL expression profiles than their adult counterpart.[23]

A recent study from Gualco and collaborators, in which 16 pediatric patients with nodal DLBCL were studied, again showed GCB predominance with better outcome in this series, independent of the presence of *MYC* translocation or TCL1 expression.[24] Specifically, when the expression pattern of BCL2, TCL1,

Table 8.1. Molecular differences between ABC and GCB-DLBCL and PMBCL.

Molecular characteristic	ABC-DLBCL	GCB-DLBCL	PMBCL
t(14;18) (%)	0	35	0
3q gain (%)	26		5
9p gain/ *JAK2* and *PDL2* amplif (%)	6		25
Ongoing *IG* mutations	No	Yes	No
REL amplification (%)	0	15	50
TP53 inactivation			
INK4a inactivation			
SOCS1 inactivation	—	—	Yes
A20 inactivation	24	2	
CARD11 inactivation	11	7	36
NF-KB activation	Yes	No	Yes
NF-KB pathway differentially expressed genes	*IRF4*, ***c-FLIP***, *CCND2*, ***CD44***, *C4orf9*, ***IL6***, *IL2RA*, *EGR1*, *BCL2*, *LITAF*, *CCR7*, ***SLC2A5***, ***CCL22***, ***NCF2***	— —	*IkB*, *FAS*, *CD31*, *TRAF1*, *IER3*, *TNIP2*, *VIM*, *SDC4*, *JUNB*, *IRF1*, *EMR1*, *CCR7*, *A20*, *SMAD7*, *CCL3*, *TNFRSF5*, *BCL2A1*, ***c-FLIP***, ***NCF2***, ***IL6***, *IL4RA*, *RAFTLIN*, *BCL2L1*, *SOD2*, *CCL4*, *PRKCD*, ***CD44***, ***SLC2A5***, ***CCL22***, *PASK*, *IL8*, *CD69*, *DUSP1*, *CCL2*, *CD23A*

In bold are genes shared as differentially expressed between ABC-DLBCL and PMBCL.[42]

and MUM1 was combined with the results of *MYC* translocation, the cases seemed to cluster in two groups, one composed of GCB cases with *MYC* translocation, TCL1 expression and good prognosis, and another group with non-GCB phenotype, BCL2 and MUM1 expression and worse prognosis. Interestingly, BCL2 expression did not correlate alone with prognosis in contrast with the results observed in adult cases.[25]

ALK-positive DLBCL

In the present issue of the WHO classification, DLBCL cases expressing the ALK kinase have been described as a recently identified novel subtype of DLBCL that occur in all age groups. Also, a very recent study have shown how these cases present clinicopathologic features that distinguish them from the common DLBCL, e.g. conventional therapy, as used for the typical DLBCL, is of limited efficacy.[26] Different studies have shown, by FISH and real time quantitative polymerase chain reaction (PCR), that the *ALK*-clathrin heavy polypeptide-like gene (*CLTC*) fusions are not restricted to adult forms of *ALK*-positive DLBCL, but are also recurrent in *ALK*-positive DLBCL arising in children.[27–30]

The few cases reported[27–30] so far showed, with few exceptions,[31] a granular cytoplasmic staining pattern associated with a translocation t(2;17)(p23;q23) fusing *ALK* to *CLTC*. Also cryptic insertions of 3′*ALK* gene sequences into chromosome 4q22–q24 have been described.[32]

Lymphoblastic B-cell lymphoma

Lymphoblastic B-cell lymphoma (B-LBL) is a common leukemia/lymphoma primarily occurring in children (75% of the cases). Some authors believe that B-LBL is distinct from B-cell acute lymphoblastic leukemia (B-ALL) because the lymphoma may remain localized without leukemic dissemination. Nevertheless, since the WHO classification classified these lymphomas together with B-ALL and scarce studies have been published on these lymphomas, it should be considered that these two entities present similar biological characteristics. In this sense, significant advances in the cytogenetic technology have been pivotal to the discovery of novel genetic changes, which have further contributed to our understanding of leukomagenesis in these cases.[33] Several genetic entities have been described based on the presence of different genetic hallmarks as t(9;22)(q34;q11.2), *MLL* gene rearrangements t(v;11q23), t(12;21)(p13;q22), t(5;14)(q31;q32) and t(1;19)(q23;p13.3) translocations (see Chapter 5). The genes involved in these translocations are described in Table 8.2. Also some cases have been classified due to phenomena of hyperdiploidy or hypodiploidy showing numerical increase of chromosomes or loss of one or more chromosomes respectively. The frequency of the presence of these translocations or ploidy phenomena is variable in the different age groups.

Other molecular studies have focused on the identification and characterization of B-ALL/LBL cases carrying intrachromosomal amplifications of chromosome 21.[34,35] These amplifications have been associated with a poor outcome although the reason for this relationship is unknown.[36] No point mutations in the *AML1* gene have been reported suggesting an oncogenic role of wild type *AML1* amplification.[37] Unlike other B-cell lymphomas, B-LBL has not yet been the subject of comprehensive studies on the rearranged *IG* gene.

Regarding GEP on these B-LBL groups, distinct expression profiles have been identified in each of the prognostically important leukemia/lymphoma subtypes, including B-ALL with *E2A-PBX1*, *BCR-ABL1* and

Table 8.2. Translocations described in B-LBL/ALL.

Translocation	Gene	Biological function	Oncogenic mechanism
t(9;22)(q34;q11.2)	*BCR-ABL1*	Cell cycle regulation, inhibition DNA repair	Fusion protein
t(v;11q23)	*MLL*	Cell transformation	Fusion protein
t(12;21)(p13;q22)	*TEL-AML1*	Leukemogenesis	Fusion protein
t(5;14)(q31;q32)	*IL3-IGH*	Cell growth, differentiation and apoptosis	Expression deregulation
t(1;19)(q23;p13.3)	*E2A-PBX1*	Transcription activator	Fusion protein

v: variable partner.

TEL-AML1 translocations, B-ALL carrying *MLL* rearrangements, and B-ALL with hyperdiploidy.[38] This remarkable difference in the expression profiles of the individual leukemia subtypes was unexpected since they have relatively homogeneous morphology. GEP studies on cases with chromosome 21 alterations have shown no significant differentially expressed genes, including *AML1*, to distinguish cases with chromosome 21 amplifications from other ALL patients with alterations in this chromosome.[39]

Rare B-cell lymphoma entities in CAYA

Primary mediastinal B-cell lymphoma

Primary mediastinal B-cell lymphoma (PMBCL) is an aggressive lymphoma affecting mainly young adult patients with one of the poorest survivals in the pediatric age range. It is now well recognized as a separate entity from DLBCL, based on clinical, histomorphologic, immunologic and molecular characteristics (see Chapter 4).[1]

It is unclear whether the biology of PMBCL in children and adolescents is the same as that seen in adults and whether the management should be the same in the two age groups (see Chapter 17). The majority of the published biology studies simply include the adolescent patients as part of the cohort without consideration of whether the biology of their tumors is the same. Nevertheless, the immunohistochemical data suggest biology may be similar in the two age groups.

Rearrangements of *BCL2*, *BCL6* and *MYC* are absent or rare whereas inactivations of *CDKN2A* and *TP53* as a result of mutation/deletion have been reported.[1] These lymphomas harbor inactivating mutations of the suppressor of cytokine signaling, *SOCS1*, gene and heterozygous missense mutations in *STAT6* DNA-binding domain that lead to the constitutive activation of *STAT6*. Additionally, PMBCLs have mutated, class-switched *IG* genes without evidence of ongoing somatic mutation.[40]

PMBCL have been characterized to harbor chromosomal gains in chromosome 9p associated with increased expression of *JAK2* at 9p24, as well as gains on chromosomal region 2p16 corresponding with the *REL* gene locus, both of which are commonly found in HL.[41] PMBCL has constitutively activated NF-κB and JAK-STAT pathways, frequently related to inactivating mutations of *SOCS1* and activation of *STAT6*. Aditionally, in almost all cases of PMBCL, REL protein accumulation has been found to be localized to the nucleus, consistent with activation of the NF-κB pathway. Moreover, it has been shown that when a NF-κB target gene signature is applied and compared between PMBCL and ABC-DLBCL, the PMBCL present increased levels of NF-κB targets that promote cell survival and favor TNFα signaling, whereas ABC-DLBCL presents a more restricted NF-κB target gene signature (Table 8.1).[42] Given the limitations of current combined modality therapy, the NF-κB pathway and supporting cytokine network may represent more specific treatment targets for PMBCL. In this sense, a recent study in which the molecule IκB kinase inhibitor, PS-1145, inhibited growth of a PMBCL cell line while inducing gene expression changes in a distinct group of NF-κB target genes, validating that this pathway may be a promising therapeutic target for lymphomas that depend on activity of NF-κB for survival and proliferation.[43]

In addition, GEP in PMBCL cases has shown a unique molecular signature with a striking overlap with HL.[44–46] Five of the genes included in the PMBCL signature (*MAL*, *SNFT*, *TNFRSF6*, *TARC* and *CD30*) are expressed in Reed–Sternberg cells.[45]

Only the *novo* methylation of the CpG-island within the promoter of *CDKN2A* has been evaluated in this disease, with the observation that methylation of its promoter was the most frequent mode of *CDKN2A* inactivation in these cases, more than mutations or deletions.[47]

Follicular lymphoma

Follicular lymphoma (FL) is a neoplasm composed of germinal center B cells which usually has at least a partially follicular pattern. It is genetically characterized by the t(14;18)(q32;q21) translocation and BCL2 alternative rearrangements with light *IG* chains. Abnormalities of 3q27 are found in 5–15% of FL, most commonly in grade 3b cases.[48] If diffuse areas are present in any case of FL, the case is reported as DLBCL with FL.

In addition, gene expression studies in FL have identified two outcome-related gene expression signatures, termed Immune response 1 and 2, pointing to a significant role of the microenvironment in the pathogenesis, evolution and prognosis of FL.[49]

Pediatric FL are considered to be an independent variant of FL that have many features indistinguishable from those seen in adults, but demonstrate an increased proportion that are localized, lack BCL2 expression and exhibit grade 3 histology (see Chapter 4).[1] Moreover, pediatric FL differ genetically from their adult counterpart.[50]

The t(14; 18)(q32; q21) translocation juxtaposing the BCL2 gene next to the *IGH* gene is detectable in more than 80% of adult FL, but is reported to be rare in pediatric patients with FL.[50] In fact, BCL2 translocations have been only demonstrated in two pediatric FL using a PCR technique but these results are under question since they require validation by an *in situ* technique like FISH to prove that the translocation is a feature of the lymphoma cells. In this sense, a recent study in which 25 cases of pediatric FL (age < 18 years) were studied by morphology, immunohistochemistry and FISH. In this study, the t(14;18)(q32; q21) which is the genetic hallmark of adult FL, was not detectable in any of the pediatric FL, although the BCL2 protein was overexpressed in 55% of the cases. In addition, no correlation between BCL2 protein expression and outcome was observed.[51]

Variable regions of *IG* heavy and light chains genes show extensive and ongoing somatic hypermutation.[1] Furthermore, transformation to DLBCL can involve different genetic pathways such as inactivation of *TP53* and *CDKN2A* and activation of *MYC*.[52]

Marginal zone lymphoma

Marginal zone lymphomas (MZL) are subdivided depending on their localization in extranodal MZL of mucosa associated lymphoid-tissue (MALT lymphoma) and nodal MZL (NMZL).

MALT lymphomas have an indolent course and are slow to disseminate. Most cases occur in adults and there is slight female preponderance. Chromosomal translocations associated with MALT lymphomas include t(11;18)(q21;q21), t(1;14)(p22;q32), t(14;18)(q32;q21), and t(3;14)(p14.1;q32), resulting in the production of a chimeric protein (API2-MALT1) or in transcriptional deregulation (BCL10, MALT1, FOXP1), respectively (Table 8.3). The frequencies in which these translocations occur vary markedly with the primary site of disease.

IG genes are rearranged and show somatic hypermutation of the variable regions, consistent with a post-germinal center B cell origin.[53] This entity is extremely rare in children and young adults and only isolated reports of MALT lymphoma in pediatric patients have been reported.[54] However, the true incidence of these lymphomas in young patients is not known and there are few data regarding their biological characteristics, since only few cytogenetic studies have been performed on this field. NMZL is a primary nodal B-cell neoplasm that resembles MALT lymphoma but without extranodal or splenic disease. The *IG* genes are rearranged in these lymphomas with a predominance of mutated *VH3* and *VH4* families.[55,56]

In the pediatric age group, MZL have distinctive clinical and morphological characteristics and have been classified as an independent entity in the new WHO classification (see Chapter 4). They are present predominantly in males (ratio 20:1) with asymptomatic and localized (90% of the cases are stage I) disease, have a similar immunophenotype to adult NMZL[1] and any of the alterations associated with NMZL are not detected.[57,58] Studies for clonal rearrangements of the *IGH* chain are necessary to help distinguish pediatric NMZL from atypical marginal zone hyperplasia with monotypic IG expression. *Tadesse-Heath* and collaborators described the clonality of the *IGH* gene by PCR in a series of pediatric MZL.[59] In this study, monoclonality was demonstrated by immunohistochemistry in paraffin sections and/or *IGH* gene rearrangement studies in almost all cases studied. The immunophenotypic and molecular features of these cases were distinct from those reported in reactive hyperplasia with marginal zone expansion.

T-Cell Lymphomas

Anaplastic large cell lymphoma

The fourth edition of the WHO Classification of Tumors of Hematopoietic and Lymphoid Tissues[1]

Table 8.3. Different translocations in MALT-MZL.

Translocation	Gene	Biological function	Oncogenic mechanism
t(11;18)(q21;q21)	*API2-MALT1*	NF-κB activator	Fusion protein
t(1;14)(p22;q32)	*IGH-BCL10*	NF-κB activator	Expression deregulation
t(14;18)(q32;q21)	*IGH-MALT1*	NF-κB activator	Expression deregulation
t(3;14)(p14.1;q32)	*IGH-FOXP1*	transcription factor	Expression deregulation

recognizes two types of anaplastic large cell lymphoma (ALCL), ALK-positive ALCL and ALK-negative ALCL (provisional entity) (see Chapters 2 and 4). ALCL is a distinct subtype of aggressive CD30 positive peripheral T-cell NHL that makes up about 10–15% of pediatric NHL.[60,61] In the pediatric population, primary cutaneous and ALK-negative ALCL are very rare.[62]

The majority of pediatric ALCL (90–95%) express ALK due to specific genetic events that lead to overexpression and constitutive activation of ALK.[63] In about 80% of tumors, ALK overexpression arises due to a t(2;5)(p23;q35) translocation that juxtaposes the *ALK* gene on chromosome 2p23 to the nucleophosmin (*NPM*) gene on 5q35. This fusion gene encodes a chimeric, constitutively activated tyrosine kinase, NPM-ALK, consisting of the N-terminal portion of the *NPM* fused to the catalytic domain of ALK. The fusion with NPM results in activation of the ALK kinase domain and its expression in a deregulated and ectopic manner.[60,64]

Over 13 alternative fusion partners for ALK have been identified and involve *CLTC*, non-muscle tropomyosin 3 gene (*TPM3*), non-muscle tropomyosin 4 (*TPM4*), moesin (MSN), Trk fusion gene (*TFG*), cysteinyl-tRNA synthetase (*CARS*), non-muscle myosin heavy chain (*MYH9*), RAN binding protein (*RANBP2*), and 5-aminoimidazole-4-carboxamide ribonucleotide formyltransferase/IMP cyclohydrolase gene (*ATIC*). Most of the partner proteins contain an oligomerization domain required for constitutive activation of the ALK kinase.[65]

GEP studies of ALCLs are relatively sparse due to the rarity of the disease. The largest study performed on 32 patients with systemic ALCL (25 ALK-positive and 7 ALK-negative) and five cell lines demonstrates the existence of two groups corresponding to morphologic subgroups (common vs. small cell and mixed variants).[66] Comparison of ALK-positive and negative ALCLs using supervised analysis demonstrated subsets of genes including *BCL6*, *PTPN12*, *CEBPB*, and *SERPINA1* to be overexpressed in ALK-positive ALCL. Other functional groups of genes that were overrepresented in gene ontology (GO) terms in ALK-positive ALCL included those related to immunologic functions (immune response, response to pathogen) and the NF-κB/IkB cascade, leukocyte transendothelial migration (ITGAM, PXN, JAM3), focal adhesion and adherens junction (CTNNB1/β-catenin, RAC1). Interestingly, many of these are recapitulated in the proteomic signature of ALCL.[8] The molecular signature of ALK-negative ALCLs did not provide any clues to the molecular mechanisms of the tumor subtype, suggesting that it was composed of heterogeneous molecular entities. GEP studies of ALCL-derived cell lines combined with functional RNAi screening revealed the transcription factor *C/EBPβ* and *BCL2A1* as critical genes required for cell transformation or maintenance of survival.[67,68] The downstream signaling pathways induced by variant partner gene products are not known, although GEP studies comparing TPM3-ALK positive and NPM-ALK positive ALCL indicate shared pathways.[69]

Genomic profiling of 74 ALCLs including 43 ALK-positive and 31 ALK-negative cases by comparative genomic hybridization (CGH) revealed genomic imbalances in 25 (58%) of ALK-positive ALCL and 20 (65%) of ALK-negative ALCLs.[70] Interestingly, ALK-positive cases with *NPM-ALK* or variant *ALK* translocations showed a similar profile of secondary genetic alterations, including gains of 17p and 17q24-qter, losses of 4q13-q21 and 11q14 (Fig. 8.3). ALK-negative cases demonstrated more frequent gains of 1q and 6p21. Some abnormalities such as gains of chromosome 7 and 6q and loss of 13q were observed in both ALK-positive and ALK-negative cases. It is unknown whether there were specific alterations seen in pediatric ALCLs vs. adult cases. Importantly, although ALK-negative patients exhibited significantly worse prognosis than ALK-positive patients, no specific chromosomal alterations were associated with survival.

Somatic mutations are rare in anaplastic large cell lymphoma. Monoallelic and bi-allelic mutations of the perforin (*PRF1*) gene have been reported in some cases of childhood lymphomas. Direct sequencing identified six different mutations in 12 patients (27.3%) of 44 patients with t(2;5)-positive ALCL. Two of the mutations were novel mutations: 529C > T and I471 > G while four were previous described. The incidence of *PRF1* mutations was found to be significantly higher in patients with ALCL compared with 400 control subjects, among whom only heterozygous A91V was observed in 41 subjects (10.2%) (chi-square test, 10.9; $P < 0.01$).[71] *PRF1* mutations have been described in other NHL and are thought to result in defective perforin-mediated cytotoxicity due to abnormal conformational changes induced by the A91V mutation.[72] The amplification of the sonic hedgehog (SHH) gene in a subset of ALK-positive ALCL[73] has been shown to lead to the deregulation of the SHH signaling pathway.

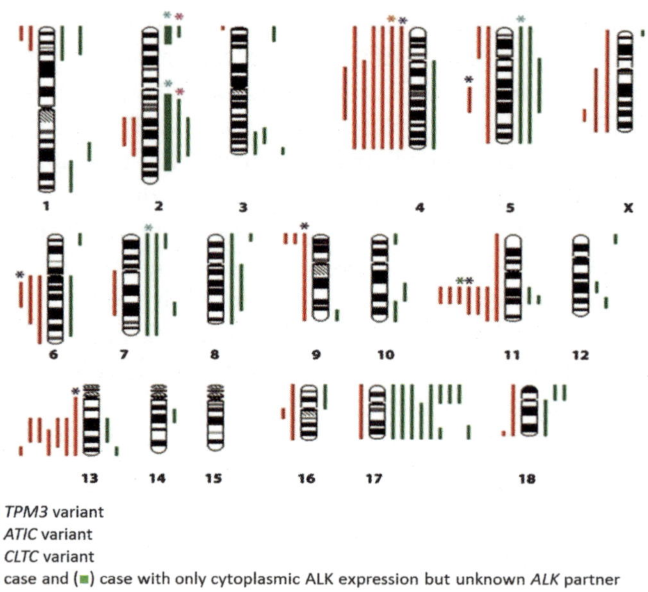

Fig. 8.3. Ideogram of the distribution of gains and losses of genetic material detected by comparative genomic hybridization (CGH) in 43 anaplastic lymphoma kinase (ALK)-positive anaplastic large cell lymphoma (ALCL) cases. Left-sided red bars correspond to genetic losses whereas right-sided green bars indicate genetic gains. Bold bars indicate genetic gains of more than one copy and amplifications. This research was originally published in Salaverria I, Beà S, Lopez-Guillermo A, Lespinet V, Pinyol M, Burkhardt B, Lamant L, Zettl A, Horsman D, Gascoyne R, Ott G, Siebert R, Delsol G, Campo E. Genomic profiling reveals different genetic aberrations in systemic ALK-positive and ALK-negative anaplastic large cell lymphomas. *Br J Haematol.* 2008; 140: 516–526.

Mass spectrometry (MS)-based proteomic studies of ALCL have been recently described. Annotation of a large-scale database of proteins comprising the proteome of the NPM/ALK-positive ALCL[74,75] resulted in a comprehensive list of proteins expressed in the NPM/ALK-positive ALCL. Using subcellular fractions including cytoplasm, nucleus and membrane subjected to gel digestion and analyzed by liquid chromatography tandem mass spectrometry (LC-MS/MS), a total of 623 proteins consisting of 210 membrane, 229 cytoplasm, and 184 nuclear proteins were identified with a $\leq 5\%$ error rate. Extensive annotation and PubMed investigation of a subset of 209 proteins indicated that 19.9% were previously reported to be expressed in T cells and 44.7% were reported to have important function in cancers. Notably, only 2.4% of the proteins have been previously reported in the literature to be implicated in ALCL pathogenesis. GoMiner™[76] protein function analysis on the ALCL proteome revealed a highly complex system and identified proteins involved in diverse cellular functions such as catalytic, enzyme, signaling, motor, translation, transcription, structural, and motor. MS-based proteomic strategy was used to determine the identity of proteins that interact with NPM/ALK (interactome).[77] Among the over 40 proteins identified in the ALK interactome, 9 proteins had been previously reported to be important mediators of the ALK signal pathway and interacted with ALK. These include phospholipase C-gamma (PLCγ1), phosphoinositide-3-kinase (PI3-K), Jak2, Jak3, STAT3, and IRS. More importantly, many proteins previously not recognized to be associated with NPM/ALK, but with potential NPM/ALK-interacting protein domains were identified. These included adaptor molecules (SOCS, Rho-GTPase activating protein, RAB35), kinases (MEK kinase 1 and 4, PKC, MLCK, cyclin G-associated kinase, EphA1, EphB, JNK kinase, MAP kinase 1), phosphatases (meprin, PTPK, protein phosphatase 2 subunit) and heat shock proteins (Hsp60 precursor). A comprehensive interactome map of NPM/ALK is illustrated using GeneGo (http://www.genego.com/) (Fig. 8.4A), an integrated systems level analysis tool for high-throughput MS and genomic data. Although the specific nature of the protein interactions needs to be functionally validated, these approaches represent a high-throughput method for the identification of proteins within a complex, and provide insights into the fundamental basis of their biological activities.

Quantitative proteomic analyses of NPM/ALK-positive and NPM/ALK-negative cells have been carried out using tandem mass spectrometry.[8,78] Proteins from nearly every cellular compartment including the

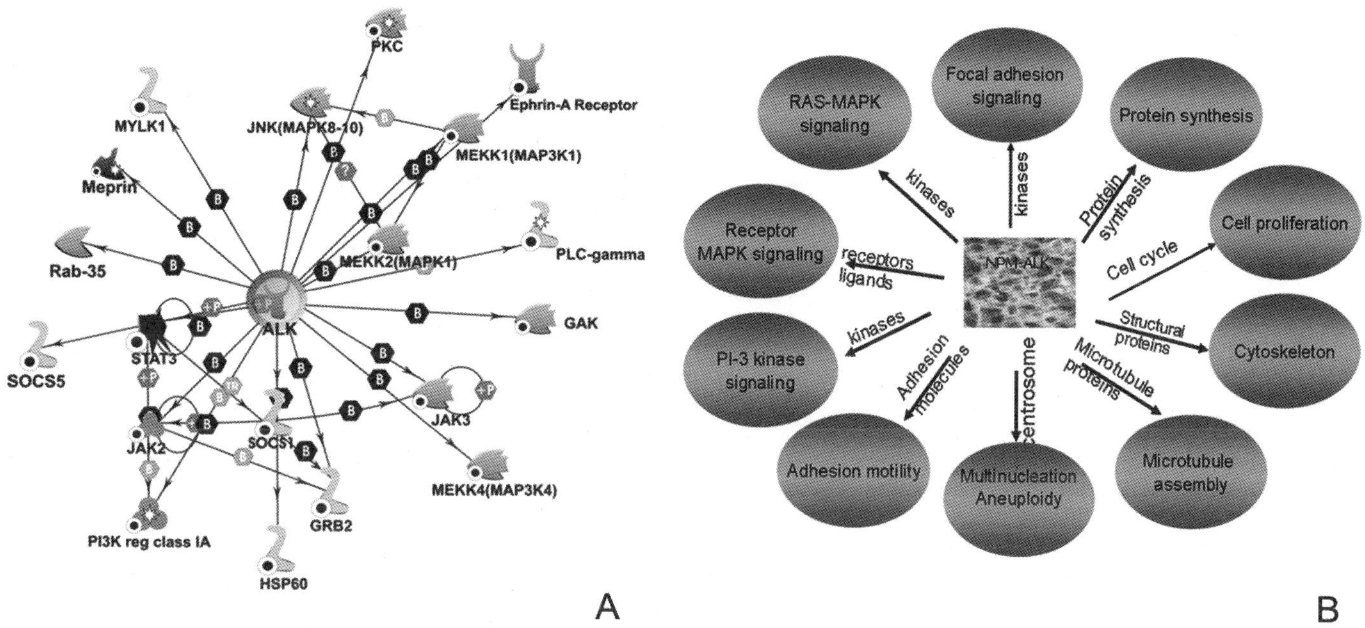

Fig. 8.4. (A) Proteins identified within the NPM/ALK protein network. The proteins identified within the NPM/ALK immunocomplex are visualized using GeneGO software analysis. (B) NPM/ALK induces the expression of proteins that are involved in diverse cellular functions. The expression of NPM/ALK induced the expression of proteins implicated in multiple signaling pathways and cellular functions such as cell motility, microtubule assembly, protein synthesis, invasion, and proliferation. *MAPK* mitogen-activated protein kinase, *PI* phosphatidylinositol. This research was originally published in *Mol. Cell Proteomics.* Lim MS and Elenitoba-Johnson KSJ. 2006 5:1787–1798. The American Society for Biochemistry and Molecular Biology, Inc.

reg: regulated; *PKC*: protein kinase C; *GAK*: cyclin G-associated kinase.

nucleus, cytoplasm, membrane and secretome were identified to be differentially expressed. Analyses of differentially expressed proteins revealed them to belong to a variety of functional groups. The common functional groups of proteins, which were upregulated, were those that belong to kinases, cell adhesion, migration and cytoskeletal function and those associated with proliferation and protein synthesis. The others represent phosphatases, small GTPases and proteins associated with centrosome assembly. As shown in Fig. 8.4B our quantitative proteomic studies reveal that NPM/ALK deregulates the expression of numerous proteins within previously described and novel signaling modules important for cell proliferation, survival, apoptosis evasion, and tumor dissemination. These data show that comprehensive analysis of the proteomic changes produced by a singular molecular alteration such as NPM/ALK facilitates the understanding of tumor pathobiology and enables the identification of novel biomarkers and therapeutic targets. A comparison of cell lines representative of two morphologic subtypes of NPM/ALK-positive ALCLs, namely the common type (SUDHL-1) and the small cell variant (COST), using two-dimensional gel electrophoresis and MALDI-TOF MS revealed distinct set of proteins which were selectively differentially expressed within each category.[79] Furthermore, the relative overexpression of one protein, carbonic anhydrase II, in the small cell variant was validated in tissue biopsy samples of small cell variants of ALCL.

Lymphoblastic T-cell lymphoma

Lymphoblastic T-cell Lymphomas (T-LBL) represent genetically and clinically heterogeneous neoplasms of immature or precursor lymphoid cells that comprise approximately 30% of the NHLs that occur in children and young adults. The majority of LBLs arise from immature T-cells.[80,81] Chromosomal translocations are the most frequent cytogenetic abnormalities that occur in T-LBL. These chromosomal translocations frequently juxtapose promoter and enhancer elements from TCR genes next to transcription factors genes such as *HOX11*, *TAL1* and *LYL1*, which are normally transcriptionally silent in normal T-lymphocytes.[82–85] The most common translocations in T-LBL involve *TCRA@* (14q11.2), *TRB@* (7q34) and *TARP* (7p14.1), with the more immature cellular phenotypes favoring the TCRγ or TCRδ loci. While the prognostic significance of these cytogenetic features is unknown in LBL, many of these same cytogenetic findings have not been shown to have prognostic significance in pediatric T-ALL.[82]

GEP of T-ALL have been extensively analyzed and is covered in Chapter 6. Very few studies have reported on the gene expression profiles of T-LBL and analyses of a limited number of cases have highlighted genes involved in cell proliferation (*PCNA, CDC2, E2F1, CDKN2A, Ki67, MADH2, MAX, MYC, CDK2, CDK4, CDK10, CDK8*), cell cycle (*TP53BP2, TP53, CCNA1, CCND2*) and cytoskeletal biology (tubulins *A1, B, B4, G1*) in T-LBL using a cDNA microarray containing 8016 clones.[86] The gene expression profiles of T-LBL formed a distinct group from peripheral T-cell lymphomas and other well-characterized entities such as ALCL and angioimmunoblastic T-cell lymphoma. Another study evaluated a common loss of heterozygosity (LOH) at chromosome 6q in a cohort of pediatric T-ALL and T-LBL.[23] A set of 25 microsatellite markers on 6q14-q24 were used to evaluate 108 T-LBL patients. LOH was detected in 21 T-LBL patients with a clear association between LOH at 6q and an increased risk of relapse. LOH was identified in 16 patients of T-ALL but was not associated with increased rate of relapse. Furthermore, the patterns of LOH at 6q were distinct between the two disease entities, providing support for the notion that they represent distinct biological entities.

To elucidate the genetic basis for T-LBL, *Raetz* and coworkers[87] compared the global gene expression profiles of 10 T-ALL and nine T-LBL using Affymetrix U133A genechip composed of over 22.283 probe sets. Unsupervised hierarchical clustering of 10 T-ALL bone marrow samples and nine T-LBL tissue samples lead to complete segregation of T-ALL and T-LBL, into distinct groups. Furthermore, they identified over 200 genes able to differentiate diseases using significance analysis of microarrays. The results indicate the clear differences in the gene expression profiles between T-ALL and T-LBL, suggesting the underlying differences in the biology of the two entities. Defects in cell cycle control due to genetic loss of *INK4* locus (*P16/P14*) and aberration of *RB1* and *TP53* are common in T-LBL.[88,89] In addition, gene rearrangements can result in deregulated expression of transcription factors that lead to aberrant cell cycle control. For example, CALM-AF10 T-ALLs overexpress BMI1 that leads to P16 suppression. Another frequent underlying genetic event in T-LBL is the dysregulation of *TAL1* (1p32), which is estimated to occur with a frequency of 30%.[90,91] Adaptation of a T cell receptor-based classification of T-ALL to 41 cases T-LBL using T cell receptor genotyping, immunohistochemistry and oncogene expression allowed the identification of three categories of T-LBL.[92] Immature LBL showed no *TCR* or only incomplete *TCRD DJ* rearrangement. These were restricted to adults with extrathymic disease and bone marrow involvement. Intermediate-LBL showed complete *TCRD VDJ* and *TCRG VJ* rearrangement with expression of *HOX11/TLX1* or *HOXA9* transcription. Intermediate LBLs were found in children and adults with predominantly thymic disease. Mature $TCRD^{del}$-LBL demonstrated bi-allelic *TCRD* deletions and both *TCRG* and *TCRB* rearrangements.

Rare T-cell lymphoma entities in CAYA

Peripheral T-cell lymphomas

Peripheral T-cell lymphomas (PTCL) other than ALCL are rare in young patients.[93] They include PTCL, not otherwise specified, hepatosplenic T-cell lymphoma, subcutaneous panniculitis-like T-cell lymphoma, extranodal natural killer/T-cell lymphoma of nasal type and enteropathy-type T-cell lymphoma. More recently, EBV-negative T-cell lymphomas with features consistent with hepatosplenic T-cell lymphomas have been reported in patients receiving infliximab for inflammatory bowel disease.[94]

GEP of γ/δ T-cell lymphoma[95] revealed that genes of NK cell-associated molecules such as killer cell Ig-like receptor (KIR) genes and killer cell lectin-like receptors were found to be overexpressed relative to other PTCL with α/β phenotype. Gene ontology analysis of differentially expressed genes showed enrichment of those involved in cellular defense response, signal transduction activity, receptor activity, transmembrane receptor activity, and IgG binding. The data support the notion that hepatosplenic γ/δ T-cell lymphomas are a distinct entity in PTCLs.

Future Directions

The rare occurrence of distinct subsets of pediatric NHL presents a challenge in our efforts in understanding the molecular and genetic abnormalities of these tumors. Specifically in T-cell malignancies such as ALCL, cellular heterogeneity can be problematic as most biopsies contain numerous infiltrating reactive lymphocytes and histiocytes.

How distinct are NHL in children and young adults from those that occur in adults? Which is the age threshold between adult and children diseases? With few exceptions (PMBCL), no specific molecular studies in young adults have been performed. Most clinical correlations are made without distinguishing patient age. Future studies will need to focus on evaluating molecular characteristics of NHLs specifically from this age group. Moreover, studies in young adult lymphomas would help in the definition of the real border between adult and pediatric diseases. Moreover, determination of the clinical impact of specific molecular abnormalities will be important to pursue.

ALK-positive ALCLs comprise the great majority of systemic ALCLs in children and young adults, thus the biological differences between ALK-negative ALCLs may be difficult to ascertain. Future international clinical trials, composed of large patient cohorts, will be necessary to carry out statistically valid studies.

Implications of novel technologies

The application of high throughput DNA sequencing, epigenetic analysis, microRNA profiling and methylation profiling will undoubtedly add complexity to the currently existing molecular genetic features. The recently identified mutations involving *A20*,[96] *CARD11*,[97] and *EZH2*[98] in adult NHLs will be of interest to pursue in pediatric cases.

Implications of novel therapeutic agents

Clinical use of small molecule ALK tyrosine kinase inhibitors, which are currently in clinical trials, may lead to the development of kinase resistant mutations and/or secondary genetic abnormalities in patients with ALCLs. Peptide inhibitors of BCL6 in NHL derived from the germinal center origin are also potential therapeutic agents for CAYA (see Chapter 22).[99]

Acknowledgments

The authors own studies on the genetics of CAYA Lymphoma were supported by Deutsche Krebshilfe, Kinderkrebsinitative Buchholz/Holm-Seppensen and Alexander Von Humboldt Foundation.

References

1. Swerdlow SH, Campo E, Harris NL, Jaffe ES, Pileri SA, Stein H, Thiele J, Vardiman JW (eds). (2008) *WHO Classification of Tumours of Haematopoietic and Lymphoid Tissues.* Lyon: IARC Press.
2. Alizadeh AA, Eisen MB, Davis RE, Ma C, Lossos IS, Rosenwald A, *et al.* (2000) Distinct types of diffuse large B-cell lymphoma identified by gene expression profiling. *Nature* **403**(6769): 503–511.
3. Dave SS, Fu K, Wright GW, Lam LT, Kluin P, Boerma EJ, *et al.* (2006) Molecular diagnosis of Burkitt's lymphoma. *N Engl J Med* **354**(23): 2431–2442.
4. Hummel M, Bentink S, Berger H, Klapper W, Wessendorf S, Barth TF, *et al.* (2006) A biologic definition of Burkitt's lymphoma from transcriptional and genomic profiling. *N Engl J Med* **354**(23): 2419–2430.
7. Lim MS, Elenitoba-Johnson KS. (2006) Mass spectrometry-based proteomic studies of human anaplastic large cell lymphoma. *Mol Cell Proteomics* **5**(10): 1787–1798.
8. Lim MS, Carlson ML, Crockett DK, Fillmore GC, Abbott DR, Elenitoba-Johnson OF, *et al.* (2009) The proteomic signature of NPM/ALK reveals deregulation of multiple cellular pathways. *Blood* **114**(8): 1585–1595.
12. Klapper W, Szczepanowski M, Burkhardt B, Berger H, Rosolowski M, Bentink S, *et al.* (2008) Molecular profiling of pediatric mature B-cell lymphoma treated in population-based prospective clinical trials. *Blood* **112**(4): 1374–1381.
15. Martin-Subero JI, Kreuz M, Bibikova M, Bentink S, Ammerpohl O, Wickham-Garcia E, *et al.* (2009) New insights into the biology and origin of mature aggressive B-cell lymphomas by combined epigenomic, genomic, and transcriptional profiling. *Blood* **113**(11): 2488–2497.
18. Einerson RR, Law ME, Blair HE, Kurtin PJ, McClure RF, Ketterling RP, *et al.* (2006) Novel FISH probes designed to detect IGK-MYC and IGL-MYC rearrangements in B-cell lineage malignancy identify a new breakpoint cluster region designated BVR2. *Leukemia* **20**(10): 1790–1799.
22. Oschlies I, Klapper W, Zimmermann M, Krams M, Wacker HH, Burkhardt B, *et al.* (2006) Diffuse large B-cell lymphoma in pediatric patients belongs predominantly to the germinal-center type B-cell lymphomas: A clinicopathologic analysis of cases included in the German BFM (Berlin-Frankfurt-Munster) Multicenter Trial. *Blood* **107**(10): 4047–4052.
23. Burkhardt B, Moericke A, Klapper W, Greene F, Salzburg J, Damm-Welk C, *et al.* (2008) Pediatric precursor T lymphoblastic leukemia and lymphoblastic lymphoma: Differences in the common regions with loss of heterozygosity at chromosome 6q and their prognostic impact. *Leuk Lymphoma* **49**(3): 451–461.
24. Gualco G, Weiss LM, Harrington WJ Jr., Bacchi CE. (2009) Nodal diffuse large B-cell lymphomas in children and adolescents: Immunohistochemical expression pat-

terns and c-MYC translocation in relation to clinical outcome. *Am J Surg Pathol* **33**(12): 1815–1822.

27. de Paepe P, Baens M, van Krieken H, Verhasselt B, Stul M, Simons A, *et al.* (2003) ALK activation by the CLTC-ALK fusion is a recurrent event in large B-cell lymphoma. *Blood* **102**(7): 2638–2641.
29. Gesk S, Gascoyne RD, Schnitzer B, Bakshi N, Janssen D, Klapper W, *et al.* (2005) ALK-positive diffuse large B-cell lymphoma with ALK-Clathrin fusion belongs to the spectrum of pediatric lymphomas. *Leukemia* **19**(10): 1839–1840.
32. Stachurski D, Miron PM, Al-Homsi S, Hutchinson L, Lee Harris N, Woda B, *et al.* (2007) Anaplastic lymphoma kinase-positive diffuse large B-cell lymphoma with a complex karyotype and cryptic 3′ ALK gene insertion to chromosome 4 q22–24. *Hum Pathol* **38**(6): 940–945.
33. Harrison CJ. (2009) Cytogenetics of paediatric and adolescent acute lymphoblastic leukaemia. *Br J Haematol* **144**(2): 147–156.
35. Soulier J, Trakhtenbrot L, Najfeld V, Lipton JM, Mathew S, Avet-Loiseau H, *et al.* (2003) Amplification of band q22 of chromosome 21, including AML1, in older children with acute lymphoblastic leukemia: An emerging molecular cytogenetic subgroup. *Leukemia* **17**(8): 1679–1682.
37. Busson-Le Coniat M, Nguyen Khac F, Daniel MT, Bernard OA, Berger R. (2001) Chromosome 21 abnormalities with AML1 amplification in acute lymphoblastic leukemia. *Genes Chromosomes Cancer* **32**(3): 244–249.
39. Strefford JC, van Delft FW, Robinson HM, Worley H, Yiannikouris O, Selzer R, *et al.* (2006) Complex genomic alterations and gene expression in acute lymphoblastic leukemia with intrachromosomal amplification of chromosome 21. *Proc Natl Acad Sci U S A* **103**(21): 8167–8172.
41. Bentz M, Barth TF, Bruderlein S, Bock D, Schwerer MJ, Baudis M, *et al.* (2001) Gain of chromosome arm 9p is characteristic of primary mediastinal B-cell lymphoma (MBL): Comprehensive molecular cytogenetic analysis and presentation of a novel MBL cell line. *Genes Chromosomes Cancer* **30**(4): 393–401.
42. Feuerhake F, Kutok JL, Monti S, Chen W, LaCasce AS, Cattoretti G, *et al.* (2005) NFkappaB activity, function, and target-gene signatures in primary mediastinal large B-cell lymphoma and diffuse large B-cell lymphoma subtypes. *Blood* **106**(4): 1392–1399.
43. Lam LT, Davis RE, Pierce J, Hepperle M, Xu Y, Hottelet M, *et al.* (2005) Small molecule inhibitors of IkappaB kinase are selectively toxic for subgroups of diffuse large B-cell lymphoma defined by gene expression profiling. *Clin Cancer Res* **11**(1): 28–40.
44. Savage KJ, Monti S, Kutok JL, Cattoretti G, Neuberg D, de Leval L, *et al.* (2003) The molecular signature of mediastinal large B-cell lymphoma differs from that of other diffuse large B-cell lymphomas and shares features with classical Hodgkin lymphoma. *Blood* **102**(12): 3871–3879.
45. Rosenwald A, Wright G, Leroy K, Yu X, Gaulard P, Gascoyne RD, *et al.* (2003) Molecular diagnosis of primary mediastinal B cell lymphoma identifies a clinically favorable subgroup of diffuse large B cell lymphoma related to Hodgkin lymphoma. *J Exp Med* **198**(6): 851–862.
49. Dave SS, Wright G, Tan B, Rosenwald A, Gascoyne RD, Chan WC, *et al.* (2004) Prediction of survival in follicular lymphoma based on molecular features of tumor-infiltrating immune cells. *N Engl J Med* **351**(21): 2159–2169.
50. Lorsbach RB, Shay-Seymore D, Moore J, Banks PM, Hasserjian RP, Sandlund JT, *et al.* (2002) Clinicopathologic analysis of follicular lymphoma occurring in children. *Blood* **99**(6): 1959–1964.
51. Oschlies I, Salaverria I, Mahn F, Meinhardt A, Zimmermann M, Woessmann W, *et al.* (2010) Pediatric follicular lymphoma — a clinico-pathological study of a population-based series of patients treated within the Non-Hodgkin's Lymphoma — Berlin-Frankfurt-Munster (NHL-BFM) multicenter trials. *Haematologica* **95**(2): 253–259.
54. Mo JQ, Dimashkieh H, Mallery SR, Swerdlow SH, Bove KE. (2004) MALT Lymphoma in Children: Case Report and Review of the Literature. *Pediatr Dev Pathol* **7**(4): 407–413.
57. Dierlamm J, Wlodarska I, Michaux L, Stefanova M, Hinz K, van Den Berghe H, *et al.* (2000) Genetic abnormalities in marginal zone B-cell lymphoma. *Hematol Oncol* **18**(1): 1–13.
58. Traverse-Glehen A, Felman P, Callet-Bauchu E, Gazzo S, Baseggio L, Bryon PA, *et al.* (2006) A clinicopathological study of nodal marginal zone B-cell lymphoma: A report on 21 cases. *Histopathology* **48**(2): 162–173.
59. Taddesse-Heath L, Pittaluga S, Sorbara L, Bussey M, Raffeld M, Jaffe ES. (2003) Marginal zone B-cell lymphoma in children and young adults. *Am J Surg Pathol* **27**(4): 522–531.
62. Tomaszewski MM, Moad JC, Lupton GP. (1999) Primary cutaneous Ki-1(CD30) positive anaplastic large cell lymphoma in childhood. *J Am Acad Dermatol* **40**(5 Pt 2): 857–861.

63. Kutok JL, Aster JC. (2002) Molecular biology of anaplastic lymphoma kinase-positive anaplastic large-cell lymphoma. *J Clin Oncol* **20**(17): 3691–3702.
66. Lamant L, de Reynies A, Duplantier MM, Rickman DS, Sabourdy F, Giuriato S, *et al.* (2007) Gene-expression profiling of systemic anaplastic large-cell lymphoma reveals differences based on ALK status and two distinct morphologic ALK+ subtypes. *Blood* **109**(5): 2156–2164.
68. Piva R, Pellegrino E, Inghirami G. (2007) Identification and validation of the anaplastic large cell lymphoma signature. *Adv Exp Med Biol* **604**: 129–136.
69. Bohling SD, Jenson SD, Crockett DK, Schumacher JA, Elenitoba-Johnson KS, Lim MS. (2008) Analysis of gene expression profile of TPM3-ALK positive anaplastic large cell lymphoma reveals overlapping and unique patterns with that of NPM-ALK positive anaplastic large cell lymphoma. *Leuk Res* **32**(3): 383–393.
70. Salaverria I, Bea S, Lopez-Guillermo A, Lespinet V, Pinyol M, Burkhardt B, *et al.* (2008) Genomic profiling reveals different genetic aberrations in systemic ALK-positive and ALK-negative anaplastic large cell lymphomas. *Br J Haematol* **140**(5): 516–526.
71. Cannella S, Santoro A, Bruno G, Pillon M, Mussolin L, Mangili G, *et al.* (2007) Germline mutations of the perforin gene are a frequent occurrence in childhood anaplastic large cell lymphoma. *Cancer* **109**(12): 2566–2571.
74. Crockett DK, Seiler CE III, Elenitoba-Johnson KS, Lim MS. (2005) Annotated proteome of a human T-cell lymphoma. *J Biomol Tech* **16**(4): 341–346.
75. Sjostrom C, Seiler C, Crockett DK, Tripp SR, Elenitoba Johnson KS, Lim MS. (2007) Global proteome profiling of NPM/ALK-positive anaplastic large cell lymphoma. *Exp hematol* **35**(8): 1240–1248.
77. Crockett DK, Lin Z, Elenitoba-Johnson KS, Lim MS. (2004) Identification of NPM-ALK interacting proteins by tandem mass spectrometry. *Oncogene* **23**(15): 2617–2629.
81. Uckun FM, Sather HN, Gaynon PS, Arthur DC, Trigg ME, Tubergen DG, *et al.* (1977) Clinical features and treatment outcome of children with myeloid antigen positive acute lymphoblastic leukemia: A report from the Children's Cancer Group. *Blood* **90**(1): 28–35.
82. Heerema NA, Sather HN, Sensel MG, Kraft P, Nachman JB, Steinherz PG, *et al.* (1998) Frequency and clinical significance of cytogenetic abnormalities in pediatric T-lineage acute lymphoblastic leukemia: A report from the Children's Cancer Group. *J Clin Oncol* **16**(4): 1270–1278.
84. Ferrando AA, Look AT. (2003) Gene expression profiling in T-cell acute lymphoblastic leukemia. *Semin Hematol* **40**(4): 274–280.
86. Ballester B, Ramuz O, Gisselbrecht C, Doucet G, Loi L, Loriod B, *et al.* (2006) Gene expression profiling identifies molecular subgroups among nodal peripheral T-cell lymphomas. *Oncogene* **25**(10): 1560–1570.
87. Raetz EA, Perkins SL, Bhojwani D, Smock K, Philip M, Carroll WL, *et al.* (2006) Gene expression profiling reveals intrinsic differences between T-cell acute lymphoblastic leukemia and T-cell lymphoblastic lymphoma. *Pediatr Blood Cancer* **47**(2): 130–140.
90. Baer R. (1993) TAL1, TAL2 and LYL1: A family of basic helix-loop-helix proteins implicated in T cell acute leukaemia. *Semin Cancer Biol* **4**(6): 341–347.
91. Bash RO, Hall S, Timmons CF, Crist WM, Amylon M, Smith RG, *et al.* (1995) Does activation of the TAL1 gene occur in a majority of patients with T-cell acute lymphoblastic leukemia? A pediatric oncology group study. *Blood* **86**(2): 666–676.
92. Baleydier F, Decouvelaere AV, Bergeron J, Gaulard P, Canioni D, Bertrand Y, *et al.* (2008) T cell receptor genotyping and HOXA/TLX1 expression define three T lymphoblastic lymphoma subsets which might affect clinical outcome. *Clin Cancer Res* **14**(3): 692–700.
95. Miyazaki K, Yamaguchi M, Imai H, Kobayashi T, Tamaru S, Nishii K, *et al.* (2009) Gene expression profiling of peripheral T-cell lymphoma including gammadelta T-cell lymphoma. *Blood* **113**(5): 1071–1074.

9

Pharmacogenetics and Drug Resistance in ALL

Monique L. den Boer and Rob Pieters

Introduction

Cellular drug resistance is predictive for both short- and long-term clinical outcomes in pediatric and adult acute lymphoblastic leukemia (ALL) (see Chapters 11 and 12). A classic example is the observation that *in vitro* resistance to prednisolone measured at initial diagnosis is predictive for an unfavorable outcome in pediatric ALL; a >1500-fold difference in resistance to prednisolone is associated with a 5-year probability of disease-free survival of 40% compared to >80% for sensitive cases.[1,2] Also, clinically poor responders to a therapeutic window with systemically administered prednisone and intrathecally given methotrexate are *in vitro* more resistant to prednisolone. Amongst good window responders, *in vitro* prednisolone resistance discriminates the cases with an unfavorable long-term clinical outcome.[3] A similar association between *in vitro* (cellular) resistance, *in vivo* (clinical) window response and unfavorable long-term clinical outcome has been found for L-asparaginase.[4] Hence, cellular drug resistance, as measured with *in vitro* drug cytotoxicity assays can serve as a tool to discriminate patients at low and high risks of treatment failure.[5–9] This information can be used to stratify patients in risk-adapted treatment protocols, like that performed by the German co-operative ALL (COALL) study group.[10,11] As important, studying patients' cellular response to single agents can yield important insights into causes of cellular drug resistance. Elucidating mechanisms of drug resistance may point to ways to circumvent or modulate resistance in leukemic cells. In this chapter, we will address the putative causes of cellular drug resistance in the context of cytogenetic subtypes and pharmacogenetics in pediatric precursor B-ALL.

Cytogenetics and Cellular Drug Resistance

Leukemic cells of pediatric ALL patients are often cross-resistant to multiple drugs, suggesting a common mechanism causing the resistance.[3] However, expression levels of multidrug efflux pumps such as P-glycoprotein, multidrug resistance-associated protein (MRP) and breast cancer resistance protein (BCRP) are not linked to resistance to different classes of drugs in pediatric ALL.[12,13] In general, resistant cells have a reduced apoptotic potential compared to sensitive cells when tested under similar drug exposure conditions. However, if one raises the drug concentration, the resistant cells will ultimately be killed, suggesting that resistance is more associated with a mechanism of reduced sensitivity than with total unresponsiveness to the drug.[14] This relative resistance may be inherent to the differentiation status of malignant lymphoid cells. (e.g. immature pro-B-ALL cells are more resistant to glucocorticoids than the more mature common/pre-B cells).[15,16] This may reflect the fact that pro-B cells are more closely related to senescent and less drug responsive hematopoietic stem cells than common/pre-B cells.

Leukemic cells, derived from adults with ALL, are generally more resistant to glucocorticoids and L-asparaginase than those of children with ALL.[17,18] This can be explained by an age-related difference in the frequency of genetic subtypes (see Chapter 5) that have altered sensitivity towards these drugs. For example, *BCR-ABL1*-positive ALL is found in approximately 25% of adults compared to < 5% in children[19] whereas, in general, *BCR-ABL1*-positive ALL cases are *in vitro* and *in vivo* more resistant to prednisolone.[18,20] In contrast, the frequency of *TEL-AML1*-positive ALL is ~25% in children compared to < 5% in adults,[19] whereas *TEL-AML1* positivity is associated with sensitivity towards L-asparaginase.[21]

The activated intracellular signaling pathways as well as the complex crosstalk between leukemic cells and their microenvironment most likely determines the responsiveness to drugs. These pathways and networks vary with maturation of normal lymphoid cells since differentiation and proliferation-associated genes have to be switched on and off in a controlled fashion to ensure proper B-cell receptor (BCR) and T-cell receptor (TCR) formation.[22,23] The lineage and differentiation status-related activity of signaling pathways also implies that the mechanism of resistance cannot be similar for all subtypes but differs between cytogenetic subtypes of ALL.

MLL-rearranged ALL: deoxynucleoside analogs sensitivity and glucocorticoid resistance

Rearrangements of the *MLL*-gene (located at chromosome 11q23) are found in > 80% of infants (< 1 year of age) with ALL (see Chapters 3 and 5). The *MLL*-rearrangements in infant ALL are mainly associated with the immature pro-B immunophenotype.[24–26] *In vitro* drug cytoxicity testing revealed that *MLL*-rearranged/pro-B cases are resistant to most classes of drugs, including glucocorticoids and L-asparaginase (Table 9.1), which reflects the poor prognosis of these cases.[16,26–28] An exception is the relative sensitivity to the deoxynucleoside analogs, cytarabine (AraC) and 2-chloro-deoxyadenosine (2CdA).[15,16,28]

Sensitivity towards deoxynucleoside analogs

(1) Metabolism of AraC

Initially, research focused on mechanisms related to the metabolism of AraC into AraCTP as the driving cause of sensitivity towards deoxynucleoside analogs (see Fig. 9.1 for an overview) since the triphosphate nucleotide is required for incorporation into the DNA.[29] However, the expression of metabolizing enzymes was not altered in AraC-sensitive infant ALL cells with the inconsistent exception of a twofold lower expression level for the AraC–AraCMP-converting enzyme deoxycytidine kinase dCK.[30] In contrast, sensitive cells turned out to have an elevated expression of the equilibrative nucleoside transporter ENT1 (or SLC29A1), which facilitates the uptake of cytosines into the cell.[30] High levels of AraCTP were found in sensitive cells that correlated with ENT1 expression levels.[30,31] Moreover, it was demonstrated that an inhibitor of the ENT1 transporter could block the uptake of AraC into leukemic cells.[32]

Table 9.1. **Differential sensitivity and resistance to commonly used drugs in pediatric precursor B-ALL.**

Subtype	Sensitive	Resistant
MLL-rearranged ALL/infant ALL	Cytarabine (AraC) 2-chlorodeoxyadenosine (2-CdA)	Glucocorticoids L-asparaginase
TEL-AML1-positive ALL	L-asparaginase	Vincristine
Hyperdiploid ALL	Cytarabine Thiopurines Methotrexate	

(2) DNA methylation

It has been demonstrated that AraCTP needs to be incorporated into the DNA to be toxic.[29] However, *in vitro*-cultured primary patients' leukemia cells do not divide, whereas these cells are still sensitive to AraC. This phenomenon raises the question whether other mechanisms may be active in these cells besides those involved in metabolism and incorporation into DNA. Gutierrez *et al.* demonstrated that *MLL*-rearranged cases are more often hypermethylated than other types of precursor B-ALL.[33] The MLL fusion product is known to alter the chromatine configuration by tri- and di-methylation of histone 3 at lysine positions K4 and K79 (H3K4me3 and H3K79me2), respectively.[34] The resulting opening of the chromatine may affect the degree of promoter methylation of genes in both the positive and negative direction. In correspondence, recent work shows that *MLL*-rearranged ALL displays both hyper- and hypomethylation of

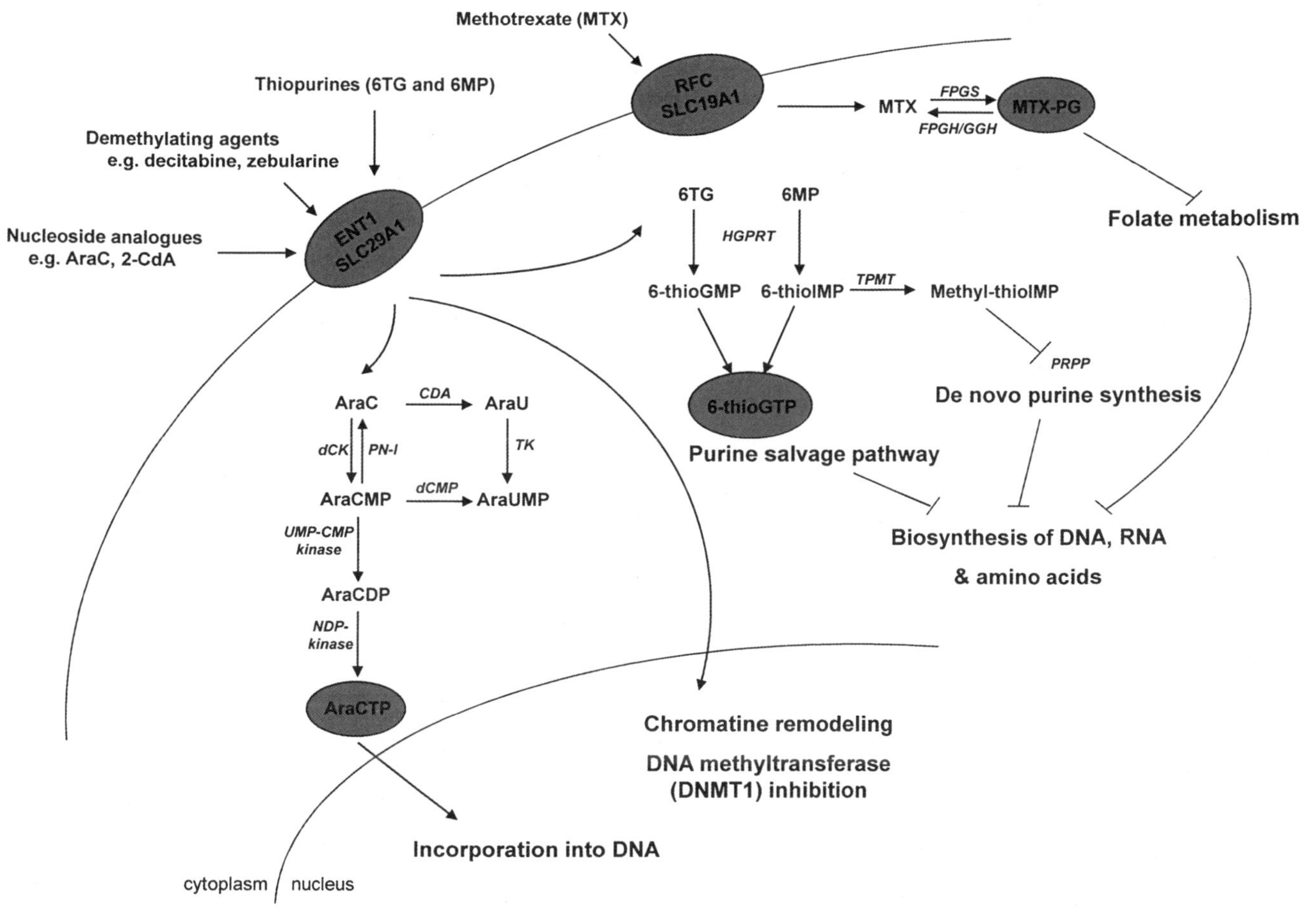

Fig. 9.1. Schematic overview of biological pathways affected by anti-metabolites and de-methylating agents. Nucleoside analogs like cytarabine (AraC) and 2-chloro-deoxyadenosine (2-CdA), thiopurines (6-thioguanine, 6TG and 6-mercaptopurine, 6MP), methotrexate (MTX) and presumable certain demethylating agents (e.g. decitabine) enter the cell via specific carriers present on the plasma membrane such as the equilibrative nucleoside transporter ENT1 and the reduced folate carrier RFC. Intracellularly, drugs are metabolized via the indicated pathways resulting in inhibition of DNA replication, epigenetic de-silencing and altered biosynthesis of DNA, RNA and amino acids components. Pediatric ALL cells sensitive to anti-metabolites have altered expression and/or activities of genes and/or metabolites that are indicated in red. Further details are described in text.

CDA: cytidine deaminase; dCMP: deoxycytidine deaminase; dCK: deoxycytidine kinase; FPGS: folypolyglutamate synthetase; FPGH/GGH: folypolyglutamate hydrolase/γ-glutamyl hydrolase; HGPRT: hypoxanthine-guanine phosphoribosyltransferase; MTX-PG: polyglutamated methotrexate; NDP-kinase: nucleoside diphosphate kinase; PN-I: pyrimidine nucleotidase I; PRPP: phosphoribosyl pyrophosphate amidotransferase; TK: thymidylate kinase; TPMT: thiopurine methyltransferase; UMP-CMP kinase: uridine monophosphate-cytidine monophosphate kinase;

genes that are respectively hypo- and hypermethylated in normal bone marrow cells.[35] One of the first genes in infant ALL that was shown to be silenced by DNA methylation was the fragile histidine triad gene *FHIT*. Re-expression of this gene by exposure to demethylating agents (decitabine) or by enforced expression resulted in the apoptosis of ALL cells,[36] confirming the earlier assigned tumor suppressor activity of *FHIT*.[37,38] Subsequent studies showed many more genes hypermethylated in *MLL*-rearranged ALL.[35,39] Remarkably, the degree of genome-wide CpG island methylation is predictive for the clinical outcome of *MLL*-rearranged cases; a part of t(4;11)/*MLL*-AF4-positive cases have a high methylation signature that is associated with a more unfavorable outcome than a less methylated signature.[35] This aberrant hypermethylation pattern may be potentially reversed by nucleoside analogs and/or demethylating agents such as AraC, 2CdA, decitabine, zebularine and others. The fact that *MLL*-rearranged cases have an elevated expression of ENT1 may facilitate the uptake of these classes of agents.

Resistance to glucocorticoids

(1) Glucocorticoid receptor-mediated pathway

In contrast to sensitivity towards nucleoside analogs, *MLL*-rearranged ALL cases are generally more resistant to the glucocorticoids prednisolone and dexamethasone (Table 9.1).[28] Figure 9.2 summarizes the mechanisms of action of glucocorticoids and potential causes of resistance in pediatric ALL. The glucocorticoids need to bind to the glucocorticoid receptor (GCR or NR3C1) to exert their function. A low number of GCRs and low expression level of the functional isoform GCRα is predictive for glucocorticoid resistance in pediatric ALL.[40,41] Functional studies indicate that an upregulation of GCR levels is not sufficient to sensitize towards glucocorticoids, suggesting that associated molecules and/or complexes are essential to induce sensitivity.[42,43] Glucocorticoids were shown to induce the expression levels of the B-cell translocation gene *BTG-1*, *GCRα* and other glucocorticoid-responsive genes (e.g. serum glucocorticoid-regulated kinase *SGK1* and FK506-binding protein *FKBP5*) in pediatric ALL.[43–45] Enforced expression of *BTG-1* sensitized otherwise resistant precursor B-ALL cells to prednisolone. In contrast, silencing of *BTG-1* made cells more resistant to prednisolone and reduced the transactivation of glucocorticoid-responsive genes. The impaired

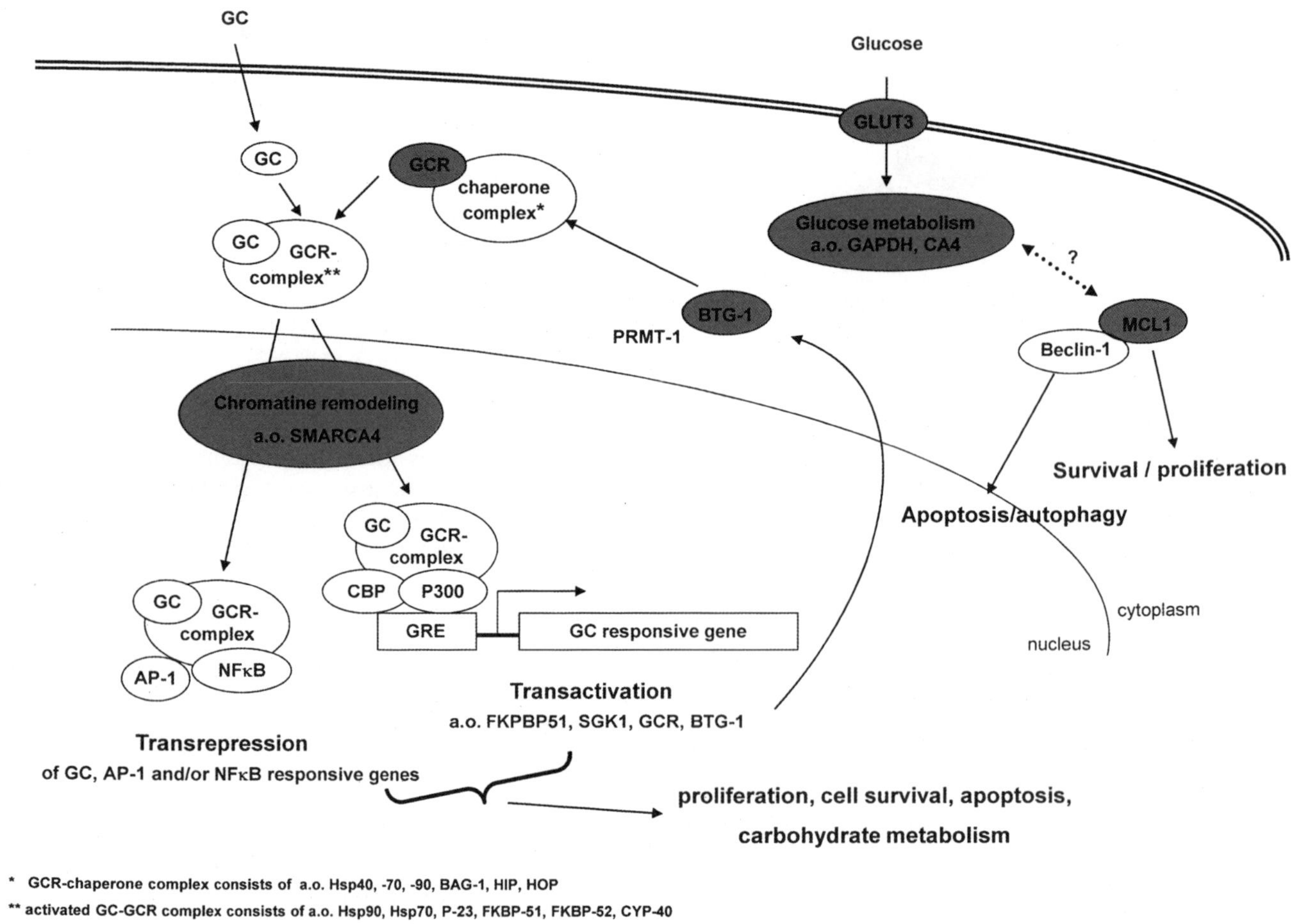

Fig. 9.2. The intracellular pathway activated by glucocorticoids and potential mechanisms of resistance in pediatric ALL. Glucocorticoids (GC) such as prednisolone and dexamethasone enter the cell by passive diffusion and bind to the glucocorticoid receptor (GCR). Upon receptor dimerization, the GC-GCR complex translocates to the nucleus to transactivate glucocorticoid responsive genes via binding to glucocorticoid responsive elements (GRE) in promoters of GC-responsive genes. In addition, the GC-GCR complex can repress other genes via scavenging of the transcription factors, AP-1 and NFκB. Resistance to glucocorticoids has been attributed to genes and/or processes that are indicated in red. Details on potential causes of resistance in subtypes of pediatric ALL are described in text.

CBP: CREB binding protein; P300: nuclear protein P300; AP-1: activating protein 1; NFκB: nuclear factor-κB; BTG-1: B-cell translocation gene 1; MCL1: myeloid cell leukemia gene 1.

transactivation of glucocorticoid-responsive genes could not be rescued by ectopic expression of *GCR*, confirming the need for functional GCR complexes to drive proper regulation of gene transcription.[43] Chaperone molecules such as heat-shock proteins *HSP40*, *HSP70* and *HSP90*, HSP70-interacting protein (*HIP*), HSP70/HSP90 organizing protein (*HOP*), BCL2-associated gene product 1 (*BAG1*) and *FKBP5* family members facilitate the binding of glucocorticoids to GCRs and enable the translocation of the glucocorticoid-bound GCR complex to the nucleus.[46] However, expression levels of these chaperone genes are not altered in resistant ALL cells.[47,48] Alternatively, inactivating mutations in GCR may occur as have been found in prednisolone-resistant ALL cell lines.[49–51] However, in patients' primary ALL cells, no such inactivating mutations nor polymorphisms have been found in GCRs of resistant cases, suggesting other causes of glucocorticoid resistance in pediatric ALL, as demonstrated for other non-leukemia patients.[52,53]

(2) Chromatin remodeling

Glucocorticoids and GCRs also contribute to chromatin unwinding, thereby facilitating the binding of other transcription factors to promoter regions of glucocorticoid-responsive genes. Glucocorticoid-GCR complexes can phosphorylate histone H1 and activate the SWI/SNF chromatin remodeling complex.[54] Expression levels of components of the SWI/SNF chromatin remodeling complex are lower in prednisolone-resistant ALL cells.[55,56] In correspondence, silencing of one of these components (i.e. SMARCA4) made cells resistant to prednisolone, indicating the direct relationship between chromatine remodeling and prednisolone resistance in ALL.[56] The role of this complex in prednisolone resistance of *MLL*-rearranged cases is unknown but deserves further studies since the epigenetics of *MLL*-rearranged ALL is highly peculiar as reflected by simultaneous histone modifications and altered CpG-island methylation patterns in the promoter regions of genes.[34,35] The altered configuration of chromatin may evoke the silencing of genes involved in mediating glucocorticoid sensitivity and/or facilitate the expression of resistance-mediating genes. One such resistance-associated gene for which the expression can be downregulated by demethylating agents is MCL1.[57]

(3) MCL1 and glucose metabolism

High expression levels of the anti-apoptotic gene MCL1 have been reported in both *MLL*-rearranged and non-*MLL* precursor B-ALL cases that are predictive for glucocorticoid resistance.[55,58–60] Functional studies show that downregulation of MCL1 by RNA interference and inhibitors (e.g. obatoclax and rapamycin) sensitize ALL cells to glucocorticoids.[58,61,62] A (cytogenetic) subtype-specific difference in the working action of MCL1 may reside in the fact that certain cells are responsive to caspase-dependent apoptosis whereas others trigger necroptosis, a form of autophagy-related programmed cell death which is caspase independent.[62]

The expression level of MCL1 highly correlates with the expression levels of glucose-metabolizing enzymes in a genome-wide analysis of genes associated with prednisolone resistance in pediatric ALL.[55] The glucose consumption was confirmed to be elevated in prednisolone-resistant ALL cells. Silencing of the glucose-metabolizing enzyme glyceraldehyde-3-phosphate dehydrogenase (GAPDH) sensitized leukemic cells to prednisolone.[63] Moreover, interference with the glucose metabolism by the non-hydrolyzable glucose-analoge 2-deoxy-D-glucose and other competitive inhibitors (lonidamine and 3-bromopyruvate) also reversed the resistance of cells, both in leukemic cell lines and in primary patients' cells being resistant to prednisolone.[63] These data suggest that interference with MCL1 and/or the glucose metabolism may be a way to circumvent resistance to glucocorticoids in pediatric ALL.

TEL-AML1-positive ALL: L-asparaginase sensitivity and vincristine resistance

The *TEL-AML1* fusion can be found in 20–25% of children with precursor B-ALL and is associated with a favorable long-term clinical outcomes (Chapter 11).[64,65] The favorable prognosis is reflected by a favorable response to a therapeutic window with L-asparaginase as well as *in vitro* sensitivity of *TEL-AML1*-positive ALL cells to L-asparaginase.[4,21] Interestingly, *TEL-AML1*-positive ALL is relatively resistant to vincristine (Table 9.1).[21,66] The discordant responsiveness to L-asparaginase and vincristine is intriguing since it rules out the role of general cross-resistance mechanisms like multidrug-efflux pumps, DNA repair or apoptotic defects in *TEL-AML1*-positive ALL.

Resistance to vincristine

- Cytoskeleton and extracellular matrix

Vincristine resistance may be caused by altered cytoskeleton composition in resistant cells (Fig. 9.3), e.g. the ratio between polymerized and non-polymerized tubulin was increased in vincristine-resistant ALL xenografts.[67] In addition, the actin components of the cytoskeleton may differ in vincristine-resistant ALL patients, as demonstrated by increased gelsolin and decreased γ-actin in vincristine-resistant ALL xenografts.[68]

Sensitivity to L-asparaginase

(1) Protein synthesis

At present, the nature of the discordant vincristine resistant/L-asparaginase sensitivity of pediatric *TEL-AML1*-positive ALL is unclear. Gene expression profiling studies in precursor B-ALL indicated that resistance to vincristine is associated with increased expression levels of extracellular matrix and cytoskeleton genes including desmocollin 3 (DSC3), ephrin-B2 (EFNB2), and myotubularin related protein 9 (MTMR9) and decreased expression levels of several ribosomal protein-S and large-P family members.[55] Remarkably, sensitivity to L-asparaginase in these precursor B-ALL cells is attributed to decreased expression levels of another class of ribosomal protein family members, i.e. the L-class.[55] Gene expression profiling of vincristine-sensitive/L-asparaginase-resistant and vincristine-resistant/L-asparaginase sensitive cases revealed a unique expression signature that was also associated with an unfavorable outcome in children with precursor B-ALL (Fig. 9.4).[69] More specifically, gene expression profiling of discordant vincristine-sensitive/L-asparaginase-resistant *TEL-AML1*-positive ALL cells confirmed the differential expression of ribosomal proteins (L, S and large P-family members), extracellular matrix (e.g. stromal antigen 3, STAG3) and actin components (e.g. gelsolin).[69] In addition, different translation initation and elongation factors (EIF and EEF-family members) were expressed in vincristine-resistant and L-asparaginase-sensitive *TEL-AML1*-positive cells. The high abundance of

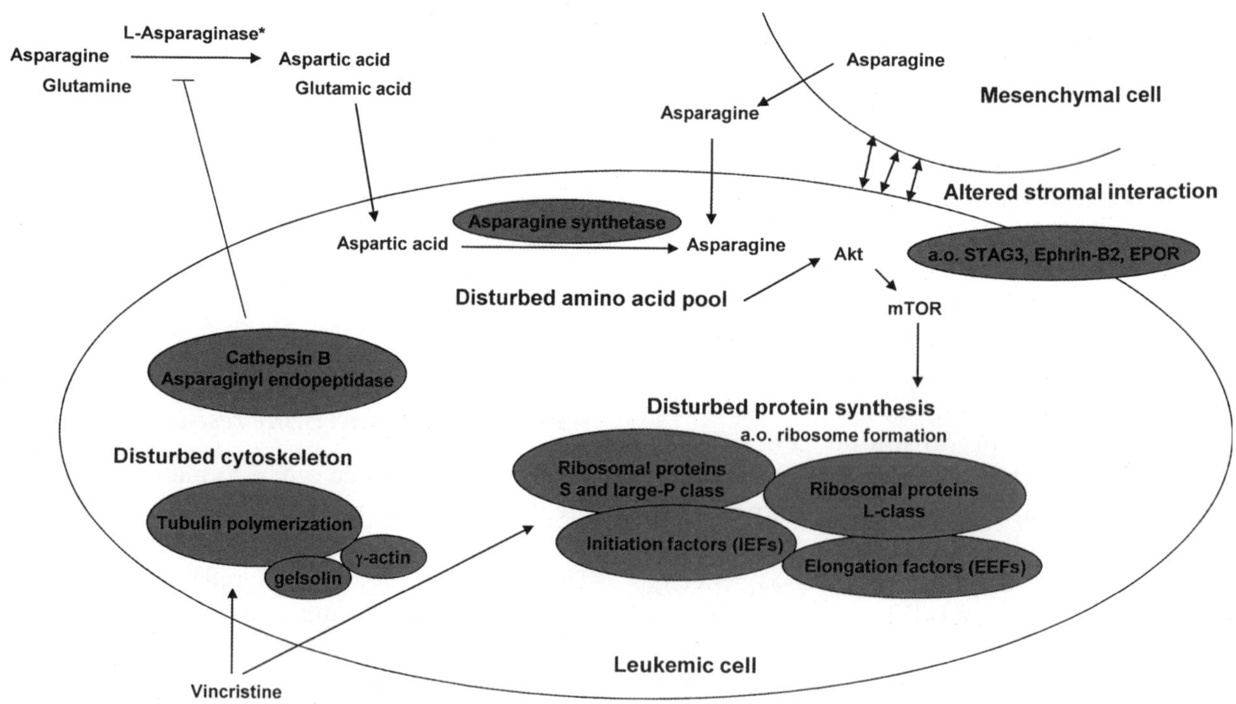

Fig. 9.3. Potential mechanisms of action of L-asparaginase and vincristine in pediatric ALL. L-asparaginase converts aspargine into aspartic acid, thereby depleting extracellular (plasma) levels of aspargine that can be taken up by cells. Intracellularly, resynthesis of asparagine is catalyzed by asparagine synthetase. Indicated in red are genes and/or processes that are affected in resistant pediatric ALL cells exposed to L-asparaginase and vincristine such as the synthesis of proteins and cytoskeleton structure, respectively. See text for further detailed information.

*L-asparaginase also has 3–4% glutaminase activity resulting into the conversion of glutamine into glutamic acid.

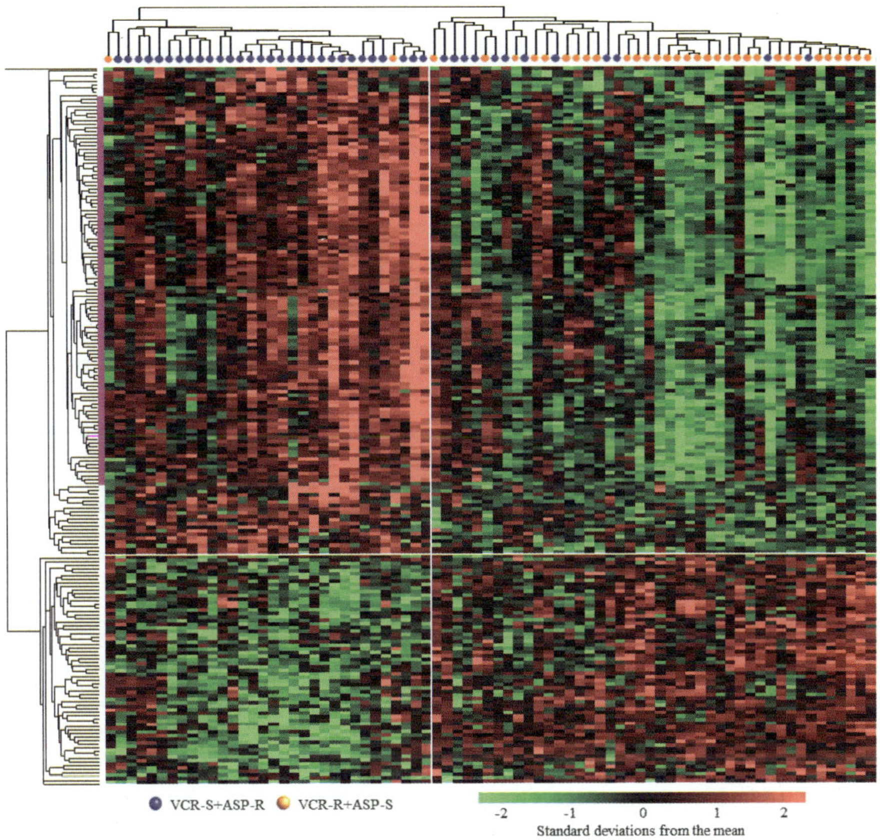

Fig. 9.4. Hierarchical clustering discriminates discordant resistance to vincristine and L-asparaginase in pediatric precursor B-ALL cases by unique gene expression signatures. Gene expression profiling in 42 vincristine-sensitive/L-asparaginase–resistant (blue symbols) and 34 vincristine-resistant/L-asparaginase sensitive (orange symbols) pediatric precursor B-ALL cases revealed a signature of 200 gene probes (representing 139 fully annotated genes and 13 cDNAs) discriminating both groups of patients. Each row represents a gene probe and each column represents a patient sample. The heatmap illustrates which genes are overexpressed (in red) and which genes are relatively under-expressed (in green) compared to the mean of all expression levels across all 76 patients. The magenta bar at the left dendrogram points to genes predominantly involved in protein synthesis. Reproduced from Lughthart *et al.*, Cancer Cell 7, 375–386 (2005) with permission from Elsevier Ltd.

aberrant ribosomal protein family members and translation factors suggests that causes of the discordant drug response may reside into changes in the pathways involved in protein synthesis. In correspondence, functional studies showed that L-asparaginase interferes with the synthesis of ribosomal proteins.[70]

(2) Amino acid metabolism

In general, resistance to L-asparaginase has been attributed to upregulated activities of the asparagine synthetase gene.[71] This asparagine synthetase catalyzes the formation of asparagine out of aspartic acid and in this way counteracts the asparagine-depleting effect of L-asparaginase (Fig. 9.3). Albeit this rescue mechanism has been advocated by many people, this statement is still part of debate. *TEL-AML1*-positive ALL cells are more sensitive to L-asparaginase compared to negative cases.[21] However, *TEL-AML1*-positive cases have higher mRNA expression levels of asparagine synthetase than other precursor B-ALL cases.[72,73] These levels are even higher than in normal bone marrow hematopoietic cells that are highly resistant to L-asparaginase.[73] These findings suggest that among *TEL-AML1*-positive cases, asparagine synthetase is not the key explanation for resistance to L-asparaginase, which is underlined by the fact that expression levels of asparagine synthetase did not correlate with the degree of L-asparaginase resistance.[73] In contrast, asparagine synthetase may contribute to resistance in *TEL-AML1*-negative precursor B-ALL cases since expression levels are linked to the degree of L-asparaginase resistance and, moreover, enforced expression of asparagine synthetase in non-*TEL-AML1*-positive leukemia cells induced resistance to L-asparaginase.[74–76] Resistance to L-asparaginase was recently also attributed to increased activity of cathepsin B and asparaginyl endopeptidase, two enzymes present in lymphoid cells that degrade L-asparaginase.[77] In line with this functional study, *BCR-ABL1*-positive ALL express high levels of asparaginyl endopeptidase[78] which may explain the relative *in vivo* resistance to L-asparaginase observed in these patients.[4]

(3) Microenvironment

- Asparagine rescue

A third explanation for the apparent resistance to L-asparaginase may be a rescue mechanism coordinated by the microenvironment. A single dose of L-asparaginase given upfront of combination chemotherapy results in increased aspartic acid and glutamic acid levels in circulating leukemic cells compared to control cells.[4] This suggests that L-asparaginase has worked efficiently since both aspartic acid and glutamic acid are the products of L-asparaginase activity (Fig. 9.3). However, intracellular asparagine and glutamine levels were not simultaneously reduced in these leukemic cells. In contrast, *in vitro* exposure to L-asparaginase reduced intracellular asparagine and glutamine levels to below detection limits within hours of exposure.[4] Taken together, these data strongly suggest that a rescue mechanism exists, feeding ALL cells with asparagine in the *in vivo* situation. In correspondence with this hypothesis, mesenchymal cells were shown to produce and secrete asparagine which may be consumed by leukemic cells present in the direct vicinity of these producing cells.[79] At present, however, it needs to be proven whether the degree of rescue by mesenchymal cells differentiates between sensitive and resistant leukemic cells since, *in vivo*, no difference was observed in intracellular aspargine, glutamine, aspartic acid and glutamic acid levels between clinically good and poor responders to a therapeutic window with L-asparaginase.[4]

- Stromal interaction

The microenvironment may play another role in facilitating the toxic response of L-asparaginase. *TEL-AML1*-positive ALL is being characterized by aberrant expression levels of different cell adhesion and stromal interaction genes, amongst others, the erythropoietin receptor (EPOR).[80–84] Enforced expression of this receptor in *TEL-AML1*-positive cells triggered the proliferation of cells which may increase the demand for essential amino acids such as asparagine and glutamine.[85] Remarkably, the gene encoding GATA3-binding protein is less expressed in vincristine-resistant and L-asparaginase-sensitive ALL cases.[69] The GATA3-binding protein represses the expression of erythropoietin, the ligand of erythropoietin receptor, in a promoter binding assay.[86] A reduced expression, of GATA3-binding protein may therefore abolish the negative regulatory effect on erythropoietin expression, thereby facilitating the activation of the erythropoietin receptor and subsequent proliferation of *TEL-AML1*-positive cells; whether this occurs in patients' leukemic cells needs to be demonstrated.

- Secreted factors

The microenvironment may produce factors that enable resistant cells to escape from L-asparaginase-induced metabolic stress by autophagy, a form of cellular senescence that can be reversed into cell growth (of resistant cells) or can result in programmed apoptosis and necrosis (necroptosis) leading to cell death (of sensitive cells). Interference with the mTOR-mediated pathway of protein synthesis by everolimus (RAD001) triggered the autophagy pathway in xenografts established from pediatric ALL cells.[87] Interestingly, everolimus also synergized with vincristine in these mice.[88] This observation needs confirmation but may point to a way to modulate the vincristine-resistant and L-asparaginase-sensitive phenotype of *TEL-AML1*-positive ALL.

Hyperdiploid ALL: sensitivity to anti-metabolites and L-asparaginase

Chromosomal copy number changes are frequently found in pediatric ALL. In ~25% of precursor B-ALL cases, gains in at least 5 chromosomes can be found per leukemic cell. Hyperdiploidy, defined by >50 chromosomes per cell, is characterized especially by gains in chromosomes 4, 10 and 17 and is associated with a highly favorable 5-year event-free survival of ≥90%.[89] The favorable prognosis of hyperdiploid cases can be attributed to a remarkable cellular sensitivity for anti-metabolites (AraC, thiopurines and methotrexate) and L-asparaginase (Table 9.1).[90]

Sensitivity to anti-metabolites

(1) Uptake and metabolism

Sensitivity to the deoxycytidine nucleoside analog AraC (cytarabine) and thiopurines (6-thioguanine and

6-mercaptopurine) presumably largely resides in the increased amount of DNA in hyperdiploid ALL cells. The phosphorylated form of AraC (AraCTP) competes with normal dCTP for incorporation into the DNA, thereby inhibiting further DNA synthesis, inducing apoptosis.[30] As shown in Fig. 9.1, thiopurines interfere with the purine salvage pathway (6-thioguanine and 6-mercaptopurine) and *de novo* purine synthesis (6-mercaptopurine), thereby reducing the amount of purines (guanines and adenosines) available for DNA and RNA synthesis, resulting in apoptosis.[91] A number of key enzymes play a role in the metabolism of thiopurines. 6-Thioguanine and 6-mercaptopurine are both metabolized into the nucleotide derivatives 6-thioGMP and 6-thioIMP, respectively by hypoxanthine guanine phosphoribosyltransferase (HGPRT), which are further processed into thioguanine nucleotides that interfere with the purine salvage pathway. In addition, 6-thioIMP can be converted into methyl-thioIMP by thiopurine methyltransferase (TPMT) which interferes with *de novo* purine synthesis by inhibiting the phosphoribosyl pyrophosphate amidotransferase PRPP. The synthesis of methyl-thioIMP and interference with the *de novo* purine synthesis pathway competes with the direct metabolism of 6-mercaptopurines into thioguanine nucleotides as part of the purine salvage pathway and hence, 6-mercaptopurine is a less efficient prodrug for anti-metabolites production. This is also reflected by the fact that higher *in vitro* concentrations are needed for 6-mercaptopurine to exert a similar cytotoxic effect as for 6-thioguanine.[16]

As mentioned earlier, the proliferative capacity of *in vitro* cultured primary patients' ALL cells is limited, suggesting that the remarkable cellular sensitivity of hyperdiploid cases towards AraC and thiopurines is predominantly caused by elevated intracellular accumulation of anti-metabolite derivatives and/or effective interference with survival mechanisms, requiring these products for RNA synthesis, amino acid metabolism and other processes (epigenetic regulation of histone and DNA methylation, base excision DNA repair etc.). In pediatric ALL, sensitivity towards 6-mercaptopurine is associated with the formation of thioguanine nucleotides.[92–94] The uptake of thiopurines is, amongst others, facilitated by the equilibrative nucleoside transporter (ENT1 of SLC29A1) that also facilitates cytarabine uptake in cells.[30,95,96] Inhibition of ENT1 by the nitrobenzylmercaptopurine ribonucleoside NBMPR significantly reduced the intracellular amount of 6-mercaptopurine-derived thioguanine nucleotides in ALL cell lines.[97] High ENT1 levels were also associated with a higher accumulation of thioguanine nucleotides upon *in vivo* 6-mercaptopurine treatment of pediatric ALL cases.[97] At present, it is unknown whether a high ENT1 level contributes to the sensitivity to anti-metabolites in hyperdiploid ALL.

Polymorphisms in TPMT, which diminish the activity of TPMT, have been found. These polymorphisms predict a favorable clinical outcome in pediatric ALL since they foster conversion into thioguanine nucleotides.[98,99] However, sensitivity towards 6-mercaptopurine in hyperdiploid ALL cases cannot be explained by a decreased TPMT activity since the majority of cases have a wild type TPMT.[99]

The intracellular metabolism by HGPRT does, in contrast to cell lines and animal models, not differ between sensitive and resistant ALL patients.[100] More downstream enzymes, such as adenosine deaminase and purine nucleoside phosphorylase, were also not discriminative for thiopurine-resistant ALL cases, nor was the case for thiopurine-degrading enzymes like cytoplasmic 5′-nucleotidase and acid and alkaline phosphatases.[101] These studies were performed in pediatric precursor B-lineage ALL cells without further knowledge of karyotype. A gene expression profiling study showed that the baseline (untreated) level of adenosine deaminase gene expression is higher in cases with high thioguanine nucleotide accumulation upon *in vivo* 6-mercaptopurine treatment of pediatric ALL cases.[97] This observation may indirectly imply a more favorable clinical outcome for those with high adenosine deaminase expression but the causal relationship with sensitivity to thiopurines of hyperdiploid cases awaits further investigation.

(2) Methotrexate metabolism

The relative sensitivity to the anti-folate methotrexate may reside in altered activities of enzymes involved in the folate metabolism that generates co-factors required for DNA, RNA and amino acid synthesis.[102] Methotrexate is actively transported into the cell by the reduced folate carrier (RFC or SLC19A1) but can be pumped out of the cell by drug efflux pumps including the multidrug resistance-associated protein family (MRP1–4), P-glycoprotein and breast cancer resistance protein (BCRP). Intracellularly, a polyglutamate tail is added to methotrexate, increasing its intracellular retention. Two enzymes determine the efficacy of methotrexate retention in the cell; the polyglutamate tail is being formed by folylpolyglutamate synthetase (FGPS) whereas this tail is being broken down by folypolyglutamate hydrolase/γ-glutamyl hydrolase (FPGH or GGH).[103] Hyperdiploid cells retain higher levels of polyglutamated methotrexate compared to non-hyperdiploid ALL cells (a.o. *TEL-AML1*-positive ALL).[104–106] Gene expression profiling for folate pathway-associated genes indicates that the RFC membrane transporter expression is increased whereas the drug efflux pumps (MRP1, BCRP, P-glycoprotein) and glutamate-metabolizing enzymes (FPGS and FPGH/GGH) are not differentially expressed in hyperdiploid ALL cells compared to non-hyperdiploid cells.[106] The elevated mRNA expression of RFC in hyperdiploid cases can partly be explained by additional copies of chromosome 21 on which the RFC gene is located.[107,108] All together, these data suggest that an efficient accumulation and retention of methotrexate may explain the relative sensitivity of hyperdiploid cases to methotrexate.

Polymorphisms in folate-metabolizing enzymes, including methylenetetrahydrofolate reductase (MTHFR), methionine synthase reductase MTRR and serine hydroxymethyl transferase (SHMT1), decrease the sensitivity towards methotrexate in pediatric ALL.[109] So far, these polymorphisms have not been investigated in hyperdiploid cells. Polymorphisms in the reduced folate carrier (RFC), thymidylate synthase (TS) and dihydrofolate reductase (DHFR) gene have also been found in ALL cells but these polymorphisms do not affect sensitivity towards methotrexate (RFC and TS)[109] or are associated with an unfavorable prognosis (DHFR)[110] in pediatric ALL and hence are unlikely to contribute to methotrexate sensitivity in hyperdiploid ALL.

Sensitivity to L-asparaginase

Apoptosis and TNF

The nature of L-asparaginase sensitivity of hyperdiploid cases is yet unclear. The expression levels of several pro-apoptotic genes are elevated in hyperdiploid ALL, such as caspases 3 and 8. This points to the capacity of hyperdiploid cells to respond to apoptotic signals, as was confirmed by functional assays.[14,59] An interesting observation that awaits further proof by functional studies is the fact that both the tumor necrosis factor (TNF) and its receptor TNFR1 are more expressed in hyperdiploid and L-asparaginase-sensitive cases.[59] The TNF pathway contributes to cytokine-mediated apoptosis which may be supported by factors released by the microenvironment, perhaps also contributing to L-asparaginase sensitivity, as postulated for *TEL-AML1*-positive ALL.

Perspectives

The relative sensitivity to anti-leukemic drugs differs between genetic subtypes of precursor B-ALL. To tailor therapy and circumvent or modulate drug resistance, knowledge of pharmacodynamics and elucidating which genes contribute to drug metabolism in each genetic subtype is essential. This is exemplified by *MLL*-rearranged infant ALL, for which laboratory results indicated that these cases are highly sensitive to cytarabine and 2-chloro-deoxyadenosine and moreover, that this type of leukemia harbors both lymphoid and myeloid characteristics.[16,60,111,112] Addition of low and high dosages of cytarabine has improved the clinical outcome of infant ALL.[26] The discovery of high level FLT3 expression in *MLL*-rearranged ALL has given rise to the inclusion of FLT3-inhibitors in ongoing trials.[113] In addition, the hypermethylated status of t(4;11)-positive ALL indicates that epigenetics drugs may target this type of leukemia more specifically.

The marked sensitivity of *TEL-AML1*-positive ALL to L-asparaginase implies a profound role for this enzymatic drug in the treatment of this prognostically favorable type of leukemia. Further treatment strategies should take into account that *TEL-AML1*-positive cases are relatively resistant to vincristine, and hence dose reductions for this drug are not recommended if one considers to include this drug in new treatment protocols.

The relative sensitivity of hyperdiploid cases to thiopurines and methotrexate may be used to optimize treatment by these drugs and to exclude agents for which they are less sensitive and which have significant side effects (e.g. anthracyclines). A recent study showed that this concept of tailored treatment with antimetabolites (6-mercaptopurine and methotrexate) was highly effective in children with hyperdiploid ALL (Chapter 11).[114]

In summary, cytogenetics and pharmacogenetics are important determinants of cellular drug resistance in pediatric ALL. Studies addressing these issues will contribute to a better tailored treatment of children with ALL which may result in more effective therapy and reduction of short- and long-term side effects. Besides improved clinical response rates, this will also foster the quality of life of adult survivors of pediatric leukemia (see Chapter 24).

References

1. Pieters R, Huismans DR, Loonen AH, Hählen K, van der Does-van den Berg A, van Wering ER, Veerman AJP. (1991) Relation of cellular drug resistance to long-term clinical outcome in childhood acute lymphoblastic leukaemia. *Lancet* **338**: 399–403.
5. Hongo T, Yamada S, Yajima S, Watanabe C, Fujii Y, Kawasaki H, Yazaki M, Hanada R, Horikoshi Y. (1999) Biological characteristics and prognostic value of *in vitro* three-drug resistance to prednisolone, L-asparaginase, and vincristine in childhood acute lymphoblastic leukemia. *Int J Hematol* **70**: 268–277.
6. Frost BM, Nygren P, Gustafsson G, Forestier E, Jonsson OG, Kanerva J, Nygaard R, Schmiegelow K, Larsson R, Lonnerholm G. (2003) Increased *in vitro* cellular drug resistance is related to poor outcome in high-risk childhood acute lymphoblastic leukaemia. *Br J Haematol* **122**: 376–385.
7. Schmiegelow K, Nyvold C, Seyfarth J, Pieters R, Rottier MM, Knabe N, Ryder LP, Madsen HO, Svejgaard A, Kaspers GJ. (2001) Post-induction residual leukemia in childhood acute lymphoblastic leukemia quantified by PCR correlates with *in vitro* prednisolone resistance. *Leukemia* **15**: 1066–1071.
8. Lonnerholm G, Thorn I, Sundstrom C, Frost BM, Abrahamsson J, Behrendtz M, Heldrup J, Jacobsson S, Li A, Olofsson T, Porwit A, Soderhall S, Larsson R, Forestier E. (2009) *In vitro* cellular drug sensitivity at diagnosis is correlated to minimal residual disease at end of induction therapy in childhood acute lymphoblastic leukemia. *Leuk Res* **33**: 46–53.
10. Janka-Schaub GE, Harms DO, den Boer ML, Veerman AJP, Pieters R. (1999) *In vitro* drug resistance as independent prognostic factor in study COALL-05-92 for treatment of childhood acute lymphoblastic leukemia; basis for treatment stratification according to traditional risk factors and drug sensitivity in study COALL-06-97. *Klin Padiatr* **211**: 233–238.
19. Pui CH, Evans WE. (1998) Acute lymphoblastic leukemia. *N Engl J Med* **339**: 605–615.
20. Aricò M, Valsecchi MG, Camitta B, Schrappe M, Chessells JM, Baruchel A, Gaynon P, Silverman L, Janka-Schaub G, Kamps W, Pui CH, Masera G. (2000) Outcome of treatment in children with Philadelphia chromosome-positive acute lymphoblastic leukemia. *N Engl J Med* **342**: 998–1006.
22. van Zelm MC, van der Burg M, de Ridder D, Barendregt BH, de Haas EF, Reinders MJ, Lankester AC, Revesz T, Staal FJ, van Dongen JJ. (2005) Ig gene rearrangement steps are initiated in early human precursor B cell subsets and correlate with specific transcription factor expression. *J Immunol* **175**: 5912–5922.
24. Heerema NA, Sather HN, Ge J, Arthur DC, Hilden JM, Trigg ME, Reaman GH. (1999) Cytogenetic studies of infant acute lymphoblastic leukemia: Poor prognosis of infants with t(4;11) — a report of the Children's Cancer Group. *Leukemia* **13**: 679–686.
27. Kosaka Y, Koh K, Kinukawa N, Wakazono Y, Isoyama K, Oda T, Hayashi Y, Ohta S, Moritake H, Oda M, Nagatoshi Y, Kigasawa H, Ishida Y, Ohara A, Hanada R, Sako M, Sato T, Mizutani S, Horibe K, Ishii E. (2004) Infant acute lymphoblastic leukemia with MLL gene rearrangements: Outcome following intensive chemotherapy and hematopoietic stem cell transplantation. *Blood* **104**: 3527–3534.
29. Prakasha Gowda AS, Polizzi JM, Eckert KA, Spratt TE. (2010) Incorporation of Gemcitabine and Cytarabine into DNA by DNA Polymerase beta and Ligase III/XRCC1. *Biochemistry* **49**: 4833–4840.
38. Rocco A, Schandl L, Chen J, Wang H, Tulassay Z, McNamara D, Malfertheiner P, Ebert MP. (2003) Loss of FHIT protein expression correlates with disease progression and poor differentiation in gastric cancer. *J Cancer Res Clin Oncol* **129**: 84–88.
41. Tissing WJ, Lauten M, Meijerink JP, den Boer ML, Koper JW, Sonneveld P, Pieters R. (2005) Expression of the glucocorticoid receptor and its isoforms in relation to glucocorticoid resistance in childhood acute lymphocytic leukemia. *Haematologica* **90**: 1279–1281.
44. Tissing WJE, den Boer ML, Meijerink JPP, Menezes RX, Swagemakers S, van der Spek PJ, Sallan SE, Armstrong SA, Pieters R. (2007) Genomewide identification of prednisolone-responsive genes in acute lymphoblastic leukemia cells. *Blood* **109**: 3929–3935.
46. Tissing WJ, Meijerink JP, den Boer ML, Pieters R. (2003) Molecular determinants of glucocorticoid sensitivity and resistance in acute lymphoblastic leukemia. *Leukemia* **17**: 17–25.
48. Tissing WJ, Meijerink JP, den Boer ML, Brinkhof B, Pieters R. (2005) mRNA expression levels of (co)chaperone molecules of the glucocorticoid receptor are not involved in glucocorticoid resistance in pediatric ALL. *Leukemia* **19**: 727–733.
50. Hillmann AG, Ramdas J, Multanen K, Norman MR, Harmon JM. (2000) Glucocorticoid receptor gene mutations in leukemic cells acquired *in vitro* and *in vivo*. *Cancer Res* **60**: 2056–2062.
51. Catts VS, Farnsworth ML, Haber M, Norris MD, Lutze-Mann LH, Lock RB. (2001) High level resistance to

glucocorticoids, associated with a dysfunctional glucocorticoid receptor, in childhood acute lymphoblastic leukemia cells selected for methotrexate resistance. *Leukemia* **15**: 929–935.

53. Koper JW, Stolk RP, de Lange P, Huizenga NA, Molijn GJ, Pols HA, Grobbee DE, Karl M, de Jong FH, Brinkmann AO, Lamberts SW. (1997) Lack of association between five polymorphisms in the human glucocorticoid receptor gene and glucocorticoid resistance. *Hum Genet* **99**: 663–668.
54. Deroo BJ, Archer TK. (2001) Glucocorticoid receptor-mediated chromatin remodeling *in vivo*. *Oncogene* **20**: 3039–3046.
57. Saito Y, Suzuki H, Tsugawa H, Nakagawa I, Matsuzaki J, Kanai Y, Hibi T. (2009) Chromatin remodeling at Alu repeats by epigenetic treatment activates silenced microRNA-512-5p with downregulation of Mcl-1 in human gastric cancer cells. *Oncogene* **28**: 2738–2744.
60. Armstrong SA, Staunton JE, Silverman LB, Pieters R, den Boer ML, Minden MD, Sallan SE, Lander ES, Golub TR, Korsmeyer SJ. (2002) MLL translocations specify a distinct gene expression profile that distinguishes a unique leukemia. *Nat Genet* **30**: 41–47.
64. Kamps WA, van der Pal-de Bruin KM, Veerman AJ, Fiocco M, Bierings M, Pieters R. (2010) Long-term results of Dutch Childhood Oncology Group studies for children with acute lymphoblastic leukemia from 1984 to 2004. *Leukemia* **24**: 309–319.
65. Moricke A, Zimmermann M, Reiter A, Henze G, Schrauder A, Gadner H, Ludwig WD, Ritter J, Harbott J, Mann G, Klingebiel T, Zintl F, Niemeyer C, Kremens B, Niggli F, Niethammer D, Welte K, Stanulla M, Odenwald E, Riehm H, Schrappe M. (2010) Long-term results of five consecutive trials in childhood acute lymphoblastic leukemia performed by the ALL-BFM study group from 1981 to 2000. *Leukemia* **24**: 265–284.
66. Stams WA, Beverloo HB, den Boer ML, R.X. DM, Stigter RL, van Drunen E, Ramakers-van-Woerden NL, Loonen AH, van Wering ER, Janka-Schaub GE, Pieters R. (2006) Incidence of additional genetic changes in the TEL and AML1 genes in DCOG and COALL-treated t(12;21)-positive pediatric ALL, and their relation with drug sensitivity and clinical outcome. *Leukemia* **20**: 410–416.
71. Haskell CM, Canellos GP, Leventhal BG, Carbone PP, Block JB. (1969) L-Asparaginase resistance in human leukemia-asparagine synthetase. *Biochem Pharmacol* **18**: 2578– 2580.
72. Krejci O, Starkova J, Otova B, Madzo J, Kalinova M, Hrusak O, Trka J. (2004) Upregulation of asparagine synthetase fails to avert cell cycle arrest induced by L-asparaginase in TEL/AML1-positive leukaemic cells. *Leukemia* **18**: 434–441.
75. Aslanian AM, Fletcher BS, Kilberg MS. (2001) Asparagine synthetase expression alone is sufficient to induce l-asparaginase resistance in MOLT-4 human leukaemia cells. *Biochem J* **357**: 321–328.
78. Strefford JC, van Delft FW, Robinson HM, Worley H, Yiannikouris O, Selzer R, Richmond T, Hann I, Bellotti T, Raghavan M, Young BD, Saha V, Harrison CJ. (2006) Complex genomic alterations and gene expression in acute lymphoblastic leukemia with intrachromosomal amplification of chromosome 21. *Proc Natl Acad Sci U S A* **103**: 8167–8172.
80. Yeoh EJ, Ross ME, Shurtleff SA, Williams WK, Patel D, Mahfouz R, Behm FG, Raimondi SC, Relling MV, Patel A, Cheng C, Campana D, Wilkins D, Zhou X, Li J, Liu H, Pui CH, Evans WE, Naeve C, Wong L, Downing JR. (2002) Classification, subtype discovery, and prediction of outcome in pediatric acute lymphoblastic leukemia by gene expression profiling. *Cancer Cell* **1**: 133–143.
82. Fine BM, Stanulla M, Schrappe M, Ho M, Viehmann S, Harbott J, Boxer LM. (2004) Gene expression patters associated with recurrent chromosomal translocations in acute lymphoblastic leukemia. *Blood* **103**: 1043–1049.
83. van Delft FW, Bellotti T, Luo Z, Jones LK, Patel N, Yiannikouris O, Hill AS, Hubank M, Kempski H, Fletcher D, Chaplin T, Foot N, Young BD, Hann IM, Gammerman A, Saha V. (2005) Prospective gene expression analysis accurately subtypes acute leukaemia in children and establishes a commonality between hyperdiploidy and t(12;21) in acute lymphoblastic leukemia. *Br J Haematol* **130**: 26–35.
84. den Boer ML, van Slegtenhorst M, de Menezes RX, Cheok MH, Buijs-Gladdines JG, Peters ST, van Zutven LJ, Beverloo HB, van der Spek PJ, Escherich G, Horstmann MA, Janka-Schaub GE, Kamps WA, Evans WE, Pieters R. (2009) A subtype of childhood acute lymphoblastic leukaemia with poor treatment outcome: A genome-wide classification study. *Lancet Oncol* **10**: 125–134.
87. Crazzolara R, Bradstock KF, Bendall LJ. (2009) RAD001 (Everolimus) induces autophagy in acute lymphoblastic leukemia. *Autophagy* **5**: 727–728.
91. Cheok MH, Pottier N, Kager L, Evans WE. (2009) Pharmacogenetics in acute lymphoblastic leukemia. *Semin Hematol* **46**: 39–51.
93. Lennard L, Lilleyman JS. (1989) Variable mercaptopurine metabolism and treatment outcome in childhood lymphoblastic leukemia. *J Clin Oncol* **7**: 1816–1823.
94. Schmiegelow K, Schroder H, Gustafsson G, Kristinsson J, Glomstein A, Salmi T, Wranne L. (1995) Risk of relapse in

childhood acute lymphoblastic leukemia is related to RBC methotrexate and mercaptopurine metabolites during maintenance chemotherapy. Nordic Society for Pediatric Hematology and Oncology. *J Clin Oncol* **13**: 345–351.

96. Kong W, Engel K, Wang J. (2004) Mammalian nucleoside transporters. *Curr Drug Metab* **5**: 63–84.
102. Rots MG, Pieters R, Kaspers GJ, Veerman AJ, Peters GJ, Jansen G. (2000) Classification of ex vivo methotrexate resistance in acute lymphoblastic and myeloid leukaemia. *Br J Haematol* **110**: 791–800.
104. Whitehead VM, Payment C, Cooley L, Lauer SJ, Mahoney DH, Shus JJ, Vuchich MJ, Bernstein ML, Look AT, Pullen DJ, Camitta B. (2001) The association of the TEL-AML1 chromosomal translocation with the accumulation of methotrexate polyglutamates in lymphoblasts and with ploidy in childhood B-progenitor cell acute lymphoblastic leukemia: A Pediatric Oncology Group study. *Leukemia* **15**: 1081–1088.
107. Zhang L, Taub JW, Williamson M, Wong SC, Hukku B, Pullen J, Ravindranath Y, Matherly LH. (1998) Reduced folate carrier gene expression in childhood acute lymphoblastic leukemia: Relationship to immunophenotype and ploidy. *Clin Cancer Res* **4**: 2169–2177.
108. Belkov VM, Krynetski EY, Schuetz JD, Yanishevski Y, Masson E, Mathew S, Raimondi S, Pui CH, Relling MV, Evans WE. (1999) Reduced folate carrier expression in acute lymphoblastic leukemia: A mechanism for ploidy but not lineage differences in methotrexate accumulation. *Blood* **93**: 1643–1650.
112. Stam RW, den Boer ML, Pieters R. (2006) Towards targeted therapy for infant acute lymphoblastic leukaemia. *Br J Haematol* **132**: 539–551.

10

Minimal Residual Disease

Lara Mussolin, Dario Campana and Angelo Rosolen

Introduction

In children with hematologic malignancies, examination of the bone marrow at diagnosis and during therapy is an integral part of their clinical management. In patients with acute leukemia, the degree of leukemia cytoreduction in response to chemotherapy is assessed by periodic examination of bone marrow smears to identify residual leukemic blasts and assess the status of normal hematopoiesis. In patients with lymphoma, the staging of the disease at diagnosis is determined by the presence of lymphoma infiltration of the bone marrow, which is typically examined in aspirates as well as biopsies.

Although the results of the bone marrow examination are critical in informing therapeutic decisions, the process is rather subjective and highly dependent of the expertise of the hemopathologist in charge. In fact, identifying individual malignant cells among normal bone marrow cells is challenging even for an experienced hemopathologist. This is particularly true in the case of acute lymphoblastic leukemia (ALL) or most lymphomas where the morphology of the malignant cells is often indistinguishable from that of immature lymphoid precursors and/or that of activated mature lymphocytes. When bone marrow examination is performed after cessation of chemotherapy or transplant, the distinction between malignant and normal cells is even more difficult, owing to the high proportion of lymphoid precursors typically present in such specimens.

The fact that many patients with acute leukemia achieving morphologic remission still had undetectable leukemic cells, i.e. minimal residual disease (MRD), was clearly shown by the occurrence of leukemia relapse. The advent of assays to detect MRD provided definitive proof that patients in complete clinical and morphologic remission might harbor residual leukemic cells in their bone marrow. The initial efforts of MRD investigators were focused on developing robust methods that could be applied in routine studies of clinical samples. As soon as these methods became available (although in forms not as refined as those used today), the clinical significance of MRD was elucidated in ALL first, followed by acute myeloid leukemia (AML). Parallel studies applied methods mostly derived from studies in ALL to determine the degree of disease dissemination at diagnosis in patients with non-Hodgkin lymphoma and assess the importance of MRD during treatment. Although the field of MRD in NHL is still at its inception, recent new developments have occurred despite the challenge posed by difficulties in obtaining representative primitive tumors.

In this chapter, we discuss the methods for detecting MRD in pediatric acute leukemias and lymphomas, and the clinical importance of this endeavor. As the experience of MRD studies in acute promyelocytic leukemia and chronic myelogenous leukemia in children is very limited, it will not be discussed here.

Acute Lymphoblastic Leukemia

Methods for MRD detection

One set of targets that can be used to identify residual ALL cells are the clonal rearrangement of immuno-globulin (Ig) and T-cell receptor (TCR) genes, which consists of variable, constant and junctional regions; the latter are unique to the leukemic clone. Investigators screen for these rearrangements at diagnosis in each case, and after identifying the leukemia-specific junctional sequences, design junctional region-specific oligonucleotides, also called allele-specific oligonucleotides, which will be used as primers for the PCR assay to MRD during treatment.[1,2] More than 95% of B-lineage ALL cases have Ig gene rearrangements and up to 90% have TCR gene rearrangements. Most cases of T-ALL have TCR gene rearrangements, while Ig gene rearrangements occur in approximately 20% of T-ALL cases.[1] Quantitation of MRD is most frequently performed using "real-time" quantitative PCR (RQ-PCR);[2] a sensitivity of detection of 1 leukemic cell in 10^5 normal cells can be achieved in approximately 90% of cases with rearrangements.[3] Ig and TCR genes in ALL might undergo continuing or secondary rearrangements, resulting in oligoclonality,[1] which has led experts to recommend the targeting of two or more different rearrangements.[2] However, this criterium may be too stringent as multiple targets that allow detection of MRD with a high sensitivity (e.g. 0.01%) are not identifiable in approximately 30% of cases.[4]

The second set of targets is represented by cell marker profiles detectable by flow cytometry. These leukemia-associated immunophenotypes, which are identified at diagnosis, are usually formed by cell markers expressed in abnormal combinations in leukemic cells, termed by some investigators as "asynchronous" or "aberrant" immunophenotypes.[5] Standard 4-antibody staining allows a sensitivity of 1 in 10,000 in approximately 95% of cases. The availability of contemporary flow cytometers capable of detecting six or more markers, together with the identification of new markers of leukemia through global gene expression studies, should further facilitate the distinction between ALL and normal cells and might improve sensitivity. Investigators should be aware that certain immunophenotypes may be undetectable in bone marrow samples from healthy adult donors but they may become apparent in samples collected from children, particularly after cessation of chemotherapy or during treatment interruptions. Only immunophenotypes truly restricted to leukemia should be used for MRD. Although some fluctuations in the intensity of marker expression during chemotherapy are to be expected,[6] the use of multiple markers helps prevent false negative results.

The final set of markers to monitor MRD in ALL is represented by mRNA transcripts derived from gene fusions, such as *BCR-ABL1*, *MLL-AFF1*, *TCF3-PBX1*, and *ETV6-RUNX1*.[7] The sensitivity of these markers, as detected by reverse transcriptase PCR, is approximately 1 in 10,000. A limitation of this approach is its lack of precision in estimating levels of MRD because the amount of transcripts per leukemic cell may vary from patient to patient with the same genetic subtype of ALL, and their expression could be predictably affected by chemotherapy and degradation.[7] Although recurrent abnormalities are present in only approximately 40% of children with ALL,[7] with the uncovering of genetic abnormalities afforded by the application of whole-genome screening technologies,[8] it is likely that additional genetic targets will become routinely available.

Several studies have shown a good level of concordance between MRD tests performed by PCR amplification of Ig and TCR genes and by flow cytometry,[9–11] but similar comparisons between these two techniques and PCR amplification of fusion transcripts are lacking. In general, PCR amplification of Ig and TCR genes has a higher sensitivity than flow cytometry (i.e. beyond 0.01%) but flow cytometry provides information not only about the percentage of MRD, but also about the status of normal hematopoiesis, and it is more widely applicable. Flow cytometry is particularly well suited for MRD studies during the early phases of therapy, e.g. during the first 2 weeks of remission induction therapy, as it is difficult to develop a patient-specific PCR assay in such a short time. On the other hand, PCR might be more informative in studies performed at the end of therapy because of its higher sensitivity. Finally, preleukemic clones in patients with *ETV6-RUNX1* may be detectable by PCR targeting of the fusion transcript but not by monitoring Ig/TCR gene rearrangements or aberrant phenotypes; *BCR-ABL1* stem cell populations may be undetectable by methods not targeting the gene fusion. The existence of these scenarios and their clinical significance needs to be ascertained using multiple methods simultaneously.

Results of clinical studies

The persistence of lymphoblasts in bone marrow or peripheral blood samples taken from patients with ALL during remission induction therapy indicates a suboptimal response and is associated with a significantly increased risk of relapse. The advent of MRD assays extended and refined this earlier observation. Indeed, measuring early treatment response has proven to be the most clinically useful application of MRD assays in ALL (see Chapter 11).

Morley and colleagues[12] studied samples from 88 children with ALL by PCR amplification of Ig/TCR genes and detected MRD in the first remission marrow of 38, a finding that predicted subsequent relapse. Ig/TCR genes were also targeted in subsequent studies that consolidated the value of MRD detection by this method. In 178 patients enrolled in a European Organization for Research and Treatment of Cancer (EORTC) protocol, the presence or absence of MRD and its level during the first 6 months of therapy significantly predicted the risk of relapse.[13] Patients with ≥ 1% MRD after remission induction therapy, or ≥ 0.1% or higher at subsequent time points had a particularly high risk of relapse. In 240 patients treated on the International BFM Study Group protocols, combined information from MRD measurements performed on days 33 and 78 were particularly informative,[14] allowing the identification of three different risk groups: a standard-risk group (43% of patients) with a 3-year relapse rate of 2%; a high-risk group (15%) with a relapse rate of 75%; and an intermediate-risk group (43%) with a 3-year relapse rate of 23%, and a 10-year event-free survival (EFS) of 93% for standard, 16% for the high, and 74% for the intermediate risk group.[4] Among 3341 patients studied, two or more targets that allow PCR analysis with a 1 in 10,000 sensitivity or better were found in 2365 (71%), while an additional 671 (20%) had only one such target.[4] Among patients with B-lineage ALL (n = 3184), those considered to have standard-risk by MRD criteria (42%) had a 5-year EFS of 92.3%. The EFS rates were 50.1 for the high-risk patients (6%) and 77.6% was those with intermediate-risk ALL (52%).[15] In 284 children with B-lineage ALL studied by the Dana-Farber Cancer Institute ALL Consortium, the 5-year risk of relapse was 5% in 176 children with no detectable MRD at the end of remission induction therapy and 44% in the 108 with detectable MRD.[16]

Flow cytometry was used at St. Jude Children's Research Hospital to prospectively monitor MRD in 195 children with newly diagnosed ALL enrolled in the Total XIII study.[17–19] Detectable MRD (i.e. ≥ 0.01%) at any of the point during treatment predicted a higher risk of relapse, and that MRD ≥ 1% at the end of remission induction therapy was associated with a particularly poor outcome. By contrast, MRD < 0.01% on day 19 of remission induction therapy was strongly associated with subsequent continuous complete remission: the 3-year cumulative incidence of relapse for patients with this finding was only 1.9%. The Children's Oncology Group also used flow cytometry to monitor MRD in bone marrow collected on day 29 (end of remission induction therapy) in 2143 children with B-lineage ALL.[20] MRD ≥ 0.01% was associated with shorter EFS in all risk groups. The Italian cooperative group AIEOP studied bone marrow samples from 830 patients on day 15, after 14 days of steroids, and one dose of intrathecal methotrexate, vincristine, daunorubicin, and asparaginase and identified 3 risk groups: standard (<0.1% MRD; 42%), intermediate (0.1% < 10% MRD; 47%), and high (≥ 10%; 11%) with a 5-year cumulative incidence of relapse of 7.5%, 17.5%, and 47.2%, respectively.[21]

Levels of MRD during induction therapy are associated with genetic features of the disease. Thus, patients with BCR-ABL1 leukemia, IKAROS mutations and early T-cell precursor ALL have a high prevalence of MRD, whereas those with *TCF3-PBX1* and *ETV6-RUNX1* most commonly have lower levels or undetectable MRD.[8,22,23] Levels of MRD have also been associated with gene expression profiles of leukemia cells at diagnosis,[24–26] and with somatic polymorphisms in drug-metabolizing enzymes (see Chapter 9).[27] Despite these associations, MRD was an independent prognostic indicator in all the above studies. In addition, MRD was significantly associated with outcome in studies limited to specific subtypes of ALL. For example, in a recent study of 99 infant patients enrolled in the Interfant-99 protocol, all patients with levels of MRD (detected by PCR of Ig/TCR and MLL genes) ≥ 0.01% at the end of consolidation relapsed, while only 13% of patients with MRD < 0.01% at both the end of induction and end of consolidation relapsed; the remaining patients had a relapse rate of 31%.[28]

Because of their strong predictive power, measurements of early treatment response according to MRD have been incorporated into clinical trials, in efforts to refine risk-assignment.[4,29] Thus, MRD studies by flow cytometry or PCR Ig/TCR were performed in all 498 evaluable patients enrolled in the St. Jude Total XV study, where MRD testing was a key part of the risk classification schema.[29] This study yielded 5-year EFS and overall survival probabilities of 85.6% and 93.5%, respectively, suggesting that the use of MRD contributed to improve outcome. However, despite treatment intensification for MRD-positive patients, high MRD (≥ 1%) at the end of induction remained an independent predictor of poor EFS.

MRD is also a strong predictor of second relapse in patients with first relapse ALL who achieve a second remission, especially in patients with a first relapse off-therapy. This was shown by early studies performed using PCR amplification of Ig/TCR genes,[30] or flow cytometry.[31] More recent data from the Children's Oncology Group also using flow cytometry has confirmed the importance of MRD as a prognostic factor in these patients: 12-month EFS was 80% for patients with MRD ≥ 0.01% at the end of the first block of reinduction vs. 58% for those who were MRD-negative.[32] There is strong evidence that MRD levels before allogeneic hematopoietic stem cell transplantation strongly predict relapse post-transplant (see Chapter 20).[33]

Acute Myeloid Leukemia

Methods for MRD detection

Since rearrangements of Ig/TCR genes occur in less than 10% of patients with AML, these targets cannot be used to monitor MRD. By contrast, aberrant immunophenotypes can be identified in nearly 95% of patients at diagnosis, allowing the use of flow cytometry for monitoring MRD.[34] However, the sensitivity that can be routinely achieved in AML is typically inferior to that of ALL, owing to the more heterogeneous cell marker expression in leukemia myeloblasts which can partially overlap with that of normal immature myeloid cells. Hence, the sensitivity of flow cytometric MRD detection in AML ranges from 0.1–0.01%.[34] Finally, approximately 40% of cases have nonrandom genetic abnormalities, such as *RUNX1-RUNX1T1* (or *AML1-ETO*), *CBFB/MYH11* and *MLL* gene rearrangements, which are suitable for molecular studies of MRD (see Chapter 6).[34]

In addition to flow cytometric detection of aberrant immunophenotypes and PCR amplification of fusion transcripts, other options have emerged to study MRD in AML. One option is to target nucleophosmin (*NPM1*) mutations which can be used to monitor MRD by PCR in approximately one-third of adult patients but in less than 10% of childhood AML cases.[35] The second option is to targets *WT1*, which is overexpressed in the majority of cases of AML,[36] although the precise percentage of childhood AML cases with levels of overexpression useful for MRD studies remains unclear. Because normal CD34+ progenitor cells express *WT1*, the setting where WT1 measurements are more informative needs to be carefully established.[37]

Results of clinical studies

Large clinical studies of MRD in childhood AML have mostly been performed by flow cytometry (see Chapter 13). Flow cytometric detection of aberrant immunophenotypes was used by investigators of the Children's Oncology Group to study MRD in 252 children with AML.[38] Occult leukemia was detected in 16% of the patients who responded to initial induction therapy; these patients were approximately 5 times more likely to relapse than those with negative MRD findings. In another study by flow cytometry performed with samples collected from children enrolled in the St. Jude Children's Research Hospital AML97 protocol, it was found that 61 of 230 bone marrow samples from 46 patients during therapy had MRD levels of 0.1% or higher.[34] Mean 2-year overall survival was 33.1% for patients with MRD ≥ 0.1% after induction therapy and 72.1% for those with undetectable MRD. MRD-positive patients were more likely to relapse within the 6 months following the test and MRD was the only significant prognostic indicator in this cohort. Langebrake *et al.*[39] also used flow cytometry to study MRD in 150 children with AML. These investigators found that MRD was significantly associated with a lower EFS but the finding lost statistical significance when assessed in combination with other parameters.

The St. Jude AML02 protocol, which succeeded AML97, used MRD measurements at various time points to aid treatment decisions in a multicentric setting.[40] MRD studies were successful in 99% of samples received. Negative MRD was achieved in 129 of 199 (64.8%) patients studied after Induction I and in 154 of 193 (80%) patients after Induction II. Presence of MRD on day 22 was significantly associated with adverse outcome: 3-year EFS rates were 71.8% ± 5.6% for MRD-negative patients ($n = 129$) and 41.8% ± 7.5% for MRD-positive patients ($n = 70$, $P < 0.0001$). Among patients with high-risk AML, those with negative MRD after Induction I had a significantly better 3-year EFS (64.2% ± 12.1%) than those with detectable MRD (33.0% ± 9.0%, p = 0.008). Multivariate analysis identified day 22 MRD ≥ 1% and *CBF* abnormalities as independent factors for EFS and day 22 MRD ≥ 1%, age at diagnosis and M7 without t(1;22) for survival.[40]

Recent data indicate that detection of MRD before allogeneic stem cell transplantation in childhood AML predicts relapse post-transplant (see Chapter 20). One study investigated the prognostic value of *WT1* expression in peripheral blood 2 weeks prior to transplant in 36 children with AML. Eleven patients had *WT1* levels higher than those measured in healthy controls and seven relapsed post-transplant, while none of the 25 patients with levels within the normal range did.[41] Another study used flow cytometry to identify 10 MRD-positive patients among 63 studied pretransplant while in morphologic remission.[42] Actuarial overall survival for patients with MRD was 15% vs. 67% for those without MRD, with a corresponding relapse rate 65% and 17%, respectively.

Burkitt's Lymphoma (BL) and Mature B-Cell Leukemia (B-ALL)

Method for MRD detection

Genetically, Burkitt's lymphoma (BL) and mature B-cell leukemia (B-ALL) are characterized by the presence of chromosomal translocations involving the *c-myc* gene on chromosome 8 and the immunoglobulin heavy- or light-chain genes on chromosome 14, 22 or 2.[43] The most common translocation, accounting for about 75% of the total, is the t(8;14)(q24;q32) which juxtaposes the *c-myc* gene to the immunoglobulin heavy chain (*IGH@*) locus on chromosome 14 in divergent orientation (see Chapter 7). The breakpoint locations vary considerably depending on the geographic distribution of the disease and the likely presence or absence of the Epstein–Barr virus (EBV) genome. On chromosome 8, breakpoints are usually located upstream of the *c-myc* gene in the endemic (African) BL and within exon 1 or intron 1 in the sporadic (Caucasian) BL. The breakpoints in the *IGH@* locus are distributed over a region of at least 100 kb, but they are preferentially located in the *IGH@* joining region (JH) or in the switch regions in the endemic and the sporadic BL, respectively.[44] The *myc-IGH@* rearrangement is detectable only at the genomic DNA level because no fusion transcript originates from this genetic alteration. In the great majority of sporadic BL, the t(8;14) translocation can be detected by a long-distance polymerase chain reaction (LD-PCR) assay which relies on the use of one primer specific for *c-myc* exon 2 combined, in different reactions, with four primers for the *IGH@* locus[44,45] The LD-PCR assay is useful not only for the molecular characterization of the primary disease, but it can also be applied to detect MRD because the LD-PCR product detecting the *myc-IGH@* rearrangements is specific for each individual tumor. The assay has a sensitivity approaching 10^{-4} both *in vitro* and *in vivo*. Notably, it is not possible to study endemic BL by this technique due to the wide chromosomal region involved.

In addition to the t(8;14), another marker for MRD detection in BL and mature B-ALL is represented by Ig rearrangements, as described in the ALL section.

Results of clinical studies

The prognostic impact of MRD in pediatric BL was studied only recently. The Italian Association of Pediatric Hematology-Oncology Group (AIEOP) used a LD-PCR-based assay to prospectively study 78 BL patients and found a specific *myc-IGH@* PCR marker in 52 of them.[46] MRD was positive in 36% of patients. The comparative analysis of sensitivity of morphologic examination of BM aspirate or BM trephine and LD-PCR in t(8;14)-positive patients demonstrated a superiority of the molecular approach in the assessment of MRD. An analysis on whether a negative BM status at diagnosis, defined by a negative LD-PCR, might impact the probability of maintaining a complete remission status was conducted. Two children among 12 BM-positive patients had a progression of disease and died, whereas none of the 21 BM-negative patients suffered disease progression (p = 0.011, by the one-tailed Z test), suggesting that a positive MRD might bear a negative prognostic impact. The study of a larger cohort of patients (134 BL specimens) showed that most of the molecular positive patients (85%) at diagnosis belonged to the R4 Risk Group according to BFM definition (stage III or stage IV according to St. Jude staging classification and LDH ≥ 1000 U/l). The 3-year progression-free survival (PFS) was 68% (±10%) in MRD positive R4 patients compared with 93% (± 5%) in MRD negative R4 patients (p = 0.03),[47] whereas there was no difference in PFS between children with morphological BM involvement at diagnosis and those who had negative BM (PFS = 67% ± 14% vs. PFS = 87% ± 6%, respectively, p = 0.12). Busch *et al.* reported a study of 18 patients with t(8;14) positive BL using a PCR assay that combined the LD-PCR with a nested PCR.[48] The sensitivity range of this approach was 10^{-3}–10^{-5}. In 8 of the 18 patients, the specific *c-myc-IGH@* rearrangement was detected not only in BM (4/19) but also in PB samples (6/15). In 2 of the 4 BM positive cases, the PB was also positive, whereas in the remaining two cases, no PB was available. In contrast, in 3 of the 6 PB-positive cases, the BM was negative, thus suggesting that analysis of both BM and PB appear relevant for MRD monitoring in BL patients.

The application of the LD-PCR assay has some limitations because in approximately one-fourth of patients the t(8;14) translocation cannot be detected, mostly because a variant chromosomal translocation is present.[49] This obstacle can be, at least in part, overcome as suggested by a recent study of a series of BL and B-ALL pediatric patients using clone-specific Ig gene rearrangements.[50] Overall, 36 B-ALL and 19 BL cases were analyzed. In 88% of the cases, a sensitivity of at least 10^{-4} was achieved. By the application of this assay, molecular BM involvement at diagnosis was detected in 6/19 BLs and persistent MRD positivity during chemotherapy in 6/36 children affected by B-ALL. Overall, 32/36 B-ALLs and 12/19 BLs were positive for t(8;14). In most patients, LD-PCR and Ig gene rearrangements-based methods detected MRD with similar results. Thus, both methods can be successfully used for MRD analysis in mature B-ALL and BL patients, each with their own advantages and disadvantages. The LD-PCR method is simple, fast and relatively inexpensive, but the t(8;14) translocation cannot be detected in all the cases. Ig rearrangements are near-universal targets for MRD studies in B-cell malignancies and provide accurate quantitation of MRD but their detection is laborious and can be expensive.[51]

Recently, Agsalda *et al.*[52] studied MRD on follow-up specimens from B-NHL cases, relying on monoclonality defined by IGVH gene rearrangements, rather than on the identification of lymphoma clono-specific Ig rearrangements that needs the availability of primary tumor tissue. They hypothesized that MRD could be screened in specimens using primer pools made up of IGV_H oligomers from respective V_{H1} to V_{H7} families. The study was limited to 14 patients but their findings support the feasibility of this approach to analyze MRD because a previous study using patient-specific primers on the same cohort of children gave completely concordant results.

Despite the large number of MRD studies conducted in childhood ALL, there are very limited information on the prognostic relevance of MRD in B-ALL, possibly due to the rarity of B-ALL as compared with B-cell precursor ALL and due to the difficulty of conducting prospective studies on a significant number of cases. An analysis on the prognostic role of MRD in B-ALL was recently published by the AIEOP group.[53] The authors studied 68 BM at diagnosis from children affected by *de novo* B-ALL for the presence of t(8;14) by LD-PCR. Sixty-nine percent were positive for t(8;14) and MRD response kinetics was determined in 39 patients. The 3-year RFS was 38% ± 7% in MRD-positive after the first chemotherapy cycle compared with 84% ± 7% in MRD-negative patients ($p = 0.0005$) (Fig. 10.1). An update of this study extended to 81 patients confirmed these results.[54]

As a whole, results of MRD studies in BL and B-ALL may contribute to design better risk-adapted therapies that may include novel anti-cancer drugs such as the anti-CD20 monoclonal antibody, in selected groups of BL and B-ALL patients (see Chapters 21 and 22).

Anaplastic Large Cell Lymphoma

Methods for MRD detection

Anaplastic large cell lymphoma (ALCL) is frequently associated with the t(2;5)(p23;q35) chromosomal translocation, which gives rise to the fusion gene NPM-ALK (see Chapter 7).[55] In the last decade, variant rearrangements at the 2p23 ALK locus other than t(2;5) have been identified in ALCL, in which partner genes other than NPM are involved.[56–61] The fusion gene transcript can be readily and sensitively detected by PCR (Fig. 10.2A).[62] In experiments testing mixtures of the translocation-positive Karpas-299 ALCL cell line with the translocation-negative Jurkat T-cell line, a sensitivity of 10^{-6} for this RT-PCR assay could be demonstrated (Fig. 10.2B).[63] More recently, a quantitative RQ-PCR for NPM-ALK was developed according to the standardized protocol of the EAC (Europe Against Cancer) program for TaqMan-based RQ-PCR.[7] The NPM-ALK fusion transcript copy number is normalized to the copy numbers of the ABL that was selected as the control gene to compensate for variations in RNA integrity. The normalized copy number is expressed as copy numbers of NPM-ALK per 10^4 copies ABL. In serial cell dilution experiments with

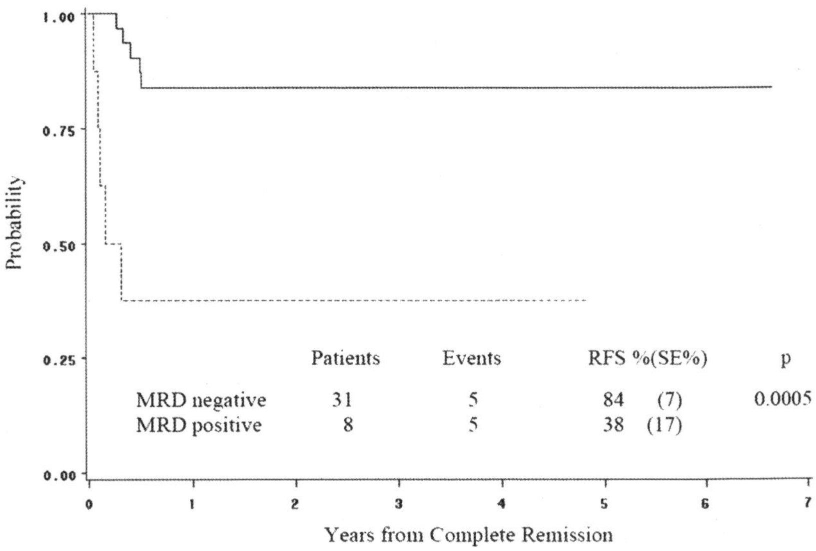

Fig. 10.1. Survival analysis. Relapse-free survival (RFS) analysis in 39 pediatric B-ALL patients according to the MRD status, determined by LD-PCR for t(8;14) in BM, after the first chemotherapy cycle: positive = broken line; negative = solid line. Used with permission from American Society of Clinical Oncology. Mussolin L, Pillon M, Conter V, Piglione M, Lo Nigro L, Pierani P, Micalizzi C, Buffardi S, Basso G, Zanesco L, Rosolen A. *J Clin Oncol* 25, 2007: 5254–5261.

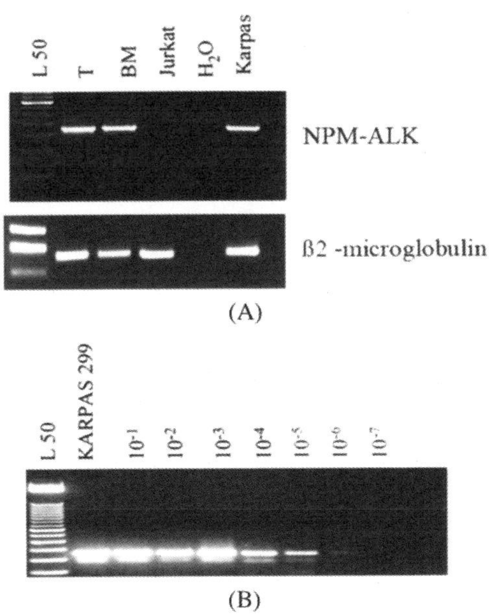

Fig. 10.2. RT-PCR detection of NPM-ALK transcript. (A) NPM-ALK expression in tumor (T) and bone marrow (BM) samples at diagnosis and in negative (Jurkat) and positive (Karpas) control cells. (B) RT-PCR detection of NPM-ALK in increasing dilutions of NPM-ALK positive Karpas-299 cells in leukemic blasts showed a sensitivity of 10^{-6}.

Karpas 299 cells in NPM-ALK-negative DG75 cells, the method detected fewer than 10 NPM-ALK-positive cells/10^6 control cells, indicating a sensitivity at least 10^{-5} at the cellular level.[64]

Results of clinical studies

Until recently, BM involvement was considered an uncommon event in ALCL, but this assumption may have been influenced by the subtle nature of the BM involvement and by the difficulty of its detection based on routine morphological examination (see Chapter 4). The first data on the prognostic impact of MRD, studied by RT-PCR in 52 pediatric ALCL patients, was reported in 2005 (see Chapter 16).[63] In that study 61% of patients presented with submicroscopic BM involvement at diagnosis. Survival analysis demonstrated a 5-year PFS of 41% for patients with molecularly positive BM versus 100% for patients with negative BM ($p = 0.001$). In addition, a significant association between molecular BM involvement and clinical risk groups was observed. Absence of BM involvement at diagnosis was an independent predictor of good prognosis. The prognostic role of MRD was also confirmed by a quantitative PCR approach.[64] BM from 80 and PB from 52 ALCL patients were analyzed. Qualitative and quantitative PCR findings in BM and PB strongly correlated. A clear relationship among qualitative BM PCR, clinical risk features, and atypical histologic subtypes was found. In particular, 16 patients with more than 10 copies number of NPM-ALK in BM, detected by quantitative PCR, was associated with a cumulative incidence of relapses (CI-Rs) of 71% ± 14% compared with a CI-R of 18% ± 6% for 59 patients with 10 or fewer copies number of NPM-ALK.

The characteristic expression of surface CD30 and cytoplasmatic and nuclear ALK can be used to quantify circulating tumor cells at the submicroscopic level in BM and PB also by a flow cytometric assay.[65] This method was tested in 11 ALCL patients and the comparative analysis of the flow cytometric assay and quantitative PCR for NPM-ALK showed a good correlation. It is worth noting that ALCL cells may have differing CD30 or ALK protein expression levels, leading to an underestimate of positive cells by flow cytometry.[65] Flow cytometry has the advantage of being less time consuming and may be less expensive, but the sensitivity of the PCR methods exceeds that of flow cytometry by at least one log, as it has been shown for leukemia MRD measurements (please see above). Further studies will be necessary to determine whether flow cytometry can be used as a substitute for PCR assays.

It is known that ALK overexpression may induce a host immune reaction, giving rise to autologous anti-ALK antibodies.[66] A recent study based on 28 ALCL children showed a strong relationship between MRD and anti-ALK antibody titer.[67] Low antibody titer and MRD positivity with more than 10 copies of NPM-ALK could identify a group of patients at greater risk of relapse (Fig. 10.3). An update of the study including a larger cohort of patients showed a relative risk of relapse of 4.7 for patients with low antibody titer, and 5.3 for patients with more than 10 copies of NPM-ALK in PB; but when the two variables were combined, the relative risk of relapse was 19.3 (Rosolen, personal communication). Thus, the combination of MRD and antibody titer represents a new prognostic indicator that may be considered in the design of new ALCL trials.

Lymphoblastic Lymphoma

Method for MRD detection

Lymphoblastic T-cell lymphoma (T-LBL) and T-ALL are often considered to be part of a spectrum of a single disease.[68] The malignant cells in T-ALL and T-LBL are morphologically indistinguishable, and the immunophenotype as well as genetic abnormalities of the cells are similar (see Chapter 4). The sensitive and specific methodologies used for MRD monitoring in T-ALL — such as PCR amplification of specific genetic abnormalities and clonal Ig/TCR gene rearrangements, previously described in this chapter, and also flow cytometric analysis — can be used to detect submicroscopic disseminated disease in patients with T-LBL.

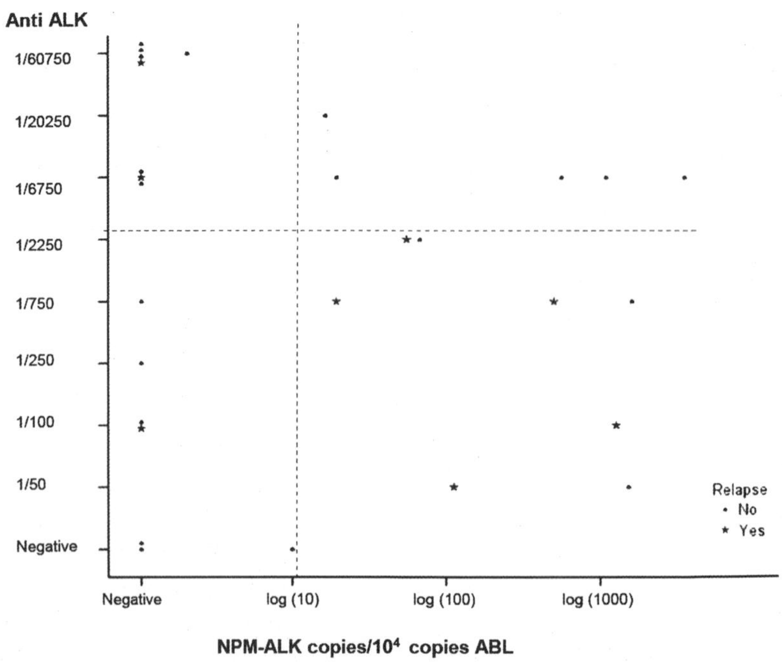

Fig. 10.3. Relationship of quantitative NPM-ALK PCR results in peripheral blood and antibody titers of the 28 ALCL patients at diagnosis. Reprinted from Mussolin L, Bonvini P, Ait-Tahar K, Pillon M, Tridello G, Buffardi S, Lombardi A, Pulford K, Rosolen A. (2009) Kinetics of humoral response to ALK and its relationship with minimal residual disease in pediatric ALCL. *Leukemia* **23**: 400–402.

Results of clinical studies

Flow cytometry and RQ-PCR for TCR gene rearrangements have been shown to identify minimal disseminated disease with a sensitivity of 0.01%. A recent retrospective study of 17 stage III T-LBL patients, analyzed at diagnosis, showed MRD positivity in the BM of 88% and 80% of the cases when evaluated by flow cytometry and RQ-PCR, respectively.[69] The concordance between the two methods was 67% at the highest sensitivity level, with 5/17 cases with discordant results (positive by RQ-PCR, negative by flow cytometry or vice versa). The very first data on the prognostic impact of minimal disease at diagnosis, evaluated by flow cytometry, was reported recently by Coustan-Smith *et al.* in 99 pediatric T-LBL patients.[70] Submicroscopic disease was detected in 72% of BM studied (71/99), with T-LBL blasts ranging from 0.01% to 31.6%. Detection of T-LBL cells was more frequent among younger patients (< 10 years; p = 0.046) and among patients with lower LDH (p = 0.0027), but was not significantly related to other features, such as gender, CNS involvement or stage. In most of the patients, a PB sample at diagnosis was also studied and every patient with detectable disease in the BM also had detectable disease in blood (r = 0.86, p < 0.0001) (Fig. 10.4). In eight T-LBL patients cells were found in PB but not in BM, suggesting that examination of PB might allow a more sensitive detection of disseminated disease. Two-year EFS was 52% for patients with ≥ 5% T-LBL cells by flow cytometry vs. 89% for the remaining patients (p = 0.009). Using a cutoff level of 1%, the 2-year EFS was 68% for patients with higher levels of disease dissemination vs. 91% for those with lower levels. These results indicate that flow-cytometric assay, which is at least 100-fold more sensitive than morphology, could allow a better stratification of patients for therapeutic purposes. Patients with no detectable disease dissemination at diagnosis and persistent MRD negativity may be candidates for reduction in treatment intensity, whereas patients with MRD positivity during remission induction therapy should be closely monitored and may be eligible for intensified therapy.

The overall scenario indicates that similar approaches used for MRD studies in ALL may be applied to analyze MRD in LBL. However, the possibility to run significant prospective MRD studies in LBL are limited by the different nature of the primary disease, which implies almost invariably the availability of unfixed bioptic material.

Summary (Table 10.1)

In this chapter, we discuss immunologic and molecular methods for detecting MRD in acute leukemias and non-Hodgkin lymphomas of childhood, adolescents

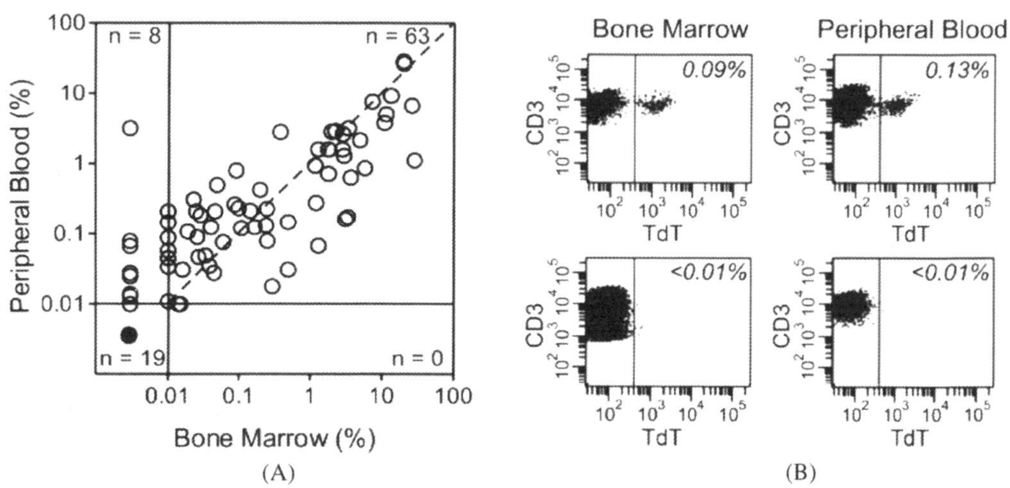

Fig. 10.4. Detection of T-ALL cells in peripheral blood. (A) Relation between percentage of T-ALL cells detected by flow cytometry in paired bone marrow and peripheral blood samples at diagnosis (r = 0.8699; P < 0.0001 by Spearman's rank correlation). The dashed line indicates the line of identity. (B) Flow cytometric dot plots illustrate findings in two representative marrow/blood paired samples, one with T-ALL cells (top panels) the other with no detectable disease (bottom panels). Percentage of TdT+ CD3+ cells among mononuclear cells is shown. Used with permission from American Society of Clinical Oncology. Coustan-Smith E, Sandlund JT, Perkins SL, Chen H, Chang M, Abromowitch M, Campana D. *J Clin Oncol* **27**, 2009:3533–3539.

Table 10.1. Key points.

ALL

- In ALL, MRD can be studied by PCR amplification of antigen-receptor genes and of fusion genes (sensitivity = 0.01–0.001%), and by flow cytometry (sensitivity = 0.01%).
- In nearly all cases, cells have immunoglobulin and/or T-cell receptor gene rearrangements or express leukemia-associated immunophenotypes. Gene fusions suitable for PCR studies are present in approximately 40% of cases.
- Numerous correlative studies demonstrated that measurements of MRD during the early phases of therapy (e.g. during and at the end of remission induction therapy) provide the most powerful prognostic indicator in childhood ALL.
- Patients who achieved MRD < 0.01% during remission induction therapy have a particularly favorable outcome with contemporary chemotherapy, while those with MRD ≥ 1% at the end of induction therapy have a very high risk of relapse.
- Risk classification schemas based on MRD are being incorporated in most major childhood ALL trials.

AML

- In AML, MRD can be studied by PCR amplification of fusion genes (sensitivity, 0.01–0.001%), and by flow cytometry (sensitivity, 0.1–0.01%). Preliminary results indicate the measurements of *WT1* gene levels could also be useful.
- Aberrant immunophenotypes can be identified in nearly 95% of patients at diagnosis. Gene fusions suitable for PCR studies are present in approximately 40% of cases.
- MRD levels after each phase of therapy were independent predictors of relapse in several studies.
- A recent MRD-based clinical trial, AML02, resulted in high event-free and overall survival rates.

BL and B-ALL

- BL and B-ALL are characterized by t(8;14) translocation accounting for about 75% of the total, which juxtaposes the *c-myc* gene to the immunoglobulin heavy chain (*IGH@*) locus on chromosome 14 in divergent orientation.
- LD-PCR and IgH rearrangement assay can be successfully used for MRD analysis in mature B-ALL and BL patients.
- MRD studies showed a negative prognostic impact in BL and B-ALL.
- MRD studies in BL and B-ALL may contribute to design better risk-adapted therapies, which may include novel anti-cancer drugs such as the anti-CD20 monoclonal antibody, in selected group of BL and B-ALL patients.

ALCL

- Anaplastic large cell lymphoma (ALCL) is frequently associated with the t(2;5)(p23;q35) chromosomal translocation, which gives rise to the fusion gene NPM-ALK.
- The fusion gene transcript can be readily and sensitively detected by RT-PCR and real-time quantitative PCR.
- Qualitative and quantitative PCR findings in BM and PB strongly correlated. A clear relationship among qualitative BM PCR, clinical risk features, and atypical histologic subtypes was found in these patients.
- ALK overexpression may induce a host immune reaction, giving rise to autologous anti-ALK antibodies.
- The combination of MRD and antibody titer represents a new prognostic indicator that may be considered in the design of new ALCL trials.

LYMPHOBLASTIC LYMPHOMA

- Lymphoblastic T-cell lymphoma (T-LBL) and T-ALL are often considered to be part of a spectrum of a single disease.
- Similar approaches used for MRD studies in ALL may be applied to analyze MRD in LBL.
- Detection of disseminated disease at diagnosis by flow cytometry was more frequent among younger patients (< 10 years) and among patients with lower LDH, but was not significantly related to other features, such as gender, CNS involvement or stage.
- Patients with higher levels of disseminated disease (i.e. ≥ 1%) had significantly lower event-free survival rates.
- The possibility to run significant prospective MRD studies in LBL using molecular methods is hampered by the limited availability of unfixed bioptic material for the primary tumor.

and young adults, and the potential impact of their clinical application. MRD testing with techniques that can detect 1 leukemia/lymphoma cell in up to 100,000 normal cells has provided definitive proof that patients, who are in complete clinical remission, can harbor significant levels of disease in bone marrow and peripheral blood. The clinical relevance of this finding has been convincingly demonstrated. In patients with ALL and AML, MRD — during the early phases of therapy — is a powerful prognostic indicator. Consequently, risk classifications based on MRD have been incorporated in many recent acute leukemia protocols. Disease dissemination at diagnosis and/or MRD during treatment were shown to be prognostically important in T-LBL, BL and ALCL.

These findings indicate that it should be beneficial to apply MRD assays to measure disease dissemination in the initial assessment of patients with NHL and to evaluate response to treatment.

References

2. van der Velden VH, Cazzaniga G, Schrauder A, Hancock J, Bader P, Panzer-Grumayer ER, Flohr T, Sutton R, Cave H, Madsen HO, Cayuela JM, Trka J, Eckert C, Foroni L, Zur Stadt U, Beldjord K, Raff T, van der Schoot CE, van Dongen JJ. (2007) Analysis of minimal residual disease by Ig/TCR gene rearrangements: Guidelines for interpretation of real-time quantitative PCR data. *Leukemia* **21**: 604–611.
3. Stow P, Key L, Chen X, Pan Q, Neale GA, Coustan-Smith E, Mullighan CG, Zhou Y, Pui CH, Campana D. (2010) Clinical significance of low levels of minimal residual disease at the end of remission induction therapy in childhood acute lymphoblastic leukemia. *Blood* **115**: 4657–4663.
4. Flohr T, Schrauder A, Cazzaniga G, Panzer-Grumayer R, van der Velden V, Fischer S, Stanulla M, Basso G, Niggli FK, Schafer BW, Sutton R, Koehler R, Zimmermann M, Valsecchi MG, Gadner H, Masera G, Schrappe M, van Dongen JJ, Biondi A, Bartram CR. (2008) Minimal residual disease-directed risk stratification using real-time quantitative PCR analysis of immunoglobulin and T-cell receptor gene rearrangements in the international multicenter trial AIEOP-BFM ALL 2000 for childhood acute lymphoblastic leukemia. *Leukemia* **22**: 771–782.
5. Campana D. (2008) Status of minimal residual disease testing in childhood haematological malignancies. *Br J Haematol* **143**: 481–489.
7. Gabert J, Beillard E, van der Velden VH, Bi W, Grimwade D, Pallisgaard N, Barbany G, Cazzaniga G, Cayuela JM, Cave H, Pane F, Aerts JL, de Micheli D, Thirion X, Pradel V, Gonzalez M, Viehmann S, Malec M, Saglio G, van Dongen JJ. (2003) Standardization and quality control studies of 'real-time' quantitative reverse transcriptase polymerase chain reaction of fusion gene transcripts for residual disease detection in leukemia — a Europe against cancer program. *Leukemia* **17**: 2318–2357.
8. Mullighan CG, Su X, Zhang J, Radtke I, Phillips LA, Miller CB, Ma J, Liu W, Cheng C, Schulman BA, Harvey RC, Chen IM, Clifford RJ, Carroll WL, Reaman G, Bowman WP, Devidas M, Gerhard DS, Yang W, Relling MV, Shurtleff SA, Campana D, Borowitz MJ, Pui CH, Smith M, Hunger SP, Willman CL, Downing JR. (2009) Deletion of IKZF1 and prognosis in acute lymphoblastic leukemia. *N Engl J Med* **360**: 470–480.
10. Neale GA, Coustan-Smith E, Stow P, Pan Q, Chen X, Pui CH, Campana D. (2004) Comparative analysis of flow cytometry and polymerase chain reaction for the detection of minimal residual disease in childhood acute lymphoblastic leukemia. *Leukemia* **18**: 934–938.
12. Brisco MJ, Condon J, Hughes E, Neoh SH, Sykes PJ, Seshadri R, Toogood I, Waters K, Tauro G, Ekert H, *et al.* (1994) Outcome prediction in childhood acute lymphoblastic leukaemia by molecular quantification of residual disease at the end of induction. *Lancet* **343**: 196–200.
13. Cave H, van der Werff ten Bosch J, Suciu S, Guidal C, Waterkeyn C, Otten J, Bakkus M, Thielemans K, Grandchamp B, Vilmer E. (1998) Clinical significance of minimal residual disease in childhood acute lymphoblastic leukemia. European Organization for Research and Treatment of Cancer — Childhood Leukemia Cooperative Group. *N Engl J Med* **339**: 591–598.
14. van Dongen JJ, Seriu T, Panzer-Grumayer ER, Biondi A, Pongers-Willemse MJ, Corral L, Stolz F, Schrappe M, Masera G, Kamps WA, Gadner H, van Wering ER, Ludwig WD, Basso G, de Bruijn MA, Cazzaniga G, Hettinger K, van der Does-van den Berg A, Hop WC, Riehm H, Bartram CR. (1998) Prognostic value of minimal residual disease in acute lymphoblastic leukaemia in childhood. *Lancet* **352**: 1731–1738.
15. Conter V, Bartram CR, Valsecchi MG, Schrauder A, Panzer-Grumayer R, Moricke A, Arico M, Zimmermann M, Mann G, de Rossi G, Stanulla M, Locatelli F, Basso G, Niggli F, Barisone E, Henze G, Ludwig WD, Haas OA, Cazzaniga G, Koehler R, Silvestri D, Bradtke J, Parasole R, Beier R, van Dongen JJ, Biondi A, Schrappe M. (2010) Molecular response to treatment redefines all prognostic factors in children and adolescents with B-cell precursor acute lymphoblastic leukemia: Results in 3184 patients of the AIEOP-BFM ALL 2000 study. *Blood* **115**: 3206–3214.
16. Zhou J, Goldwasser MA, Li A, Dahlberg SE, Neuberg D, Wang H, Dalton V, McBride KD, Sallan SE, Silverman LB, Gribben JG. (2007) Quantitative analysis of minimal residual disease predicts relapse in children with B-lineage acute lymphoblastic leukemia in DFCI ALL Consortium Protocol 95-01. *Blood* **110**: 1607–1611.
17. Coustan-Smith E, Behm FG, Sanchez J, Boyett JM, Hancock ML, Raimondi SC, Rubnitz JE, Rivera GK, Sandlund JT, Pui CH, Campana D. (1998) Immunological detection of minimal residual disease in children with acute lymphoblastic leukaemia. *Lancet* **351**: 550–554.
18. Coustan-Smith E, Sancho J, Behm FG, Hancock ML, Razzouk BI, Ribeiro RC, Rivera GK, Rubnitz JE, Sandlund JT, Pui CH, Campana D. (2002) Prognostic importance of measuring early clearance of leukemic cells by flow cytometry in childhood acute lymphoblastic leukemia. *Blood* **100**: 52–58.

19. Coustan-Smith E, Sancho J, Hancock ML, Boyett JM, Behm FG, Raimondi SC, Sandlund JT, Rivera GK, Rubnitz JE, Ribeiro RC, Pui CH, Campana D. (2000) Clinical importance of minimal residual disease in childhood acute lymphoblastic leukemia. *Blood* **96**: 2691–2696.
20. Borowitz MJ, Devidas M, Hunger SP, Bowman WP, Carroll AJ, Carroll WL, Linda S, Martin PL, Pullen DJ, Viswanatha D, Willman CL, Winick N, Camitta BM. (2008) Clinical significance of minimal residual disease in childhood acute lymphoblastic leukemia and its relationship to other prognostic factors: A Children's Oncology Group study. *Blood* **111**: 5477–5485.
21. Basso G, Veltroni M, Valsecchi MG, Dworzak MN, Ratei R, Silvestri D, Benetello A, Buldini B, Maglia O, Masera G, Conter V, Arico M, Biondi A, Gaipa G. (2009) Risk of relapse of childhood acute lymphoblastic leukemia is predicted by flow cytometric measurement of residual disease on day 15 bone marrow. *J Clin Oncol* **27**: 5168–5174.
23. Coustan-Smith E, Mullighan CG, Onciu M, Behm FG, Raimondi SC, Pei D, Cheng C, Su X, Rubnitz JE, Basso G, Biondi A, Pui CH, Downing JR, Campana D. (2009) Early T-cell precursor leukaemia: A subtype of very high-risk acute lymphoblastic leukaemia. *Lancet Oncol* **10**: 147–156.
28. van der Velden VH, Corral L, Valsecchi MG, Jansen MW, de Lorenzo P, Cazzaniga G, Panzer-Grumayer ER, Schrappe M, Schrauder A, Meyer C, Marschalek R, Nigro LL, Metzler M, Basso G, Mann G, den Boer ML, Biondi A, Pieters R, van Dongen JJ. (2009) Prognostic significance of minimal residual disease in infants with acute lymphoblastic leukemia treated within the Interfant-99 protocol. *Leukemia* **23**: 1073–1079.
29. Pui CH, Campana D, Pei D, Bowman WP, Sandlund JT, Kaste SC, Ribeiro RC, Rubnitz JE, Raimondi SC, Onciu M, Coustan-Smith E, Kun LE, Jeha S, Cheng C, Howard SC, Simmons V, Bayles A, Metzger ML, Boyett JM, Leung W, Handgretinger R, Downing JR, Evans WE, Relling MV. (2009) Treating childhood acute lymphoblastic leukemia without cranial irradiation. *N Engl J Med* **360**: 2730–2741.
30. Eckert C, Biondi A, Seeger K, Cazzaniga G, Hartmann R, Beyermann B, Pogodda M, Proba J, Henze G. (2001) Prognostic value of minimal residual disease in relapsed childhood acute lymphoblastic leukaemia. *Lancet* **358**: 1239–1241.
31. Coustan-Smith E, Gajjar A, Hijiya N, Razzouk BI, Ribeiro RC, Rivera GK, Rubnitz JE, Sandlund JT, Andreansky M, Hancock ML, Pui CH, Campana D. (2004) Clinical significance of minimal residual disease in childhood acute lymphoblastic leukemia after first relapse. *Leukemia* **18**: 499–504.
32. Raetz EA, Borowitz MJ, Devidas M, Linda SB, Hunger SP, Winick NJ, Camitta BM, Gaynon PS, Carroll WL. (2008) Re-induction platform for children with first marrow relapse of acute lymphoblastic Leukemia: A Children's Oncology Group Study [corrected]. *J Clin Oncol* **26**: 3971–3978.
33. Krejci O, van der Velden VH, Bader P, Kreyenberg H, Goulden N, Hancock J, Schilham MW, Lankester A, Revesz T, Klingebiel T, van Dongen JJ. (2003) Level of minimal residual disease prior to haematopoietic stem cell transplantation predicts prognosis in paediatric patients with acute lymphoblastic leukaemia: A report of the Pre-BMT MRD Study Group. *Bone Marrow Transplant* **32**: 849–851.
34. Coustan-Smith E, Ribeiro RC, Rubnitz JE, Razzouk BI, Pui CH, Pounds S, Andreansky M, Behm FG, Raimondi SC, Shurtleff SA, Downing JR, Campana D. (2003) Clinical significance of residual disease during treatment in childhood acute myeloid leukaemia. *Br J Haematol* **123**: 243–252.
36. Cilloni D, Renneville A, Hermitte F, Hills RK, Daly S, Jovanovic JV, Gottardi E, Fava M, Schnittger S, Weiss T, Izzo B, Nomdedeu J, van der Heijden A, van der Reijden BA, Jansen JH, van der Velden VH, Ommen H, Preudhomme C, Saglio G, Grimwade D. (2009) Real-time quantitative polymerase chain reaction detection of minimal residual disease by standardized WT1 assay to enhance risk stratification in acute myeloid leukemia: A European LeukemiaNet study. *J Clin Oncol* **27**: 5195–5201.
37. Willasch AM, Gruhn B, Coliva T, Kalinova M, Schneider G, Kreyenberg H, Steinbach D, Weber G, Hollink IH, Zwaan CM, Biondi A, van der Velden VH, Reinhardt D, Cazzaniga G, Bader P, Trka J. (2009) Standardization of WT1 mRNA quantitation for minimal residual disease monitoring in childhood AML and implications of WT1 gene mutations: A European multicenter study. *Leukemia* **23**: 1472–1479.
38. Sievers EL, Lange BJ, Alonzo TA, Gerbing RB, Bernstein ID, Smith FO, Arceci RJ, Woods WG, Loken MR. (2003) Immunophenotypic evidence of leukemia after induction therapy predicts relapse: Results from a prospective Children's Cancer Group study of 252 patients with acute myeloid leukemia. *Blood* **101**: 3398–3406.
39. Langebrake C, Creutzig U, Dworzak M, Hrusak O, Mejstrikova E, Griesinger F, Zimmermann M,

Reinhardt D. (2006) Residual disease monitoring in childhood acute myeloid leukemia by multiparameter flow cytometry: The MRD-AML-BFM Study Group. *J Clin Oncol* **24**: 3686–3692.

40. Rubnitz JE, Inaba H, Dahl G, Ribeiro RC, Bowman WP, Taub J, Pounds S, Razzouk BI, Lacayo NJ, Cao X, Meshinchi S, Degar B, Airewele G, Raimondi SC, Onciu M, Coustan-Smith E, Downing JR, Leung W, Pui CH, Campana D. (2010) Minimal residual disease-directed therapy for childhood acute myeloid leukaemia: Results of the AML02 multicentre trial. *Lancet Oncol* **11**: 543–552.
41. Jacobsohn DA, Tse WT, Chaleff S, Rademaker A, Duerst R, Olszewski M, Huang W, Chou PM, Kletzel M. (2009) High WT1 gene expression before haematopoietic stem cell transplant in children with acute myeloid leukaemia predicts poor event-free survival. *Br J Haematol* **146**: 669–674.
42. Rosenberg AR, Leisenring W, Sanders JE, Woolfrey AE, Carpenter PA, Wells DA, Loken MR, Meshinchi S. (2009) Sub-morphologic evidence of disease prior to stem cell transplantation correlates with inferior post transplant outcome in childhood acute myeloid leukemia. *Blood* **114**: 328.
43. Dalla-Favera R, Bregni M, Erikson J, Patterson D, Gallo RC, Croce CM. (1982) Human c-myc onc gene is located on the region of chromosome 8 that is translocated in Burkitt lymphoma cells. *Proc Natl Acad Sci U S A* **79**: 7824–7827.
44. Basso K, Frascella E, Zanesco L, Rosolen A. (1999) Improved long-distance polymerase chain reaction for the detection of t(8;14)(q24;q32) in Burkitt's lymphomas. *Am J Pathol* **155**: 1479–1485.
48. Busch K, Borkhardt A, Wossmann W, Reiter A, Harbott J. (2004) Combined polymerase chain reaction methods to detect c-myc/IgH rearrangement in childhood Burkitt's lymphoma for minimal residual disease analysis. *Haematologica* **89**: 818–825.
52. Agsalda M, Kusao I, Troelstrup D, Shiramizu B. (2009) Screening for residual disease in pediatric burkitt lymphoma using consensus primer pools. *Adv Hematol* **2009**: 412163.
53. Mussolin L, Pillon M, Conter V, Piglione M, Lo Nigro L, Pierani P, Micalizzi C, Buffardi S, Basso G, Zanesco L, Rosolen A. (2007) Prognostic role of minimal residual disease in mature B-cell acute lymphoblastic leukemia of childhood. *J Clin Oncol* **25**: 5254–5261.
54. Mussolin L, Pillon M, Tridello G, Conter V, lo Nigro L, Micalizzi C, Lombardi A, Piglione M, Mura R, Arcamone G, Rosolen A. (2009) Analysis update of the prognostic role of minimal residual disease in B-cell acute lymphoblastic leukemia of childhood treated in the AIEOP protocols. *Hematolgy Meeting Reports* **3**: 24.
55. Lamant L, Meggetto F, al Saati T, Brugieres L, de Paillerets BB, Dastugue N, Bernheim A, Rubie H, Terrier-Lacombe MJ, Robert A, Rigal F, Schlaifer D, Shiuta M, Mori S, Delsol G. (1996) High incidence of the t(2;5)(p23;q35) translocation in anaplastic large cell lymphoma and its lack of detection in Hodgkin's disease. Comparison of cytogenetic analysis, reverse transcriptase-polymerase chain reaction, and P-80 immunostaining. *Blood* **87**: 284–291.
62. Downing JR, Shurtleff SA, Zielenska M, Curcio-Brint AM, Behm FG, Head DR, Sandlund JT, Weisenburger DD, Kossakowska AE, Thorner P, *et al.* (1995) Molecular detection of the (2;5) translocation of non-Hodgkin's lymphoma by reverse transcriptase-polymerase chain reaction. *Blood* **85**: 3416–3422.
63. Mussolin L, Pillon M, d'Amore ES, Santoro N, Lombardi A, Fagioli F, Zanesco L, Rosolen A. (2005) Prevalence and clinical implications of bone marrow involvement in pediatric anaplastic large cell lymphoma. *Leukemia* **19**: 1643–1647.
64. Damm-Welk C, Busch K, Burkhardt B, Schieferstein J, Viehmann S, Oschlies I, Klapper W, Zimmermann M, Harbott J, Reiter A, Woessmann W. (2007) Prognostic significance of circulating tumor cells in bone marrow or peripheral blood as detected by qualitative and quantitative PCR in pediatric NPM-ALK-positive anaplastic large-cell lymphoma. *Blood* **110**: 670–677.
65. Damm-Welk C, Schieferstein J, Schwalm S, Reiter A, Woessmann W. (2007) Flow cytometric detection of circulating tumour cells in nucleophosmin/anaplastic lymphoma kinase-positive anaplastic large cell lymphoma: Comparison with quantitative polymerase chain reaction. *Br J Haematol* **138**: 459–466.
66. Pulford K, Falini B, Banham AH, Codrington D, Roberton H, Hatton C, Mason DY. (2000) Immune response to the ALK oncogenic tyrosine kinase in patients with anaplastic large-cell lymphoma. *Blood* **96**: 1605–1607.
67. Mussolin L, Bonvini P, Ait-Tahar K, Pillon M, Tridello G, Buffardi S, Lombardi A, Pulford K, Rosolen A. (2009) Kinetics of humoral response to ALK and its relationship with minimal residual disease in pediatric ALCL. *Leukemia* **23**: 400–402.
68. Moricke A, Zimmermann M, Reiter A, Gadner H, Odenwald E, Harbott J, Ludwig WD, Riehm H, Schrappe M. (2005) Prognostic impact of age in children and adolescents with acute lymphoblastic leukemia: Data

from the trials ALL-BFM 86, 90, and 95. *Klin Padiatr* **217**: 310–320.

69. Stark B, Avigad S, Luria D, Manor S, Reshef-Ronen T, Avrahami G, Yaniv I. (2009) Bone marrow minimal disseminated disease (MDD) and minimal residual disease (MRD) in childhood T-cell lymphoblastic lymphoma stage III, detected by flow cytometry (FC) and real-time quantitative polymerase chain reaction (RQ-PCR). *Pediatr Blood Cancer* **52**: 20–25.
70. Coustan-Smith E, Sandlund JT, Perkins SL, Chen H, Chang M, Abromowitch M, Campana D. (2009) Minimal disseminated disease in childhood T-cell lymphoblastic lymphoma: A report from the children's oncology group. *J Clin Oncol* **27**: 3533–3539.

11

Childhood ALL

Paul Gaynon and Martin Schrappe

Introduction

Acute lymphoblastic leukemia (ALL), a malignant disorder of lymphoid progenitor cells, affects both children and adults and is the most common childhood malignancy. Remarkable progress has been made in our understanding and treatment of ALL since the early 1960s. Studies in childhood ALL have provided a paradigm for clinical and laboratory research well beyond pediatric hemato-oncology.

Childhood ALL can now be successfully treated with a 5-year survival rate of about 80–90% by the application of intensive combination chemotherapy regimes in combination with radiation therapy and/or allogeneic hematopoietic stem cell transplantation (SCT) in specific patient subsets (see Chapter 20).[1–4] Presenting clinical and laboratory prognostic features and early response to treatment are employed to allocate risk-adapted therapy.[5–7] Although almost all patients achieve remission, disappearance of microscopically detectable leukemia blasts with recovery of peripheral blood counts, leukemia returns or relapses in about 1 patient in 7, usually in the bone marrow but also in extramedullary sites (see Chapter 10). Outcome after relapse remains poor, unfortunately and most of these patients die.[8] Furthermore, a small but significant number of patients succumb, usually from infection while neutropenic from therapy. Late effects like avascular necrosis of bone and subtle neurocognitive damage are seen in some patients. Late cardiomyopathy, neuroendocrine abnormalities, and secondary malignant neoplasms (SN) remain concerns (see Chapter 24).[9–11] Thus, future research in childhood ALL will focus on (1) the reduction of acute and long-term toxicity in selected patient groups with favorable prognosis, (2) the improvement of outcome in poor-risk groups, and (3) better means to estimate a patient's risk of relapse more precisely.

Incidence and Epidemiology

ALL represents only about 12% of all leukemia cases in the general population; more than 60% of patients diagnosed with ALL are children. Childhood ALL, the most common malignancy in children, represents approximately 25–30% of childhood malignancies and 80% of childhood leukemias (see Chapter 1).[12]

The annual incidence rates of childhood ALL vary worldwide with between 1 and 4 new cases per 100,000 children younger than 15 years old per year.[13–15] Incidence is higher in more affluent countries like the United States of America (USA), Germany, Italy, Switzerland and Costa Rica as compared to developing countries, e.g. India or Cuba.[12] In addition, incidence varies among ethnic groups within countries. In USA, rates are highest in Hispanic children, and white children have a higher incidence rate than African American children.[16] Reasons are still unclear but this variability has led to speculation that factors associated with socioeconomic status may play an important role in the etiology of ALL.[14]

Incidence also varies by gender with a slightly higher incidence in males at ages > 1 year and a higher incidence in females at ages < 1 year. Incidence is highest at the age of 2–5 years with a median age of 4 years and 10 months.[1]

Etiology and Pathogenesis

Many questions regarding pathogenesis remain to be answered but much has been. In ALL, a progenitor cell becomes genetically and/or epigenetically altered and undergoes dysregulated proliferation, survival and clonal expansion. Spontaneous somatic mutations are the most important developmental factors in pathogenesis of childhood ALL. A two-hit hypothesis is proposed with a relatively rare first genetic change followed by a much rarer second hit. This proposal is supported most strongly by the data for prenatal appearance of *ETV6/RUNX1* (also known as *TEL/AML1*) with breakthrough of leukemia in about 1% of patients with the translocation at birth (see section "Chromosomal translocations and somatic genetic aberrations" below).[17] Only a small proportion of all cases (< 5%) can be attributed to a genetic predisposition such as Down syndrome (DS), the most common abnormality in ALL, Bloom syndrome, ataxia telangiectasia, or Nijmegen breakage syndrome, which have a clearly increased risk.[5]

The temporal and geographical variation of incidence, perhaps linked to the level of socioeconomic development, suggests a significant role for environmental factors in the pathogenesis of ALL. In addition, multiple lines of evidence support a role for infection or lack of infection in the first years of life.[5,18] However, no proximate cause is identified for a large majority of patients. Parents' guilt is common. Friends and relatives all too often share their theories as to how the parents erred and the physician should try to assuage parents' unneeded suffering (see Chapter 28).

Genetics and syndromes

In a small proportion, up to 5% of acute leukemias, a predisposing genetic syndrome exists. Often, these syndromes are characterized by an aberrant function of genes relevant for genomic stability and DNA repair mechanisms such as ataxia telangiectasia or Nijmegen breakage syndrome.[19] DS represents the most frequent syndrome predisposing for ALL with a 10- to 20-fold increased risk.[18] Other genetic syndromes with an increased ALL risk are neurofibromatosis type I, Fanconi anemia, and Bloom syndrome. However, recent data from genome-wide association studies suggest a genetic susceptibility for the development of ALL, independent of known genetic syndromes.[20,21]

Environmental factors

Certain environmental factors have been implicated in the development of leukemia. Exogenic factors like ionizing radiation, certain chemicals such as benzene and/or chemotherapeutic drugs, all may contribute to leukemogenesis.[18] Ionizing radiation is most thoroughly explored. An X-ray examination during pregnancy or a postnatal radiation may have a mutagenic effect. Famous examples include Marie Curie and her daughter Irene who died of leukemia, likely caused by exposure to ionizing radiation.[19]

Proximity to a nuclear power station remains controversial. A case control study from the German Childhood Cancer Registry examined 593 patients with acute leukemia and 1766 controls and found a link to living in the vicinity of a nuclear power plant. Within a 5-km zone, the odds ratio for development of leukemia was 2.19 compared to living further away. However, radiation is unlikely the simple cause as the differences in local background radiation exposure in Germany are larger than the increased radiation exposure from proximity to nuclear power plants.[22]

Epidemiological data indicate associations between infant leukemia and maternal alcohol intake, high birth weight, marijuana smoking and exposure to benzene and petrol in pregnancy. Other durable factors are a fetal loss of two or more, which might increase the relative risk of developing leukemias up to 25 times, a maternal reproductive history, maternal diet and prenatal vitamin use.[18]

ALL subsequent to radiotherapy and chemotherapy

Radiotherapy and chemotherapeutic drugs induce DNA damage and are genotoxic. Their impact on SN depends on dose, schedule, and additional treatment elements.[19] Examples are inhibitors of topoisomerase type I and II like etoposide, which was shown to induce *MLL* rearrangement-positive ALL.[23] The majorities of SN, however, are acute myeloid leukemias (AML) and myelodysplastic syndromes.[11,24]

Infections

The association of industrialization in modern or affluent societies with an increased prevalence of ALL, as well as repeated clustering of cases in "new" towns, is believed to reflect a correlation of ALL with infection or lack of infection at critical ages. The peak age of onset of childhood ALL is 2–5 years, suggesting that infections in the first years of life influence the risk of common childhood ALL. Two infection-based hypotheses are discussed. One hypothesis, the delayed infection hypothesis, suggests some susceptible individuals with a prenatally acquired preleukemic clone had low or no exposure to common infections early in life because they lived in an affluent hygienic environment. Such infectious naiveté then predisposes the immune system to aberrant or pathological responses after later delayed exposure to common infections.[25] To date, specific infectious agents like viruses remain to be identified. The second hypothesis asserts that clusters of cases result from exposure of susceptible (non-immune) individuals to common but fairly non-pathological infections after population mixing with carriers.[26]

Chromosomal translocations and somatic genetic aberrations

ALL is a progressive clonal disorder driven by mutations which, at least in some cases, already occur *in utero*. For instance, some chromosomal translocations associated with precursor-B-cell ALL (pB-ALL) have been detected in neonatal specimens. Often, these translocations can be detected before the onset of leukemia, thus they seem to be primary events in the development of the disease (see Chapter 5). However, differences exist. In ALL, characterized by translocations involving the *MLL* gene on chromosome 4, there is a very short latency to the development of ALL: *MLL* rearrangements have been identified in neonatal blood spots of patients who develop leukemia and *MLL*-positive ALL is predominantly found in very young infants.[27] In ALL, characterized by an *ETV6/RUNX1* (also known as *TEL/AML1*) rearrangement, a comparison between blood samples at diagnosis and neonatal blood spots (Guthrie samples) again showed that in this subgroup, ALL is frequently initiated by the occurrence of the translocational event *in utero*.[28] Moreover, studies on concordant twins with *TEL/AML1*-positive ALL, in whom the disease appeared at a different age, have shown an identical genomic sequence of DNA for the *TEL/AML1* rearrangement, indicating a common origin of ALL *in utero*.[28] Otherwise, the rare concordance rate of only about 5% for the development of a *TEL/AML1*-positive ALL in twins, the variable incubation period, the clinical outcome of such cases, and transgenic models suggest that an additional postnatal event is required for the development of ALL.[29] Moreover, the presence of a *TEL/AML1* rearrangement in the cord blood of newborns is 100-times higher than the prevalence of ALL defined by this fusion gene. All of these data support the classical "two-hit" model for non-inheritable cancers in the childhood.[28,30] The postnatal event providing the second hit remains to be identified. Here, again infections may play an important role.

Chromosomal translocations, when present, are defining characteristics as for other human leukemias. Large studies of genome-wide gene expression of newly diagnosed leukemias have substantiated that specific chromosomal translocations identify unique subtypes of the disease.[31] Important chromosomal translocations and their respective gene rearrangements in childhood ALL are t(12;21) and *TEL/AML1*, t(9;22) and *BCR/ABL*, t(1;19) and *E2A/PBX1*, and translocations involving the *MLL* gene on chromosome 11. The detection of some of these translocations is used for risk stratification. Moreover, the fusion of the BCR signaling protein to the ABL non-receptor kinase in *BCR/ABL*-positive ALL, results in a constitutive tyrosine kinase activation which serves as a molecular target for the treatment with the specific tyrosine kinase inhibitor imatinib. Very recently, a substantial number of additional chromosomal translocations, as well as other genetic aberrations, have been described.[32,33] However, their clinical relevance still has to be determined. Importantly, comparative genomic hybridization shows that patients sharing a specific translocation may have differing associated genetic changes.[34]

Diagnosis/Classification

Morphology

Morphologic and histochemical criteria have guided the classification of leukemia since the late 19th century (see Chapters 2 and 4). Although newer techniques like flow cytometry as well as classical and molecular cytogenetics have supplemented morphology over recent years, the French–American–British (FAB) classification is still a critical method used to establish the diagnosis from bone marrow (BM) or peripheral blood (PB) smears. According to the FAB classification, ALL can be divided into three subtypes: L1, L2, and L3 (Table 11.1, Fig. 11.1). Most importantly, the subtype L3 must be distinguished from L1 and L2, as therapy differs. L3 morphology is characterized by blast cells of moderate to large size with

Table 11.1. Morphological classification of acute lymphoblastic leukemia.[a]

	Morphology			
FAB	**Cells**	**Nucleus**	**Nucleoli**	**Cytoplasm**
L1	Small, uniform	Round, homogeneous	Not visible	Scanty, moderate basophilic
L2	Varying size	Irregular, inhomogeneous	One or more	Variable
L3	Large, uniform	Round to oval, homogeneous	One or more, vesicular	Abundant, basophilic

[a]Morphological classification according to the French-American-British (FAB) classification.

From Bennett JM, Catovski D, Daniel MT, Flandrin G, Galton DAG, Gralnick HR, Sultan C. (1976) Proposals for the classification of the acute leukaemias. French-American-British (FAB) cooperative group. *Br J Haematol* **33**: 451–458.[35]

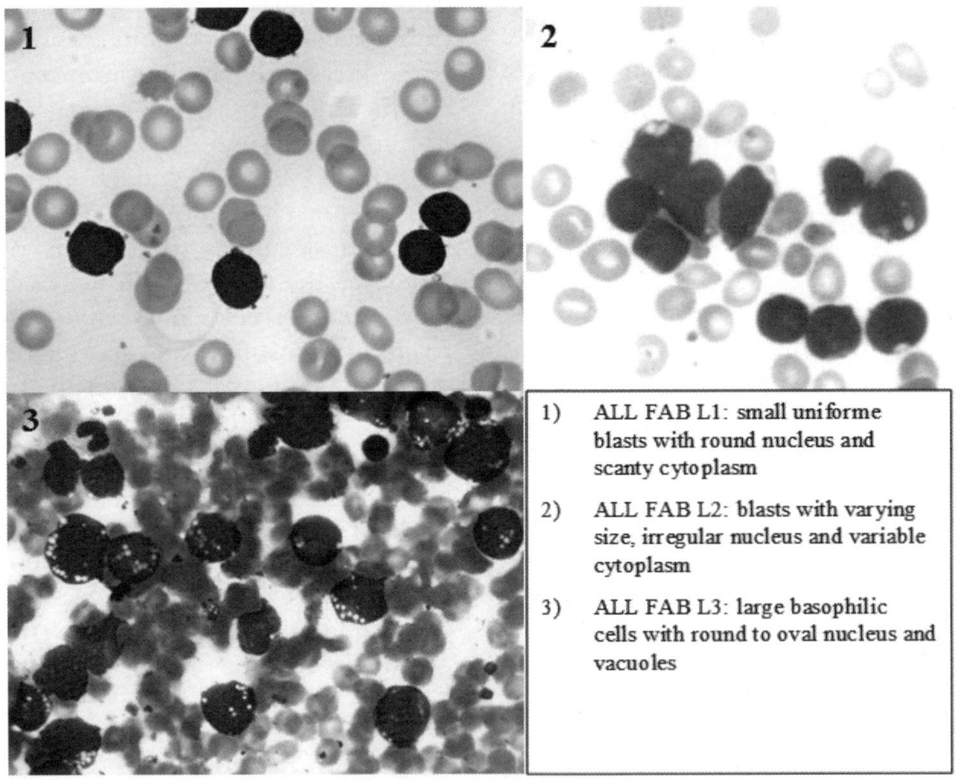

Fig. 11.1. Morphological classification of acute lymphoblastic leukemia. Morphological classification of acute lymphoblastic leukemia from bone marrow according to the French-American-British (FAB) classification is illustrated.

From Bennett JM, Catovski D, Daniel MT, Flandrin G, Galton DAG, Gralnick HR, Sultan C. (1976) Proposals for the classification of the acute leukaemias. French-American-British (FAB) cooperative group. *Br J Haematol* **33**: 451–458.[35]

regular nuclei, fine-to-slightly coarse chromatin, frequent multiple nucleoli and basophilic cytoplasm. Vacuolization is frequent but not a defining characteristic.[35] FAB L3 corresponds to the mature B-cell ALL immunophenotype (Burkitt's leukemia) and is associated with chromosomal rearrangements involving the *MYC* gene on chromosome 8q24. This subtype, which represents approximately 2% of all ALL cases, possesses the same biological traits and chemotherapy sensitivity as Burkitts lymphomas. Thus, patients with this specific form of ALL must be treated according to protocols for Burkitts lymphoma.

Cytochemistry

ALL blasts are periodic acid-schiff (PAS)-positive in about 50% of cases, usually in the form of coarse granules and myeloperoxidase (MPO) negative, which may be used to distinguish ALL from AML.

Immunophenotyping

Immunophenotyping of leukemic lymphoblasts by multiparameter flow cytometry is essential to establish the correct diagnosis by distinguishing ALL from AML and by defining the correct immunophenotypic subtype of ALL (Fig. 11.2).[36,37] In Europe, the EGIL Classification (European Group for the Immunological Classification of Leukemia's) is well accepted.[38] Precursor B-cell ALL (pB-ALL) cells are typically CD79a, CD19, CD10, CD34 and TdT positive. Precursor B-cell blasts do not express surface immunoglobulin (slg). Cytoplasmic μ heavy chain proteins are found in the pre-B cell subtype. For T-cell ALL, the immunophenotype also varies, but most are cyCD3, CD7, TdT and CD34 positive (Table 11.2). T-cell ALL originating from early T-cell precursors (ETPs) are characterized by a distinctive immunophenotype (CD1a(–), CD8(–), CD5(weak) with stem cell or myeloid markers) and an ETP typical gene expression signature. These cases show an increased genomic instability, in terms of number and size of genetic lesions, compared to those with typical T-ALL. Patients with ETP-ALL have a high risk for remission failure and for hematological relapse (up to 72% cumulative incidence of relapse at 10 years vs. 10% at 10 years for patients with typical T-ALL).[39]

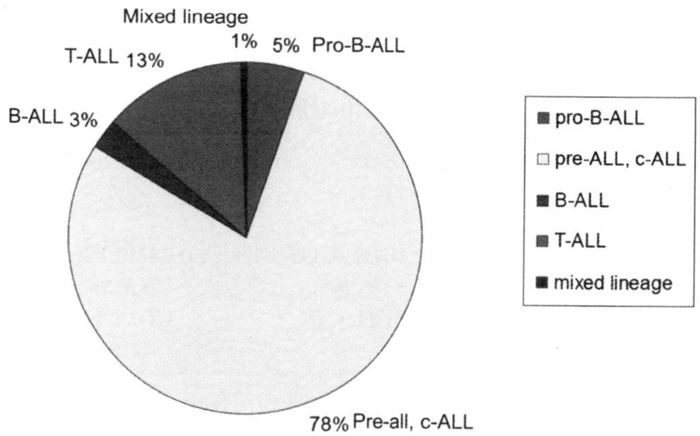

Fig. 11.2. Distribution of immunological subtypes in childhood ALL. From Ludwig WD, Teichmann JV, Sperling C, Komischke B, Ritter J, Reiter A, Odenwald E, Sauter S, Riehm H. (1990) Incidence, clinical markers and prognostic significance of immunologic subtypes of acute lymphoblastic leukemia (ALL) in children: experiences of the ALL-BFM 83 and 86 studies. *Klin Pediatr* **202**: 243–252.[37]

A scoring system has been devised to distinguish the rare, true biphenotypic acute leukemia from the more common single lineage acute leukemia with co-expression of markers from other lineages (Table 11.3).[40] Flow cytometry may also be used to assess response to therapy.[41–46]

Table 11.2. Classification of acute lymphoblastic leukemia by immunophenotype.[a]

	B-cell precursor ALL				T cell lineage ALL			
	Pro-B	**Common**	**Pre-B**	**B**	**Pro-T**	**Pre-T**	**Cortical**	**Mature**
Progenitor-Antigens								
TdT	+	+	+	–	+	+	+	+/–
HLA-DR	+	+	+	+	+/–	–	–	–
CD10	–	+	+/–	+/–	+/–	+/–	+/–	–
B-cell-Antigens								
CD19	+	+	+	+	–	–	–	–
CD22	+	+	+	+	–	–	–	–
CD79a	+	+	+	+	–	–	–	–
cylgM	–	–	+	–	–	–	–	–
slg	–	–	–	+	–	–	–	–
T-cell-Antigens								
cyCD3	–	–	–	–	+	+	+/–	–
CD7	–	–	–	–	+	+	+	+
CD2	–	–	–	–	–	+	+	+
CD1a	–	–	–	–	–	–	+	–
mCD3	–	–	–	–	–	–	+/–	+

[a]Immunphenotypic classification of acute lymphoblastic leukemia is shown according to the criteria of the European Group (EGIL).

From Bene MC, Castoldi G, Knapp W, Ludwig WD, Matutes E, Orfao A, van't Veer MB. (1995) Proposals for the immunological classification of acute leukaemias. European group for the immunological characterisation of leukaemias (EGIL). *Leukemia* **9**(10): 1783–1786.[38]

Table 11.3. EGIL scoring system for biphenotypic acute leukemia.[a]

Points	B-cell markers	T-cell markers	Myeloid markers
2	CD79α Cyt IgM Cyt CD22	CD3 TCR	Anti-MPO
1	CD19, CD10, CD20	CD2, CD5, CD8, CD10	CD13, CD33, CD65, CD117
0.5	TdT, CD24	TdT, CD7, CD1a	CD14, CD15, CD64

[a]Score must be >2 points for the myeloid as well as for one of the lymphatic phenotype.

cyt: cytoplasmatic, m: membranous.

From Bene MC. (2009) Biphenotypic, bilineal, ambiguous or mixed lineage: strange leukemias! *Haematologica* **94**: 891–893.[40]

Cyto- and molecular genetics

As already mentioned, most cases of ALL are characterized by clonal genetic abnormalities such as translocations, deletions, and additions. The detection of these leukemia-specific characteristics based on various techniques, such as fluorescence *in situ* hybridization (FISH) and polymerase chain reaction (PCR) has become an essential part of the diagnostic evaluation for acute leukemias. It is not only relevant for making the diagnosis of an ALL but also has important implications with respect to the treatment subsequently given: The characterization of the molecular subtype is essential to identify both patients with a higher risk of treatment failure and those with a low risk of relapse (Table 11.4) in order to choose the appropriate therapy.

Specific genetics

In more than 70% of ALL cases, specific genetic aberrations can be found in the ALL blasts. The majority of chromosomal aberrations are balanced, mostly translocations, rarely inversions. Other aberrations are changes in the number of chromosomes of blasts like hyper- and hypodiploidy.

Number of chromosomes

Hyperdiploidy, defined by > 50 chromosomes per cell or a DNA index ≥ 1.16 and ≥ 1.6, is characterized by additional copies of whole chromosomes. The number of chromosomes varies between 51 and 63, while trisomies or tetrasomies are preferentially found for chromosomes 4, 10, 17, 18 and 21. Hyperdiploidy occurs in 20–25% of pB-ALL cases and is rarely found in T-cell ALL. It is usually associated with a favorable outcome.[47] Hypodiploidy occurs when the chromosome number ≤ 45 chromosomes. The majority of hypodiploid leukemias show exactly 45 chromosomes and have a significantly better outcome than cases with fewer than 45 chromosomes. In general, there seems to be a trend for a progressively worse outcome with a decreasing number of chromosomes in hypodiploid ALL.[48] In some cases, the predominant clone is hyperdiploid, representing a duplication of the near haploid hypodiploid clone, e.g. a modal clone with 50 chromosomes masking the subclone with 25 chromsomes.[49]

Chromosomal translocations

The detection of ALL-specific chromosomal translocations by FISH or RT-PCR is an essential part of the

Table 11.4. Frequency and prognosis of chromosome aberrations in acute lymphoblastic leukemia.[a]

Chromosome Ab.	Molecular Gen.	Frequency	Leukemia	Prognosis
t(1;19)(q23;p13)	*E2A/PBX1*	5%	Pre-B ALL	Intermediate-good
t(4;11)(q21;q23)	*MLL/AF4*	4%	Pro-B ALL	Poor
t(11;19)(q23;p13)	*MLL/ENL*	4%	Pro-B ALL	Poor
t(12,21)(p13;q22)	*TEL/AML1*	20–25%	Common ALL	Good
Hyperdiploidy >50	diverse	20–25%	Common ALL	Good
t(9;22)(q34;q11)	*BCR/ABL*	3%	Common ALL	Poor
Hypodiploidy <45	diverse	1%	Common ALL	Poor
14q11-Aberration	TCRα/TCRβ	5–10%	T-cell ALL	Intermediate
t(10;14)(q24q11)	*HOX11*	5–10% (of T-cell ALL)	T-cell ALL	Not unfavorable
t(8;14)(q24;q11)	*MYC*	2% (of T-cell ALL)	T-cell ALL	Unclear
t(1;14)(p32;q11)	*TAL1*	3% (of T-cell ALL)	T-cell ALL	Unclear

[a]www.infobiogen.fr/services/chromcancer/

Ab.: Aberration; Gen.: Genetics.

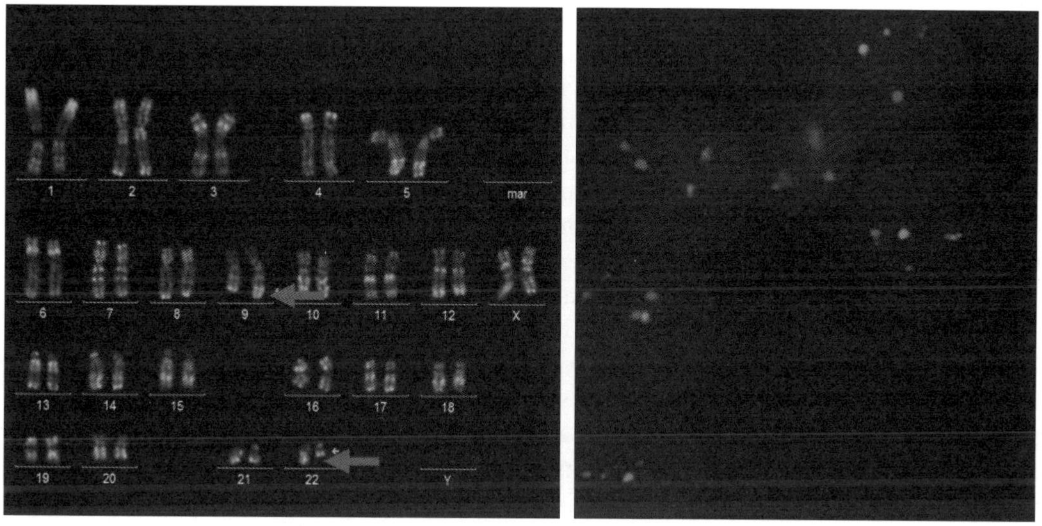

(A) (B)

Fig. 11.3. Cytogenetic and FISH results of a Philadelphia positive acute lymphoblastic leukemia. (A) cytogenetic report: 46,XX,t(9;22)(q34;q11). (B) FISH report: nuc ish 9q34 (ABL × 3), 22q11 (BCR × 3)(ABL con BCR × 2). Kindly provided by L. Harder, Institute of Human Genetics, University of Kiel and University Medical Center, Germany.

diagnostic panel. Karyotype alone may miss a substantial number of patients with abnormalities.[50] The panel includes the detection of the translocation t(9;22) and *BCR/ABL* rearrangement (Fig. 11.3), the detection of *MLL* rearrangements on chromosome 11q23 (e.g. translocation t(4;11)), and the detection of the translocation t(12;21) and *TEL/AML1* rearrangement. The translocation t(1;19) and *E2A/PBX1* rearrangement, respectively, is often included in the screening panel. The frequency of chromosomal translocations in ALL is about 3% for translocation t(9;22), 4% for translocation t(4;11), 5% for translocation t(1;19) and 20–25% for translocation t(12;21).[51] The outcome of cases with intrachromosomal amplication of AML1 on chromosome 21 is a matter of current debate.[52]

Whereas both the *BCR/ABL* and the *MLL/AF4* rearrangements have been associated with a poor prognosis, B-precursor ALL with translocation t(12;21) have a very favorable prognosis with survival rates of more than 90%. When treated according to modern therapeutic regimen, the *E2A/PBX1* rearrangement seems to be associated with a favorable outcome as well.[51,53,54]

Clinical Presentation and Diagnosis

The initial clinical presentation of a child with ALL depends on the extent of the leukemic infiltration of the BM and any extramedullary sites. Because leukemic blasts replace normal BM, symptoms result from anemia, thrombocytopenia, and granulocytopenia with or without concomitant leukocytosis. Typical clinical signs are fever, pallor, petechiae, bleeding, fatigue, and an enlargement of lymph nodes, especially cervical and neck lymph nodes. Abdominal pain can be attributed to an enlargement of the liver and spleen, an invagination or an ileus, associated with an abdominal lymph node bulge. Bone pain results from infiltration of blasts in the bone and periostium. Children aged 2–4 years may present with a sudden aversion to walking. Bone pain may lead to the consideration of osteomyelitis or rheumatoid arthritis. The compression of the trachea or bronchi due to an enlargement of the mediastinal lymph nodes and thymus may result in orthopnea or dyspnea. This presentation is especially common in T-cell ALL and can be life threatening. Headache and cerebral nerve palsies may be symptoms of CNS involvement; painless enlargement of the testes may indicate substantial testicular infiltration.

The diagnosis of ALL is usually made by the cytomorphological examination of PB or BM smears. The diagnosis is established when at least 25% lymphoblasts are present in the BM. In some cases, BM aspiration can fail and a Jamshidi needle biopsy may be needed if diagnosis cannot be made on PB smears. In some situations, preliminary diagnosis may follow the examination of a pleural effusion. However, a BM examination is still required to distinguish leukemia from lymphoma. Initial evaluation is further complemented by flow cytometric immunophenotyping and cytogenetics,

FISH and/or molecular genetic techniques to verify the diagnosis and to define the biological subgroup.

Successful treatment of childhood ALL requires sufficient central nervous system (CNS)-directed therapy to treat any occult or overt CNS leukemia as well as to prevent later relapses originating from the CNS. The intensity of CNS-directed therapy depends on the degree of initial CNS infiltration. By definition, overt CNS involvement (CNS3) is diagnosed if more than 5 cells/μl are counted in the cerebrospinal fluid (CSF) and blasts are present on the CSF cytospin. If CSF cell count is ≤ 5 cells/μl (with presence of blasts) the disease is classified as CNS2. In case of a traumatic lumbar puncture (TLP), as defined by either visual blood contamination or ≥ 10 erythrocytes/μl CSF, one has to distinguish those with and without identifiable blasts: The CNS status is categorized as TLP+ if blasts are present and as TLP– if blasts are not present. Intracerebral infiltrates, detected by the magnetic resonance imaging (MRI) and cerebral nerve palsies, are also used as proof of CNS involvement; however, isolated occurrence without abnormal CSF is rare. Known risk factors for CNS involvement include T-cell immunophenotype, a high white blood cell (WBC) count, and presence of translocations t(9;22) and t(4;11). Very recently, a high *IL-15* gene expression was found to be associated with CNS involvement at diagnosis and with CNS relapse in ALL.[55]

An early chest X-ray is mandatory to exclude mediastinal mass and the threat of respiratory compromise as previously mentioned. Ultrasound examination may be useful to assess leukemic involvement of abdominal organs and lymph nodes, to exclude a post-renal obstruction, and to assess the involvement of testes.

Treatment of Primary Childhood ALL

Introduction

Since the early 1960s, treatment results in childhood ALL have improved continuously, reaching an overall cure rate of about 80–90% in developed countries (Fig. 11.4). National and international multicenter clinical trials have addressed important treatment questions in randomized trials with adequate patient numbers. The drugs in current use were developed between 1950 and 1970. Better usage has led to better outcomes over 40 years. Major efforts to identify new antileukemic agents continue.

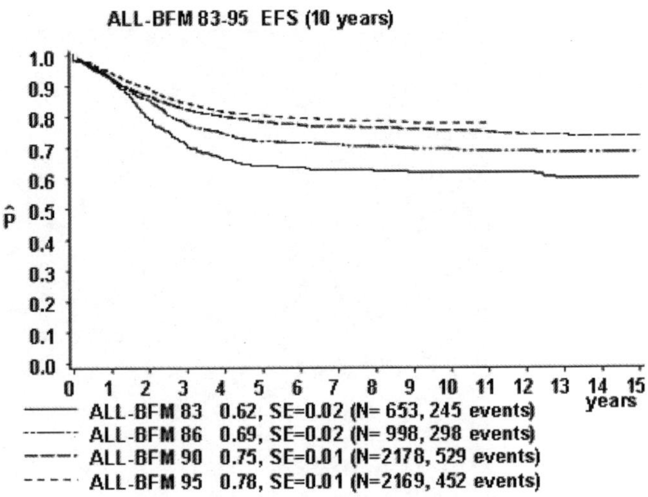

Fig. 11.4. Kaplan-Meier estimate of event-free survival of patients included in trials ALL-BFM 83, 86, 90, and 95.

Treatment is allocated according to an estimate of a patient's individual risk of relapse, as determined by presenting clinical features, extramedullary disease, immunophenotype, and cytogenetics, and response to treatment. Higher risk patients receive more aggressive therapy. Although a large majority of children and adolescents are now being cured, a significant number of patients still suffer disease recurrence and treatment toxicity. Most patients with ALL and relapse ultimately succumb to the disease, despite high second remission rates and intensive treatments including hematopoietic stem cell transplant.

Stratification strategies

The reasons for treatment failure remain to be elucidated but a wide range of leukemic biological features correlate with outcome. Less well-defined host factors also likely influence treatment success. A variety of different treatment regimens provide similar outcomes for similar patients. With the current exceptions of Burkitts lymphoma therapy for FAB L3 leukemia and a tyrosine kinase inhibitors for Philadelphia chromosome positive ALL, therapy remains rather uniform despite the vast heterogeneity of childhood ALL. In modern protocols, patients are stratified into different risk groups based on their estimated risk of relapse and assigned to treatments of varying intensity. For some patients with an exceptionally high risk of CNS relapse, radiotherapy may be applied. Patients, at very high risk for relapse despite the most intensive conventional chemotherapy, may be referred for HSCT in first remission. These may include translocations t(9;22) and t(4;11), severe hypodiploidy and an inadequate response to therapy such as induction failure or persistence of high levels of occult leukemia beyond 3 months into therapy. Less consensus exists for the following potential indications, namely, T-cell ALL, translocation t(9;11), CNS involvement/and or a TLP+, WBC ≥ 50,000/μl, age ≥ 10 years and an age < 1 year.[56]

In the German-Italian-Austrian-Swiss AIEOP-BFM ALL 2000 protocol risk-adapted treatment stratification (standard- (SR), intermediate- (IR), or high-risk (HR)) was performed using cytogenetic markers (t(9;22), t(4;11)) or their molecular equivalents (*BCR/ABL* and *MLL/AF4*) and the *in vivo* response to treatment.[7] Response was assessed by microscopy, looking at the initial peripheral blood (PB) cytoreduction after intrathecal methotrexate (MTX) and 7 days of prednisone ("prednisone response", PR) and BM blast clearance after induction therapy on treatment day 33, and by PCR, assessing the level of submicroscopic "minimal residual disease" (MRD) on treatment-day 33 and after week 12.[57] Besides positivity for *BCR/ABL* or *MLL/AF4* rearrangements, patients are assigned to the HR group by a poor PR, a non-response on treatment day 33 and a high MRD load after induction consolidation at week 12 (see Chapter 10). Table 11.5 summarizes the prognostic factors and Table 11.6 the event-free survival (EFS) of clinical subgroups treated according to the previous trial ALL-BFM 95.[4]

The Children's Oncology Group (COG) in the USA stratifies patients at diagnosis based on age and presenting WBC count. At the end of induction, risk stratification is then refined based on the presence of extramedullary disease, chromosomal aberrations, early treatment response as assessed cytomorphologically on days 7 and 14, and by end-induction MRD measurement by flow cytometry on day 29.[3] Future COG trials will use day 8 PB and end of induction BM response only, assessed by flow cytometry. The Dutch Childhood Leukemia Study Group (DCLSG) stratifies patients in their protocol ALL-9 (1997–2004) into a non-high risk (NHR) and an HR group. NHR patients have an initial WBC count < 50,000/μl, no mediastinal mass, no initial CNS involvement, no testicular disease, no T-cell immunophenotype, no translocation t(9;22) or *BCR/ABL* rearrangement and absence of 11q23 abnormalities with *MLL* rearrangement.[58] The Dana-Farber Cancer Institute (DFCI) ALL Consortium Protocols (1985–2000) stratifies patients into three groups. SR-, HR, VHR-group based on age, WBC count, immunophenotype, presence of initial CNS disease, mediastinal mass or translocation t(9;22).[59]

Treatment

Successful treatment of children with ALL requires the control of systemic and extramedullary disease, particularly the involvement of the CNS. Standard therapy regimes include four phases: an *induction*

Table 11.5. Prognostic factors in childhood acute lymphoblastic leukemia.

Factor	Favorable prognostic factors	Unfavorable prognostic factors
Age at diagnosis	≥ 1 and < 10 years	< 1 or ≥ 10 years
Gender	Female	Male
WBC at diagnosis	< 50,000/μl	> 50,000/μl
Immunophenotype		
	CD10+ precursor B-cell ALL	CD10− precursor B-cell ALL
CNS status	CNS negative	CNS positive, TLP+
Genetic features	Hyperdiploidy	Hypodiploidy
	TEL/AML1 positivity	t(9;22) or *BCR/ABL* positivity
		t(4;11) or *MLL/AF4* positivity
Prednisone response	< 1000/μl blasts in peripheral blood	≥ 1000/μl blasts in peripheral blood
Remissions status[a]	< 5% blasts	≥ 5%
MRD[b]	≤ 10^{-4} after 5 weeks of treatment	≥ 10^{-3} after 12 weeks of treatment

[a]After 4 to 5 week of treatment.
[b]Minimal residual disease in the bone marrow assessed by molecular genetic techniques.

CNS: central nervous system; MRD: minimal residual disease; TLP+: traumatic lumbar puncture with identifiable blasts; WBC: white blood cells.

Table 11.6. Six-year event-free survival (EFS) of clinical subgroups treated according to the ALL-BFM 95 protocol.

Age	n	%	EFS	Initial WBC count (/μl)	n	%	EFS
< 1 year	34	1.6	40%	< 10,000	1071	49.4	84%
1–6 years	1255	57.9	84%	10,000–< 20,000	319	14.7	84%
6–< 10 years	447	20.6	80%	20,000–< 50,000	362	16.7	79%
10–< 15 years	340	15.7	71%	50,000–< 100,000	180	8.3	74%
15 years and older	93	4.3	58%	100,000–< 200,000	111	5.1	63%
				200,000 and over	126	5.8	53%
CNS Status				**Gender**			
CNS1	1717	90,7	81%	Male	1226	56.5	78%
CNS2	112	5.9	80%	Female	943	43.5	81%
CNS3	64	3.4	58%				
Immunophenotype				**Prednisone response**			
Precursor B-cell ALL	1708	86.5	80%	Good	1963	91.4	82%
T-cell ALL	277	13.3	75%	Poor	184	8.6	55%
Genetics				**Therapy response**			
TEL/AML1 positive	916	78.6	91%	BM day 15 M1	880	61.5	87%
TEL/AML1 negative	250	21.4	75%	BM day 15 M2	365	25.5	76%
				BM day 15 M3	186	13.0	47%
BCR/ABL positive	42	2.1	26%				
BCR/ABL negative	1918	97.9	80%	Nonremission day 33	49	2.3	36%
				Remission day 33	2120	97.7	81%
MLL/AF4 positive	25	2.1	40%				
MLL/AF4 negative	1154	97.9	77%				

BM: bone marrow; CNS: central nervous system; n: number of patients; WBC: white blood count.

Adapted from Moricke A, Reiter A, Zimmermann M, Gadner H, Stanulla M, Dordelmann M, Loning L, Beier R, Ludwig WD, Ratei R, Harbott J, Boos J, Mann G, Niggli F, Feldges A, Henze G, Welte K, Beck JD, Klingebiel T, Niemeyer C, Zintl F, Bode U, Urban C, Wehinger H, Niethammer D, Riehm H, Schrappe M. (2008) Risk-adjusted therapy of acute lymphoblastic leukemia can decrease treatment burden and improve survival: Treatment results of 2169 unselected pediatric and adolescent patients enrolled in the trial ALL-BFM 95. *Blood* **111**: 4477–4489.[4]

phase aiming at the disappearance of all obvious leukemia and recovery of peripheral counts; the consolidation/extracompartment treatment phase; the re-induction phase and finally the maintenance phase to further stabilize achieved remission by suppressing re-emergence of drug resistant clones through continuing repression of residual leukemic cells. Overall, the intensive treatment period takes about 6–9 months, the less intensive maintenance treatment phase lasts between 1.5 and 3 years.

Treatment elements

Induction

The aim of the induction phase is to induce a complete remission (CR), i.e. less than 5% marrow blasts with a restoration of normal hematopoiesis within 4–6 weeks, and to achieve a stable general state of health. A CR is achieved in about 98% of patients with rare deaths from infection or bleeding and rare induction failures. Three drugs, vincristine (VCR), a glucocorticoid (GC, prednisone (PRED) or dexamethasone (DEX)), and asparaginase (ASP), comprise induction. In some regimens, an anthracycline, is added as a fourth drug. Based on the lack of efficacy of daunomycin for standard risk (SR) patients receiving Protocol II or delayed intensification on CCG-105, COG utilizes a three drug regimen (DEX, VCR and ASP) for standard-risk B precursor patients, while HR patients receive an anthracycline and PRED instead of DEX.[60] In other protocols like the Berlin-Frankfurt-Münster (BFM) protocols, anthracyclines are a part of induction therapy for all patients. The contribution of anthracyclines in lower risk patients remains controversial.[1] Cyclophosphamide (CP) and an intensive use of ASP may be beneficial for patients with T-cell immunophenotype.[5]

The BFM protocols start with one intrathecal dose of MTX on treatment day 1 and 7 days of oral or intravenous (IV) PRED "monotherapy" which may diminish complications of tumor lysis syndrome. Moreover, the "prednisone response" (PR) on treatment day 8 is used for later regimen assignment. Treatment then continues with a 4-drug induction followed by early intensification with IV CP and cytarabine (ARA-C), and oral 6-mercaptopurine (6-MP).

The choice of the better GC (PRED vs. DEX) in induction and the truly equivalent doses are still controversial. Many regimens have tested induction DEX; results from diverse trials indicate patients treated with DEX may have a better EFS due to a lower number of systemic and CNS relapses.[3,58,59,61] The CNS effect is attributed to DEX's longer half-life and better CNS penetration. Table 11.7 summarizes three randomized trials comparing DEX and PRED.[62–64] While DEX may be more effective than PRED, data also suggest that DEX is associated with an increased toxicity, especially in the context of 4-drug induction regimens. Reports showed patients treated with DEX have an increased frequency of bacterial and fungal infections in the induction phase with an increasing mortality, especially in adolescent patients.[65] DEX half-life may be increased in adolescents, contributing to excess morbidity.[66] An increased risk of severe symptomatic osteonecrosis with a cumulative incidence of 8.9% among young people older than 10 years seems to be an important late side effect of extensive GC in general.[67]

Similar to the use of GC, the preparation of asparaginase (ASP) utilized differs among protocols. Several forms of ASP (native and pegylated *E. coli* L-ASP, native Erwinia L-ASP) are available and have different pharmacokinetics. Several preparations are provided by more than one manufacturer and have differing pharmacokinetics. However, with respect to disease control, appropriate dose intensity and the duration of treatment are more important than the type of the drug used. PEG-ASP is an alternative form of ASP in which the *E. coli* enzyme is modified by the covalent attachment of polyethylene glycol. PEG-ASP has a 4–5-fold longer serum half-life than native *E. coli*-ASP, with commensurate asparagine depletion. In case of neutralizing and/or an allergic reaction, many switch to an alternative product (typically from naïve *E. coli*-ASP to PEG-ASP to Erwinia-ASP). Some recommend that ASP activity be monitored to assure adequate dosing.[68] Table 11.8 summarizes a number of randomized trials examining ASP. Two trials, EORTC 58881[69] and DFCI 95–01, found inferior EFS when shorter half-life Erwinia-ASP was used at the same dose and scheduled as longer half-life *E. coli*-ASP. Erwinia was associated with fewer ASP-related side effects. Subsequently, the Medical Research Council of the United Kingdom mandated a change to native *E. coli*-ASP and outcomes improved.[61] Two trials, DFCI 91–01 and CCG-1962, compared native and pegylated *E. coli*-ASP and found similar outcomes. Intramuscular PEG *E. coli*-ASP was associated with a reduced risk of hypersensitivity. In COG, PEG *E. coli*-ASP has safely and effectively replaced native *E. coli*-ASP, avoiding about 100 intramuscular injections a day for the 2000 COG ALL patients per year.[3,70] The current DFCI study 2005–01 compares weekly intramuscular native *E. coli*-ASP with intravenous biweekly PEG *E. coli*-ASP.[59,71]

Table 11.7. Randomized studies comparing prednisone vs. dexamethasone.

Trial	n	GC administration in protocol	GC dose	Outcome (%) EFS	Outcome (%) CNS[a]	Ref.
CALGB 7111 (1971–1974)	646	Induction: days 1–28 (or days 1–21, 1–28) Maintenance: 7-day pulses	PRED 40 ($mg/m^2/d$) DEX 6 ($mg/m^2/d$)	— —	25.5 14.3	62
CCG 1922 (1993–1995)	1060	Induction: days 1–28 Consolidation: 5-day pulses Maintenance: 5-day pulses	PRED 40 ($mg/m^2/d$) DEX 6 ($mg/m^2/d$)	6y: 77 6y: 82	7.1 3.7	63
UK MRC ALL97 and ALL97/99 (1997–2002)	1603	Induction: days 1–28 (ALL97) Induction: days 1–29 (ALL97/99) Interim-Maintenance: 5-day pulses Maintenance: 5-day pulses	PRED 40 ($mg/m^2/d$) DEX 6.5 ($mg/m^2/d$)	5y: 76 5y: 83	5.3 2.2	64

[a]Isolated CNS relapse rates.

CNS: central nervous system; DEX: dexamethasone; EFS: event-free survival; GC: glucocorticoids; PRED: prednisone; Ref.: Reference; n: number of patients included in the study.

Table 11.8. Selected randomized trials comparing the type of asparaginase.

Trial	Risk group/n	ASP administration	Outcome	Ref.
EORTC 58881 (1990–1993)	All patients, n = 700	*E. coli* ASP 25,000 IU/m^2 weekly Erwinia ASP 25,000 IU/m^2 weekly	6yEFS: 73.4% 6yEFS: 59.8%	69
DFCI 91–01 (1991–1996)	All patients, n = 198	*E. coli* ASP 25,000 IU/m^2 weekly PEG ASP 2,500 IU/m^2 biweekly	5yEFS: 84% 5yEFS: 79%	59
DFCI 95–01 (1996–2000)	All patients, n = 286	*E. coli* ASP 25,000 IU/m^2 weekly Erwinia ASP 25,000 IU/m^2 weekly	5yEFS: 88% 5yEFS: 78%	59
CCG-1962 (1997–1998)	SR patients, n = 118	*E. coli* ASP 6000 IU/m^2 3 times per week (9 doses in induction, 6 doses in each DI) PEG ASP 2500 IU/m^2 day 3 of induction and each of 2 DI phases	3yEFS: 85% 3yEFS: 88%	70

ASP: asparaginase; DI: delayed intensification; EFS: event-free survival; Ref.: Reference; n: number of patients SR: standard risk.

Unlike many adult ALL regimens, most pediatric regimens provide early intrathecal therapy, starting in induction. Patients usually receive either MTX alone or in combination with ARA-C and hydrocortisone as a "triple therapy". COG protocols employ day 1 intrathecal ARA-C as MTX excretion may be delayed by renal impairment from tumor lysis syndrome.

Approximately 2–4% patients do not reach a CR after treatment induction within 4–6 weeks, either having a non-responsive resistant disease or having died due to disease complications or treatment toxicity. Patients with a resistant disease have a poor prognosis and must receive a more intensive therapy to have a chance to be cured. Some of these patients may have a benefit from SCT once a CR is achieved.[72]

Consolidation/extracompartment therapy and reinduction

Although most patients are in morphologic remission at the end of induction, most have detectable residual leukemia by PCR and all will relapse if therapy is halted. In the past, simply extending the two most effective induction agents, VCR and GC, did not delay relapse substantially.[73] Improvements in the first 6 months of post-induction therapy are responsible for most of the gains of the last 30 years. Post-induction intensification improves disease control in extramedullary sites. On CCG-105 replacement of cranial irradiation with extended intrathecal MTX was possible only with intensified post-induction therapy.[74]

Post-induction intensification differs among cooperative groups in terms of chemotherapeutic drugs, dose, number of doses, the application time and the overall treatment context.[1] Most protocols include some form of parenteral MTX. COG has employed escalating-dose intravenous MTX to good effect.[75,76] Others have employed higher dose parenteral MTX 1–5 g/m^2 with folinic acid (leukovorin) rescue. The leucovorin rescue must not be given too soon after the application of MTX or at too high dosage because it may counteract its antileukemic effect. Parallel to the IV MTX, children receive intrathecal MTX to assure prolonged cytotoxic levels in the CSF. In addition to MTX, patients often receive 6-MP and/or 6 months of continuous ASP administration, depending on the protocol.[3,6,58,59,77,78] Currently, COG is comparing escalating dose and high-dose MTX for T-cell and higher risk B-precursor patients.

Reinduction

This phase, termed Protocol II or Delayed Intensification (DI), represents a modified repetition of the initial induction phase and contributes greatly to successful ALL treatment.[79–81] Introduced by the BFM group in trial ALL-BFM 76, it has been employed successively around the world for over one-third of a century. An attempt to omit the reinduction in low-risk patients resulted in a clear decrease of EFS.[6,82]

The Children's Cancer Group built on this experience. CCG-1882 showed an advantage for longer and stronger post-induction intensification for higher risk patients with a slow day 7 response.[83] Hospital days saved by prevented relapses more than made up for the additional hospital days incurred by "Augmented" therapy.[84] Two recent randomized trials suggest that the strength of intensification may be more important than length.[76] With better outcomes for adolescents and young adults,[85] osteonecrosis has emerged as a major challenge.[10] Dexamethasone exposure in DI has been decreased to two 7-day courses, 1 week apart, for older children with preservation of outcomes and halving the incidence of clinical osteonecrosis.[76]

Maintenance

Childhood ALL is unique in its requirement for prolonged therapy. The aim of the maintenance therapy is preventing re-emergence of a drug-resistant clone through continuous repression of potential residual leukemic cells. The duration of maintenance therapy differs depending on the study protocol and lasts between 2–3 years.[3,6,58,59,78]

For the past 50 years, daily oral 6-MP and weekly oral MTX have comprised the most commonly employed maintenance therapy. These drugs act synergistically as MTX inhibits the *de novo* synthesis of purines, leading to a higher intracellular availability and increased incorporation of phosphorylated thiopurines in DNA and RNA.[86] Doses of 6-MP and MTX are adjusted according to the total leukocyte or absolute neutrophil count and platelet cell counts. Many investigators target a leukocyte count below 3000/μl and neutrophil counts between 500 and 1500/μl to ensure optimal dose intensity. 6-MP is best given in the evening hours, for unknown reasons, and not in proximity to milk as milk's xanthine oxidase activity can decrease the bioavailability. Relling *et al.* found EFS improved with increased intensity of 6-MP therapy. Therapy interruptions for neutropenia-eroded intensity more than under-dosing.[87]

Homozygous polymorphmisms of thiopurine S-methyltransferase (TPMT), an enzyme that catabolizes 6-MP, results in severe toxicity with conventional dosage (Chapter 9). Thus, the dose of 6-MP must be substantially lower in these patients as compared to those with wild type or those heterozygous for mutant TPMT alleles. Patients who are heterozygous generally tolerate 6-MP without serious toxicity but also receive, on average, lower doses than patients who have a normal enzyme activity.[88] Unfortunately, patients with normal TPMT may still have excessive myelosuppression with conventional dosage.

6-thioguanine (6-TG) is about one log more active than 6-MP *in vitro* and provides potentially useful CSF penetration. With isotoxic dosing, red cell levels of 6-TG nucleotide are 4–6-fold higher with 6-TG than those with 6-MP. This striking but irrelevant difference follows red cell's lack of inosine monophosphate dehydrogenase, the enzyme that converts 6-MP to 6-TG. This enzyme is present in leukocytes. 6-TG is included in Protocol II. Several trials compared 6-MP and 6-TG in maintenance. Only CCG-1952 found any outcome advantage, which seemed restricted to boys. The use of 6-TG leads to an increased risk of hepatic complications. Table 11.9 summarizes three randomized trials comparing 6-MP and 6-TG. Hepatic complications including veno-occlusive disease and portal hypertension, profound thrombocytopenia and an increased risk of death in remission were seen in patients who received 6-TG.[2,89–91] Thus, 6-MP remains the thiopurine of choice.

Pulses of VCR and corticosteroids are often added to 6-MP and MTX, however, any effect on treatment outcome remains controversial. A large randomized multicenter "prospective meta-analysis" trial revealed no

Table 11.9. Selected randomized trials comparing 6-mercaptopurine and 6-thioguanine.

Trial	Risk group/n	Dose (mg/m²/d)	Outcome	Toxicity of 6-TG	Ref.
COALL-92	All patients, n = 474	6-MP 75	6.6yEFS: 79%		89
(1992–1997)		6-TG 50/40[a]	6.6yEFS: 78%	Prolongated myelosuppression with thrombocytopenia	
CCG-1952	SR patients, n = 2026	6-MP 75	7yEFS: 79% OS: 91%		90
(1996–2000)		6-TG 50/40[a]	7yEFS: 84% OS: 92%	VOD: 20% of patients	
UK MRC ALL97	All patients, n = 1498	6-MP 75	6.6yEFS: 81%		91
and ALL97/99 (1997–2002)		6-TG 40	6.6yEFS: 80%	Features of VOD: 11% of patients Increased risk of death due to infections	

[a]Dose reduction during trial due to side-effects.

6-MP: 6-mercaptopurine; 6-TG: 6-thioguanine; EFS: event-free survival; OS: overall survival; Ref.: Reference; n: number of patients; SR: standard risk; VOD: veno-occlusive disease.

benefit in the context of modern BFM-based therapy.[92] Curiously, a smaller conventional European randomized study found benefit,[93] keeping this long simmering question alive.

The duration of the maintenance therapy is about 2–3 years. Reduction of the therapy to less than 2 years was associated with an increased risk of relapse.[6] Longer therapy seems more advantageous for standard risk than higher risk patients, B-precursor than T-cell patients, and boys than girls. Any advantage for three over two years of maintenance remains uncertain for any subgroup in the context of contemporary therapy.[1]

Treatment of the extramedullary disease

Only approximately 3–5% of patients have a detectable CNS involvement at presentation. However, before the introduction of CNS-directed therapy in the 1960s, more than 50% suffered from CNS relapse as the first site of treatment failure.[2] Therefore, all children with ALL now receive a CNS-directed therapy. Intrathecal MTX alone or in combination with ARA-C and hydrocortisone (triple intrathecal therapy, TIT), the systemic application of chemotherapeutic drugs with adequate CNS penetration like high-dose MTX, DEX and high-dose ARA-C and in some subgroups, cranial irradiation keep the CNS relapse rate below 5%.[3–5,58,59,77] The CCG-1952 trial compared intrathecal MTX alone with intrathecal triples (MTX, ARA-C and hydrocortisone) as presymptomatic CNS treatment for SR patients. Following remission induction, patients were randomized to receive MTX alone or TIT. Whereas the rate of relapses originating from the CNS was significantly lower in patients receiving TIT compared to those with MTX alone (3.4% ± 1.0 vs. 5.9% ± 1.2), significantly more BM and testes were observed in the TIT arm. Because the salvage rate after BM relapse is inferior to that after CNS relapse, the 6-year overall survival was 90.3% ± 1.5% for patients treated with TIT vs. 94.4% ± 1.1% for patients treated with MTX alone. Thus, TIT improved CNS control but did not improve overall outcome in the context of that study, which included no parenteral MTX.[3,94] More aggressive CNS-directed therapy, especially cranial irradiation, is associated with an increased acute toxicity (e.g. strokes, seizures, paralysis) and with more long-term sequals (e.g. leukoencephalopathy, impaired intellectual and psychomotor functioning, neuroendocrine system abnormalities, and secondary malignancies). Although the percentage of patients for whom cranial irradiation is currently applied has been reduced to 5–20%, further reduction without increasing the risk of CNS relapse is a major challenge (see Chapter 24).[95]

In present protocols, the intensity of the CNS-directed treatment is adjusted according to the risk of CNS relapse. T-cell ALL phenotype and hyperleucocytosis at diagnosis, the chromosomal aberrations t(9;22) or t(4;11), and the TLP+ status are associated with an increased risk of CNS involvement at presentation and subsequent CNS relapse.[1,2,95,96] The early intrathecal chemotherapy is critical for the prevention of CNS relapse and usually starts at the onset of induction therapy. Intrathecal therapy increases in the second month of therapy and often continues during reinduction and maintenance therapy. Patients with overt CNS disease at diagnosis and those with a high risk for CNS relapses, e.g. HR patients and T-cell ALL patients with a high WBC count, may receive cranial irradiation at a dose of 12 or 18 Gy (dose is dependent on the age of the patients and the individual risk profile). Patients at lesser risk with CNS2 status or patients with a TLP+ status may receive additional intrathecal therapy.

The reduction in the number of children receiving whole brain irradiation has been a major theme over the past 25 years. Very recently, results from the St. Jude Children's Research Hospital have shown that by applying an effective risk-adjusted chemotherapy prophylactic, cranial irradiation can be safely omitted.[97] However, only 14% of patients in the study reported on by Pui *et al.* would have received cranial irradiation in previous trials and randomized trials with larger numbers of patients and a longer follow-up period are needed.[98]

Treatment in subgroups

Over the years, therapy has been optimized over the entire population of young people with ALL. Several patient subgroups stand out with consistently inferior outcomes.

Philadelphia chromosome positive (Ph+) ALL

Overall, *BCR/ABL*-positive ALL accounts for only approximately 3% of children with ALL but these patients have a very poor prognosis.[4,51,59,99,100] The group of Ph+ ALL is heterogeneous with a different treatment sensitivity and different outcome. A good response to the PRED prophase, a low initial WBC count and a younger age at diagnosis are associated with a better prognosis. Allogeneic SCT from an HLA-matched related donor offered greater benefits than intensive chemotherapy alone (relative risk, 0.3; 95% confidence interval, 0.2 to 0.5; $P < 0.001$) before the advent of tyrosine kinase inhibitors but results were still not satisfactory.[99]

Tyrosine kinase inihibitors, like imatinib, appear to hold promise (see Chapter 22). Imatinib, an inhibitor of the protein tyrosine kinase, shows selectivity for the ABL protein tyrosine kinase, which is activated as a result of the *BCR/ABL* rearrangement. Imatinib has revolutionized the treatment of chronic myelogenous leukemia (CML). Imatinib therapy results in clinically relevant hematological response rates in relapsed or refractory Ph+ acute ALL patients as well.[101] Currently, a large international randomized trial of imatinib in Ph+ ALL is underway. Very recently, results from the COG showed an improved outcome in a cohort of 50 patients with cytoxic chemotherapy and continuous imatinib exposure plus. The 3-year EFS was 80% ± 11%, more than twice of the historical controls (35% ± 4%; $P < .0001$). Earlier cohorts, with the same cytotoxic chemotherapy and lesser imatinib were no better than historical controls. Interestingly, the 3-year EFS was higher for patients treated with chemotherapy plus imatinib (88% ± 11%) as compared to those with sibling donor BMT (57% ± 22%).[102]

ALL in infants

ALL in infants aged younger than 12 months is rare and comprises about 4% of childhood ALL (see Chapter 3). Although the CR rate is about 90%, the overall outcome is poor with an EFS between 30% and 45%.[6,61,77] Relapse, often early, is the major cause of treatment failure. Infant ALL is usually characterized by a high WBC count at diagnosis, a high frequency of an immature precursor B-cell immunophenotype characterized by the lack of CD10 expression (pro-B ALL), and the presence of *MLL* gene rearrangements. *In vivo*, blasts show a greater *in vitro* resistance to chemotherapeutic drugs like PRED and ASP.[103] Within the subgroup of infant ALL, several adverse prognostic factors are identified, namely, age younger than 3 or 6 months at diagnosis, a WBC count with more than 300,000/μl, overt CNS involvement, presence of a *MLL* gene rearrangement, lack of CD10 expression, and the co-expression of myeloid markers, and prednisone poor response (PPR).[104]

Because of distinctive biological characteristics, unique dosing due to patients' young age, and high risk of relapse, some study groups treat infants on specifically designed protocols. Two large collaborative efforts — a COG study and the "Interfant study", involving many European and several non-European groups, address this population. Treatment is risk based and include elements designed to treat both ALL and AML. *In vitro* studies suggest infant blasts are sensitive to high-dose ARA-C. The role of allogeneic SCT remains unclear and is under study in the current Interfant-06 trial.[104] SCT has been beneficial for the highest risk infant patients in trial INTERFANT-99.[105]

High-risk or very high-risk ALL

Other subsets remain at high risk of treatment failure such as severe hypodiploidy. Criteria used by different study groups vary (see Chapter 6.2). In general, patients are stratified as HR when ALL with *BCR/ABL* is diagnosed. In the BFM group, all *MLL/AF4* patients are included in HR while in COG only those who remain MRD positive. *In vitro* or *in vivo* treatment resistance, e.g. PPR, MRD persistence, etc. may be employed to define (very) high risk ALL.[4,58,75,100,106]

The ALL-BFM 90 study replaced Protocol II, so crucial in initial therapy, with rotational intensification blocks derived from the BFM relapse studies for these high-risk patients without benefit.[96] Outcomes actually improved on ALL-BFM 95 with the reintroduction of Protocol II, which achieved an improved 6-years EFS of 53%, higher than ALL-BFM 86 and 90 (BFM-86: 45%; BFM-90: 32%). Although all patients received the same intensified chemotherapy, outcome was very different within different subgroups (6-years EFS in *BCR/ABL*-positive ALL: 26%; in patients with nonresponse day 33:36%, *MLL/AF4*-positive patients: 40% and for PPR: 55%).[4] Very intensive therapy entails substantial side effects. Some patients may benefit from SCT (see Chapter 8).[72,107]

Treatment of Relapsed Childhood ALL

Relapses

Despite the successful treatment of the majority of children with ALL, about 15% of patients still die. Only a small proportion of deaths occur due to disease complications, treatment-related toxicity, or nonresponse to the primary treatment (Fig. 11.5). About 20% of patients with ALL suffer from a relapse; relapsed ALL is still the fourth most common malignancy in childhood. Despite continuous improvement of the risk stratification in frontline trials, the majority of relapses still

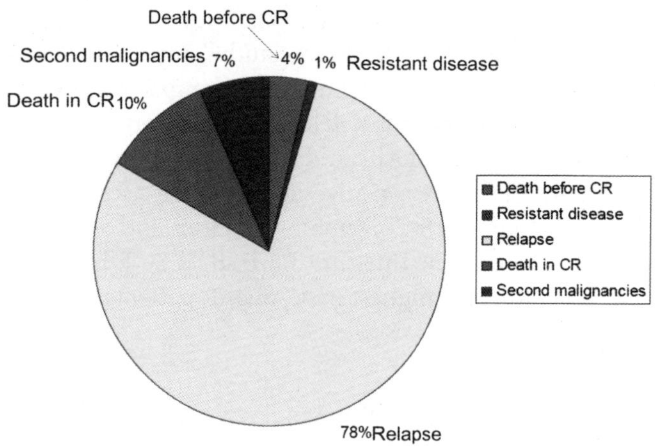

Fig. 11.5. Relative frequency of events in patients included in the ALL BFM-95 trial.[4]

Table 11.10. Distribution of relapses in patients (n = 2169) treated according to the trial ALL BFM 95.

Relapses	n	CI[b]	Risk group	Relapses/ patients	CI[b]
All	356	16.2	SR (35% of all patients)	62/758	7.8
Isolated					
BM	232	10.5	MR (53% of all patients)	197/1157	16.8
CNS	39	1.8			
Testes	12	0.5	HR (12% of all patients)	97/254	38.6
Combined					
CNS/BM	48	2.2			
Combined BM/other[a]	22	1.0			
Other relapse	3	0.1			

[a]Without CNS.
[b]Cumulative incidences.

BM: bone marrow; CNS: central nervous system; HR: high risk; MR: medium risk; n: number of Patients; SR: standard risk.

Data from Moricke A, Reiter A, Zimmermann M, Gadner H, Stanulla M, Dordelmann M, Loning L, Beier R, Ludwig WD, Ratei R, Harbott J, Boos J, Mann G, Niggli F, Feldges A, Henze G, Welte K, Beck JD, Klingebiel T, Niemeyer C, Zintl F, Bode U, Urban C, Wehinger H, Niethammer D, Riehm H, Schrappe M. (2008) Risk-adjusted therapy of acute lymphoblastic leukemia can decrease treatment burden and improve survival: Treatment results of 2169 unselected pediatric and adolescent patients enrolled in the trial ALL-BFM 95. *Blood* **111**: 4477–4489.[4]

occur in patients stratified as non-HR (Table 11.10). Although second remission rates can be achieved for most patients, the majority of children with relapse ultimately die.[108]

As effectively all patients achieve remission, relapse occurs from a re-accumulation of residual blasts. Blasts may survive because of innate resistance or failure to deliver adequate therapy to a sanctuary site such as the CNS or testes. At relapse, the leukemia blasts are usually quite similar to the blasts at presentation. *In vitro*, glucocorticoid resistance is most striking among relapse patients[109] but represents the recurrence of resistant cases rather than evolution (see Chapter 9). Gene expression arrays examining paired diagnosis and relapse specimens link early relapse with changes in cell cycle regulation, DNA repair, and apoptosis. No common patterns emerged for late relapse.[110] ALL is an oligoclonal disease. Comparative genomic hybridization offers new insights into relapse.[111] The predominant clone at relapse derives from the predominant clone at presentation or a common ancestral clone. Relapse occurs when cell proliferation outpaces cell death for a subclone or a disappearing subclone undergoes further evolution and escapes control.

Relapses can occur in one or more sites. Isolated BM relapse is most common, followed by combined and isolated CNS relapses (Table 11.10). In patients with isolated extramedullary relapse, the BM remains the most common site of second relapse. In many cases of conventional isolated extramedullary relapse, submicroscopic marrow involvement may be documented with PCR or flow cytometry.

Similar to diagnosis, a number of consistent prognostic factors are known. Shorter first remission, bone marrow vs. extramedullary relapse, T-cell immunophenotype, and t(9;22) are associated with poor prognosis.[108,112,113] In addition, MRD levels after the initial induction treatment have predictive value.[114,115]

The diagnostic work-up is similar to primary diagnosis. The BM relapse is unequivocally established when at least 25% BM lymphoblasts are present, a CNS relapse requires > 5 cells/mL of CSF and unequivocal blasts on cytospin. Flow cytometry is gradually supplementing microscopy. If a patient has extramedullary relapse with marrow blasts ≥ 5%, the relapse is termed a combined relapse. A testicular relapse is confirmed by open-wedge biopsy and a subclinical involvement of the contralateral testis has to be excluded. In rare cases of an involvement of any other extramedullary sites such as lymph nodes and/or mediastinum, eye and bone, a histological examination should be done.[116] The initial diagnostics is complemented by flow cytometry and molecular genetic and/or cytogenetic analysis. A chest X-ray is routine. A cranial MRI, and the ultrasound of the abdomen, lymph nodes and testes may be necessary to characterize the organ involvement comprehensively.

Treatment of relapses

During the last decades, prospective treatment trials for children with relapsed ALL have been conducted.[8,113,116–120] Until the early 1980s, relapse was regarded as an almost incurable disease. With current salvage protocols, approximately 85% of patients achieve a second CR and cure rates of 30–40% are reported. Identification of risk factors have allowed the establishment of risk-adapted treatment strategies. As mentioned before, the prognosis depends on the site of relapse, the duration of the initial remission, and the immunophenotype.[113,116,119] By site of relapse, 5-year survival rates (± standard error) after isolated BM, isolated CNS, and isolated testis relapse in COG patients treated between 1988 and 2002, are 24.1% ± 2.1% (n = 1123), 58.7% ± 3.2% (n = 409), and 58.0% ± 8.0% (n = 104), respectively. By time to relapse, survival after early (CR1 < 18 months), intermediate (18–36 months), and late (> 36 months) isolated BM relapse are 11.5% ± 1.9% (n = 412), 18.4% ± 3.1% (n = 324), and 43.5% ± 5.2% (n = 387), respectively. Higher risk patients have an inferior survival after relapse (23%) compared to standard risk patients after relapse (50%). Outcomes are best for children aged 1–9 years as compared to < 1 year and ≥ 10 years, 45%, 20%, and 18%, respectively and better for B-precursor than T-cell disease, 37% vs. 23%.[8] Curiously, outcomes were similar after relapse for CCG-1961 patients, who relapsed either with inferior "standard" or superior "stronger" post-induction intensification.[121]

Based on these data, risk groups are defined: In COG, three groups are defined by outcome, namely (1) early/intermediate marrow relapse, (2) late marrow relapse and early extramedullary relapse, and (3) intermediate/late extramedullary relapse. Risk group assignment of the German ALL-BFM-REZ study group, shared by a number of other investigators, is shown in Table 11.11.

A second complete remission (CR2) is the first goal of therapy, which can be achieved in approximate 85% of cases. The same drugs employed in initial therapy are usually employed more aggressively after relapse with a higher tolerance for side effects. The incidence of toxic complications and deaths is higher as compared to primary treatment. Approximate 15% of patients die from either toxicity during induction or induction failure.[113] Patients with a persistent disease (nonresponse) at the end of the first month of the induction treatment have an extremely poor prognosis despite subsequent therapy, later complete remissions, and SCT. Similar to the first line therapy, patients need additional CNS-directed therapy to protect children from later CNS relapse. By conventional intensive therapy, perhaps one third of children with relapsed ALL can be cured. In a substantial number of patients, allogeneic SCT may be indicated.

Table 11.11. Risk group assignment for relapsed non–T-cell and T-cell ALL according to the ALL-BFM-REZ strategy.

Time point	Extramedullary	Combined	BM (isolated)
Non-T-cell ALL			
Very early	S2	S4	S4
Early	S2	S2	S3
Late	S1	S2	S2
T-cell ALL			
Very early	S2	S4	S4
Early	S2	S4	S4
Late	S1	S4	S4

BM: bone marrow.
Very early: < 18 months from diagnosis and < 6 months from completion of therapy, early: ≥ 18 months from diagnosis and < 6 months from completion of therapy, late: ≥ 6 months from completion of therapy.

Stem Cell Transplantation

Allogeneic hematopoietic SCT allows administration of brief marrow ablative chemotherapy and total body irradiation therapy. The allograft offers an opportunity of further disease control via a graft vs. leukemia affect (see Chapter 20). Assessment is difficult because of variable patient eligibility, patient selection for SCT from among eligible patients, and variable treatment regimens. Results from conventional frontline and relapse protocols have improved over time, but SCT may be indicated for distinct patient subsets. With decreased transplant-related mortalities (TRM) through the progress in the understanding, prevention, and management of graft-vs.-host disease and the more effective utilization of the graft-vs.-leukemia effect, as well as an increasing number of registered donors, allogeneic BM- or PB-SCT is a relevant therapeutic option for an increasing number of patients with a high risk or very high risk disease in first, second, or third remission.

In CR1, current BFM guidelines restrict matched related or unrelated donor SCT to specific patient subsets; namely, patients not in remission at the end of induction treatment on day 33, those with a persistent high MRD load despite further intensive treatment, and those with translocations t(9;22) or t(4;11).[72] However, considering the early risk of TRM as well as late treatment morbidity, continuing the re-examination of these recommendations is required. Any benefit of transplant for infants remains controversial.[105,122] For the Ph+ ALL, the COG recently found a better 3-year EFS with chemotherapy plus a continuous imatinib exposure (88% ± 11%) compared to those receiving a sibling donor SCT (57% ± 22%).[102]

Allogeneic SCT is widely accepted as an appropriate therapy for patients in second remission after a marrow relapse.[118] In addition to site of relapse, time to relapse, immunophenotype, and cytogenetic abnormalities, pre-transplant therapy, response to this treatment, and time to transplant are important selection factors.[123] The overall disease-free survival after SCT from a matched sibling donor in second CR has been reported to range from 40–60%. The most commonly used conditioning regimen consists of a combination of TBI and CP or etoposide. For patients with a very early BM relapse (within 18 months of achieving first CR), allogeneic SCT in CR2 from an HLA-identical sibling or unrelated matched donor is currently considered as the treatment of choice. For other subgroups of relapsed ALL (later marrow relapses, extramedullary disease), the role of allogeneic SCT remains controversial and prospective trials are needed.[124,125]

Complications

The most important "side effect" of current ALL therapy is lack of efficacy. About 20% of patients still suffer relapse. In addition, the treatments employed have both acute and long-term complications, which may become apparent years after therapy has ceased.

Acute complications

Approximately 1% of patients succumb to complications before achieving a first CR.[96] Extreme hyperleukocytosis (> 400,000/µl) constitutes a high risk factor for early complications like hemorrhage in the CNS and pulmonary or neurological events due to the leucostasis. Thrombocytopenia can be associated with bleeding, especially into the CNS. A mediastinal mass, which is often seen in T-cell ALL, can cause an acute pulmonary failure by compressing the air passages. Pulmonary symptoms can also result from pleural effusion. A tumor lysis syndrome is a complication of high leukemic cell burden (see Chapter 30). Here, the rapid release of intracellular contents with treatment leads to hyperuricemia due to the metabolism of purines and leads to hyperphosphatemia, hypocalcemia and hyperkalemia with potentially lethal consequences. Infection is the most common cause of death in the early weeks before achieving first CR (see Chapter 25). In the context of 4-drug induction, severe infections seem more common with DEX than with PRED.[65] Older patients are at higher risk than younger patients. Bacteria cause approximately 70% of lethal infections. Thus, vigilance and prompt, effective antimicrobial therapy is needed. Other acute complications may be severe but not life threatening, namely, hyperglycemia from GC's and ASP, CNS toxicity from CNS-directed chemotherapy and cranial irradiation, pancreatitis from ASP, and peripheral neuropathy from VCR. ASP and GC's contribute to thromboses including sinus venous thrombosis. The incidence of fatal complications is highest in the highest risk patients. After induction, infection remains the most common causes of death. Other complications are massive bleeding and organ failure such as cardiomyopathy, hepatopathy, and encephalopathy.[4,96]

Late effects of treatment

With the overall improvement in cure and survival rates, long-term adverse effects of treatment have become more apparent. These late side effects include neuropsychological and endocrinological deficits, cardiac complications, osteonecrosis as well as SN (see Chapters 24 and 28).

SN result from mutagenic effect of chemotherapeutic drugs and/or radiation and to date approximately 1–2% of successfully treated ALL patients will develop a SN.[3,6,58,100] Among these, AML and myelodysplastic syndrome as well as brain tumors in patients having received cranial irradiation are most frequent. Other secondary tumors include Hodgkin lymphomas and Ewing sarcomas.[4,11,78] To evaluate the rate and type of SN after BFM-treatment, the study group analyzed the data from 5006 children with ALL from 5 ALL-BFM multicenter trials (1979–1995). 52 SN were documented including 16 AMLs, 13 CNS tumors and 23 other neoplasms.[11]

CNS-directed therapy was introduced in the early 1970s and consisted initially of a 24 Gy radiation to the CNS, including the spinal cord. As mentioned before, the introduction of systemic high-dose MTX and intrathecal injections of MTX (with or without ARA-C and hydrocortisone) has allowed reduction independent on brain irradiation. The dosage of radiation has been reduced to 12–18 Gy without an increase of relapses, and has been limited to cranial irradiation. Currently, cranial radiation is reserved for subgroups of patients with an especially high risk for CNS relapses which should lead to a further reduction of serious late side effects.[95,126]

Cardiomyopathy, a toxic effect of anthracyclines, has been well described for moderate to high cumulative doses of more than 350 mg/m^2. Very recently, long-term follow-up studies showed that patients treated with doses of 300 mg/m^2 or less may also show a measurable decline of cardiac function over time.[9] Cardiomyopathy can appear many years after treatment, thus it is important to include echocardiography in follow-up examinations. To reduce the incidence of cardiomyopathy, several study groups are trying to reduce the cumulative doses of anthracyclines or alter its schedule of administration. The DFCI protocol 91-01 compared doxorubicin (30 mg/m^2) as a bolus and as a 48-hour continuous infusion every 3 weeks in HR patients to a total cumulative dose of 360 mg/m^2. Prolonged infusion offered no protection from cardiotoxicity and no EFS advantage.[127] In the DFCI protocol 95-01, patients were randomized to receive bolus doxorubicin (30 mg/m^2) every 3 weeks with or without dexrazoxane (300 mg/m^2), a "cardioprotectant". EFS was equivalent but patients treated without dexrazoxane were more likely to have elevated troponin T levels (50% vs. 21%, $P < 0.001$) and extremely elevated troponin T levels (32% vs. 10%, $P < 0.001$).[128] Treponin T is a marker for myocardial injury.

Another serious late effect of ALL treatment is the appearance of osteonecrosis, mainly related to the treatment with GC. Adolescents, females and patients with extensive exposure to DEX seem at highest risk. Where the incidence of symptomatic cardiotoxicty is less than 1%, the incidence of symptomatic osteonecrosis was 0.2% for children younger than 10 years and 8.9% for young people older than 10 years.[67]

Conclusion

Many have noticed the increasing challenge of late effects as EFS has improved. The emergence of long-term adverse effects depends on an individual's health status and the specific treatment received. Leukemia survivors should receive regular examinations by healthcare professionals, who are familiar with leukemia treatment and its associated long term risks. They can provide detailed recommendations for screening and management of any late effects. Long-term follow-up approaches will not only improve the health and quality of life for survivors, but they also will provide an improved infrastructure for systematic studies of the long-term consequences of childhood ALL treatment and, hopefully, their future prevention. A child suffering long-term disability as a result of life-saving treatment is not cured.

Prognosis and Outcome of Childhood ALL

Fifty years ago, survival rates for children with ALL were less than 30%; they improved to approximately 50% in the 1970s and to more 80% in the 1990s.[129] This success derives from the continuing work of dedicated researchers and multi-center study groups, which could accrue adequate patient numbers for statistically potent trials. The first chemotherapeutic agents appeared about 50 years ago, namely, MTX, steroids, and 6-MP. However, the durations of remissions were short and most patients died within a year. In the 1960s, VCR was discovered, and investigators noted longer remission rates when VCR was used *in combination* with ASP and PRED. CNS relapse emerged as the most common site of initial treatment failure. The emergence of effective presymptomatic CNS-directed therapy in the late 1960s and the early 1970s offered cure for about one half of patients. The introduction of CNS-directed treatment in addition to the systemic combinational therapy resulted in an improved cure rate with EFS at 5 years of 55% (± 6%) in the BFM study 1970–1976.[79] Over time, cranial irradiation with intrathecal MTX replaced craniospinal irradiation. In the 1980s, risk-adapted therapy was introduced and SCT became an option for children with relapsed or refractory leukemia. Intrathecal MTX with better systemic chemotherapy spared most children from CNS irradiation all together. The results of a number of international and national clinical trials in developed countries are presented in Table 11.12 and outcomes are quite similar with 5-year EFS rates of 70–85%. However, outcomes in ALL subsets remain heterogeneous, i.e. some patients are cured and some are lost in each subgroup.

Table 11.12. Overall treatment results for childhood acute lymphoblastic leukemia treated according to different study protocols.

Trial (country)	Years	No. of patients	5 years EFS	Reference
AIEOP-ALL 95 (Italy)	1995–2000	1743	76 ± 1%	77
ALL-BFM 95[a]	1995–2000	2169	80 ± 1%	6
CCG-1900 series (USA)	1996–2002	4464	76 ± 1%	3
DCOG ALL-9 (NL)	1997–2004	859	81 ± 1%	58
DFCI 95–01 (USA)	1996–2000	491	82 ± 2%	59
NOPHO ALL-2000[b]	2002–2007	1023	79 ± 0%	100
SJCRH Study 14 (USA)	1998–1999	53	77 ± 6%	78
UK MRC ALL 97 (UK)	1997–1999	997	74 ± 1%	61
UK MRC ALL 97/99 (UK)	1999–2002	938	81 ± 2%	61

[a] Germany, Austria, Switzerland.
[b] Denmark, Finland, Iceland, Norway, Sweden.

AIEOP: Italian Association of Pediatric Hematology and Oncology; ALL-BFM: acute lymphoblastic leukemia–Berlin–Frankfurt-Münster; CCG: Children's Cancer Group; DCOG: Dutch Childhood Oncology Group; DFCI: Dana Farber Cancer Institute; EFS: event-free survival; NOPHO ALL: Nordic Society of Pediatric Hematology and Oncology acute lymphoblastic leukemia; SJCRH: St Jude's Children's Research Hospital; UK MRC ALL: United Kingdom Medical Research Council acute lymphoblastic leukemia.

Prognosis by clinical presentation and properties of leukemia

Age at diagnosis is a strong prognostic factor reflecting different age dependent biological features in childhood ALL. Best results have been achieved in the age group 2–5 years with an EFS of approximate 85%. This group represents 60% of all children with ALL. Outcomes are worse for adolescents and even worse for infants, less than 1 year old.[4,104] Infant ALL often shows poor prognosis in both clinical and laboratory features known such as hyperleukocytosis or *MLL* gene rearrangements. The prognosis of adolecents older than 10 years, however remains unsatisfying with an EFS of approximate 65%.[3,6,77,78] Adolescents are less likely to have favorable hyperdiploidies or translocation t(12;21) and more likely to have unfavorable translocation t(9;22) (see Chapters 3 and 5). Leukemic cell burden at diagnosis is still an important prognostic parameter despite more intensified therapy regimens. A higher *WBC count at diagnosis* is associated with an increased risk of treatment failure. Moreover, the risk of poor outcome increases continuously with an increasing WBC count, especially in patients with pB-ALL. The group of patients with a high WBC > 200,000/µl has only an EFS of 35–40% (BFM-95 study).[4] Patients with an extreme hyperleukocytosis (>400,000/µl) are additionally at a high risk for early complications such as CNS hemorrhage or pulmonary and neurological events due to leucostasis. Moreover, a high WBC is often associated with other prognostic factors, for instance unfavorable chromosomal translocations t(4;11), or t(9;22) or CNS involvement.[130] The group of patients with a low WBC count less than 10,000/µl has an EFS of approximate 85% (BFM-95 study).[4] As shown in Table 11.13, treatment results according to age and WBC count at diagnosis are very similar across different clinical study groups despite differences in treatment regimen.

The National Cancer Institute (NCI) risk classification was developed to define more uniform criteria for risk-based treatment assignment. Patients with < 50,000 leukocytes/µl and an age between 1 and 9 years at diagnosis are defined as standard risk patients; patients with an age <1 year or ≥ 10 years with any WBC or WBC count >50,000/µl at any age, are HR patients. Today, this classification is especially useful when comparing treatment results across different study groups.[131,132]

Treatment outcome also differs dependent on *gender and ethnicity*. The outcome of boys is consistently inferior to that of girls with an EFS of 79% vs. 82% (BFM-95 study).[4] This difference cannot be explained by testes relapses, as boys also show an inferior response to initial treatment with a higher rate of PPR.[96] EFS for white children are higher compared to that of black or Hispanic children (77% vs. 65% for black and 68% for Hispanic children),[133] though this difference may be diminishing.[3]

Approximately 1.5% of patients with ALL are children with *Down's syndrome* (DS). Patients with and without DS do not differ with respect to gender, WBC count at diagnosis, CNS leukemia or cytogenetic abnormalities. Children with DS are slightly older and the T-cell immunophenotype is very rare. EFS is slightly worse in children with DS (58 ± 8% vs. 70 ± 1%), mainly due to late BM recurrences. However, EFS in DS patients is comparable to the non-DS group once they either receive treatment with no major modifications (65 + 9% vs. 70 ± 1%) or if they are < 6 years of age, irrespectively of therapy modifications (73 ± 9% vs. 74 ± 1%). Thus, majority of DS patients can be successfully treated if they receive intensive antileukemic treatment with no major modifications; however, they require an optimal supportive management.[134]

Table 11.13. 5-Year event-free survival (EFS) according to prognostic factors for patients treated according to different study protocols.

	CCG trials (3)	DFCI 95–01 (59)	UK MRC ALL 97/99 (61)
	1996–2002 n = 4464 EFS (%) ± SE	1996–2000 n = 491 EFS (%) ± SE	1997–2002 n = 1935 EFS (%) ± SE
Age at diagnosis			
1–9 years	79.4 ± 0.8	84.8 ± 1.9	79.9 ± 1.0
≥ 10 years	70.9 ± 1.4	74.5 ± 4.6	65.4 ± 2.4
Gender			
Male	73.8 ± 3.8	79.9 ± 2.5	77.4 ± 1.3
Female	78.9 ± 1.0	83.8 ± 2.6	76.2 ± 1.5
WBC (per μl)			
< 10,000	80.6 ± 0.9	86.2 ± 2.3	81.8 ± 1.3
10–< 50,000	77.0 ± 1.3	80.8 ± 3.2	78.0 ± 1.7
50–< 100,000	70.6 ± 2.1	78.9 ± 6.3	70.1 ± 3.3
≥ 100,000	63.6 ± 2.1	66.0 ± 6.5	62.6 ± 3.0
Immunophenotype			
B-lineage	76.0 + 0.9	81.3 + 1.9	77.8 ± 1.0
T-lineage	72.8 + 2.1	84.6 + 5.0	68.6 ± 3.2

CNS: central nervous system; CCG: Children's Cancer Group; DFCI: Dana-Farber Cancer Institute; SE: standard error; UK MRC: United Kingdom Medical Research Council; WBC: white blood cells.

Symptomatic CNS disease at the onset of ALL is rare and CNS involvement is usually diagnosed in asymptomatic patients. The CNS status is mainly determined by the analysis of CSF and fewer than 5% of children with ALL have overt CNS disease at the time of diagnosis as defined by a CNS3 status. However, leukemic blasts in CSF are identified in about 15–30% of patients at diagnosis. An initial involvement of the CNS is associated with a reduced EFS as compared to CNS negative patients (CNS1 6-years EFS: 81%, CNS2: 80%, CNS3: 58%) (BFM-95 study).[4] Patients with a CNS involvement often show other unfavorable characteristics like male gender, a high initial WBC at diagnosis, T-cell immunophenotype and an age > 10 years. The CNS remains the most common site of extramedullary relapse, but CNS involvement at primary diagnosis is also associated with an increased number of marrow relapses. Moreover, a blood contamination of the CSF with identifiable blasts due to a traumatic lumbar puncture (TLP+) constitutes an unfavorable prognostic risk factor with an EFS of approximate 70% (Table 11.14).[4,59,135–137] Consequentially, patients with CNS3, CNS2, or TLP+ status may receive graduated and more intensive CNS-directed therapy than those with CNS1 status.

Prognosis in childhood ALL differs by the immunophenotype as well. In pB-ALL approximately three-quarters of patients are positive for the common ALL antigen CD10 without surface or cytoplasmic immunoglobulin expression (common ALL). In contrast, the pro-B ALL (CD10 negative) phenotype, which is most common in young infants, is often associated with a translocation t(4;11) and a high WBC count, and confers a poor prognosis as compared to the common ALL phenotype. The T-cell ALL immunophenotype is also often considered to be associated with a high risk of relapse and is often associated with other unfavorable factors like male gender, higher age, a high WBC count and CNS involvement. However, outcome depends, in a great extent, on the treatment applied and on the treatment response, and has clearly improved over the last years.[4,59,107,138] Meanwhile, the EFS of patients with a common ALL immunophenotype and those with T-cell ALL are similar when treated according to the BFM regimen (6-year EFS of pB-ALL: 80%, T-cell ALL: 75%).[4] Patients with early T precursor-ALL with its distinctive gene expression signature or immunophenotype (CD1a–, CD8–, CD5(weak) with stem cell or myeloid markers have high risk of relapse.[39] However, outcomes after relapse of patients with T-cell

Table 11.14. 5-Year event-free survival (EFS) of patients treated according to different study protocols depending on CNS status.

	DFCI 95–01 (59)	ALL BFM 95 (4)	SJCRH Study 14 (78)	TPOG-2002 (137)
	1996–2000 n = 491 EFS (%) ± SE	1995–2000 n = 2169 EFS (%) ± SE	1998–1999 n = 53 EFS (%) ± SE	2002–2007 n = 793 EFS (%) ± SE
CNS status				
CNS1	83 ± 2	81 ± 1	83 ± 4	80 ± 2
CNS2	72 ± 7	80 ± 4	71 ± 7	59 ± 13
CNS3	75 ± 13	58 ± 6	50 ± 18	45 ± 11
Traumatic				
TLP +	68 ± 11	69 ± 4	69 ± 11	68 ± 10

BFM: Berlin Frankfurt Münster; CNS: central nervous system; DFCI: Dana-Farber Cancer Institute; SE: standard error; SJCRH: St. Jude Children Research Hospital; TLP: traumatic lumbar puncture; TPOG: Taiwan Pediatric Oncology Group.

disease are unequivocally worse than for patients with B-precursor disease.[119]

During the last decades, a number of leukemia-specific genetic aberrations have been identified and analyzed for prognostic relevance. Often, the frequency was found to be age dependent. *TEL/AML1*, which is found predominantly in pB-ALL in 20–25% of cases and rarely observed in T-cell ALL, occurs mostly in children aged 2–9 years and is very rare in adolescents or adults. It is associated with a favorable prognosis with a long-term EFS of approximately 85%.[4,7,59,78] Patients with the *E2A/PBX1* rearrangement and a contemporary treatment have a favorable overall outcome but may have an increased risk of CNS relapse.[54,139]

The translocation t(9;22) and its *BCR/ABL* rearrangement, respectively which is present with a frequency of approximately 3% in childhood ALL, compared to about 25% in adults, confers to an unfavorable prognosis with an EFS of 25–30% in children when treated with conventional chemotherapy, prior to the TKI-era.[99,140] Outcome is particularly poor if the patients show additional unfavorable features like a high WBC count or a poor response to the early therapy. Rearrangements involving the *MLL* gene are also associated with an increased risk of treatment failure and are detected with a frequency of around 4% in the entire ALL group but are present in a majority of infants. The translocation t(4;11) and its *MLL/AF4* rearrangement, respectively, is the most frequent MLL aberration in children, and is predominantly found in very young children, mainly in infants younger than 1 year. This translocation is also often associated with other poor risk factors such a high WBC count at diagnosis, poor response to early therapy, and CNS involvement.[103,141]

Response to treatment

Response to therapy is determined by the interaction of leukemic-cell specific biological features, such as intrinsic drug sensitivity, host factors such as pharmacogenetic and pharmacodynamic features, the treatment regimen administered and finally treatment adherence (see Chapter 9). Response to therapy remains a consistent prognostic factor when assessed in any of a number of ways. The extent of blast clearance is defined by the number of persisting blasts: CR is defined by < 5% blasts (M1 marrow), nonresponse by ≥ 5% blasts (M2: 5–< 25%, M3: ≥ 25%).

The outcome of patients with more than 5% blasts after 4–5 weeks of induction therapy is very poor compared to the vast majority of patients with CR. Failure is only observed in approximately 2–3% of children.[4] In the United States in 1975, the CCG began examining marrow aspirates on day 15 of induction therapy.[142] Patients who show a rapid blast clearance have a more favorable prognosis compared to those with slower blast clearance.[143] An M3-BM at treatment day 15 (> 25% residual blasts) was associated with an EFS of approximate 50%, and a nonremission (> 5% blasts) on treatment day 33 after treatment induction is associated with a prognosis of approximate 35%.[4] Results from other study groups are similar. In 1981, the CCG began examining a marrow aspirate on day 8 of therapy and also found prognostic significance. Results from the CCG showed a

4-year EFS of 47% and 77% for higher risk patients with marrow blasts greater or fewer than 25% on day 8 of induction therapy.[144] For standard risk patients, the 5-year EFS was 67% and 84% for patients with greater or fewer than 5% marrow blasts on day 15 of induction therapy.[60] However, the vast majority of relapses still occur in the large group of patients with an adequate morphological response to treatment. Cytomorphological evaluation with a threshold of sensitivity of about 1–5% blasts is not sufficient.

In Europe in 1983, the BFM study group started to assess the prognostic value of the response to the initial administration of prednisone over seven days and one intrathecal dose of MTX by analyzing the number of blasts in PB on treatment day 8 (PR). The prednisone good response (PGR) is characterized by less than 1000 blasts/μl and is observed in about 90% of patients. The prednisone poor response (PPR), as defined by peripheral blasts ≥ 1000/μl, is associated with a significantly worse EFS as compared to PGR.[145] Patients with a PPR on day 8 as determined in PB have a 6-years EFS of only 55% when treated according to the BFM-95 trial.[4]

PCR and flow cytometry lower the threshold for blast detection to at least 0.01% or 1 cell in 10,000. Leukemia below the level of microscopic detection is termed minimal residual disease (MRD) (see Chapter 10). In the last 2 decades, MRD has emerged as one of the strongest predictors of outcome. PCR analysis allows detection of leukemic clone-specific immunoglobulin and/or T-cell receptor gene rearrangements with a sensitivity of the equivalent of one malignant cell per 10^3–10^6 normal cells. Several groups clearly demonstrated that such assessments might be done promptly for a large majority of patients with compelling prognostic value.[57,146] A 10-year update on the I-BFM-SG MRD study demonstrated an EFS of 93% for MRD negativity at weeks 5 and 12 of treatment (standard risk group (MRD-SR)), 74% for low MRD positivity $< 10^{-3}$ at week 5 and/or 12 of treatment (the intermediate risk group (MRD-IR)) and 16% for high MRD load $\geq 10^{-3}$ at week 12 of treatment (the high risk group (MRD-HR)).[57] Results from the AIEOP-BFM ALL 2000 study are similar.[7] Flow cytometric methods provide an alternative approach.[41,45,147] MRD measurement after induction may contribute to individual treatment decisions, e.g. the allocation to SCT.

The outcome after first relapse depends on the site of relapse, the duration of the first CR and the immunophenotype (Tables 11.15 and 11.16). Although second remission rates are high, the majority of relapsed patients cannot be cured yet. The overall probability of an EFS and OS is approximately 30% and 37%, respectively, when treated according to the BFM-REZ protocol.[113,119] Whereas 6-years OS is approximately 70% in patients with isolated testes relapse, overall survival is 50% in patients with an isolated CNS relapse and only 20% in patients with an isolated BM relapse (Table 11.15).[116]

Perspective and New Treatment Strategies

Further improvement of childhood ALL treatment will mainly be based on further understanding of the molecular mechanisms of emergence of leukemia and the development of treatment resistance. Risk assessment may become more precise and novel anticancer agents shall be provided to appropriate patient subsets, e.g. tyrosine kinase inhibitors in Ph+ ALL. However, new strategies are also needed to improve the quality of life for our patients. A patient requiring hip replacement surgery at 14 years of age is not cured.

The causative factors in the development of ALL are still unknown. Only a few cases may be attributed to inherited genetic syndromes like the DS or an exposure to known leukemogenic agents. However, the introduction of high-resolution genomic fine mapping tools opened new perspectives with respect to the discovery

Table 11.15. 6-Year event-free survival (EFS) and 6-year survival by site and time to first relapse of patients treated according to CCG-100 series trials.

Adverse event	EFS (%) ± SE	Survival (%) ± SE
Isolated marrow	16 ± 2	20 ± 2
Early	5 ± 2	6 ± 2
Intermediate	10 ± 2	11 ± 4
Late	33 ± 4	43 ± 4
Combined marrow	29 ± 4	29 ± 5
Early	9 ± 5	9 ± 5
Intermediate	11 ± 6	11 ± 6
Late	48 ± 7	49 ± 8
Isolated CNS	37 ± 3	48 ± 4
Early	24 ± 4	33 ± 5
Intermediate	44 ± 5	59 ± 5
Late	59 ± 9	72 ± 8
Isolated Testes	64 ± 5	70 ± 5
Early	48 ± 11	52 ± 11
Intermediate	44 ± 11	57 ± 10
Late	76 ± 6	81 ± 5

Early: 0–17 months; intermediate: 18–35 months; late: ≥ 36 months.

Adapted from Gaynon PS, Qu RP, Chappell RJ, Willoughby ML, Tubergen DG, Steinherz PG, Trigg ME. (1998) Survival after relapse in childhood acute lymphoblastic leukemia: impact of site and time to first relapse — the Children's Cancer Group Experience. *Cancer* **82**: 1387–1395.[116]

Table 11.16. Long-term event-free survival (EFS) by site, time and immunophenotype for patients with first relapse treated according ALL-REZ BFM 90.

Characteristics of relapse	No. of patients	10y-EFS (%) ± SE
Time of Relapse		
Very Early	136	14 ± 3
Early	172	20 ± 3
Late	217	47 ± 3
Site of Relapse		
BM isolated	324	23 ± 2
BM combined	117	35 ± 4
EM isolated	84	50 ± 6
EM sites (combined + isolated)		
CNS	95	39 ± 5
Testes	71	53 ± 6
Other EM sites	29	28 ± 8
Immunophenotype		
Pro-B ALL	36	17 ± 6
Common-ALL	303	33 ± 3
Pre-B ALL	89	27 ± 5
Pre-T-cell ALL	17	18 ± 9
Cortical-T-cell ALL	17	5 ± 6
Mature-T-cell ALL	39	21 ± 7

BM: bone marrow; CNS: central nervous system; EM: extramedullary; SE: standard error.
Very early: within 18 months after initial diagnosis.
Early: more than 18 months from initial diagnosis and less than 6 months after cessation of frontline therapy.
Late: after 6 months of cessation of frontline treatment.

Adapted from Tallen G, Ratei R, Mann G, Kaspers G, Niggli F, Karachunsky A, Ebell W, Escherich G, Schrappe M, Klingebiel T, Fengler R, Henze G, von Stackelberg A. (2010) Long-term outcome in children with relapsed acute lymphoblastic leukemia after time-point and site-of-relapse stratification and intensified short-course multidrug chemotherapy: results of trial ALL-REZ BFM 90. *J Clin Oncol* **28**: 2339–2347.[119]

of factors associated with an increased susceptibility for leukemia development (see Chapter 6). Very recently, first genome-wide studies discovered several susceptibility loci.[20,21,148] High-throughput sequencing allows the description of the complete leukemic genome and may lead to the identification of new recurrent genetic lesions. Future clinical research may focus on distinct biological subgroups as those with common genetic lesions such as *BCR/ABL*, *MLL/AF4* or *TEL/AML1* rearrangement.[5] One of these newly identified subgroups with poor prognosis is characterized by an aberrant expression of the cytokine receptor-like factor 2 (CRLF2).[149,150]

The drugs currently used currently were developed between 1950 and 1970. Two generations of researchers have sharpened our use. In large genome-wide gene expression array studies, common signatures of distinct biological subgroups have emerged. Moreover, candidate treatment targets have been identified, e.g. Jak-2, which, paired with appropriate agents, may in the future complement or — in some situations — even replace standard chemotherapy.[151] The inhibition of certain key enzymes such as tyrosine kinases, DNA methyltransferases, or histone deacetylases might be an effective goal of treatment for specific patient subsets. For example, the tyrosine kinase inhibitor imatinib improved the outcome of *BCR/ABL* positive leukemia in adults; however, its effect was limited by the rapid development of drug resistance.[152] The combination of imatinib with new ABL-kinase inhibitors might help to overcome that problem.[5] Other candidates for targeted treatment are FLT3 inihibitors (lestaurtinib), DNA methyltransferase inhibitors (azacytidine), and the histone deacetylase inhibitors (romidepsin) (see Chapter 22).

The targeting of leukemia specific surface antigens is another promising approach. Antibodies against these targets can be mono- or bispecific, unconjugated or conjungated with chemotherapeutic agents, immunotoxins or radioactive molecules. Examples already used in clinical practice are rituximab, a humanized anti-CD20 antibody, epratuzumab that targets CD22, alemtuzumab, a humanized antibody that is reactive with CD52 (see Chapter 21).

In addition to novel treatment approaches, new formulations of standard chemotherapeutic drugs may hold promise. A well-established drug already widely employed is the polyethylene glycol-conjugated asparaginase (PEG-ASP). Encapsulating drugs into liposomes is one strategy to improve the therapeutic potency. Others drugs with a modified formulation include liposomal VCR, which might have higher tissue concentration and a reduced neurotoxicity and liposomal anthracyclines with the potential advantage of a reduced cardiotoxicity.[101] Novel nucleoside analogs like clofarabine or nelarabine and the alkylating agent, bendamustine, offer promise.

In summary, contemporary methods of risk classification in childhood ALL including standard MRD analyses provide excellent tools for clinical treatment stratification. However, current insights into the molecular mechanisms of resistance and treatment failure are sorely deficient. In ALL, multidrug resistance seems to emerge in one step, focusing attention on shared cell death pathways. Drug development is like "cutting a key" and then beginning a search for the elusive lock that this candidate key just might open. A more rational approach might begin with a careful study of the "locks", i.e. patients' leukemia cells, followed by the design of more likely keys. Given the heterogeneity of childhood ALL, more than one key will most likely be required. The real success — of science and human organization — of the past half century, combined with the burgeoning expansion of biological understanding, make the next half century promising indeed.

References

1. Stanulla M, Schrappe M. (2009) Treatment of childhood acute lymphoblastic leukemia. *Semin Hematol* **46**: 52–63.
2. Pui CH, Evans WE. (2006) Treatment of acute lymphoblastic leukemia. *N Engl J Med* **354**: 166–178.
3. Gaynon PS, Angiolillo AL, Carroll WL, Nachman JB, Trigg ME, Sather HN, Hunger SP, Devidas M. (2010) Long-term results of the children's cancer group studies for childhood acute lymphoblastic leukemia 1983–2002: A Children's Oncology Group report. *Leukemia* **24**: 285–297.
4. Moricke A, Reiter A, Zimmermann M, Gadner H, Stanulla M, Dordelmann M, Loning L, Beier R, Ludwig WD, Ratei R, Harbott J, Boos J, Mann G, Niggli F, Feldges A, Henze G, Welte K, Beck JD, Klingebiel T, Niemeyer C, Zintl F, Bode U, Urban C, Wehinger H, Niethammer D, Riehm H, Schrappe M. (2008) Risk-adjusted therapy of acute lymphoblastic leukemia can decrease treatment burden and improve survival: Treatment results of 2169 unselected pediatric and adolescent patients enrolled in the trial ALL-BFM 95. *Blood* **111**: 4477–4489.
5. Pui CH, Robison LL, Look AT. (2008) Acute lymphoblastic leukaemia. *Lancet* **371**: 1030–1043.
6. Moricke A, Zimmermann M, Reiter A, Henze G, Schrauder A, Gadner H, Ludwig WD, Ritter J, Harbott J, Mann G, Klingebiel T, Zintl F, Niemeyer C, Kremens B, Niggli F, Niethammer D, Welte K, Stanulla M, Odenwald E, Riehm H, Schrappe M. (2010) Long-term results of five consecutive trials in childhood acute lymphoblastic leukemia performed by the ALL-BFM study group from 1981 to 2000. *Leukemia* **24**: 265–284.
7. Conter V, Bartram CR, Valsecchi MG, Schrauder A, Panzer-Grumayer R, Moricke A, Arico M, Zimmermann M, Mann G, de Rossi G, Stanulla M, Locatelli F, Basso G, Niggli F, Barisone E, Henze G, Ludwig WD, Haas OA, Cazzaniga G, Koehler R, Silvestri D, Bradtke J, Parasole R, Beier R, van Dongen JJ, Biondi A, Schrappe M. (2010) Molecular response to treatment redefines all prognostic factors in children and adolescents with B-cell precursor acute lymphoblastic leukemia: Results in 3184 patients of the AIEOP-BFM ALL 2000 study. *Blood* **115**: 3206–3214.
8. Nguyen K, Devidas M, Cheng SC, La M, Raetz EA, Carroll WL, Winick NJ, Hunger SP, Gaynon PS, Loh ML. (2008) Factors influencing survival after relapse from acute lymphoblastic leukemia: A Children's Oncology Group study. *Leukemia* **22**: 2142–2150.
20. Trevino LR, Yang W, French D, Hunger SP, Carroll WL, Devidas M, Willman C, Neale G, Downing J, Raimondi SC, Pui CH, Evans WE, Relling MV. (2009) Germline genomic variants associated with childhood acute lymphoblastic leukemia. *Nat Genet* **41**: 1001–1005.
31. Yeoh EJ, Ross ME, Shurtleff SA, Williams WK, Patel D, Mahfouz R, Behm FG, Raimondi SC, Relling MV, Patel A, Cheng C, Campana D, Wilkins D, Zhou X, Li J, Liu H, Pui CH, Evans WE, Naeve C, Wong L, Downing JR. (2002) Classification, subtype discovery, and prediction of outcome in pediatric acute lymphoblastic leukemia by gene expression profiling. *Cancer Cell* **1**: 133–143.
39. Coustan-Smith E, Mullighan CG, Onciu M, Behm FG, Raimondi SC, Pei D, Cheng C, Su X, Rubnitz JE, Basso G, Biondi A, Pui CH, Downing JR, Campana D. (2009) Early T-cell precursor leukaemia: A subtype of very high-risk acute lymphoblastic leukaemia. *Lancet Oncol* **10**: 147–156.
45. Basso G, Veltroni M, Valsecchi MG, Dworzak MN, Ratei R, Silvestri D, Benetello A, Buldini B, Maglia O, Masera G, Conter V, Arico M, Biondi A, Gaipa G. (2009) Risk of relapse of childhood acute lymphoblastic leukemia is predicted by flow cytometric measurement of residual disease on day 15 bone marrow. *J Clin Oncol* **27**: 5168–5174.
51. Moorman AV, Ensor HM, Richards SM, Chilton L, Schwab C, Kinsey SE, Vora A, Mitchell CD, Harrison CJ. (2010) Prognostic effect of chromosomal abnormalities in childhood B-cell precursor acute lymphoblastic leukaemia: Results from the UK Medical Research Council ALL97/99 randomised trial. *Lancet Oncol* **11**: 429–438.
52. Attarbaschi A, Mann G, Panzer-Grumayer R, Rottgers S, Steiner M, Konig M, Csinady E, Dworzak MN, Seidel M, Janousek D, Moricke A, Reichelt C, Harbott J, Schrappe M, Gadner H, Haas OA. (2008) Minimal

residual disease values discriminate between low and high relapse risk in children with B-cell precursor acute lymphoblastic leukemia and an intrachromosomal amplification of chromosome 21: The Austrian and German acute lymphoblastic leukemia Berlin-Frankfurt-Munster (ALL-BFM) trials. *J Clin Oncol* **26**: 3046–3050.

53. Jeha S, Pei D, Raimondi SC, Onciu M, Campana D, Cheng C, Sandlund JT, Ribeiro RC, Rubnitz JE, Howard SC, Downing JR, Evans WE, Relling MV, Pui CH. (2009) Increased risk for CNS relapse in pre-B cell leukemia with the t(1;19)/TCF3-PBX1. *Leukemia*

55. Cario G, Izraeli S, Teichert A, Rhein P, Skokowa J, Moricke A, Zimmermann M, Schrauder A, Karawajew L, Ludwig WD, Welte K, Schunemann HJ, Schlegelberger B, Schrappe M, Stanulla M. (2007) High interleukin-15 expression characterizes childhood acute lymphoblastic leukemia with involvement of the CNS. *J Clin Oncol* **25**: 4813–4820.

57. Flohr T, Schrauder A, Cazzaniga G, Panzer-Grumayer R, van der Velden V, Fischer S, Stanulla M, Basso G, Niggli FK, Schafer BW, Sutton R, Koehler R, Zimmermann M, Valsecchi MG, Gadner H, Masera G, Schrappe M, van Dongen JJ, Biondi A, Bartram CR. (2008) Minimal residual disease-directed risk stratification using real-time quantitative PCR analysis of immunoglobulin and T-cell receptor gene rearrangements in the international multicenter trial AIEOP-BFM ALL 2000 for childhood acute lymphoblastic leukemia. *Leukemia* **22**: 771–782.

60. Schultz KR, Pullen DJ, Sather HN, Shuster JJ, Devidas M, Borowitz MJ, Carroll AJ, Heerema NA, Rubnitz JE, Loh ML, Raetz EA, Winick NJ, Hunger SP, Carroll WL, Gaynon PS, Camitta BM. (2007) Risk- and response-based classification of childhood B-precursor acute lymphoblastic leukemia: A combined analysis of prognostic markers from the Pediatric Oncology Group (POG) and Children's Cancer Group (CCG). *Blood* **109**: 926–935.

63. Bostrom BC, Sensel MR, Sather HN, Gaynon PS, La MK, Johnston K, Erdmann GR, Gold S, Heerema NA, Hutchinson RJ, Provisor AJ, Trigg ME. (2003) Dexamethasone versus prednisone and daily oral versus weekly intravenous mercaptopurine for patients with standard-risk acute lymphoblastic leukemia: A report from the Children's Cancer Group. *Blood* **101**: 3809–3817.

66. Yang L, Panetta JC, Cai X, Yang W, Pei D, Cheng C, Kornegay N, Pui CH, Relling MV. (2008) Asparaginase may influence dexamethasone pharmacokinetics in acute lymphoblastic leukemia. *J Clin Oncol* **26**: 1932–1939.

68. Schrey D, Borghorst S, Lanvers-Kaminsky C, Hempel G, Gerss J, Moricke A, Schrappe M, Boos J. (2010) Therapeutic drug monitoring of asparaginase in the ALL-BFM 2000 protocol between 2000 and 2007. *Pediatr Blood Cancer* **54**: 952–958.

69. Duval M, Suciu S, Ferster A, Rialland X, Nelken B, Lutz P, Benoit Y, Robert A, Manel AM, Vilmer E, Otten J, Philippe N. (2002) Comparison of Escherichia coli-asparaginase with Erwinia-asparaginase in the treatment of childhood lymphoid malignancies: Results of a randomized European Organisation for Research and Treatment of Cancer-Children's Leukemia Group phase 3 trial. *Blood* **99**: 2734–2739.

72. Balduzzi A, Valsecchi MG, Uderzo C, de Lorenzo P, Klingebiel T, Peters C, Stary J, Felice MS, Magyarosy E, Conter V, Reiter A, Messina C, Gadner H, Schrappe M. (2005) Chemotherapy versus allogeneic transplantation for very-high-risk childhood acute lymphoblastic leukaemia in first complete remission: Comparison by genetic randomisation in an international prospective study. *Lancet* **366**: 635–642.

74. Tubergen DG, Gilchrist GS, O'Brien RT, Coccia PF, Sather HN, Waskerwitz MJ, Hammond GD. (1993) Prevention of CNS disease in intermediate-risk acute lymphoblastic leukemia: Comparison of cranial radiation and intrathecal methotrexate and the importance of systemic therapy: A Childrens Cancer Group report. *J Clin Oncol* **11**: 520–526.

76. Seibel NL, Steinherz PG, Sather HN, Nachman JB, Delaat C, Ettinger LJ, Freyer DR, Mattano LA Jr., Hastings CA, Rubin CM, Bertolone K, Franklin JL, Heerema NA, Mitchell TL, Pyesmany AF, La MK, Edens C, Gaynon PS. (2008) Early postinduction intensification therapy improves survival for children and adolescents with high-risk acute lymphoblastic leukemia: A report from the Children's Oncology Group. *Blood* **111**: 2548–2555.

83. Nachman J, Sather HN, Cherlow JM, Sensel MG, Gaynon PS, Lukens JN, Wolff L, Trigg ME. (1998) Response of children with high-risk acute lymphoblastic leukemia treated with and without cranial irradiation: A report from the Children's Cancer Group. *J Clin Oncol* **16**: 920–930.

84. Gaynon PS, Bostrom BC, Hutchinson RJ, Lange BJ, Nachman JB, Steinherz PG, Sensel MG, Lee MK, Stram DO, Sather HN. (2001) Duration of hospitalization as a measure of cost on Children's Cancer

Group acute lymphoblastic leukemia studies. *J Clin Oncol* **19**: 1916–1925.

85. Nachman JB, La MK, Hunger SP, Heerema NA, Gaynon PS, Hastings C, Mattano LA Jr., Sather H, Devidas M, Freyer DR, Steinherz PG, Seibel NL. (2009) Young adults with acute lymphoblastic leukemia have an excellent outcome with chemotherapy alone and benefit from intensive postinduction treatment: A report from the Children's Oncology Group. *J Clin Oncol* **27**: 5189–5194.
89. Harms DO, Gobel U, Spaar HJ, Graubner UB, Jorch N, Gutjahr P, Janka-Schaub GE. (2003) Thioguanine offers no advantage over mercaptopurine in maintenance treatment of childhood ALL: Results of the randomized trial COALL-92. *Blood* **102**: 2736–2740.
90. Stork LC, Matloub Y, Broxson E, La M, Yanofsky R, Sather H, Hutchinson R, Heerema NA, Sorrell AD, Masterson M, Bleyer A, Gaynon PS. (2010) Oral 6-mercaptopurine versus oral 6-thioguanine and veno-occlusive disease in children with standard-risk acute lymphoblastic leukemia: Report of the Children's Oncology Group CCG-1952 clinical trial. *Blood* **115**: 2740–2748.
91. Vora A, Mitchell CD, Lennard L, Eden TO, Kinsey SE, Lilleyman J, Richards SM. (2006) Toxicity and efficacy of 6-thioguanine versus 6-mercaptopurine in childhood lymphoblastic leukaemia: A randomised trial. *Lancet* **368**: 1339–1348.
92. Conter V, Valsecchi MG, Silvestri D, Campbell M, Dibar E, Magyarosy E, Gadner H, Stary J, Benoit Y, Zimmermann M, Reiter A, Riehm H, Masera G, Schrappe M. (2007) Pulses of vincristine and dexamethasone in addition to intensive chemotherapy for children with intermediate-risk acute lymphoblastic leukaemia: A multicentre randomised trial. *Lancet* **369**: 123–131.
94. Matloub Y, Lindemulder S, Gaynon PS, Sather H, La M, Broxson E, Yanofsky R, Hutchinson R, Heerema NA, Nachman J, Blake M, Wells LM, Sorrell AD, Masterson M, Kelleher JF, Stork LC. (2006) Intrathecal triple therapy decreases central nervous system relapse but fails to improve event-free survival when compared with intrathecal methotrexate: Results of the Children's Cancer Group (CCG) 1952 study for standard-risk acute lymphoblastic leukemia, reported by the Children's Oncology Group. *Blood* **108**: 1165–1173.
97. Pui CH, Campana D, Pei D, Bowman WP, Sandlund JT, Kaste SC, Ribeiro RC, Rubnitz JE, Raimondi SC, Onciu M, Coustan-Smith E, Kun LE, Jeha S, Cheng C, Howard SC, Simmons V, Bayles A, Metzger ML, Boyett JM, Leung W, Handgretinger R, Downing JR, Evans WE, Relling MV. (2009) Treating childhood acute lymphoblastic leukemia without cranial irradiation. *N Engl J Med* **360**: 2730–2741.
99. Arico M, Valsecchi MG, Camitta B, Schrappe M, Chessells J, Baruchel A, Gaynon P, Silverman L, Janka-Schaub G, Kamps W, Pui CH, Masera G. (2000) Outcome of treatment in children with Philadelphia chromosome-positive acute lymphoblastic leukemia. *N Engl J Med* **342**: 998–1006.
102. Schultz KR, Bowman WP, Aledo A, Slayton WB, Sather H, Devidas M, Wang C, Davies SM, Gaynon PS, Trigg M, Rutledge R, Burden L, Jorstad D, Carroll A, Heerema NA, Winick N, Borowitz MJ, Hunger SP, Carroll WL, Camitta B. (2009) Improved early event-free survival with imatinib in Philadelphia chromosome-positive acute lymphoblastic leukemia: A Children's Oncology Group study. *J Clin Oncol* **27**: 5175–5181.
104. Pieters R, Schrappe M, de Lorenzo P, Hann I, de Rossi G, Felice M, Hovi L, LeBlanc T, Szczepanski T, Ferster A, Janka G, Rubnitz J, Silverman L, Stary J, Campbell M, Li CK, Mann G, Suppiah R, Biondi A, Vora A, Valsecchi MG. (2007) A treatment protocol for infants younger than 1 year with acute lymphoblastic leukaemia (Interfant-99): An observational study and a multicentre randomised trial. *Lancet* **370**: 240–250.
105. Mann G, Attarbaschi A, Schrappe M, de Lorenzo P, Peters C, Hann I, de Rossi G, Felice M, Lausen B, Leblanc T, Szczepanski T, Ferster A, Janka-Schaub G, Rubnitz J, Silverman LB, Stary J, Campbell M, Li CK, Suppiah R, Biondi A, Vora A, Valsecchi MG, Pieters R. (2010) Improved outcome with hematopoietic stem cell transplantation in a poor prognostic subgroup of infants with mixed-lineage-leukemia (MLL)-rearranged acute lymphoblastic leukaemia: Results from the Interfant-99 Study. *Blood* **116**: 2644–2650.
107. Schrauder A, Reiter A, Gadner H, Niethammer D, Klingebiel T, Kremens B, Peters C, Ebell W, Zimmermann M, Niggli F, Ludwig WD, Riehm H, Welte K, Schrappe M. (2006) Superiority of allogeneic hematopoietic stem-cell transplantation compared with chemotherapy alone in high-risk childhood T-cell acute lymphoblastic leukemia: Results from ALL-BFM 90 and 95. *J Clin Oncol* **24**: 5742–5749.
110. Bhojwani D, Kang H, Moskowitz NP, Min DJ, Lee H, Potter JW, Davidson G, Willman CL, Borowitz MJ, Belitskaya-Levy I, Hunger SP, Raetz EA, Carroll WL. (2006) Biologic pathways associated with relapse in

childhood acute lymphoblastic leukemia: A Children's Oncology Group study. *Blood* **108**: 711–717.

113. Einsiedel HG, von Stackelberg A, Hartmann R, Fengler R, Schrappe M, Janka-Schaub G, Mann G, Hahlen K, Gobel U, Klingebiel T, Ludwig WD, Henze G. (2005) Long-term outcome in children with relapsed ALL by risk-stratified salvage therapy: Results of trial acute lymphoblastic leukemia-relapse study of the Berlin-Frankfurt-Munster Group 87. *J Clin Oncol* **23**: 7942–7950.

115. Bader P, Kreyenberg H, Henze GH, Eckert C, Reising M, Willasch A, Barth A, Borkhardt A, Peters C, Handgretinger R, Sykora KW, Holter W, Kabisch H, Klingebiel T, von Stackelberg A. (2009) Prognostic value of minimal residual disease quantification before allogeneic stem-cell transplantation in relapsed childhood acute lymphoblastic leukemia: The ALL-REZ BFM Study Group. *J Clin Oncol* **27**: 377–384.

119. Tallen G, Ratei R, Mann G, Kaspers G, Niggli F, Karachunsky A, Ebell W, Escherich G, Schrappe M, Klingebiel T, Fengler R, Henze G, von Stackelberg A. (2010) Long-term outcome in children with relapsed acute lymphoblastic leukemia after time-point and site-of-relapse stratification and intensified short-course multidrug chemotherapy: Results of trial ALL-REZ BFM 90. *J Clin Oncol* **28**: 2339–2347.

121. Freyer DR, Seibel NL, La MK, Devidas M, Carroll WL, Hunger SP, Gaynon PS. (2008) Survival after relapse in higher risk acute lymphoblastic leukemia (ALL) in children and adolescents is independent of prior treatment intensity: A report from the Children's Oncology Group (COG). *Blood* **112**: 917.

135. Burger B, Zimmermann M, Mann G, Kuhl J, Loning L, Riehm H, Reiter A, Schrappe M. (2003) Diagnostic cerebrospinal fluid examination in children with acute lymphoblastic leukemia: Significance of low leukocyte counts with blasts or traumatic lumbar puncture. *J Clin Oncol* **21**: 184–188.

136. Gajjar A, Harrison PL, Sandlund JT, Rivera GK, Ribeiro RC, Rubnitz JE, Razzouk B, Relling MV, Evans WE, Boyett JM, Pui CH. (2001) Traumatic lumbar puncture at diagnosis adversely affects outcome in childhood acute lymphoblastic leukemia. *Blood* **96**: 3381–3384.

139. Jeha S, Pei D, Raimondi SC, Onciu M, Campana D, Cheng C, Sandlund JT, Ribeiro RC, Rubnitz JE, Howard SC, Downing JR, Evans WE, Relling MV, Pui CH. (2009) Increased risk for CNS relapse in pre-B cell leukemia with the t(1;19)/TCF3-PBX1. *Leukemia* **23**: 1406–1409.

147. Borowitz MJ, Devidas M, Hunger SP, Bowman WP, Carroll AJ, Carroll WL, Linda S, Martin PL, Pullen DJ, Viswanatha D, Willman CL, Winick N, Camitta BM. (2008) Clinical significance of minimal residual disease in childhood acute lymphoblastic leukemia and its relationship to other prognostic factors: A Children's Oncology Group study. *Blood* **111**: 5477–5485.

148. Sherborne AL, Hosking FJ, Prasad RB, Kumar R, Koehler R, Vijayakrishnan J, Papaemmanuil E, Bartram CR, Stanulla M, Schrappe M, Gast A, Dobbins SE, Ma Y, Sheridan E, Taylor M, Kinsey SE, Lightfoot T, Roman E, Irving JA, Allan JM, Moorman AV, Harrison CJ, Tomlinson IP, Richards S, Zimmermann M, Szalai C, Semsei AF, Erdelyi DJ, Krajinovic M, Sinnett D, Healy J, Neira AG, Kawamata N, Ogawa S, Koeffler HP, Hemminki K, Greaves M, Houlston RS. (2010) Variation in CDKN2A at 9p21.3 influences childhood acute lymphoblastic leukemia risk. *Nat Genet* **42**: 492–494.

152. Ottmann OG, Druker BJ, Sawyers CL, Goldman JM, Reiffers J, Silver RT, Tura S, Fischer T, Deininger MW, Schiffer CA, Baccarani M, Gratwohl A, Hochhaus A, Hoelzer D, Fernandes-Reese S, Gathmann I, Capdeville R, O'Brien SG. (2002) A phase 2 study of imatinib in patients with relapsed or refractory Philadelphia chromosome-positive acute lymphoid leukemias. *Blood* **100**: 1965–1971.

12

Treatment of Adolescents and Young Adults with Acute Lymphoblastic Leukemia in the Modern Era

James Nachman and Hagop Kantarjian

Introduction

Modern chemotherapy regimens produce long-term survival rates of 80–95% for children and young adults with acute lymphoblastic leukemia (ALL).[1,2] Chemotherapy regimens for adult ALL result in complete response (CR) rates of 90% and long-term survival rates are only 30–50%.[3,4] Children less than 10 years of age have a better prognosis than patients 10–21 years of age when treated with pediatric regimens and young adults 16–30 have a better outcome compared to older adults when treatment is given according to adult protocols.

For the purposes of this review, we will consider adolescent and young adult patients (AYA) to be between the ages of 16 and 30 years of age at diagnosis (see Chapter 3). A rationale for this definition comes from a report of a Spanish trial utilizing a "pediatric" type regimen for adults with ALL which showed no difference in outcome for patients 15–18 years old (n = 35) compared with patients 19–30 years old (n = 46). Within this AYA group, there is a subgroup of patients between 16 and 21–25 years of age who may be treated by either pediatric or medical oncologists.

Since the primary care physician generally determines the referral to an oncologist, AYA patients who continue to see a pediatrician are referred to pediatric oncologists while AYA patients whose primary care is given by an internist are generally referred to a medical oncologist. Some AYA patients live at home with parents and are likely covered by parental insurance; such patients are more likely to be seen by a pediatric oncologist. Other AYA patients live on their own and may or may not have insurance. Living status and insurance status may play a role in determining outcome for these AYA patients.

Biological and Clinical Features of ALL with Increasing Age — Impact on Defining Prognosis in AYAs

T-cell ALL is more frequent in AYA patients with ALL (25%) than in children or adults with ALL (10–15%).[5] The incidence of Philadelphia chromosome (Ph)+ ALL is only 2–3% in childhood ALL, about 5–10% in AYA ALL (higher in the 22–30 age group than the 16–21 year age group), and increases to 15–25% in adult ALL (see Chapter 5).[6] In children with ALL, the two most common cytogenetic abnormalities are the TEL-AML1 translocation and high hyperdiploidy. Among patients 1–9 years of age, with white blood cell (WBC) counts less than 50×10^9/L at diagnosis, more than 50% have either a high hyperdiploid karyotype or a TEL-AML1 translocation. A hyperdiploid karyotype is noted in 10–15% of AYA patients with ALL, but the TEL-AML1 translocation is rarely seen in this age group.[7,8] Lymphoblasts from older adolescents have decreased *in vitro* sensitivity to vincristine, prednisone, and asparaginase compared with younger patients.[9] ALL blasts from older patients show significantly more promoter methylation and a higher incidence of CRLF2 rearrangements compared with younger patients. AYA patients with ALL have higher hemoglobin levels at diagnosis and a lower incidence of lymphomatous features compared with younger patients despite the increased incidence of T-cell ALL. There are no significant differences in clinical or biological features of ALL among patients 10–15 years old and those 16–21 years old.

In a group of 262 AYA patients 16–21 years of age with ALL treated on the Children's Cancer Group (CCG) 1961 study, 21% had T-cell ALL, and 26% had an initial WBC greater than 50×10^9/L. Seven percent of patients had Ph+ ALL, 1.4% had t(4;11), 6.3% had t(1;19), and 6.9% had hyperdiploid karyotypes with trisomies of chromosomes 4, 10, and 17. TEL-AML1 translocation testing was not performed for patients on this study.[10]

Why do Children have a Better Prognosis Than Adults with ALL?

Adults with ALL have a worse outcome compared with children. The worse outcome can be attributed to several factors listed in Table 12.1 which include biological factors (see Chapters 4, 5 and 6), medical factors, treatment-related factors, and psychosocial factors (see Chapter 28).

Table 12.1. Potential reasons for differences in the prognosis of childhood and adult ALL.

- Differences in the biology (cytogenetic-molecular) in different age groups
- Intensive use of non-myelosuppressive agents such as steroids, vincristine, and asparaginase
- Earlier and more intensive use of intrathecal central nervous system prophylaxis (e.g. 16–20 intrathecals in pediatric regimens compared with 2–16 intrathecals in adult regimens).
- Longer duration of maintenance therapy with 6-mercaptopurine, vincristine, methotrexate, and prednisone (POMP maintenance), typically 2–2 and a half years in pediatric regimens compared with < 1 to up to 2 years in adult regimens.
- Adherence to treatment regimen by both physicians and patients, in particular as it relates to insurance under parent versus patient own insurance and/or lack of insurance; socioeconomic status of adolescents or young adults at the time of disease diagnosis.

Table 12.2. Differences in the incidences and outcome of cytogenetic-molecular abnormalities in children and adults with ALL.

Cytogenetic/ molecular group	Pediatric Pts	Cure	Adolescent/ young adult	Cure
PH Positive	< 5%	28%	20–30%	< 5%
Hyperdiploid >50 Chromosomes	28%	> 80%	< 5%	No available data
TEL-AML-1 t(12:21)	25–30%	90%	< 5%	No available data

Biological factors

The TEL-AML translocation is present in 25–30% of children with ALL but only in 2% of adult ALL. Similarly, a hyperdiploid karyotype (> 50 chromosomes) is noted in 28% of childhood ALL but only in 2–3% of adult ALL. Both the TEL-AML1 translocation and high hyperdiploidy are associated with an excellent prognosis. In contrast, Ph+ ALL is noted in 20–30% of adult ALL cases but only in 5% of childhood ALL cases (Table 12.2). Ph+ ALL historically carries a poor prognosis. There is a higher incidence of promoter methylation and CRLF2 mutations in adult ALL and both abnormalities are associated with a poor prognosis.

Medical factors

The presence of comorbidities in older adults may adversely impact the ability to give intensive ALL therapy. It is well known that both treatment-related mortality and morbidity increase with age. Adults may have significantly greater toxicity associated with asparaginase administration compared to younger patients. The salvage rate for older patients who experience ALL relapse is significantly lower compared to the salvage rates for younger patients.[11,12]

Treatment factors

Until recently, significant treatment differences existed between adult and pediatric ALL protocols and likely accounts for some of the outcome differences for children and adults.

Treatment — Evolution of Pediatric and Adult Regimens Over Time

Evolution of pediatric regimens

Pediatric regimens for ALL feature higher cumulative doses of the non-myelosuppressive agents vincristine, asparaginase, and steroids compared to adult treatment protocols. Adult ALL protocols utilize higher cumulative doses of myelosuppressive agents including anthracyclines, cytarabine, and cyclophosphamide.

The original CCG studies for AYA patients utilized a Berlin-Frankfurt-Munster (BFM) type backbone therapy which included an intensive induction-consolidation followed by an interim maintenance and delayed reinduction-reconsolidation phases, before proceeding with 1–2 years of maintenance therapy. CNS prophylaxis consisted of cranial or cranio-spinal radiation and intrathecal therapy. Over time, the use of craniospinal radiation has been eliminated and the use of cranial radiation has decreased significantly. For patients who still require radiation, the dose of radiation has been reduced.

In the late eighties, BFM investigators reported that patients who had more than 10^9 peripheral blasts/L following a 7-day prednisone prophase (approximately 10% of patients) had an EFS rate of 40% with BFM-type therapy. Similarly, CCG reported that patients with more than 25% marrow blasts on day 7 of 4-drug induction therapy (slow early response) had an EFS rate of less than 50%. Based on these findings, the German BFM research group introduced regimen modifications for prednisone poor responder patients that utilized post-induction blocks of intensive intermittent chemotherapy featuring high-dose methotrexate, high-dose cytarabine, ifosfamide, and vindesine. No delayed intensification was given. These modifications did not improve the results compared with standard BFM therapy.[13]

CCG investigators chose a different approach in treating slow early responder patients. The hypothesis behind the modified CCG regimen, called "augmented" BFM, was that treatment failure in such patients resulted from a relative rather than an absolute resistance to the standard drugs used in ALL therapy. Augmented BFM maintained the basic BFM backbone but markedly increased the dose intensity of vincristine and asparaginase. In addition, intravenous methotrexate was used without leucovorin rescue in interim maintenance phases.[14]

The consolidation phase in BFM protocols consists of cyclophosphamide, cytarabine, and 6-mercaptopurine. In the Children's Oncology Group (COG) studies, cyclophosphamide is given on days 1 and 14, cytarabine is given for 4 days every week × 4, and 6-mercaptopurine is given daily for 28 days. However, by day 14 of therapy, many patients are neutropenic and often febrile, and chemotherapy is generally held until blood counts recover. Therefore, the CCG augmented regimen added a 2-week course of non-myelosuppressive chemotherapy consisting of weekly vincristine and 6 doses of asparaginase beginning on day 14 of the consolidation course. A second course of cyclophosphamide, cytarabine, and 6-mercaptopurine followed by vincristine and asparaginase was started on day 28. During delayed intensification, vincristine and asparaginase was given on day 14 of reconsolidation.

Interim maintenance on CCG protocols had consisted of daily oral 6-mercaptopurine and weekly oral methotrexate. In the augmented BFM regimen, interim maintenance consisted of courses of vincristine and escalating dose intravenous methotrexate without leucovorin rescue on day 1, and asparaginase on day 2. Courses were repeated at 10-day intervals for a total of five courses. To further intensify chemotherapy, a second interim maintenance and delayed intensification were given prior to starting maintenance therapy.

In the first year of therapy, the augmented BFM regimen delivered twice as many doses of vincristine and three times as many doses of asparaginase compared with standard BFM. The augmented BFM regimen also delivered 10 courses of intravenous methotrexate without rescue and additional doses of cyclophosphamide, cytarabine, and steroids. The total doses delivered on augmented BFM compared to other regimens are shown in Table 12.3.

In the pilot trial of augmented BFM therapy, toxicity was manageable. Many patients required dose reductions of vincristine. There was a relatively high incidence of asparaginase allergy. Following completion of the pilot trial, National Cancer Institute (NCI) high-risk patients with slow early response were randomized to receive either augmented BFM or standard BFM. Patients receiving augmented BFM had a statistically significant improvement in both EFS and survival compared with patients receiving standard BFM.[14]

In the successor CCG 1961 study, conducted from 1996–2002, CCG investigated whether the incorporation of elements of augmented BFM therapy would improve the outcome for NCI high-risk patients who

Table 12.3. Dose intensity of induction and consolidation maintenance in Children Cancer Group (CCG) vs. common acute leukemia group B (CALGB) regimens.[15]

A. Induction with CCG vs. CALGB

Agent/Therapy	CCG	CALGB
Prednisone (mg/m^2)	1680	1260
Vincristine (mg)	8	8
L-asparaginase (U/m^2)	54,000	36,000
Daunorubicin (mg/m^2)	100	135
Cyclophosphamide (mg/m^2)	—	1200
IT-methotrexate	Day 14	—
IT-cytarabine	Day 0	—

B. Consolidation with CCG-BFM (Berlin–Frankfurt Muster) vs. augmented BFM vs. CALGB

Agent/Therapy	CCG-BFM	A-BFM	CALGB
Dexamethasone (mg/m^2)	210	420	140
Vincristine (mg/m^2)	22.5	45	14
L-asparaginase (U/m^2)	90,000	318,000	48,000
Doxorubicin (mg/m^2)	75	150	90
Cyclophosphomide (mg/m^2)	3000	4000	3000
IT methotrexate (mg/m^2), Cranial XRT [cGy]	132 + XRT or 216, no XRT	132 [1800]	105 [2400]

This research was originally published in *Blood.* Stock, W., La, M., Sanford, B., Bloomfield, C.D., Vardiman, J.W., Gaynon, P., Larson, R.A. and Nachman, J. What determines the outcomes for adolescents and young adults with acute lymphoblastic leukemia treated on cooperative group protocols? A comparison of Children's Cancer Group and Cancer and Leukemia Group B studies. *Blood.* 2001;112:1646–1654. © The American Society of Hematology.

showed a rapid response to induction therapy. The basic question was whether increasing the dose intensity of therapy — additional vincristine and asparaginase — during consolidation/reconsolidation courses and the use of intravenous methotrexate without rescue during interim maintenance phases or the addition of a second interim maintenance and delayed intensification, or both interventions would improve outcome. For rapid responders, the study was conducted according to a 2 by 2 design — patients were concurrently randomized to increase or standard strength chemotherapy, and to one or two interim maintenance and delayed intensification phases. The study was only powered to detect differences for the two randomized therapeutic strategies.[19] Patients with slow early response received full augmented BFM and were randomized to receive or not receive idarubicin and cyclophosphamide courses during re-induction phases. All AYA patients were entered on this protocol.

Two hundred and sixty-two patients 16–21 years of age were entered on this study. One hundred and

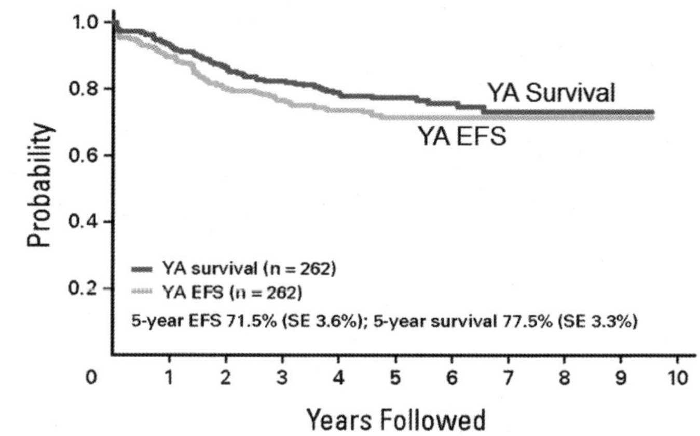

Fig. 12.1. Event-free survival (EFS) and overall survival for young adult (YA) patients treated on Children's Cancer Group 1961 (n = 262).

Originally published by the American Society of Clinical Oncology. [Nachman, J.B., La, M.K., Hunger, S.P., Heerema, N.A., Gaynon, P.S., Hastings, C., Mattano, L.A., Jr, Sather, H., Devidas, M., Freyer, D.R., Steinherz, P.G., Seibel, N.L: *J Clin Oncol* 27(31), 2009: 5189–5194].

seventy-seven patients were rapid responders, 75 patients were slow responders and 10 patients had no day 7-marrow performed. Seventy-one patients experienced adverse events (induction death: 6; remission death: 7; induction failure: 6; relapse: 46; second malignancy: 5). The 5-year EFS and survival for patients 16–21 years old were 71.5% (SE 3.6%) and 77.5% (SE 3.3%), respectively (Fig. 12.1). The 5 year EFS was 82% (SE 5.4%) for young adult rapid responders who were randomized to augmented intensity therapy, vs. 67% (SE 6.7%) for patients randomized to standard intensity therapy (P = .07). The study was not powered to adequately assess differences in EFS by treatment arm in the young adult population, but the magnitude of the EFS difference between standard and augmented intensity therapy was similar to that seen for the overall study population for whom the difference in outcome was statistically significant. There was no statistical difference in EFS for young adults rapid responder patients, randomized to 1 or 2 delayed intensification phases. For slow early responders, the 5-year EFS was 71% (SE 7.3%). There were no significant prognostic factors for patients with T lineage ALL. For patients with B-precursor ALL, WBC $\geq 50 \times 10^9$/L (Fig. 12.2) and unfavorable cytogenetics (t(9;22); t(4;11); hypodiploid karyotypes with < 44 chromosomes) were unfavorable prognostic factors.

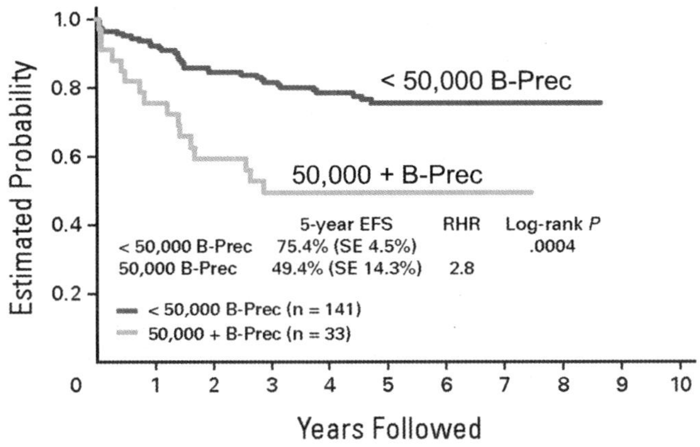

Fig. 12.2. Prognostic significance of WBCs more than 50,000/μL in young adult patients with B-precursor (B-Prec) acute lymphoblastic leukemia. EFS, event-free survival; RHR, relative hazard rate.

Originally published by the American Society of Clinical Oncology. [Nachman, J.B., La, M.K., Hunger, S.P., Heerema, N.A., Gaynon, P.S., Hastings, C., Mattano, L.A., Jr, Sather, H., Devidas, M., Freyer, D.R., Steinherz, P.G., Seibel, N.L: *J Clin Oncol* 27(31), 2009: 5189–5194].

Evolution of adult regimens

Most adult regimens have included induction with vincristine, steroids, and anthracyclines; multiple consolidations with high doses of cytarabine, methotrexate, plus or minus asparaginase, and maintenance therapy with POMP in conjunction with CNS prophylaxis. In contrast to the evolution of pediatric regimens, many adult ALL protocols began investigating myelosuppressive or ablative therapies (allogeneic and autologous transplant in first remission). At the same time, the intensity of non-myelosuppressive therapies and intrathecal therapy was reduced. The duration of maintenance therapy was also shortened. The adoption of more intensive myelosuppressive treatment components and shortening the duration of maintenance therapy generally followed the principles of adult AML therapy protocols.

The major differences between pediatric and adult ALL regimens may account, in part, for the significant differences in outcomes for AYA patients treated on pediatric vs. adult ALL regimens (summarized in Table 12.4). Dosages of chemotherapeutic agents utilized in the CCG vs. CALGB regimens are shown in Table 12.3.

Comparison of Outcome for AYA Patients Treated on Pediatric vs. Adult Protocols

The first study comparing AYA patients, treated on either a pediatric or an adult ALL trial, was reported by Stock *et al.* (see Chapter 11).[15] Patients 16–21 years of age at diagnosis were included. The investigators performed a retrospective comparison of 321 AYA patients treated on CCG and CALGB studies from 1988–2001. There were no significant differences in either presenting clinical features or cytogenetics between the two patient groups, but the majority of CCG patients were either 16 or 17 years of age while the majority of CALGB patients were 18–21 years of age. While the CR

Table 12.4. Comparison of adult vs. pediatric regimens in adolescents and young adults with ALL.

Country (Reference)	Regimen	Age	No.	% CR	% EFS (Years)
• United States (15)	CCG (Peds)	16–21	197	90	63 (7)
	CALGB (Adult)		124	90	34 (7)
• France (13)	FRALLE 93 (Peds)	15–20	77	94	67 (5)
	LALA94 (Adult)		100	83	41 (5)
• Holland (14)	DGOG (Peds)	15–18	47	98	69 (5)
	HVON (Adult)		44	91	34 (5)
• United Kingdom (17)	ALL97 (Peds)	15–17	61	98	65 (5)
	UKALLXII (Adult)		67	94	49 (5)
• Italy (18)	AIEOP (Peds)	14–18	150	94	80 (2)
	GIMEMA (Adult)		95	89	71 (2)
• Finland (19)	NOPHO (Peds)	10–25	128	96	67 (5)
	ALL (Adult)		97	97	60 (5)
• M. D. Anderson	Hyper CVAD (Adult)	13–30	175	97	70 (3)
	Augmented BFM	14–36	48	95	82 (2)
Cancer Center (21, 27)	(Peds)				

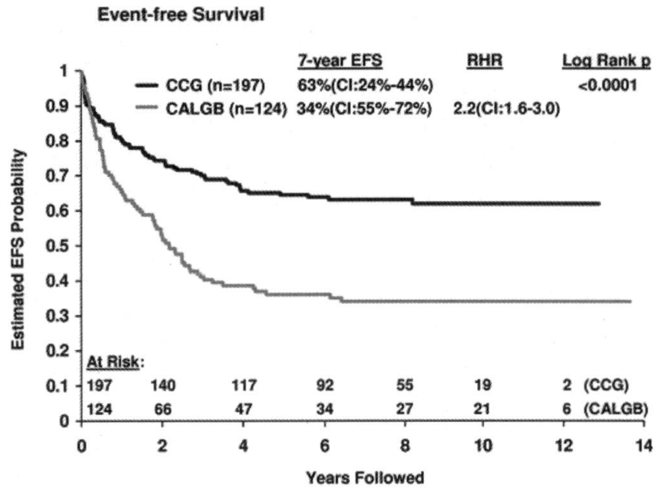

(A)

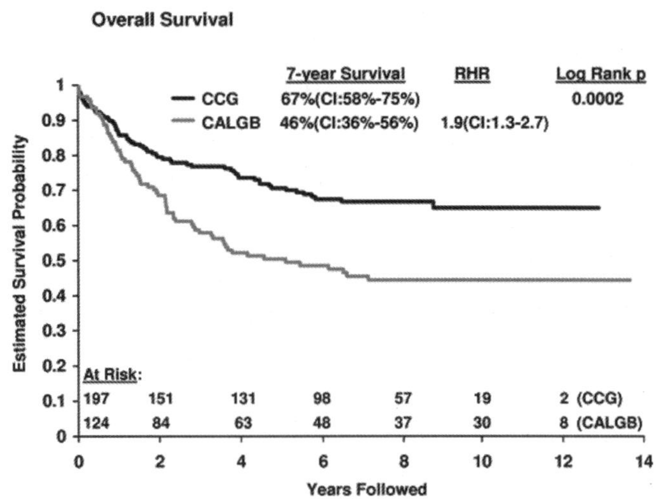

(B)

Fig. 12.3. Comparison of EFS and OS. (A) Comparison of EFS among CALGB (gray line) and CCG (black line) patients. The 7-year RHR for CALGB patients was 2.2 (Cl, 1.6–3.0; *P* < .001). (B) Comparison of OS among CALGB (gray line) and CCG (black line) patients. The 7-year relative hazard ratio (RHR) for death in CALGB patients was 1.9 (Cl, 1.3–2.7; *P* < .001).

This research was originally published in *Blood.* Stock, W., La, M., Sanford, B., Bloomfield, C.D., Vardiman, J.W., Gaynon, P., Larson, R.A. and Nachman, J. What determines the outcomes for adolescents and young adults with acute lymphoblastic leukemia treated on cooperative group protocols? A comparison of Children's Cancer Group and Cancer and Leukemia Group B studies. *Blood.* 2001;112:1646–1654. © The American Society of Hematology.

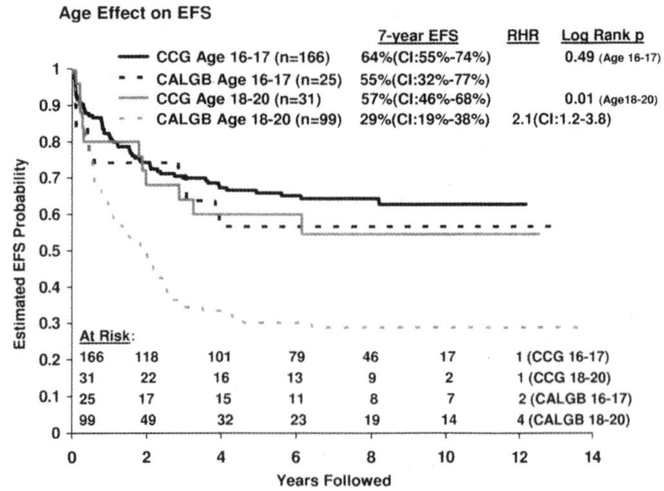

Fig. 12.4. Age effect on outcome. CALGB patients aged 16 to 17 years had a 7-year EFS of 55%, which was similar to a 64% EFS for 16- to 17-year-old CCG patients (*P* = .49). CALGB patients aged 18 to 20 years old had a 7-year EFS of 29%, which was significantly worse than that for the younger CALGB patients and the 57% EFS for 18- to 20-year-olds on CCG trials (*P* = .01; RHR, 2.1 [Cl, 1.2–3.8]).

This research was originally published in *Blood.* Stock, W., La, M., Sanford, B., Bloomfield, C.D., Vardiman, J.W., Gaynon, P., Larson, R.A. and Nachman, J. What determines the outcomes for adolescents and young adults with acute lymphoblastic leukemia treated on cooperative group protocols? A comparison of Children's Cancer Group and Cancer and Leukemia Group B studies. *Blood.* 2001;112:1646–1654. © The American Society of Hematology.

rates were identical (90%) patients treated on CCG protocols had a significantly higher 7-year EFS rate (63% vs. 34%) and survival rate (67% vs. 46%) (Fig. 12.3A–B). While outcome was similar among patients 16–17 years old, patients 18–20 years old had a 7-year EFS of 55% treated on the CCG protocol vs. only 29% for patients treated on the CALGB protocol (Fig. 12.4). As noted in Table 12.2, the CCG regimen provided significantly higher doses of dexamethasone (about twofold), vincristine (about twofold), and asparaginase (about threefold), as well as earlier and more intensive CNS prophylaxis.

French investigators compared AYA patients (age 15–20 years old) treated on a pediatric regimen, FRALLE-93 (n = 77) and those treated on an adult protocol, LALA-94 (n = 100). The CR rates were 94% vs. 83% and the estimated 5-year EFS rates were 67% vs. 41%. In a multivariate analysis, treatment regimen was an independent prognostic factor for outcome. In these studies, the pediatric regimens delivered a fivefold higher cumulative dose of prednisone, a threefold higher cumulative dose of vincristine, and a 20-fold higher cumulative dose of asparaginase. On pediatric protocols, asparaginase was administered during induction while in the adult regimen, asparaginase was begun during consolidation.[13]

Similar studies conducted in the Netherlands, Italy, Sweden, and the UK all showed better outcomes for AYA patients treated on pediatric protocols.[14,16–18]

In contrast, a study from Finland showed similar results for AYA patients treated on the pediatric NOPHO (n = 128; age 10–16 years) protocol compared to patients treated utilizing an adult ALL regimen (n = 97; age 17–25 years). The CR rates were 96% and 97% and the estimated 5-year EFS rates were 67% and 60%, respectively. In this particular study, the investigators emphasized that the cumulative doses of non-myelosuppressive agents (steroids, vincristine, asparaginase) were similar in the pediatric and adult protocols, perhaps explaining the similar outcome of AYA patients in this particular analysis.[19]

Why do Pediatric Regimens Produce Better Outcomes for AYA Patients

Analyses of the above trials suggest many possible reasons for the better results observed utilizing pediatric protocols: (1) dose intensity and cumulative dosage of non-myelosuppressive agents; (2) administration of long term maintenance therapy; (3) less utilization of allogeneic SCT in first CR, which, in the case of AYAs, may increase mortality without improving outcome; (4) earlier and more intensive use of intrathecal therapy for CNS prophylaxis and (5) a cluster of less tangible factors including expertise in caring for younger patients with ALL, better familiarity with supportive care measures, compliance to therapy on the part of both physicians and patients (and the multiple reasons behind it), and possibly, in the United States, the insurance status of AYA patients.[13–21]

The intensity of central nervous system (CNS) prophylaxis has been mentioned as one reason for the better success of pediatric regimens which generally utilize 16 or more intrathecal chemotherapy injections. Eradicating early CNS disease potentially reduces the incidence of reseeding and systemic relapse.

Many adult ALL regimens have either omitted maintenance with 6-mercaptopurine, vincristine, methotrexate and prednisone (POMP maintenance) or utilized it for shorter periods of time (1–2 years) than in pediatric regimens (2–2 and one half years). It is now well known from Japanese pediatric experience that shorter durations of POMP maintenance are associated with significantly worse outcome.[22]

Many adult ALL regimens offer allogeneic stem cell transplant (SCT) in first remission if a suitable donor is available. In some studies, patients without a suitable donor have been randomized to autologous SCT vs. chemotherapy. In a recent joint Medical Research Council (MRC) and Eastern Cooperative Oncology Group (ECOG) study, the 5-year survival for 234 Ph– patients younger than 20 years of age was only 43%. In a group of patients considered as having "standard" risk ALL — age less than 35 years, no t(9;22), B precursor and WBC count less than 100×10^9/L or T and WBC less than 30×10^9/L — a significant survival advantage was observed among patients with a suitable donor for allogeneic SCT. The 5-year survival rate was 62% for patients with a donor vs. 52% for patients without a donor (P = .02). However, these patients constituted only about 12–15% of the total study group. In contrast, the remaining patients (age 35 years or older, Ph+ ALL, other high-risk features) did not benefit from allogeneic SCT. In addition, this MRC-CCG study reported a significantly worse survival with autologous SCT compared with maintenance therapy, except in the subset of T-cell ALL in which the two approaches appeared equivalent. Within the COG 1961 trial, 16–21-year-old patients meeting the standard risk criteria of the MRC-ECOG had a 5-year EFS and survival rate of 73% and 80%, respectively. This suggests that pediatric regimens are effective for AYA patients with favorable prognostic features and preclude the need for allogeneic SCT in first remission.

The current COG trial for NCI high-risk ALL includes patients 16–30 years old. Patients are initially randomized to receive either dexamethasone (10 mg/m^2 for 14 days) or prednisone (60 mg/m^2 for 28 days) during induction, and either escalating doses of methotrexate without rescue or high dose methotrexate with leucovorin rescue. The induction steroid randomization was discontinued because of a high rate of avascular bone necrosis in the dexamethasone arm. The methotrexate randomization is ongoing.

An adult trial for AYA patients, which utilizes one of the arms of the COG trial, is also ongoing.

Outcome of AYA patients with ALL treated by medical oncologists utilizing pediatric-like regimens

Based on the better outcome for young adult ALL patients treated on pediatric protocols, several adult groups have begun to treat AYA, as well as older patients (up to the age of 50 years), on pediatric regimens in an attempt to improve outcome and to gain insight into the toxicities observed when adults are treated on pediatric protocols.

French investigators recently reported the outcome of 215 patients with ALL aged 15–60 years old treated on a pediatric-based regimen, GRALL-2003. The overall CR rate was 93% and the 42-month EFS rate was 55% and survival rate 60%. In this study, the cumulative dose of prednisone was 8.6-fold higher than in the previous adult protocols, the vincristine cumulative dose was 3.7-fold higher, and the cumulative dose of asparaginase was 16-fold higher. The best results were among patients 15–45 years old. In patients 45–60 years old, the regimen was associated with a high incidence of chemotherapy-related death compared with the LALA94 regimen (23% vs. 5%).[23]

As part of a large scale analysis of 844 patients aged 1–18 years treated on Dana Farber Cancer Institute (DFCI) protocols, Barry *et al.* reported the outcome of 51 AYA (age 15–18 years old) accrued on these studies. The 5-year EFS rate for this particular group was 78%, similar to the outcome of 108 younger patients (age 10–15 years) treated on the same protocols. Of note, the 5-year EFS rate of 78% is similar to that of patients of similar age treated on CCG protocols.[24] Recently, the DFCI adult consortium reported the results of the same regimen, now used in adults (age 18–50 years). In this protocol, the emphasis was on an extended course of asparaginase for 30 weeks. Among 74 patients treated, the CR rate was 82%, the 2-year EFS was 72%, and the 2-year survival was 73%. Toxicities related particularly to non-myelosuppressive agents were significant, including severe pancreatitis in 13% and thromboembolic events in 19% of patients.[25] A modified DFCI pediatric regimen used by Canadian investigators in 68 patients (age 17–71 years) yielded a CR rate of 85%, a 3-year disease-free survival rate of 77% and a 3-year survival rate of 65%.[26]

Outcome for AYA patients and possibly adults with ALL is improved using pediatric-inspired regimens that emphasize higher dose intensity of non-myelosuppressive agents, in particular asparaginase. When pediatric regimens are used to treat adults with ALL, complications are observed including pancreatitis, renal dysfunction, thromboembolic events and neurotoxicity; these may be significant enough to nullify the potential benefit of pediatric type regimens among patients 45 years or older. Allogeneic stem cell transplant in first remission for AYA patients should not be utilized for all patients with a suitable donor. The use of maintenance for 1 and a half to 2 years for AYA and adult patients may improve outcome.

Some currently utilized adult regimens more closely resemble pediatric protocols. The hyper-CVAD regimen developed at M. D. Anderson Cancer Center continues to use dose intensive non-myelosuppressive therapy and prolonged POMP maintenance but has de-emphasized asparaginase intensification because of the potential neurotoxicity among older patients. The hyper-CVAD regimen has accrued 175 patients aged 13–30 years (83 patients aged 13–21 years, 92 patients aged 22–30 years). The overall CR rate was 97%, the 3-year survival rate was 69% and 3-year disease-free survival rate 70%.[21] These results are not different from those reported by DeAngelo *et al.* and Storring *et al.*[25,26] An ongoing study at M. D. Anderson Cancer Center utilizes the pediatric augmented BFM regimen among AYA with ALL. So far, 48 patients (median age 20 years; range 14 to 36 years) have been treated. The CR rate was 95% and the estimated 2-year survival rate 82%.[27] The results of this study will be compared to similarly aged patients treated with hyper-CVAD. It appears that the general consensus in the evolution of adult ALL regimens is to utilize more non-myelosuppressive agents during induction, consolidation and maintenance, with particular emphasis on asparaginase.

Specific Subgroups

About 10% of AYA with ALL demonstrate a hyperdiploid karyotype with additional copies of chromosomes 4 and 10. As in younger patients, AYAs with hyperdiploid karyotype have a good prognosis with current therapies.

About 5–8% of AYAs with precursor B-ALL have Ph+ ALL. Until recently, standard Ph+ ALL therapy resulted in EFS rates of less than 30–50%. Rapid early response to induction, younger age, and WBC $< 50 \times 10^9$/L were favorable prognostic features. Most groups recommended allogeneic SCT in first remission for patients with Ph+ ALL if suitable donors were available. A recent COG study combined chemotherapy with a BCR-ABL tyrosine kinase inhibitor, imatinib, for the treatment of Ph+ ALL. The preliminary results were encouraging with an estimated 3-year EFS rates of 80% without the use of allogeneic SCT. Thus, it is not clear whether allogeneic SCT in first remission is the best option for patients with Ph+ ALL who have a rapid early response to chemotherapy and imatinib. A longer follow-up is required to assess whether chemotherapy and imatinib will prevent or only delay relapse.

About 2–3% of patients 16–21 years old have t(4;11). These patients generally present with a high WBC count and have CD10-negative blasts by flow cytometry.

Patients with t(4:11) and a rapid response to induction therapy generally have a reasonable outcome. However, slow responders have a poor outcome and may benefit from allogeneic SCT in first remission.

The TEL-AML1 translocation occurs in less than 5% of AYA with ALL. There is no data concerning the outcome in this small subgroup of patients. Patients with a hypodiploid karyotype (with less than 44 chromosomes) are rare. It is generally accepted that these patients have a poor prognosis and should be offered allogeneic SCT in first remission when possible.

Treatment Complications

In all pediatric cooperative group trials, AYA patients have experienced increased treatment-related morbidity and mortality compared to children with ALL. In the CCG 1961 study, AYA patients had significantly higher incidence of side effects including hyperglycemia, stroke, encephalopathy, and avascular necrosis (AVN) compared to children.

AVN has been recognized as a complication of long-term steroid use and was first reported as a significant complication of ALL therapy on CCG 1882. Interestingly, this was the first CCG study to use an age criterion of 10 years or older as an indicator of high risk. The incidence of AVN was 0.9% for patients less than 10 years of age and 14.2% for patients 10 years of age or older. In this trial, the CCG compared standard and augmented BFM therapies for slow responder patients (more than 25% blasts on a day 7 marrow aspirate). For patients 10 years or older with slow early response, the incidence of AVN was 16.4% with standard BFM and 23.2% with augmented BFM. Thus, AVN was identified as a significant complication for patients 10 years or older.

In the CCG 1961 trial, patients receiving discontinuous dexamethasone (days 1–7 and 14–21) during each of two delayed intensification courses had approximately half the incidence of AVN compared with patients receiving continuous dexamethasone during a single delayed intensification course (days 1–21). Thus, discontinuous dexamethasone during delayed intensification was adopted for ALL patients over 12 years old entered on the next generation high-risk ALL trial.

In the ongoing AALL0232 study, NCI high-risk patients randomized to dexamethasone at 10 mg/m^2 for 14 days during induction had a significantly higher incidence of AVN compared with patients randomized to prednisone at 60 mg/m^2 for 28 days. Therefore, the dexamethasone arm was discontinued for patients greater than 10 years of age and these patients are assigned to prednisone therapy during induction.

Despite these measures — discontinuous dexamethasone for all patients 10 years and older during delayed intensification and prednisone during induction — the incidence of AVN in AYA remains in the 10–20% range. The incidence of AVN is lower in patients younger than 10 years and older than 21 years.

The high incidence of AVN has led some trial groups to consider MRI screening for AVN at defined time points during therapy for ALL. At the present time, this is not the standard of care. The COG is planning a randomized comparison of pravastatin vs. no specific anti-AVN therapy in an attempt to reduce the incidence of AVN.

Adolescent and Young Adults with Acute Lymphoblastic Leukemia: Future Considerations

Determination of the presence of minimal residual disease (MRD), either by flow cytometry or PCR techniques, in conjunction with cytogenetic analysis (both standard and molecular) is the basis for post-induction risk stratification in most current ALL trials. MRD at end induction, alone or in combination with MRD at the end of consolidation, has been shown to be a highly significant prognostic factor in both adult and pediatric ALL trials. Many groups use MRD determinations, usually at a post-consolidation time point to determine which patients should receive an allogeneic SCT in first remission (see Chapter 20).

Gene profiling may identify different subgroups with differing prognoses and may be instrumental in determining new therapeutic targets (see Chapter 22). Ikaros gene deletions and rearrangement in CRLF2 are examples of genetic mutations associated with poor outcome for which targeted therapy may soon exist (see Chapter 6).[28]

New drugs have become available which may impact EFS and overall survival. These include clofarabine in precursor B-ALL and nelarabine for T-cell ALL.[29,30]

The development of new tyrosine kinase inhibitors has the potential to further improve cure rates in patients with Ph+ ALL. Combinations of the more potent BCR-ABL inhibitors, e.g. dasatinib, with chemotherapy as initial treatment for Ph+ ALL are under investigation.[31]

Monoclonal antibodies with or without an attached cytotoxic molecule show promise in the treatment of

ALL (see Chapter 21). Investigators at M.D. Anderson Cancer Center have incorporated rituximab into treatment protocols for patients with CD20+ ALL, demonstrating positive results in mature B ALL and in CD20+ ALL.[32,33] Additional studies are planned to evaluate epritzumab, an anti-CD22 antibody, in the treatment of patients with high-risk B precursor ALL.

References

1. Pui CH, Robison LL, Look AT. (2008) Acute lymphoblastic leukaemia. *Lancet* **371**: 1030–1043.
2. Pulte D, Gondos A, Brenner H. (2008) Trends in 5- and 10-year survival after diagnosis with childhood hematologic malignancies in the United States, 1990–2004. *J Natl Cancer Inst* **100**: 1301–1309.
3. Gokbuget N, Hoelzer D. (2009) Treatment of adult acute lymphoblastic leukemia. *Semin Hematol* **46**: 64–75.
4. Larson S, Stock W. (2008) Progress in the treatment of adults with acute lymphoblastic leukemia. *Curr Opin Hematol* **15**: 400–407.
5. Pullen J, Shuster JJ, Link M, Borowitz M, Amylon M, Carroll AJ, Land V, Look AT, McIntyre B, Camitta B. (1999) Significance of commonly used prognostic factors differs for children with T cell acute lymphocytic leukemia (ALL), as compared to those with B-precursor ALL. A Pediatric Oncology Group (POG) study. *Leukemia* **13**: 1696–1707.
6. Secker-Walker LM, Craig JM, Hawkins JM, Hoffbrand AV. (1991) Philadelphia positive acute lymphoblastic leukemia in adults: Age distribution, BCR breakpoint and prognostic significance. *Leukemia* **5**: 196–199.
7. Aguiar RC, Sohal J, van Rhee F, Carapeti M, Franklin IM, Goldstone AH, Goldman JM, Cross NC. (1996) TEL-AML1 fusion in acute lymphoblastic leukaemia of adults. M.R.C. Adult Leukaemia Working Party. *Br J Haematol* **95**: 673–677.
8. Harrison CJ. (2009) Cytogenetics of paediatric and adolescent acute lymphoblastic leukaemia. *Br J Haematol* **144**: 147–156.
9. Pieters R, den Boer ML, Durian M, Janka G, Schmiegelow K, Kaspers GJ, van Wering ER, Veerman AJ. (1998) Relation between age, immunophenotype and *in vitro* drug resistance in 395 children with acute lymphoblastic leukemia — implications for treatment of infants. *Leukemia* **12**: 1344–1348.
10. Nachman JB, La MK, Hunger SP, Heerema NA, Gaynon PS, Hastings C, Mattano LA Jr., Sather H, Devidas M, Freyer DR, Steinherz PG, Seibel NL. (2009) Young adults with acute lymphoblastic leukemia have an excellent outcome with chemotherapy alone and benefit from intensive postinduction treatment: A report from the children's oncology group. *J Clin Oncol* **27**: 5189–5194.
11. Malempati S, Gaynon PS, Sather H, La MK, Stork LC. (2007) Outcome after relapse among children with standard-risk acute lymphoblastic leukemia: Children's Oncology Group study CCG-1952. *J Clin Oncol* **25**: 5800–5807.
12. Thomas DA, Kantarjian H, Smith TL, Koller C, Cortes J, O'Brien S, Giles FJ, Gajewski J, Pierce S, Keating MJ. (1999) Primary refractory and relapsed adult acute lymphoblastic leukemia: Characteristics, treatment results, and prognosis with salvage therapy. *Cancer* **86**: 1216–1230.
13. Boissel N, Auclerc MF, Lheritier V, Perel Y, Thomas X, Leblanc T, Rousselot P, Cayuela JM, Gabert J, Fegueux N, Piguet C, Huguet-Rigal F, Berthou C, Boiron JM, Pautas C, Michel G, Fiere D, Leverger G, Dombret H, Baruchel A. (2003) Should adolescents with acute lymphoblastic leukemia be treated as old children or young adults? Comparison of the French FRALLE-93 and LALA-94 trials. *J Clin Oncol* **21**: 774–780.
14. de Bont JM, Holt B, Dekker AW, van der Does-van den Berg A, Sonneveld P, Pieters R. (2004) Significant difference in outcome for adolescents with acute lymphoblastic leukemia treated on pediatric vs adult protocols in the Netherlands. *Leukemia* **18**: 2032–2035.
15. Stock W, La M, Sanford B, Bloomfield CD, Vardiman JW, Gaynon P, Larson RA, Nachman J. (2008) What determines the outcomes for adolescents and young adults with acute lymphoblastic leukemia treated on cooperative group protocols? A comparison of Children's Cancer Group and Cancer and Leukemia Group B studies. *Blood* **112**: 1646–1654.
16. Hallbook H, Gustafsson G, Smedmyr B, Soderhall S, Heyman M. (2006) Treatment outcome in young adults and children >10 years of age with acute lymphoblastic leukemia in Sweden: A comparison between a pediatric protocol and an adult protocol. *Cancer* **107**: 1551–1561.
17. Ramanujachar R, Richards S, Hann I, Goldstone A, Mitchell C, Vora A, Rowe J, Webb D. (2007) Adolescents with acute lymphoblastic leukaemia: Outcome on UK national paediatric (ALL97) and adult (UKALLXII/E2993) trials. *Pediatr Blood Cancer* **48**: 254–261.
18. Testi AM, Valsecchi MG, Conter V, Vignetti M, Paoloni F, Giona F, Moleti ML, Nigro LL, Locatelli F, la Dogana S, Specchia G, Fabiano F, Recchia A, Mandelli F, Foa' R, Masera G. (2004) Difference in Outcome of Adolescents with Acute Lymphoblastic Leukemia (ALL) Enrolled in

Pediatric (AIEOP) and Adult (GIMEMA) Protocols. *Blood* **104**: 1954.

19. Usvasalo A, Raty R, Knuutila S, Vettenranta K, Harila-Saari A, Jantunen E, Kauppila M, Koistinen P, Parto K, Riikonen P, Salmi TT, Silvennoinen R, Elonen E, Saarinen-Pihkala UM. (2008) Acute lymphoblastic leukemia in adolescents and young adults in Finland. *Haematologica* **93**: 1161–1168.
20. Schiffer CA. (2003) Differences in outcome in adolescents with acute lymphoblastic leukemia: A consequence of better regimens? Better doctors? Both? *J Clin Oncol* **21**: 760–761.
21. Thomas DA, Rytting M, O'Brien S, Faderl S, Wierda WG, Franklin A, Garris R, Ravandi F, Cortes J, Kantarjian HM. (2009) Outcome for Adolescents and Young Adults (AYA) with the Hyper-CVAD (with or without Rituximab) Regimens for *De Novo* Acute Lymphoblastic Leukemia (ALL) or Lymphoblastic Lymphoma. *Blood* **114**: 3084.
22. Toyoda Y, Manabe A, Tsuchida M, Hanada R, Ikuta K, Okimoto Y, Ohara A, Ohkawa Y, Mori T, Ishimoto K, Sato T, Kaneko T, Maeda M, Koike K, Shitara T, Hoshi Y, Hosoya R, Tsunematsu Y, Bessho F, Nakazawa S, Saito T. (2000) Six months of maintenance chemotherapy after intensified treatment for acute lymphoblastic leukemia of childhood. *J Clin Oncol* **18**: 1508–1516.
23. Huguet F, Leguay T, Raffoux E, Thomas X, Beldjord K, Delabesse E, Chevallier P, Buzyn A, Delannoy A, Chalandon Y, Vernant JP, Lafage-Pochitaloff M, Chassevent A, Lheritier V, Macintyre E, Bene MC, Ifrah N, Dombret H. (2009) Pediatric-inspired therapy in adults with Philadelphia chromosome-negative acute lymphoblastic leukemia: The GRAALL-2003 study. *J Clin Oncol* **27**: 911–918.
24. Barry E, DeAngelo DJ, Neuberg D, Stevenson K, Loh ML, Asselin BL, Barr RD, Clavell LA, Hurwitz CA, Moghrabi A, Samson Y, Schorin M, Cohen HJ, Sallan SE, Silverman LB. (2007) Favorable outcome for adolescents with acute lymphoblastic leukemia treated on Dana-Farber Cancer Institute Acute Lymphoblastic Leukemia Consortium Protocols. *J Clin Oncol* **25**: 813–819.
25. DeAngelo DJ, Silverman LB, Couban S, Dahlberg S, Amrein PC, Seftel MD, Turner AR, Wadleigh M, Sirulnik LA, Galinsky I, Sallan SE, Stone RM. (2006) A multicenter phase II study using a dose intensified pediatric regimen in adults with untreated acute lymphoblastic leukemia. *Blood* **108**: 1858.
26. Storring JM, Brandwein J, Gupta V, Schuh AC, Schimmer A, Yee K, Wells RA, Lipton JH, Messner HA, Xu W, Minden MD. (2006) Treatment of Adult Acute Lymphoblastic Leukemia (ALL) with a Modified DFCI Pediatric Regimen — The Princess Margaret Experience. *Blood* **108**: 1875.
27. Rytting M, Thomas DA, Franklin AR, Jabbour E, Wierda W, Faderl S, Wells R, Kadia T, Ravandi F, Ferrajoli A, Cortes J, O'Brien S, Kantarjian H. (2009) Pediatric-based therapy for young adults with newly diagnosed lymphoblastic leukemia. *Blood* **114**: 2037.
28. Martinelli G, Iacobucci I, Storlazzi CT, Vignetti M, Paoloni F, Cilloni D, Soverini S, Vitale A, Chiaretti S, Cimino G, Papayannidis C, Paolini S, Elia L, Fazi P, Meloni G, Amadori S, Saglio G, Pane F, Baccarani M, Foa R. (2009) IKZF1 (Ikaros) deletions in BCR-ABL1-positive acute lymphoblastic leukemia are associated with short disease-free survival and high rate of cumulative incidence of relapse: A GIMEMA AL WP report. *J Clin Oncol* **27**: 5202–5207.
29. Faderl S, Thomas DA, Koller CA, Ravandi F, Burger J, O'Brien S, Dara S, Kantarjian HM. (2008) Hyper-CVAD plus nelarabine: A pilot study for patients with newly diagnosed T cell Acute Lymphoblastic Leukemia (ALL)/Lymphoblastic Lymphoma (LL). *Blood* **112**: 3960.
30. Jeha S, Gandhi V, Chan KW, McDonald L, Ramirez I, Madden R, Rytting M, Brandt M, Keating M, Plunkett W, Kantarjian H. (2004) Clofarabine, a novel nucleoside analog, is active in pediatric patients with advanced leukemia. *Blood* **103**: 784–789.
31. Ravandi F, Kantarjian HM, Thomas DA, Faderl S, Jones D, Koller CA, Dara S, Garris R, Kebriaei P, Champlin R, Borthakur G, Wierda WG, Burger JA, Cortes J, O'Brien S. (2009) Phase II study of combination of the hypercvad regimen with dasatinib in the front line therapy of patients with Philadelphia Chromosome (Ph) Positive Acute Lymphoblastic Leukemia (ALL). *Blood* **114**: 837.
32. Thomas DA, Faderl S, O'Brien S, Bueso-Ramos C, Cortes J, Garcia-Manero G, Giles FJ, Verstovsek S, Wierda WG, Pierce SA, Shan J, Brandt M, Hagemeister FB, Keating MJ, Cabanillas F, Kantarjian H. (2006) Chemoimmunotherapy with hyper-CVAD plus rituximab for the treatment of adult Burkitt and Burkitt-type lymphoma or acute lymphoblastic leukemia. *Cancer* **106**: 1569–1580.
33. Thomas DA, Kantarjian HM, Faderl S, Wierda WG, Cortes J, Burger JA, Ferrajoli A, Estrov Z, Koller C, Konopleva M, Borthakur G, Jabbour E, Ravandi F, Kadia T, Garcia-Manero G, Kornblau SM, Andreeff M, Garris R, Keating MJ, O'Brien S. (2009) Chemoimmunotherapy with a modified hyper-CVAD and rituximab regimen improves outcome for patients with *de novo* philadelphia negative precursor B-cell Acute Lymphoblastic Leukemia (ALL). *Blood* **114**: 836.

13

Childhood, Adolescent and Young Adult Acute Myeloid Leukemias

Robert J. Arceci, Soheil Meshinchi, Todd L. Rosenblat, Joseph G. Jurcic and Martin S. Tallman

Definitions

Acute myeloid leukemia (AML) is a molecularly heterogeneous hematologic malignancy characterized by the clonal proliferation and accumulation of variably differentiated bone marrow-derived myeloid precursors. The molecular heterogeneity is furthermore manifested by nearly every aspect of the physiology, clinical presentation, prognostic factors, treatments, and outcomes.

Epidemiology

The incidence of AML in children less than 20 years old in the United States is approximately 7 per million per year or approximately 600 new cases per year, accounting for 19% of leukemia in childhood (see Chapter 1).[1] From 1975 to 2004, the incidence of AML in children 0 to 19 years of age in the United States increased at a rate of 1.3% per year. With the exception of an increased incidence of AML in infants, the incidence of AML is relatively constant until early adolescence when it continues to slowly rise through young adulthood; after 50 years of age, the incidence rises dramatically, mostly due to secondary, high risk MDS/AML until after about 80 years of age, when the incidence declines (Fig. 13.1).[2]

The incidence of AML varies according to race and ethnicity. For example, in the United States, the annual incidence of AML in Hispanic children and young adults is 9 per million, which is mainly secondary to the increase of acute promyelocytic leukemia (APL).[3,4] The United States Surveillance, Epidemiology and End Results (SEER) database demonstrates similar incidence rates between Caucasian and African American youth.[5] The rates of AML cases from Japan, Australia and Zimbabwe are 8, 8 and 11 per million annually.[6]

Several environmental factors have also been linked to the development of AML, including specific genotoxic exposures. For example, ionizing radiation exposure after the atomic bomb detonations in Hiroshima and Nagasaki during World War II resulted in a 20-fold increase in the incidence of AML that peaked 6–8 years after exposure.[7–10] No increased risk was demonstrated in children following prenatal exposure of mothers to that ionizing radiation.[11] No substantial evidence has been presented for a link between paternal ionizing radiation exposure and increased incidence of childhood leukemia.[12] Prenatal exposure to diagnostic X-rays has not been definitively linked to an increased

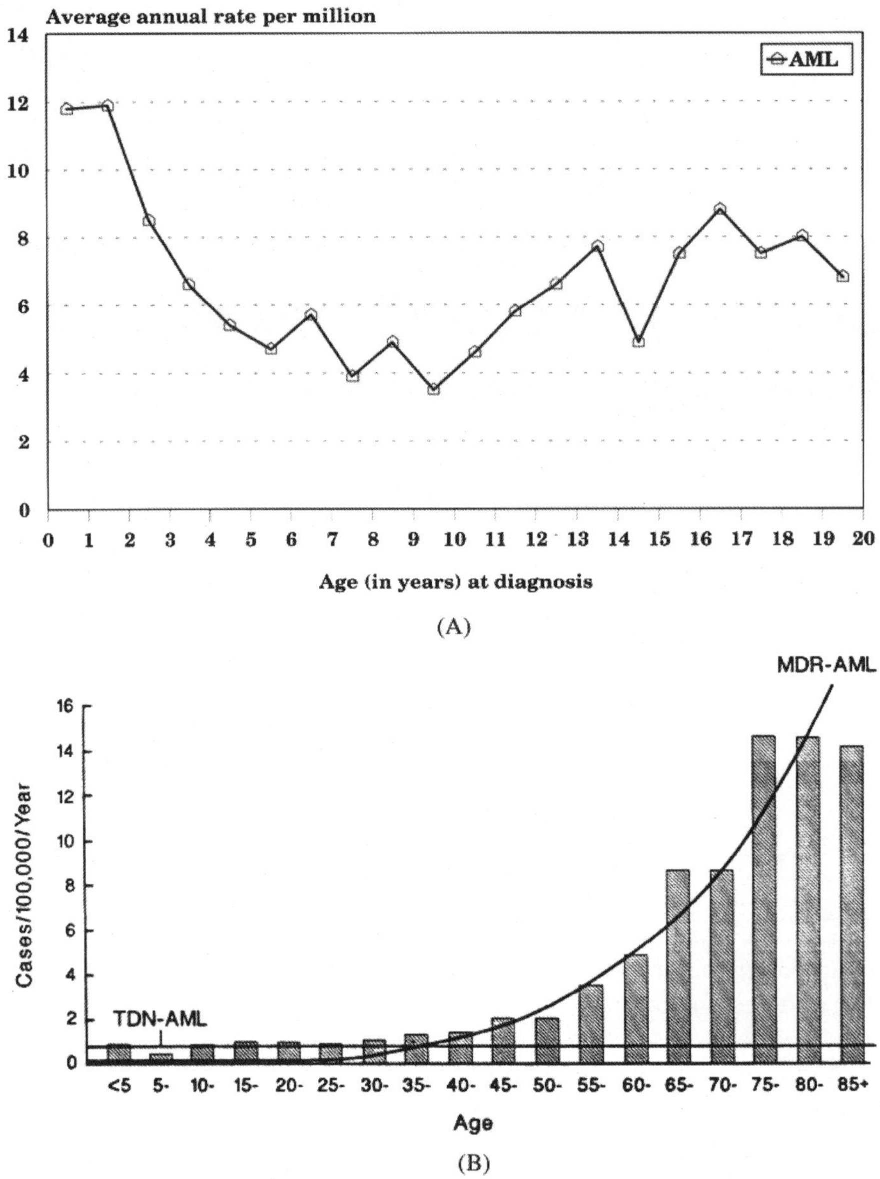

Fig. 13.1. Frequency of AML at different ages, (A) showing a peak during infancy and (B) a gradual increase occurring with age. From Head DR. (1996) Revised classification of acute myeloid leukemia. *Leukemia* 10: 1826–1831.[387]

incidence of AML in offspring.[12] Of note, there has also been no definitive evidence that exposure to ultrasound or electromagnetic fields, such as observed from electrical power lines, increases the incidence of AML.[13,14]

A variety of chemical exposures have been linked to the development of AML. Prenatal exposure of marijuana, cigarette smoking or alcohol has been linked to the development of AML in offspring in some studies but other reports have not confirmed those observations.[15–19] However, a stronger association has been reported for increased infant AML characterized by chromosome 11q23 rearrangements and maternal use of substances that contain topoisomerase II inhibitors, such as flavonoids and catechins present in green tea, caffeine as well as quinolones in some classes of antibiotics.[20–22] Such observations are consistent with the induction of chromosome 11q23 and MLL rearrangements by *in vitro* exposure of CD34+ hematopoietic precursors to bioflavonoids.[22]

Environmental chemical exposures, including petroleum products, benzene, herbicides and pesticides have also been associated with increased likelihood of developing MDS and AML.[22–26] Not unexpectedly, secondary AML arising from the treatment of patients with cancer, and sometimes non-malignant disorders, with genotoxic chemotherapeutic agents has been extensively documented.[27–31] Usually, alkylating agents, as well as ionizing radiation, result in MDS/AML 5–7 years from exposure; these leukemias are commonly associated with monosomies or deletions of chromosome 7 and (sometimes) 5. Topoisomerase II inhibitors have a shorter latency period of around 2 years from exposure and, as noted above, commonly lead-to-lead to AML characterized by chromosome 11q23 abnormalities, although other subtypes, including acute promyelocytic leukemia (APL) have also been described.[32–35] While cumulative dose and timing of alkylating agents, particularly, etoposide, are important considerations in the development of AML, minimal exposures have also been linked to the early development of 11q23 AML.[36–38]

Inherited Predisposition

Several inherited syndromes demonstrate an increased incidence of AML and have helped define some of the key molecular etiologic pathways (Table 13.1). For example, Down syndrome (DS) represents the most common predisposing condition with the highest incidence of developing leukemia. There is a 10- to 20-fold increased risk of leukemia in children with DS, particularly the development of megakaryoblastic subtype (AMKL, FAB M7) of AML during the first 3 years of life.[39] Of note, approximately 10% of neonates with DS have a transient myeloproliferative disorder (TMD) that mimics the AMKL but resolves spontaneously in 4–6 weeks; however, about 20–30% of these patients subsequently develop true AMKL. While it is unclear how the presence of trisomy 21 increases the risk of leukemia in these patients, both TMD and AMKL share similar somatic mutations of the GATA1 transcription factor in nearly all cases.[40] The presence of GATA1 mutations can be used to follow patients with DS and TMD for subsequent development of AML. Several bone marrow failure syndromes (BMFS) also demonstrated increased risks of developing AML. These include Fanconi anemia (defects in DNA repair), Kostmann syndrome (defects in neutrophil elastase *ELA2*), Schwachman–Diamond syndrome (ribosomal processing *SBDS* gene), Diamond–Blackfan anemia (defects in ribosomal small and large subunit proteins) and dyskeratosis congenita (X-lined mutations in the dyskerin or autosomal recessive forms with mutations in genes regulating telomere maintenance and RNA processing). Other rare inherited disorders with a propensity to develop AML include congenital amegakaryocytic thrombocytopenia (defects in the *CFFA2* gene and thrombopoietin receptor gene, *c-mpl*), autosomal dominant macrothrombocytopenia (Fechtner syndrome, *MYH9* gene), familial platelet disorder with propensity to myeloid malignancy (FPD/AML, germline mutations in the *RUNX1/CEPB*α-gene).[41–48] In addition, mutations in the neurofibromin gene, encoding a RAS-inactivating GTPase, is responsible for neurofibromatosis type I and an increased incidence of juvenile myelomonocytic leukemia (JMML) and AML.[49,50] Mutations in the *PTPN11* gene, which encodes a SHP-2 tyrosine phosphatase, leads to Noonan syndrome and increased predisposition to JMML.[51,52] Mutations in *CBL*, encoding an E3 ubiquitin ligase, have been reported to be associated with a dominant inheritance of a developmental disorder and predisposition to JMML (see Chapter 14).[53–55] Patients with Li-Fraumeni syndrome and Bloom syndrome, involving defects in *p53* and the *BLM* helicase gene, respectively, have also been reported to have a propensity to develop leukemia, including AML.[41,56–59]

The increased incidence of AML in a twin or sibling of a patient with AML (or ALL) can vary from nearly 100% concordance in monozygotic or identical twins to approximately 20% in fraternal twins up until about 6 years of age, when the incidence decreases to that of the general population.[60–62] Non-twin, familial cases of AML are rare and often associated with constitutional translocations, such as t(7;20 and t(3;6) or monosomy 7.[63–65]

Acquired Predisposition

As in the case of inherited predispositions, the development of AML arising from acquired disorders has also shed light on etiologic factors. For example, patients with severe aplastic anemia (SAA) treated with immunosuppressive agents, such as cyclosporin A (CsA) and anti-thymocyte globulin (ATP) or cyclophosphamide, often along with recombinant human granulocyte colony-stimulating factor (G-CSF) have been reported to have up to a 20% risk of developing myelodysplastic syndrome (MDS) or AML.[66–68] A similar disorder, paroxysmal nocturnal hemoglobinuria (PNH), is also associated with an increased risk of developing MDS and AML although less frequently than SAA.[69] While AML arising in patients with MDS is a relatively common event in adults, MDS is relatively rare in children and may differ in biological and clinical characteristics from that observed in adults.[70] This is an area that requires more comparative studies.[67,68,71[2–4]]

Table 13.1. Pediatric disorders with a leukemia predisposition syndrome.

Disorder	Inheritance	Associated myeloid malignancy	Clinical features	Molecular genetic features
Fanconi anemia	AR	MDS, AML (cumulative risk up to 50%)	Characteristic congenital abnormalities (skeletal, renal, mental retardation), progressive bone marrow failure	Mutations in one of several components of FA/BRCA multi-protein complex involved in homology-directed DNA repair, resulting in chromosomal instability, increased sensitivity to genotoxic agents (mitomycin C, diepoxybutane), cancer risk
Bloom syndrome	AR	AML	Characteristic congenital abnormalities (dwarfism, facies), sun sensitivity	*BLM* (a RecQ helicase family member) mutations, resulting in chromosomal instability, sister chromatid exchanges, cancer risk (many types)
Dyskeratosis congenita	XR, AD, AR	MDS, AML	Abnormal skin pigmentation, nail dystrophy, leukoplakia, progressive bone marrow failure	*DKC1* (XR) or *TERC* (AD) (components of telomerase complex) mutations, resulting in defective telomere maintenance
Li-Fraumeni syndrome	AD	AML	Cancer predisposition (mostly solid tumors, leukemia less common)	*P53* mutations
Neurofibromatosis type 1	AD	JMML, MDS, AML	Characteristic neurocutaneous syndrome	*NF1* mutations, resulting in enhanced RAS signaling
Noonan syndrome	AD	JMML, MDS, AML	Characteristic congenital abnormalities (cardiac, short stature, facies, webbed neck)	*PTPN11* mutations, resulting in enhanced RAS signaling
Kostmann syndrome	AR	MDS, AML	Severe congenital neutropenia	*ELA2* mutations, resulting in agranulocytosis; secondary activating mutations of G-CSF receptor often responsible for progression to AML
Congenital amegakaryocytic thrombocytopenia	AR	MDS, AML	Congenital thrombocytopenia, progressive bone marrow failure	*MPL* (thrombopoietin receptor) mutations
Familial platelet disorder with predisposition to AML	AD	AML	Qualitative and quantitative platelet defects	*AML1* mutations
Diamond-Blackfan anemia	AD	AML	Pure red cell aplasia, characteristic congenital abnormalities (facial, skeletal, genitourinary)	*RPS19* mutations
Schwachman-Diamond syndrome	AR	MDS, AML	Neutropenia, exocrine pancreatic insufficiency, skeletal abnormalities	*SBDS* mutations

(Adapted from Brown P, Arceci RJ. Acute Myelogenous Leukemia, Myelodysplasia and Myeloproliferative Syndromes in Children. In: Carroll W, Finlay J, eds. *Pediatric Oncology* (2010)[389].)

Etiology

The heterogeneity of AML at the morphological, immunophenotypic and especially molecular levels has made unifying causes initially difficult to conceptualize. However, evidence from both cellular and molecular studies have led to a model of AML etiology that links genetic defects, caused by environmental and/or inherited predisposition abnormalities, affecting cellular self-renewal and differentiation.[72] For example, an initial transforming event in so-called type II mutations involving transcription factors such as core-binding factor (CBF) proteins or the histone methyltransferase MLL (mixed lineage leukemia) may confer self-renewal properties to hematopoietic stem or progenitor cells. Subsequent Type I mutations, involving such genes as tyrosine kinases receptors (e.g. FLT3/ITD and c-KIT), can result in the activation of these receptor-mediated pathways and a profound proliferative signal to hematopoietic progenitors. Depending on which stem or progenitor cells such mutations occur, as well as the identity of the specific mutations, a different subtype of AML can be derived. Thus, while normal hematopoiesis is characterized by a hierarchical progression from a hematopoietic stem cell (HSC) which possesses both self-renewal and differentiation potential, leukemia stem cells (LSC) or leukemia-initiating cells (LIC) may also have a hierarchical progression, but with limited or restricted differentiation capacity.[73] Such models have led to the important considerations for targeting therapeutics toward both the leukemia-initiating cells, as well as the majority of the leukemia, represented by the LIC progeny. Historically, clinical trials in patients with AML have involved cytotoxic agents, which have not been necessarily designed to target selected populations of leukemia cells. However, the detailed analysis of mutated genes and the physiological changes they generate have led to a greater understanding of the etiology of the different types of AML as well as the ability to risk stratify patients and test the therapeutic targeting of those same prognostic pathways.[74]

Clinical Manifestations

Most symptoms and signs of AML in children and young adults are the result of the leukemia cells, ability to replace the bone marrow instead of normal progenitors as well as infiltrate multiple other organs throughout the body. Approximately one trillion leukemia cells have been estimated to be present at the time of diagnosis.

Replacement of normal bone marrow with leukemic blasts leads to alterations in blood counts, which in most cases include neutropenia, anemia and thrombocytopenia. The total white blood cell count may be low, normal or high, depending upon the number of circulating leukemic cells and the residual normal cells. The absolute neutrophil count less often than 500 per microliter and is associated with an increased risk of serious, life-threatening infection. Blood cultures and broad spectrum intravenous antibiotic coverage are indicated in any newly diagnosed leukemia patient with fever. Anemia results in fatigue, lethargy, decreased exercise tolerance, headache and pallor. While uncommon at the time of presentation, congestive heart failure (CHF) may occur, particularly with severe anemia; the transfusion of packed red blood cells should usually be done slowly to avoid worsening or precipitating CHF. Thrombocytopenia often leads to bruising and petechiae, and occasionally over the morrhage into the gastrointestinal track, lungs, or central nervous system. Platelet transfusions should be expeditiously given for very low platelet counts of less than 10,000 per microliter or higher if a patient shows signs of infection. Patients with concomitant coagulopathy due to disseminated intravascular coagulation (DIC) are at particularly high risk for bleeding complications.[75] The leukemia subtype most commonly associated with DIC and life-threatening bleeding is acute promyelocytic leukemia (APL, or M3 AML).[76] This association is due in part to the release of thromboplastin from the cytoplasmic granules in promyelocytic blasts. Aggressive blood product support and early treatment with the differentiation-inducing agent all-trans retinoic acid (ATRA) has been shown to decrease the risk of bleeding in APL.[77,78] Despite these measures, however, up to 10% of patients with APL will die of bleeding complications during the initial weeks of therapy; other permanent sequelae include visual impairment from retinal hemorrhages and other neurologic problems from non-fatal central nervous system hemorrhages.[79,80]

Hyperleukocytosis becomes a potential clinical problem when the WBC rises above 100,000 per microliter.[81] Circulating blood can become hyperviscous with markedly elevated WBC, leading to sludging of blood in brain, lungs, kidneys, and other organs. The risk of hyperviscosity is higher with AML than ALL, since myeloblasts are generally larger and more adherent than lymphoblasts. Management consists of treating the leukemia as soon as possible and exchange transfusion or leukapheresis in cases where initial symptoms are prominent.[82]

A rare but important presentation of AML is spinal cord compression, which results from a chloroma (a solid tumor resulting from the localized proliferation of myeloblasts) in the paraspinal/epidural region.[83] Chloromas, most commonly, are present in the skin or bones, but can occur anywhere in the body. They are most frequently seen in FAB M2 AML, and, in particular, cases with the t(8;21) translocation that results in the AML1/ETO fusion gen (Fig. 13.2).[84] Chloromas are

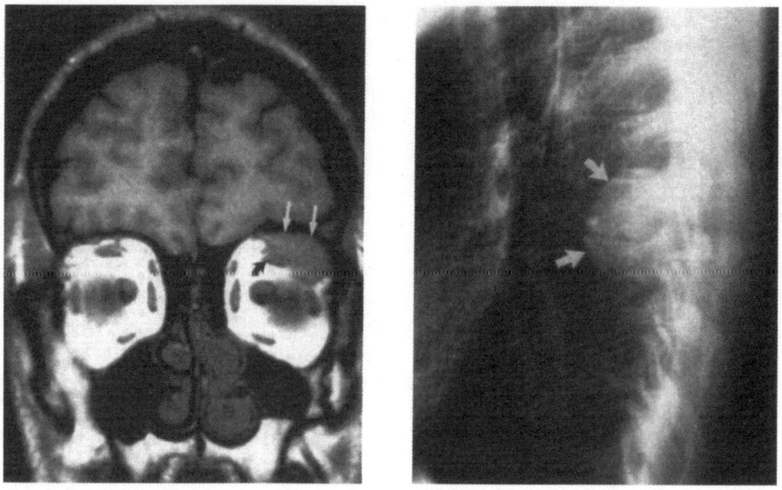

(A) (B)

Fig. 13.2. Panel (A) shows a T1 weighted, coronal MR scan demonstrating a left orbital chloroma; Panel (B) demonstrates a lateral chest radiograph revealing a large right paraspinal pleural-based chloroma.

From Tallman MS, Hakimian D, Shaw JM, Lissner GS, Russell EJ, Variakojis D. (1993) Granulocytic sarcoma is associated with the 8;21 translocation in acute myeloid leukemia. *J Clin Oncol* 11: 690–697.[84]

also commonly observed in patients with FAB M4 and M5 subtypes. Chloromas may occur in approximately 10% of patients with AML. Rarely, patients can present with a chloroma in the absence of detectable bone marrow or other systemic involvement.[85,86] The terms myeloid sarcoma or granulocytic sarcoma are often used to refer to these myeloid neoplasms. In nearly all such cases, the AML will become systemic if the patient is not treated with conventional AML therapy. The management of chloromas has been addressed in a report from CCG in which the EFS and local recurrence rates were not found to be different for patients who received local irradiation to a chloroma along with systemic therapy compared to those who only received systemic therapy.[87] Thus, irradiation is reserved for situations in which a chloroma is not responding to intensive combination therapy or when the chloroma runs the risk of causing significant morbidity, such as loss of vision or spinal cord compression.[87]

Tumor lysis syndrome (TLS) is a complication resulting from the rapid lysis of large numbers of tumor cells, releasing intracellular contents (see Chapter 30). While TLS is seen most often after initial treatment with chemotherapy, it may also be present prior to the initiation of therapy due to spontaneous lysis. Risk factors include high WBC, lymphadenopathy, hepatosplenomegaly, high mitotic index, and a diagnosis of ALL (especially Burkitt leukemia/lymphoma and T-cell ALL), although both spontaneous and treatment-associated TLS is a significant problem in AML, as well. TLS is characterized by hyperuricemia, hyperkalemia, and hyperphosphatemia (with secondary hypocalcemia). Renal insufficiency may develop due to the nephrotoxic effects of precipitated urate crystals in the renal tubules; in severe cases, dialysis may be necessary. Management consists of aggressive hydration to reduce tubular uric acid concentration; some also advocate alkalinization of urine to promote solubility of urate crystals. Frequent electrolyte monitoring with standard management of abnormal levels is essential. Allopurinol is a xanthine oxidase inhibitor routinely used at the outset of leukemia management to decrease the production of uric acid. Rasburicase (recombinant urate oxidase) is an enzymatic agent used in severe cases of TLS to rapidly convert uric acid to the more soluble allantoin.[88]

Prognostic Factors

Risk stratification in the treatment of leukemia has become part of standard practice largely by the success of this approach in improving the overall outlook for children with acute lymphoblastic leukemia (ALL). The rationale underlying risk stratification is that patients known to have a high risk of relapse might benefit from more intensive, albeit potentially more toxic, treatment, and patients who have a lower risk of relapse could be successfully treated with lower intensity regimens and lower treatment-related toxicity. The classification of patients into various risk groups has historically been based on prognostic factors, which were identified by retrospective analysis followed by prospective. Since many of these factors have been interdependent, multivariate analyses are routinely employed to adjust for other contributions of other prognostic factors. Furthermore, the impact of specific prognostic factors may vary based on leukemia subtypes, age groups, and different treatment regimens. Prognostic factors in AML can be based on host and disease characteristics.

Host characteristics

Gender, age, race and constitutional abnormalities have been associated with outcome in young patients with AML. Females tend to have a slightly better prognosis than males, although this association has not been so strong as to be included in treatment stratification. While some reports have described inferior outcomes for infants with AML, most current studies treat infants in a fashion similar to older children with approximately equal outcomes.[89,90] Racial variation appears to have a significant impact on outcomes. For example, non-white patients appear to have a worse outcome than Caucasians treated with identical chemotherapy regimens. An analysis of 1600 children treated on the CCG 2891 and 2961 trials showed that African American and Hispanic patients had an overall survival of approximately 35% vs. 48% for the Caucasians.[91]

Patients with Down syndrome (constitutional trisomy 21) and AML, particularly those under the age of 4 years, usually have megakaryoblastic leukemia that is extremely sensitive to cytotoxic therapy, particularly cytarabine; these patients, even when their marrow shows mosaicism for the trisomy 21, thus have significantly improved outcome with less intensive therapy with remission rates of approximately 90% and an overall survival of 80%. These patients are now treated with significantly intensity-reduced regimens.[92–94]

The body weight of patients with AML has been reported to influence clinical outcome. Patients with AML treated on the CCG-2961 study who were either underweight (≤ 10th percentile) or overweight (> 95th percentile) at diagnosis had an approximately twofold higher risk of death. The increased death rate was secondary to excess treatment-related mortality as opposed to excess relapse risk in both underweight and overweight patients.[95]

Inherited alterations in the detoxification enzyme, GST theta, which result in a null protein phenotype, are associated with a significantly decreased survival due to excess toxicity. This association of toxicity with GST genotype may reflect host metabolic responses to specific drug combinations and may also result in a predisposition for developing leukemia.[96]

Disease characteristics

Historically, prognostic factors have included diagnostic WBC count, morphologic classification (FAB subtype) and biological characteristics such as cytogenetics (see Chapters 4–6). With advances in molecular diagnostics and genomic profiling, additional prognostic factors are being used to further refine risk stratification groups as well as further define the immense heterogeneity of AML.

WBC and morphology

Diagnostic WBC has been demonstrated to be a prognostic factor in AML. The diagnostic WBC appears to be a continuous variable for outcome with increasing WBC being associated with decreased survival. Such a continuous variable has thus far been difficult to incorporate into risk stratification strategies in AML. Thus, cutoff points have been used. For example, a WBC less than 20,000 cells/μL has been associated with improved prognosis and WBC of greater than 100,000 cells/μL has been linked to an unfavorable outcome.[97] Identification of the underlying biological mechanisms responsible for leukemic proliferation and survival leading to a leukocytosis, such as FLT3/ITD mutations, are beginning to provide a more definitive understanding of the key prognostic factors contributing to WBC.

AML has been classified based on morphologic appearance using the French American British (FAB) classification. However, due to the subjective nature of such a classification scheme and lack of strict correlation with underlying biology, The World Health Organization (WHO) developed a system for AML classification based on clinical characteristics, cytogenetics and biology.[98] This has demonstrated, for instance, that FAB subtypes associated with poor outcome (e.g. M6/M7) have revealed that high-risk cytogenetics are seen significantly more frequently in those subtypes. Those FAB subtypes associated with a better prognosis (e.g. M1/M2) have a higher representation of good risk cytogenetic changes.

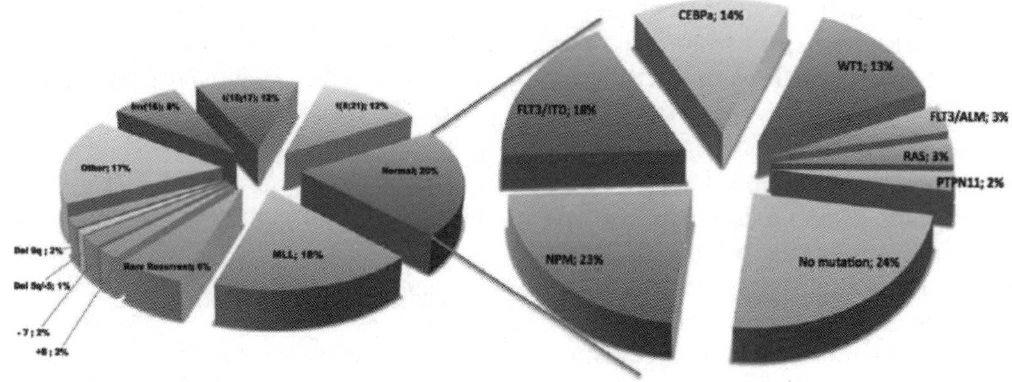

Fig. 13.3. Genetic abnormalities in AML. Left panel demonstrates the most common karyotypic alterations. Eighty percent of all children have disease-associated genomic structural alterations. Mutation profile in those without cytogenetic abnormalities (normal karyotype) is shown in the right panel. Seventy-six percent of those in the normal karyotype population have one of the known mutations; thus, > 95% of all children with AML have at least one known genomic abnormality.

From Childhood Leukemias, ed. Gregory Reaman and Frank Smith, Springer, 2010.

Cytogenetic and molecular abnormalites (Fig. 13.3)

Chimeric transcription factors

Chimeric transcription factors are generally produced as a result of chromosomal translocations that fuse a DNA-binding domain of a transcriptional activator to a transcriptional repressor. The transcriptionally active domain is thereby redirected to target genes of the transcriptional activator, many of which function in myeloid differentiation.

The t(8;21) translocation involves the DNA-binding domain of the transcriptional activator AML1 (RUNX1, CBFA2) on chromosome 21q22 that is fused to the transcriptional repressor ETO on chromosome 8q22. The t(8;21) translocation is associated with characteristic clinical, morphologic, and immunophenotypic features such as chloromas that can occur in about 20% of cases.[83,99] Over 80% of t(8;21) cases are classified as FAB type M2. However, of cases classified as FAB M2, approximately 40% will be found to harbor t(8;21).[100] The immunophenotype of cases with t(8;21) also commonly includes the expression of the B-cell antigen CD19 and the natural killer (NK) cell antigen CD56.[101] In both adults and children, t(8;21) is associated with a favorable prognosis. Improved outcome for adult patients with AML and t(8;21) have been shown to be associated with dose intensity of cytarabine treatment.[102]

Chromosomal abnormalities involving inv(16) or t(16;16) have the CBFB gene at chromosome band 16q22 fused to the MYH11 gene at chromosome band 16p13. CBFB encodes the β subunit of the core binding factor (CBF) transcriptional complex, which normally heterodimerizes with AML1 (or CBFA2, which encodes the α subunit of CBF). The fusion of CBFB with the multimerization domain of the myosin heavy chain gene MYH11 results in decreased CBF transcriptional activity. The inv(16) and t(16;16) abnormalities are closely linked to the FAB M4Eo subtype, and both confer a favorable prognosis for both adults and children with AML.[103,104]

AML with t(15;17) is associated with M3 FAB subtype or APL. The t(15;17) translocation leads to the production of a fusion protein involving the retinoid acid receptor alpha and PML, that in turn confers an increased sensitivity to the differentiating effects of all-trans retinoic acid (ATRA). Outcomes for patients with APL have improved significantly to approximately 75% overall survival with the use of targeted differentiation therapies in combination with conventional chemotherapy. Other much less common translocations involving the retinoic acid receptor alpha can also result in APL (e.g. t(11;17) involving the PLZF gene).[105] Identification of cases with the t(11;17) is important because of their decreased sensitivity to ATRA.

AML with MLL gene rearrangements

MLL-rearranged AML comprise a diverse group of leukemias with variable outcomes depending on the type of rearrangement.[106] Translocations of chromosomal band 11q23 involving the MLL gene, including most AML secondary to epipodophyllotoxin, are associated with monocytic differentiation (FAB M4 and M5) and frequently have an unfavorable prognosis.[106] In an international study examining outcomes for a large number of young patients, overall survival was 100%, 63%, 27%, and 22% for patients with the t(1;11), the t(9;11), the t(4;11), and the t(6;11), respectively.[107] AML with t(10;11) may also have fusion of the CALM gene on chromosome 11 with the AF10 gene.[108] Prognosis appears poor for cases with t(10;11) regardless of the type of gene fusion present.[109] The variability in outcomes and lack of definitive data that demonstrate the superiority of HSCT have led to most cooperative trials not to include patients with *MLL*-rearranged AML in the high-risk group requiring allogeneic HSCT in first remission.[110,111]

The t(1;22)(p13;q13) translocation is restricted to acute megakaryoblastic leukemia (AMKL) and occurs in as many as one-third of AMKL cases in children. In leukemias with t(1;22), the OTT (RBM15) gene on chromosome 1 is fused to the MAL (MLK1) gene on chromosome 22.[112,113] Once associated with a very poor prognosis,[114] AMKL with the t(1;22) has improved outcome with contemporary treatment, and HSCT may not be indicated in these patients.[115,116]

Miscellaneous chromosomal abnormalities

Chromosomal abnormalities associated with poorer prognosis in patients with AML include those involving chromosome 7 (monosomy 7 and del(7q)), chromosome 5 (monosomy 5 and del(5q)) and the long arm of chromosome 3 (inv(3)(q21;q26) or t(3;3)(q21;q26)).[117,118] These cytogenetic subgroups are also associated with poor prognosis in both children and adults with AML, although abnormalities of the long arm of chromosome 3q and 5q are extremely rare in children with AML.[119]

1. Subkaryotypic chromosomal abnormalities

Small structural alterations, including deletions or duplications, can escape detection by conventional cytogenetics but can be detected using specialized techniques such as fluorescence *in situ* hybridization (FISH). Loss of heterozygosity (LOH) that is generally associated with deletions can lead to haploinsufficiency, that in turn may contribute to malignant transformation. SNP genotyping and copy number evaluation of the leukemic genome shave the capacity to detect genomic alterations of even smaller magnitude. For example, these methodologies have identified regions of copy-neutral LOH (CN-LOH), also referred to as acquired uniparental disomy (aUPD).[120–122] The importance of aUPD is underscored by its underlying cause; it arised from a homologous recombination-mediated process by which a homozygous state is achieved after an initial acquisition of a heterozygous mutation. Thus, during the DNA repair process, a mutant allele is used as a template, and the wild type allele is converted to that of the mutant, resulting in a homozygous state, thus altering the gene dosage of a particular mutation. aUPD has been described in specific populations of AML including FLT3/ITD and CEBPA mutations.[123,124]

2. Oncogene mutations

Internal tandem duplication (ITD) mutations of FLT3 occur in approximately 25% of adults with AML and are associated with poor prognosis, particularly when both alleles are mutated or there is a high ratio of the mutant allele to the normal allele.[125–128] FLT3-ITD mutations occur with lower frequency (10–15%) in childhood AML, but have a similar negative prognostic impact.[126,129–133] Mutations in the kinase domain (KD) of FLT3 have also been identified in about 7% of adults and children with AML but these are not negative prognostic factors.[126,134,135] FLT3 mutations occur in 30–40% of children and adults with APL; they are strongly associated with the microgranular variant (M3v) and hyperleukocytosis. However, it is unclear whether FLT3/ITD mutations are associated with poorer prognosis in patients with APL who are treated with modern therapy that includes ATRA.[129,136,137]

c-KIT is another type III tyrosine kinase and receptor for stem cell factor (SCF). Mutations of *c-KIT*, most commonly observed in CBF AML, have been reported to portend a poor prognosis in some studies,[138,139] but not in a recent COG study.[140]

RAS (N-RAS or K-RAS) mutations occur in approximately 20% AML,[141,142] but have not been associated alone with an altered prognosis; thus, patients with RAS-mutated AML are usually treated with chemotherapy and not allogeneic HSCT.

NPM mutations convey both increased chemosensitivity and improved outcome.[143,144] However, whether or not the presence of *NPM* mutations can partially abrogate the adverse affect of co-expressed *FLT3-ITD* is controversial.[144] *CEBPA* mutations are often associated with normal karyotype AML and improved overall survival.[145] Thus, HSCT in first remission is not recommended for pediatric and young adult patients with isolated *NPM* or *CEBPA* mutations. *WT1* mutations appear to have an independent, poor prognostic impact in one study,[146] but not in another (except in patients with co-expression of *FLT3-ITD*).[147] Most clinical trials do not recommend allogeneic transplantation based on isolated *WT1* mutations at this time.

GATA-1 mutations are present in nearly all children with Down syndrome and either transient myeloproliferative disease (TMD) or AMKL, but not in patients without Down Syndrome and AMKL.[148–151] GATA-1 is a transcription factor that is required for normal development of erythroid cells, megakaryocytes, eosinophils, and mast cells. GATA-1 mutations confer increased sensitivity to cytarabine, possibly by decreasing cytidine deaminase expression and thus providing an explanation for the superior outcome of children with Down syndrome and M7 AML when treated with cytarabine-containing regimens.[152]

The presence of the Philadelphia chromosome and/or BCR-ABL fusion in children and young adults with AML most likely represents chronic myelogenous leukemia (CML) that has transformed to AML rather than *de novo* AML.

Genomic alterations in *TET2* gene (4q24) have been demonstrated in myeloid malignancies in adults. The prevalence of these mutations appears to be approximately 20% in MDS, 10–20% in myeloproliferative disease and 12% in adult AML. Data from COG studies show that these mutations are uncommon with a prevalence of 3%. In adults, *TET2* mutations have been associated with decreased overall survival compared with wild type patients;[153] however, the prognostic impact is unclear in children (Fig. 13.4). Similarly, mutations of genes affecting other cellular pathways in AML, such as *SHIP*, *PTPN11*, *RUNX1* and *IDH1* and *IDH2*, are relatively rare in young patients with AML (Fig. 13.4). Mutations in *IDH1* and *IDH2* in adults with AML are particularly intriguing in that they confer a new enzymatic activity on the enzyme product thus resulting in altered cellular metabolism; these mutations have been associated with a neutral or somewhat poorer prognosis.[154–156]

3. Altered chromatin structure and gene expression

In addition to gene mutations and chromosome abnormalities, an increasing body of evidence has demonstrated that epigenetic modifications may contribute to the pathogenesis of leukemia (see Chapter 7). The term epigenetics refers to heritable changes of DNA and chromatin that modify gene expression and cellular physiology other than alterations in the DNA sequence. Epigenetic changes that underlie the development of leukemia can be in one of two major categories: changes in the DNA methylation state and alterations in histone or chromatin modifying proteins. These two processes work together and can lead to activation or repression of gene expression. Emerging evidence shows altered methylation, as well as changes in histone modifications, regulate both normal and malignant hematopoiesis.[157–161]

Evidence linking alterations in DNA methylation in malignancies has prompted comprehensive evaluations of DNA methylation patterns in AML in an attempt to identify specific methylation profiles that can be used for risk identification as well as identification of potential targets for epigenetically directed therapies. One study in adult AML used DNA methylation patterns to group patients into 16 different cohorts based on their methylation pattern.[159] The methylation pattern segregated with specific mutation and cytogenetic groups. This study also identified a 15-gene methylation classifier that appeared to predict overall survival. Contribution of alterations in DNA methylation patterning and its clinical significance is not yet well defined in childhood AML, but such evaluations are currently underway.

Histone acetylation is catalyzed by histone acetyltransferases (HATs) and associated with transcriptionally active chromatin. Several transcriptional coactivators, including CREB binding protein (CBP), have been shown to possess HAT activity. Transcriptional corepressor complexes, such as nuclear corepressor 1 (NCOR1), have been shown to exist in protein complexes containing histone deacetylase (HDAC) activity. As acetylation and methylation status of the histone lysine residues help to determine whether chromatin is in the transcriptionally active or repressed state, altered histone modification patterns could mediate malignant transformation by altering expression of oncogenes. As alterations in methylation and acetylation status have significant contribution to myeloid transformation and proliferation, they pose attractive targets epigenetic therapy.[162]

Mutations in transcription factors and signal transduction molecules can have far reaching effects on the regulation of expression of multiple genes that in turn

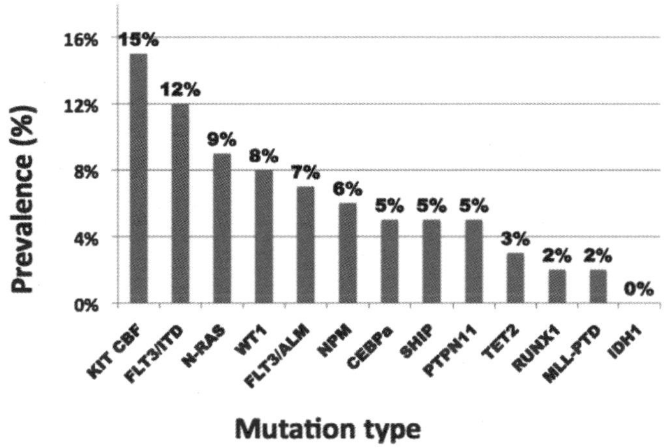

Fig. 13.4. Prevalence of disease-associated mutations in pediatric AML. From Childhood Leukemia, Heidelberg, Germany, eds. GH Reaman, FO Smith, Springer-Verlag, 2010.

affect a variety of key cellular pathways. Multidrug resistance has been associated with rapid drug efflux mediated by a family of drug transporters, including the multidrug resistance gene 1 (MDR1) encoding P-glycoprotein (PgP) as well as other proteins of the same family of multidrug resistance such as MRP1 (multidrug resistance-associated protein 1) and LRP (lung resistance protein). Unlike evidence in adults with AML, MDR gene expression in pediatric patients has not been definitively associated with poor clinical outcomes. Sievers *et al.* demonstrated a prevalence of 13% for the expression of PgP in a group of 130 pediatric AML patients treated on CCG-2891, but the expression of this transporter was not significantly correlated with outcome.[163] Another pediatric study demonstrated MDR1 expression was not higher in patients with relapsed AML.[164] The POG 9421 trial randomized the use of cyclosporine A as an inhibitor of MDR1 but was not able to demonstrate any advantage in terms of clinical.[165]

The expression level of the Wilms tumor gene (WT1) has been implicated in the pathogenesis and prognosis in AML. Although WT1 expression level, at the time of diagnosis and during remission, has been correlated with clinical outcome, such findings have not been uniformly observed.[166,167] Telomerase activity has been implicated in leukemogenesis and there are data to suggest telomerase activity may have prognostic significance in pediatric AML.[168] BAALC (brain and acute leukemia, cytoplasmic) is a gene whose elevated expression has also been implicated in the adverse outcome in adults with acute myeloid leukemia.[169] High levels of expression of AF1q, a MLL fusion partner whose expression regulates hematopoietic development, has been reported to be associated with poor outcome.[170] High levels of expression of vasoactive endothelial growth factor (VEGF) ligand have been reported to predict outcome.[171] At this time, these associations have not been definitively validated and are thus not used in current cooperative group clinical trials for risk group stratification.

Similarly, although total cellular RNA signatures, including microRNA expression, can accurately discriminate cases with specific chromosomal translocations and identify novel subsets of AML,[107,172–175] independent pediatric studies were not able to identify an expression pattern with consistent prognostic significance.[176,177] Some of the differences observed in gene expression studies are also beginning to be understood in terms of epigenetic regulation of chromatin function. The finding of a similar expression profile between an AML subset with the methylation and silencing of the *CEBPA* promoter and another characterized by *CEBPA* mutations demonstrates the critical relationship between epigenetic changes and gene expression play in AML.[178,179] As an example, the distinctive myeloid/T-lymphoid characteristics of this subtype has been linked to the finding that decreased CEBPA expression leads to increased expression of T lineage genes in hematopoietic precursors.[161,179] Larger prospective studies using gene expression profiling for prognostic determination from pediatric cooperative group studies are likely to be required to establish the role of genomic profiling in risk identification in pediatric AML. Such studies may also lead to the identification of therapeutic targets.

Response to Therapy and Prognosis

Primary induction failure (PIF)

Achieving a complete morphological remission at the end of induction has been shown to be an important prognostic factor. Failure to achieve such a CR portends a poor prognosis even if a subsequent remission is achieved with additional therapy.

The MRC 10 trial evaluated the response to therapy as a part of the MRC 10 AML trials, where they demonstrated that patients with >15% marrow blast prior to the start of second induction course had a significantly worse outcome than those with <15% disease.[90,180] They established this clinical cutoff by demonstrating that patients with partial remission (5–15% blast) at the end of induction had a survival rather similar to those with <5% blast whereas the survival for those with greater than 15–20% blast was poor and mirrored the outcome for those with >20% marrow blast. Based on these findings, the MRC subsequently used the threshold of 15% morphologically evident disease to define refractory disease. COG pediatric AML trials also have used 15% leukemic blasts, detected by morphology, at the end of induction therapy to define primary induction failure (PIF).

However, it is becoming clearer with the use of immunophenotypic flow cytometric detection of AML that a significant percentage of patients with 5–15% leukemic blasts represented recovering bone marrows, which can be confused morphologically with the presence of disease. Thus, patients with truly resistant AML after the initial course of induction therapy are being re-evaluated in terms of their outcome and alternative approaches to treatment.

Minimal residual disease (MRD) detection by PCR and flow cytometric techniques

Based on the discussion in the previous section and in Chapter 10 and on the longstanding observation that although the majority of children and young adults with AML achieve a complete remission, as assessed by morphologic evaluation of the marrow at the end of induction therapy, nearly half of these patients suffer a relapse of their disease. Therefore, identification of occult disease in patients in morphologic remission has been sought after as a means of identifying those patients at high risk of relapse, with the hope of offering alternative treatments. In contrast, if patients can be identified, who would not have a high chance of AML relapse, then potentially less toxic therapies could be offered to them, such as not offering HSCT in first remission.

While a substantial amount of information on MRD detection in AML has been generated using PCR-based methods to detect the persistence of genetic changes, the utility of PCR methods has been limited because of the heterogeneity and frequent instability of such changes. For instance, the t(8;21) translocation-generated fusion product has been reported to be sometimes present in the general population as well as remain detectable for many years in patients with AML in morphologic remission.[181,182] However, other reports have shown that an increasing, quantitative RT-PCR detection of t(8;21) transcripts can effectively predict relapse.[182–184] Other mutations, such as FLT3/ITD, have been shown to be discordant between diagnosis and relapse and thus may not provide stable defects to detect MRD.[185] Mutations in NPM1 have proven to be more stable and usually present in what is considered to be an AML-initiating cell, thus making it potentially more useful for MRD detection and prediction of relapse. However, taken together, PCR-based methods for detecting MRD in AML appears to be able to account for about 50% of patients.[186]

In contrast, APL detection of persistent t(15;17) fusion product is significantly associated with a high risk of relapse, and early therapeutic intervention, prior to morphologic relapse, has been shown to improve outcome.[187,188] Thus, in APL, molecular status in terms of detection of the PML-RAR alpha fusion transcript, is routinely used to modify treatment alternatives.[189–191]

Thus, a more universally applicable approach to detection of meaningful values of MRD would be useful. Flow cytometric immunophenotyping exploits that leukemic blast express aberrant surface antigen patterns that differ from the pattern observed in normal progenitors. Multiparameter flow cytometry (MPFC) can detect multiple antigens and patterns of expression and detect one leukemic cell in 1000 to 10,000 normal nucleated cells on a routine basis and in at least 85% of all patients with AML.

Several studies have used flow cytometry to detect residual AML in patients in morphologic remission and have shown that the presence of MRD correlates strongly with an adverse clinical outcome. In evaluation of 126 adult AML patients in clinical remission, San Miguel *et al.* demonstrated that patients with occult disease detected by flow cytometry had a significantly greater relapse rate than patients without measurable

MRD.[192] In a CCG study of 252 pediatric patients with AML in morphologic remission, Sievers *et al.* demonstrated, using a multivariate analysis, that MRD was the strongest prognostic factor predicting outcome.[193] In that study, 16% of the patients in complete remission who were identified as having occult AML had a five-fold higher risk of relapse (35% relapse-free survival) than patients who were MRD negative (65% relapse-free survival). This study also showed that the median time to relapse for the MRD-positive population was 173 days, more than adequate for intervention. Rubnitz *et al.* reported that patients with less than 0.1% MRD at the end of the second course of induction therapy had a 17% relapse rate; a 1% or greater MRD level was the only significant independent prognostic factor for EFS and OS.[116] van der Velden *et al.* have reported from the MRC AML 12 and the Dutch COG ANLL97 trials that, at the end of the first course of chemotherapy, less than 0.1% MRD was associated with a RFS of $85 \pm 8\%$, $64 \pm 10\%$ for those with MRD $\geq 0.1\%$ but $< 0.5\%$ and $14 \pm 9\%$ for those with $\geq 0.5\%$; all of these comparisons were statistically significant.[186] Of note, this study was able to detect MRD by flow cytometry in 94% of patients, and, although antigenic drift was observed with discordant surface immunophenotyping in 91% of samples between diagnosis and relapse, this did not interfere with MRD analysis.[186] An exception to such studies has been the results from the BFM trials, which reported that MRD detection did not provide additional prognostic information compared to that provided by more traditional risk factors.[194] Potential issues regarding this study included a relatively small numbers of patients analyzed, a significant percentage of patients who did not have samples analyzed, and the inclusion of morphologically evident disease in the analysis.

The issue of how to utilize MRD information in order to optimize treatment and outcomes for the majority of patients with AML is still uncertain. Nevertheless, the next COG trial for newly diagnosed patients with AML will use, for the first time, the combination of MRD status, as well as cytogenetic and molecular information, to risk stratify patients into two groups. Low-risk AML will include mutations involving *CBF*, *CEBPA*, *NPM* and those with no MRD at the end of induction therapy; from retrospective analyses, this group represents about 73% of patients with a predicted survival close to 75%. The high-risk AML, representing the remaining 27% of patients having a survival less than 35%, includes patients with adverse cytogenetic abnormalities, such as monosomy 7, del(5q)-, –5, high FLT3-ITD to wild type allelic ratio, or MRD at the end of induction. This group of patients will be offered HSCT in first remission with the most appropriate available donor. Patients in the low risk group will not be offered HSCT in first remission.

Treatment: Risk-Adapted Approaches with Conventional and Experimental Approaches

Newly diagnosed AML

Remission induction (Please see Table 13.2 for CR rates using different regimens)

Children and young adults with newly diagnosed AML will usually receive, essentially, a common induction chemotherapy regimen, with some variations depending in what part of the world they live and what clinical trials are open for enrollment. During this period of induction therapy, as well as at the end of induction, risk factors are usually determined which, as noted above, may impact subsequent treatment recommendations.

The first significant successful remission, inducing treatment for patients with AML, included the use of 7 days of Ara-C at 100 mg/m^2 by continuous infusion and 3 initial days of an anthracycline, such as daunorubicin, at 45 mg/m^2 per day. The continuous infusion of Ara-C was deliberate with the knowledge of its S phase-specific effects on the cell cycle. This regimen resulted in remission rates of between 60–70% in children and young adults.[195,196] The "7 and 3" combination is still a standard in the treatment of adults with AML. Several approaches have been utilized to test the improvement on these remission rates, including altering the schedule and doses of Ara-C and anthracyclines, introduction of additional agents, and supportive care measures such as the preemptive use of broad-spectrum antibiotics, blood product transfusions, and hematopoietic cytokines.

The introduction of several different types of anthracyclines or anthracenediones have not resulted in a significantly clear advantage in remission rates or overall outcome. The BFM AML 93 study randomized patients to idarubicin vs. daunorubicin in combination with Ara-C and etoposide. The group of patients who received idarubicin experiences a more rapid clearing of leukemic blasts at day 15 of induction, although the 5-year EFS and DFS were similar in the two groups. CCG-2941 was a pilot study that attempted to deliver two consecutive cycles of idarubicin as part of the

Table 13.2. Characteristics and treatment results from selected clinical trials in children and adolescents.

Study[a]	Years of study	No. of patients[b,c]	Early deaths (%)	CR rate (%)	Time of CR evaluation	Anthracyclines[d] mg/m²	Cytarabine g/m²	Etoposide g/m²	EFS 5 yr ± SE	OS 5 yr ± SE	Data source
POG 8821	1988–1993	511	3.9	77	2 courses	360	55.7	2.25	31 ± 2	40.4 ± 2	Ravindranath *et al.*[260]
CCG 2891	1989–1995	750	4	77	2 courses	350	28.3	1.9	34 ± 3	45 ± 3	Smith *et al.*[210]
MRC-AML 10	1988–1995	303	4	93	4 courses	550	10.6	0.5–1.5	49	58	Gibson *et al.*[201]
PINDA-92	1992–1998	151	21	74	Not specified	350	7.64	0.45	36	37	Quintana *et al.*[322]
LAME-91[e]	1991–1998	247	6.4	91	2 courses	460	9.8–13.4	0.4	48 ± 4	62.3 ± 4	Perel *et al.*[202]
TCCSG M91–13/M96–14	1991–1998	192	3.6	88	Not specified	495	69.4–99.4	3.75–5.75	56	62	Tomizawa *et al.*[321]
BFM-93	1993–1998	427	7.4	82	4 courses	300–400	23–41	0.95	50 ± 2	57 ± 2	Creutzig *et al.*[211]
POG 9421	1995–1999	565	10.5	88–91	2 courses	360	55.7	2.25	36.3 ± 2.2	53.6 ± 2.2	Becton *et al.*[166]
CCG 2961	1996–1999	901	6	83	2 courses	360	15.2–19.6	1.6	42 ± 3	52 ± 4	Lange *et al.*[104]
EORTC-CLG 58921	1993–2000	166	1	84	2 courses	380	23–29	1.35	49 ± 4	62 ± 4	Entz-Werle *et al.*[320]
GATLA-AML90	1993–2000	179	20	70	Not specified	300	41.1	1.45	31 ± 4	41 ± 4	Armendariz *et al.*[319]
AIEOP LAM-92	1992–2001	160	6	89	2 courses	Not Provided	Not Provided	Not Provided	54 ± 4	60 ± 4	Pession *et al.*[318]
NOPHO-AML 93	1993–2001	223	2	92	3 courses	300–375	49.6–61.3	1.6	50 ± 3	66 ± 3	Lie *et al.*[103]
MRC-AML 12	1994–2002	455	4	92	4 courses	300–610	4.6–34.6	1.5	56	66	Burnett *et al.*[16]/ Gibson *et al.*[201]
AML99	2000–2002	260	1.7	94	2 courses	300–375	59.4–78.4	3.15–3.2	61 ± 3	75 ± 3	Tsukimoto *et al.*[323]
BFM-98	1998–2003	473	3	88	4 courses	420	41–47	0.95	49 ± 3	62 ± 3	Creutzig *et al.*[211]
SJCRH AML02[f]	2002–2008	230	1	94	2 courses	300–550	34–48	1–1.5	63 ± 4	71 ± 4	Rubnitz *et al.*[116]
COG AAML03P1[f,g]	2003–2005	350	2.6	83	2 courses	300–480	21.6–45.6	1–1.75	53 ± 6	66 ± 5	Cooper *et al.*[390]

[a]Results are reported for only those trials that had ≥ 150 patients and information provided for each of the column headings. The AIEOP LAM-92 did not allow for definitive dose calculations of drugs because consolidation therapy was given based on the treating physician's judgement, but usually included anthracyclines, etoposide and high dose cytarabine.

[b]No. of patients excludes patients with Down Syndrome.

[c]Ages include patients from 0 up to and including age 15 years: BFM-98 included patients from 0 to less than 17 years of age; CCG-2961 included patients from 0 to < 21 years.

[d]Anthracycline conversions were according to daunorubicin equivalents including idarubicin 5×, mitoxantrone 5×, doxorubicin 1×. Another conversion factor for idarubicin and mitoxantrone that has been used is 3×.

[e]LAME-91 also used 450 mg/m² of amsacrine; MRC-10 and MRC-12 both also included 500 mg/m² of amsacrine.

[f]SJCRH AML02 and the COG AAML03P1 have EFS and OS at 3-year follow-up.

[g]COG AAML03P1 enrolled patients ≥ 1 month and ≤ 21 years of age.

AIEOP: Associazione Italianadi Ematologiaed Oncologia Pediatrica; BFM: Berline-Frankfurt-Munster; CCG: Children's Cancer Group; COG: Children's Oncology Group; EFS: event-free survival; LAM: Leucemia Acuta Meiloide; MRC AML: United Kingdom's Medical Research Council Acute Myelogenous leukemia study; OS: overall survival; POG: Pediatric Oncology Group; SJCRH: Saint Jude Children's Research Hospital; TCCSG: Tokyo Children's Cancer Study Group. Adapted from Pui, C., Carroll, W., Meshinchi, S and Arceci, R.J., Biology, Risk Stratification, and Therapy of Pediatric Leukemias: An Update, *J Clin Oncol*, January 10, 2011.[391]

CCG-2891 DCTER/DCTER regimen. The results showed that the combination of this combination chemotherapy with idarubicin was too toxic, leading to the alternative of IDA/DCTER in the first course followed by DCTER/DCTER in consolidation, which was the remission induction regimen for the CCG-2961 study.[104,197]

A meta-analysis of several randomized trials comparing idarubicin, mitoxantrone and daunorubicin suggested remission rates were highest with idarubicin, intermediate with mitoxantrone and lowest with daunorubicin; however, such trials may not have compared equitoxic doses of the different anthracyclines and no significant differences were observed in DFS.[198]

In an intention-to-treat analysis in patients 17–60 years of age with newly diagnosed AML, Fernandez *et al.* reported that 90 mg/m^2 of daunorubicin taken for 3 days along with standard Ara-C at 100 mg/m^2/day for 7 days was superior to the 45 mg/m^2 for 3 days of daunorubicin both in remission induction (70.6% vs. 57.3% $p < 0.001$) and overall survival (median months of 23.7 vs. 15.7, $p = 0.003$). They concluded that the use of the increased dose intensity with daunorubicin should be used as a standard induction practice in young adults with AML. The issue of adverse late cardiotoxic events in such patients was not evaluated.[199,200]

Analogous clinical trials have investigated the doses and schedules of Ara-C during induction. The CALGB 7921 study used a "10 and 3" schedule and noted improved CR rates compared to the "7 and 3" regimen.[200] A subsequent trial testing a more prolonged exposure to Ara-C was the MRC AML 9 study which demonstrated that a "10 and 3" schedule of Ara-C plus daunorubicin with thioguanine resulted in improved remission rates of 91% compared to MRC AML 8 study, which had used a "5 and 1" schedule.[202] The French LAME 89 and 91 studies used 7 days of Ara-C at a higher dose of 200 mg/m^2 per day by continuous infusion along with 5 days of mitoxantrone at 12 mg/m^2 per day with CR rates of 85% and 90%, respectively.[203] Similarly, the Nordic NOPHO-AML 88 and 93 studies used Ara-C at 200 mg/m^2 per day and mitoxantrone and achieved CR rates of 83% and 92%, respectively.[103] However, in direct randomized comparisons of different Ara-C dosing regimens (ranging from 100 mg/m^2 per day as a continuous infusion for 7 days to 3000 mg/m^2 per day divided every 12 hours usually for 5 days), no significant differences have been observed in remission rates.[204–206] Two strictly pediatric trials, the POG 9421 and a more recent SJCRH, compared a low dose to a high dose Ara-C schedule during induction and showed no significant different in remission rates, both achieving remission rates in the 85–95% range.[116,165]

The timing and scheduling of chemotherapeutic agents has been the subject of considerable interest as well, in large part as a response to the limited number of effective drugs available. Based on both theoretical and laboratory-based studies designed to optimize the timing of sequential drug exposures in leukemia, several studies tested such approaches in patients with AML.[207,208]

The small LAME SP study attempted to improve remission induction rates by using timed sequential therapy including Ara-C at 200 mg/m^2 per day on days 1–4 by continuous infusion along with mitoxantrone at 12 mg/m^2 per day on days 1–3 followed by 8–14 days later with 3 days of the Ara-C and 2 days of mitoxantrone. The CR rate for 32 patients was 84% with 3% induction deaths; however, this study observed significant delays in starting consolidation therapy because of prolonged delays in hematopoietic recovery.[203]

The CCG-2891 trial attempted to test whether compressing the timing chemotherapy would lead to improved remission rates and overall outcomes. Thus, the trial randomized standard timing that gave the second cycle of chemotherapy only after upon marrow recovery compared to an intensively timed approach, which gave a second cycle given on days 10–13 following the first course of treatment regardless of the status of the bone marrow. In each arm, the five-drug DCTER (dexamethasone, cytarabine, thioguanine, etoposide, and rubidomycin) regimen was used for each treatment cycle.[209,210] The CR rates for the intensive and standard timing arm were 78% and 74% and not significantly different.[209,210] However, the overall survival and EFS proved to be significantly better for patients who received the intensively timed induction therapy. This held up regardless of whether post-remission therapy was chemotherapy, autologous HSCT or allogeneic HSCT.[210,211] These results, furthermore, supported the concept that the depth of the initial complete remission was critically important, which has been confirmed with subsequent analyses of MRD and its impact on outcome. In contrast, the BFM AML 93 trial showed, in a randomized trial, that idarubicin led to a more rapid and lower level of leukemia compared to daunorubicin during induction therapy, but did not result in improved EFS.[212] This latter result raises an issue as to what the most important aspects of induction treatment are that result in a sufficiently more robust remission that can translate into more patients experiencing an improved outcome.

Testing the addition of other chemotherapeutic agents to the "7 and 3" or other two drug combinations has not always been done in a prospective, randomized fashion. There are, however, some exceptions. The MRC AML 10 trial randomized patients during induction to receive either thioguanine or etoposide along with daunorubicin and Ara-C (DAT vs. ADE regimens, respectively). The results showed no difference in remission rate (81% for DAT and 83% for ADE); however, ADE resulted in a slightly higher death rate during induction and more mucositis.[213] Overall survival at 6 years was approximately 40% for both induction regimens.[213] The introduction of novel nucleoside inhibitors, such as clofarabine, has been tested in combination with other chemotherapeutic drugs, based in part on its single agent responses as well as its ability to inhibit DNA repair pathways.[214–217] While still being tested in ALL, testing in AML in children and young adults has been halted. The use of liposomal anthracyclines may represent another approach to improve a conventional agent through chemical modification that potentially reduces its toxicity while improving its cytotoxic effects.[218–220]

A sometimes overlooked key element contributing to the success of induction therapy for patients with AML is intensive supportive care. Most patients remain hospitalized until hematopoietic recovery is evident and severe cytopenias resolved. In addition, the use of broad-spectrum antibiotics and antifungal agents along with blood product support are now routine and life-saving aspects of the care for patients with AML. The use of hematopoietic cytokines has been more controversial.

Several studies have tested whether G-CSF (granulocyte colony-stimulating factor) can improve outcomes by reducing the period of profound neutropenia following induction or even post-remission therapy.[221–223] Some of these studies have demonstrated that the time the length of neutropenia can be significantly reduced by several days but this gain has not translated into significant improvements in survival.[221–223] A non-randomized addition of G-CSF to the intensely timed regimen of the CCG-2891 trial was reported to reduce the number of deaths due to infections, leading to an improved CR rate of 82% vs. 78% without G-CSF; however, the result was modest and the lack of a prospective randomized design prevented this from being a definitive study that changed conventional practice approaches.[224] In the BFM AML 98 trial, patients were randomized to receive or not receive G-CSF during the first two cycles of therapy.[225,226] Although the period of neutropenia was decreased from 23 to 18 days in the first course and from 16 to 11 days in the second course for the group receiving G-CSF, there were no differences in relapse rates, EFS, incidence of secondary malignancies or infection-associated mortality.[225,226] Thus, while one could argue that the expense of G-CSF is worth a slight to modest potential gain in reduced neutropenia and possible infection, Ehlers *et al.* have reported from the BFM study follow-up that the subset of patients whose AML expressed the G-CSF receptor isoform IV had a significantly higher rate of relapse.[227] These results raise important warnings for the use of supportive measures that do not have proven and significant benefit.

While the limits of intensification have essentially been reached in terms of risk/benefit, alternative strategies for improving the rate of complete remission as determined by morphology along with measurement of MRD are being tested. These have included the addition of agents that demonstrate non-cross-resistance as well as non-overlapping toxicities with conventional chemotherapy.[228] Examples of these agents include immunotargeted monoclonal antibodies, such as the anti-CD33/calicheamicin conjugate (gemtuzumab ozogamicin, Mylotarg),[229–231] or inhibitors of signaling or apoptosis regulatory pathways, such as tyrosine kinase inhibitors of FLT3/ITD (CEP701 and midostaurin),[232,233] or c-KIT mutant receptors,[234] anti-BCL2 antisense oligomers,[5,235,236] farnesyl transferase inhibitors directed toward the RAS signaling pathway (tipifarnib/R115777),[228,237–239] proteasome inhibitors (bortezemib)[240–243] and multidrug resistance ABC transporter inhibition (PSC833, cyclosporine)[165] or chromatin-modifying agents (demethylating drugs and histone deacetylase inhibitors)[244–248] to sensitize AML cells to conventional drugs. Thus far, none of these agents have resulted in a significantly improved remission induction rate or overall outcome. Some of them, such as gemtuzumab ozogamicin, CEP701 and tipifarnib, have not met satisfactory expectations and had FDA approval revoked or denied as well as the cessation of efforts on the part of the companies developing them. Whether agents, such as the tyrosine kinase inhibitors sorafenib and midostaurin, or chromatin-remodeling active drugs can improve remission induction rates and overall outcomes is being tested in ongoing phase III, randomized trials.

Optimal post-remission approaches (Please see Table 13.2 for survival using different regimens)

Key elements and questions for patients who achieve a complete remission is what to do next. Although the answer to this question remains controversial, it is quite clear that without any post-remission therapy, nearly all patients will have a relapse of their disease. The types as well as the length of post-remission therapy have been the subject of key clinical trials which have begun to provide optimal, risk-adapted approaches.

Duration vs. intensity

Aside from the treatment of patients with APL, the use of relatively low-dose maintenance chemotherapy in patients with AML has not proven to be a successful strategy. Several key trials illustrate this point.

A pivotal study by the Cancer and Leukemia Group B (CALGB) examined three dose levels of cytarabine given for four cycles as post-remission therapy. This study clearly demonstrated that outcomes following high-dose cytarabine (HiDAC, 3 gm/m^2 q12 hours on days 1, 3, and 5) were superior to intermediate-dose (400 mg/m^2 continuous IV infusion, days 1–5) or standard-dose cytarabine (100 mg/m^2 continuous IV infusion, days 1–5) in patients under the age of 60 years. Cerebellar toxicity was the most frequently observed in patients over the age of 40 and with renal or hepatic dysfunction.[249] In a subgroup analysis, it was demonstrated that this benefit was most pronounced in core-binding factor [(CBF), i.e. t(8;21), inv16, t(16;16)] AML patients and, to a lesser extent, in patients with a normal karyotype.[250]

The CCG-213 trial randomized patients after 4 months of post-remission intensification treatments to either receive 2 years of maintenance therapy with the PATCO regimen (prednisolone, Ara-C, 6-thioguanine, cyclophosphamide and vincristine) or no further therapy.[251] This study showed that treatment with only 4 months of intensification resulted in a 5-year survival of 68% vs. 44% for the group that received maintenance chemotherapy.[211,251] The LAME 91 trial randomized patients after post-remission intensification to either receive an 18-month maintenance regimen of daily 6-mercaptopurine and monthly 4-day pulses of subcutaneous Ara-C vs. no maintenance; the results were similar to the CCG-213 trial in that DFS was 62% in the group which received intensification and 51% in the group which received maintenance therapy.[203,252] In contrast, the BFM AML 87 trial reported a benefit of maintenance therapy for a low-risk group of patients who did not receive a HSCT.[212,253] The BFM trials continue to include a maintenance phase in the post-remission period. Another important finding from such studies has been that the ability to cure patients who received prolonged maintenance therapy following a relapse is less effective than if they had not received maintenance treatment, suggesting that additional drug resistance develops during treatment. Whether more targeted therapies will change the role of maintenance therapy, as has been observed in APL, remains untested.

What are the optimal number of intensification cycles?

If maintenance therapy is not required in most patients with AML, then an important issue is how many courses of therapy are needed to achieve optimal cure rates. There are few examples of randomized trials to address this question.

The CCG-2961 study gave patients a total of three courses of intensive chemotherapy with an overall survival of 52%, which is comparable to other studies of that period, suggesting that more courses may not be necessary.[253] Of interest, the survival improved over the course of the study, with an overall survival of approximately 42% for patients treated during the period from 1996 to 1998 in contrast to approximately 57% for those treated in the period from 2000 to 2002.[254] This trend to improve survival has been observed in other trials without a clear explanation, although a possibility may be a positive learning curve on the part of caretakers in terms of the delivery of treatment and supportive care of patients.

The MRC AML 12 study randomized four compared to five total courses of chemotherapy is preferable. Preliminary results from this study suggested no difference between four and five courses, with an overall survival of 81% for four courses compared to 78% for five courses ($p = 0.5$).[202] Subsequent publication of matured data confirmed the preliminary data in that four courses of chemotherapy were as good as five.[255] Although these results might suggest that four courses of MRC 12 therapy is better than three courses of CCG-2961 therapy, it is impossible to definitively compare the two sets of results and additional conclusions will need to await further direct comparisons. However, with overall survival rates of approximately 50% or less overall and worse in the very high risk groups of patients, testing whether three courses is better than four courses of therapy would be able to be justified possibly only for patients with favorable risk AML.

For whom and when should HSCT be used?

Advances in chemotherapy-based treatment of patients with AML have decreased the need for all patients being considered for allogeneic HSCT. In addition, several studies have demonstrated no advantage to autologous HSCT compared to chemotherapy; most trials have therefore omitted such transplants in order to avoid potentially greater short- and long-term toxicities (see Chapter 20).[210,213,256,257] However, with equivalency of overall outcome between autologous HSCT and chemotherapy, one might also conclude that either approach would be a reasonable, evidence-based recommendation.[110] In addition, alternative approaches to transplantation, such as the use of nonablative or intensity reduced allogeneic or haploidentical HSCT, remain experimental strategies and have not be yet extensively compared prospectively to conventional chemotherapy-based ablative HSCT.

In order to balance the short- and long-term adverse consequences of ablative allogeneic HSCT, an increasing emphasis has been placed on recommending HSCT for solely those patients who are significantly likely to benefit more from it than treatment with solely chemotherapy. Thus, a key question has been how to best define such groups of patients. In addition, it has been particularly difficult to conduct randomized trials for patients with matched sibling donors in part because of physician and likely patient or guardian bias. Thus, most trials have analyzed outcomes based on whether patients had or did not have an HLA-matched donor. However, with an increasing ability to perform matched unrelated donor HSCT, the analysis of outcomes based on family member HLA-matched donor availability has been appropriately questioned.[255]

Overall, most trials have demonstrated improved disease-free survival following allogeneic HSCT compared to chemotherapy or autologous HSCT.[110,210,255,256,258,259] However, while such data suggest that an ablative preparative regimen, along with an allogeneic anti-leukemic effect, may play important roles in controlling leukemic relapse, event-free and overall survival have not commonly demonstrated an advantage for HSCT, in part because of increased treatment-related mortality. However, in light of the potential for improved disease control as well as balancing treatment-related toxicities, the role of allogeneic HSCT in specific subgroups of patients needs to be carefully considered.[255,258–260]

In order to better address this issue, significant effort has gone into defining subgroups of patients who show a true survival advantage when treated with allogeneic HSCT or have such a poor outcome with chemotherapy alone that in the context of a clinical trial, HSCT is used.

The MRC AML 10 trial analyzed outcome based on whether or not a donor was available. Of the 85 children with donors, 61 received HSCT, including 12 of 21 classified as good risk.[202] Although the relapse rate was significantly lower for those with a donor (30% vs. 45%), there was no statistically significant difference in overall survival between those children with (68%) or without (59%) a donor ($p = 0.3$) at 10 years. Of note, survival at 5 years from the time of relapse was 57%, 14%, and 8% for good, standard and poor risk groups respectively, leading to the recommendation that patients with good risk AML receive allogeneic HSCT only in CR2. For patients in the standard and poor risk groups, the data suggested that an allogeneic HSCT in first remission might be advantageous. However, when data from MRC AML 10 and 12 studies were combined, allogeneic HSCT was not shown to provide a statistically significant survival advantage for any of these other risk groups.[202] Similar results and conclusions were reported from the BFM trials,[212] as well as the POG 8821 and 9421 studies, although no detailed subgroup analyses were reported in the latter two trials.[165,261]

In contrast, analysis of post-remission treatment of 1464 children less than age 21 years on five consecutive CCG trials from 1979 to 1996 has shown an advantage to patients assigned a HSCT in terms of overall survival ($p = 0.026$), disease free survival ($p = 0.005$) and relapse rate ($p < 0.001$).[262] Subgroup analysis demonstrated that HSCT was associated with improved survival for patients with WBC greater than 50,000/μL and for those with normal karyotype, but was not beneficial for patients with AML characterized by good risk cryogenics, such as inv(16) or t(8;21). In support of such data, a report from the CCG 2961 trial showed no statistically significant advantage of having a HSCT donor in terms of OS or DFS in the subgroup of patients with inv(16) or t(8;21) chromosomal translocations.[254] A detailed analysis of the effect of donor availability on patients with standard and poor risk features was not reported although no advantage of having a HSCT matched family member donor was observed compared to chemotherapy for the entire study population. Overall, these results appear to be consistent with those reported from the MRC AML trials.

A more detailed analysis of the MRC AML 12 outcomes has reported no advantage of HSCT for patients in the good and intermediate groups, but a statistically significant advantage for relapse-free survival and overall survival for a subset of patients with high risk AML; for example, in the 12% of patients defined as having poor risk AML, HSCT was associated with an overall survival of 41% compared to 10% for those who received only chemotherapy ($p = 0.001$).[255]

This raises an important question as to whether patients with other subtypes of AML might also benefit from receiving an allogeneic HSCT. A high FLT3/ITD mutant to normal allele frequency has been uniformly associated with a poor prognosis when patients are treated with standard chemotherapeutic regimens alone.[128,133,263] A significant question is whether more intensive allogeneic HSCT is able to improve outcomes.

Some studies have strongly suggested an advantage of HSCT for patients with a high mutant allele frequency of FLT3/ITD mutations.[135,263–266] The CCG 2941 and 2961 trials showed a borderline significant difference for the relapse rate for patients with FLT3/ITD positive AML who received a allogeneic matched sibling donor HSCT (27% ± 27%) compared to those treated with only chemotherapy (65% ± 15%, $p = 0.05$). However, overall survival at 4 years from the end of the second course of treatment was not significantly different; results showed 64% ± 29% for those with FLT3/ITD AML who received an allogeneic HSCT and 48% ± 17% for those treated only with chemotherapy, but this was not significantly different ($p = 0.4$).[135,263] The MRC AML 10 and 12 trials reported on 1135 young adult patients concluded that there was no strong evidence that FLT3 status should be considered as to whether to perform a HSCT or not.[267] This conclusion was based on the lack of statistically significant differences in DFS or OS when patients with FLT3/ITD AML who did or did not receive a transplant were compared. Essentially, OS was not found to be significantly improved by having a donor in patients with FLT3/ITD positive or negative AML, suggesting that allogeneic HSCT is not able to overcome the chemoresistance or radiation resistance that characterizes FLT3/ITD positive AML. Thus, whether allogeneic HSCT can improve outcomes for patients with FLT3/ITD remains open with no randomized prospective data available to resolve the question. Nevertheless, most ongoing clinical trials for children and young adults recommend allogeneic HSCT for patients with AML characterized by a high mutant FLT3/ITD to normal allelic ratio, often in the context of additional targeted therapy directed towards inhibition of the mutant receptor.

Current strategies for determining which patients should receive matched or single mismatched family donor or alternative donor HSCT are based on risk assessment and stratification. Patients with AML, characterized by alternations in core binding, transcription factors (e.g. t(8;21 and inv(16)) have an approximately 80% overall survival with chemotherapy alone; thus, HSCT is recommended only in CR2. Of note, it has been demonstrated that that while patients with t(8;21) are likely to have a higher relapse rate than those with inv(16) AML, such patients, HSCT in CR2 results in a similar overall survival.[138] Similarly, children and young adults with APL have an overall survival of 75–90%, depending on risk group, with chemotherapy accompanied by the use of ATRA and, more recently, arsenic.[190,268] Thus, HSCT is not usually recommending in CR1 for these patients, but instead following CR2, in which case allogeneic, and in some instances autologous, HSCT result in an approximately 70% overall survival.[269,270]

MLL-rearranged AML represents an extremely heterogeneous group of leukemias associated with variable outcomes. For example, an international trial has reported that survival is 100%, 63%, 27%, and 22% for patients with the t(1;11), the t(9;11), the t(4;11), and the t(6;11), respectively.[107] Because of the wide variability of outcomes along with small numbers of patients with MLL subtypes, as well as no prospective definitive data demonstrating that HSCG improves outcome in this group of patients, most cooperative group clinical trials have not mandated allogeneic HSCT in first remission.[110]

Patients with AML, characterized by a normal karyotype, represent an important challenge in risk classification as this group represents the majority of patients with AML. However, this group of patients, with normal cytogenetic AML, is subdivided by molecular markers that may help direct treatment. For example, *NPM1* mutations are associated with an improved outcome, although whether the presence of mutated *NPM1* can alter the poor prognosis of high mutant FLT3/ITD to normal allelic ratio is somewhat controversial.[143,144] AML with *CEBPA* mutations is usually associated with normal karyotype AML and improved overall survival.[145] Thus, HSCT in first remission is not recommended for children and young adults with isolated *CEBPA* mutations. Whether other molecular alterations, such as mutations in IDH1 and IDH2[155] or DNMT3a,[271] increased expression of BAALC[169] or aberrant RNA expression and epigenetic patterns,[159,175,272,273] will be used to further risk stratify this group of patients, will take further prospective confirmatory studies. Most pediatric trials do not currently recommend allogeneic HSCT in CR1 for patients with normal cytogenetic AML who are rapid responders to induction therapy and have no adverse features such as a high FLT3-ITD to normal allele ratio or persistence of MRD. However, in young adults, allogeneic HSCT is still sometimes recommended when a related HLA-matched donor is available.

As discussed above, AML with a high mutant FLT3/ITD to wild type allelic ratio is associated with an overall survival of (usually) less than 30%.[125] In addition, there are some data suggesting that HSCT might improve outcome. Thus, the use of various FLT3 inhibitors is often tested in preceding or after allogeneic HSCT in this group of patients. In the next COG trial for newly diagnosed AML, patients with a high FLT3-ITD to wild type allelic ratio will be offered an allogeneic HSCT from the best available donor in CR1. Point mutations involving *c-KIT, RAS or WT1*, have yet been definitively shown to improve outcome with allogeneic HSCT, which is not usually recommended for these patients in first remission.[140,146,147] Furthermore, patients with AML having high-risk cytogenetics, such as monosomy 7 or del(5q)- and −5, are recommended to have HSCT in CR1. Patients who demonstrate MRD positivity at then end of induction represent a high-risk group and often have HSCT recommended as part of their post-remission therapy.

The use of a matched unrelated donor (MUD) for allogeneic HSCT in CR1 is not as clearly defined, since the majority of published trials are retrospective comparisons. The only study to prospectively address this issue is the German AML 01/99 trial. Patients with high-risk disease, defined as having unfavorable cytogenetics or residual disease on day 15 post-induction, were treated with allogeneic HSCT from a matched sibling if available, a MUD HSCT if such a donor could be identified, or autologous HSCT otherwise. Survival at 4 years was 68% for patients with an HLA-matched sibling donor, 56% for patients with a MUD, and 23% for patients allocated to autologous transplantation.[274] A retrospective analysis reported by the Fred Hutchinson Cancer Research Center (FHCRC) showed that 5-year survival rates were equivalent between matched sibling and unrelated allografts in AML CR1 at 63% and 61%, respectively for all risk groups.[275] These data suggest that indications for HSCT in AML using a matched related or 10 of 10 matched unrelated donor should be similar although the patients in this analysis were likely selected and further studies will need to be done. The Center for International Blood and Marrow Transplant Research however, demonstrated only a 30% 5-year survival for poor-risk AML patients in CR1 after transplant with a MUD.[276] Nevertheless, given the high risk for relapse for patients with unfavorable cytogenetics, allogeneic HSCT from either a matched sibling or MUD should be pursued in CR1 (see below).

The optimal timing for allogeneic HSCT after induction therapy has not been determined. In part, because of timing to perform HLA typing, assessment of risk and planning for a HSCT, most cooperative groups recommend doing the HSCT following the second or third course of chemotherapy, i.e. a remission induction course followed by one or two post-remission courses. However, this issue has not been determined in a prospective randomized manner. In an attempt to get a more definitive answer to this question, Tallman *et al.* retrospectively analyzed pre-transplant treatment in a cohort of adult patients and did not show a difference in outcome whether transplant was done directly after induction or following a course of consolidation therapy with standard or higher dose Ara-C.[277] In part, because of the retrospective nature of this report and the heterogeneity of patients examined, it has not defined a standard of HSCT after only induction chemotherapy. In contrast, because of data that has demonstrated improved outcomes for patients who undergo HSCT with no MRD, the addition of one or two post-induction courses have become more standard approaches.[278,279] Unfortunately, the issue of disease status at the time of HSCT has not been addressed in a prospective randomized trial.

Combinatorial approaches to risk classification and treatment stratification

Based on the above considerations, most cooperative groups recommend HSCT in first remission for patients with high-risk AML defined by the disease having high-risk cytogenetics or molecular features along with a poor response to induction therapy. In the pediatric population, patients with good risk and intermediate risk AML are treated similarly with chemotherapy alone. For young adults, however, some studies have demonstrated an overall survival benefit of allogeneic HSCT in first remission for patients with normal cytogenetics and lack of either favorable or unfavorable molecular markers. Moreover, a meta-analysis of clinical trial that prospectively assigned allogeneic HSCT vs. consolidation chemotherapy vs. autologous HSCT in an intent-to-treat donor vs. no donor fashion showed a clear overall survival advantage for patients with intermediate and high-risk AML.[280–283] The question of whether to transplant in CR1 is best answered on an individual basis, taking into account cytogenetic and molecular risk factors, predicted treatment-related mortality, and availability of a suitable donor.

The COG has adopted this type of combinatorial approach, but has defined risk groups into only two groups with the intent of risk-directing treatment. A low-risk group will include patients with AML characterized by mutations involving *CBF*, *CEBPA*, *NPM* and those with no MRD at the end of induction therapy. This group represents about 73% of all patients and has an approximately 75% survival. A high-risk group, representing the remaining 27% of patients and having an approximately 35% survival, will include patients whose AML is characterized by adverse cytogenetic abnormalities, such as monosomy 7, del(5q)- or −5, high FLT3-ITD to wild type allelic ratio or MRD at the end of induction. HSCT in first remission with the most suitable donor will be recommended for this group of patients.

As noted above, along with the discussion of special groups to follow, there are many commonly shared characteristics between pediatric patients and young adults with AML. However, significant differences also exist in some of the biological, clinical and treatment approaches (Table 13.3).

Special groups

Down syndrome

The superior outcome of patients with Down syndrome (DS) with AML has been documented since the 1990s with overall survival rates in the 85–95% range.[94,119,284–288] Several important observations have emerged from such studies.

The first is that these excellent outcomes were the result of using less intense therapy than that used in patients without DS. In particular, patients with DS and AML do not usually require a HSCT in first remission. The CCG 2891 studied showed that children with DS and AML who received intensive timing chemotherapy only had a 60% CR rate compared to 90% for the standard timing arm; the difference was due to an approximately 30% toxic death rate. In addition, children with DS and AML who underwent an allogeneic HSCT had a DFS of 33% compared to 89% for those treated only with chemotherapy.[288] In contrast, children without DS, who received standard timing, had only a 38% relapse-free survival.[93,288]

Age at diagnosis has also emerged as an important prognostic factor. For example, children greater than 4 years of age, who account for less than 10% of patients with DS and AML, have a significantly worse prognosis with a 4-year EFS of only 28%.[93,288] Unfortunately, there is currently no optimized therapeutic strategy for these older children with DS and they are usually being treated according to regimens used for patients without DS and AML. For patients with DS and AML, who are less than four years of age, the goal of current clinical trials is to continue to determine ways to decrease exposure to cytotoxic agents, particularly anthracyclines.

TMD, characteristic of infants with DS, is usually a self-limited condition, which tends to resolve within weeks to months of onset. However, because infants with TMD can experience significant morbidity and mortality from complications, such as hydrops fetalis, massive hepatomegaly, hepatic fibrosis, hepatorenal syndrome, and liver failure as well as respiratory distress and DIC.[93,289] While the initial therapy for these patients should primarily involve support care only, some patients who experience progression of signs and symptoms may require therapeutic intervention, including exchange transfusion or low dose AraC.[93,288,290] Approximately 25–30% of infants who survive TMD will develop AML, so these patients need to be closely followed through their early childhood years, particularly up to age 3 years. Further, the nearly universal presence of GATA1 mutations in patients with DS and TMD or AML provides a potentially molecular measure by which to follow these patients.

Acute promyelocytic leukemia

The introduction of ATRA along with ATRA plus antimetabolite chemotherapy in maintenance into chemotherapy-based treatment regimens for patients with APL markedly improved outcomes with 5-year

Table 13.3. Comparison of AML in pediatric vs. adult patients.

Characteristic	Pediatric ≤ 21 years	Adults > 21 and < 55–60 years
Cytogenetics	Higher frequency favorable risk cytogenetics	Greater percent of unfavorable cytogenetics and drug-resistant markers
Antecedent disease evolution to AML	Rare (some inherited predisposition)	Common (MDS, MPN and therapy-related)
Subtype	More M4/M5, DS, TMD	Less M4/M5, no DS or TMD
Extramedullary disease	More CNS disease/leukemia cutis	Uncommon except in monocytic lineage
Induction	ADE most used	"7&3" still standard
Remission rates (after 2 courses)	85–90%	60–80%
CNS prophylaxis	Yes	Not routine
HSCT	Only for high-risk patients	For some intermediate and most high risk patients
APL treatment	ATRA at 25 mg/m^2	ATRA at 45 mg/m^2
Overall survival	Approximately 60–65%	Approximately 40%
Late complications	Growth, endocrine, cardiac, neurocognitive, secondary malignancies	Secondary malignancies less well studied

overall survival in the 75–90% range depending on risk characteristics.[189,268]

Although ATRA alone or in combination with chemotherapy result in a CR rate of greater than 90%, approximately 3% of patients, representing around half of induction failures, still die from hemorrhagic complications.[291] In some studies, the use of ATRA in maintenance has also contributed to superior overall survival.[291–293] Although ATRA is clearly effective in the treatment of patients with APL, there are significant toxicities associated with it. Patients younger than 20 years of age have a higher incidence of pseudotumor cerebri.[294] There are some evidence that smaller doses may be as effective clinically[295] and many pediatric hematologists recommend starting this group of patients with doses of 25 mg/m^2 daily. In addition, some adults groups also use a dose of 25 mg/m^2 given the evidence of equal efficacy and less toxicity.[296]

Historically, approximately 25% of APL patients receiving ATRA during induction develop the "APL differentiation syndrome" or "retinoic acid syndrome". APL differentiation syndrome is characterized by fever, respiratory distress, pulmonary infiltrates, pleural or pericardial effusions, weight gain due to fluid overload, episodic hypotension, and acute renal failure. Although hyperleukocytosis is frequently associated with APL differentiation syndrome, the reaction may occur with a normal leukocyte count.[297] Several mechanisms for the development of this syndrome have been proposed, including the release of vasoactive cytokines, the expression of adhesion molecules on myeloid cell surfaces, and the ability of malignant promyelocytes to gain chemotactic properties as they undergo differentiation. The progression of APL differentiation syndrome can be abated by early intervention with high-dose dexamethasone. Anticipation, immediate recognition and appropriate intervention are critical, since delayed treatment is associated with significant morbidity and mortality. In uncontrolled trials, a low mortality and morbidity rate was reported as a result of differentiation syndrome after ATRA treatment when corticosteroids were administered prophylactically in patients presenting with WBC counts >5000/μL.[298] As a consequence, this approach has been adopted more frequently. While the vast majority of APL is characterized by the ATRA-sensitive t(15;17) translocation, other less common translocations involving the retinoic acid receptor alpha can also occur (e.g. t(11;17)) but tend to show decreased sensitivity to ATRA.[105] A presenting WBC > 10×10^9/L, is associated with an event-free survival of about 60%.[268] APL, characterized as a microgranular variant (M3v) with a bcr3 PML breakpoint and the presence of FLT3-ITD, have also been associated with a poor prognosis; such patients usually present with an increased presenting WBC.[232,291,299–301] In most studies, patients are considered low risk or high risk based on WBC ≤ or > 10×10^9/L, respectively.

Given that ATRA combined with chemotherapy for induction followed by anthracycline-based postremission therapy, provides as favorable results in children with APL as in adults, it remains the reference first-line treatment in both age groups.[302] An important issue in the treatment of children and young adults with APL, however, is the commonly used cumulative doses of anthracyclines in the range of 400–750 mg/m^2.[189] Therefore, the use of arsenic trioxide, which has achieved as a single agent remission rates in patients with relapsed APL of up to 85%, has been investigated in the upfront treatment of APL.[303–306] A recent North American Intergroup trial (C9710) showed that the addition of two cycles of consolidation with ATO to two cycles of ATRA-daunorubicin consolidation significantly increased 3-year event-free survival (77% vs. 59%, p = 0.0013) and OS (86% vs. 77%, p = 0.029), compared to consolidation with ATRA-daunorubicin alone, suggesting a role in the initial management of APL.[306] Alternative approaches have included ATRA in combination with arsenic or with gemtuzumab ozogamicin.[307–310] In a small randomized study from China, induction with ATRA and ATO resulted in prolonged disease-free survival compared to induction with either ATRA or ATO alone.[296] Similarly, a study from the MD Anderson Cancer Center showed that durable remission could be seen in some patients receiving induction and consolidation with ATRA and ATO alone.[311] Mathews *et al.* treated 72 patients, including both adults and children with single-agent ATO for induction followed by a 28-day consolidation. Patients then received ATO for 10 days/month for 6 months. Sixty-two patients (86%) achieved hematologic remission. With median follow-up of 58 months, the estimated 5-year overall, event-free, and disease-free survival rates for the entire group were 74%, 69%, and 80%, respectively.[311,312] Furthermore, a role for the use of Ara-C in APL treatment has been reported and can serve as an alternative approach to provide effective treatment that is not anthracycline based.[303]

The current COG trial, thus, replaces a course of anthracycline-containing chemotherapy with arsenic, thereby reducing anthracycline exposure to 355 mg/m^2 of daunorubicin equivalents for standard-risk patients with negative MRD at the end of induction and to 455 mg/m^2 for high-risk patients and standard-risk patients who have MRD after the third treatment course. This trial also includes high-dose Ara-C based on the survival advantage observed in a European trial.[303] Maintenance therapy with ATRA plus antimetabolites will also be given to all patients for approximately 2 years.

Despite the significant improvement in remission and survival rates since the incorporation of ATRA in the treatment of APL, historically, 15–20% of patients have relapsed, particularly those with intermediate- or high-risk disease. As a result of its high efficacy and safety profile, ATO is now used as standard therapy in patients with relapsed APL.[314] Patients who achieve a second remission, irrespective of the salvage regimen used, however, will need additional therapy to achieve long-term remissions. Among the 20 patients treated with ATO induction followed by additional courses of ATO consolidation and maintenance, 10 (50%) are alive with median follow-up of over 2 years. In contrast, 14 of 18 patients (78%) who underwent either allogeneic or autologous SCT after reinduction with ATO achieved long-term remission,[315] suggesting that patients in second or greater remission who are eligible should be referred for HSCT.

The outcome of patients receiving either allogeneic or autologous SCT in second remission after salvage with ATRA and chemotherapy was reported by the European APL Group.[269] Although allogeneic HSCT was associated with a decreased risk of relapse compared to autologous HSCT, the 7-year OS rate was significantly better for the autologous group than the allogeneic group (60% vs. 52%; p = 0.04), due to treatment-related toxicity. For patients undergoing autologous SCT, RT-PCR status for PML-RARα at the time of transplant is an important consideration. Meloni *et al.* reported that among seven patients whose cells used in the graft were RT-PCR-positive, all relapsed in less than 9 months post-transplant.[316] In contrast, only one of the eight patients whose graft was RT-PCR-negative relapsed. More recently, an estimated 5-year EFS of 83.3% was reported in patients who underwent autologous SCT in second molecular remission after autologous SCT compared to 34.5% (p = 0.001) for patients who received only maintenance therapy.[270] These data support autologous SCT for patients in second molecular remission and allogeneic SCT for patients who remain RT-PCR-positive after reinduction and consolidation with ATO.

Congenital and infant acute myelogenous leukemia

Congenital leukemia is defined by presentation within the first month of life. It is characterized by high numbers of myeloid, lymphoid or erythroid precursor cells, infiltration of clonal, immature hematopoietic cells into non-hematopoietic tissues and the absence of other etiologies.[317] There is a predominance of monocytic and myelomonocytic subtypes. Approximately two thirds of these patients will show signs of leukemia cutis along with marked hepatosplenomegaly and lymphadenopathy.[318] CNS involvement may occur in approximately 50% of these patients.[318] A significant proportion of these patients have 11q23 chromosomal abnormalities.[202,317,318]

Because spontaneous remissions have been reported more frequently in the neonate age group, the first treatment recommendation is usually to initially observe such patients and provide supportive measures, such as transfusions or antibiotics as indicated clinically. In addition, if cytoreduction is indicated, an exchange transfusion is usually recommended. However, AML-directed therapy with dosing adjustments for size is usually required. Outcome in this age group is worse than that in older children despite similar therapy due to both treatment toxicities and resistant disease.[317]

In contrast to neonates, infants more than one month old appear to do as well as older children when treated with current, intensive regimens.[103,116,202,203,211,212,254,255,261,319–324] The role of transplantation in infants is controversial because it has not been shown to definitely improve outcome and has significant adverse sequelae.

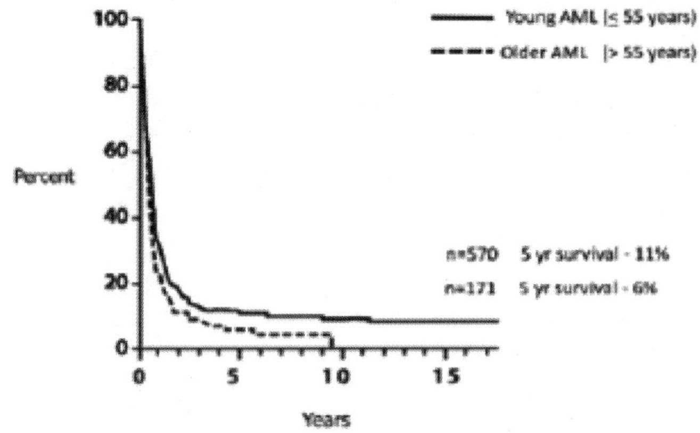

Fig. 13.5. Survival from relapse of 2441 patients entered on 8 consecutive ECOG studies.

From Rowe JM, Tallman MS. (2010) How I treat acute myeloid leukemia. *Blood* **116**: 3147–3156. Rowe JM, Li X, Cassileth PA, *et al.* (2005) Very poor survival of patients with AML who relapse after achieving a first complete remission: The Eastern Cooperative Oncology Group Experience. *Blood* **106**: 162a.[332,389]

Relapsed/refractory disease

The outcome for patients with relapsed AML is not uniformly poor, but depends upon several key factors, such as cytogenetics, previous therapy, time to relapse from first remission, host comorbidities and the site of relapse.[325,326]

For example, patients with inv(16) or t(8;21) who relapsed after having been treated on the MRC AML10 trial and who subsequently received reinduction chemotherapy followed by allogeneic HSCT experienced a 5-year survival from relapse of 57%. By comparison, patients in the standard and poor risk groups who relapsed experienced an overall survival of 14% and 8%, respectively.[202,327] Patients who relapse on therapy or within 6 months after obtaining an initial remission are reported to have less than 20% survival at 5 years.[325,328–330] Two key prognostic factors were reported from the 1988–2003 NOPHO results, including duration of the first remission and whether a patient relapsed after having already had a HSCT.[331] This analysis reported that patients having a less than 1-year remission had a 5-year survival of 21% vs. 48% for those with relapses greater than a year. For patients who relapsed after having received either an autologous or allogeneic HSCT, survival was less than 20% at 5 years compared to 41% for those who relapsed after having received only chemotherapy.[331] For adults less than or equal to age 55 years or those greater than 55 years of age treated on ECOG studies, the 5-year survival has been reported as less than 20% (Fig. 13.5).[332]

A variety of reinduction regimens have been successfully used, although remission rates following relapse are significantly lower than initial treatment. Such combinations include mitoxantrone and high dose Ara-C, fludarabine and high dose Ara-C plus G-CSF (FLAG), and idarubicin with FLAG (IDA-FLAG).[333–338] In addition, immunotargeted agents, such as anti-CD33/calicheamicin (gemtuzumab ozogamicin), either alone or in combination with chemotherapy, has reasonable safety profiles and activity; however, this agent has not been approved by the FDA and will be unavailable in the US.[229,230] Modified forms of specific classes of drugs, such as clofarabine in combination with high dose Ara-C or other agents, are also being tested to reduce the exposure of patients to further anthracycline exposure as well as to introduce a novel agent.[214,217,339–341] Clinical trials using other novel agents are also underway as discussed below, including novel tyrosine kinase inhibitors, such as sorafenib alone or in combination with chemotherapy,[233,342,343] another FLT3 inhibitor AC220,[344] proteosome inhibitors,[241,345] disruption of microenvironmental/leukemia interactions,[346–350] as well as a chromatin-modifying agents, used alone, in combination with conventional chemotherapy or following HSCT.[244,245,351–354]

The overall strategy for most patients with relapsed or refractory AML is to attempt to achieve a CR and then proceed to an ablative allogeneic HSCT with the best available donor.[355] Patients who relapse after HSCT have a nearly 100% mortality, although survival after a second HSCT has been reported.[356,357] The role for non-ablative, allogeneic HSCT for relapsed AML has not been established, but may provide an approach to deliver an allogeneic anti-leukemic effect while reducing toxicity in certain patients with significant comorbidities.[358] Patients who have a relapse of AML after HSCT have a nearly 100% mortality, although survival after a second HSCT has been reported.[356,357]

Hyperleukocytosis and leukostasis

Patients presenting with hyperleukocytosis, defined as a WBC greater than 100,000/μL, have an increased risk of peri-induction mortality due to hemorrhagic events, tumor lysis syndrome, and infection.[359] Hyperleukocytosis with symptoms of leukostasis, such as pulmonary infiltrates, retinal hemorrhage, or cerebral hemorrhage, requires immediate attention. While leukapheresis can rapidly improve these symptoms, it has not been shown to improve long-term survival.[360] In general, hydroxyurea at doses of 50–60 mg/kg, is recommended to lower the WBC to 10,000–20,000/μL, with prompt initiation of definitive induction chemotherapy. Until the WBC has been reduced, excessive red blood cell transfusions should be avoided, since this can result in increased blood viscosity.

Central nervous system involvement

Involvement of the CNS is rare at presentation in AML. Therefore, in the absence of neurologic symptoms, routine examination of the cerebrospinal fluid and prophylactic intrathecal chemotherapy has not been proven to be indicated.[361] However, intrathecal prophylaxis may be considered in patients with high numbers of circulating leukemic blasts and monocytic disease, where CNS disease is more common.[362] In patients with CNS involvement, cytarabine at a dose of 50–70 mg should be given intrathecally or intraventricularly via an Ommaya reservoir, 2–3 times weekly, until cerebrospinal fluid (CSF) blasts are cleared, followed by at least three additional doses given every 2–4 weeks. Alternatively, methotrexate at a dose of 12 mg may be given using the same schedule of administration. A change in agents should be considered in patients who fail to clear CSF blasts within two treatments. Alternatively, liposomal cytarabine at a dose of 50 mg every other week for approximately six cycles may be given. Dexamethasone (4 mg three times daily) can be given on the days of intrathecal therapy for the prevention of arachnoiditis.

Radiotherapy can be used alone or occasionally in combination with intrathecal chemotherapy, particularly in patients who fail to respond to or relapse after intrathecal chemotherapy.[363] Radiotherapy should consist of 1800 to 2400 cGy in 150- to 200-cGy fractions administered to the whole brain. Higher doses should be avoided because of the risk of late toxicity and the possible later use of total body irradiation as conditioning for HSCT. Despite encouraging results in children, spinal radiotherapy should be avoided in adults unless overt disease is noted on magnetic resonance imaging, since the radiation dose to marrow-bearing areas can result in significant myelosuppression and limit the ability to deliver systemic therapy.

Extramedullary leukemia

AML cells may diffusely infiltrate any organ of the body or form tumor masses, known as myeloid sarcoma (or granulocytic sarcoma, chloroma, or extramedullary myeloid tumor). Myeloid sarcomas may present *de novo*, preceding AML, concurrently with AML, prior to systemic relapse, or as blastic transformation of MDS or myeloproliferative neoplasms. Often myeloid sarcomas will exhibit myelomonocytic or monoblastic features and are associated with hyperleukocytosis, (8;21) translocation, and CD56 expression.[364,365] *De novo* myeloid sarcoma heralds the development of overt AML and should be treated as such. While some studies suggest that myeloid sarcoma is a poor prognostic feature, others report similar outcomes to patients with AML when treated with conventional chemotherapy or allogeneic SCT.[366]

Diffuse leukemic involvement of the skin is referred to as leukemia cutis and should be distinguished from Sweet syndrome, which is infiltration of the skin by neutrophils. Like myeloid sarcoma, leukemia cutis should be treated with systemic therapy for AML. Although, external electronic beam therapy has been used for local disease control, particularly in relapsed or refractory patients, it has been associated with fatal dermatitis in patients had previously received anthracyclines.[367]

Pregnancy

AML during pregnancy should be managed jointly by a hematologist, obstetrician, and neonatologist. Pregnant women with AML have a higher incidence of abortion, intrauterine growth restriction, and perinatal mortality. In general, treatment should start as quickly as possible after the diagnosis of leukemia is made, as delays can compromise maternal outcome.[368] Combination chemotherapy, however, given during the first trimester of pregnancy is associated with a high incidence of fetal abnormalities or loss. One study reported fetal death, malformation, or spontaneous abortion rates of 4%, 11%, and 7%, respectively, when anthracyclines were given during the first trimester.[369] Since idarubicin is more lipophilic than daunorubicin, and thus has a greater chance of placental transfer, daunorubicin is preferred in this setting.[370] Given the risk of teratogenicity, therapeutic termination of pregnancy during the first trimester followed by treatment of the leukemia is advisable. There have been many reports of patients safely treated with chemotherapy in the second and third trimesters, although stillbirths and low birthweights have been described.[371–372] There have been no reports of leukemia occurring in children, nor an increased incidence of fetal abnormalities in infants who have been exposed to full-dose antileukemia chemotherapy during the later stages of gestation. Delivery during cytopenic episodes should be avoided.

Late Effects and Long-Term Monitoring of Patients with AML

Although several studies have reported on the late effects in childhood AML,[374–378] population-based studies following recent intensive therapies are beginning to become available.[379–381] Further, with the overall survival of children and adolescents continuing to improve (Fig. 13.6), the need to appropriate long-term follow-up has become increasingly important (see Chapter 24).

Common late effects included growth delay, endocrine abnormalities, cataracts, secondary malignancies, and cardiac abnormalities.[374,382] Increasing radiation dose and younger age at diagnosis and initiation of radiation therapy were risk factors for growth delay, infertility, academic difficulties, cataracts, and hypothyroidism. Patients receiving total body irradiation had lower cumulative anthracycline doses (204 mg/m^2 vs. 335 mg/m^2), but did not have a lower rate of cardiomyopathy, which was approximately 1% but still 10-fold higher than expected in the general population. Thus, HSCT and radiation exposure stand out as significant risk factors for subsequent adverse late sequelae.[374,378,382] Dyslipidemias have also been

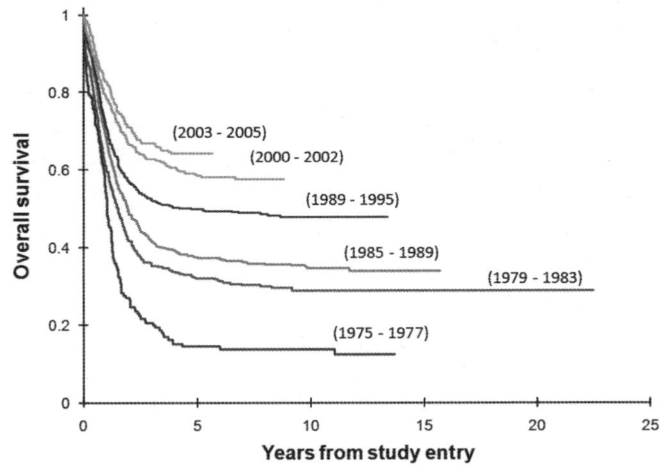

Fig. 13.6. The overall survival is shown based on successive CCG/COG trials (Figure kindly supplied by Drs. William Woods, Alan Gamis and Todd Alonzo). Data from groups from other international, cooperative groups show similar outcomes (please see text for more details).

noted as an adverse late effect, particularly for children less than 3 years of age.[383] In a report from BFM AML studies, Creutzig *et al.* showed that approximately 5% of patients who had received 300–450 mg/m^2 of anthracyclines 11 years following the cessation of treatment.[384] In an analysis of COG AML trial outcomes, Neglia *et al.* reported that with an approximately 20-year follow-up (range: 5–33 years), about half of the survivors reported a chronic medical condition and had a 16% increased risk of having a severe or life-threatening chronic medical condition compared to their siblings. There was also evidence that survivors of AML had significantly less socioeconomic achievement than others within their family unit, but not significantly different than the general population.[385] A study from the same group on health risk behaviors reported that about a quarter of survivors, regardless of the type of AML treatment they received, demonstrated tobacco/marijuana use as well as binge drinking.[386] Quality of life has also begun to be examined in survivors of AML; here again, one of the key factors of adverse sequelae was HSCT (see Chapter 28).[387]

Important resources for details on follow-up and risks for survivors of cancer have been developed by the Children Oncology Group's *Long-Term Follow-Up Guidelines for Survivors of Childhood, Adolescent, and Young Adult Cancers* (available at www.survivorshipguidelines.org) and the *National Comprehensive Cancer Network* or NCCN (available at www.nccn.com). Furthermore, an increasingly recognized important component of long-term follow-up for cancer survivors is to have access to their past medical history that can be shared with subsequent medical providers. Templates to address this issue are being developed, such as those from the Cancer Survivor's Treatment Record available at www.patientcenters.com and the Cancer Survivor's Medical Treatment Summary available at www.livestrong.org.

References

2. Juliusson G, Antunovic P, Derolf A, Lehmann S, Mollgard L, Stockelberg D, Tidefelt U, Wahlin A, Hoglund M. (2009) Age and acute myeloid leukemia: Real world data on decision to treat and outcomes from the Swedish Acute Leukemia Registry. *Blood* **113**: 4179–4187.
39. Ross JA, Spector LG, Robison LL, Olshan AF. (2005) Epidemiology of leukemia in children with Down syndrome. *Pediatr Blood Cancer* **44**: 8–12.
40. Wechsler J, Greene M, McDevitt MA, Anastasi J, Karp JE, Le Beau MM, Crispino JD. (2002) Acquired mutations in GATA1 in the megakaryoblastic leukemia of Down syndrome. *Nat Genet* **32**: 148–152.
72. Gilliland DG, Jordan CT, Felix CA. (2004) The molecular basis of leukemia. *Hematology (Am Soc Hematol Educ Program)* 80–97.
73. Bonnet D, Dick JE. (1997) Human acute myeloid leukemia is organized as a hierarchy that originates from a primitive hematopoietic cell. *Nat Med* **3**: 730–737.
79. Stein E, McMahon B, Kwaan H, Altman JK, Frankfurt O, Tallman MS. (2009) The coagulopathy of acute promyelocytic leukaemia revisited. *Best Pract Res, Clin Haematol* **22**: 153–163.
91. Aplenc R, Alonzo TA, Gerbing RB, Smith FO, Meshinchi S, Ross JA, Perentesis J, Woods WG, Lange BJ, Davies SM. (2006) Ethnicity and survival in childhood acute myeloid leukemia: A report from the Children's Oncology Group. *Blood* **108**: 74–80.
93. Gamis AS. (2005) Acute myeloid leukemia and Down syndrome evolution of modern therapy — state of the art review. *Pediatr Blood Cancer* **44**: 13–20.
98. (2007) *WHO Classification of Tumours of Haematopoietic and Lymphoid Tissues.* Albany, NY: WHO Publications Center.
104. Lange BJ, Smith FO, Feusner J, Barnard DR, Dinndorf P, Feig S, Heerema NA, Arndt C, Arceci RJ, Seibel N, Weiman M, Dusenbery K, Shannon K, Luna-Fineman S, Gerbing RB, Alonzo TA. (2008) Outcomes in CCG-2961, a children's oncology group phase 3 trial for untreated pediatric acute myeloid leukemia: A report from the children's oncology group. *Blood* **111**: 1044–1053.
107. Balgobind BV, Raimondi SC, Harbott J, Zimmermann M, Alonzo TA, Auvrignon A, Beverloo HB, Chang M, Creutzig U, Dworzak MN, Forestier E, Gibson B, Hasle H, Harrison CJ, Heerema NA, Kaspers GJ, Leszl A, Litvinko N, Nigro LL, Morimoto A, Perot C, Pieters R, Reinhardt D, Rubnitz JE, Smith FO, Stary J, Stasevich I, Strehl S, Taga T, Tomizawa D, Webb D, Zemanova Z, Zwaan CM, van den Heuvel-Eibrink MM. (2009) Novel prognostic subgroups in childhood 11q23/MLL-rearranged acute myeloid leukemia: Results of an international retrospective study. *Blood* **114**: 2489–2496.
116. Rubnitz JE, Inaba H, Dahl G, Ribeiro RC, Bowman WP, Taub J, Pounds S, Razzouk BI, Lacayo NJ, Cao X, Meshinchi S, Degar B, Airewele G, Raimondi SC, Onciu M, Coustan-Smith E, Downing JR, Leung W, Pui CH, Campana D. (2010) Minimal residual disease-directed therapy for childhood acute myeloid leukaemia: Results of the AML02 multicentre trial. *Lancet Oncol* **11**: 543–552.
117. Grimwade D, Walker H, Oliver F, Wheatley K, Harrison C, Harrison G, Rees J, Hann I, Stevens R, Burnett A, Goldstone A. (1998) The importance of diagnostic cytogenetics on outcome in AML: Analysis of 1,612 patients entered into the MRC AML 10 trial. The Medical Research Council Adult and Children's Leukaemia Working Parties. *Blood* **92**: 2322–2333.
118. Lugthart S, Groschel S, Beverloo HB, Kayser S, Valk PJ, van Zelderen-Bhola SL, Jan Ossenkoppele G, Vellenga E, van den Berg-de Ruiter E, Schanz U, Verhoef G, Vandenberghe P, Ferrant A, Kohne CH, Pfreundschuh M, Horst HA, Koller E, von Lilienfeld-Toal M, Bentz M, Ganser A, Schlegelberger B, Jotterand M, Krauter J, Pabst T, Theobald M, Schlenk RF, Delwel R, Dohner K, Lowenberg B, Dohner H. (2010) Clinical, molecular, and prognostic significance of WHO type inv(3)(q21q26.2)/t(3;3)(q21;q26.2) and various other 3q abnormalities in acute myeloid leukemia. *J Clin Oncol* **28**: 3890–3898.
119. Stevens RF, Hann IM, Wheatley K, Gray RG. (1998) Marked improvements in outcome with chemotherapy alone in paediatric acute myeloid leukemia: Results of the United Kingdom Medical Research Council's 10th AML trial. MRC Childhood Leukaemia Working Party. *Br J Haematol* **101**: 130–140.
126. Meshinchi S, Alonzo TA, Stirewalt DL, Zwaan M, Zimmerman M, Reinhardt D, Kaspers GJ, Heerema NA,

Gerbing R, Lange BJ, Radich JP. (2006) Clinical implications of FLT3 mutations in pediatric AML. *Blood* **108**: 3654–3661.

127. Schnittger S, Schoch C, Dugas M, Kern W, Staib P, Wuchter C, Loffler H, Sauerland CM, Serve H, Buchner T, Haferlach T, Hiddemann W. (2002) Analysis of FLT3 length mutations in 1003 patients with acute myeloid leukemia: Correlation to cytogenetics, FAB subtype, and prognosis in the AMLCG study and usefulness as a marker for the detection of minimal residual disease. *Blood* **100**: 59–66.
128. Thiede C, Steudel C, Mohr B, Schaich M, Schakel U, Platzbecker U, Wermke M, Bornhauser M, Ritter M, Neubauer A, Ehninger G, Illmer T. (2002) Analysis of FLT3-activating mutations in 979 patients with acute myelogenous leukemia: Association with FAB subtypes and identification of subgroups with poor prognosis. *Blood* **99**: 4326–4335.
143. Hollink IH, Zwaan CM, Zimmermann M, Arentsen-Peters TC, Pieters R, Cloos J, Kaspers GJ, de Graaf SS, Harbott J, Creutzig U, Reinhardt D, van den Heuvel-Eibrink MM, Thiede C. (2009) Favorable prognostic impact of NPM1 gene mutations in childhood acute myeloid leukemia, with emphasis on cytogenetically normal AML. *Leukemia* **23**: 262–270.
144. Brown P, McIntyre E, Rau R, Meshinchi S, Lacayo N, Dahl G, Alonzo TA, Chang M, Arceci RJ, Small D. (2007) The incidence and clinical significance of nucleophosmin mutations in childhood AML. *Blood* **110**: 979–985.
145. Ho PA, Alonzo TA, Gerbing RB, Pollard J, Stirewalt DL, Hurwitz C, Heerema NA, Hirsch B, Raimondi SC, Lange B, Franklin JL, Radich JP, Meshinchi S. (2009) Prevalence and prognostic implications of CEBPA mutations in pediatric acute myeloid leukemia (AML): A report from the Children's Oncology Group. *Blood* **113**: 6558–6566.
146. Hollink IH, van den Heuvel-Eibrink MM, Zimmermann M, Balgobind BV, Arentsen-Peters ST, Alders M, Willasch A, Kaspers GJ, Trka J, Baruchel A, de Graaf SS, Creutzig U, Pieters R, Reinhardt D, Zwaan CM. (2009) Clinical relevance of Wilms tumor 1 gene mutations in childhood acute myeloid leukemia. *Blood* **113**: 5951–5960.
147. Ho PA, Zeng R, Alonzo TA, Gerbing RB, Miller KL, Pollard JA, Stirewalt DL, Heerema NA, Raimondi SC, Hirsch B, Franklin JL, Lange B, Meshinchi S. (2010) Prevalence and prognostic implications of WT1 mutations in pediatric acute myeloid leukemia (AML): A report from the Children's Oncology Group. *Blood* **116**: 702–710.
153. Abdel-Wahab O, Manshouri T, Patel J, Harris K, Yao J, Hedvat C, Heguy A, Bueso-Ramos C, Kantarjian H, Levine RL, Verstovesk S. (2010) Genetic analysis of transforming events that convert chronic myeloproliferative neoplasms to leukemias. *Cancer Research* **70**(2): 447–452.
154. Abbas S, Lugthart S, Kavelaars FG, Schelen A, Koenders JE, Zeilemaker A, van Putten WJ, Rijneveld AW, Lowenberg B, Valk PJ. (2010) Acquired mutations in the genes encoding IDH1 and IDH2 both are recurrent aberrations in acute myeloid leukemia: Prevalence and prognostic value. *Blood* **116**: 2122–2126.
155. Marcucci G, Maharry K, Wu YZ, Radmacher MD, Mrozek K, Margeson D, Holland KB, Whitman SP, Becker H, Schwind S, Metzeler KH, Powell BL, Carter TH, Kolitz JE, Wetzler M, Carroll AJ, Baer MR, Caligiuri MA, Larson RA, Bloomfield CD. (2010) IDH1 and IDH2 gene mutations identify novel molecular subsets within de novo cytogenetically normal acute myeloid leukemia: A Cancer and Leukemia Group B study. *J Clin Oncol* **28**: 2348–2355.
156. Paschka P, Schlenk RF, Gaidzik VI, Habdank M, Kronke J, Bullinger L, Spath D, Kayser S, Zucknick M, Gotze K, Horst HA, Germing U, Dohner H, Dohner K. (2010) IDH1 and IDH2 mutations are frequent genetic alterations in acute myeloid leukemia and confer adverse prognosis in cytogenetically normal acute myeloid leukemia with NPM1 mutation without FLT3 internal tandem duplication. *J Clin Oncol* **28**: 3636–3643.
157. Ji H, Ehrlich LI, Seita J, Murakami P, Doi A, Lindau P, Lee H, Aryee MJ, Irizarry RA, Kim K, Rossi DJ, Inlay MA, Serwold T, Karsunky H, Ho L, Daley GQ, Weissman IL, Feinberg AP. (2010) Comprehensive methylome map of lineage commitment from haematopoietic progenitors. *Nature* **467**: 338–342.
165. Becton D, Dahl GV, Ravindranath Y, Chang MN, Behm FG, Raimondi SC, Head DR, Stine KC, Lacayo NJ, Sikic BI, Arceci RJ, Weinstein H. (2006) Randomized use of cyclosporin A (CsA) to modulate P-glycoprotein in children with AML in remission: Pediatric Oncology Group study 9421. *Blood* **107**: 1315–1324.
189. Sanz MA, Grimwade D, Tallman MS, Lowenberg B, Fenaux P, Estey EH, Naoe T, Lengfelder E, Buchner T, Dohner H, Burnett AK, Lo-Coco F. (2009) Management of acute promyelocytic leukemia: Recommendations from an expert panel on behalf of the European LeukemiaNet. *Blood* **113**: 1875–1891.
190. Sanz MA, Montesinos P, Rayon C, Holowiecka A, de la Serna J, Milone G, de Lisa E, Brunet S, Rubio V, Ribera JM, Rivas C, Krsnik I, Bergua J, Gonzalez J, Diaz-Mediavilla J, Rojas R, Manso F, Ossenkoppele G, Gonzalez JD,

Lowenberg B. (2010) Risk-adapted treatment of acute promyelocytic leukemia based on all-trans retinoic acid and anthracycline with addition of cytarabine in consolidation therapy for high-risk patients: Further improvements in treatment outcome. *Blood* **115**: 5137–5146.

191. Grimwade D, Vyas P, Freeman S. (2010) Assessment of minimal residual disease in acute myeloid leukemia. *Curr Opin Oncol* **22**: 656–663.

193. Sievers EL, Lange BJ, Alonzo TA, Gerbing RB, Bernstein ID, Smith FO, Arceci RJ, Woods WG, Loken MR. (2003) Immunophenotypic evidence of leukemia after induction therapy predicts relapse: Results from a prospective Children's Cancer Group study of 252 patients with acute myeloid leukemia. *Blood* **101**: 3398–3406.

194. Langebrake C, Creutzig U, Dworzak M, Hrusak O, Mejstrikova E, Griesinger F, Zimmermann M, Reinhardt D. (2006) Residual disease monitoring in childhood acute myeloid leukemia by multiparameter flow cytometry: The MRD-AML-BFM Study Group. *J Clin Oncol* **24**: 3686–3692.

201. Preisler H, Bjornsson S, Henderson ES, Hryniuk W, Higby D, Freeman A, Naeher C. (1979) Remission induction in acute nonlymphocytic leukemia: Comparison of a seven-day and ten-day infusion of cytosine arabinoside in combination with adriamycin. *Med Pediatr Oncol* **7**: 269–275.

202. Gibson BE, Wheatley K, Hann IM, Stevens RF, Webb D, Hills RK, de Graaf SS, Harrison CJ. (2005) Treatment strategy and long-term results in paediatric patients treated in consecutive UK AML trials. *Leukemia* **19**: 2130–2138.

209. Woods WG, Kobrinsky N, Buckley JD, Lee JW, Sanders J, Neudorf S, Gold S, Barnard DR, DeSwarte J, Dusenbery K, Kalousek D, Arthur DC, Lange BJ. (1996) Timed-sequential induction therapy improves postremission outcome in acute myeloid leukemia: A report from the Children's Cancer Group. *Blood* **87**: 4979–4989.

210. Woods WG, Neudorf S, Gold S, Sanders J, Buckley JD, Barnard DR, Dusenbery K, DeSwarte J, Arthur DC, Lange BJ, Kobrinsky NL. (2001) A comparison of allogeneic bone marrow transplantation, autologous bone marrow transplantation, and aggressive chemotherapy in children with acute myeloid leukemia in remission. *Blood* **97**: 56–62.

211. Smith FO, Alonzo TA, Gerbing RB, Woods WG, Arceci RJ. (2005) Long-term results of children with acute myeloid leukemia: A report of three consecutive Phase III trials by the Children's Cancer Group: CCG 251, CCG 213 and CCG 2891. *Leukemia* **19**: 2054–2062.

212. Creutzig U, Zimmermann M, Ritter J, Reinhardt D, Hermann J, Henze G, Jurgens H, Kabisch H, Reiter A, Riehm H, Gadner H, Schellong G. (2005) Treatment strategies and long-term results in paediatric patients treated in four consecutive AML-BFM trials. *Leukemia* **19**: 2030–2042.

268. Ortega JJ, Madero L, Martin G, Verdeguer A, Garcia P, Parody R, Fuster J, Molines A, Novo A, Deben G, Rodriguez A, Conde E, de la Serna J, Allegue MJ, Capote FJ, Gonzalez JD, Bolufer P, Gonzalez M, Sanz MA. (2005) Treatment with all-trans retinoic acid and anthracycline monochemotherapy for children with acute promyelocytic leukemia: A multicenter study by the PETHEMA Group. *J Clin Oncol* **23**: 7632–7640.

269. de Botton S, Fawaz A, Chevret S, Dombret H, Thomas X, Sanz M, Guerci A, San Miguel J, de la Serna J, Stoppa AM, Reman O, Stamatoulas A, Fey M, Cahn JY, Sotto JJ, Bourhis JH, Parry A, Chomienne C, Degos L, Fenaux P. (2005) Autologous and allogeneic stem-cell transplantation as salvage treatment of acute promyelocytic leukemia initially treated with all-trans-retinoic acid: A retrospective analysis of the European acute promyelocytic leukemia group. *J Clin Oncol* **23**: 120–126.

270. Thirugnanam R, George B, Chendamarai E, Lakshmi KM, Balasubramanian P, Viswabandya A, Srivastava A, Chandy M, Mathews V. (2009) Comparison of clinical outcomes of patients with relapsed acute promyelocytic leukemia induced with arsenic trioxide and consolidated with either an autologous stem cell transplant or an arsenic trioxide-based regimen. *Biol Blood Marrow Transplant* **15**: 1479–1484.

291. Fenaux P, Chastang C, Chevret S, Sanz M, Dombret H, Archimbaud E, Fey M, Rayon C, Huguet F, Sotto JJ, Gardin C, Makhoul PC, Travade P, Solary E, Fegueux N, Bordessoule D, Miguel JS, Link H, Desablens B, Stamatoullas A, Deconinck E, Maloisel F, Castaigne S, Preudhomme C, Degos L. (1999) A randomized comparison of all transretinoic acid (ATRA) followed by chemotherapy and ATRA plus chemotherapy and the role of maintenance therapy in newly diagnosed acute promyelocytic leukemia. The European APL Group. *Blood* **94**: 1192–1200.

306. Powell BL, Moser B, Stock W, Gallagher RE, Willman CL, Stone RM, Rowe JM, Coutre S, Feusner JH, Gregory J, Couban S, Appelbaum FR, Tallman MS, Larson RA. (2010) Arsenic trioxide improves event-free and overall survival for adults with acute promyelocytic leukemia: North American Leukemia Intergroup Study C9710. *Blood* **116**: 3751–3757.

332. Rowe JM, Tallman MS. (2010) How I treat acute myeloid leukemia. *Blood* **116**: 3147–3156.
384. Creutzig U, Diekamp S, Zimmermann M, Reinhardt D. (2007) Longitudinal evaluation of early and late anthracycline cardiotoxicity in children with AML. *Pediatr Blood Cancer* **48**: 651–662.
385. Mulrooney DA, Dover DC, Li S, Yasui Y, Ness KK, Mertens AC, Neglia JP, Sklar CA, Robison LL, Davies SM. (2008) Twenty years of follow-up among survivors of childhood and young adult acute myeloid leukemia: A report from the Childhood Cancer Survivor Study. *Cancer* **112**: 2071–2079.
386. Schultz KA, Chen L, Chen Z, Zeltzer LK, Nicholson HS, Neglia JP. (2010) Health and risk behaviors in survivors of childhood acute myeloid leukemia: A report from the Children's Oncology Group. *Pediatr Blood Cancer* **55**: 157–164.
390. Brown P, Arceci RJ. (2010) Acute Myelogenous Leukemia, Myelodysplasia and Myeloproliferative Syndromes in Children. In: W Carrol, J Finlay, (eds). *Pediatric Oncology*. Sudbury, MA: Jones and Bartlett Publishers, Inc.
392. Pui CH, Carroll WL, Meshinchi S, Arceci RJ. (2011) Biology, Risk Stratification, and Therapy of Pediatric Acute Leukemias: An Update. *J Clin Oncol.* epub 10.1200/JCO.2010.30.7405

14

Juvenile Myelomonocytic Leukemia

Mignon L. Loh and Franco Locatelli

Introduction

Myeloid neoplasms derive from the pathologic clonal expansion of an abnormal stem cell and span a diverse spectrum of phenotypes including acute myeloid leukemia (AML), myeloproliferative neoplasms (MPN), and myelodysplastic syndromes (MDS). Expansion of myeloid blasts with suppression of normal hematopoiesis is the hallmark of AML, whereas MPN is associated with the overproliferation of one or more lineages that retain the capacity to differentiate, and MDS is characterized by peripheral blood cytopenias and aberrant/impaired differentiation of hematopoietic stem cells. MPN and MDS can progress to AML, which is likely due to the acquisition of cooperative mutations.

Juvenile myelomonocytic leukemia (JMML) is an aggressive myeloid neoplasm of childhood that is clinically characterized by the overproduction of monocytic cells that can infiltrate organs, including the spleen, liver, GI tract, and lung. JMML is categorized as an overlap MPN/MDS by the World Health Organization and also shares some clinical and molecular features with chronic myelomonocytic leukemia (CMML), a similar disease in adults. While the current standard of care for patients with JMML relies on allogeneic hematopoietic stem cell transplantation, relapse is the most frequent cause of treatment failure.

Major progress in understanding the pathogenesis of JMML has been achieved by mapping out the genetic lesions that occur in patients. The spectrum of mutations described thus far in JMML occur in genes that encode proteins that signal through the Ras/MAPK pathways, thus providing potential new opportunities for both diagnosis and therapy. These genes include *NF1*, *NRAS*, *KRAS*, *PTPN11*, and, as most recently demonstrated, *CBL*.

Rarely, spontaneous resolution of JMML can occur, but, so far, there are neither clinical nor biological reliable markers to predict this event. This review outlines our understanding of the genetic underpinnings of JMML with a recent update on the discovery of novel *CBL* mutations, as well as a brief review on current therapeutic approaches.

Juvenile Myelomonocytic Leukemia (JMML)

JMML is an aggressive MPN of early childhood that occurs with an estimated incidence of 1.2 cases per million (see Chapter 1).[1,2] JMML predominates in infants, with the median age at diagnosis being 2 years. About 9% of patients are diagnosed by the age of 4 months, whereas only 8% are 6 years or older. Because of the rarity of the disease and the heterogeneous nature of the clinical manifestations, the diagnosis of JMML is frequently challenging for the average general practitioner. Physicians are usually asked to consult on a young child (more frequently a male, the male/female ratio of affected subjects being 2–3:1) with fever, splenomegaly (present in most but not all patients at diagnosis), and a high white blood cell count with a peripheral monocytosis (above 1.000 elements/μl) and a few circulating myeloid precursor cells. Anemia and thrombocytopenia are also common findings. An intermittent erythematous rash, cough, or bloody stools may be present and the child may have previously exhibited poor growth.

At presentation, a rare circulating nucleated red blood cell can also usually be found in the peripheral blood smear and approximately 50% of patients will present with an elevated hemoglobin F corrected for age.[3] Most patients will present with significant splenomegaly; the 7% of patients who do not display a large spleen at the initial presentation will frequently develop this in the first several weeks to months after diagnosis (Niemeyer C., personal communication). Bone marrow examination must display fewer than 20% myeloblasts by definition (Table 14.1), can display varying degrees of aberrant myelopoiesis or megakaryopoiesis, and must also be negative for the *BCR/ABL* translocation. The main karyotypic abnormality is monosomy 7, which can be detected in up to 25% of patients.[4] One of the hallmark laboratory features of JMML — hypersensitivity of myeloid progenitor cells to granulocyte–macrophage colony stimulating factor (GM-CSF) in colony forming assays (i.e. CFU-GM)[5] — can be present in certain viral infections, thus providing a sensitive, but nonspecific and laborious adjunctive diagnostic tool.[6] Table 14.1 lists both currently accepted and recently updated criteria for making the diagnosis of JMML.

The current standard treatment of patients with JMML is allogeneic hematopoietic stem cell transplantation (HSCT) from either an HLA-identical sibling or an unrelated donor (see Chapter 20). Through this approach more than 50% of patients can be definitively cured; relapse is the most frequent cause of treatment failure.[7] Rarely, spontaneous resolution of this disorder can occur but is unpredictable.[8–10]

Major progress in understanding the pathogenesis of JMML has been achieved by deciphering the genetic lesions that occur in patients (Table 14.2). Children affected by specific congenital syndromes are at a higher risk of developing JMML or a related transient myeloproliferative disorder in infancy, and the identification of genes associated with these syndromes have provided unique insights into the pathogenesis of this intriguing myeloid malignancy. Recent discoveries have advanced our ability to make a firm molecular diagnosis of JMML in 85–90% of children (Fig. 14.1).[3,11] The spectrum of mutations described thus far in JMML occur in genes that encode proteins that signal through the Ras/MAPK pathways, thus providing potential new opportunities for both diagnosis and treatment.

Molecular genetics implicate initiating lesions in the Ras/MAPK pathway

In 1978, it was noted that children affected by neurofibromatosis type 1 (NF1) were particularly prone to developing a "chronic myeloid leukemia" or acute myelomonocytic leukemia in the first decade of life.[12] NF1 is an autosomal dominant disorder although, less

Table 14.1. Current diagnostic criteria for JMML.

Category 1 (All of the following)[a]	Category 2 (at least one of the following)[b]	Category 3 (two of the following if no category 2 criteria are met)[a]
Absence of the *BCR/ABL* fusion gene	Somatic mutation in RAS or PTPN11	White blood cell count > 10,000 (10×10^9/uL)
> 1000 (1×10^9/uL) circulating monocytes	Clinical diagnosis of NF1 or NF1 gene mutation	Circulating myeloid precursors
< 20% blasts in the bone marrow	Monosomy 7	Increased hemoglobin F for age
Splenomegaly[b]		Clonal cytogenetic abnormality excluding monosomy 7[b]
		GM-CSF hypersensitivity

[a]Current World Health Organization (WHO) criteria.

[b]Proposed additions to the WHO criteria that were discussed by participants attending the JMML Symposium in Atlanta, GA, 2008.[49] Note that *CBL* mutations have since been discovered and should be screened for in the workup of a patient with suspected JMML. Patients who are found to have a category 2 lesion need to meet criteria in category 1 but do not need to meet category 3 criteria. Patients who are not found to have a category 2 lesion must meet the category 1 and 3 criteria. Only 7% of patients with JMML will not present with splenomegaly but virtually all patients develop this within several weeks to months of initial presentation (Niemeyer, personal communication).

Table 14.2. Spectrum of genetic alterations in *de novo* JMML.

Gene	Location and type of mutation	Associated germline syndrome	Abnormality seen in malignant cells on SNP array	Percentage
NF1	Varied for the inherited allele (can be missense, nonsense, or frameshift), and always LOH for the contralateral wildtype allele in the JMML cells of affected NF1 children	Neurofibromatosis type I[a]	Copy-neutral LOH of chromosome 17q (with associated clinical NF1)	10–15%
NRAS *KRAS*	Exon 1 and 2, in codons 12, 13, or 61	No	None	25%
PTPN11	Exon 3, 4 (rarely) or 13	Possibly[b]	None	35%
CBL	Intron 7 or 8 splice sites Exon 8 or 9	Yes[c]	Copy-neutral LOH of chromosome 11q	10%

[a]In general, the NF1 lesions are seen in patients with NF1; however a small number of patients may harbor heterozygous lesions in NF1 with associated other lesions in the Ras pathway.

[b]Note that germline mutations in *PTPN11* occur in patients with Noonan syndrome and that some of these mutations are associated with transient myeloproliferation in infancy and patients with this syndrome are generally not considered to have *de novo* JMML, though some may require low-dose chemotherapy similar to Down syndrome patients with TMD. However, there are two mutations detected in patients with NS that have been reported to occur in aggressive JMML: D61G and E139D.

[c]Most, but not all, reported cases of JMML with *CBL* mutations first occur as germline events; however a small number may be somatically acquired with duplication of the mutant allele. The presence of copy-neutral LOH of chromosome 11 does not automatically define a patient to have a germline mutation as this event can also occur in cancer via somatic acquisition.

LOH: loss of heterozygosity; NF: neurofibromatosis.

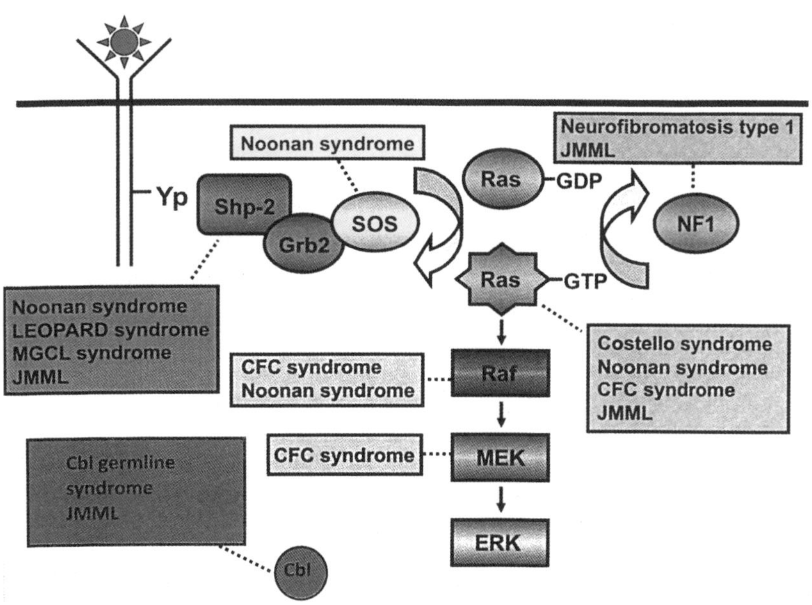

Fig. 14.1. Schematic diagram showing ligand-stimulated Ras activation, the Ras-MAPK pathway, and the gene mutations reported to date contributing to the neuro-cardio-facio-cutaneous congenital disorders, a newly defined CBL germline syndrome, and *de novo* JMML.

CFC: cardia-facio-cutaneous; JMML: juvenile myelomonocytic leukemia; NL/MGCL: Noonan-like/multiplegiant cell lesion.

Modified from Chan RJ, Cooper T, Kratz CP, Weiss B, Loh ML. (2009) Juvenile myelomonocytic leukemia: A report from the 2nd International JMML Symposium. *Leuk Res* **33**: 355–362 and used with permission from Elsevier.

frequently, it can arise spontaneously in the germline. World Health Organization criteria for NF1 include ≥ 6 *café au lait* macules, ≥ 2 neurofibromas or 1 plexiform neurofibroma, Lisch nodules, axillary or inguinal freckling, and/or optic gliomas.

In 1990, the *NF1* gene was cloned and the encoded neurofibromin protein was identified to function as a GTPase-activating protein (GAP) for Ras, which greatly enhances the hydrolysis of the active, GTP-bound conformation of Ras to the inactive, GDP-bound conformation.[13] In 1994, Shannon *et al.* demonstrated the loss of the wild type allele in bone marrow cells of children with JMML affected by NF1, thus establishing *NF1* as a classic tumor suppressor gene.[14] In subsequent mouse models engineered to conditionally delete the Nf1 allele, MPN develops and elevated levels of Ras-GTP occur, thus validating the hypothesis that the absence of normal neurofibromin, then, would result in a relative increase in Ras-GTP.[15,16] In additional reports in 1994, Kalra and Miyauchi separately identified somatic, oncogenic mutations in *NRAS* or *KRAS2* (*RAS*) occurring in a second, independent cohort of patients with JMML, thus providing additional genetic evidence to support that hyperactivation of the Ras/MAPK pathway was essential for the pathogenesis of this disease.[17,18] Animal models have been developed and reveal that Kras mutant mice also develop fatal myeloid disorders that resemble JMML *in vivo* and *in vitro*.[19,20] This observation strongly supports a role for hyperactivation of the Ras/MAPK pathway-initiating JMML in contrast to most subtypes of AML, where it may be a cooperating event.[21]

Noonan syndrome (NS) is another congenital disorder that can either be inherited in an autosomal dominant fashion or arise spontaneously.[22] NS is characterized by facial dysmorphism, short stature, webbed neck, and cardiac anomalies (typical the stenosis of pulmonary artery), as well as varying levels of impaired cognition. Interestingly, some children with NS also display hematological anomalies, including a self-resolving myeloproliferative disorder in early infancy that resembles JMML, as well as bleeding diatheses. In 2001, Tartaglia and Gelb identified germline mutations in *PTPN11*, a gene encoding the non-receptor tyrosine phosphatase protein SHP-2, as causative in approximately 50% of children with NS.[23] Based on the observation that children with NS can display myeloproliferative features, mutations in *PTPN11* were subsequently found to occur as somatic lesions in *de novo*, non-syndromic JMML in as many as 35% of patients in some series.[24,25]

SHP2 phosphatase includes two Src homology 2 (SH2) domains (termed N-SH2 and C-SH2) and a catalytic protein tyrosine phosphatase (PTP) domain.[26] Analysis of the crystal structure of SHP-2 revealed that the N-SH2 domain functions to directly block the active site of the PTP domain, thereby resulting in a catalytically inactive SHP-2 protein. The SHP-2 PTPase is activated when the SH-2 domains bind to an appropriately tyrosine phosphorylated ligand; this results in a conformational shift that allows the active site to interact with target molecules. SHP-2 participates in signal transduction downstream of growth factor receptors to regulate multiple cellular responses including proliferation, differentiation, and migration.

A comparison of the *PTPN11* mutations in *de novo* vs. syndromic JMML (namely that occurring in NS patients) reveals that many, but not all, of the same codons in exon 3, 4, and 13 are affected.[27] However, the codon substitutions are largely different in NS-MPN than in JMML, leading investigators to hypothesize that the transforming ability of mutations in NS are "weaker" and, thus, may be tolerated as germline events. Indeed, the most common *PTPN11* mutation in *de novo* JMML is 226G > A, resulting in E76K, an alteration that has never been documented as a germline lesion in NS. Studies of the E76K protein reveal that it displays the highest phosphatase activity, induces profound hypersensitivity to GM-CSF in fetal liver cells, and transforms transduced BaF3 cell lines to cytokine independence.[25,28,29] The D61G mutation is the only one reported to occur in both NS and *de novo* JMML. Transgenic mouse models with this lesion develop a mild MPN with a latency of 5 months in contrast to the D61Y, which is a lesion only occurring in JMML and in which transplanted mice develop a fatal JMML-like aggressive disease by 6–7 months.[30,31] By developing these *in vivo* models, researchers continue to study disordered hematopoiesis associated with these lesions and can also test novel molecules for improved therapeutic targets in JMML.

Recently, high-density single nucleotide polymorphism (SNP) arrays have revolutionized the ability to identify regions of copy number gain and loss in a variety of human cancers. Comparison of tumor with germline tissues also allows detection of copy neutral loss of heterozygosity, otherwise known as acquired uniparental isodisomy (aUPD). In cancer, this arises as a duplication of a region containing a mutation that frequently, but not always, behaves as a tumor suppressor gene, as has recently been shown to occur in cases of NF1-associated JMML.[32,33]

To determine if additional regions of aUPD existed in JMML, an Affymetrix SNP 6.0 array analysis was performed on samples from 27 JMML patients with and without known *PTPN11*, *RAS*, or *NF1* abnormalities.[11] Through this approach, it was possible to identify a region of 11q UPD in five of these cases. Importantly, recent reports uncovered similar lesions in adults with atypical chronic myelogenous leukemia (CML), CMML, and MDS, and, in these contexts, subsequent molecular analysis identified homozygous *c-CBL* (*CBL*) mutations.[34–36] All five of the JMML patients also displayed homozygous *CBL* lesions. In collaboration with investigators from the European Working Group on Childhood Myelodysplastic Syndromes (EWOG-MDS), a total of 27 *CBL* mutations in a group of 68 JMML patients with no other known lesions were subsequently detected. The most common mutation is the c.1111T > C transversion, resulting in a substitution of a histidine for a key tyrosine residue at codon 371 in the alpha linker region of the protein. Other investigators have subsequently confirmed these findings.[37,38]

Cbl is an E3 ubiquitin ligase that is known to mark activated receptor tyrosine kinases and other proteins for degradation by ubiquitination, but also retains important adaptor functions.[39] Most of the mutant Cbl proteins reported to occur thus far in myeloid malignancies result from missense mutations or splice site variants in which the majority have been shown to result in an encoded protein. It has been shown that defective E3 ligase activity results from specific substitutions at this region (Y371H, Y371S) only in the absence of the wild type protein.[36,40] Initial review of the medical records of 21 children with JMML harboring these homozygous mutations revealed that a number of them also shared other phenotypic features, suggesting that these lesions might first occur as germline events. Indeed, further investigation of the germline tissues from 17 of these patients revealed heterozygous lesions, and additional studies of parental DNA, when available, indicate that these mutations are autosomally inherited in a dominant fashion approximately 50% of the time, while they arise spontaneously in the other cases.[41,42]

Other mutations recently reported to occur rarely in JMML, include AXSL1.[43] In contrast to other MPNs of adulthood, *JAK2* mutations do not occur in JMML. A single case report of a *FLT3* mutation has been reported to date.[44] Taken together, these data would suggest that the current spectrum of commonly occurring mutations in *NF1*, *RAS*, *PTPN11*, and *CBL* converge on the Ras/MAPK pathway in a highly specific way that remains to be fully elucidated.

Chromosomal abnormalities

JMML lacks the Philadelphia chromosome and the *BCR-ABL* fusion gene. Chromosomal studies of leukemic cells show monosomy 7 in about 25% of patients, other abnormalities in 10%, and a normal karyotype in 65%.[4,45] When monosomy 7 is present, it is generally the sole karyotypic abnormality. Clinical characteristics of patients with monosomy 7 usually do not differ from those of patients with a normal karyotype. However, patients with monosomy 7 display some characteristic hematologic features. They present with a lower median WBC, but similar absolute monocyte count, explained by a higher percentage of monocytes on the differential count. Red blood cells are often macrocytic, and erythropoiesis is more pronounced than in cases with a normal karyotype. In addition, patients with monosomy 7 present with a normal or only moderately elevated HbF, which is often elevated in patients with normal karyotype. Among the chromosomal abnormalities other than monosomy 7, loss of material on the long arm of chromosome 7 is frequent. Interestingly, patients with *CBL* mutations have not been reported to harbor monosomy 7, in contrast to all of the other Ras pathway lesions, which have been reported to occur in conjunction with monosomy 7.

Prognostic factors in JMML

While the current standard of care for JMML is allogeneic HSCT, continued controversy exists about identifying those patients who need to be moved quickly to HSCT vs. those rare patients who might be observed. Certainly, now it is possible to anticipate that most patients with NS who present with a JMML-like MPN in the neonatal period will spontaneously resolve over the first year of life, somewhat akin to the transient myeloproliferative syndrome (TMD) of patients with Down syndrome (DS) (though NS-MPN is slower to resolve than DS-TMD). Rare NS patients may require some low or intermediate dose chemotherapy to improve splenomegaly and control uncomfortably high white blood cell counts, but there is no longer the expectation that these children will require HSCT if they show clinical improvement in the first year of life. In addition, unlike patients with DS, individuals with

NS who suffer from transient MPN of infancy do not appear to be at an increased risk of myeloid malignancies later in childhood.

For patients without NS, there have been multiple case reports in the literature describing a phenomenon of "self-resolving" JMML. Matsuda *et al.* observed that three children with JMML bearing *N-* or *KRAS*^{G12S} demonstrated a milder clinical course with spontaneous clinical improvement.[10] Flotho *et al.* were unable to confirm in the EWOG-MDS database the observation that patients harboring *RAS*^{G12S} benefited from long-term survival in the absence of HSCT.[9] However, it was noted that among 12 patients observed without HSCT for more than 3 years from diagnosis, there were five patients experiencing long-term survival who harbored various *RAS* mutations. Of great interest in both series is the observation that spontaneously resolving patients all presented with the well-known favorable prognostic factors: young age at diagnosis, platelet counts >33,000/uL and relatively low age-adjusted hemoglobin F levels.[2,45]

We now know that patients with homozygous *CBL* mutations have a high rate of spontaneous resolution, though this is not a uniform occurrence, as some children with *CBL* lesions have progressed and relapsed after HSCT. In addition, of the five patients reported with spontaneously resolving JMML and the germline Cbl syndrome, four developed signs consistent with serious vasculitis by the end of their second decade of life, as evidenced by optic atrophy, hypertension, cardiomyopathy, or arteritis.[40]

As stated above, certain clinical factors have been associated with a poorer prognosis, and, thus, should sway investigators towards earlier HSCT. Such factors include older age at diagnosis (>2 years), increased fetal hemoglobin for age (Hgb F), and/or a platelet count < 33,000/uL at presentation, as well as female sex in some series.[2,45] These factors consistently correlate with a poor outcome (reduced event-free and overall survival [EFS, OS]) following allogeneic HSCT.[7]

Several published series have also examined the hypothesis that mutational status may correlate with JMML clinical features and prognosis, however this remains controversial, as well. Yoshida and colleagues evaluated the clinical course and laboratory findings of 49 JMML patients, 32 of whom harbored mutations in *NF1*, *KRAS*, *NRAS*, or *PTPN11*.[46] In their series, the mutation of *PTPN11* was associated with older age at diagnosis (>24 months), increased Hgb F (>10%), reduced overall survival, and, importantly, appeared to be an unfavorable prognostic factor predicting relapse following transplantation.

Recently, Bresolin *et al.*, reported that gene expression signatures could segregate JMML patients into those who displayed an AML-type signature vs. those who did not.[47] These signatures were significantly associated with outcome, as children who displayed an AML-type signature experienced a 10-year EFS of only 6% in contrast to 63% of those without the AML-type signature. Of interest was the statistically significant correlation between an AML-type signature and known prognostic variables at diagnosis predicting a dismal outcome, including older age, lower platelet count, and higher Hgb F levels. However, in the multivariate analysis, only the AML-type gene expression signature retained significance, though the levels of Hgb F and platelet count in this model were not defined at the same levels as previously determined to carry prognostic significance.

Taken together, the lack of prognostic significance of specific genetic mutations, as well as the lack of correlation between the AML-type signature and genetic lesions suggests that additional, as yet unidentified factors are responsible for disease modulation and subsequent progression. Additional work to identify these events are ongoing. In this regard, high methylation of CpG islands in some genes in JMML seem to predict a particularly dismal outcome (unpublished results).

Approaches to therapy prior to HSCT

Another area of controversy surrounding the care of JMML patients is the type of therapy to be delivered prior to HSCT. To date, no standard chemotherapy regimens used prior to transplantation has been shown to impact on the incidence of relapse post-HSCT.[4] A wide variety of approaches have been used, from watchful waiting to high dose AML-type chemotherapy. The Children's Oncology Group (COG) sponsored a phase II trial, AAML0122 that incorporated a window phase of a farnesyl-transferase inhibitor (FTI) followed by cis-retinoic acid (cis-RA) and cytatarabine/fludarabine prior to HSCT. The majority of JMML patients treated had partial clinical responses defined by decreased white blood count and organomegaly prior to transplantation; however, EFS was not impacted by FTI treatment[48] (unpublished data). Indeed, the promise of FTI therapy as "Ras" inhibitors is misleading, as alternative geranylation can substitute for prenylation, a critical step in the activation of Ras at the cell membrane. With a median follow up of 4 years, the

EFS of patients enrolled in the AAML0122 trial was 40%, while overall survival was 55% (Cooper, personal communication).

Similarly, the EWOG-MDS/EBMT JMML trial showed that patients who received either no pre-HSCT therapy or low-dose chemotherapy pre-HSCT in comparison to high-dose AML-like chemotherapy had identical EFS (52% vs. 50%), relapse incidence (RI, 35% vs. 38%), and transplantation-related mortality (TRM, 13% vs. 13%).[7] Given the heterogeneity of disease burden at presentation in children with JMML, it is not possible to draw definitive conclusions about the patients who were given various pretreatment therapies and the impact of these treatments on ultimate outcome.

Finally, pre-transplant splenectomy is also controversial. The previous COG trial for JMML mandated splenectomy for all children prior to HSCT. However, the EWOG-MDS/EBMT JMML trial demonstrated that, when comparing children with a spleen size < 5 cm or > 5 cm, children undergoing splenectomy had no statistical benefit in EFS (61% vs. 44% vs. 48%, respectively), RI (24% vs. 45% vs. 39%, respectively), or TRM (15% vs. 11% vs. 13%, respectively).[7] Therefore, neither splenectomy nor high-dose chemotherapy can be routinely recommended prior to a patient receiving conditioning for an allogeneic HSCT unless clinically indicated for symptomatic relief. In particular, the indication to perform splenectomy has to be evaluated for each single patient, the presence of massive splenomegaly with evidence of hypersplenism and/or refractoriness to platelet transfusions being an argument for considering this procedure in order to promote engraftment, to hasten neutrophil and platelet recovery and to lower the risk of hemorrhagic complications after HSCT.

There is growing consensus for watchful waiting for those patients who are asymptomatic while identifying an appropriate donor. For patients with very high WBC counts, pulmonary problems (dry cough, tachypnea and interstitial infiltrates on chest X-rays are signs of peribronchial and interstitial pulmonary infiltrates), and/or prominent organomegaly, one can consider oral 6-mercaptopurine (50 mg/m^2/day) +/− cis-RA (100 mg/m^2/day), a differentiating agent potentially able to control expansion of clonal CFU-GM which proved to be effective in some patients with JMML (in particular in children below the age of 12 months who, nevertheless, are known to have a less aggressive disease course). For severely ill children, or those children who progress on less intensive therapies, low-dose intravenous cytarabine (40 mg/m^2/day × 5 days) can be administered. If this fails, the combination of high-dose cytarabine (2 g/m^2/day × 5 days) plus fludarabine (30 mg/m^2/day × 5 days) (both agents were dose adjusted for patients < 12 kg) can also be utilized and is generally well tolerated. To assess the efficacy of such therapies, clinical response criteria have been further defined.[49] In addition to such criteria, allele-specific PCR-based strategies have been developed to track specific mutations in patients on therapy and to monitor minimal residual disease; their role will be tested prospectively in future clinical trials.[50]

Targeted therapies in JMML

Future targeted therapies are being intensely investigated in a variety of laboratories worldwide. Inhibition of activated Ras would appear to be a logical therapeutic strategy in JMML, however, there are several caveats to this approach.[51,52] The importance of Ras signaling in diverse physiologic processes in normal cells raises the concern of nonspecific systemic toxicities with any therapies in which normal Ras proteins or their effectors are inhibited. However, active investigation is ongoing in this area and extend not only to effectors of the Ras pathway but additional pathways, including PI3K and the JAK/STAT signaling cascade (see Chapter 22).

Approaches to HSCT

As mentioned above, allogeneic HSCT is the only curative approach for children with JMML, resulting in long-term survival in a significant proportion of patients given the allograft. In the most recent study, which included the largest number of patients with JMML given allogeneic HSCT from either a histocompatible relative or from an HLA-matched/1-antigen disparate donor, the probability of EFS was above 50%.[7] In multivariate analysis, age greater than 4 years and female sex predicted poorer outcome. An update of this study substantially confirmed those results (see also Fig. 14.2 for further details). The outcome of children with JMML given allogeneic HSCT reported in studies published the last decade is shown in Table 14.3. Available incidence[7,53–55] indicate that, in the more recent years, the use of an unrelated volunteer as donor offers minimal or possibly no significant disadvantage as compared to employing an HLA-identical sibling. Umbilical cord blood transplantation is a suitable option for children with JMML lacking an HLA-compatible relative; the search for an unrelated cord blood unit should be initiated at

Table 14.3. Studies analyzing outcome of children with JMML given allogenic HSCT in the last 10 years.

Study	No of patients analyzed (M/F)	Type of donor	Stem cell source	LFS	TRM	OS	Relapse	Factors influencing outcome
Manabe *et al.* (2002)[54]	27 (20/7)	MRD(12) MMRD (4) MUD (10) MMUD (1)	BM (23) PB (3) CB (1)	54.2 ± 11.2% (4 years)	3/27 (11%)	57.9 ± 11% (4 years)	7/24	Abnormal karyotype Age > 1 year at diagnosis Absence of grade 0–1 acute GvHD or absence of chronic GvHD (In multivariate analysis, karyotype remained the only significant risk factor)
Smith *et al.* (2002)[55]	46	MUD (29) MMUD (17)	TCD BM (15) No TCD BM (31)	24% (2 years)	18% (2 years)	42% (2 years)	58% (2 years)	Absence of chronic GvHD
Locatelli *et al.* (2005)[7]	100 (67/33)	MRD (48) MUD (52)	BM (79) PB (14) CB (7)	52% (5 years): MRD 55% MUD 49%	13% (5 years): MRD 10%, MUD: 16%	64% (5 years)	35% (5 years)	Age > 4 years both at diagnosis and at HSCT, femal sex
Korthof *et al.* (2005)[53]	23 (15/8)	MRD (11) MMRD (3) MUD (4) MMUD (5)	TCD BM (5) no TCD BM (18)	Not described (9/23 pts are alive after 1 or 2 HSCT)	4/23	43.5 ± 10% at 5 and 10 years	8/23 + 2/23 with persistent disease	TCD Intensive chemotherapy before HSCT TBI-containing regimen

BM: bone marrow; CB: cord blood; LFS: leukemia-free survival; MRD: matched related donor; MMRD: mismatched related donor; MUD: matched unrelated donor; MMUD: mismatched unrelated donor; OS: overall survival; PB: peripheral blood; TCD BM: T-cell depleted bone marrow; TRM: transplant-related mortality.

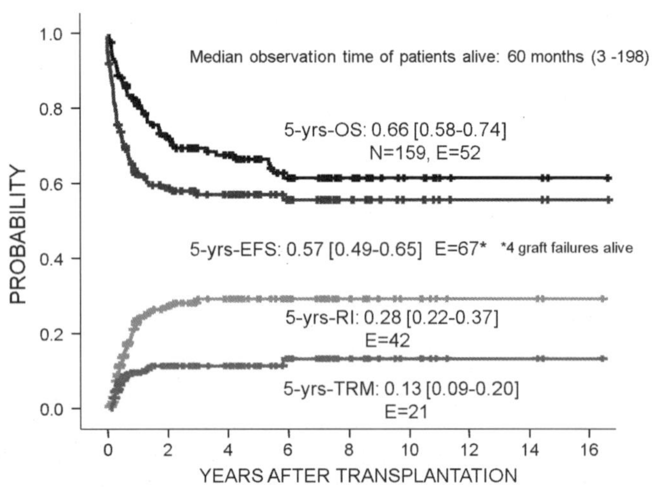

Fig. 14.2. Probability of overall and event-free survival, as well as cumulative incidence of relapse and transplant-related mortality in children with JMML after a conditioning regimen including busulfan, cyclophosphamide and melphalan enrolled in the EWOG-MDS study.

the same time as that for an unrelated BM donor. Cord blood offers the advantage of prompter availability of stem cells and allows to perform HSCT even in the presence of donor HLA disparities.

There is controversy over current conditioning regimens prior to HSCT for JMML. Preparative regimens without total body irradiation (TBI) are particularly attractive for children with JMML since radiation-induced late effects, such as severe growth retardation, cataracts, hypothyroidism and neuropsychologic sequels may be especially deleterious for very young children. Moreover, in a retrospective analysis of the EWOG-MDS, busulfan-based myeloablative therapy offered a greater anti-leukemic efficacy than TBI.[56] Chemotherapy-based conditioning regimens, such as the one published by the EWOG-MDS utilize busulfan, cytoxan, and melphalan with reasonable transplantation-related mortality and morbidity.[7,57] The use of TBI is now generally reserved for second transplants and should be used cautiously in these young patients, who may experience substantial late effects from TBI. In order to reduce the risk of disease recurrence, rapid taper of immunosuppression after HSCT should be initiated as quickly as possible, as a graft-vs.-leukemia effect in JMML has been documented. In addition, novel methods of detecting relapse early post-transplantation beyond traditional donor chimerism include sorted cell donor chimerism, quantitative PCR to assess chimerism, as well as allele-specific PCR strategies to detect mutation specific clones.[50,58] Such sensitive measurements may facilitate earlier and more rapid withdrawal of immunosuppression or the initiation of novel targeted therapies. There is minimal data on the utility of donor lymphocyte infusions for prevention of disease recurrence.[58,59]

Finally, for children with JMML experiencing leukemia relapse after allogeneic HSCT, donor lymphocyte infusions was proved to be largely ineffective,[58] whereas a second allograft, from either the same or a different donor, together with reduction of the intensity of GVHD prophylaxis aimed at optimizing the GVL effect, is able to render about one third of the patients cured of their original disease.[60]

Summary and Directions for Future Work

In summary, JMML is a rare MPN of childhood in which a firm molecular diagnosis can now be made in approximately 90% of patients. The majority of JMML patients require to be treated with HSCT for having the chance to be cured by this life-threatening aggressive neoplasm; controversy continues to exist over the identification of rare patients who may be observed. Certain clinical factors may aid in that decision, such as older age, lower platelet count, and higher Hgb F levels at diagnosis. In addition, some patients with *RAS* or *CBL* mutations may experience spontaneous resolution but it remains challenging to identify exactly who will do well without HSCT. Indeed, patients with *CBL* mutations who resolve spontaneously may develop serious complications later in life related to vasculitis, though further studies are needed in larger cohorts of patients to validate these early findings, as well as to determine if patients with *CBL* mutations who have undergone HSCT are spared from developing this late complication. Finally, a stepwise approach to treating patients with JMML with chemotherapy prior to definitive HSCT can now be considered, as data remain elusive about the benefits of such chemotherapy prior to transplant.

Future studies will focus on refining prognostic risk factors and optimizing therapy for these patients. Ongoing investigations of targeted therapies centering on the biochemical consequences of the genetic lesions occurring in JMML will mandate fruitful collaborations between basic, translational, and clinical scientists.

References

2. Passmore SJ, Chessells JM, Kempski H, Hann IM, Brownbill PA, Stiller CA. (2003) Paediatric myelodysplastic syndromes and juvenile myelomonocytic leukaemia in the UK: A population-based study of incidence and survival. *Br J Haematol* **121**: 758–767.
3. Niemeyer CM, Kratz CP. (2008) Paediatric myelodysplastic syndromes and juvenile myelomonocytic leukaemia: Molecular classification and treatment options. *Br J Haematol* **140**: 610–624.
4. Bergstraesser E, Hasle H, Rogge T, Fischer A, Zimmermann M, Noellke P, Niemeyer CM. (2007) Non-hematopoietic stem cell transplantation treatment of juvenile myelomonocytic leukemia: A retrospective analysis and definition of response criteria. *Pediatr Blood Cancer* **49**: 629–633.
5. Emanuel PD, Bates LJ, Castleberry RP, Gualtieri RJ, Zuckerman KS. (1991) Selective hypersensitivity to granulocyte-macrophage colony stimulating factor by juvenile chronic myeloid leukemia hematopoietic progenitors. *Blood* **77**: 925–929.
7. Locatelli F, Nollke P, Zecca M, Korthof E, Lanino E, Peters C, Pession A, Kabisch H, Uderzo C, Bonfim CS, Bader P, Dilloo D, Stary J, Fischer A, Revesz T, Fuhrer M, Hasle H, Trebo M, van den Heuvel-Eibrink MM, Fenu S, Strahm B, Giorgiani G, Bonora MR, Duffner U, Niemeyer CM. (2005) Hematopoietic Stem Cell Transplantation (HSCT) in children with Juvenile Myelomonocytic Leukemia (JMML): Results of the EWOG-MDS/EBMT trial. *Blood* **105**: 410–419.
9. Flotho C, Kratz CP, Bergstrasser E, Hasle H, Stary J, Trebo M, van den Heuvel-Eibrink MM, Wojcik D, Zecca M, Locatelli F, Niemeyer CM. (2008) Genotype-phenotype correlation in cases of juvenile myelomonocytic leukemia with clonal RAS mutations. *Blood* **111**: 966–967; author reply 967–968.
10. Matsuda K, Shimada A, Yoshida N, Ogawa A, Watanabe A, Yajima S, Iizuka S, Koike K, Yanai F, Kawasaki K, Yanagimachi M, Kikuchi A, Ohtsuka Y, Hidaka E, Yamauchi K, Tanaka M, Yanagisawa R, Nakazawa Y, Shiohara M, Manabe A, Kojima S. (2007) Spontaneous improvement of hematologic abnormalities in patients having juvenile myelomonocytic leukemia with specific RAS mutations. *Blood* **109**: 5477–5480.
11. Loh ML, Sakai DS, Flotho C, Kang M, Fliegauf M, Archambeault S, Mullighan CG, Chen L, Bergstraesser E, Bueso-Ramos CE, Emanuel PD, Hasle H, Issa JP, van den Heuvel-Eibrink MM, Locatelli F, Stary J, Trebo M, Wlodarski M, Zecca M, Shannon KM, Niemeyer CM.

(2009) Mutations in CBL occur frequently in juvenile myelomonocytic leukemia. *Blood* **114**: 1859–1863.

12. Bader JL, Miller RW. (1978) Neurofibromatosis and childhood leukemia. *J Pediatr* **92**: 925–929.
13. Xu GF, Lin B, Tanaka K, Dunn D, Wood D, Gesteland R, White R, Weiss R, Tamanoi F. (1990) The catalytic domain of the neurofibromatosis type 1 gene product stimulates ras GTPase and complements ira mutants of S. cerevisiae. *Cell* **63**: 835–841.
14. Shannon KM, O'Connell P, Martin GA, Paderanga D, Olson K, Dinndorf P, McCormick F. (1994) Loss of the normal NF1 allele from the bone marrow of children with type 1 neurofibromatosis and malignant myeloid disorders. *N Engl J Med* **330**: 597–601.
15. Largaespada DA, Brannan CI, Jenkins NA, Copeland NG. (1996) *Nf1* deficiency causes Ras-mediated granulocyte-macrophage colony stimulating factor hypersensitivity and chronic myeloid leukemia. *Nat Genet* **12**: 137–143.
16. Bollag G, Clapp DW, Shih S, Adler F, Zhang Y, Thompson P, Lange BJ, Freedman MH, McCormick F, Jacks T, Shannon K. (1996) Loss of *NF1* results in activation of the Ras signaling pathway and leads to aberrant growth in murine and human hematopoietic cells. *Nat Genet* **12**: 144–148.
17. Kalra R, Paderanga D, Olson K, Shannon KM. (1994) Genetic analysis is consistent with the hypothesis that *NF1* limits myeloid cell growth through $p21^{ras}$. *Blood* **84**: 3435–3439.
18. Miyauchi J, Asada M, Sasaki M, Tsunematsu Y, Kojima S, Mizutani S. (1994) Mutations of the N-*ras* gene in juvenile chronic myelogenous leukemia. *Blood* **83**: 2248–2254.
19. Braun BS, Tuveson DA, Kong N, Le DT, Kogan SC, Rozmus J, le Beau MM, Jacks TE, Shannon KM. (2004) Somatic activation of oncogenic Kras in hematopoietic cells initiates a rapidly fatal myeloproliferative disorder. *Proc Natl Acad Sci U S A* **101**: 597–602.
20. Chan IT, Kutok JL, Williams IR, Cohen S, Kelly L, Shigematsu H, Johnson L, Akashi K, Tuveson DA, Jacks T, Gilliland DG. (2004) Conditional expression of oncogenic K-ras from its endogenous promoter induces a myeloproliferative disease. *J Clin Invest* **113**: 528–538.
22. Rauen KA, Schoyer L, McCormick F, Lin AE, Allanson JE, Stevenson DA, Gripp KW, Neri G, Carey JC, Legius E, Tartaglia M, Schubbert S, Roberts AE, Gelb BD, Shannon K, Gutmann DH, McMahon M, Guerra C, Fagin JA, Yu B, Aoki Y, Neel BG, Balmain A, Drake RR, Nolan GP, Zenker M, Bollag G, Sebolt-Leopold J, Gibbs JB, Silva AJ, Patton EE, Viskochil DH, Kieran MW, Korf BR, Hagerman RJ, Packer RJ, Melese T. (2010) Proceedings from the 2009 genetic syndromes of the Ras/MAPK pathway: From bedside to bench and back. *Am J Med Genet A* **152A**: 4–24.
23. Tartaglia M, Mehler EL, Goldberg R, Zampino G, Brunner HG, Kremer H, van der Burgt I, Crosby AH, Ion A, Jeffery S, Kalidas K, Patton MA, Kucherlapati RS, Gelb BD. (2001) Mutations in PTPN11, encoding the protein tyrosine phosphatase SHP-2, cause Noonan syndrome. *Nat Genet* **29**: 465–468.
24. Loh ML, Vattikuti S, Schubbert S, Reynolds MG, Carlson E, Lieuw KH, Cheng JW, Lee CM, Stokoe D, Bonifas JM, Curtiss NP, Gotlib J, Meshinchi S, le Beau MM, Emanuel PD, Shannon KM. (2003) Somatic mutations in PTPN11 implicate the protein tyrosine phosphatase SHP-2 in leukemogenesis. *Blood.*
25. Tartaglia M, Niemeyer CM, Fragale A, Song X, Buechner J, Jung A, Hahlen K, Hasle H, Licht JD, Gelb BD. (2003) Somatic mutations in PTPN11 in juvenile myelomonocytic leukemia, myelodysplastic syndromes and acute myeloid leukemia. *Nat Genet* **34**: 148–150.
27. Kratz CP, Niemeyer CM, Castleberry RP, Cetin M, Bergstrasser E, Emanuel PD, Hasle H, Kardos G, Klein C, Kojima S, Stary J, Trebo M, Zecca M, Gelb BD, Tartaglia M, Loh ML. (2005) The mutational spectrum of PTPN11 in juvenile myelomonocytic leukemia and Noonan syndrome/myeloproliferative disease. *Blood* **106**: 2183–2185.
28. Schubbert S, Lieuw K, Rowe SL, Lee CM, Li X, Loh ML, Clapp DW, Shannon KM. (2005) Functional analysis of leukemia-associated PTPN11 mutations in primary hematopoietic cells. *Blood* **106**: 311–317.
30. Araki T, Mohi MG, Ismat FA, Bronson RT, Williams IR, Kutok JL, Yang W, Pao LI, Gilliland DG, Epstein JA, Neel BG. (2004) Mouse model of Noonan syndrome reveals cell type- and gene dosage-dependent effects of Ptpn11 mutation. *Nat Med* **10**: 849–857.
31. Mohi MG, Williams IR, Dearolf CR, Chan G, Kutok JL, Cohen S, Morgan K, Boulton C, Shigematsu H, Keilhack H, Akashi K, Gilliland DG, Neel BG. (2005) Prognostic, therapeutic, and mechanistic implications of a mouse model of leukemia evoked by Shp2 (PTPN11) mutations. *Cancer Cell* **7**: 179–191.
32. Flotho C, Steinemann D, Mullighan CG, Neale G, Mayer K, Kratz CP, Schlegelberger B, Downing JR, Niemeyer CM. (2007) Genome-wide single-nucleotide polymorphism analysis in juvenile myelomonocytic leukemia identifies uniparental disomy surrounding the NF1 locus in cases associated with neurofibromatosis but not in cases with mutant RAS or PTPN11. *Oncogene* **26**: 5816–5821.
33. Stephens K, Weaver M, Leppig KA, Maruyama K, Emanuel PD, le Beau MM, Shannon KM. (2006) Interstitial uniparental isodisomy at clustered breakpoint intervals is a

frequent mechanism of NF1 inactivation in myeloid malignancies. *Blood* **108**: 1684–1689.

34. Dunbar AJ, Gondek LP, O'Keefe CL, Makishima H, Rataul MS, Szpurka H, Sekeres MA, Wang XF, McDevitt MA, Maciejewski JP. (2008) 250K single nucleotide polymorphism array karyotyping identifies acquired uniparental disomy and homozygous mutations, including novel missense substitutions of c-Cbl, in myeloid malignancies. *Cancer Res* **68**: 10349–10357.
35. Grand FH, Hidalgo-Curtis CE, Ernst T, Zoi K, Zoi C, McGuire C, Kreil S, Jones A, Score J, Metzgeroth G, Oscier D, Hall A, Brandts C, Serve H, Reiter A, Chase AJ, Cross NC. (2009) Frequent CBL mutations associated with 11q acquired uniparental disomy in myeloproliferative neoplasms. *Blood* **113**: 6182–6192.
36. Sanada M, Suzuki T, Shih LY, Otsu M, Kato M, Yamazaki S, Tamura A, Honda H, Sakata-Yanagimoto M, Kumano K, Oda H, Yamagata T, Takita J, Gotoh N, Nakazaki K, Kawamata N, Onodera M, Nobuyoshi M, Hayashi Y, Harada H, Kurokawa M, Chiba S, Mori H, Ozawa K, Omine M, Hirai H, Nakauchi H, Koeffler HP, Ogawa S. (2009) Gain-of-function of mutated C-CBL tumour suppressor in myeloid neoplasms. *Nature* **460**: 904–908.
37. Muramatsu H, Makishima H, Jankowska AM, Cazzolli H, O'Keefe C, Yoshida N, Xu Y, Nishio N, Hama A, Yagasaki H, Takahashi Y, Kato K, Manabe A, Kojima S, Maciejewski JP. Mutations of an E3 ubiquitin ligase c-Cbl but not TET2 mutations are pathogenic in juvenile myelomonocytic leukemia. *Blood* **115**: 1969–1975.
38. Makishima H, Cazzolli H, Szpurka H, Dunbar A, Tiu R, Huh J, Muramatsu H, O'Keefe C, Hsi E, Paquette RL, Kojima S, List AF, Sekeres MA, McDevitt MA, Maciejewski JP. (2009) Mutations of e3 ubiquitin ligase cbl family members constitute a novel common pathogenic lesion in myeloid malignancies. *J Clin Oncol* **27**: 6109–6116.
39. Schmidt MH, Dikic I. (2005) The Cbl interactome and its functions. *Nat Rev Mol Cell Biol* **6**: 907–918.
41. Niemeyer CM, Kang MW, Shin DH, Furlan I, Erlacher M, Bunin NJ, Bunda S, Finklestein JZ, Sakamoto KM, Gorr TA, Mehta P, Schmid I, Kropshofer G, Corbacioglu S, Lang PJ, Klein C, Schlegel PG, Heinzmann A, Schneider M, Stary J, van den Heuvel-Eibrink MM, Hasle H, Locatelli F, Sakai D, Archambeault S, Chen L, Russell RC, Sybingco SS, Ohh M, Braun BS, Flotho C, Loh ML. (2010) Germline CBL mutations cause developmental abnormalities and predispose to juvenile myelomonocytic leukemia. *Nat Genet.*
42. Perez B, Mechinaud F, Galambrun C, Ben Romdhane N, Isidor B, Philip N, Derain-Court J, Cassinat B, Lachenaud J, Kaltenbach S, Salmon A, Desiree C, Pereira S, Menot ML, Royer N, Fenneteau O, Baruchel A, Chomienne C, Verloes A, Cave H. (2010) Germline mutations of the CBL gene define a new genetic syndrome with predisposition to juvenile myelomonocytic leukaemia. *J Med Genet.*
43. Sugimoto Y, Muramatsu H, Makishima H, Prince C, Jankowska AM, Yoshida N, Xu Y, Nishio N, Hama A, Yagasaki H, Takahashi Y, Kato K, Manabe A, Kojima S, Maciejewski JP. (2010) Spectrum of molecular defects in juvenile myelomonocytic leukaemia includes ASXL1 mutations. *Br J Haematol.*
45. Niemeyer CM, Arico M, Basso G, Biondi A, Cantu Rajnoldi A, Creutzig U, Haas O, Harbott J, Hasle H, Kerndrup G, Locatelli F, Mann G, Stollmann-Gibbels B, van't Veer-Korthof ET, van Wering E, Zimmermann M. (1997) Chronic myelomonocytic leukemia in childhood: A retrospective analysis of 110 cases. European Working Group on Myelodysplastic Syndromes in Childhood (EWOG-MDS). *Blood* **89**: 3534–3543.
46. Yoshida N, Yagasaki H, Xu Y, Matsuda K, Yoshimi A, Takahashi Y, Hama A, Nishio N, Muramatsu H, Watanabe N, Matsumoto K, Kato K, Ueyama J, Inada H, Goto H, Yabe M, Kudo K, Mimaya J, Kikuchi A, Manabe A, Koike K, Kojima S. (2009) Correlation of clinical features with the mutational status of GM-CSF signaling pathway-related genes in juvenile myelomonocytic leukemia. *Pediatr Res* **65**: 334–340.
47. Bresolin S, Zecca M, Flotho C, Trentin L, Zangrando A, Sainati L, Stary J, de Moerloose B, Hasle H, Niemeyer CM, Te Kronnie G, Locatelli F, Basso G. (2010) Gene expression-based classification as an independent predictor of clinical outcome in juvenile myelomonocytic leukemia. *J Clin Oncol* **28**: 1919–1927.
48. Castleberry RP, Loh ML, Jayaprakash N, Peterson A, Casey V, Chang M, Widemann B, Emanuel PD. (2005) Phase II Window Study of the Farnesyltransferase Inhibitor R115777 (Zarnestra(R)) in Untreated Juvenile Myelomonocytic Leukemia (JMML): A Children's Oncology Group Study. *Blood (ASH Annual Meeting Abstracts)* **106**: 2587.
49. Chan RJ, Cooper T, Kratz CP, Weiss B, Loh ML. (2009) Juvenile myelomonocytic leukemia: A report from the 2nd International JMML Symposium. *Leuk Res* **33**: 355–362.
50. Archambeault S, Flores NJ, Yoshimi A, Kratz CP, Reising M, Fischer A, Noellke P, Locatelli F, Sedlacek P, Flotho C, Zecca M, Emanuel PD, Castleberry RP, Niemeyer CM, Bader P, Loh ML. (2008) Development of an allele-specific minimal residual disease assay for patients with juvenile myelomonocytic leukemia. *Blood* **111**: 1124–1127.
51. Le DT, Shannon KM. (2002) Ras processing as a therapeutic target in hematologic malignancies. *Curr Opin Hematol* **9**: 308–315.

52. Flotho C, Kratz C, Niemeyer CM. (2007) Targeting RAS signaling pathways in juvenile myelomonocytic leukemia. *Curr Drug Targets* **8**: 715–725.
54. Manabe A, Okamura J, Yumura-Yagi K, Akiyama Y, Sako M, Uchiyama H, Kojima S, Koike K, Saito T, Nakahata T. (2002) Allogeneic hematopoietic stem cell transplantation for 27 children with juvenile myelomonocytic leukemia diagnosed based on the criteria of the International JMML Working Group. *Leukemia* **16**: 645–649.
55. Smith FO, King R, Nelson G, Wagner JE, Robertson KA, Sanders JE, Bunin N, Emaunel PD, Davies SM. (2002) Unrelated donor bone marrow transplantation for children with juvenile myelomonocytic leukaemia. *Br J Haematol* **116**: 716–724.
56. Locatelli F, Niemeyer C, Angelucci E, Bender-Gotze C, Burdach S, Ebell W, Friedrich W, Hasle H, Hermann J, Jacobsen N, Klingebiel T, Kremens B, Mann G, Pession A, Peters C, Schmid HJ, Stary J, Suttorp M, Uderzo C, van't Veer-Korthof ET, Vossen J, Zecca M, Zimmermann M. (1997) Allogeneic bone marrow transplantation for chronic myelomonocytic leukemia in childhood: A report from the European Working Group on Myelodysplastic Syndrome in Childhood. *J Clin Oncol* **15**: 566–573.
58. Yoshimi A, Niemeyer CM, Bohmer V, Duffner U, Strahm B, Kreyenberg H, Dilloo D, Zintl F, Claviez A, Wossmann W, Kremens B, Holter W, Niethammer D, Beck JF, Kontny U, Nollke P, Klingebiel T, Bader P. (2005) Chimaerism analyses and subsequent immunological intervention after stem cell transplantation in patients with juvenile myelomonocytic leukaemia. *Br J Haematol* **129**: 542–549.
59. Yoshimi A, Bader P, Matthes-Martin S, Stary J, Sedlacek P, Duffner U, Klingebiel T, Dilloo D, Holter W, Zintl F, Kremens B, Sykora KW, Urban C, Hasle H, Korthof E, Revesz T, Fischer A, Nollke P, Locatelli F, Niemeyer CM. (2005) Donor leukocyte infusion after hematopoietic stem cell transplantation in patients with juvenile myelomonocytic leukemia. *Leukemia* **19**: 971–977.
60. Yoshimi A, Mohamed M, Bierings M, Urban C, Korthof E, Zecca M, Sykora KW, Duffner U, Trebo M, Matthes-Martin S, Sedlacek P, Klingebiel T, Lang P, Fuhrer M, Claviez A, Wossmann W, Pession A, Arvidson J, O'Marcaigh AS, van den Heuvel-Eibrink MM, Stary J, Hasle H, Nollke P, Locatelli F, Niemeyer CM. (2007) Second allogeneic hematopoietic stem cell transplantation (HSCT) results in outcome similar to that of first HSCT for patients with juvenile myelomonocytic leukemia. *Leukemia* **21**: 556–560.

15

Myeloproliferative and Myelodysplastic Disorders in Children, Adolescents and Young Adults

Shalini Shenoy and Michael Deininger

Introduction

Myelodysplastic syndromes (MDS) and myeloproliferative neoplasms (MPN) are rare in children, adolescents and young adults (herein referred to as the CAYA population). While the biological mechanisms that drive these disorders are generally similar irrespective of age group, associations with genetic disorders are more common among the young. Clinical manifestations, approaches to management, supportive care, and therapy can vary considerably according to age. Small numbers of patients in the pediatric/young adult age groups preclude large trials, and treatment strategies adopted from trials in older patients largely drive the field. Consensus regarding the standard of care is lacking in many cases. This chapter will provide an overview of the biology as well as clinical management of MDS and MPN in children and young adults, with particular emphasis on the special features pertinent to this age group.

Myleoproliferative Neoplasms (MPN)

MPN are a heterogeneous group of hematopoietic disorders that encompass the "classical" entities of chronic myeloid leukemia (CML), essential thrombocythemia (ET), polycythemia vera (PV) and primary myelofibrosis (PMF) as well as "atypical" MPN such as chronic myelomonocytic leukemia (CMML), chronic neutrophilic leukemia and systemic mastocytosis (SM), amongst others (Table 15.1) (see Chapter 2).[1] Of these, CML, ET and PV are the most common disorders that afflict the CAYA population. MPN exclusive to the pediatric population include juvenile myelomonocytic leukemia (JMML), and disorders associated with Down syndrome, including transient myeloproliferative disorder (DS-TMD) and acute megakaryocytic leukemia (DS-AMKL). JMML and related diseases are discussed in Chapter 14.

MPN share several common features, including the expansion of one or more of the myeloid lineages, the capacity to proliferate at extramedullary sites (usually those of fetal hematopoiesis), and a biphasic clinical course that consists of an indolent chronic phase (CP) followed by progression to an aggressive acute phase. Although common to all MPN in principle, these disease features are extremely variable in their incidence and penetrance, depending on the specific disease entity.

Current thinking holds that at least two types of genetic events are required to induce acute leukemia.[2] Type I mutations activate signaling pathways that

Table 15.1. Diagnostic criteria for the classical MPN.

Disease	Diagnostic criteria
Chronic myeloid leukemia	Presence of BCR-ABL in the context of an MPN
Polycythemia vera	**Major criteria** 1. Hemoglobin > 18.5 g/dL in men, 16.5 g/dL in women or other evidence of increased red cell volume[a] 2. Presence of *JAK2* V617F or other functionally similar mutation such as *JAK2* exon 12 mutation **Minor criteria** 1. Bone marrow biopsy showing hypercellularity for age with trilineage growth (panmyelosis) with prominent erythroid, granulocytic and megakaryocytic proliferation 2. Serum erythropoietin level below the reference range for normal 3. Endogenous erythroid colony formation *in vitro* [a]Hemoglobin or hematocrit > 99th percentile of method-specific reference range for age, sex, altitude of residence or hemoglobin >17 g/dL in men, 15 g/dL in women if associated with a documented and sustained increase at least 2 g/dL from an individual's baseline value that cannot be attributed to correction of iron deficiency, or elevated red cell mass > 25% above mean normal predicted value.
Primary myelofibrosis	**Major criteria** 1. Presence of megakaryocyte proliferation and atypia,[a] usually accompanied by either reticulin and/or collagen fibrosis, or in the absence of significant reticulin fibrosis, the megakaryocyte changes must be accompanied by an increased bone marrow cellularity characterized by granulocytic proliferation and often decreased erythropoiesis (i.e. prefibrotic cellular-phase disease). 2. Not meeting WHO criteria for polycythemia vera,[b] *BCR-ABL1*+ chronic myelogenous leukemia,[c] myelodysplastic syndrome,[d] or other myeloid neoplasms 3. Demonstration of *JAK2* V617F or other clonal marker (e.g. *MPL* W515K/L), or in the absence of a clonal marker, no evidence that the bone marrow fibrosis or other changes are secondary to infection, autoimmune disorder or other chronic inflammatory condition, hairy cell leukemia or other lymphoid neoplasm, metastatic malignancy, or toxic (chronic) myelopathies[e] **Minor criteria** 1. Leukoerythroblastosis[f] 2. Increase in serum lactate dehydrogenase level[f] 3. Anemia[f] 4. Splenomegaly[f] [a]Small to large megakaryocytes with an aberrant nuclear/cytoplasmic ratio and hyperchromatic, bulbous, or irregularly folded nuclei and dense clustering. [b]Requires the failure of iron replacement therapy to increase hemoglobin level to the polycythemia vera range in the presence of decreased serum ferritin. Exclusion of polycythemia vera is based on hemoglobin and hematocrit levels, and red cell mass measurement is not required. [c]Requires the absence of *BCR-ABL1*. [d]Requires absence of dyserythropoiesis and dysgranulopoiesis. [e]Patients with conditions associated with reactive myelofibrosis are not immune to PMF, and the diagnosis should be considered in such cases if other criteria are met. [f]Degree of abnormality could be borderline or marked.

(*Continued*)

Table 15.1. (*Continued*)

Disease	Diagnostic criteria
Essential thrombocythemia	1. Sustained[a] platelet count $\geq 450 \times 10^9$/L 2. Bone marrow biopsy specimen showing proliferation mainly of the megakaryocytic lineage with increased numbers of enlarged, mature megakaryocytes. No significant increase or left-shift of neutrophil with granulopoiesis or erythropoiesis 3. Not meeting WHO criteria for polycytemia vera,[b] primary myelofibrosis,[c] *BCR-ABL1*+ chronic myelogenous leukemia[d] or myelodysplastic syndrome[e] or other myeloid neoplasm 4. Demonstration of *JAK2* V617F or other clonal marker, or in the absence of *JAK2* V617F, no evidence for reactive thrombocytosis[f] [a] Sustained during the work-up process. [b] Requires the failure of iron replacement therapy to increase hemoglobin level to the polycythemia vera range in the presence of decreased serum ferritin. Exclusion of polycythemia vera is based on hemoglobin and hematocrit levels and red cell mass measurement is not required. [c] Requires the absence of relevant reticulin fibrosis, collagen fibrosis, peripheral blood leukoerythroblastosis, or markedly hypercellular marrow accompanied by megakaryocyte morphology that is typical for primary myelofibrosis including small to large megakaryocytes with an aberrant nuclear/cytoplasmic ratio and hyperchromatic, bulbous or irregularly folded nuclei and dense clustering. [d] Requires the absence of *BCR-ABL1*. [e] Requires absence of dyserythropoiesis and dysgranulopoiesis. [f] Causes of reactive thrombocytosis include iron deficiency, splenectomy, surgery, infection, inflammation, connective tissue disease, metastic cancer, and lymphoproliferative disorders. However, the presence of a condition associated with reactive thrombocytosis may not exclude the possibility of ET if the first three criteria are met.

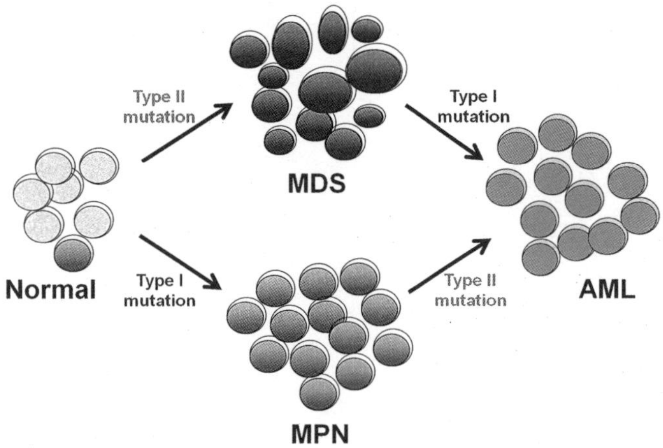

Fig. 15.1. Schematic showing the role of type I and type II mutations in leukemogenesis. Type I mutations primarily increase cell proliferation and reduce apoptosis, resulting in the accumulation of cells that retain differentiation, consistent with the clinical phenotype of a myeloproliferative neoplasm (MPN). Type II mutations primarily impair differentiation, and in isolation are thought to lead to myelodysplasia. The combination of a type I and a type II mutation produces the clinical phenotype of acute myeloid leukemia, either *de novo* or as blastic transformation of a pre-existing MPN.

primarily increase proliferation, frequently inducing a state of cytokine hypersensitivity, while type II mutations impair or abrogate coordinated cell differentiation and maturation (Fig. 15.1). It is believed that type I mutations are sufficient to induce the CP of MPN, while type II mutations cause progression to the acute phase. Thus, what are seemingly simultaneous events in acute leukemia are sequential events in MPN. Activated tyrosine kinase alleles such as BCR-ABL, $JAK2^{V617F}$ and gene fusions involving the platelet-derived growth factor receptors (PDGFRs) are by far the most common type I mutations in MPN, followed by mutations in K-RAS or N-RAS and mutations in growth factor receptors, such as the thrombopoietin (TPO) receptor MPL.[3–7] A well-documented consequence of type I mutations is genomic instability that promotes the acquisition of type II mutations, which in turn lead to transformation to the acute phase, a phenomenon studied extensively in CML.[8] MPNs exhibit a surprising range of phenotypic divergence or convergence, the etiology of which remains largely elusive. For example, the $JAK2^{V617F}$ allele occurs in almost all patients with PV and approximately 50% of patients with ET and PMF, but also in several of the atypical MPNs, including CMML.[4,9–11] On the other hand, there are no consistent clinical features that would distinguish $JAK2^{V617F}$-positive from $JAK2^{V617F}$-negative PMF, suggesting that as yet unknown mutations precisely phenocopy the $JAK2^{V617F}$ — positive disease. Another area of great interest is the contribution of heritable factors to MPN pathogenesis. While familial occurrence is very rare in CML, large epidemiologic studies have demonstrated a significantly increased risk for other classical MPN in first-degree relatives of affected individuals.[12,13] Consistent with this, there is a strong association between a certain JAK2 haplotype and the acquisition of the $JAK2^{V617F}$ mutation.[14–16]

Chronic myeloid leukemia

Epidemiology

CML, a disease of older individuals, accounts for only 2% of all pediatric leukemias and is exceptionally rare in infancy. The Germans reported a median age of 60.3 years at diagnosis. Less than 10% of cases occurred in children.[17,18] A Japanese study reported that CML accounts for 0.2% of leukemias in the 1–4-year group, 2.2% in the 5–9-year group, 3.7% in the 10–14-year group, and 8.3% in the 15–19-year group.[19] The US incidence rate reported from 11 SEER (Surveillance, Epidemiology and End Result Program of the National Cancer Institute) reporting areas is 0.1 per 100,000 in the 0–19-year age group irrespective of race, compared to an overall incidence of $1.8/10^5$ (see Chapter 1). There are no significant differences between ethnicities, and no hereditary predisposition, but there is a slight male preponderance.[20]

Pathogenesis

CML is caused by the BCR-ABL tyrosine kinase, the result of the t(9;22)(q34;q11) reciprocal translocation, cytogenetically visible as the Philadelphia chromosome (Ph).[21] Ph is demonstrable in approximately 95% of CML patients, while the remainder have cryptic translocations that are invisible by conventional chromosomal banding techniques, but detected by fluorescence *in situ* hybridization (FISH). Apart from CML, BCR-ABL is found in a subset of patients with B-cell acute lymphoblastic leukemia (B-ALL). In the context of a myeloproliferative neoplasm, the presence of BCR-ABL is sufficient to establish the diagnosis of CML.

1. Molecular anatomy of the BCR-ABL translocation

The breakpoints within the ABL gene occur upstream of exon 1b, downstream of the alternative exon 1a, or, more frequently, between the two (Fig. 15.2).[22] Regardless of the exact location of the breakpoint, splicing of the primary

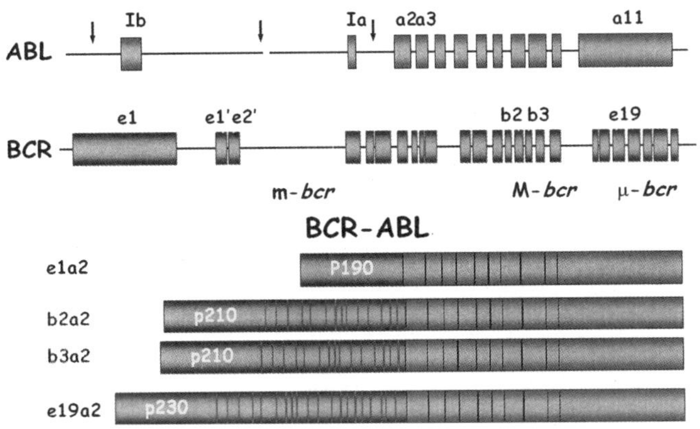

Fig. 15.2. Molecular anatomy of the BCR-ABL translocation. The two upper panels show the genomic organization of the BCR and ABL genes. Arrows denote breakpoints in ABL. The lower panel shows the structure of BCR-ABL variants generated as a result of the various breakpoints. Adapted from Deininger *et al.* (2000). The molecular biology of chronic myeloid leukemia. Blood 15;96(10):3343–3356.

hybrid transcript yields an mRNA molecule in which BCR sequences are fused upstream of the ABL exon a2. Breakpoints within BCR localize to one of three so-called breakpoint cluster regions (*bcr*). More than 90% of CML patients and one-third of Ph+ B-cell ALL (B-ALL) patients express the 210-kDa isoform of BCR-ABL. In the case of this isoform, the break within BCR occurs within the major breakpoint cluster region (M-*bcr*), a 5.8-kilobase (kb) area spanning exons e12–e16 (formerly exons b1–b5). Alternative splicing gives rise to hybrid transcripts with either e13a2 (b2a2) or e14a2 (b3a2) junctions. Apart from a well-established association between e14a2 transcript type and higher platelet counts, there is little evidence that these transcript types are clinically relevant. In rare cases of CML, and commonly in ALL, the breakpoints are further upstream in the 54.4-kb minor breakpoint cluster region (m-*bcr*) between two alternative second exons of BCR, e2′ and e2. This generates an e1a2 transcript that translates into p190$^{BCR\text{-}ABL}$. A third genomic breakpoint of the BCR gene was identified downstream of exon 19, referred as the micro-breakpoint cluster region (μ-*bcr*). This translocation gives rise to an e19a2 BCR-ABL mRNA encoding a 230-kDa fusion protein (p230$^{BCR\text{-}ABL}$), which is associated with neutrophilia.[23]

2. Structure of the fusion protein and constitutive activation of the ABL kinase

Depending on the BCR-ABL type, smaller or larger portions of BCR are preserved in the fusion protein. In contrast, the majority of ABL is retained, including the Src homology (SH) domains 1–3, a praline-rich region and the large C-terminus that carries DNA binding, nuclear localization and actin binding functions (Fig. 15.3). The SH3 and SH2 domains and the proline-rich region are critical for the docking of other proteins, while the SH1 domain carries tyrosine kinase activity. Recent data from several laboratories have revealed that the N-terminal "Cap" of ABL is central to the regulation of kinase activity through an intramolecular clamp that stabilizes the kinase in an inactive conformation.[24–26] The replacement of ABL exon 1 with BCR sequences disrupts this autoinhibited conformation through formation of multimers. In BCR-ABL, this is afforded by the dimerization domain (DD) of BCR, but other sequences can substitute for BCR. An example is the ETV6-ABL fusion gene found in some cases of ALL and MPN.[27] It is thought that transphosphorylation of kinase regulatory tyrosines is the initiating step, followed by incremental phosphorylation of other residues. Remarkably, despite the fact that many point mutations can activate ABL *in vitro*, none of these have been seen in patients, suggesting that BCR sequences play a crucial role for the induction of the disease in addition to activating the kinase.

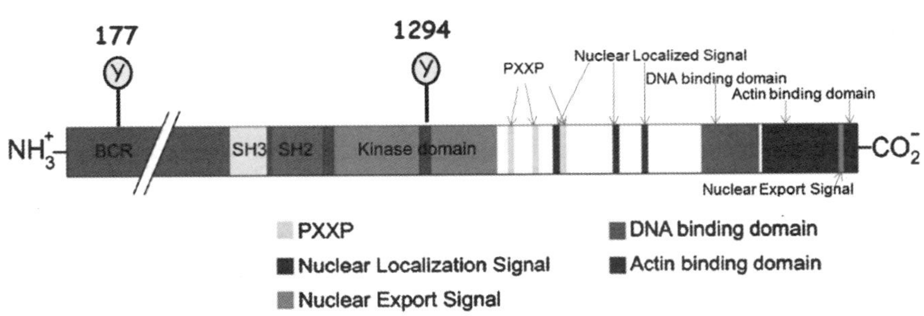

Fig. 15.3. Structural domains of the ABL tyrosine kinase. Adapted from Nagar *et al.* (2003) Structural basis for the autoinhibition of c-Abl tyrosine kinase. Cell. 2003 Mar 21;112(6):859–871.

3. Stem cell origin of CML and organization of leukemic hematopoiesis

BCR-ABL is demonstrable in cells of all hematopoietic lineages, including subsets of B-lymphocytes and pre-T cells, indicating that CML originates in a pluripotent hematopoietic stem cell.[28] Despite the ubiquitous expression of BCR-ABL, for unknown reasons, the proliferative drive conferred by BCR-ABL predominantly targets the granulocyte-megakaryocyte progenitor cells (GMP), clinically evident as left-shifted neutrophilic leukocytosis and frequently also thrombocytosis.[29] With this in mind, one can understand the superficially surprising finding that the stem cell compartment of many newly diagnosed CML patients is predominantly Ph–.[30] Furthermore, there is compelling evidence that BCR-ABL, unlike some acute myeloid leukemia (AML)-related oncogenes, does not confer self-renewal capacity, which implies that the translocation must occur in a cell that is already endowed with this capacity.[31] These findings have two important clinical implications. Firstly, suppression of the CML clone will allow Ph– hematopoiesis to be restored, as long as there is a sufficient reserve of normal stem cells. Secondly, at least in CP, the organization of leukemic hematopoiesis is highly hierarchical and as such liable to therapeutically targeting its roots.

4. Signal transduction in BCR-ABL–expressing cells

CML is arguably the most extensively studied human cancer, with thousands of publications on signal transduction in BCR-ABL-expressing cells. Much of this work is based on studies in cell lines, either human lines derived from patients in blast crisis or murine lines transformed to growth factor independence as a result of BCR-ABL expression, while research on primary CML cells has lagged behind. A complicated and highly redundant transformation network has emerged, a comprehensive review of which would go much beyond the scope of this chapter. What is clear, however, despite this complexity is that BCR-ABL kinase activity is *conditio sine qua non* for cellular transformation.[3] BCR-ABL is thought to impact several essential cellular functions, including the regulation of cell cycle, the threshold for the initiation of apoptosis, adhesion to extracellular matrix, and DNA repair.[21] In contrast to their normal counterparts, $CD34^+$ CML cells are capable of entering the S-phase of the cell cycle in the absence of cytokines.[32] Various signaling events are likely to contribute to this, particularly the activation of RAS/mitogen-activated protein kinase (MAPK) and phosphatidyl inositol kinase (PI3K) signaling, which lead to inactivation of cell cycle inhibitors such as p27.[33] Additionally, autocrine cytokine loops can contribute to reduced growth factor requirements. Another major effect of BCR-ABL is an increase of the apoptotic threshold, which is due to upregulation of anti-apoptotic proteins such as BCL-X_L and MCL-1 and as well as inactivation of pro-apoptotic proteins such as Bad.[34–36] It appears that the anti-apoptotic effects of BCR-ABL are mostly mediated through PI3K. CML progenitor cells exhibit decreased adhesion to extracellular matrix, including integrins as well as increased migration. This is thought to result in part from the phosphorylation of cell adhesion molecules such as paxillin and focal adhesion kinase (FAK). Interestingly, unlike the effects on proliferation and apoptosis, migration and adhesion defects are partially independent of BCR-ABL kinase activity.[37] Lastly, BCR-ABL impairs DNA repair through numerous mechanisms, which cause genomic instability and the acquisition of additional mutations, eventually leading to blastic transformation.[38] A variety of mutations can lead to or contribute to blast crisis.[39] Transcription factor mutations typical of AML, such as AML1-ETO and MYH11-CBFbeta, are rare in CML transformation, suggesting that the block in differentiation must be caused by different mechanisms. One particularly interesting finding is that BCR-ABL-mediated dysregulation of ribonucleoprotein hnRNP E2 inhibits translation of the key myeloid transcription factor CAAT enhancer-binding protein alpha (CEBPα).[40] Thus, the increased expression of BCR-ABL that is seen with disease progression may itself cause a differentiation block. Recent studies have shown that lymphoid blastic transformation, which accounts for approximately 30% of cases, is biologically similar to Ph+ ALL, and involves inactivation of the IKAROS transcription factor.[41]

Clinical presentation

1. Clinical course

CML has three clinically recognizable phases — CP, accelerated (AP) and blastic phase (BP). The initial CP is typically indolent and often asymptomatic. Prognostic scoring systems have been developed taking into consideration variables in presentation. The widely used Sokal score is based on age, spleen size, platelet count, and peripheral blood blasts to segregate patients into three risk groups. Four-year survival with busulfan-based chemotherapy was 62% (low risk), 43% (intermediate risk), and 33% (high risk), respectively.[42] In younger patients (< 45 years), sex and hematocrit were included as additional prognostic indicators. Cytogenetic abnormalities were associated with adverse outcomes in all groups.[43] The Sokal risk groups correlate with response to imatinib as well.[44] The Hasford score, a prognostication system developed specifically for patients treated with IFN-α, additionally takes into consideration eosinophil and basophil percentages.[45] In view of the fact that older age is one of the adverse factors included in the Sokal risk score, one might surmise that CML may be clinically more benign in younger patients.[42] However, there is little evidence to suggest major differences in the clinical behavior according to age, although the data is limited due to the rarity of CML in children, and older reports may be misleading due to the inclusion of patients with JMML. In a study of 40 children and adolescents treated at 16 centers in France, the presenting signs and symptoms were identical to those seen in adults.[46] There was a 1.5:1 predominance of boys over girls, with 45% of patients reporting asthenia, 20% splenic discomfort and 17.5% weight loss.[46] The only peculiar feature was a median white blood cell count of 242×10^9, which is higher than described in adults and consistent with another pediatric study which reported a median WBC of 192×10^9.[47] Interestingly, this study also found a significantly higher frequency of the e13a2 transcript type in males compared to females (51% vs. 27%), while e14a2 transcripts were more common in females (45% vs. 25%). This data is in contrast to the experience in adults, but it is doubtful whether it has significant clinical implications. All in all, it appears that the biology of CML in children and adults is not different, and the adverse effect of higher age in the Sokal score reflects reduced tolerance to now largely obsolete treatments like IFN-α and busulfan. Consistent with this, the results of imatinib are independent of age.[48]

2. Initial evaluation and staging

All patients with suspected CML must undergo a complete diagnostic workup, including detailed physical examination (with documentation of spleen size and any other sites of suspected extramedullary disease), complete blood count with white blood cell differential, routine serum chemistries, bone marrow aspirate, and marrow karyotyping. Fluorescence *in situ* hybridization (FISH) and RT-PCR to detect BCR-ABL are not mandatory for diagnosis except in cases of clinically typical CML with a normal karyotype. Bone marrow trephines are sometimes helpful to detect focal accumulations of blasts, but their use as a diagnostic routine is not universally accepted. Thorough staging is important to exclude progression to accelerated or blastic phase and to calculate the Sokal risk score as an easily accessible risk stratification tool.[42] Patients with high white counts should be started on hydroxyurea, with supportive hydration and allopurinol. Leukapheresis is indicated in cases of circulatory impairment (leukostasis), such as neurological symptoms or priapism. There is no indication for imatinib until the diagnosis of CML has been established and staging has been completed.

Therapy

1. Tyrosine kinase inhibitors

Imatinib was approved for use in children in 2003 and until recently was the initial therapy of choice for CML in all stages (see Chapter 22). Imatinib was initially met with considerable skepticism in parts of the pediatric community, out of concerns about the durability of responses, as well as side effects of a therapy, that is indeed almost lifelong in young patients.[49] With the studies in adults demonstrating stable responses in most patients started on imatinib in CP and a low incidence of late toxicities, confidence has grown in the use of imatinib as first-line therapy for all patients.[44] Data in the pediatric population are sparse, and less than 100 children have been entered on prospective studies. Champagne and colleagues reported the results of imatinib in 31 children who had failed interferon-α.[50] All 14 patients treated in CP achieved CHR, and 10 of 12 patients evaluable for cytogenetic response attained CCyR. Activity was also seen in advanced disease, but responses were less profound and durable, just like in adults. In contrast to the flat dosing used in adults, imatinib dosing in children is based on body surface area. The recommended imatinib doses are 260 mg/m^2 for second-line therapy of CP, 340 mg/m^2 for newly diagnosed CP, 400–500 mg/m^2 for accelerated phase, and 500–800 mg/m^2 for blastic phase. Pharmacokinetics are similar to those in adults.[51]

- Side effects

Side effects of imatinib in children are not fundamentally different from those in adults and occur with roughly the same frequency and severity. They include fluid retention with peripheral edema, specifically periorbital edema, nausea and diarrhea, musculoskeletal pain, skin rashes, hepatotoxicity, as well as laboratory abnormalities such hypomagnesemia and hypocalcemia.[49] Clinically, the most important side effect is myelosuppression, while grade 3/4 non-hematologic toxicity is relatively rare. Side effects specific to the CAYA population include perturbation of prepubertal growth velocity. This has been attributed to inhibition of PDGFR β signaling, which may lead growth plate changes and decreased longitudinal bone growth. Careful monitoring of growth is therefore mandatory in children on imatinib therapy.[52,53] In addition to inhibition of ABL and PDGFR α/β, imatinib also inhibits c-kit and c-fms. Some of these have important roles in gonadal development, implantation, and germ cell function.[54] Both oligospermia and primary ovarian failure have been described after starting imatinib, necessitating the consideration of cryopreservation of sperm, oocytes or embryos prior to starting therapy.

2. Imatinib in pregnancy

Though there are rare reports of fetal abnormalities and fetal loss in partners of men on imatinib, there are many more normal pregnancies and deliveries reported after imatinib use in men, suggesting that imatinib does not affect spermatogenesis. However, of the 125 women that conceived while on imatinib, three had elective abortions following detection of fetal abnormalities, 18 had spontaneous abortions, and 9 had babies with abnormalities. Thus, pregnancy is a strong contraindication to the use of imatinib, especially during the first trimester. Fetal abnormalities reported include exomphalos (in three patients), bony defects, meningocele, hydrocephalus, cerebellar hypoplasia, hypospadias, pyloric stenosis and cardiac defects.[49] Imatinib induced inhibition of PDGFR α may be to blame, although this remains to be proven. Interferon α is considered to be a safe alternative during pregnancy.[49] Women who plan a pregnancy on treatment must be advised to withdraw imatinib several days prior to unprotected intercourse and to plan the pregnancy shortly after stopping the drug (given that the patient will also be off the drug for the duration of the pregnancy). Breast feeding is also contraindicated as imatinib is freely excreted in breast milk.[55] Interruption of therapy puts patients at risk of relapse, but imatinib usually reinduces remissions upon rechallenge. Chemotherapy is inevitable for advanced phase disease and any pregnancy at this juncture puts the fetus at risk for congenital malformations and is better terminated, especially during the first trimester.[49]

Table 15.2. Monitoring the response to imatinib.

Response	Description of monitoring
Hematologic	At diagnosis, then every 15 days until CHR has been achieved and confirmed, then at least every 3 months or as required.
Cytogenetic	At diagnosis, at 3 months, and at 6 months; then every 6 months until a CCgR has been achieved and confirmed, then every 12 months if regular molecular monitoring cannot be assured; always for occurrences of treatment failure (primary or secondary resistance), and for occurrences of unexplained anemia, leucopenia, or thrombocytopenia
Molecular by RT-Q-PCR	Every 3 months until MMolR has been achieved and confirmed, then at least every 6 months
Molecular by mutational analysis	In occurrences of suboptimal response or failure; always required before changing to other TKIs or other therapies

Note: Cytogenetics should be performed by chromosome-banding analysis of marrow cell metaphases until CCgR has been achieved and confirmed. Interphase fluorescent *in situ* hybridization cannot be used to assess a less-than-complete response, but it can substitute for chromosome banding analysis to monitor the completeness of a CCgR, provided that *BCR-ABL1* extrasignal, dual color, dual fusion, or *in situ* hybridization probes are used and that at least 200 nuclei are scored.

CHR: complete histologic response; CCgR: complete cytogenetic response; MMolR: major molecular response; RT-Q-PCR: real-time quantitative polymerase chain reaction.

- Monitoring response to imatinib

Careful monitoring of response is essential to fully exploit the therapeutic benefit of imatinib (Table 15.2). An expert panel convened by the European Leukemia Net (ELN) has formulated recommendations with respect to response milestones on standard dose imatinib.[56] While these widely accepted recommendations are based on studies in adults, it is reasonable to apply them to the pediatric population. The key feature of the ELN recommendations is that response as a time-dependent variable is categorized as optimal, suboptimal, or failure. An optimal response implies that a good outcome is likely if imatinib is continued. A suboptimal response implies that a good outcome with imatinib is uncertain and alternatives should be considered, although they are not mandatory and more observation is reasonable. Lastly, failure indicates that continuation of imatinib is unlikely to result in a good outcome, and a change of therapeutic strategy is required (Table 15.3). In addition to these definitions, there are "warning signs" that suggest that the risk of failure is increased and closer monitoring is required. It is important to realize these are recommendations rather than

Table 15.3. Evaluation of overall response to imatinib first-line in early chronic phase.

	Response			
Evaluation time (Months)	**Optimal**	**Suboptimal**	**Failure**	**Warnings**
Baseline	NA	NA	NA	High risk; CCA/Ph+[a,b]
3	CHR and at least minor CgR (Ph+ ≤ 65%)	No CgR (Ph+ > 95%)	Less than CHR	NA
6	At least PCgR (Ph+ ≤ 35%)	Less than PCgR (Ph+ > 35%)	No CgR (Ph+ > 95%)	NA
12	CCgR	PCgR (Ph+ 1–35%)	Less than PCgR (Ph+ > 35%)	Less than MMoIR[b]
18	MMoIR[b]	Less than MMoIR[b]	Less than CCgR	NA
Any time during treatment	Stable of improving MMoIR[b]	Loss of MMoIR;[b] mutations[c]	Loss of CHR; loss of CCgR; mutations;[e] CCA/Ph+	Increase in transcript levels;[d] CCA/Ph-

Note: With respect to prior recommendations, a new definition of optimal response was introduced; an earlier definition of suboptimal response is recommended at 3 months in instances of cytogenetic resistance; an earlier definition of failure is recommended at 3 months in instances of hematologic resistance and at 5 months in instances of cytogenetic resistance; clonal progression (i.e. CCA/Ph+) during treatment was identified as treatment failure; a deletion of the long arm of chromosome 9 (del9q+) is no longer recognized as a warning.

NA: not applicable; CCA: clonal chromosome abnormalities; Ph+: Philadelphia chromosome positive; CHR: complete hematologic response; CgR: cytogenetic response; PCgR: partial cytogenetic response; MMoIR: major molecular response; CCgR: complete cytogenetic response; Ph–: Philadelphia chromosome negative.

[a]CCA/Ph+ is a warning factor at diagnosis, although its occurrence during treatment (i.e. clonal progression) is a marker of treatment failure. Two consecutive cytogenetic tests are required and must show the same CCA in at least two Ph+ cells.

[b]MMoIR indicates a ratio of *BCR-ABL1* to *ABL1* or other housekeeping genes of ≤ 0.1% on the international scale.

[c]*BCR-ABL1* kinase domain mutations still sensitive to imatinib.

[d]*BCR-ABL1* kinase domain mutations poorly sensitive to imatinib.

[e]The significance of the increase may vary by a factor of 2 to 10, depending on the laboratories.

rules, and that the individual patient's circumstance must be taken into account. Thus, in a child with an excellent allograft option, the demands on the quality of response at any given time will be higher compared to an elderly patient with multiple comorbidities. A comprehensive review of the monitoring strategies and their pitfalls is beyond the scope of this chapter and the reader is referred to a recent review.[57] Clearly, the fact that blood rather than bone marrow can be used for qPCR monitoring is of particular advantage in the pediatric population. An important development is the expression of qPCR results on the "international scale" (IS), which allows for comparison of results between different laboratories.[57]

- Imatinib failure

Primary imatinib resistance implies that a patient fails to achieve a desired level of response, while secondary resistance refers to a loss of response from any level. It is important to consider imatinib resistance as a diagnosis that is based on established criteria, has very significant prognostic implications, and should trigger a systematic resistance workup.[56,58] An important component of such a workup is to exclude noncompliance or drug interactions, before drawing any far-reaching conclusions. Point mutations in the kinase domain of BCR-ABL that impair or prevent imatinib binding to its target are the best characterized mechanisms of resistances. More than 50 different mutations have been described, with clusters in the ATP-binding loop, activation loop and the gatekeeper residue threonine 315.[57] While some mutations such as M351T or M244V confer only a minor degree of resistance, others like the gatekeeper mutation T315I render the kinase impervious to imatinib. Although kinase domain mutations are clearly important, many patients with imatinib resistance have no demonstrable mutations, and the mechanisms driving resistance in these patients remain largely elusive. From a practical point of view, however, screening for BCR-ABL mutations is important as certain mutations can inform the choice of one second-line inhibitor (dasatinib or nilotinib, discussed below) over the other.[59] For example, the presence of an F359V mutation predicts a poor response to nilotinib, while F317L is associated with resistance to dasatinib. T315I confers resistance to all currently approved TKIs, and patients with this mutation are candidates for an allogeneic transplant or experimental therapies.

- Dasatinib and nilotinib

Very limited data are available on the use of the second-line TKIs in the CAYA population. Results for dasatinib have been presented as abstracts. In one study of children (median age of 11, range 2–20) with refractory malignancies, there were significant responses in 5 out of 6 patients with CML. Toxicities were similar to those observed in adults.[60] Sixteen CML patients were entered in the CA180018 study of dasatinib in childen and adolescents with relapsed/refractory leukemia. Six of eight CP patients achieved CCyR.[61] No data are currently available on nilotinib in the pediatric population. Nilotinib has some activity in CML patients with resistance to or intolerance of imatinib and dasatinib. In one study where patients ranged in age from 19 to 78 years, nilotinib induced hematologic response rates in 79% and 29% of patients with CP and AP, respectively, with an overall survival rate of over 80% at 18 months in both groups.[62] Imatinib failure in a CAYA patient should be taken extremely seriously. All patients with AP or BC should be offered an allogenetic transplant. If failure occurs in CP, a second-line TKI may be justifiable, as long as the response is closely monitored.

3. Allogeneic stem cell transplant

Prior to the introduction of TKIs, allogeneic transplant was the standard of care for young patients with CML and a compatible donor, and provided proof of the efficacy of immunotherapy associated with allogenicity. In the 1990s, CML was the most frequent indication for allogeneic transplants worldwide (see Chapter 20). However, allografts for CML declined after the introduction of imatinib. More than 1000 transplants for CML were reported to the European Blood and Marrow Transplantation Group (EBMT) registry in 1999, but only 434 in 2007, of which only 228 were for first CP.

The era of transplantation for CML identified risk factors that predicted poor survival and included older age, infusion of a low nucleated cell dose, absence of cytogenetic response at transplant, advanced disease stage, interval from diagnosis of more than 1 year, unrelated or mismatched donor, and donor/recipient sex mismatch.[63,64] Registry studies, the largest being from the EBMT, showed an overall long-term survival post-transplant of 55–75%.[65–67] Although the results of allografting in the CAYA population are generally more favorable than in adults, mortality and morbidity are still significant, particularly in recipients of unrelated donor transplants. The prognostic parameters of the EBMT risk score apply equally to young patients.[68] In an EBMT report on pediatric patients, the 3-year overall survival was 75% for CP recipients of matched related donor (MRD) transplants and 65% for recipients of matched unrelated donor (URD) transplants.[65] In patients transplanted in advanced phase, overall survival was 46% and 39% for MRD and URD, respectively. The difference in survival was largely due to transplant-related mortality (TRM), which was 20% with sibling donors and 35% with unrelated donors. The only prospective trial, which used biological randomization between allografting and drug therapy according to donor availability, reported a 5-year overall survival rate of 87% for recipients of matched related, but only 52% for recipients of matched unrelated donors.[69] This study was initiated in 1995 and stopped in 2004 due to lack of recruitment. The interpretation of these data from a 2010 perspective is problematic in view of the fact that they do not reflect the progress in transplant technologies that was made since the start of this study.

Myeloablative regimens have been the standard approach to transplants for CML. However, myeloablative transplants predispose to late systemic complications in pediatric recipients. These include cataracts (47%), avascular necrosis (10%), pulmonary disease (15%), endocrine impairment, visual loss, motor and sensory impairment, need for special education, and behavioral problems.[70] Reduced intensity conditioning (RIC) was adopted in children to offset toxicities and TRM. Children with comorbid conditions may also benefit from an RIC approach. Only a small number of CAYA with CML have received RIC prior to transplantation and more data is required to evaluate this treatment option in this population. While TRM was reduced with RIC regimen, mixed chimerism/graft rejection rates were higher and the incidence of GVHD was similar to myeloablative transplants.[71–73] One report of CAYA and adults with CML undergoing RIC described a TRM of only 20% at 2 years even in advanced disease but donor lymphocyte infusions (DLI) became necessary in 23% for relapse or mixed chimerism.[71] Post-transplant imatinib has been shown to reduce or delay relapse in the RIC setting and may be beneficial when incorporated into the transplant plan preemptively.[74] In conjunction with the RIC approach, peripheral blood stem cells as the donor source may be associated with enhanced engraftment and reduce the risk of relapse but the trade-off is an increased risk of chronic graft versus host disease (GVHD).[75,76] In general, myeloablative transplants are indicated for AP/BC, whereas RIC can be considered in CP CML to offset toxicity but needs to be studied in a formal trial setting.

The single most frequent cause of death, and a major deterrent to transplant still remains GVHD for both ablative and reduced intensity transplants.[73] Improvements in transplant evaluation and predictors of risk factors, conditioning regimen, and supportive care serve to improve transplant outcomes both from toxicity and engraftment perspectives and have reduced TRM to less than 10%.[77] For example, a recent report suggested that high levels (> 9 mg/L) of C-reactive protein pretransplant in conjunction with a comorbidity index score > 0 predicts poor survival post transplant after imatinib failure.[78] Other developments that have contributed to improvements in outcome are intravenous busulfan with better pharmacokinetic predictability, less toxic newer agents such as treosulphan, expansion of donor registries enhancing high resolution HLA compatible transplants, and better supportive care (infection prophylaxis and GVHD therapy). With these tools, the 2-year probability of survival of patients transplanted more recently in first CP pre- or post-imatinib failure was over 85%. In the advanced phase, TRM was 15% and survival following transplant was 50%.[79,80]

Relapse rates after transplant for CML range between 7% and 20% in the first 5 years, depending on the stage of the disease, and decreased to 2–8% beyond this time.[69,77,81] Relapses have been reported as late as 18 years post-transplant. Donor lymphocyte infusions (DLI) or TKI alone or in combination have been used to reinduce remission and are most successful after cytogenetic or molecular relapse.[82,83] Cytogenetic and molecular response rates of over 80% and 60% have been described. Response rates were lower (50–70%) but still encouraging in advanced phase recurrence.[84] DLI, however, was associated with the development of acute and secondary or *de novo* chronic GVHD in as many as 38% of patients treated, resulting in a mortality of 11%, especially in those with acute or early onset symptoms.[85] Risk factors for GVHD included a high T-cell dose at first infusion, unrelated donor DLI, and a short time interval between transplant and infusion. DLI is less likely to be successful if relapse occurs within 6 months of transplant.[86] Second-line TKIs can be considered instead of imatinib in post-transplant relapse following previous history of imatinib resistance or intolerance. The immunoregulatory effects of TKIs via inhibition of T-cell receptor-mediated functions have raised questions about the use of TKIs in post-transplant relapse and a theoretical inhibition of the graft vs. leukemia effect.[87] Along these lines, there is no consensus on the durability of remission with post-transplant TKIs. For patients with relapsed or advanced disease more than 1 year after a previous transplant, retransplantation is an option, and is likely to be better tolerated by younger patients.

What is the role of allogeneic transplant for CAYA newly diagnosed CML patients in 2010? It has been argued that the approach to young CML patients should be more aggressive compared to adults, given that the results of allogeneic transplant are generally more favorable, and TKIs are indicated over a long period. This implies that one may consider defining more aggressive therapeutic goals than stipulated in accepted recommendations for adult patients. Given the paucity of data, such decisions are by necessity individual and must take into account the patient's disease features, therapeutic alternatives and personal preferences. Altogether, there is now consensus that for CP allografting should be considered only in case of imatinib failure. The assessment is fundamentally different if there is progression to advanced phase CML, where allotransplant continues to be the standard of care.[88] In this situation, TKIs serve as a bridge to transplant, with the aim of inducing a second CP, which in turn is associated with reduced relapse risk and reduced TRM. Allografting must be considered for patients who fail imatinib, although second-line TKIs are an option if the patient continues to be in CP. Cytogenetic response at 3 months is a good indicator of benefit bestowed by the switch to second-line TKI.[89] For patients with the T315I mutation or who fail second-line TKIs, allogeneic transplant is the treatment of choice. A difficult situation can arise when a patient with transformed disease achieves a very profound response to TKIs, raising the question whether one should proceed to transplant or not. The best approach is to avoid this conundrum by discussing upfront what to do in this case.

Polycythemia vera, essential thrombocythemia and primary myelofibrosis

Epidemiology

PV is a disease of older individuals, with an overall incidence of 10–20/10^6. One percent of patients with PV present before the age 25 and 0.1% are younger than 20. PV has been described in children as young as 7 months.[90] ET is also very rare in children (estimated incidence of 1/10^7), but slightly more common in young adults.[91,92] A review of 402 cases of ET revealed an age range from 5 to 91 years, with 43% of patients over 60 years of age.[93] Approximately 50 cases of childhood PMF have been reported in the English literature, generally as case reports.[94] Secondary myelofibrosis has been described in CAYA more frequently and occurs in hematologic and lymphoid malignancies, as well as solid tumors that infiltrate the bone marrow such as neuroblastoma, collagen-vascular disease, pure red cell aplasia, Fanconi anemia, and disorders of bone and bone metabolisms such as vitamin D deficiency, renal osteodystrophy, osteopetrosis and osteomalacia, amongst others.[95] For obvious reasons, it is critical to distinguish between these secondary causes and PMF.

Pathogenesis

Compared to CML, the elucidation of the molecular pathogenesis of other classical MPNs had been lagging behind, reflecting the lack of consistent chromosomal markers to provide investigative clues. This changed radically when the laboratory of William Vainchencker reported the discovery of an activating mutation in the JAK2 tyrosine kinase ($JAK2^{V617F}$) in more than 90% of patients with PV and approximately 50% of patients with ET and PMF.[4] These findings were subsequently confirmed by several other groups. Since then, $JAK2^{V617F}$ has been described in several nonclassical MPN, albeit at lower frequencies. Additionally, mutations in exon 12 of JAK2 were detected in the few PV patients without $JAK2^{V617F}$.[96] Interestingly, the disease in these patients is characterized by very high hemoglobin levels in the absence of thrombocytosis and leukocytosis. Activating mutations of MPL have been detected in some patients with PMF and ET that are similar to the $JAK2^{V617F}$-positive disease,[7] consistent with downstream activation of JAK2 as the critical event. Given the phenotypic similarities, it is likely that JAK2 is activated by as yet unidentified mechanisms in PMF and ET patients without detectable JAK2 or MPL mutations.

1. Mechanism of JAK2 activation by the V617F mutation

JAK2 is a non-receptor tyrosine kinase that is involved in signal transduction downstream of many cytokine receptors. Interestingly, in analogy to ABL, activation of JAK2 by N-terminal fusion of ETV6 had been observed in isolated cases of ALL. The V617F mutation is localized in the so-called pseudokinase domain of JAK2, a regulatory domain that evolutionarily resulted from a duplication of the kinase domain and is common to all JAK2 family kinases. It is still unknown how exactly $JAK2^{V617F}$ disrupts JAK2 autoinhibition. Compared to BCR-ABL, $JAK2^{V617F}$ has weaker transformation potency and transformation of factor-dependent cells requires the presence of a type I cytokine receptor to induce cytokine independence.[11,97] Mutational analysis revealed that the FERM domain of JAK2 is required for transformation.[98] The discovery of $JAK2^{V617F}$ has enhanced the interest in the role of JAK kinases as oncogenes, and mutations in JAK1 and JAK3 have since been described in acute lymphoblastic leukemia and acute megakaryoblastic leukemia, respectively,[99,100] along with different types of JAK2 mutations in patients with Down syndrome-associated ALL.[43] A puzzling finding is the strong, sometimes exclusive correlation between the different point mutations and certain disease entities and on the other hand the association of $JAK2^{V617F}$ with a variety of different disease phenotypes.

2. Molecular and biological features of $JAK2^{V617F}$-positive MPN

Studies in purified hematopoietic cells from MPN patients have demonstrated that $JAK2^{V617F}$ is present in all hematopoietic lineages, consistent with disease origin in a hematopoietic stem cell.[101] Although experimental proof is incomplete, it is likely that $JAK2^{V617F}$ does not confer self-renewal capacity, similar to BCR-ABL. The canonical biological consequences of $JAK2^{V617F}$ signaling may be very similar to those of BCR-ABL: increased proliferation with preserved differentiation, reduced apoptosis, altered adhesion, and genetic instability. Despite these similarities, $JAK2^{V617F}$ apparently activates a unique array of pathways that lead to a divergent phenotype. Hypersensitivity to growth factors, specifically erythropoietin, has been used for a long time to distinguish between MPN and reactive conditions, in assays referred to as erythropoietin-independent erythroid colonies (EEC).[102] Studies of individual EEC have revealed that most, but not all of these express $JAK2^{V617F}$, suggesting that as yet unidentified mechanisms drive EEC growth in some cases. $JAK2^{V617F}$-expressing cells exhibit increased resistance to apoptosis in response to DNA damage, which is due to increased expression of anti-apoptotic BCL-2 family proteins, such as $BCL\text{-}X_L$.[103] Perturbed adhesion and trafficking of PMF cells has been documented in many studies. The most intriguing question is how $JAK2^{V617F}$ induces the diverse phenotypes of PV, ET, and PMF. There are two obvious explanations: either the mutation is acquired by a cell already committed to a specific differentiation program or acquired events must influence phenotype selection. At the moment, there is more evidence in favor of the latter explanation, as studies in humans, as well as animal models, have found that a high allelic ratio ($JAK^{V617F}/JAK2^{WT}$) promotes PV over ET.[104] The normal JAK2 allele is frequently deleted in PV, while the mutant allele is duplicated (a phenomenon referred to as uniparental disomy), while this is not the case in most patients with ET.[105] This implies that some patients may progress from ET to PV through acquisition of a second mutated allele. Whether this actually happens or whether there are ET patients who have a "form fruste" of PV due to iron deficiency is a matter of debate. Furthermore, it is unclear how PMF fits into this picture. As ET and PV can evolve to MF, it has been suggested that MF represents a disease state akin to the accelerated phase of CML; however, this would imply that an undetected, indolent CP predates PMF, which is not the case in most of these patients.[1]

Is JAK^{V617F} of equal importance for PV, ET and PMF as BCR-ABL for CML? Several lines of evidence suggest that this is not the case. Most compelling is the observation that approximately half of the MPN patients who progress to acute myeloid leukemia have $JAK2^{V617F}$-negative blasts, indicating that the AML clone is not in immediate succession of the $JAK2^{V617F}$-positive MPN clone.[106] In fact, a recent manuscript has reported that multiple abnormal clones may coexist in the same patient, which may or may not be clonally related.[107] In contrast, while some cases of Ph– blast crisis have been reported in CML, overall this is a very rare event. Another important point is the much stronger familial predisposition in first degree relatives of MPN patients.[12] Lastly, while BCR-ABL inhibitors are extremely effective in CML, data from studies of JAK2 inhibitors in MPN are less impressive, suggesting $JAK2^{V617F}$ may play a less important role. Clearly, the MPN data are early and should be interpreted with caution as results may improve with better drug design.

Clinical presentation

1. Polycythemia vera

A recent literature survey identified 36 patients diagnosed with PV at the age of 18 or younger. The median hematocrit at diagnosis was 61%, leukocyte count 13.2×10^9/L and platelet count 600×10^9/L and thus comparable to adult patients.[90] Molecular features, where available, were also similar to those in adult PV patients. Clinically, these patients had a high incidence of severe thrombotic complications, including Budd-Chiari syndrome in 7 patients (19%). These data are in line with previous publications that reported an up to 30% incidence of Budd-Chiari syndrome in adults below the age of 40.[108,109] A fairly large study of patients below the age of 50 diagnosed with PV also found a high incidence of thrombotic events (14% before the diagnosis of PV, and 11% during follow-up), although not Budd-Chiari syndrome.[110] The latter study found a 5.3-fold increased age- and gender-adjusted mortality rate, mainly due to leukemic transformation or progression to myelofibrosis. Given the rarity of PV in CAYA patients, there are insufficient data to know whether the biology differs according to the patient's age. What is presumably different are disease-modifying factors, mainly cardiovascular risk factors, which are more prevalent in older patients. However, as discussed above, young age may not be uniformly protective against thromboembolic events, which needs to be taken into account when making therapeutic choices. Leukocytosis seems to be directly proportional to the complication rate. A white count of > 15 × 10 E9/L heralds an increased risk of DVTs and hemorrhagic complications while patients with lower leukocyte numbers seem better protected. Additional complications of PV described in the young include gangrene, pulmonary embolism, gastrointestinal hemorrhage, epistaxis, headache, hypertension, nausea, syncope, lassitude, dizziness, pruritus, impaired vision, arthralgia, and tinnitus.[90]

While the presence of $JAK2^{V617F}$ or equivalent mutations in conjunction with an elevated red cell mass or hematocrit is diagnostic of PV,[1] in cases without JAK2 mutations, it is important to consider alternative diagnoses. These include primary familial and congenital polycythemia (PFCP) and congenital secondary erythrocytosis. PFCP is due to mutations of the erythropoietin (Epo) receptor that confer hypersensitivity to Epo due to impaired binding of negative regulators. Secondary congenital erythrocytosis may be caused by high oxygen affinity in hemoglobin variants, 2,3-bisphosphoglycerate deficiency, or mutations in the *von Hippel-Lindau* (VHL) gene that lead to an oxygen-sensing defect, best known in the Chuvash polycythemia.[111] In contrast to PV, hematopoiesis in these patients is always polyclonal; a specialized laboratory is required to make the correct diagnosis. WHO revised diagnostic criteria are applicable to children and young adults with PV, accepting either the presence of both major criteria + 1 minor criterion or 1 major and 2 minor criteria to establish the diagnosis.[112] A normal Epo level does not rule out a diagnosis of PV.

Epo-independent erythroid colony growth was seen in 4 of 13 (8 sporadic and 5 familial) pediatric PV cases in one study and in 8 of 8 patients in a second study.[113] Secondary polycythemia can be associated with malignancies, e.g. acute lymphoblastic leukemia and lymphoma, either during relapse or after completion of therapy.[114,115] The etiopathogenesis that drives this proliferation is unknown, but clinical manifestations closely resemble PV.

2. Essential thrombocythemia

Clinical manifestations of ET in CAYA patients are variable. In one study, more than 60% of young adults were asymptomatic at diagnosis. Others noted vasomotor symptoms such as headache, dizziness and visual disturbances. Major thrombotic or minor hemorrhagic events were present in 9% and 3%, respectively. Palpable splenomegaly was noted in 10%. The median platelet and leukocyte counts at diagnosis were 830×10^9/L and 8.7×10^9/L, respectively.[116–119] The largest study reported 126 patients, 43% of whom were positive for $JAK2^{V617F}$, with a median age of 31 (range 5–40) years. There was a significantly increased risk for stroke (odds ratio 50, 95% CI 21.5–115) and venous thrombosis (OR 5.3, 95% CI 3.9–10.6) compared to age-matched controls. Thrombosis-free survival at 10 years was 84%, and 92% remained free of a major bleeding event.[116] Transformation to acute leukemia occurred in only one patient and transformation to myelofibrosis was also rare at 5%. Young ET patients have a risk of thromboembolic events that are not predicted by the usual overt risk factors such as the platelet count, smoking, cardiovascular risk factors, the presence of JAK2 mutations, or leukocytosis.[90] An important consideration in young women with ET is pregnancy. It is generally thought that the rate of miscarriage in considerably higher than in age-matched controls. In a study of 74 women, 50 years or younger, 34 pregnancies occurred. Only 17 were normal, while 14 resulted in miscarriages, 2 in induced abortions, and 1 in an ectopic pregnancy.[118] Another study in patients younger than 40 reported that 13 normal babies were born in 16 pregnancies.[117] Managing young women with ET who want to conceive can pose significant therapeutic challenges.

Similar to patients with erythrocytosis, the differential diagnostic considerations in young patients with thrombocytosis are different from those in adults. Most cases of thrombocytosis in children are reactive and commonly due to infections.[120] Essential thrombocythemia must be distinguished from hereditary thrombocytosis, which encompasses two pathogenetically different types of diseases with autosomal-dominant inheritance. The first is caused by germline mutations in the 5′ untranslated region of the *Tpo* gene that cause the deletion of an untranslated open reading frame, and consequently more efficient translation.[121,122] The second type is due to germline mutations in the Tpo receptor MPL that affect MPL function by one of two distinct mechanisms. Mutations in the transmembrane domain such as S505N lead to constitutive dimerization of the receptor and consequently activation of signal transduction.[123,124] In contrast, the K39N polymorphism in the ligand-binding domain is thought to impair Tpo binding, resulting in increased availability of ligand to stimulate thrombopoiesis.[125]

The strictly hereditary forms of erythrocytosis and thrombocytosis that are caused by germline transmission of disease-inducing mutations such as the VHL mutations in Chuvash polycythemia or MPL^{S505N} in hereditary thrombocytosis must be distinguished from familial myeloproliferative neoplasms, where an as yet unknown predisposition for MPN is transmitted through the germline. Many of these familial cases exhibit JAK2 mutations, and the clinical presentation of these patients is not different from sporadic cases.

Therapy

1. Polycythemia vera

Given the rarity of PV in the CAYA population, the management of these disorders is less standardized than in adults, but it seems reasonable to formulate similar therapeutic goals to minimize the risk of thromboembolic complications. Low-dose aspirin is indicated, but caution is warranted in the young due to the association with Reye's syndrome. Acquired von Willebrand disease is a contraindication to aspirin and should be ruled out. In PV, the target hematocrit is 42% in female and 45% in male patients. In many cases, this can be achieved with phlebotomy only. However, the non-hematologic side effects of the therapeutic iron depletion can be limiting. Hydroxyurea (HU), which is frequently used in adults, is an alternative to phlebotomy in such cases. However, the long-standing debate whether HU is leukemogenic has not been settled completely, and naturally the issue is particularly relevant to pediatric patients with their prospect of life-long therapy. Based on encouraging results in adults, consideration should be given to interferon (IFN)-α, which can frequently be used at low and well-tolerated doses. In contrast to HU, IFN has been shown to restore normal (polyclonal) hematopoiesis in a subset of patients, implying a much more profound effect on disease pathogenesis. Since IFN is neither mutagenic nor teratogenic, it is the treatment of choice in young women who plan to start a family.

2. Essential thrombocythemia

There is no uniform approach to the management of ET in the CAYA population. With the restrictions stated above for PV, all patients should receive low dose aspirin. Platelet-lowering agents are indicated in patients with platelet counts of more than 1.5×10^9/L or with thrombembolic complications. However, given the significant incidence of such complications in CAYA patients discussed above, an argument can be made for a more aggressive approach. As in PV, options include HU and IFN, while anagrelide should not be used any longer, based on inferior results in a randomized comparison with HU.[126] We believe that IFN is the treatment of choice for CAYA patients with ET, given its ability to restore normal hematopoiesis and the lack of mutagenicity or teratogenicity. Other agents such as alkylators (melphalan or busulfan), radiophosphorus, and folate antagonists have been tried, but are nowadays reserved for severe unresponsive cases, given their leukemogenic potential and other major toxicities.[119]

3. Primary myelofibrosis

PMF in children has variable outcomes ranging from spontaneous remission to an indolent course with shortened survival, or evolution to a hematologic malignancy (in 6 of 46 reported cases).[94] As in adults, there is no standard of care and treatment includes blood transfusions, intravenous immunglobulins, corticosteroids, and HU. Many children are diagnosed with PMF following presentation with chronic hematologic manifestations such as unresponsive anemia or mild thrombocytopenia and require no therapeutic or supportive care interventions over many years of follow up.[127] Spontaneous erythropoietic recovery has also been described in children 2–3 years after diagnosis, suggesting that different pathogenetic mechanisms may underlie PMF in children.[128]

Stem cell transplantation is a treatment option in patients that fail conservative management and successful related, as well as unrelated, donor transplantation has been reported in both PV and PMF. The decision to transplant is generally made based on suspicion or evidence of progression to myelofibrosis or leukemia. The number of children transplanted is small and described as case reports. Myeloablative transplants, with chemotherapy-based conditioning have been the norm using the best available stem cell source — bone marrow, peripheral blood (related and unrelated), or cord blood cells. In a report of transplantation for PMF in two young children, successful engraftment was reported with transfusion independence and resolution of marrow fibrosis 3–12 months post transplant. Another report ot transplant for PV described the successful use of DLI following decreasing chimerism at 3 months post-transplant indicating barriers to engraftment that need to be factored in as transplant plans are formulated.[127,129,130] Transplant-related morbidity and mortality attributable to GVHD and organ toxicity, such as pulmonary hypertension, remain deterrents to transplant. Transplant is not indicated in asymptomatic patients or those responsive to conservative therapy, especially as some children with PMF may eventually have spontaneous remission, and the incidence of progression to leukemia is low.

Myelodysplastic Disorders

Transient myeloproliferative disorder (TMD) and acute megakaryoblastic leukemia (AMKL) in Down syndrome

Epidemiology

Down syndrome (DS) is the most common chromosomal abnormality in humans (1.2/1000 live births). Children with DS have an increased susceptibility for the neonatal preleukemic transient myeloproliferative disorder (DS-TMD) as well as acute leukemia of megakaryoblastic origin (AMKL) and acute lymphoblastic leukemia (ALL). The risk of leukemia is increased 10–36-fold in DS. The risk of developing AMKL is increased 46–83-fold and the risk of ALL is increased 10–27-fold. About 10% of babies with DS are diagnosed with TMD.[131]

Pathogenesis

TMD develops during fetal hematopoiesis, implicating liver hematopoietic stem cells in the pathogenesis. Significant hepatic infiltration with proliferating hematopoietic cells and relative sparing of the bone marrow are hallmarks of TMD. In murine xenograft models, there is enhanced erythroid and megakaryocytic engraftment of trisomy 21 fetal liver $CD34^+$ cells. TMD is associated with GATA1 mutations that are thought to synergize with the altered DNA dosage from chromosome 21, although the mechanisms are unclear. Acquired cytogenetic abnormalities are rare. All GATA1 mutations result in N-terminal truncations in the gene and the production of a shorter GATA1 protein. In murine models and human DS primary hematopoietic cells, this results in an impaired ability to regulate excess proliferation of megakaryocyte progenitors via a number of downstream transcription factors including GATA2, MYC, MYB, GATA1 itself, BACH1 and SON in humans.[132] Human chromosome 21 encodes a microRNA (miR-125b-2) that is overexpressed in DS-AMKL/TMD. This microRNA has been shown to increase proliferation of megakaryocytic/erythroid progenitors and perturb myeloid differentiation and may work in synergy with the proliferative potential afforded by GATA1 mutations.[133] Additionally, the oxidative stress and aberrant folate metabolism caused by trisomy 21 has been implicated in the development of GATA1 mutations and impaired DNA repair capacity, driving leukemogenesis in DS.[134]

Clinical presentation

Hydrops fetalis can be a manifestation of TMD *in utero.* TMD after birth is characterized by circulating peripheral blast cells and dysplasia in the erythroid and megakaryocytic series. The median age at diagnosis is 3–7 days and TMD is always diagnosed within 2 months of age. Ten percent of babies have no symptoms, and the diagnosis is made by circulating blasts with or without leukocytosis. The incidence of myeloproliferation may thus be higher than recognized and can be missed in the absence of routine hematologic follow up in DS babies. Systemic manifestations include hepatomegaly (59%), splenomegaly (39%), serous pleural and pericardial effusions (10–20%), ascites, obstructive jaundice, anemia or polycythemia, low or high platelet counts, and skin rashes. Clinical intervention is often required for manifestations of hyperviscosity with respiratory distress, congestive heart failure, disseminated intravascular coagulation and renal dysfunction. Ten percent of DS babies with TMD develop liver fibrosis due to blast cell infiltration of the liver which can progress to fulminant hepatic failure.

Circulating blasts detected on the peripheral smear is a diagnostic hallmark of DS-TMD but is not exclusive of this diagnosis. DS-TMD must be differentiated from systemic manifestations of sepsis, cardiac failure, and alternate causes of hepatorenal dysfunction. TMD may be diagnosed and monitored by peripheral blood examination and analysis of GATA1 mutations. A bone marrow evaluation is unnecessary. Most babies need no chemotherapy and spontaneous resolution is the norm within approximately 3–6 months after birth. Chemotherapy with low-dose cytarabine is recommended for babies with hepatomegaly, hepatic or renal dysfunction, or high numbers of circulating blasts and leukocytosis $> 100 \times 10^9$/L, in an effort to prevent liver fibrosis and associated morbidity and mortality. TMD blasts are highly sensitive to cytarabine, perhaps due to an increased gene dose of cystathionine-β-synthetase and similar genes localized on chromosome 21. Clearance of peripheral blood blasts is usually evident by 1 week of therapy. It is unclear whether therapy for TMD influences the risk of development of AMKL, but continued monitoring on a 3-month basis is recommended to monitor the development of leukemia.

The prognosis of TMD is variable. Overall, there is a 20% mortality associated with TMD despite therapy. Patients with high-risk features have a 3-year mortality as high as 20–40%. Mortality is associated with rising transaminases, cholestatic jaundice, and leukocytosis of $> 100 \times 10^9$/L. An outcome analysis from the Children's Oncology Group differentiated good-risk (no hepatomegaly and liver dysfunction) and intermediate-risk (hepatomegaly and mild liver dysfunction) babies from the high-risk group (hepatomegaly with severe liver dysfunction). The EFS for these three groups were 83, 64 and 36%, respectively.[135] Of the majority that recover from TMD, 20–30% subsequently develop leukemia, often within the first 4 years of life, presumably due to the survival of selectively advantaged subclones of TMD blasts. Overall, DS children have a 50-fold increased risk of leukemia during the first 5 years, and a 10-fold increased risk between 5 and 29 years, which then becomes comparable to that of the general population with age.

A prolonged indolent pre-phase of thrombocytopenia and marrow fibrosis with dysplasia often heralds the development of AMKL. The morphologic, immunophenotypic and cytochemical profile of the blasts are similar to those seen in TMD. The presence of the same GATA1 mutations as seen in TMD suggest that AMKL is a progression from TMD but trisomy and GATA1 mutations alone are insufficient to cause progression to AMKL. Clonal evolution, often involving additional copies of chromosome 8 and/or

21 (10–15%), monosomy 7 and –5/5q (10–20%) is frequently present in AMKL. However, unlike in MDS that is not associated with DS, they have no adverse prognostic significance. Several additional candidate genes have been implicated in progression including JAK2, JAK3, FLT3, and TP53. The 5-year disease-free survival following AML therapy for DS-AMKL is 70–80% in contrast to non-DS-AMKL with 22–28%.[136]

Myelodysplastic syndromes

Epidemiology

Myelodysplastic syndromes (MDS) comprise a group of clonal hematopoietic stem cell disorders characterized by ineffective hematopoiesis, cytopenias, qualitative cellular defects, and a predisposition to acute leukemia (see Chapter 1). Pediatric MDS is rare with an incidence 0.5 to $4.0/10^6$ and accounts for 3–9% of pediatric hematologic malignancies. The diagnosis is usually made between 6 and 8 years of age. Twenty percent of pediatric AML cases and 56% of pediatric AML cases in DS are associated with myelodyplasia.[137]

Pathogenesis and clinical considerations

Primary pediatric MDS differs from the adult variety in clinical features, associated chromosomal aberrations and genetic abnormalities. In 24–54% of children, MDS is associated with a constitutional disorder such as DS, Naxos disease, Dandy-Walker syndrome or Lowe syndrome, amongst others. The underlying genetic predisposition has a profound impact on prognosis.[138] Other bone marrow disorders associated with MDS include Schwachman-Diamond syndrome, Fanconi anemia and other conditions associated with bone marrow failure, as well as neurofibromatosis I, and mitochondrial cytopathies. MDS associated with heritable disorders is more frequent (86%) in the first 2 years of life and is associated with longer survival and a lesser propensity to progress to acute leukemia than idiopathic MDS. Mutations in RUNX1 (14%) and CEBPA (4%) have been identified in childhood MDS, but overall, the pathogenesis of MDS in children is not well understood due to the rarity of the disorder. Less than 10% of childhood MDS is therapy related, such as that associated with immunosuppressive therapy for acquired aplastic anemia.[137] Secondary MDS occurs following chemo- or radiotherapy, familial disorders, congenital bone marrow failure syndromes or acquired aplastic anemia.[139]

A detailed review of pediatric MDS classification has been published recently.[137] The key consideration is that the International Prognostic Scoring System (IPSS) is of limited value in children.[140,141] Broadly, three diagnostic groups are recognized in pediatric MDS: Refractory cytopenia (< 5% blasts), refractory anemia with excess blasts (RAEB) (5–20%) and RAEB-T (in transformation) (20–30% blasts). A two-lineage dysplasia in a minimum of 10% of cells is required to establish a diagnosis of dysplasia. Multilineage cytopenias are more common in the young. In a pediatric study of 34 patients with primary and secondary MDS, 85% had dysplastic features in the erythroid, 50% the granulocytic and 90% in the megakaryocytic lineage; bone marrow cellularity was decreased in 60%; in contrast, hypoplastic MDS is fairly uncommon in adults.[142] A hypocellular bone marrow, typical for pediatric MDS especially of the RA subtype, must be distinguished from aplastic anemia, congenital bone marrow failure syndromes, infectious etiologies (EBV, HHV6, chronic parvovirus), heavy metal poisoning, and nutritional deficiencies. Chromosomal abnormalities were reported in 30% of children with MDS, and there are differences compared to adults.[142] For example, 19% of cases exhibited monosomy 7, in contrast to 10% of adults. The clinical course of these patients is no less aggressive than that of the adult population, with a median time to progression to AML of only 2 years. Young patients with other karyotypes such as trisomy 8 can experience a stable course for a long period. In analogy to adults, patients with RA have a relatively good prognosis. Thus, in one study, while none of the patients with RA progressed to leukemia over a median follow up period of 3.5 years, 62% of RAEB/RAEB-T underwent leukemic transformation at a median of 1.7 years.[143] Myelodysplasia and AML associated with Down syndrome are grouped together as DS-AML, a separate entity from pediatric MDS as their clinical behaviors differ vastly. These are summarized in Table 15.4.

Treatment

There is no standard of care for the management of MDS in CAYA patients, but considerations are analogous to those in adults and involve a careful assessment of procedure- vs. disease-related risks. Given the rarity of MDS in young patients, data are very limited and most treatment decisions must be individualized. For obvious reasons, the fact that allogeneic stem cell transplantation is the only known curative option carries great weight in the pediatric population.

Table 15.4. Differences between MDS in children and Down syndrome-associated MDS/AML.

	MDS in children	MDS/AML in Down syndrome
Incidence	4% of hematologic malignancies	10–20% in DS children
Median age at diagnosis (years)	7.5	1.8
FAB AML subtype	M1/M2 (41%); M4/M5 (37%)	M7 (62%)
Common karyotype abnormality	−7; 7q− (30%)	+8 (14%)
Prognostic significance of −7/7q−	Poor	No significance
Hematologic presentation	Refractory cytopenias (neutrophils, platelets) +/− increased blasts	Anemia, thrombocytopenia
Sensitivity to chemotherapy	No	Yes
Preferred therapy	Stem cell transplant	Low-dose chemotherapy
EFS (4 years)	35%	68%

AML: acute myeloid leukemia; FAB: French–American–British classification.

Supportive care and drug therapy

Some patients may be managed with supportive care only, which includes blood and platelet transfusions, erythropoietin and myeloid growth factors, prophylactic antimicrobials in neutropenic patients, and iron chelation in patients with significant transfusion requirements. Drug therapy is based either on immunosuppression using anti-thymocyte globulin (ATG) combined with cyclosporine, or hypomethylating agents such as 5-azacytidine or 5-aza-2-deoxycytidine (decitabine) or lenalidomide. Myelosuppression is a frequent side effect of the hypomethylating agents (azacytidine and decitabine) and is seen in nearly half of the patients after multiple treatment cycles. Other side effects range from fatigue, muscle pain, and GI disturbances to more serious but rare complications of severe infections, organ failure, and thrombosis. Teratogenicity is of concern in the CAYA population but data with these agents is scarce due to the rarity of long-term use in the young. Some of these drugs or drug combinations have efficacy in specific MDS subgroups such as 5q-(lenalidomide) and immunosuppression in patients with HLADR15 or a paroxysmal nocturnal hemoglobinuria subclone. Some patients achieve major and durable responses though time to response is often several months. Emerging data from adults suggest that hypomethylating agents prolong survival even in the absence of complete responses, and that maintenance therapy is beneficial; it is likely that this will be similar in the pediatric population.

Allogeneic stem cell transplant

Allogeneic stem cell transplantation is the only curative therapy for MDS and should be seen as the treatment of choice in eligible patients, although timing will depend on individual patient risk factors (see Chapter 20). Transplant may be delayed in low risk patients to optimize results of drug therapy whereas in high risk patients early transplant is indicated. In low-risk patients 3-year survival post-transplant is 50–70%.[144,145] In high-risk patients, nonrelapse mortality (32–42%) and relapse risk (25%) result in lower long-term event-free survival (33–45%).[144,146,147] Secondary therapy-related MDS has poor prognosis and is almost uniformly fatal with nontransplant therapy. In contrast, allogeneic transplantation has resulted in 40% EFS in the case of secondary MDS developing after alkylating agent/radiotherapy, while EFS is only 11% if MDS is related to topoisomerase II inhibitors.[145] Although tolerability of full-dose myeloablative therapy is not usually an issue in young patients, late toxicities are considerable. Thus, there is a need to evaluate reduced intensity approaches that reduce long-term sequelae, while avoiding an increased relapse risk. As in adults, the RIC approach is better suited for low-risk patients (for example those with RA and a normal karyotype), whereas high-risk disease is an indication for myeloablative conditioning due to an aggressive course. RIC transplants may also have a role in patients transplanted in remission (defined as < 5% marrow blasts). In one report of such patients, TRM was 15% and EFS was 60% at 12 months.[148] There is evidence that peripheral blood stem cells may provide an advantage over bone marrow products, and based on the adult experience one may surmise that this will be most useful in high risk patients.[146,149]

Conclusions

Compared to adults, MDS and MPN are infrequent in the CAYA population. While some diseases such as CML are almost always sporadic, there is a higher incidence of associated congenital or familial predisposition syndromes in the CAYA population with MDS/MPN that impact disease biology. Important clinical considerations are that the differential diagnosis is different from that in adults, and that the transient nature of some conditions can pose considerable diagnostic difficulties.

In some diseases such as MDS, classification schemes that are well established and validated in adults have limited utility in CAYA patients. However, the biggest challenge is the lack of large and well-controlled therapeutic studies, an inevitable consequence of the rarity of MPN and MDS in this group of patients. As a result, clinical management is less well standardized and more dependent on individual experience and preference. For the "classical" MPN CML, ET and PV therapy is mostly modeled on the experience in adults, while TMD and AMKL associated with Down syndrome have their own specific treatment approaches. Overriding considerations are that CAYA patients are more likely to tolerate aggressive interventions such as allogeneic stem cell transplant and that any noncurative approach needs to take into account its truly lifelong duration. Bearing this in mind, the threshold to intervene aggressively is lower in CAYA patients than in adults. The flipside is long-term and late adverse effects specific to children, such as developmental delays and organ toxicities in recipients of allogeneic transplants.

The past several years have seen profound advances in our understanding of the molecular biology of MPN, and to a lesser degree MDS. In the case of CML, this has led to the development of imatinib and subsequently second-line TKIs that have revolutionized therapy. The hope is that this paradigm will be applicable to other hematologic malignancies. As in adults, the key tasks ahead are to improve risk stratification through discovery of new biomarkers, develop novel therapies based on improved understanding of molecular disease pathogenesis and minimize the toxicity of allogeneic stem cell transplantation. Achieving these goals will require continued collaborative efforts in a small patient population.

Acknowledgment

Supported in part by NHLBI grant HL082978-01 (MWD) and the Leukemia and Lymphoma Society (MWD). MWD is a Scholar in Clinical Research of the Leukemia and Lymphoma Society.

References

12. Landgren O, Goldin L, Kristinsson S, Helgadottir E, Samuelsson J, Bjorkholm M. (2008) Increased risks of polycythemia vera, essential thrombocythemia, and myelofibrosis among 24,577 first-degree relatives of 11,039 patients with myeloproliferative neoplasms in Sweden. *Blood* **112**: 2199–2204.
21. Deininger M, Goldman J, Melo J. (2000) The molecular biology of chronic myeloid leukemia. *Blood* **96**: 3343–3356.
44. Druker B, Guilhot F, O'Brien S, Gathmann I, Kantarjian H, Gattermann N, *et al.* (2006) Five-year follow-up of patients receiving imatinib for chronic myeloid leukemia. *N Engl J Med* **355**: 2408–2417.
46. Millot F, Traore P, Guilhot J, Nelken B, Leblanc T, Leverger G, *et al.* (2005) Clinical and Biological Features at Diagnosis in 40 Children With Chronic Myeloid Leukemia. *Pediatrics* **116**: 140–143.
49. Apperley J. (2009) CML in pregnancy and childhood. *Best Pract Res Clin Haematol* **22**: 455–474.
50. Champagne M, Capdeville R, Krailo M, *et al.* (2004) Imatinib mesylate (STI571) for treatment of children with Philadelphia chromosome-positive leukemia: Results from a Children's Oncology Group phase I study. *Blood* **104**: 2655–2660.
57. Hughes T, Deininger M, Hochhaus A, Branford S, Radich J, Kaecla J, *et al.* (2006) Monitoring CML patients responding to treatment with tyrosine kinase inhibitors: Review and recommendations for harmonizing current methodology for detecting BCR-ABL transcripts and kinase domain mutations and for expressing results. *Blood* **108**: 28–37.
60. Aplenc R, Strauss L, Shusterman S, *et al.* (2008) Pediatric phase I trial and pharmacokinetic (PK) study of dasatinib: A report from the Children's Oncology Group phase I consortium. *J Clin Oncol* **26**: 20–25.
64. Muramatsu H, Kojima S, Yoshimi A, Atsuta Y, Nagatoshi Y, Inoue M, *et al.* (2010) Outcome of 125 children with chronic myelogenous leukemia who received transplants from unrelated donors: The Japan Marrow Donor Program. *Biol Blood Marrow Transplant* **16**: 231–238.
65. Cwynarski K, Roberts I, Iacobelli S, *et al.* (2003) Stem cell transplantation for chronic myeloid leukemia in children. *Blood* **102**: 1224–1231.
69. Suttorp M, Claviez A, Bader P, Peters C, Gadner H, Ebell W, *et al.* (2009) Allogeneic stem cell transplantation for pediatric and adolescent patients with CML: Results from the prospective trial CML-paed I. *Klin Pediatr* **221**: 351–357.

71. Crawley C, Szydlo R, Lalancette M, *et al.* (2005) Outcomes of reduced intensity transplantation for chronic myeloid leukemia: An analysis of prognostic factors from the Chronic Leukemia Working Party of the EBMT. *Blood* **106**: 2969–2976.
80. Holowiecki J, Giebel S, Wojnar J, Krawczyk-Kulis M, Markiewicz M, Holowiecka-Goral A, *et al.* (2008) Treosulfan and fludarabine low-toxicity conditioning for allogeneic hematopoietic stem cell transplantation in chronic myeloid leukemia. *Br J Haematol* **42**: 284–292.
89. Deininger M, Schleuning M, Greinix H, Sayer H, Fischer T, Martinez J, *et al.* (2006) The effect of prior exposure to imatinib on transplant-related mortality. *Haematologica* **91**: 452–459.
90. Cario H, McMullin M, Pahl H. (2009) Clinical and hematological presentation of children and adolescents with polycythemia vera. *Ann Hematol* **88**: 713–719.
91. Millard F, Hunter C, Anderson M, Edelman M, Kosty M, Luiken G, *et al.* (1990) Clinical manifestations of essential thrombocythemia in young adults. *Am J Hematol* **33**: 27–31.
92. Randi M, Rossi C, Fabris F, Girolami A. (2000) Essential thrombocythemia in young adults: Major thrombotic complications and complications during pregnancy — a followup study in 68 patients. *Clin Appl Thromb Hemost* **6**: 31–35.
96. Scott L, Tong W, Levine R, Scott M, Beer P, Stratton M, *et al.* (2007) JAK2 exon 12 mutations in polycythemia vera and idiopathic erythrocytosis. *N Engl J Med* **356**: 459–468.
113. Cario H, Schwarz K, Herter J, *et al.* (2008) Clinical and molecular characterization of a prospectively collected cohort of children and adolescents with polycythemia vera. *Br J Haematol* **142**: 622–626.
116. Alvarez-Larran A, Cervantes F, Bellosillo B, Giralt M, Julia A, Hernandez-Boluda J, *et al.* (2007) Essential thrombocythemia in young individuals: Frequency and risk factors for vascular events and evolution to myelofibrosis in 126 patients. *Leukemia* **21**: 1218–1223.
119. Palandri F, Polverelli N, Ottaviani E, Castagnetti F, Baccarani M, Vianelli N. (2010) Long-term follow-up of essential thrombocythemia in young adults: Treatment strategies, major thrombotic complications and pregnancy outcomes. A study of 76 patients. *Haematologica* **95**: 1038–1040.
123. Ding J, Komatsu H, Wakita A, Kato-Uranishi M, Ito M, Satoh A, *et al.* (2004) Familial essential thrombocythemia associated with a dominant-positive activating mutation of the c-MPL gene, which encodes for the receptor for thrombopoietin. *Blood* **103**: 4198–4200.
126. Harrison C, Campbell P, Buck G, Wheatley K, East C, Bareford D, *et al.* (2005) Hydroxyurea compared with anagrelide in high-risk essential thrombocythemia. *N Engl J Med* **353**: 33–45.
127. Sekhar M, Prentice H, Popat U, Anderson D, Janmohammed R, Roberts I, Britt R. (1996) Idiopathic myelofibrosis in children. *Br J Haematol* **93**: 394–397.
134. Cabelof D, Patel H, Chen Q, van Rammen H, Matherly L, Ge Y, Taub J. (2009) Mutational spectrum at GATA1 provides insights into mutagenesis and leukemogensis in Down syndrome. *Blood* **114**: 2753–2763.
136. Roy A, Roberts I, Norton A, Vyas P. (2009) Acute megakaryoblastic leukaemia (AMKL) and transient myeloproliferative disorder (TMD) in Down syndrome: A multi-step model of myeloid leukaemogenesis. *Br J Haematol* **147**: 3–12.
139. Niemeyer C, Kratz CP, Hasle H. (2005) Pediatric myelodysplastic syndromes. *Curr Treat Options Oncol* **6**: 209–214.
141. Hasle H, Niemeyer C, Chessells J, *et al.* (2003) A pediatric approach to the WHO classification of myelodysplastic and myeloproliferative disorders. *Leukemia* **17**: 277–282.
143. Novitzky N, Prindull G. (2000) Myelodysplatic syndromes in children: A critical review of clinical manifestations and management. *Am J Hematol* **63**: 212–222.

16

Childhood Non-Hodgkin Lymphoma

Ross Pinkerton and Mitchell S. Cairo

Introduction

The dramatic improvement in outcome for childhood lymphoma over the past 2 decades is testament to the value of collaborative multicenter studies investigating innovative chemotherapy regimens and treatment strategies.[1–4] The range of histological types of non-Hodgkin lymphomas (NHLs) in children is narrower than in adults and the majority are high-grade lymphoma with low-grade lymphoma such as classical follicular lymphoma being extremely rare. The commonest subtype, Burkitt lymphoma (BL), is curable in over 80% of cases. Treatment protocols based on immunological and morphological classifications are now standard, unlike in the past when similar regimens were used for all high-grade NHL. As a highly chemosensitive tumor, BL in childhood has been curable in those with localized diseases for many years using simple cyclophosphamide/doxorubicin-based chemotherapy. With dose intensification and enhanced central nervous system (CNS)-directed therapy, the outcome for those with bone marrow (BM) involvement and CNS disease has improved dramatically and is now around 80%. For very localized disease the treatment duration has been reduced to as short as 6 weeks.

The second largest group, T lymphoblastic lymphoma (TLL), now has outcome similar to T-cell acute lymphoblastic leukemia (ALL) using an almost identical treatment approach usually lasting up to 2 years. The third group, anaplastic large cell lymphoma (ALCL), which has come to prominence in the last decade as a result of more sophisticated immunophenotyping and cytogenetic studies, remains an enigmatic disease possibly consisting of a number of as yet undetermined subgroups. The optimum treatment remains to be defined but overall outcome has improved and is currently around 80% survival. Diffuse large B-cell lymphoma (DLBCL), including primary mediastinal B-cell lymphoma (PMBL), has generally been included on protocols designed for mature B NHL. With the larger numbers recruited on international collaborative studies, it has become feasible to address more specific questions for this subgroup.

The least common high-grade lymphoma in childhood is precursor B lymphoblastic lymphoma, which is treated in the same manner as the precursor B leukemia, with comparably good outcome. The recent demonstration of the value of monoclonal antibody in DLBCL in adults has excited interest in the application of immunotherapy in childhood BL and DLBCL; studies are underway to determine the precise role in various histological subtypes.

With the impressive overall long-term cure rates, emphasis is now on further definition of prognostic subgroups seeking to reduce both treatment duration and potential late sequelae in those with favorable outcome. This has led to reevaluation of traditional staging systems which have served well over many years but may now be of more value as simple descriptors of disease extent are used to allocate patients into specific prognostic groupings upon which treatment is based.

Historical Perspective

Early treatment regimens for childhood NHL mirrored those used in adults with a common strategy for all high-grade childhood NHLs. A number of protocols based on cyclophosphamide, doxorubicin, vincristine, and prednisolone (COMP), in some cases with blocks of treatment derived from either leukemia or adult NHL protocols, were evaluated. In the early eighties, with the development of immunophenotyping and clearer histopathological distinction of tumor types, it became clear that lymphoblastic lymphoma (LL) behaved very differently to BL. The LSA2L2 regimen was devised for ALL and comprised induction, intensification (asparaginase-based), and multiagent maintenance therapy. It appeared to also be effective in NHL. However, a Children's Cancer Group (CCG) randomized trial provided the rationale for treatment based on immunophenotype. This study showed clearly the superior outcome for BL when treated with the COMP regimen compared to LSA2L2 and, conversely, LL fared better with the LSA2L2 "leukaemia" approach compared to the shorter COMP regimen.[2,5] These differences applied mainly to those with nonlocalized disease and the issue of the best treatment strategy for those with localized disease has remained contentious. In the CCG trial, the survival for this group was 89% and 84% with COMP and LSA2L2, respectively.[5]

In contrast, for nonlocalized disease with LL, relapse-free survival (RFS) was 76% with LSA2L2 vs. 26% with COMP, and for undifferentiated (Burkitt), the reverse was observed; 57% RFS with COMP and 28% with LSA2L2.[6]

A subsequent study by the Pediatric Oncology Group (POG) compared a more intensive six drug ACOP (doxorubicin, cyclophosphamide, vincristine, prednisone) regimen with LSA2L2 specifically in LL and again showed no difference between regimens for localized disease but a nonstatistical advantage for leukemia-based regimen in stage 3 disease. The question of duration of treatment was also considered and irrespective of histological subtype for localized disease, there was no difference between 6 months and 18 months treatment duration.[6] The argument for a COMP-type regimen is the short duration and simplicity; a leukemia-based regimen has the advantage of less anthracycline and alkylating agent, but the total duration is much longer.

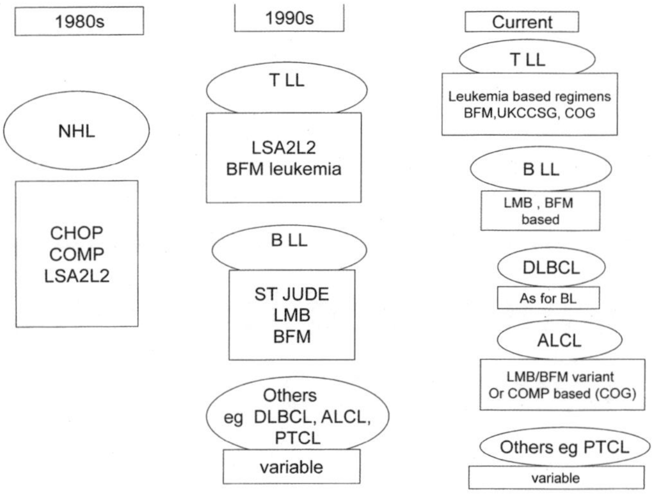

Fig. 16.1. Outline of the evolution of treatment strategies over recent decades (see text for description of regimens).

Figure 16.1 outlines the move from regarding pediatric NHL as a single entity with a common treatment approach, to a more refined strategy based on pathological subtype. Over the past 20 years, a series of randomized trials have addressed some key issues in the treatment of childhood NHL. These have been organized primarily by the CCG and POG (now combined as the Children's Oncology Group [COG]) in the USA during the 1980s and, subsequently, the French Society of Pediatric Oncology (SFOP), United Kingdom Children's Cancer Study Group (UKCCSG), and the Berlin-Frankfurt-Munster (BFM) Group. More recently, international collaboration between the USA, France and the UK led to the French–American–British/large mature B (FAB/LMB) study.

For LL, the main focus has been on the intensification of treatment, initially using the COMP regimen and subsequently leukemia-based protocols such as LSA2L2 or BFM strategy (see Chapter 12). Intensification of COMP with asparaginase and doxorubicin failed to show any significant benefit. Intensified asparaginase consolidation did, however, improve survival in a combined study of T-ALL and advanced LL. This trial was marred by an unexpected high incidence of second malignancy.[7] The addition of high-dose cytarabine to high-dose methotrexate (MTX) failed to lead to any advantage either in the instance of CNS relapse or systemic recurrence. *Erwinia* asparaginase was compared with *E. coli* asparaginase in another combined study of leukemia and lymphoma. This demonstrated a higher event-free survival (EFS) with *E. coli* asparaginase but an increased incidence of toxicity.[6]

In studies combining subtypes of non-LL, predominantly BL and DLBCL, a number of issues have been addressed. The SFOP Group demonstrated that reducing treatment duration to 4 months from 7 months maintained overall RFS. The St. Jude Group compared the total B protocol, which was the forerunner of many current regimens introducing very high doses of cytarabine and MTX, vs. traditional COMP regimen and demonstrated a significant advantage to the total B regimen. In contrast, modest alterations to the basic COMP regimen with the addition of doxorubicin failed to show an advantage.

Several trials have been carried out by the POG; the first failed to show any advantage to adding cyclophosphamide to the basic APO (doxorubicin, prednisone, vincristine, 6-mercaptopurine [6-MP]) regimen and, similarly, intensification of the maintenance phase of standard protocol adding intermediate-dose MTX and high-dose cytarabine did not significantly improve outcome.[6] It is of note, however, that in both those studies, a wide range of pathological subtypes were included and conclusions may not be applicable to a more defined group.

Treatment Strategies for Advanced Burkitt Lymphoma (BL)

In the mid 1980s, the St. Jude Group introduced the Total B protocol with the concept of significantly escalating the dose of cyclophosphamide with fractionation over a number of days, combined with both high-dose MTX and high-dose cytarabine. This high-dose intensity, short duration strategy was further developed by the BFM and LMB groups and the UKCCSG "MACHO" (cyclophosphamide, vincristine, adriamycin, MTX, cytosine arabinoside, triple intrathecal [IT]) protocol based on the St. Jude approach confirmed the initial encouraging results. The largest number of patients initially reported using this treatment approach was by the SFOP group, who demonstrated a clear improvement in the outcome of patients with advanced stage 3 disease and stage 4 or B-ALL. Initially, the outcome for those with CNS disease at presentation remained relatively poor despite the use of craniospinal irradiation and high-dose chemotherapy with BM rescue. A marked improvement in the outcome of this prognostic subgroup came with both the SFOP and BFM utilization of more aggressive triple IT therapy and escalation of the dose of both MTX and cytarabine.[3,8,9] This led to one of the most dramatic improvements in cure rate of any children's cancer, from virtually incurable in the 1980s to 70% cure at present time. The superiority of the total B protocol compared to cyclophosphamide, doxorubicin, vincristine and prednisone (CHOP) was demonstrated in a randomized trial and similarly the LMB approach was superior to the more conventional "Orange" regimen. A number of ultra short protocols have been developed e.g. the Milan protocol, where treatment is completed within a 45-day period.[10] Experience with this approach is limited but published data on 60 patients, including 14 with CNS and or BM disease, report an overall EFS of 81%. The BFM and LMB protocols are summarized in Figs. 16.2A–B and the Milan regimen in Figs. 16.3A–C. One significant difference between these regimens is the use of intraventricular chemotherapy in children with initial CNS disease in the BFM protocol. With this approach, around 60% of patients with initial CNS disease survive compared to 80% with stage 4 or B-ALL that are CNS negative. This does not seem significantly different from that recorded from the LMB group and the value of intraventricular as opposed to repeat IT therapy remains unproven.

With the overall excellent outcome for most risk groups, an important question has been how to further refine treatment in order to reduce morbidity in better risk patients but define more precisely poor risk groups in whom more intensive strategies may be appropriate. In the SFOP and subsequent LMB regimens, the initial response to cyclophosphamide, vincristine, prednisone (COP) and the failure to obtain a histologically proven complete remission (CR) after three courses of intensive chemotherapy has been an indication to intensify treatment. In the BFM 90 and 95 protocols, patients in risk groups R2 and R3 who had an incomplete response were escalated to the CC protocol including high-dose cytarabine and etoposide (Fig. 16.2A). This almost identical approach was followed in the SFOP where cytarabine and etoposide was utilized in this risk group (Fig. 16.2B). Both study groups followed a strategy of assessing any residual imageable abnormality with surgical biopsy and, in the presence of active tumor further dose escalation, was indicated. In the BFM group, this was after the intensive CC course; in the SFOP protocol, it was after CYM1. Unresectable viable tumor at this time was an indication for moving to high-dose therapy with stem cell rescue.

Risk Group	Definition	Therapy Courses
R1	Stage I+II, completely resected	A B
R2	Stage I+II, not resected Stage III and LDH < 500 U/L	V A B A B
R3	Stage III and LDH ≥500-<1000 U/L Stage IV+B-AL and LDH <1000 U/L and CNS-neg.	V AA BB CC AA BB
R4	Stage III+IV+B-AL and LDH ≥1000 U/L or/and CNS-pos.	V AA BB CC AA BB CC

Fig. 16.2A. Treatment strategy. Patients were stratified into four risk groups: R1, R2, R3, and R4. V indicates cytoreductive prephase.

A: dexamethasone, vincristine, ifosfamide, cytarabine; B: dexamethasone, vincristine, cyclophosphamide, doxorubicin; V: prophase, dexamethasone, cyclophosphamide; AA: high-dose methotrexate; CC: dexamethasone, vincristine, high-dose cytarabine, etoposide.

Used with permission Woessmann *et al.* (2005) The impact of the methotrexate administration schedule and dose in the treatment of children and adolescents with B-cell neoplasms: A report of the BFM Group Study NHL-BFM95 *Blood* **105**: 948–958.

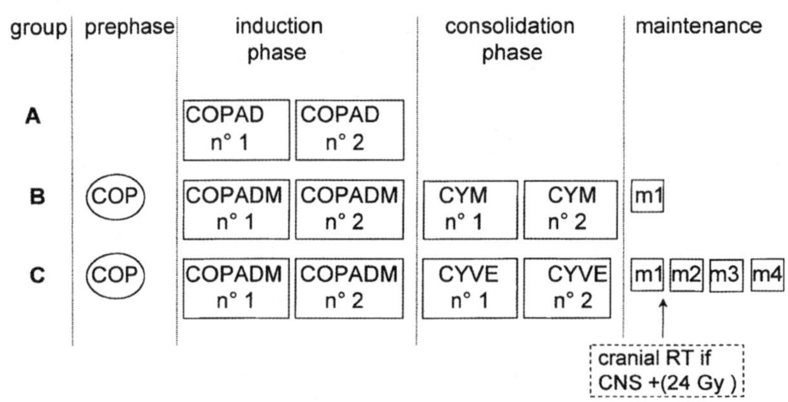

Fig. 16.2B. LMB89 protocol schedule. Patients were stratified into three risk groups: A, B, and C, depending on stage, resection status, percentage of blasts in BM, and CNS involvement.

COP: cyclophosphamide, vincristine, prednisone; COPAD: cyclophosphamide, vincristine, doxorubicin; COPADM: cyclophosphamide, vincristine, high-dose methotrexate; CYM: cytarabine, high-dose methotrexate; CYVE: high-dose cytarabine, etoposide; M1: vincristine, high-dose methotrexate, prednisone, cyclophosphamide, doxorubicin; M3: vincristine, high-dose methotrexate, prednisone, cyclophosphamide, doxorubicin minus high-dose methotrexate; M2, M4: etoposide, cytarabine.

Used with permission Patte *et al.* (2001) The Société Française d'Oncologie Pédiatrique LMB89 protocol: highly effective multiagent chemotherapy tailored to the tumor burden and initial response in 561 unselected children with B-cell lymphomas and L3 leukemia *Blood* **97**: 3370–3379.

In order to try and limit both early and late morbidity, the FABLMB trial was designed.[11,12] This was a collaboration between the UKCCSG, SFOP, and the CCG. The study recruited over a thousand patients and addressed specific issues in two risk groups with advanced disease. Group C was the high-risk group comprising patients presenting with CNS disease, B-ALL or BM involvement greater than 25%. In this group, the issues of dose level and intensity were addressed. Patients were randomized to receive full or half dose cytarabine in combination with etoposide and also deletion of the three maintenance courses M2, M3, M4. All patients with CNS disease had additional high dose MTX (8 gm/m^2) plus extra IT therapy with triple drugs. In this study, 51% of patients had BM involvement, 20% CNS involvement and 29% combined BM and CNS. One hundred and ninety patients were randomized and overall, the 4-year EFS was 79%.[11] Overall, patients with combined BM and CNS had a significantly worse outcome, 61% EFS compared to either isolated BM or CNS 88% and 83%, respectively (Fig. 16.4A). Despite intensification of treatment, it is of note that the

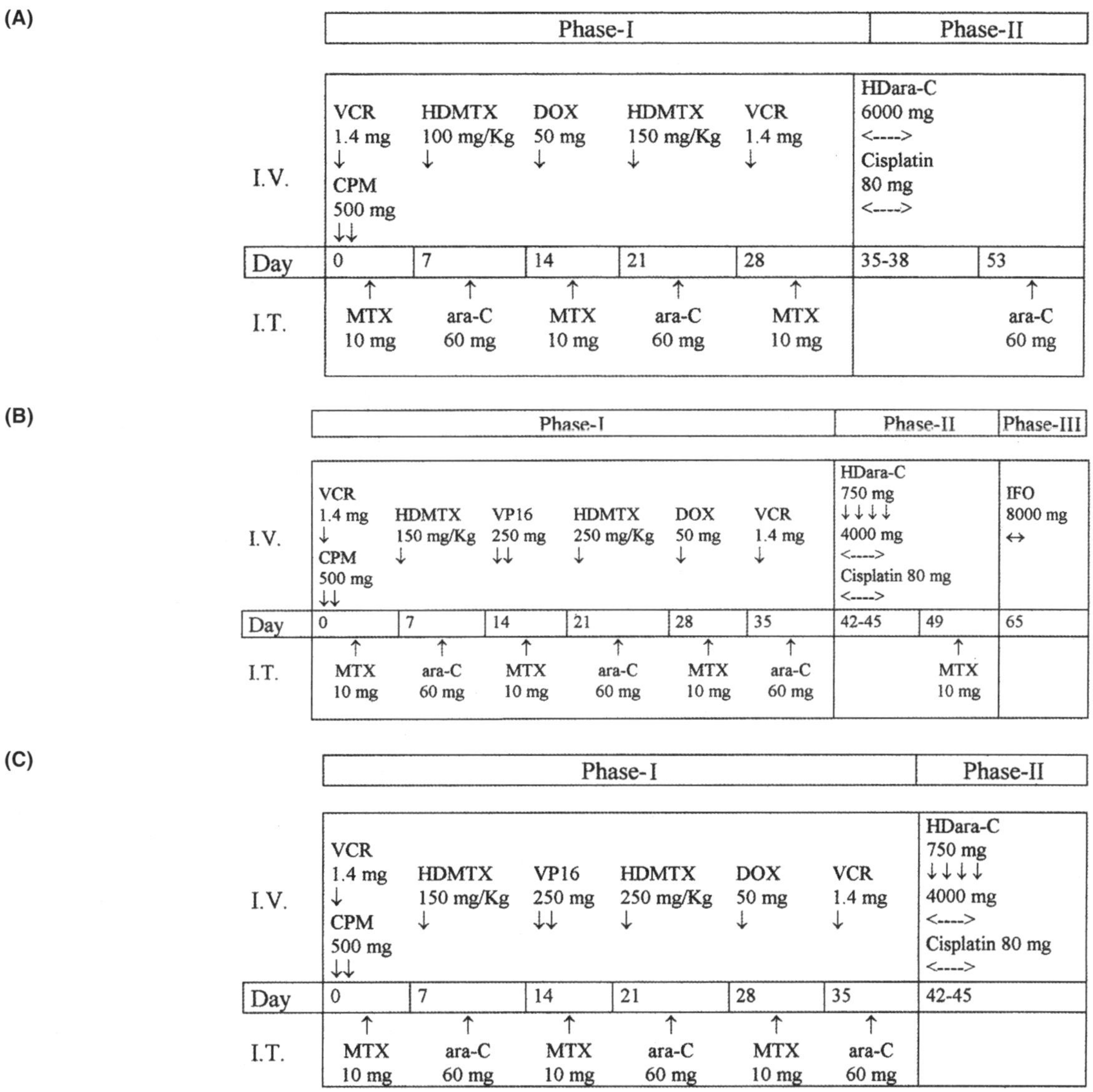

Fig. 16.3. (A) Regimen IA, used for patients with disease without bone marrow or CNS involvement (1987–1992). Drug doses are expressed as mg/m^2; for HDMTX, in mg/kg. VCR, vincristine; CPM, cyclophosphamide. (B) Regimen IB, used for patients with disease with bone marrow or CNS involvement (1987–1992). Drug doses are expressed as mg/m^2; for HDMTX, in mg/kg. (C) Regimen II, used from 1992 onward for patients with Murphy's stage III to IV Burkitt's lymphoma. Drug doses are expressed as mg/m^2; for HDMTX, in mg/kg.

Used with permission Spreafico F, Massimino M, Luksch R, Casanova M, Cefalo GS, Collini P, Ferrari A, Polastri D, Terenziani M, Gasparini M, Fossati-Bellani F. (2002) Intensive, very short-term chemotherapy for advanced burkitt's lymphoma in children. *J Clin Oncol* **20**: 2783–2788.

poor initial COP responders still had a significantly inferior outcome and alternative approaches are required for this small group (Fig. 16.4B).[11] In patients randomized to standard vs. reduced intensity treatment, the 4-year EFS was 90% vs. 80% and survival is 93% vs. 83%.[11] It was concluded that higher doses of chemotherapy with the significant increase in infection, stomatitis, and nonhematological toxicity, was justified to achieve optimal outcome.

The largest subgroup in the LMB trial was group B, which comprised those not within the very good- or very poor-risk groups, the majority of these being Murphy stage 3 or stage 4 with less than 25% BM involvement. In this study, there were four arms, two receiving half dose cyclophosphamide in the second induction course cyclophosphamide, vincristine, high-dose methotrexate (COPADM) and two not receiving the maintenance course M1.[12] A total of 657 patients were randomized

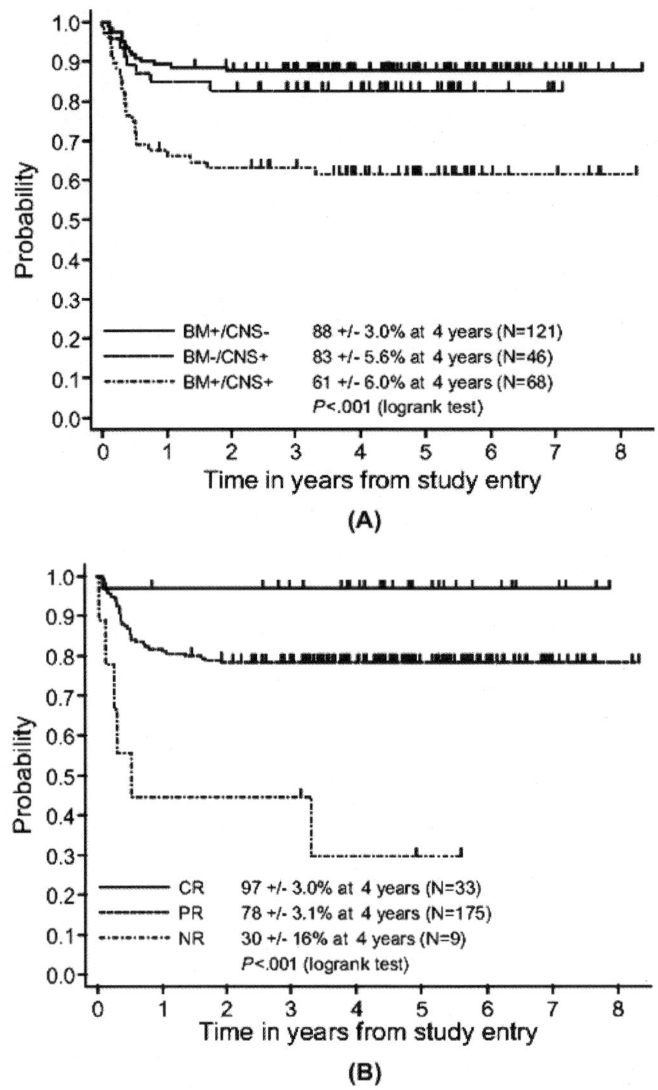

Fig. 16.4. Stratified probabilities. Probability of EFS and S stratified by (A) BM, CNS, or BM/CNS and (B) response to COP reduction. (A) Product-limit estimate of probability of EFS in patients with BM disease only (BM^+/CNS^-), CNS disease only (BM^-/CNS^+), and combined BM and CNS disease (BM^+/CNS^+) (88% ± 3.0% vs. 82 ± 5.6% vs. 61% ± 6.0%, $P < .001$). (B) Product-limit estimate of probability of EFS in patients with complete response (CR; 100%), incomplete response (IR; 20%–99%) and nonresponse (NR; < 20%) after COP reduction therapy (94% ± 3.8% vs. 78% ± 3.1% vs. 30% ± 16%, $P < .001$).

Used with permission Cairo MS, Gerrard M, Sposto R, Auperin A, Pinkerton CR, Michon J, Weston C, Perkins SL, Raphael M, McCarthy K, Patte C. (2007) Results of a randomized international study of high-risk central nervous system b non-Hodgkin lymphoma and b acute lymphoblastic leukemia in children and adolescents. *Blood* **109**: 2736–2743.

and the 4-year EFS was 93% and 90% for full dose and half dose cyclophosphamide, respectively, and 91% and 92% in the groups with and without maintenance therapy M1 (Figs. 16.5A–D).[12] For BL specifically, there was no difference in outcome between the 228 patients who received full dose cyclophosphamide and the 222 who received half dose cyclophosphamide or the 219 patients receiving or not receiving maintenance therapy. It was concluded that patients who have initial response to COP chemotherapy and have achieved CR after the third course can be cured with four-course treatment, limiting the dose of both cyclophosphamide and doxorubicin.[12]

For localized disease, relatively simple chemotherapy is highly effective and CHOP, COMP, or APO have been used by different groups. Studies in which LL (precursor B and T) and non-lymphoblastic NHL were combined have generally shown an excellent outcome

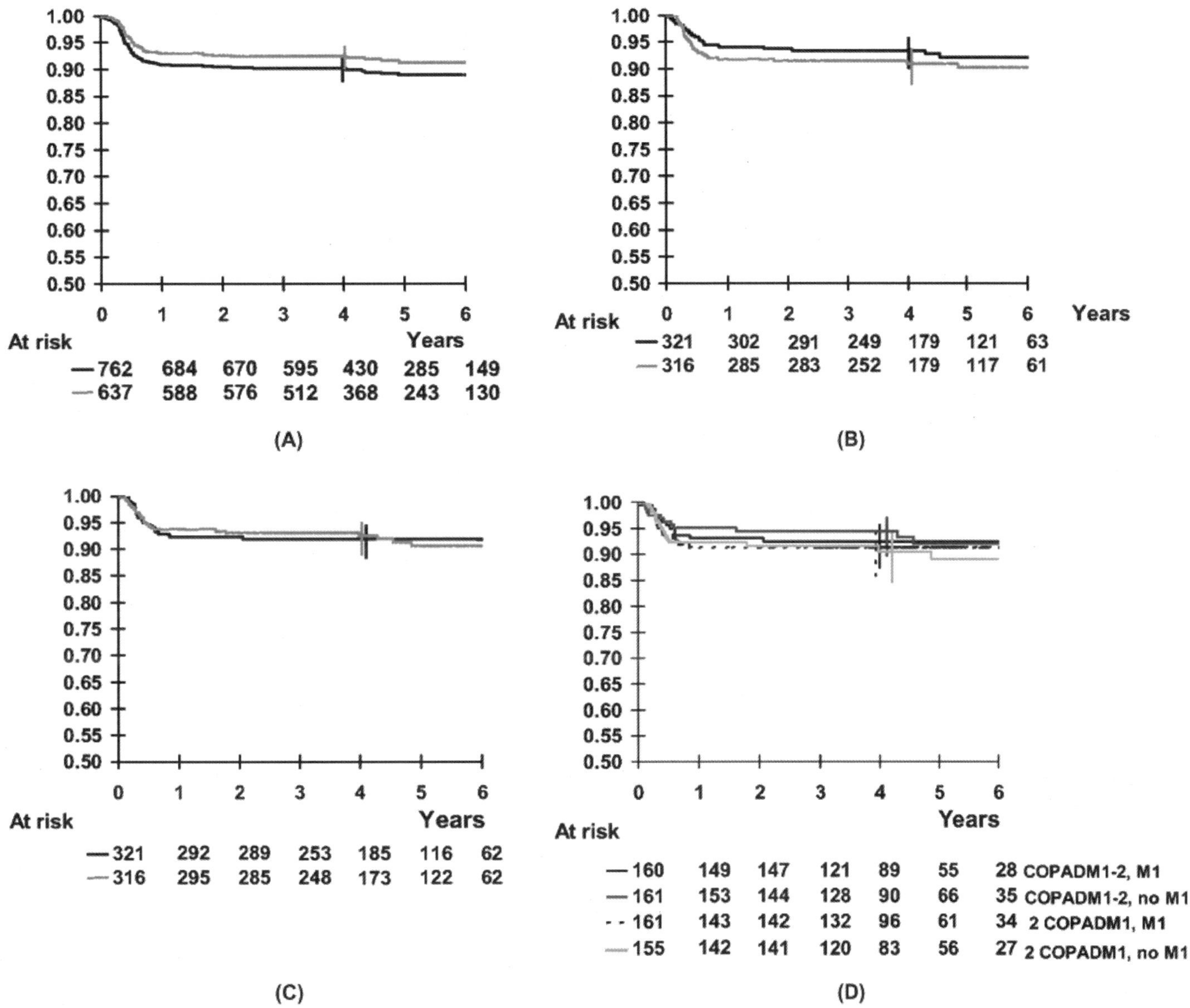

Fig. 16.5. Kaplan-Meier curves for survival, EFS, and FFS. Vertical bars denote 95% CI of the actuarial rates. (A) Kaplan-Meier estimates of EFS of all patients and of randomized patients. Solid black line indicates all patients, 4-year rate, 90.2%; dotted line, randomized patients, 4-year rate from start of treatment, 92.4% (92.2% from time of randomization). (B) Kaplan-Meier estimates of EFS according to cyclophosphamide dose randomization in the second COPADM course. Black line indicates full-dose CPM in second COPADM, 4-year rate, 93.4%; gray line, half-dose CPM in second COPADM, 4-year rate, 90.9%. (C) Kaplan-Meier estimates of EFS according to maintenance course M1 randomization. Black line indicates with M1, 4-year rate, 91.9%; gray line, without M1, 4-year rate, 92.5%. (D) Kaplan-Meier estimates of EFS according to the 4 arms of randomization. COPADM1–2, M1 (standard), 4-year rate, 92.5%; COPADM1–2, no M1, 4-year rate, 94.4%; 2 COPADM1, M1, 4-year rate, 91.3%; 2 COPADM1, no M1, 4-year rate, 90.5.

Used with permission Patte C, Auperin A, Gerrard M, Michon J, Pinkerton R, Sposto R, Weston C, Raphael M, Perkins SL, McCarthy K, Cairo MS. (2007) Results of the randomized international fab/lmb96 trial for intermediate risk B-cell non-Hodgkin lymphoma in children and adolescents: It is possible to reduce treatment for the early responding patients. *Blood* **109**: 2773–2780.

almost irrespective of the chemotherapy used. Longer follow up has, however, demonstrated that the late relapse rate is higher with LL where the shorter CHOP type protocol is used. The difference is less marked than with advanced disease; therefore, there has remained some controversy about the best approach. In general a full leukemia regimen lasting 2 years is recommended even for minimal bulk LL.

In BL, the aim of recent studies has been to determine how minimal treatment can be, avoiding late effects but maintaining effectiveness. The UKCCSG developed a regimen, which omitted cyclophosphamide to avoid the risk of impaired fertility,[13] also applied by the CCSG with the APO regimen. The SFOP group demonstrated that two courses of COPAD (cyclophosphamide, vincristine, doxorubicin) was adequate and this was confirmed in the nonrandomized component of the FAB LMB trial (group A). In the latter, 132 patients with stage 1 and 2 diseases were included with an EFS of 98%.[14]

The role of MTX scheduling has been addressed by the BFM group in a randomized trial where a prolonged 24-hour infusion was compared with a 4-hour infusion. This demonstrated that there was no difference for standard risk patients, but the outcome in the high-risk group was superior.[15]

Radiation therapy has no role in first line therapy for any type of NHL in childhood, except occasionally as an emergency treatment to relieve local tumor pressure on vital organs. This is rarely required due to the usual sensitivity of most childhood NHL to steroids and chemotherapy. In the case of a slower than anticipated response, low-dose radiotherapy may be administered to local bulky disease. In the past, patients with CNS disease at presentation were felt to be candidates for this modality but the FABLMB trial has shown clearly that with very intensive IT therapy and CNS-directed systemic therapy, the outcome is as good as when the radiation is given.[11] Consideration should however, be given to the use of local radiation as part of second-line therapy, particularly if there is a slow response to second-line therapy. Again, individualization and consideration of likely individual morbidity must be taken into consideration in each case.

In the 1980s, when the overall outcome was poor, particularly in patients with stage 4 disease, many protocols included high-dose, with either autologous or allogeneic, stem cell procedures. With the dramatic improvement of outcome, particularly in those with stage 4 or B ALL, there appears to be little, if any, indication to such an approach in the first remission. In those with a poor COP response, residual unresected active disease mid-therapy, there may be a role for autograft procedures (see Chapter 20).

Treatment for Diffuse Large B-Cell Lymphoma (DLBCL)

The prognosis for advanced DLBCL has also improved significantly over the past few decades.[16–18] In Europe, these patients are generally included in protocols for treatment of mature B-cell lymphoma such as the SFOP or BFM Burkitt regimens.[8,12] With this approach, the outcome is at least as good as for BL. In view of the much lower risk of BM or CNS disease, it seems likely that a number of patients are receiving excessive treatment. There are lessons to be learned from the American experience where less aggressive treatment regimens such as the APO protocol have been used. A randomized study run by the COG study group addressed the question whether incorporating a higher dose of MTX and cytarabine in the maintenance phase of the APO regimen would improve outcome.[19] One hundred and eighty patients were enrolled and the 4-year EFS was 67% overall. As with many other studies in large cell lymphoma (LCL) in childhood, this included a range of histological subtypes; 86 were ALCL, 10 peripheral B-cell lymphoma and only 73 were DLBCL. There was no significant differences in the EFS in the latter group of patients, with 4-year EFS for APO alone, 64% and the intensified MTX and cytarabine regimen, 70%. More recent experience in adults with DLBCL have reported excellent outcome using the dose intensive CHOP 14 rituximab protocol, but to date, there is no experience with this protocol in children.[20,21] Because of the rarity of this tumor type, international collaboration would be required to clarify the extent dose reduction may be feasible or whether the introduction of rituximab may be advantageous.

A novel approach used by the St. Jude group in an attempt to reduce late toxicity, was the introduction of the DHAP (dexamethasone, cytarabine, cisplatin) regimen which is of proven value in adults with high risk lymphoma.[22] Two courses of DAC (high-dose cytarabine, dexamethasone, carboplatin) (selected rather than cisplatin) were given prior to the conventional ACOP+ regimen (cyclophosphamide, doxorubicin, vincristine, 6-MP, and prednisone). An overall response rate of 88%, including 52% CR, was reported; overall EFS was 54%. This series, however, contained a heterogeneous group of tumors, predominantly ALCL. Of six patients with DLBCL, all were alive in remission at follow up. The relatively high doses of carboplatin and cytarabine inevitably resulted in this regimen being severely myelosuppressive with attendant complications, but has important potential with regard to sparing the dose of anthracycline and alkylating agent in both this and other histological subtypes.

Treatment for PMBL

PMBL usually presents as a large mediastinal mass perhaps involving adjacent structures in mediastinal and lung parenchyma. In general, extranodal spread to other organs such as BM or CNS is very rare (Table 16.1). The most appropriate treatment is yet to be defined in children and because of its rarity there are few large published series. A study published in 2000[23] suggested that LCL arising in mediastinum was associated with excellent outcome. In this CCG report, the 5-year EFS was 75% which compared favorably with outcome for mature B-cell lymphoma at that time. With the steady improvement in the outcome of the latter, PMBL has lagged behind and in a recent review of this pathological subgroup within the FAB/LMB trial, the outcome was clearly inferior.[24] Of 111 patients with DLBCL, 42 were PMBL. These were treated intensively with group B therapy. Two-year EFS for stage 3 PMBL was 69%, significantly less than the 91% for other DLBCL on the same regimen. Seventeen percent of the PMBL patients had a less than 20% response to initial COP treatment, although this did not have an adverse impact upon outcome.[24] In an analysis of three therapeutic studies run by the BFM Group,[25] 30 patients (1.8%) of the total population of pediatric NHL had PMBL. As for many other histological subtypes, the BFM approach was similar to that for BL with a combination of the classic AB or AA/BB/CC regimen (Fig. 16.1A). In the BFM95 study, risk group 2 were St. Jude stage 3 with lactate dehydrogenase (LDH) less than 500 who received two A blocks and 2 B blocks. Risk 3, stage 3 with LDH 500–1000 received two courses AA, two courses BB and one course CC and risk group 4 with LDH greater than 1000 received an additional CC course. Of particular interest in this analysis was the rate of patients who failed to have an initial CR. Of 22 patients with an incomplete response after two courses, five had second-look surgery and of these, all five had necrotic tissue. Of a further 15 who had residual imageable abnormality at the end of chemotherapy, three were biopsied and all again had necrotic tissue. In total, two patients received local radiation therapy but overall disease recurred in only four patients. In this series, LDH retained significant prognostic impact with LDH less than 500, 88% EFS compared to only 40% for LDH over 500.[25] In the more recent FAB/LMB trial, LDH did not appear to have significant influence. In a review combining data on 116 patients from the American, French, German, and Italian studies between 1984 and 2003, the overall survival (OS) was 79% and EFS 67%.[26] There was no difference in outcome in patients with PMBL who received radiotherapy for failure to achieve a CR in the Italian group series. This again emphasizes the high incidence of inactive imageable disease following treatment. In a review comparing outcome in pediatric and adult studies, three pediatric and four adult trials described and contrasted[27] a variety of regimens used, with improved outcome in the more intensified multi-agent regimens, in some cases including high-dose therapy and stem cell rescue. Reports of dose-adjusted EPOCH, particularly with the addition of rituximab, suggest a significant improvement with over 80% OS.[28] In most adult studies, involved-field radiation therapy was incorporated and appeared to improve outcome regardless of the type of chemotherapy; this review concluded that this modality is an important component in the treatment of PMBL. This has not, however, been generally accepted in pediatric practice. To what extent the addition of rituximab will be of benefit

Table 16.1. Comparative clinical features of diffuse large B-cell lymphoma, primary mediastinal B-cell lymphoma and Burkitt lymphoma.

	All DLBCL	PMBCL	BL
No. of patients	244	33	924
Male: female	2:1	1.06:1	4.7:1
Age, M, Range	11.4 (1.4–17.9)	14.7 (1.4–17.9)	8.6 (0.7–19.2)
Stage 1 (St. Jude)	21%	0%	9%
II	35%	0%	22%
III	41%	97%	41%
IV	4%	3%	28%[a]
BM	1%	3%	25%
CNS	3%	0%	10%
Mediastinal	14%	100%	8%
Lung	5%	36%	2%
Kidney	4%	24%	13%
Skin	1%	0%	1%
Bone	8%	3%	7%
Soft tissue	3%	3%	3%
Pleural effusion	3%	39%	14%
Ascites	6%	6%	24%
B_Symptoms	14%	36%	17%
LDH ≥ 500 U/I	14%	30%	46%

[a]Including cases with > 25% FAB-L3 blasts in the bone marrow ("B-ALL").

BL: Burkitt lymphoma; BM: bone marrow; CNS: central nervous system; DLBCL: diffuse large B-cell lymphoma; PMBCL: primary mediastinal (thymic) large B-cell lymphoma.

Adapted with permission from Reiter A, Klapper W. (2008) Recent advances in the understanding and management of diffuse large B-cell lymphoma in children. *Br J Haematol* **142**: 329–347, © John Wiley & Sons.

needs to be the subject of a future prospective randomized trial.

Treatment for ALCL

Many early reports of treatment for ALCL have included a range of other histological subtypes. It is only with the widespread application of anti-CD30 antibody and improved cytogenetics that separation of ALCL has been become clearer. Previous studies have included peripheral T-cell lymphoma (PTCL) and Hodgkin lymphoma (HL).

The presenting features of ALCL are very different for other subtypes (Table 16.2) and over the past decade, a small number of key publications have outlined a number of different treatment strategies. The BFM Group and the UKCCSG have applied a standard mature B-cell treatment program identical to that used for BL. The SFOP Group also developed a short-duration pulsed regimen incorporating some aspects of a Burkitt protocol but adding agents such as vinblastine. The approach applied by the St. Jude group and the Italian Association of Pediatric Hematology/Oncology (AIEOP) was based on the LSA2L2 program for T-cell lymphoma/leukemia and the APO regimen has formed the basis of recent COG studies.

More recent reports have applied prognostic grouping derived from a review carried out by the European Intergroup for childhood NHL.[29] This retrospective analysis of over 200 patients treated by BFM, SFOP and the UKCCSG between 1986 and 1997 demonstrated that with the use of the standard B-cell or modified SFOP protocol, a high-risk group could be identified, namely those with mediastinal involvement, visceral involvement or skin disease. In this group, the relative risk of relapse was 4.4 compared to standard risk and OS 4.8 (Fig. 16.6).

The AIEOPLNH92 protocol[30] was based on the LSA2L2 regimen with induction phase followed by consolidation and maintenance for a total of 24 months, independent of stage. This included two courses of high-dose MTX (2 gm/m^2 as a 2-hour infusion). During the latter part of the study, the maintenance was changed from weekly rotation of doublets of cyclophosphamide, MTX, 6-MP, cytarabine, VM-26,

Table 16.2. Clinical features of anaplastic large cell lymphoma.

Characteristics	Total n = 225 n (%)
Sex: Male	140 (62)
Age: ≥ 10 years	117 (52)
Positivity for ALK antibody (82 MD)	128/143 (90)
Immunophenotype	
T-markers	135 (71)
Null	55 (29)
B symptoms (1 MD)	121 (54)
Lymph nodes,	206 (92)
Lymph nodes, mediastinal involvement	81 (36)
Extranodal disease	154 (68)
Skin lesion (s)	59 (26)
Bone lesion (s)	32 (14)
Marrow involvement	17 (8)
CNS disease	3 (1)
Soft tissue mass	33 (15)
Visceral involvement including:	97 (43)
Spleen involvement	42 (19)
Liver involvement	42 (19)
Lung lesion	28 (12)
Other visceral involvement	52 (23)
St. Jude staging	
Stage 1	19 (9)
Stage 2	39 (17)
Stage 3	147 (65)
Stage 4	20 (9)

MD: missing data.

Adapted from Le Deley MC, Reiter A, Williams D, Delsol G, Oschlies I, McCarthy K, Zimmermann M, Brugieres L. (2008) Prognostic factors in childhood anaplastic large cell lymphoma: Results of a large European intergroup study. *Blood* **111**: 1560–1566.

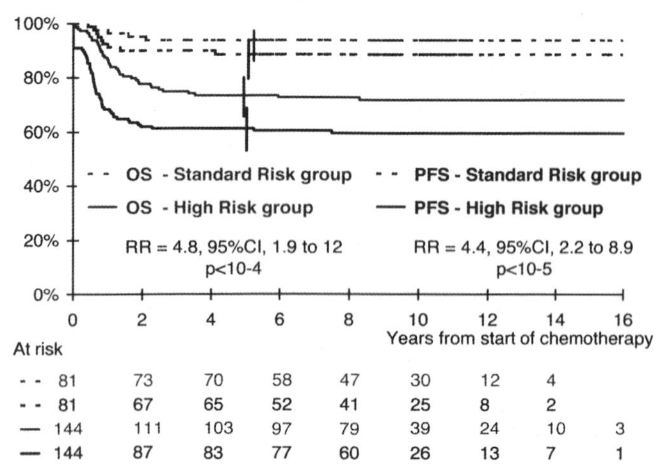

Fig. 16.6. OS and PFS according to risk group. Standard risk group indicates no risk factor (i.e. no mediastinal involvement and no lung, spleen, or liver involvement, and no skin lesion). High-risk group, at least one risk factor, mediastinal involvement, visceral involvement, or skin lesion.

Used with permission Le Deley MC, Reiter A, Williams D, Delsol G, Oschlies I, McCarthy K, Zimmermann M, Brugieres L. (2008) Prognostic factors in childhood anaplastic large cell lymphoma: Results of a large european intergroup study. *Blood* **111**: 1560–1566.

vincristine and dexamethasone, to a simpler maintenance regimen with weekly MTX and daily oral 6-MP. CR was achieved in 88% of patients and EFS was 65%, with OS 85%. The numbers were relatively small with only 34 included, but almost half of these had poor-risk features such as mediastinal mass or skin involvement.[30] Using a T-cell directed approach, the CCG 5941 protocol was used in 86 children with non-localized ALCL.[31] There were 21 relapses and four toxic deaths. Five-year EFS was 68% and only BM involvement was an independent predictor of outcome (Fig. 16.7).[31]

The UKCCSG reported 72 patients included with a standard 9003 or 9002 B-cell regimen.[32] The CR rate was 82% but the EFS at 5 years was 59%. In the larger NHL BFM 90 protocol, patients were stratified into three branches: risk group K1 stage 1 and 2 resected who received three 5-day courses of the regimen ABA as per the B NHL regimen, risk group K2 stage 2 non-resection at stage 3 received six courses alternating AB, risk group K3 for stage 4 or multiple bone involvement received a more intensive regimen including a higher dose of MTX 5 gm/m^2 given over a 24-hour period. In this study, as in the UKCCSG trial, over a third of patients had a mediastinal mass and almost one-fifth had skin disease.[33] For group K1, there was a 100% EFS, K3 79% and K2 73%. The results are better than the UKCCSG series presumable secondary to more prolonged infusions in the BFM regimen but there are also

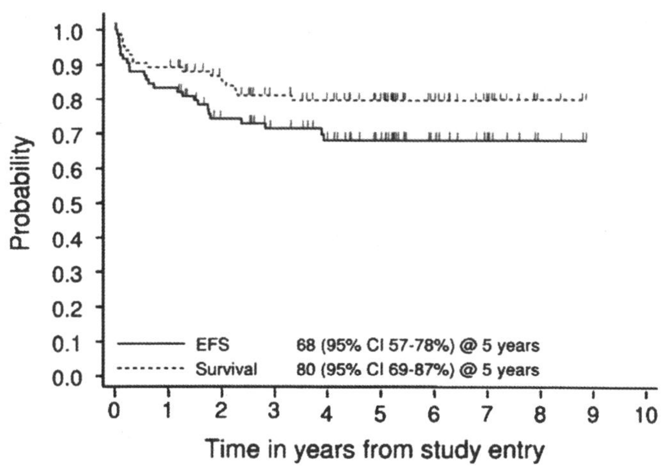

Fig. 16.7. Overall and event-free survival of 86 patients with systemic ALCL treated on CCG-5941.

Used with permission Lowe EJ, Sposto R, Perkins SL, Gross TG, Finlay J, Zwick D, Abromowitch M. (2009) Intensive chemotherapy for systemic anaplastic large cell lymphoma in children and adolescents: Final results of children's cancer group study 5941. *Pediatr Blood Cancer* **52**: 335–339.

differences such as the inclusion of dexamethasone and cytosine/etoposide. In the UKCCSG protocol, high-dose cytarabine/etoposide was only used for the rare CNS-positive patients.

The SFOP HM89 and HM91 protocols[34] resembled the LMB regimens for mature B NHL but included etoposide in the VEN block and vinblastine, etoposide and bleomycin in the VEBBP block. Eighty-two patients were reported, of whom 39% had mediastinal disease and 33% had skin disease. The EFS of the whole cohort was 66% with OS of 83%. In this report, mediastinal and visceral involvement and high LDH appear to be risk factors. When analyzed on the basis of St. Jude classification, stage 1 and 2 (17 patients) had an EFS of 100%. In this group, those with the above mentioned risk factors, the 3-year EFS was 67%. For St. Jude stage 3 and 4, the EFS for the group overall was 86%, but for those with adverse risk factors it was only 45%.[34]

In recent years, two important randomized trials have addressed key issues in ALCL in children. The COG ANHL0131 is a randomized trial comparing standard APO vs. consolidation with a regimen including vinblastine. The study was open to stage 3 and 4 patients. The duration of therapy was 1 year, initially the dose of 6 mg/m^2 of vinblastine was used but due to hematological toxicity, this was reduced to 4 mg/m^2 given weekly. Interim analysis of 119 patients revealed a 75% 2-year EFS for standard APO and 80% for patients receiving vinblastine. The APV arm was associated with more toxicity. However, there is no difference in OS which was 90% and 86%, respectively.[35] A major collaborative European study including German, Italian, French and UK groups, the EICNHL (European Intergroup Co-operation on Childhood NHL) group, have completed a study where the NHL BFM90 protocol was used in a large group of both high-and standard-risk patients.[36] The patients were classified as high risk if there was at least one risk factor, defined as the presence of skin and/or mediastinal and/or visceral involvement (defined as lung/liver/spleen involvement) and a standard risk if there are no adverse risk factors. One arm included MTX 1 gm/m^2 as a 24-hour infusion with triple IT chemotherapy; the other received a higher dose of 3 gm/m^2 given as a short 3-hour infusion but without IT injections. Additionally, high-risk patients could enter a second trial that randomly assigned patients to receive 6 mg/m^2 of vinblastine during the periods of pulsed chemotherapy and then weekly for a total duration of 1 year. Interim analysis of the latter component, reported at the Frankfurt NHL meeting, demonstrated that in 217 patients recruited to the study with a median follow up of 4.7 years, patients who received vinblastine had a low risk of events during the first year (hazard ratio 0.3), however they, had an increased risk of relapse beyond the first year and consequently EFS differed at 1 year, 74% vs. 91%, but no different at 2 years 70% vs. 73%, respectively. It appeared that the addition of vinblastine during induction and maintenance after 1 year simply delayed recurrence of relapse but did not reduce the overall risk of failure. Full analysis of the first question regarding MTX therapy demonstrated that of 375 randomized patients with median follow up of 3½ years CR rates were identical, 89% and 87%, respectively, for MTX1 and MTX3 and the EFS occurrence were also superimposed at 74% (Figs. 16.8A–C).[35] It is concluded, that the high dose over a short period was comparable to a low dose over a longer period with regard to systemic disease control and the short higher dose removed the need for additional IT therapy. Moreover, the incidence of toxicity was significantly higher in patients given the low infusion schedule with regard to neutropenia, thrombocytopenia infection, and stomatitis.

Minimal residual disease (MRD) evaluation in ALCL is emerging as an important component of prognostic grouping and is likely to be incorporated in future regimens (see Chapter 10).

Intriguing data on the favorable outcome in patients with anti-anaplastic lymphoma kinase (ALK) antibodies has raised the possibility of active immunotherapy strategies (see later in this chapter). There are, occasionally, patients presenting with unusual features such as isolated single bone lesion or isolated skin disease. These are too rare to be confidently included in specific risk groups and it is possible that these receive unnecessary intensive chemotherapy. Overall, the outcome in these subgroups has been favorable despite the sites being adverse prognostic factors as part of a multisystem disease.

Treatment for LL

The treatment of precursor T-LL and precursor B-LL are essentially the same, and improved outcome has followed that for ALL.[37] For localized diseases using simpler regimens for all histological subtypes, the outcome was poorer for LL compared to mature B-cell lymphoma. This has been the experience of both COG and the CCG, where a duration of 6 months appears to be inadequate in contrast to the full 2-year regimen that reported EFS over 80%. These patients may present with very small bulk disease and it is tempting to rely on reduced intensity chemotherapy. Although the initial

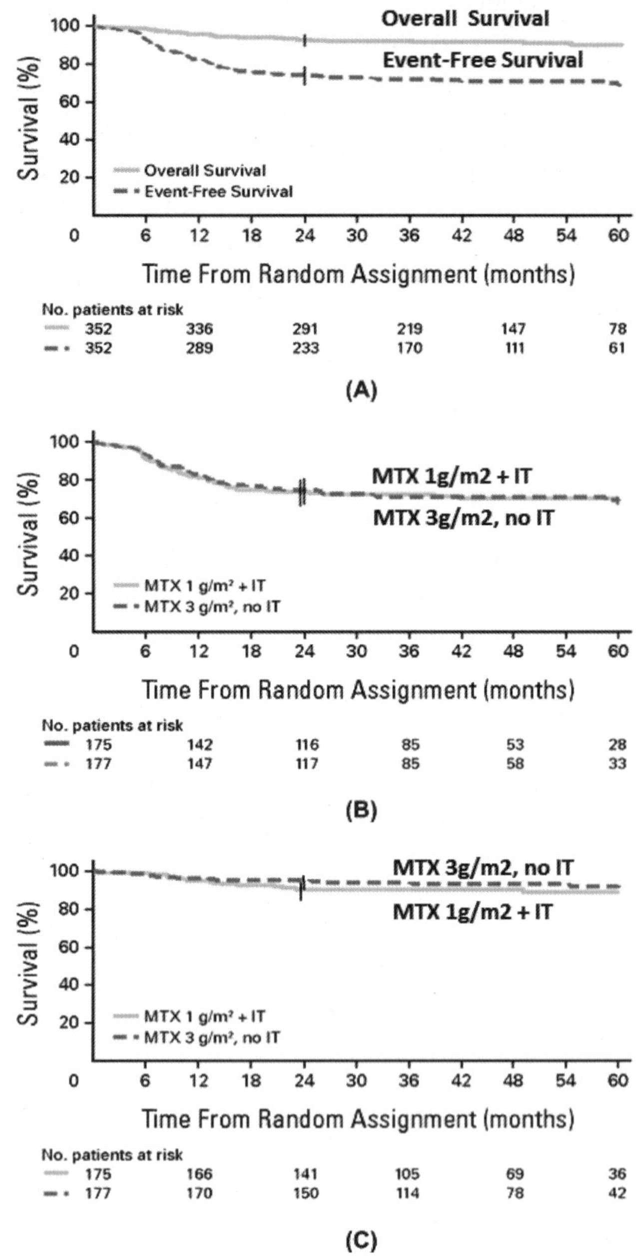

Fig. 16.8. (A) Event-free survival (EFS) and overall survival (OS) of the whole study population. (B) EFS by treatment. (C) OS by treatment. MTX, methotrexate.

Used with permission Brugieres L, Le Deley MC, Rosolen A, Williams D, Horibe K, Wrobel G, Mann G, Zsiros J, Uyttebroeck A, Marky I, Lamant L, Reiter A. (2009) Impact of the Methotrexate Administration Dose on the Need for Intrathecal Treatment in Children and Adolescents With Anaplastic Large-Cell Lymphoma: Results of a Randomized Trial of the EICNHL Group *Journal of Clinical Oncology*, **27**: 897–903.

response rates are very high, in view of the substantial relapse rate, the increased complexity and morbidity of full-dose regimens appears to be justified. Within the context of a full leukemia-type protocol, there is some place for dose modification. For example, in the BFM strategy, stage 1 and 2 patients do not have the standard reinduction regimen as used for patients with advanced disease. The outcome of patients with localized LL included on the COG-A5971 has also been reported.[38] A total of 57 with stage 1 or 2 disease received the CCG BFM protocol i.e. without high-dose MTX and in addition, fewer IT MTXs were given during maintenance therapy; the duration was 24 months. Five-year EFS was 85% with no toxic deaths.

T-LL typically presents with bulky mediastinal disease and often BM involvement (Table 16.3). With advanced disease, the demonstration in the CCG-randomized trial of the superiority of the LSA2L regimen compared to COMP led to the adoption of protocols based on the

Table 16.3. Clinical features of T-lymphoblastic lymphoma.

Characteristics	Combined NHL-BFM90/86 (n = 163)	
	No.	%
Sex		
Female	45	28
Male	118	72
Age	95	58
< 10 years	58	36
10–14 years	10	6
> 14 years		
Stage of disease		
Stage III	130	80
Stage IV	33	20
BM involvement	33	20
Mediastinal tumor	144	88
Immunophenotype Precursor		
B cell	14	9
T cell	145	89
N/A	4	2

AML: acute myeloid leukemia; BM: bone marrow; LBL: lymphoblastic lymphoma; NHL-BFM: non-Hodgkin's lymphoma–Berlin-Frankfurt-Munster; N/A: not available.

Adapted from Burkhardt B, Woessmann W, Zimmermann M, Kontny U, Vormoor J, Doerffel W, Mann G, Henze G, Niggli F, Ludwig WD, Janssen D, Riehm H, Schrappe M, Reiter A. (2006) Impact of cranial radiotherapy on central nervous system prophylaxis in children and adolescents with central nervous system-negative stage III or IV lymphoblastic lymphoma. *J Clin Oncol* **24**: 491–499.

approach used for ALL. For example, the UKCCSG studies were based on the UK ALL approach with two intensification modules and no local radiation therapy.[39,40] The best results reported to date are by the BFM group which in 2000, described a series of 101 patients with stage 3 and 4 disease who received an eight drug induction over 9 weeks followed by an 8-week consolidation including high-dose MTX (Fig. 16.9).[41] Patients with stage 1 and 2 disease went on to maintenance therapy but those with advanced disease received an eight drug intensification over several weeks and also 12 Gray cranial radiotherapy. This was followed by maintenance for a total treatment period of 2 years. If there was less than 70% tumor regression on day 33, patients were treated with the high-risk ALL regimen. If there was still residual imageable disease on day 64, surgery or biopsy was recommended and if active disease was found, treatment intensification including high-dose therapy was considered. Of 101 patients, 64 achieved CR by day 33, only 2 of which are adolescents (70% response). Of the 35 patients who had residual tumor at the end of induction, the majority who were biopsied had necrotic tissue only. The EFS did not appear to differ in relation to initial response, 95% vs. 89% for CR vs. incomplete response. From these data, it was concluded that tumor regression should not be taken as an indication for localized radiotherapy except in those with less than 70% regression on day 33. Only one patient in this series developed a CNS relapse; this very low rate led to modification in the subsequent BFM95 trial, where cranial radiotherapy was omitted for CNS negative patients. Those with CNS

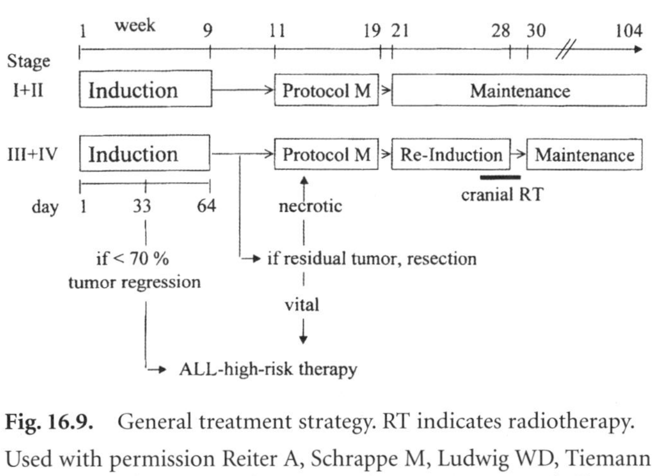

Fig. 16.9. General treatment strategy. RT indicates radiotherapy.

Used with permission Reiter A, Schrappe M, Ludwig WD, Tiemann M, Parwaresch R, Zimmermann M, Schirg E, Henze G, Schellong G, Gadner H, Riehm H, BFM group. (2000) Intensive ALL-type therapy without local radiotherapy provides a 90% event-free survival for children with T-cell lymphoblastic lymphoma: A BFM Group report *Blood* **95**: 416–421.

disease at presentation received additional IT chemotherapy and radiation following reintensification. The dose of radiation was 12 Gray for patients under 2, and 18 Gray for older children; no radiation was given to those under 1 year. In this series, there were 126 with precursor T- and 26 with precursor B-lymphoma. The 5-year EFS was 80% comparing with 88% for BFM 90, 82% for BFM 86 and 86% for BFM. There was no difference in CNS relapse rate, indicating that radiation therapy was not required (Figs. 16.10A–B).[42] The somewhat higher overall failure rate compared to the historical control role group was difficult to explain. There were some differences including higher dose intensity in BFM 90 and also a different formulation and dose of asparaginase. Nonetheless, the overall results were excellent and this remains the gold standard regimen.

Results of the LSA2L2 protocol over a 30-year period have been reviewed and are an interesting

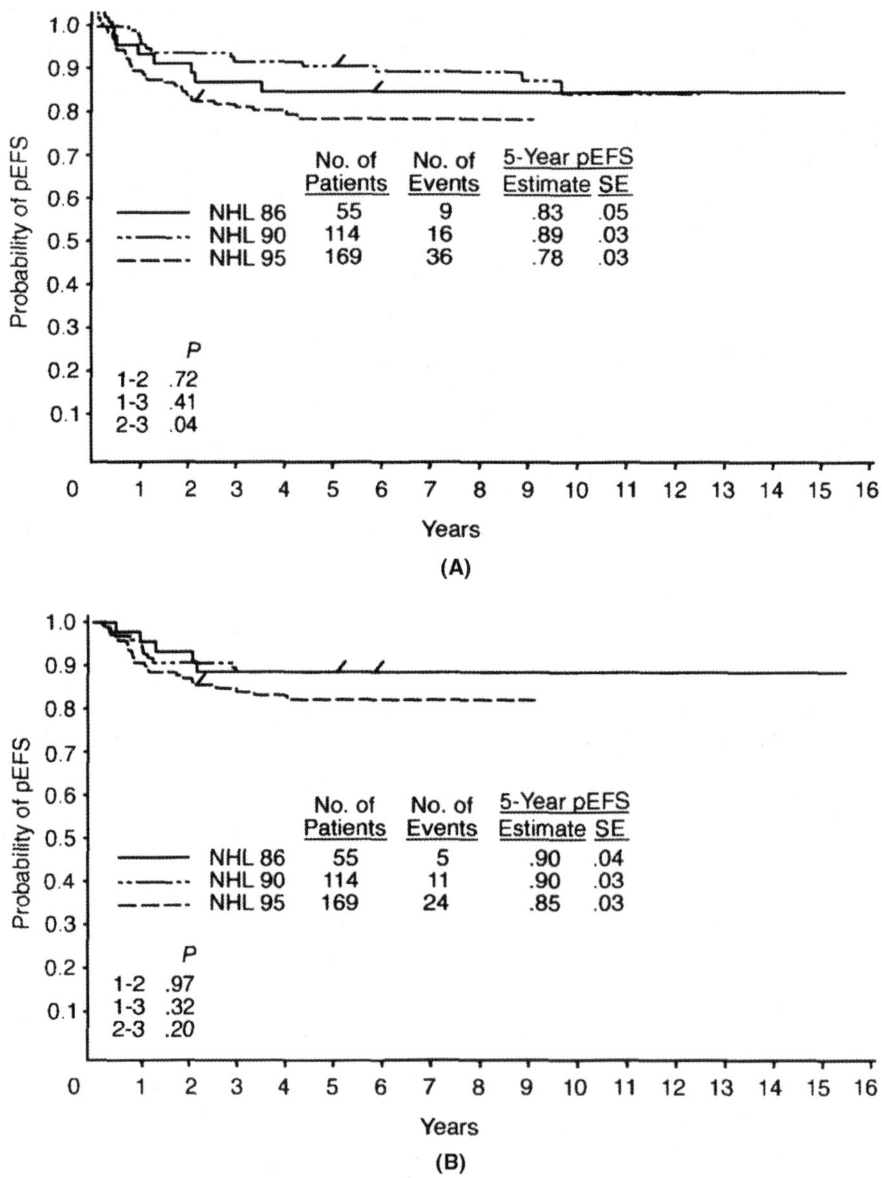

Fig. 16.10. Outcome at 5 years for all lymphoblastic lymphoma patients with stage III or IV, CNS negative disease in Non-Hodgkin's Lymphoma (NHL) –Berlin-Frankfurt-Munster trials 95, 90, and 86. (A) Event-free survival. (B) Disease-free survival.

Used with permission Burkhardt B, Woessmann W, Zimmermann M, Kontny U, Vormoor J, Doerffel W, Mann G, Henze G, Niggli F, Ludwig WD, Janssen D, Riehm H, Schrappe M, Reiter A. (2006) Impact of cranial radiotherapy on central nervous system prophylaxis in children and adolescents with central nervous system-negative stage III or IV lymphoblastic lymphoma. *J Clin Oncol* **24**: 491–499.

documentation of the evolution of treatment strategy with sequential dose modifications, reduction in duration and the omission of radiation therapy.[43] In this report the EFS for patients with stage 3 disease was 85% over a prolonged period. The Italian group have reported a modification of the LSA2L2 regimen with EFS of 69% in 55 patients.[44] It was suggested that the absence of a reinduction phase and the relatively late use of asparaginase would account for the inferior outcome. It is also of note that this regimen was of shorter duration, lasting a total of only 11 months. Another recent study that evaluated the use of aggressive shorter duration treatment is the CCG-5941, a compressed 12-month intensive multiagent regimen.[45] Granulocyte colony-stimulating factor (GCSF) was used to maintain dose intensity and the 42-week maintenance period consisted of pulses of a combination of chemotherapy including high-dose MTX rather than standard 6-MP and oral MTX. Eighty-five patients with stage 3–4 disease were enrolled and the 5-year EFS was 78%. There were four toxic deaths (5%). This compares with 3% in the BFM NHL 95 study. This report also includes an overview of studies in children reported from 1983–2008.

The most recent COG-A5971 study adopted the BFM-90 regimen, addressing the issue whether high-dose MTX was essential and whether intensification with anthracycline and cyclophosphamide would further improve disease-free survival.[46] Initial report is of 3-year EFS of 84% including high-dose MTX and 83% where this was omitted, and similarly identical outcome of 83% for additional intensification vs. none. This indicates that some components of the BFM regimen may not be essential and exemplifies the difficulty evaluating each component of a complex multiagent regimen.

The St. Jude NHL 13 regimen[47] based on the Total 13 regimen for T-ALL, included an unusual maintenance phase consisting of complex modules of mainly intravenous couplets of seven drugs given weekly for 15 weeks. Forty-one patients were reported with 95% CR rate and 5-year EFS of 82%. The incidence of secondary leukemia in the Total 13 regimen raises concerns about the use of etoposide in this regimen.

The European collaborative group EICNHL designed Euro LB02 to address the issue of treatment duration. Using the BFM backbone, treatment duration of 24 months was compared with 18 months. In addition, there was a randomization to the use of dexamethasone vs. prednisolone. Unfortunately, this trial was, however, closed prematurely due to high toxicity in the dexamethasone arm and the issue of optimal treatment duration remains to be answered.

Treatment for PTCL

PTCLs (not other specified [NOS]) other than ALCLs are composed of a diverse group of rare disease entities. In children and adolescents, PTCL-NOS occurs in approximately 1% of all cases of NHL.[48] The biological characteristics of PTCL-NOS exhibit diversity. It has been difficult to identify the normal counterpart T cells that correlate with the cellular origin of disease for PTCL-NOS. A variety of immunophenotypic subtypes have been observed across different stages of T cell differentiation with cells expressing different combinations of pan-T cell antigens as well as markers of both cytotoxic and activated T cell subtypes.[49] Similarly, although several different cytogenetic changes have been observed in cases of PTCL-NOS, a specific pattern correlating to clinically meaningful consequences has yet to be determined.[50,51]

Unfortunately, treatment strategies employed for childhood and adolescent PTCLs have been as varied as their clinical and pathological findings. It has been extremely challenging to develop and establish effective treatment regimens because the clinical experience in pediatric PTCL has been sparse and individual studies have been hampered by too few patients. The COG recently analyzed 20 childhood and adolescent patients over a 9-year period.[52] The cohort included mostly patients with PTCL-NOS, however, there were also patients with extranodal natural killer (NK)/T-cell lymphoma nasal type, subcutaneous panniculitis-like T-cell lymphoma, and enteropathy-type T-cell lymphoma. Treatment choice was based upon clinical staging. Patients with advanced stage III/IV disease were treated with a regimen of doxorubicin, prednisone, vincristine, mercaptopurine and MTX ± alternating therapy with high-dose cytarabine and intermediate-dose MTX. Patients with localized stage I/II disease were treated with CHOP-like regimen. Of 10 patients with localized disease, 2 relapsed and 9 of 10 survived. Of 10 patients with advanced stage disease, 6 relapsed and 5 of 10 survived.[52]

The experience in the UKCCSG was quite similar to that of the COG in the USA.[48,52] The UKCCSG study analyzed 25 cases of PTCL in children and adolescents over a 20-year period. They observed a similar distribution of PTCL subtypes with 68% of patients having PTCL-NOS; the remainder of cases were angiocentric

PTCL, angioimmunoblastic T-cell lymphoma, and subcutaneous panniculitis-like T-cell lymphoma. Patients were treated either with B-NHL CHOP-like regimens or with T-ALL type of treatment. Among children with PTCL-NOS, 9 of 12 survived with T-ALL therapy, while only 1 of 5 that received B-NHL therapy survived. Similar to the COG results, when analyzed based upon extent of disease, the majority of patients (9 of 12) with localized stage I/II disease survived, while only 6 of 12 children with advanced stage disease survived.[48]

High-dose chemotherapy with autologous stem cell transplantation (autoSCT) has been attempted as both salvage and front-line therapy in adults with PTCL (see Chapter 20). In the setting of refractory or recurrent disease, OS after autoSCT has been reported around 33–50%.[53,54] Attempts to treat PTCL with front-line autoSCT have yielded slightly better results, however, the biggest obstacle to achieving better outcomes was the inability to attain remission. A large study performed in Italy for patients with high-risk PTCL receiving autoSCT as upfront therapy reported long-term OS rates of 39%.[55] Of the patients that did get high-dose chemo and autoSCT, the 12-year disease-free survival rate was 55%.[55]

Many groups have also attempted allogeneic stem cell transplantation (alloSCT) for adults with PTCL. This strategy provides the advantage of infusing lymphoma-free grafts and potential for a graft-vs.-lymphoma effect. Studies have demonstrated a lower risk of relapse in patients receiving alloSCT (in comparison to autoSCT), however, the high rates of transplant-related mortality with fully ablative conditioning regimens have offset any survival advantages.[56] The Italian group has recently reported on the role of alloSCT with reduced intensity conditioning regimens. In a pilot study of 17 patients with refractory and recurrent disease (8 of whom relapsed after prior autoSCT), a 3-year progression-free survival of 64% was achieved, with only 1 of 17 patients suffering from transplant-related mortality.[57]

Treatment for Post-Transplant Lymphoproliferative Disorder (PTLD)

Children and adolescents who are immunosuppressed following solid organ transplantation (SOT) are at risk of developing PTLD. There are three major subtypes including: (a) lymphoid hyperplasia, (b) polymorphic PTLD, and (c) monomorphic or lymphomatous PTLD.[58] The less common variety, occurring in less than 10% of cases, includes plasmacytoma, myeloma, Hodgkin disease-like and T-cell PTLD.[58] The vast majority of histological subtypes express B-cell markers such as CD20.[58] Furthermore, over 90% of cases of PTLD express Epstein–Barr virus (EBV) by immunohistochemistry, *in situ* hybridization, or by coding RNA.[58,59] The highest risk groups in children and adolescents include SOT with bowel, lung, liver, heart and combined organs and also include patients who have recessive OKT-3, calcineurin inhibitors such as cyclosporine or tacrolimus and age less than 5 years.[60–64] The most prominent immune defect is a lack or reduced number of specific T-cell EBV cytotoxic T-lymphocytes (EBV-CTLs).

The primary treatment of children with PTLD following SOT has been the reduction of immunosuppression.[65,66] This therapeutic approach has excellent success in patients with lymphoid hyperplasia and moderate success in those with polymorphic PTLD subtypes and one-third of patients with monomorphic or lymphomatous PTLD will respond to reduction of immunosuppression alone.[65] Reducing immunosuppression is a double-edge sword in that it may control or eradicate PTLD but at the same time it may increase the risk of solid organ allograft rejection. Successful treatment of PTLD requires both control of EBV-induced B-cell proliferation and the increase of specific EBV-CTLs.[67]

Early studies with anti-B cell antibody (anti-CD21 and anti-CD24) demonstrate response in patients with refractory PTLD.[68,69] More recent studies in adults with PTLD have demonstrated success with anti-CD20 antibody using the chimeric antibody, rituximab.[70,71] Forty-three adult patients with PTLD following SOT who failed reduced immunosuppression, received four doses of rituximab (375 mg/m^2/weekly $\times$ 4) and had a response rate of 44% and 1-year OS of 67% (see Chapter 21).[70,71] In a retrospective review of 17 children with PTLD who received single agent rituximab, the overall response rate was similar with a 47% response rate.[72] Immunotherapy with rituximab alone only induces a 40–50% overall response rate in both children and adults and other approaches are needed.

Chemotherapy has been utilized as an alternative to immunotherapy for children with PTLD post SOT in those who develop PTLD.[65,67] Gross *et al.* studied 36 children with PTLD following SOT with a combination of low-dose cyclophosphamide and prednisone (CY/Pred).[73] The overall response rate was 83% (75% CR and 8% partial response [PR]) and 2-year OS and failure-free survival were 73% and 67%, respectively.[73] Orjuela and Cairo *et al.* piloted the combination of CY/Pred with rituximab (CPR) in a small group of children with PTLD following SOT refractory to reduced immunosuppression and demonstrated an 85–90% EFS in this small group.[74] Based on the two above mentioned studies, the COG conducted a phase II study of CPR in children with PTLD following SOT who failed reduced immunosuppression.[75] There were 50 patients with nonfulminant PTLD who received CPR (cyclophosphamide 600 mg/m^2/d × 1, prednisone 1 mg/kg bid × 5d and rituximab 375 mg/m^2/wk × 3) in cycle one and two and CY/Pred in cycles 3, 4, 5, and 6. The overall response rate was 87% (74% CR) and the estimated 1- and 2-year OS was 83 and 80%, respectively.[75] Furthermore, recent studies by Orjuela and Cairo *et al.* suggest that expression of CD20 in childhood PTLD following SOT denotes improved OS.[76]

Cellular therapy is the newest and most promising approach, especially in EBV-associated PTLD.[77] Papadopoulos first demonstrated use of donor leukocytes to treat EBV-associated PTLD following alloSCT.[78] Rooney *et al.* first demonstrated the use of specific EBV-CTLs to treat PTLD.[79] A further discussion of cellular therapy for these and other diseases is covered in this textbook by Heslop and Cooper (Chapter 23).

Monoclonal Antibody Therapy for Childhood NHL

There has been an increasing use of monoclonal antibodies in the treatment of NHL. We will focus our brief review on four surface antigens: CD20, CD22, CD30, and CD52. There are, however, many other surface antigens on B-malignant cells that are drug use targets (Fig. 16.11). Each of these antigens have antibodies either already approved for clinical use in adults or are in a late phase of development. A more comprehensive review can be found in the chapter by Satwani and Wayne (Chapter 21).

CD20

CD20 is a transmembrane protein that, in part, regulates intracellular calcium levels and may, in part, regulate cell cycle regulation and induction of apoptosis.[80] It is an ideal surface antigen that does not appear to shed, modulate or internalize and it has been demonstrated to be expressed in ≥98% of all childhood mature B-cell lymphomas including BL, BLL and DLBCL.[80] Rituximab is a naked chimeric IgG1 antibody directed at CD20 which contains variable light and heavy chains from the murine anti-CD20 and appears to mediate antibody-dependent cell-mediated cytotoxicity (ADCC), complement-dependent cytotoxicity and induce apoptosis.

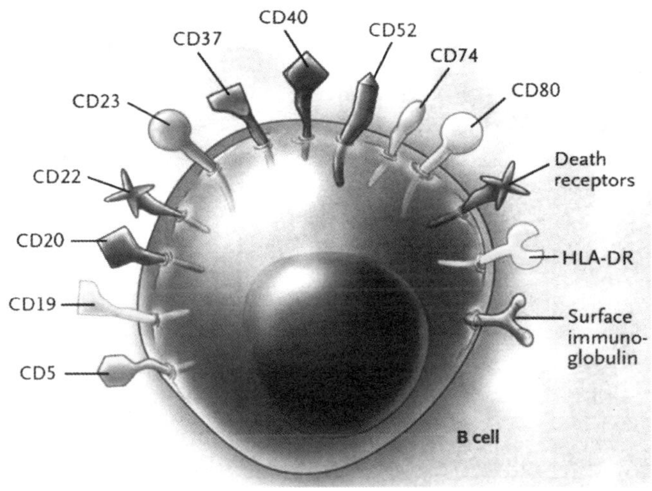

Fig. 16.11. Cell-Surface Antigens on the B Cell. The B cell has a large number of associated cell-surface antigens that can be exploited as targets for monoclonal-antibody therapy. The presence of CD5 on the surface of B cells varies according to histologic type. Used with permission from Cheson BD and Leonard JP. (2008) Monoclonal antibody therapy for B-cell non-Hodgkin's lymphoma. *N Engl J Med* **359**: 613–626.

Rituximab added to chemotherapy backbone such as CHOP, CHOP-like regimens and etoposide/vincristine/doxorubicin/cyclophosphamide/prednisone (EPOCH) has significant activity in adult DLBCL.[20,21,81] To investigate the safety and response rate of ritixumab added to ifosfamide, carboplatin and etoposide (ICE) chemotherapy in children with recurrent B-NHL,[82] Griffin *et al.* tested the addition of rituximab (375 mg/m^2/dose) in children and adolescents with recurrent/refractory B-NHL in combination with ICE chemotherapy.[83] This reinduction regimen resulted in a 60% overall response including a 6/14 response (CR/PR) in patients with BL.[83]

In children with newly diagnosed *de novo* mature B-NHL, Reiter *et al.* investigated the safety and response rate as a single dose (375 mg/m^2) as a window prior to BFM B-NHL therapy.[84] There were 136 patients entered on study and 87 were evaluable for response 5 days after one single dose.[84] There were 37 (42%) responders, including 29/68 BL patients and 6/14 DLBCL patients.[84]

The COG recently tested the use of rituximab (375 mg/m^2/dose) used as six doses in combination with FAB 84 chemotherapy backbone (COPADM$_3$) in children with newly diagnosed *de novo* mature B-NHL.[85] In this study of 48 children, the 2-year EFS and OS were 93% and 98%, respectively.[85] More recently, the results of combining rituximab with FAB group C1 chemotherapy backbone (COPADM$_8$) were reported and demonstrated in children with BM and/or CNS involvement, a 2-year EFS and OS of 86% and 88%, respectively.[86] A randomized international trial is in development to determine if rituximab improves EFS when added to the FAB chemotherapy backbone in children and adolescents with stage III/IV and BM/CNS B-NHL.

There are other antibody approaches to investigate targeting CD20, including the use of humanized anti-CD20 antibodies, antibody–drug conjugates and radioimmunoconjugates. The use of radioimmunotherapy with indium-111 ibritumomab-tiuxetan has been investigated in relapsed/refractory B-cell (CD20 positive) lymphoma in children.[87] The radioimmunotherapy was well tolerated and radiation exposure well below the limit for all organs evaluated.[87] Further studies will be required to determine its efficacy and role in childhood B-NHL.

CD22

CD22 surface antibody has been demonstrated to be expressed in 95% of BL, BLL and DLBCL in children.[80] Epratuzumab is a humanized monoclonal antibody that binds to the third extracellular domain of CD22 and after binding is rapidly internalized as antigen/antibody complex.[88,89] Epratuzumab appears to modulate B-cell signaling and activation and enhance ADCC, CD22 phosphorylation and crosslinking, leading to inhibition of B-cell proliferation.[88] Epratuzumab has been demonstrated to be efficacious in adults with both indolent and aggressive B-cell lymphomas.[90–92] CD22 is also expressed in ≥ 90% of childhood precursor B-ALL.[93] The safety of adding epratuzumab (360 mg/m^2/dose) to vincristine, prednisone, L-asparaginase and doxorubicin reinduction therapy has been demonstrated in children with CD22 positive relapsed ALL and after reinduction, 7/9 were MRD negative and in CR.[93] Further studies are required to investigate the safety and efficacy of epratuzumab in children with relapsed/refractory B-NHL.

CD30

CD30 is expressed in ≥ 95% of all childhood ALCL. CD30 is a member of the tumor necrosis factor (TNF) receptor superfamily and appears to be involved with the regulation of cell cycle and programmed cell death.[94] Several antibodies have been developed against CD30 including SGN-30 and SGN-35. SGN-30 is a chimeric antibody constructed from the variable region from the murine anti-CD30 antibody and contains human gamma 1 heavy chain and kappa light chain construct regions.[95] In an adult phase II study with ALCL, there was a 17% objective response in 28 evaluable patients.[95] A phase I/II pediatric ALCL study was attempted by T. Sandlund, MD on behalf of the COG, but the study was closed prematurely due to low accrual. SGN-35 is a second generation antibody with anti-CD30 binding sites that is conjugated to auristatin, which is a significant microtubular inhibitor. In a phase I/II study of SGN-35 in adults with relapsed/refractory ALCL, there has been 6/7 CRs (personal communication, Eric Sievers, MD). There are plans within the COG to investigate the safety and efficacy of SGN-35 in a maintenance setting in children with newly diagnosed but high-risk ALCL (personal communication E. Lowe, MD).

CD52

The expression of CD52 along with CD25, CD74 and CD80 has been recently evaluated in children and adolescents with NHL including BL, DLBCL, ALCL, T-LBL and B-LBL (Fig. 16.12).[96] CD52 was expressed in ≥ 90% in all forms of childhood NHL.[96] CD52 is a glycoprotein of unknown function presently expressed on normal cells including T, B, NK, and dendritic cells (DC) and malignant lymphomas/leukemias. There is an antibody directed at CD52 named alemtuzumab, which is a recombinant humanized monoclonal antibody that induces complement-dependent cytotoxicity, ADCC and induces apoptosis.[97–99] Alemtuzumab has been demonstrated to be active in adult leukemias including chronic lymphocytic leukemia (CLL)[100] and other B and T forms of adult NHL.[101,102] Alemtuzumab has been studied as a single agent in refractory/recurrent adults with PTCL, achieving a 36% overall response rate in a pilot study of 14 patients.[103] A more recent study examined the role of alemtuzumab in adults with PTCL in combination with CHOP chemotherapy as front-line therapy. This experience

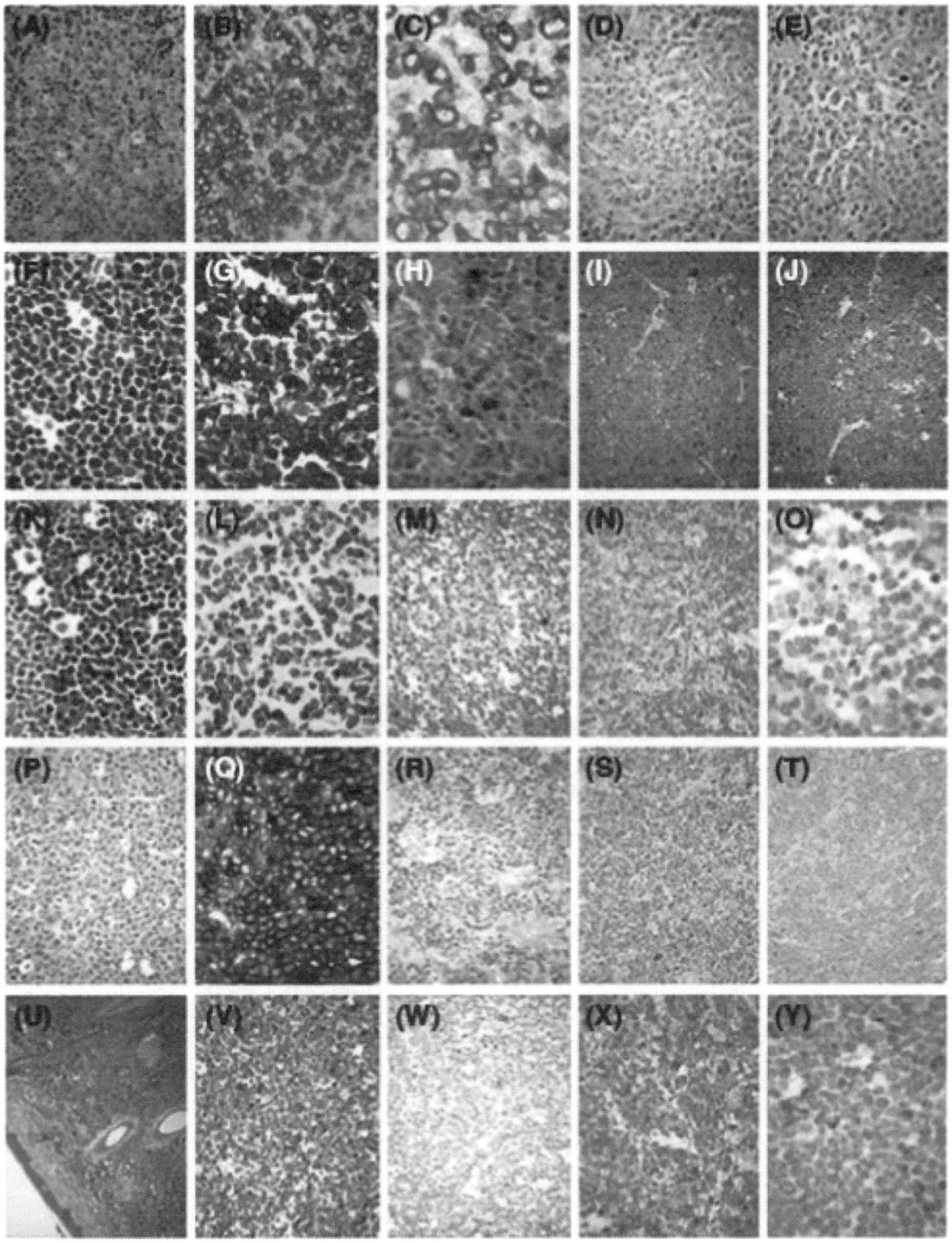

Fig. 16.12. (A–E) Classical type ALCL showing (A) large, multinucleated tumours cells (H&E, 1000×) that shows (B) strong diffuse cytoplasmic and partial membrane expression of CD52 (1000×). CD25 shows membrane and cytoplasmic staining of the (C) tumor cells, while (D) CD74 and (E) CD80 show no tumor cell staining. (F–J) T-LBL. (F) H&E stain showing the diffuse effacement of nodal architecture by blast-like cells (1000×). (G) The tumor cells show strong, diffuse staining for CD52. (H) The CD25 immunostain shows staining of reactive T cells but no staining of the neoplastic T-lymphoblasts (1000×). (I) CD74 and (J) CD80 showed staining of background lymphocytes but not tumor cells. (K–O) BL. K and L demonstrate a BL with moderately intense granular cytoplasmic staining by CD52. (K, H&E; L, CD52, 1000×). (M) CD25 stains non-neoplastic lymphocytes, but the tumor cells are negative. (N) CD74 stains > 50% of the cells (400×), and (O) CD80 shows weak staining on < 50% of tumor cells (1000×). (P–T) DLBCL. (P) DLBCL (H&E stain) with (Q) strong, diffuse cytoplasmic staining with CD52 but (R) no tumor cell staining for CD25. (S) Staining for CD74 is strong and diffuse (400×), while (T) CD80 is negative (400×). (U–Y) B-LBL. (U) B-LBL (H&E) showing (V) strong, diffuse staining for CD52, but (W) no tumor cell staining for or CD25. (X) Staining for CD74 is strong and diffuse (400×) and (Y) staining for CD80 is weak and diffuse (1000×). H&E: hematoxylin and eosin.

Used with permission from Miles RR, Cairo MS, Satwani P, Zwick DL, Lones MA, Sposto R, Abromowitch M, Tripp S, Angiolillo AL, Roman E, Davenport V, Perkins SL. (2007) Immunophenotypic identification of possible therapeutic targets in paediatric non-Hodgkin lymphomas: A Children's Oncology Group report. *Br J Haematol* **138**: 506–512.

revealed tolerable rates of toxicity and a 1-year EFS of 41%.[104] There is a paucity of data on the use of alemtuzumab in children with NHL despite the high expression of CD52 in almost all histological subtypes of childhood NHL.[96] Although alemtuzumab can be immunosuppressive and cause acute allergic reactions, future studies are required to determine its role in childhood NHL.

Treatment Following Relapse

In the case of recurrence of BL after localized disease treated with standard dose chemotherapy, retreatment with a more dose-intensive regimen such as the LMB group C protocol, is likely to achieve a second CR. Following the evidence from adult high-grade lymphoma where high-risk chemotherapy with stem cell rescue has a proven role in the second PR or CRs following relapse, it is appropriate to consider this as a component of second-line therapy, especially for early or extensive recurrence.[105] In patients with initial BM disease or B-ALL, if there is a matched sibling or matched unrelated donor, it is appropriate to consider the use of allogeneic transplantation. Although there is some evidence from adult studies of a graft-vs.-lymphoma effect this has not been demonstrated to date in pediatric BL. The individual patient characteristics and treatment-related morbidity of the respective procedures must be taken into account in making a decision regarding allograft vs. autograft. The efficacy of novel second-line therapy such as ICE or ICE+ rituximab justifies the inclusion of such combinations in any second-line regimen following initial intensive treatment.[83]

The outcome of relapse after initial stage 4 disease, particularly with CNS disease, remains bleak and although a CR may be achieved with second-line therapy, particularly using ICE+ rituximab, it is too early to conclude whether this novel reinduction strategy followed by high-dose therapy will produce a significant long-term survival. There is a need to consider novel approaches, particularly in the case of CNS disease where alternative drugs such as IT mafosfamide or IT rituximab may have their role to play.

Relapse strategies for T-NHL tend to mirror those for relapsed T-ALL with more intensive second-line therapy followed by allogeneic transplantation using either a matched sibling or a matched donor. The role of allografting in recurrent local T-NHL without BM involvement remains unclear and in general autografting may be considered. The lower morbidity associated with newer reduced intensity conditioning regimens may increase the use of donor transplants.[106]

A striking characteristic of pediatric ALCL is the high salvage rate following relapse. Early reports of PTCL describe encouraging results using alloSCT in patients whose disease had recurred. Many of these patients were subsequently shown to be ALCL. The demonstration of a clear immunological impact on this tumor type suggests that allogeneic transplantation with a potential graft-vs.-lymphoma may be a useful strategy in high risk recurrent disease. This is now being explored in current prospective studies, although disease numbers remain too small to mount a randomized trial. It is of note that earlier studies have demonstrated the administration of weekly vinblastine following third relapse produced a longer lapse-free remission than the use of autoSCT.

The number of published reports describes the effectiveness of alloSCT as a rescue therapy for the initial refractory or relapsed ALCL. In a report from the BFM group, EFS at 3 years after allograft was 75%.[107] A number of reports have also described encouraging results after a strikingly different approach, namely, the use of single dose vinblastine. The French SFOP Group reviewed data on 36 patients who were treated for either refractory or relapsed ALCL (often multiple), 15 had undergone a previous transplant procedure. Eighty-three percent of the patients achieved a CR and the OS of this group was 65%.[108] An alternative low-dose approach using pulsed dexamethasone and low dose oral etoposide given in four weekly pulses over a 2-year period may also have had some efficacy.[109]

Stem Cell Transplantation for Children with NHL

There are now few indications for SCT for childhood NHL and these include induction failure, sensitive relapse resulting in CR or PR, or the few patients with ultra high-risk features at diagnosis.[110,111] A more complete discussion of stem cell transplantation can be found in Chapter 20.

High-dose chemoradiotherapy followed by autoSCT has been a standard approach but there is increasing use of full or reduced intensity alloSCT, especially in those with B-cell lymphomas with BM

Table 16.4. Stem cell transplantation in childhood NHL.

Author	Center/Group	N	Age (yrs)	NHL histology	Donor source	Conditioning regimen	DFS/EFS
Loiseau *et al.*[115]	Institut Gustave Roussy	24	NA	16 B-NHL 8 T-NHL	Autologous	BU/CY, BU/Melphalan	33%
Won *et al.*[117]	Korea	33	1.7–16	6 B-NHL 13 LL 14 LCL	Autologous	BEAM BEAC CBV TBI regimen	59%
Philip *et al.*[116]	SFOP	15	NA	B-NHL	14 Autologous 1 Allogeneic	BEAM/BEAC, Other	27%
Ladenstein *et al.*[114]	EBMT	89	2.8–16.2	B-NHL	Autologous	BACT 31 BEAM 23 BU/CY 9 Other 26	44% sensitive relapse
Kobrinsky *et al.*[121]	CCG	50	< 21	N/A	Autologous	N/A	50%
Levine *et al.*[112]	IBMTR	128	2–67	LL	Autologous	N/A	39%
		76	5–53		Allogeneic	N/A	36%
Fanin *et al.*[122]	EBMT	64	3.2–53	ALCL	Autologous	N/A	47%
Woessmann *et al.*[107]	BFM	20	1–15.8	ALCL	Allogeneic	TBI/CY/VP-16	75%
Bureo *et al.*[123]	Spain	46	1–17	21LL 19 B-NHL 6 LCL	14 Allogeneic 32 Autologous	BEAM CY/TBI CY/TBI/ARA-C	58%

ALCL: anaplastic large cell lymphoma; BEAM: carmustine, etoposide, cytarabine, and melphalan; BEAC: carmustine, etoposide, Ara-C and cyclophosphamide; BFM: Berlin-Frankfurt-Münster; B-NHL: B-cell non-Hodgkin's lymphoma; BU: busfulfan; CBV: cyclophosphamide, carmustine, etoposide (VP-16); CY: cyclophosphamide; DFS: disease-free survival; EBMT: The European Group for Blood and Marrow Transplantation; EFS: event-free survival; CCG: Children's Cancer Group; IBMTR: International Bone Marrow Transplant Registry; LCL: large cell lymphoma; LL: lymphoblastic lymphoma; NA: not available; SFOP: Société Française di'Oncologie Pédiatrique; T-NHL: T-cell non-Hodgkin's lymphoma; N/A: not applicable; TBI: total body irradiation; NHL: non-Hodgkin's lymphoma.

Reprinted by permission from Macmillan Publishers Ltd: Bone Marrow Transplant, Bradley MB, Cairo MS. (2008) Stem cell transplantation for pediatric lymphoma: Past, present and future. *Bone Marrow Transplant* **41**: 149–158 © 2008.

involvement, LL and ALCL.[107,110–113] A summary of published reports on SCT in children with NHL is noted in Table 16.4.[107,110,112,114–117]

More recently, a retrospective CIBMTR study performed by Gross *et al.* reviewed 182 SCTs (92 auto and 92 allo) in pediatric recipients with NHL. In this retrospective analysis, alloSCT was associated with a lower rate of relapse in children with ALCL and LL, similar to Woessmann *et al.* and Levine *et al.*, respectively.[107,112,118] Overall, the results were 5-year EFS of 28% for autoSCT and 20% for alloSCT, respectively.[118] Lastly, Harris *et al.* recently reported better results in children with NHL who relapsed or progressed on front line therapy following CBV (cyclophosphamide, carmustine, etoposide) conditioning and autoSCT with a 3-year EFS of 70% (CI_{95}: 33–80%) among only six patients with NHL who achieved a CR/PR after reinduction.[119] A more novel approach has been the use of myeloablative therapy and autoSCT followed by a reduced intensity conditioning and alloSCT.[113] Future studies should focus on multicenter, prospective trials with uniform conditioning regimens and stem cell sources and focused post-SCT therapeutic approaches.[110]

Current Issues

Staging

In BL, it has become clear that the St. Jude staging system, based on the anatomical location of disease, no longer adequately defines prognostic subgroups in the context of much more effective systemic chemotherapy. For this reason, in the FAB/LMB studies, risk stratification based on group rather than stage was devised. At the 2009 International Symposium on Childhood and Adolescent NHL in Frankfurt, a proposal was put forward to amend this system with modifications including a clearer definition of BM and CNS disease (Table 16.5) (personal communication, Angelo

Table 16.5. Modified version of the St. Jude staging system, based on discussion at the Frankfurt International Symposium on Child and Adolescent Lymphoma 2009.

Stage I

Nodes and extranodal

A single tumor with the exclusion of the mediastinum and abdomen. (N: nodal; EN: extranodal; bone or skin: EN-B, EN-S or other)

BM and CSF negative

Stage II

Nodal

Two or more nodal areas on the same side of the diaphragm.
A primary gastrointestinal tract tumor (usually in the ileocecal area), with or without involvement of associated mesenteric nodes, that is completely resectable. (If ascites is present or the tumor extends to adjacent organs, it should be regarded as stage III.)

Extranodal

A single extranodal tumor with regional node involvement (EN S or EN B or other).

BM & CNS negative

Stage III

Nodal

Two or more nodal areas above and below the diaphragm.
Any mediastinal, hilar or thymic tumor).
Incompletely resected intra-abdominal disease, including liver, spleen and/or kidney localizations.

Extranodal

Two or more extranodal tumors (EN S, EN B or other).
Single bone lesion with concomitant involvement of extranodal and/or nodal sites
Any paraspinal or epidural tumor, whether or not other sites are involved
Pulmonary or pleural tumor

BM & CNS negative

Stage IV

Any of the above findings with initial involvement of the central nervous system (IV CNS), bone marrow (IV BM), or both (IV combined).

Bone marrow on morphological examination +/– immunophenotypic studies
BMm BM positive by morphology (specify the % blasts)
BMi BM positive by immunophenotypic methods (histochemical/flow cytometric analysis

CNS

Defined by presence of:

- CNS tumor mass (excluding extradural parameningeal) and/or
- cranial nerve palsy that cannot be explained by extradural lesions and/or
- blasts in CSF on morphological examination +/– immunophenotypic studies

CSFm CSF positive by morphology (specify the number of blasts/μL)
CSFi CSF positive by immunophenotypic methods (histochemical/flow cytometric analysis)

For BM & CNS, cytogenetics and molecular studies may be documented but on their own would not define stage 4 disease. (personal communication, Angelo Rosolen, MD)

Supplemental data

Bone marrow involvement

Independently of stage, type and degree of BM involvement should be specified, using the abbreviations below:
BMm BM positive by morphology (specify the % blasts)
BMi BM positive by immunophenotypic methods (histochemical/flow cytometric analysis)
BMc BM positive by cytogenetic/FISH analysis
BMmrd BM positive by PCR-based techniques

(Continued)

Table 16.5. (*Continued*)

Examples: "stage III (BMi)" (stage III disease with BM positive by immunohistochemical analysis);
"stage III (BMm 2%)" (stage III disease with BM with 2% blasts by morphological examination).

Same approach should be used for peripheral blood (PB) involvement (i.e.: PBm; PBi etc.)

Central nervous system (CNS) involvement

CNS is considered involved in cases of:
(1) any CNS tumor mass;
(2) cranial nerve palsy that cannot be explained by extra-dural lesions
(3) blasts in CSF

Condition that defines CNS positivity should be specified: CNS positive/mass; CNS positive/palsy; CNS positive/blasts

CSF status: CSF positivity is usually based on morphological examination by light microscopy
CSF should be considered positive when any number of blasts is detected.
CSF unknown

Similarly to BM, positivity of CSF based on techniques other that microscopic examination should be described whenever possible.

CSFm	CSF positive by morphology (specify the number of blasts/μL)
CSFi	CSF positive by immunophenotypic methods (histochemical/flow-cytometric analysis)
CSFc	BM positive by cytogenetic/FISH analysis
CSFmrd	CSF positive by PCR-based techniques

Note

Until sufficient data are available, Positron Emission Tomography (PET) should not be used for staging. A PET positivity should not be interpreted as tumor localization unless proven by other imaging approaches (Echo, CT, MRI) or, ideally, by biopsy.

Rosolen, MD). Although the original SFOP studies indicated that patients with less than 70% BM involvement fared as well as those with stage 3 disease, in the collaborative FAB/LMB trial the conventional cutoff of 25% BM involvement was utilized. It has been proposed that BM is defined as in ALL, e.g. M1–3, and similarly the extent of CNS disease, i.e. CNS 1–3. A number of additional features were also specified such as, initial resection, LDH, sites e.g. skin, bone, nodal or extranodal.

The aim of risk groupings is to achieve a consistent 100% EFS in the best risk group and to reliably define the patients of whom the prognosis remains poor, where there is need for improvement. The Frankfurt modifications on the St. Jude classification could be utilized by all pediatric oncology groups to enable comparisons of outcome. In the past, this has been problematic not only due to differences in the inclusion criteria based on histopathology, but also staging and risk grouping.

The majority of T-LL are either stage 3 or 4 disease, and it is clear that the traditional St. Jude classification fails to distinguish outcome between these two stages. In some recent studies, stage 3 disease has fared worse than stage 4. Most patients will present with a large mediastinal mass as the main site of disease bulk and the speed of response of mediastinal disease is likely to be a useful prognostic factor. Simple X-ray confirmation of complete mediastinal remission correlates with a favorable prognosis. Recent BFM regimens have upstaged patients who failed to respond more than 70% after remission chemotherapy. In this group of patients, there may be indication for further dose escalation or the use of radiation therapy.

In pediatrics, DLBCL has generally been included with other mature B-cell lymphoma in clinical trials and the conventional St. Jude staging system has been applied. CNS and BM involvement is much less likely in this condition. The pattern of nodal distribution is comparable to BL and therefore, a descriptive staging system devised for BL is probably appropriate. An adaptation of the staging system used in adult lymphoma with formal prognostic indices may be applicable to younger patients and should be the subject of retrospective analysis.

No histological subtype exemplifies more clearly the shortfalls of the St. Jude classification than ALCL in children. The disease distribution is completely different from either BL or DLBCL with a higher incidence of skin disease, parenchymal lung disease and bone disease. More recent clinical trials have attempted to use novel risk stratifications to achieve more appropriate allocation of treatment related to outcome. To date, in pediatric practice, there is no consensus regarding the optimal staging system and there is an urgent need for international agreement to ensure that clinical outcomes from different trials are comparable.

Initially, ALK expression was thought to be of prognostic significance as was the presence of a t2;5 translocation. More recent data have suggested this is not the case in childhood ALCL. There is a need for retrospective and prospective studies to define whether there are further subtypes related to immunophenotype or molecular genetics which may correlate with the clinical behavior of the disease both in terms of the initial disease distribution and the natural history.

Evaluation of response to treatment

In ALL, it has been demonstrated that the early response to treatment is one of the most powerful prognostic indicators and although the strategy of steroid monotherapy prephase as in the BFM leukemia protocols has not been applied in NHL, the response to COP has proven to be a useful prognostic indicator in the LMB studies. The optimal therapy for the COP poor responders remains unclear. In the FAB/LMB trial, these patients were upstaged to group C and received a more dose-intensive regimen. In the earlier SFOP studies, they may have also received high-dose chemotherapy with stem cell rescue. Despite this, the outcome remained relatively poor.

In the FAB/LMB trial, formal reassessment is also done after the four courses: COP, COPADM, COPADM, CYM. At this point, CR is required for the patient to remain on the group B regimen. In the absence of image-based CR, excision of residual imageable abnormality is recommended. In previous SFOP studies, patients with incomplete resection of residual disease at this stage were regarded as particularly poor risk and received not only group C chemotherapy but also received high-dose therapy with stem cell rescue. In the FAB/LMB trial, no patients in first remission received high-dose therapy. The contribution of minimal detectable disease monitoring or positron emission tomography (PET)/computed tomography (CT) in early response assessment remains to be demonstrated.

Role of 2-Deoxy-2-[18F]fluoro-D-Glucose (FDG) PET

PET CT now has a proven role in HL with regard to both initial staging and stratification on the basis of initial chemotherapy response. Although this modality has been increasingly introduced into pediatric practice, its precise role remains unclear. Preliminary data have indicated that the PET scan may show FDG positivity where nodal disease is undetectable on CT or magnetic resonance imaging (MRI). To date however there is, no evidence that such upstaging leads to changes in treatment or improved outcome.

It seems likely that the early PET response following COP will prove to be a useful prognostic indicator comparable to either the percentage of BM blasts following initial steroid prephase in ALL or the kinetics of blast cell reduction following initial chemotherapy. PET has also been used in an attempt to distinguish residual active disease following an initial course of chemotherapy in order to avoid the need for surgical biopsy. Potential delays in administration of chemotherapy due to either laparoscopic or laparotomy resection of tumor justifies an approach to find a noninvasive method. One concern with PET imaging in children is the relatively high false-positive rate by comparison with adult NHL or HL and at the present time outside prospective studies are evaluating its role; it is probably unreliable to conclude that PET positivity indicates residual active disease. In contrast, as in HL, a negative PET almost certainly indicates the absence of active disease if the PET scan has been positive at presentation.

PET may have a useful role in T-NHL for quantitation of early response. It is possible that comparing the standardized uptake values (SUV) at presentation vs. SUV after a short period of initial chemotherapy will prove of value. Similarly, PET may be of help to confirm complete remission in patients with some residual CT or MRI abnormalities. There is a need for prospective studies to determine the role of PET/CT rather than accept its widespread introduction on the basis of availability or commercial considerations rather than evidence of a real impact on treatment decision-making and patient outcome.[120]

Chemotherapy

In BL, with the very high cure rates currently achieved, there is some reluctance to consider alternatives which may have lesser acute morbidity, in fear of reduced effectiveness. The reduced intensity LMB regimen has doses of alkylating agents and anthracycline which should carry minimal late effects. The possibility of using rituximab in place of either of these agents has been considered but not yet evaluated. In preference, adding rituximab to standard and high-risk regimens will be investigated in a future international collaborative trial as a successor to the FAB/LMB study.

A key issue in DLBCL is whether treatment needs to be as intensive as in BL. In view of the very low incidence of CNS involvement, the intensive CNS-directed therapy in either the FAB/LMB or BFM approach is almost certainly excessive. This may be accompanied by subtle neurodevelopmental complications and therefore, it is desirable to minimize this aspect of therapy. The use of less CNS-intensive treatment in adults with this condition has not compromised outcome due to CNS recurrence. The problem has been the relatively low incidence of DLBCL in children and it has been difficult to mount prospective studies addressing treatment strategies in this specific histological subtype. Major advances in the outcomes in young adults with DLBCL using dose dense regimens such as the CHOP14 protocol, particularly with the addition of rituximab or etoposide has led to EFSs in young adults very close to that achieved in children with a more intensive BL approach. Although hospitalization for treatment and early complications is almost certainly higher using a Burkitt approach, late sequelae related to anthracycline exposure and doses of alkylating agent may be lower and therefore, there are those who advocate retention of this approach rather than moving to the less complex adult regimen. Provided a large international collaboration could recruit sufficient numbers, it would be desirable to mount a randomized trial asking this question and including specific evaluation of late sequelae such as infertility and cardiac dysfunction.

If the conventional Burkitt approach is retained for DLBCL, it would be important to clarify the role of rituximab in this histological subtype. Current randomized trials that are proposed to address the role of rituximab in BL are unlikely to have a sufficient number of DLBCL in children alone and in such studies should include young adults up to the age of 25 to try and answer this important question.

No histological subtype in childhood lymphoma has a more varied approach to treatment than ALCL. This ranges from immunophenotype-based regimens identical to those used in TLL, to short duration, low morbidity mature B-cell regimens. One of the key difficulties has been risk adaptation of chemotherapy. Recent studies indicating that certain clinical features of presentation such as skin combined with mediastinal disease are indicative of poor outcome and therefore, necessitate a more intensive approach. The overall favorable outcome from the CCSG/POG approach using less intensive treatment need to be reexamined in the context of the newer prognostic groupings to determine whether for certain subgroups this approach may be suboptimal. In contrast, the European approach of applying a more dose-intensive regimen almost certainly results in the over treatment of the better prognostic subgroups. The role of vinblastine remains unclear despite two randomized trials, as the OS does not appear to be influenced by the addition of this agent as currently used. The increase in RFS achieved with vinblastine indicates the need to further consolidate with an alternative approach, such as immunotherapy. The intriguing information emerging regarding the influence of the inherent immune response to ALCL has stimulated interest in this area. A number of studies now show a significant correlation between anti-ALK circulating antibody and outcome. Moreover, ALK appears to be a target for active antibody therapy and immunization approach. These avenues require urgent exploration.

Treatment of adolescents and young adults (AYA)

Although the upper age limit for enrollment on many paediatric trials covers the AYA group, constraints on recruitment have included trial group membership, poor communication between adult and pediatric specialists, competing trials run by adult groups and fixed views on the relative merits of different treatment approaches (see Chapters 3 and 17). Consequently, an AYA with NHL may receive very different therapy depending on where treated. With some diseases such as BL, the outstanding results achieved in pediatric studies have lead to widespread adoption of the LMB/BFM approach provided that appropriate supportive care is available for these very intensive regimens. In contrast, with DLBCL, the improvements in outcome with simpler CHOP-based regimens utilizing rituximab have lead to a debate about relative merits of this approach vs. the LMB/BFM, particularly with regard to short- and long-term morbidity. It is gratifying that the increased awareness of the psychosocial needs of AYA patients has lead to a much closer dialogue and collaboration across the specialties including greater efforts to facilitate trial recruitment to address a number of issues related to both tumor biology and therapies in the AYA lymphoma patient (see Chapter 28).

Summary

NHL is the third most common cancer in children ≤ 15 years of age. The four most common histological subtypes, including BL, DLBCL, LL and ALCL, account for ≥90% of all childhood NHL and are roughly divided into 70% aggressive and 30% intermediate histology. Currently, over 80% of children with NHL are cured today with multiagent chemotherapy. Radiation therapy has been practically eliminated from upfront childhood NHL protocols except for special circumstances such as CVC or acute neurological complication at diagnosis or local control of relapse or progressive disease. Similarly, surgery is limited to biopsy for diagnosis or relapse or local complications.

The next 10–20 years should be focused in the following areas of research in childhood NHL: (1) biology and genomics of childhood NHL subtypes, (2) reduction of broad-based chemotherapy and integration of targeted therapy, (3) emphasis on high-risk disease at diagnosis such as PMBL, BL with combined BM and CNS, patients with disseminated residual disease at diagnosis, patients with poor biological characteristics, (4) new therapeutic approaches to patients who relapse, progress or induction failures, (5) decrease both acute and long-term complications, (6) epidemiology and etiology of childhood NHL, (7) identification of unique targets and concomitant development of new targeted therapeutic approaches, and (8) international collaboration.

Although the last 40 years of research in childhood NHL have resulted in a significant increase in cure and reduction in length and complexity of therapy, the next 40 years should also be an exciting time to enhance our understanding of the biology of childhood NHL and to develop more novel and translational approaches to reduce toxicity and late effects, increase EFS, and identify approaches to prevent the development of childhood NHL.

Acknowledgments

The authors would like to thank Erin Morris, RN for her assistance in the development of this chapter.

Supported in part by the Pediatric Cancer Research Foundation, Sonia Scaramella Fund, Andrew J. Gargiso Foundation, Ashley Gaines Foundation and the National Cancer Institute (NIH U10 CA98543).

References

5. Anderson JR, Wilson JF, Jenkin DT, Meadows AT, Kersey J, Chilcote RR, Coccia P, Exelby P, Kushner J, Siegel S, Hammond D. (1983) Childhood non-Hodgkin's lymphoma. The results of a randomized therapeutic trial comparing a 4-drug regimen (COMP) with a 10-drug regimen (LSA2-L2). *N Engl J Med* **308**: 559–565.
7. Amylon MD, Shuster J, Pullen J, Berard C, Link MP, Wharam M, Katz J, Yu A, Laver J, Ravindranath Y, Kurtzberg J, Desai S, Camitta B, Murphy SB. (1999) Intensive high-dose asparaginase consolidation improves survival for pediatric patients with T cell acute lymphoblastic leukemia and advanced stage lymphoblastic lymphoma: A Pediatric Oncology Group study. *Leukemia* **13**: 335–342.
8. Reiter A, Schrappe M, Tiemann M, Ludwig WD, Yakisan E, Zimmermann M, Mann G, Chott A, Ebell W, Klingebiel T, Graf N, Kremens B, Muller-Weihrich S, Pluss HJ, Zintl F, Henze G, Riehm H. (1999) Improved treatment results in childhood B-cell neoplasms with tailored intensification of therapy: A report of the Berlin-Frankfurt-Munster Group Trial NHL-BFM 90. *Blood* **94**: 3294–3306.
9. Salzburg J, Burkhardt B, Zimmermann M, Wachowski O, Woessmann W, Oschlies I, Klapper W, Wacker HH, Ludwig WD, Niggli F, Mann G, Gadner H, Riehm H, Schrappe M, Reiter A. (2007) Prevalence, clinical pattern, and outcome of CNS involvement in childhood and adolescent non-Hodgkin's lymphoma differ by non-Hodgkin's lymphoma subtype: A Berlin-Frankfurt-Munster Group Report. *J Clin Oncol* **25**: 3915–3922.
10. Spreafico F, Massimino M, Luksch R, Casanova M, Cefalo GS, Collini P, Ferrari A, Polastri D, Terenziani M, Gasparini M, Fossati-Bellani F. (2002) Intensive, very short-term chemotherapy for advanced Burkitt's lymphoma in children. *J Clin Oncol* **20**: 2783–2788.
11. Cairo MS, Gerrard M, Sposto R, Auperin A, Pinkerton CR, Michon J, Weston C, Perkins SL, Raphael M, McCarthy K, Patte C. (2007) Results of a randomized international study of high-risk central nervous system B non-Hodgkin lymphoma and B acute lymphoblastic leukemia in children and adolescents. *Blood* **109**: 2736–2743.

12. Patte C, Auperin A, Gerrard M, Michon J, Pinkerton R, Sposto R, Weston C, Raphael M, Perkins SL, McCarthy K, Cairo MS. (2007) Results of the randomized international FAB/LMB96 trial for intermediate risk B-cell non-Hodgkin lymphoma in children and adolescents: It is possible to reduce treatment for the early responding patients. *Blood* **109**: 2773–2780.
13. Amos Burke GA, Imeson J, Hobson R, Gerrard M. (2003) Localized non-Hodgkin's lymphoma with B-cell histology: Cure without cyclophosphamide? A report of the United Kingdom Children's Cancer Study Group on studies NHL 8501 and NHL 9001 (1985–1996). *Br J Haematol* **121**: 586–591.
14. Gerrard M, Cairo MS, Weston C, Auperin A, Pinkerton R, Lambilliote A, Sposto R, McCarthy K, Lacombe MJ, Perkins SL, Patte C. (2008) Excellent survival following two courses of COPAD chemotherapy in children and adolescents with resected localized B-cell non-Hodgkin's lymphoma: Results of the FAB/LMB 96 international study. *Br J Haematol* **141**: 840–847.
15. Woessmann W, Seidemann K, Mann G, Zimmermann M, Burkhardt B, Oschlies I, Ludwig WD, Klingebiel T, Graf N, Gruhn B, Juergens H, Niggli F, Parwaresch R, Gadner H, Riehm H, Schrappe M, Reiter A. (2005) The impact of the methotrexate administration schedule and dose in the treatment of children and adolescents with B-cell neoplasms: A report of the BFM Group Study NHL-BFM95. *Blood* **105**: 948–958.
18. Reiter A, Klapper W. (2008) Recent advances in the understanding and management of diffuse large B-cell lymphoma in children. *Br J Haematol* **142**: 329–347.
19. Laver JH, Kraveka JM, Hutchison RE, Chang M, Kepner J, Schwenn M, Tarbell N, Desai S, Weitzman S, Weinstein HJ, Murphy SB. (2005) Advanced-stage large-cell lymphoma in children and adolescents: Results of a randomized trial incorporating intermediate-dose methotrexate and high-dose cytarabine in the maintenance phase of the APO regimen: A Pediatric Oncology Group phase III trial. *J Clin Oncol* **23**: 541–547.
21. Pfreundschuh M, Trumper L, Osterborg A, Pettengell R, Trneny M, Imrie K, Ma D, Gill D, Walewski J, Zinzani PL, Stahel R, Kvaloy S, Shpilberg O, Jaeger U, Hansen M, Lehtinen T, Lopez-Guillermo A, Corrado C, Scheliga A, Milpied N, Mendila M, Rashford M, Kuhnt E, Loeffler M. (2006) CHOP-like chemotherapy plus rituximab versus CHOP-like chemotherapy alone in young patients with good-prognosis diffuse large-B-cell lymphoma: A randomised controlled trial by the MabThera International Trial (MInT) Group. *Lancet Oncol* **7**: 379–391.
22. Sandlund JT, Santana VM, Hudson MM, Onciu M, Head D, Murry DJ, Ribeiro R, Wallace D, Rencher R, Pui CH. (2008) Combination of dexamethasone, high-dose cytarabine, and carboplatin is effective for advanced large-cell non-Hodgkin lymphoma of childhood. *Cancer* **113**: 782–790.
23. Lones MA, Perkins SL, Sposto R, Kadin ME, Kjeldsberg CR, Wilson JF, Cairo MS. (2000) Large-cell lymphoma arising in the mediastinum in children and adolescents is associated with an excellent outcome: A Children's Cancer Group report. *J Clin Oncol* **18**: 3845–3853.
25. Seidemann K, Tiemann M, Lauterbach I, Mann G, Simonitsch I, Stankewitz K, Schrappe M, Zimmermann M, Niemeyer C, Parwaresch R, Riehm H, Reiter A. (2003) Primary mediastinal large B-cell lymphoma with sclerosis in pediatric and adolescent patients: Treatment and results from three therapeutic studies of the Berlin-Frankfurt-Munster Group. *J Clin Oncol* **21**: 1782–1789.
27. Attias D, Hodgson D, Weitzman S. (2009) Primary mediastinal B-cell lymphoma in the pediatric patient: Can a rational approach to therapy be based on adult studies? *Pediatr Blood Cancer* **52**: 566–570.
29. le Deley MC, Reiter A, Williams D, Delsol G, Oschlies I, McCarthy K, Zimmermann M, Brugieres L. (2008) Prognostic factors in childhood anaplastic large cell lymphoma: Results of a large European intergroup study. *Blood* **111**: 1560–1566.
30. Rosolen A, Pillon M, Garaventa A, Burnelli R, d'Amore ES, Giuliano M, Comis M, Cesaro S, Tettoni K, Moleti ML, Tamaro P, Visintin G, Zanesco L. (2005) Anaplastic large cell lymphoma treated with a leukemia-like therapy: Report of the Italian Association of Pediatric Hematology and Oncology (AIEOP) LNH-92 protocol. *Cancer* **104**: 2133–2140.
31. Lowe EJ, Sposto R, Perkins SL, Gross TG, Finlay J, Zwick D, Abromowitch M. (2009) Intensive chemotherapy for systemic anaplastic large cell lymphoma in children and adolescents: Final results of Children's Cancer Group Study 5941. *Pediatr Blood Cancer* **52**: 335–339.
34. Brugieres L, le Deley MC, Rosolen A, Williams D, Horibe K, Wrobel G, Mann G, Zsiros J, Uyttebroeck A, Marky I, Lamant L, Reiter A. (2009) Impact of the methotrexate administration dose on the need for intrathecal treatment in children and adolescents with anaplastic large-cell lymphoma: Results of a randomized trial of the EICNHL Group. *J Clin Oncol* **27**: 897–903.
41. Reiter A, Schrappe M, Ludwig WD, Tiemann M, Parwaresch R, Zimmermann M, Schirg E, Henze G,

Schellong G, Gadner H, Riehm H. (2000) Intensive ALL-type therapy without local radiotherapy provides a 90% event-free survival for children with T-cell lymphoblastic lymphoma: A BFM group report. *Blood* **95**: 416–421.

42. Burkhardt B, Woessmann W, Zimmermann M, Kontny U, Vormoor J, Doerffel W, Mann G, Henze G, Niggli F, Ludwig WD, Janssen D, Riehm H, Schrappe M, Reiter A. (2006) Impact of cranial radiotherapy on central nervous system prophylaxis in children and adolescents with central nervous system-negative stage III or IV lymphoblastic lymphoma. *J Clin Oncol* **24**: 491–499.
44. Pillon M, Piglione M, Garaventa A, Conter V, Giuliano M, Arcamone G, Mura R, Cellini M, D'Amore ES, Varotto S, Mussolin L, Rosolen A. (2009) Long-term results of AIEOP LNH-92 protocol for the treatment of pediatric lymphoblastic lymphoma: A report of the Italian Association of Pediatric Hematology and Oncology. *Pediatr Blood Cancer* **53**: 953–959.
45. Abromowitch M, Sposto R, Perkins S, Zwick D, Siegel S, Finlay J, Cairo MS. (2008) Shortened intensified multi-agent chemotherapy and non-cross resistant maintenance therapy for advanced lymphoblastic lymphoma in children and adolescents: Report from the Children's Oncology Group. *Br J Haematol* **143**: 261–267.
47. Sandlund JT, Pui CH, Zhou Y, Behm FG, Onciu M, Razzouk BI, Hijiya N, Campana D, Hudson MM, Ribeiro RC. (2009) Effective treatment of advanced-stage childhood lymphoblastic lymphoma without prophylactic cranial irradiation: Results of St Jude NHL13 study. *Leukemia* **23**: 1127–1130.
48. Windsor R, Stiller C, Webb D. (2008) Peripheral T-cell lymphoma in childhood: Population-based experience in the United Kingdom over 20 years. *Pediatr Blood Cancer* **50**: 784–787.
50. Nelson M, Horsman DE, Weisenburger DD, Gascoyne RD, Dave BJ, Loberiza FR, Ludkovski O, Savage KJ, Armitage JO, Sanger WG. (2008) Cytogenetic abnormalities and clinical correlations in peripheral T-cell lymphoma. *Br J Haematol* **141**: 461–469.
51. Zettl A, Rudiger T, Konrad MA, Chott A, Simonitsch-Klupp I, Sonnen R, Muller-Hermelink HK, Ott G. (2004) Genomic profiling of peripheral T-cell lymphoma, unspecified, and anaplastic large T-cell lymphoma delineates novel recurrent chromosomal alterations. *Am J Pathol* **164**: 1837–1848.
52. Hutchison RE, Laver JH, Chang M, Muzzafar T, Desai S, Murphy S, Schwenn M, Shuster J, Link MP. (2008) Non-anaplastic peripheral t-cell lymphoma in childhood and adolescence: A Children's Oncology Group study. *Pediatr Blood Cancer* **51**: 29–33.
54. Paolo C, Lucia F, Anna D. (2007) Hematopoietic stem cell transplantation in peripheral T-cell lymphomas. *Leuk Lymphoma* **48**: 1496–1501.
55. Corradini P, Tarella C, Zallio F, Dodero A, Zanni M, Valagussa P, Gianni AM, Rambaldi A, Barbui T, Cortelazzo S. (2006) Long-term follow-up of patients with peripheral T-cell lymphomas treated up-front with high-dose chemotherapy followed by autologous stem cell transplantation. *Leukemia* **20**: 1533–1538.
57. Corradini P, Dodero A, Zallio F, Caracciolo D, Casini M, Bregni M, Narni F, Patriarca F, Boccadoro M, Benedetti F, Rambaldi A, Gianni AM, Tarella C. (2004) Graft-versus-lymphoma effect in relapsed peripheral T-cell non-Hodgkin's lymphomas after reduced-intensity conditioning followed by allogeneic transplantation of hematopoietic cells. *J Clin Oncol* **22**: 2172–2176.
59. Pickhardt PJ, Siegel MJ, Hayashi RJ, Kelly M. (2000) Posttransplantation lymphoproliferative disorder in children: Clinical, histopathologic, and imaging features. *Radiology* **217**: 16–25.
60. Cox KL, Lawrence-Miyasaki LS, Garcia-Kennedy R, Lennette ET, Martinez OM, Krams SM, Berquist WE, So SK, Esquivel CO. (1995) An increased incidence of Epstein-Barr virus infection and lymphoproliferative disorder in young children on FK506 after liver transplantation. *Transplantation* **59**: 524–529.
63. Opelz G, Henderson R. (1993) Incidence of non-Hodgkin lymphoma in kidney and heart transplant recipients. *Lancet* **342**: 1514–1516.
64. Webber SA, Naftel DC, Fricker FJ, Olesnevich P, Blume ED, Addonizio L, Kirklin JK, Canter CE. (2006) Lymphoproliferative disorders after paediatric heart transplantation: A multi-institutional study. *Lancet* **367**: 233–239.
70. Choquet S, Leblond V, Herbrecht R, Socie G, Stoppa AM, Vandenberghe P, Fischer A, Morschhauser F, Salles G, Feremans W, Vilmer E, Peraldi MN, Lang P, Lebranchu Y, Oksenhendler E, Garnier JL, Lamy T, Jaccard A, Ferrant A, Offner F, Hermine O, Moreau A, Fafi-Kremer S, Morand P, Chatenoud L, Berriot-Varoqueaux N, Bergougnoux L, Milpied N. (2006) Efficacy and safety of rituximab in B-cell post-transplantation lymphoproliferative disorders: Results of a prospective multicenter phase 2 study. *Blood* **107**: 3053–3057.

72. Messahel B, Taj MM, Hobson R, Hadzic N, Ramsay A, Hann I, Pinkerton R. (2006) Single agent efficacy of rituximab in childhood immunosuppression related lymphoproliferative disease: A United Kingdom Children's Cancer Study Group (UKCCSG) retrospective review. *Leuk Lymphoma* **47**: 2584–2589.
73. Gross TG, Bucuvalas JC, Park JR, Greiner TC, Hinrich SH, Kaufman SS, Langnas AN, McDonald RA, Ryckman FC, Shaw BW, Sudan DL, Lynch JC. (2005) Low-dose chemotherapy for Epstein-Barr virus-positive post-transplantation lymphoproliferative disease in children after solid organ transplantation. *J Clin Oncol* **23**: 6481–6488.
74. Orjuela M, Gross TG, Cheung YK, Alobeid B, Morris E, Cairo MS. (2003) A pilot study of chemoimmunotherapy (cyclophosphamide, prednisone, and rituximab) in patients with post-transplant lymphoproliferative disorder following solid organ transplantation. *Clin Cancer Res* **9**: 3945S-3952S.
79. Rooney CM, Smith CA, Ng CY, Loftin SK, Sixbey JW, Gan Y, Srivastava DK, Bowman LC, Krance RA, Brenner MK, Heslop HE. (1998) Infusion of cytotoxic T cells for the prevention and treatment of Epstein-Barr virus-induced lymphoma in allogeneic transplant recipients. *Blood* **92**: 1549–1555.
81. Wilson WH, Dunleavy K, Pittaluga S, Hegde U, Grant N, Steinberg SM, Raffeld M, Gutierrez M, Chabner BA, Staudt L, Jaffe ES, Janik JE. (2008) Phase II study of dose-adjusted EPOCH and rituximab in untreated diffuse large B-cell lymphoma with analysis of germinal center and post-germinal center biomarkers. *J Clin Oncol* **26**: 2717–2724.
83. Griffin TC, Weitzman S, Weinstein H, Chang M, Cairo M, Hutchison R, Shiramizu B, Wiley J, Woods D, Barnich M, Gross TG. (2009) A study of rituximab and ifosfamide, carboplatin, and etoposide chemotherapy in children with recurrent/refractory B-cell (CD20+) non-Hodgkin lymphoma and mature B-cell acute lymphoblastic leukemia: A report from the Children's Oncology Group. *Pediatr Blood Cancer* **52**: 177–181.
87. Cooney-Qualter E, Krailo M, Angiolillo A, Fawwaz RA, Wiseman G, Harrison L, Kohl V, Adamson PC, Ayello J, vande Ven C, Perkins SL, Cairo MS. (2007) A phase I study of 90yttrium-ibritumomab-tiuxetan in children and adolescents with relapsed/refractory CD20-positive non-Hodgkin's lymphoma: A Children's Oncology Group study. *Clin Cancer Res* **13**: 5652s–5660s.
88. Carnahan J, Stein R, Qu Z, Hess K, Cesano A, Hansen HJ, Goldenberg DM. (2007) Epratuzumab, a CD22-targeting recombinant humanized antibody with a different mode of action from rituximab. *Mol Immunol* **44**: 1331–1341.
90. Leonard JP, Coleman M, Ketas J, Ashe M, Fiore JM, Furman RR, Niesvizky R, Shore T, Chadburn A, Horne H, Kovacs J, Ding CL, Wegener WA, Horak ID, Goldenberg DM. (2005) Combination antibody therapy with epratuzumab and rituximab in relapsed or refractory non-Hodgkin's lymphoma. *J Clin Oncol* **23**: 5044–5051.
92. Strauss SJ, Morschhauser F, Rech J, Repp R, Solal-Celigny P, Zinzani PL, Engert A, Coiffier B, Hoelzer DF, Wegener WA, Teoh NK, Goldenberg DM, Lister TA. (2006) Multicenter phase II trial of immunotherapy with the humanized anti-CD22 antibody, epratuzumab, in combination with rituximab, in refractory or recurrent non-Hodgkin's lymphoma. *J Clin Oncol* **24**: 3880–3886.
93. Raetz EA, Cairo MS, Borowitz MJ, Blaney SM, Krailo MD, Leil TA, Reid JM, Goldenberg DM, Wegener WA, Carroll WL, Adamson PC. (2008) Chemoimmunotherapy reinduction with epratuzumab in children with acute lymphoblastic leukemia in marrow relapse: A Children's Oncology Group Pilot Study. *J Clin Oncol* **26**: 3756–3762.
94. Forero-Torres A, Leonard JP, Younes A, Rosenblatt JD, Brice P, Bartlett NL, Bosly A, Pinter-Brown L, Kennedy D, Sievers EL, Gopal AK. (2009) A Phase II study of SGN-30 (anti-CD30 mAb) in Hodgkin lymphoma or systemic anaplastic large cell lymphoma. *Br J Haematol* **146**: 171–179.
96. Miles RR, Cairo MS, Satwani P, Zwick DL, Lones MA, Sposto R, Abromovitch M, Tripp S, Angiolillo AL, Roman E, Davenport V, Perkins SL. (2007) Immunophenotypic identification of possible therapeutic targets in paediatric non-Hodgkin lymphomas: A children's oncology group report. *Br J Haematol* **138**: 506–512.
104. Gallamini A, Zaja F, Patti C, Billio A, Specchia MR, Tucci A, Levis A, Manna A, Secondo V, Rigacci L, Pinto A, Iannitto E, Zoli V, Torchio P, Pileri S, Tarella C. (2007) Alemtuzumab (Campath-1H) and CHOP chemotherapy as first-line treatment of peripheral T-cell lymphoma: Results of a GITIL (Gruppo Italiano Terapie Innovative nei Linfomi) prospective multicenter trial. *Blood* **110**: 2316–2323.
105. Attarbaschi A, Dworzak M, Steiner M, Urban C, Fink FM, Reiter A, Gadner H, Mann G. (2005) Outcome of children with primary resistant or relapsed non-Hodgkin lymphoma and mature B-cell leukemia after intensive first-line treatment: A population-based

analysis of the Austrian Cooperative Study Group. *Pediatr Blood Cancer* **44**: 70–76.

106. Burkhardt B, Reiter A, Landmann E, Lang P, Lassay L, Dickerhoff R, Lakomek M, Henze G, von Stackelberg A. (2009) Poor outcome for children and adolescents with progressive disease or relapse of lymphoblastic lymphoma: A report from the Berlin-Frankfurt-Muenster Group. *J Clin Oncol* **27**: 3363–3369.

107. Woessmann W, Peters C, Lenhard M, Burkhardt B, Sykora KW, Dilloo D, Kremens B, Lang P, Fuhrer M, Kuhne T, Parwaresch R, Ebell W, Reiter A. (2006) Allogeneic haematopoietic stem cell transplantation in relapsed or refractory anaplastic large cell lymphoma of children and adolescents — a Berlin-Frankfurt-Munster group report. *Br J Haematol* **133**: 176–182.

108. Brugieres L, Pacquement H, le Deley MC, Leverger G, Lutz P, Paillard C, Baruchel A, Frappaz D, Nelken B, Lamant L, Patte C. (2009) Single-drug vinblastine as salvage treatment for refractory or relapsed anaplastic large-cell lymphoma: A report from the French Society of Pediatric Oncology. *J Clin Oncol* **27**: 5056–5061.

109. Stockklausner C, Behnisch W, Mechtersheimer G, Moller P, Kulozik AE. (2008) Long-term remission of children with relapsed and secondary anaplastic large cell non-Hodgkin lymphoma (ALCL) following treatment with pulsed dexamethasone and low dose etoposide. *Pediatr Blood Cancer* **50**: 126–129.

112. Levine JE, Harris RE, Loberiza FR Jr., Armitage JO, Vose JM, van Besien K, Lazarus HM, Horowitz MM, Bashey A, Bolwell BJ, Burns LJ, Cairo MS, Champlin RE, Freytes CO, Gibson J, Goldstein SC, Laughlin MJ, Lister J, Marks DI, Maziarz RT, Miller AM, Milone GA, Pavlovsky S, Pecora AL, Rizzo JD, Schiller G, Schouten HC, Zhang MJ. (2003) A comparison of allogeneic and autologous bone marrow transplantation for lymphoblastic lymphoma. *Blood* **101**: 2476–2482.

118. Gross TG, Hale GA, He W, Camitta BM, Sanders JE, Cairo MS, Hayashi RJ, Termuhlen AM, Zhang MJ, Davies SM, Eapen M. (2009) Hematopoietic stem cell transplantation for refractory or recurrent non-hodgkin lymphoma in children and adolescents. *Biol Blood Marrow Transplant.*

120. Shankar A, Fiumara F, Pinkerton R. (2008) Role of FDG PET in the management of childhood lymphomas — case proven or is the jury still out? *Eur J Cancer* **44**: 663–673.

17

Adolescent Non-Hodgkin Lymphoma

Burgit Burkhardt and Ian Waxman

Introduction

Non-Hodgkin lymphoma (NHL) is the fourth most common cancer among adolescents in the US, accounting for 8% of all cancers in patients between the ages of 15 and 19 years (see Chapter 3).[1] Among adolescent patients (age 15–19 years), males are more commonly affected than females (M/F ratio: 1.7) and whites are more commonly adolescents affected than blacks (W/B ratio: 1.7).[2] The most commonly diagnosed NHL subtypes in adolescent patients include several subtypes found in children, Burkitt's lymphoma (BL), lymphoblastic lymphoma (LL), and anaplastic large cell lymphoma (ALCL), as well as the most common aggressive B-cell NHL subtype found in adult patients, diffuse large B-cell lymphoma (DLBCL). Recent US SEER data collected from 1996–2002 indicate that DLBCL is the most common adolescent NHL subtype, followed in decreasing order of incidence by LL, BL, and ALCL (see Chapter 1).[1] Similar incidences were reported in Europe, where DLBCL was again found to be the most common NHL subtype in adolescents (37%), followed by BL (22%), ALCL (18%), and LL (17%).[3] In addition to the four main subtypes of NHL found in adolescents, primary mediastinal large B-cell lymphoma (PMBL) is a fifth subtype of NHL diagnosed in adolescent and young adults patients. PMBL was previously classified by the World Health Organization (WHO) as a subtype of DLBCL, but is now considered to be a unique type of mature B-cell lymphoma (see Chapter 2).[3] In general, survival in adolescent NHL is not affected by race or gender. However, improved outcomes have been reported for adolescent patients treated at pediatric cooperative group sites.[4]

The incidence of non-Hodgkin lymphoma increases from birth through adulthood and into older age (Fig. 17.1). There is a higher mortality rate in adolescents compared to younger patients, with the number of deaths per million per year 160% higher in the 15–19-year-old age group than in the 10–14-year-old age group.[1]

Mature B-Cell Lymphoma

Diffuse large B-cell lymphoma (DLBCL) and Burkitt lymphoma (BL) are the most common mature B-cell lymphomas reported in adolescents, together accounting

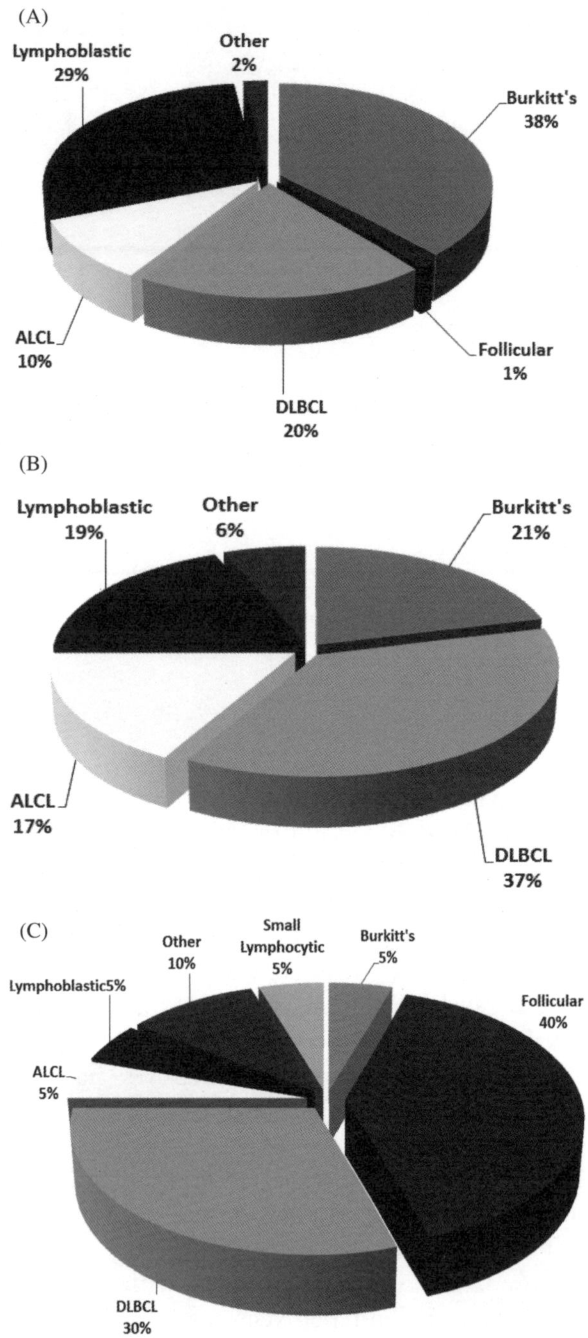

Fig. 17.1. Incidence of non-Hodgkin lymphoma subtypes in (A) 0–14-year-old age group, (B) 15–19-year-old age group, and (C) 20-year-old and older age group. Originally published Hochberg, J., Waxman, I.M., Kelly, K.M., Morris, E., Cairo, M.S. Adolescent non-Hodgkin lymphoma and Hodgkin lymphoma: State of the science. British Journal of Haematology 2009;144:24–40.

for more than half of all new diagnoses of NHL in this age group. Primary mediastinal large B-cell lymphoma (PMBL), although more rare than DLBCL and BL, occurs predominantly in adolescents and younger adults and will therefore also be discussed. While DLBCL and BL are more common in adolescent males than females, PMBL occurs equally in both sexes.[5]

Diffuse large B-cell lymphoma (DLBCL)

DLBCL accounts for approximately 40% of new NHL diagnoses in adolescent patients, making it the most common subtype in this age group.[1,6] DLBCL can be divided into subgroups based on patterns of gene expression. Activated B-cell like (ABC) and germinal center B-cell like (GCB) are the two main subtypes of DLBCL identified using gene array profiling (see Chapter 8).[7,8] ABC DLBCL, as well as PMBL (discussed later) exhibits constitutive activation of NF-κB signal transduction genes, while GCB DLBCL does not.[9] In addition, ABC DLBCL stains for MUM1, while GCB DLBCL stains for CD10 and BCL6, allowing for subtyping by immunohistochemistry.[10] While the vast majority of pediatric and adolescent DLBCL is of the better prognosis GCB-subtype, less than half of adult DLBCL patients exhibit this subtype.[10–12] Morphologically, DLBCL can be subdivided into centroblastic, immunoblastic, T-cell/histioctye–rich, anaplastic or not otherwise specified subtypes. The majority of pediatric DLBCL is of the monomorphic centroblastic variant, whereas immunoblastic variants are also commonly found in adults.[12]

Primary mediastinal large B-cell lymphoma (PMBL)

PMBL is a rare malignancy thought to arise from mature thymic B-cells. Gene expression profiling has shown PMBL to share similarities with classic Hodgkin lymphoma (cHL) and, for this reason, PMBL is thought to fall along the biological spectrum between NHL and cHL (see Chapter 8).[13,14] Further supporting a link between PMBL and cHL is the presence of several of the same chromosomal aberrations in both diseases, including gains in chromosome 9p and 2p, the gene loci for JAK-2 and c-rel, respectively.[15]

Burkitt lymphoma (BL)

BL is the most common NHL subtype in children age 5–14 years, but is less common than DLBCL in the adolescent age group, where it accounts for 21% of all NHL.[1] Gene expression profiling can be used to distinguish between BL and DLBCL, as the BL gene signature includes a high level of expression of c-myc target genes and low levels of expression of NF-κB genes (see Chapter 8).[16,17]

Clinical features of mature B-cell lymphoma in adolescents

In general, the clinical manifestations of mature B-cell lymphoma depend primarily on primary and secondary sites of involvement. Clinical presentation is more directly related to subtype of mature B-cell lymphoma (DLBCL vs. PMBL vs. BL) rather than age of patient at diagnosis.

DLBCL manifests most commonly with an abdominal mass without, while PMBL always involves a mediastinal mass. The mediastinal mass of PMBL is usually large, involves adjacent structures and the lungs, and may be accompanied by superior vena cava syndrome. DLBCL and PMBL rarely spread to the CNS or bone marrow. BL commonly presents with abdominal or head and neck disease and often involves the bone marrow or CNS. Abdominal presentation is characteristic of the sporadic type, while head and neck involvement is more commonly associated with endemic BL.

Of note, while DLBCL is more common in adults than children and BL is more common in childhood, PMBL is found most often in adolescents and young adults, with a median age of onset of 13.2 years reported for 40 PMBL patients treated on three successive pediatric protocols (up to age 18 years) in Germany.[5]

Risk stratification and treatment of adolescent mature B-cell NHL

No trials for mature B-cell NHL have taken place exclusively in an adolescent population and there is no risk stratification system that takes into account adolescent age. Adolescent patients with DLBCL, BL, and PMBL have generally been treated on pediatric protocols for mature B-cell NHL. Two pediatric B-cell NHL risk stratification strata are used: the German BFM stratification which includes four risk categories, and the FAB stratification which includes three risk strata (Table 17.1) (see Chapter 16).

Most pediatric mature B-cell NHL protocols, including the French LMB and German BFM protocols, utilize a cyclophosphamide, high-dose methotrexate, cytarabine, and triple intrathecal chemotherapy backbone for intermediate and high-risk patients.[18,19] Trials have

Table 17.1. Risk stratification groups for pediatric B-cell NHL.

	Berlin–Frankfurt–Munster (BFM)	French–American–British (FAB)
Low Risk	**R1** Stage I or II, completely resected	**Group A** Resected stage I and abdominal completely resected stage II
	R2 Stage I or II, not resected Stage III with LDH < 500 U/L	**Group B** All patients not in Group A or C
	R3 Stage III with LDH ≥ 500 to < 1000 U/L or Stage IV with LDH < 1000 U/L and CNS-negative	**Group C** Bone marrow disease (≥ 25% L3 blasts) and/or CNS-positive
High Risk	**R4** Stage III or IV with LDH ≥ 1000 U/L and/or CNS-positive	

Originally published in Waxman, I., Hochberg, J., and Cairo, M.S. Lymphoma. Nelson Textbook of Pediatrics, 19th Edition, Kliegman, R.M., Stanton, B.F., St. Geme, J., Schor, N., Behrman, R.E., eds. Elsevier, Philadelphia, 2010 (in press).

included higher dose intensity during the first month of treatment and dose intensification for lack of response after 7 days of therapy.

Adult B-cell NHL patients are generally treated as per National Comprehensive Cancer Network (NCCN) guidelines.[20] The treatment of adult DLBCL generally includes a cyclophosphamide, doxorubicin, vincristine, and prednisone (CHOP)-based regimen with rituximab. Adult patients with DLBCL are generally recommended for clinical trials after second or greater relapse. In younger adult patients, improved outcomes with the addition of rituximab to CHOP-based therapy in were reported in the MabThera International Trial (Mint).[21] In this trial, an improvement in 3 year EFS from 59% to 79% ($p < 0.0001$) was found with the addition of rituximab to six cycles of CHOP therapy (see Chapter 21).

Though NCCN guidelines acknowledge that CHOP-based regimens are widely used for PMBL, they suggest that more intense therapy may be appropriate in the first-line setting.

As BL is exceedingly rare in adult patients, accounting for only 5% of NHL in the adult population, NCCN guidelines include a recommendation for enrollment in a clinical trial at initial diagnosis. CHOP therapy is not considered adequate for adult BL, and recommended combination regimens include hyperCVAD (cyclophosphamide, vincristine, doxorubicin, and dexamethasone) alternating with high-dose methotrexate and cytarabine ± rituximab, dose-adjusted EPOCH (etoposide, prednisone, vincristine, cyclophosphamide, doxorubicin) ± rituximab, and CODOX-M (cyclophosphamide, doxorubicin, vincristine with intrathecal methotrexate and cytarabine followed by high-dose systemic methotrexate) ± rituximab with (for high-risk patients) IVAC (ifosfamide, cytarabine, etoposide, and intrathecal methotrexate).

Surgical resection is used as part of the treatment of localized mature B-cell NHL in both pediatric and adult treatment regimens.

Outcomes in adolescent mature B-cell NHL

Adult patients with mature B-cell NHL tend to have worse outcomes than pediatric and adolescent patients (except for PMBL), which may be due to a combination of factors including differences in tumor biology and therapy. Numerous examples of differences in tumor biology exist for pediatric and adult DLBCL, including a predominance of the GCB subtype in younger patients and a higher percentage of tumors expressing the t(14;18) translocation in adults compared to children and adolescents (28% vs. 7%, respectively).[22] Outcomes in children and adolescents with PMBL are worse than in pediatric patients with other mature B-cell NHL subtypes and are also inferior to those seen in adults with PMBL.

Outcomes have been reported for the FAB/LMB 96 pediatric trial in mature B-cell NHL. Sixteen percent of patients in the FAB/LMB intermediate risk treatment arm were older than age 15 years, while 12% of high-risk patients were between the ages of 15 and 19 years. Intermediate risk patients >15 years of age enrolled in the FAB/LMB 96 trial had a 4-year EFS of 92%, while higher risk patients had a 4-year EFS of 79%.[18,23] A univariate analysis of data from the French–American–British (FAB)/Lymphome Malins de Burkitt (LMB) 96 study in pediatric patients with B-cell NHL found that patients age ≥15 years had significantly lower 5-year event-free survival (EFS) and overall survival (OS) compared to patients <15 years. However, with multivariate analysis, differences in outcome by age disappeared and were explained by differences in tumor histology, stage of disease, and increased lactate dehydrogenase (LDH). In an examination of EFS by age (5-year intervals) in high-risk patients, no significant differences were found (see Chapter 16).

In a recent review of 378 adolescent NHL patients treated according to six consecutive NHL-BFM protocols from 1986 to 2007, 378 adolescent (age 15–18 years) patients were identified.[24] Among adolescent patients, 101 had BL or B-cell acute leukemia (B-AL), 55 had DLBCL (centroblastic type), and 24 had PMBL. Analysis of results from these studies revealed inferior pEFS in adolescents compared to children with BL/B-AL (82 ± 4% vs. 88 ± 1%, respectively, $p = 0.06$), as well as in adolescents compared to children with DLBCL (85 ± 5% vs. 96 ± 2%, respectively, $p = 0.002$). Although a difference in pEFS was also seen for PMBL in adolescents vs. children (57 ± 10% vs. 68 ± 8%), this difference did not approach statistical significance ($p = 0.55$). In an analysis of four consecutive Children's Cancer Group (CCG) studies, adolescents with BL or Burkitt-like lymphoma were also found to have a lower EFS when compared to younger patients (4-year EFS: 34 ± 7% vs. 59 ± 2%, respectively, $p < 0.05$).[25]

Lower risk pediatric patients have excellent outcomes with reduced duration and intensity of chemotherapy, as evidenced by the results patients enrolled in the FAB/LMB 96 study with localized B-cell NHL.[26] Among 132 patients treated with two courses of cyclophosphamide, vincristine, prednisolone, and doxorubicin (COPAD), the 4-year EFS and OS were 98% and 99%, respectively.

Prognostic factors in adolescent mature B-cell NHL

In an analysis of patients treated on three successive pediatric NHL protocols, Burkhardt *et al.* reported that adolescent females with DLBCL (centroblastic subtype) had a worse outcome than younger females with the same diagnosis, while no difference was found between adolescent and younger males with DLBCL.[5] In this same analysis, the risk ratios for PMBL and DLBCL in patients ≥15 years vs. <15 years were 3.19 and 3.62, respectively, with *p*-values trending toward statistical significance.

Prognostic factors other than age have been examined in pediatric mature B-cell NHL trials. Among high-risk patients on FAB/LMB 96, Cairo *et al.* found no significant difference in EFS by diagnosis (DLBCL vs. B-ALL) or LDH (≤ 2 vs. > 2 time ULN).[23] 4-year EFS for intermediate-risk patients on FAB/LMB 96, however, was found to depend on diagnosis. When patients were separated into BL, DLBCL and PMBL subgroups, 4-year EFS for intermediate-risk patients were 93.3%,

92.7%, and 71.5%, respectively. Among pediatric patients with PMBL treated on three successive BFM studies, those with PMBL had 5-year EFS of 65 ± 8% compared with 85 ± 1% for the entire patient cohort.[5]

Anaplastic Large Cell Lymphoma (ALCL)

Anaplastic large cell lymphoma (ALCL) was first described by Stein *et al.* in 1985.[27] It is characterized by large anaplastic cells which stain positive for CD30, which is also characteristic of Hodgkin lymphoma's Reed–Sternberg cells. The wide morphological spectrum of the lymphoma cells has allowed the identification of histological subtypes. The identification of the nonrandom translocation t(2;5)(p23;q35) in the majority of cases in 1994 marked a major advance in the characterization of ALCL.[28] This translocation leads to the fusion of the nucleophosmin (NPM) gene at chromosome 5q35 and the anaplastic lymphoma kinase (ALK) gene at 2p23, resulting in the production of a fusion protein (for details on the biology see Chapters 2, 4, 7, and 8). The identification of monoclonal antibodies directed against two formalin-resistant epitopes of ALK supported the characterization of the disease.[29] Recognition of the importance of the characterization of ALK protein expression for the biology and clinical presentation as well as ongoing elucidation of the molecular biology of ALCL led to the specification of distinct subgroups in the 2008 version of the WHO classification of tumors of the hematopoietic and lymphoid tissue: primary cutaneous CD30-positive T-cell lymphoproliferative disorders, ALK-positive anaplastic large-cell lymphoma, and ALK-negative anaplastic large cell lymphoma.

ALCL occurs more commonly in adolescent NHL patients than in patients < 14 years of age. Within pediatric NHL populations, ALCL accounts for 11% of cases compared to 20% in adolescent NHL series.[24] Median age at diagnosis was 11.8 years for 215 ALCL patients registered in the NHL-BFM study center.[5] ALK-negative ALCL was reported to occur more frequently with increasing age and to be associated with inferior outcome.[30,31] However, for the NHL-BFM studies including patients diagnosed between 1986 and 2007, it was reported that the frequency of ALK-negative ALCL did not differ between pediatric and adolescent patients, with data from immunohistochemical analysis of ALK protein expression in 211 pediatric and 52 adolescent patients showing 10% vs. 12% ALK-negative ALCL.[5] In a large pediatric multicenter trial conducted between 1999 and 2005 and including patients up to the age of 22 years, the frequency of ALK-positive cases diagnosed with modern molecular techniques was 96%.[32] Unfortunately, the rate of ALK-negative cases was not specified for the adolescent age group. However, the available data indicate that ALK-negative ALCL represents a small subgroup of ALCL in adolescents, accounting for about 10% or even less.

Clinical features of ALCL in adolescents

The clinical presentation of ALCL is heterogeneous and can vary greatly between individual patients. Extranodal lymphoma manifestations of the skin, bone or soft tissue are reported more frequently than in other adolescent NHL subtypes.[33–35] Longer periods with nonspecific symptoms such as fever and lymphadenopathy are reported in a relevant number of cases prior to the diagnosis of ALCL. Among adolescent ALCL patients, about 40% are female. Elevated lactic dehydrogenase (LDH) at diagnosis (≥ 500 U/L) is observed in less than 10% of the patients, advanced stages of disease (St. Jude stage III or IV)[36] is frequent and diagnosed in about 80% of adolescent ALCL patients, while overt BM or CNS involvement is diagnosed in 5% and < 5% of patients, respectively. About half of patients suffer from B symptoms and, roughly a quarter of adolescent ALCL patients have poor performance status according to Karnofsky scale at initial diagnosis.

Comparison of clinical characteristics in pediatric and adolescent ALCL patients enrolled in the NHL-BFM trials reveals no significant differences between the two age groups with regard to gender distribution, serum LDH level, BM and/or CNS involvement, B symptoms and Karnofsky performance status at diagnosis. The only exception is a trend towards a higher frequency of advanced stage disease according to the St. Jude staging system[36] in adolescents (80%) compared to pediatric ALCL patients (68%) ($p = 0.06$). Concerning the impact of gender within the adolescent age group, clinical characteristics do not show significant differences between male and female adolescent patients with ALCL in the NHL-BFM trials.[24]

Treatment, outcome and prognostic factors in ALCL

No clinical trials specifically focused on adolescents with ALCL have been reported to date. Treatment of adolescent ALCL patients therefore follows either pediatric or adult protocols, and the criteria for the allocation of adolescents to pediatric or internal medicine departments vary even within countries and study groups.

Adolescent ALCL patients in pediatric trials

Several pediatric clinical trials defined the upper age limit of their protocols by 18 or 21 years at diagnosis and included relevant numbers of adolescent patients. Up to the present, variable treatment approaches for anaplastic large cell lymphoma have been used. Both ALL-based regimen and short-pulse–type B-NHL strategies have resulted in comparable event-free survival rates of 65–80% and overall survival rates of 70–93%, as shown in Table 17.2 (for details see Chapter 16).[33,35,37–40]

The largest pediatric series of ALCL patients reported 352 patients enrolled in the European intergroup cooperation (EICNHL) trial ALCL 99,[32] which was open for patients less than 22 years of age at diagnosis. Chemotherapy in EICNHL trial ALCL 99 was based on the NHL-BFM 90 protocol[35] and consisted of a cytoreductive prephase and three to six intensive 5-day courses. The methotrexate (MTX) dose and administration schedule were randomly allocated into MTX1 or MTX3 before the first course. Arm MTX1 included 1-g/m^2 methotrexate in 24-hour infusion with triple intrathecal injection at day 1 and leucovorin rescue (15 mg/m^2) at least at 42, 48, and 54 hours (ending when the methotrexate level was < 0.25 μmol/L). Arm MTX3 included methotrexate 3 g/m^2 in 3-hour infusion without intrathecal injection and with leucovorin rescue (15 mg/m^2 every 6 hours) starting at 24 hours and ending when the methotrexate level was <0.25 μmol/L. Additionally, high-risk patients could enter a second randomized trial before the second course and were then randomly assigned to receive or not receive a vinblastine injection (6 mg/m^2) during the five latter

Table 17.2. Pediatric trials for anaplastic large cell lymphoma, outcome and outcome according to age.

	Whole study including children and adolescents			Data according to age groups		
Trial	Age	Pts	Outcome	Age (years)	Pts	Outcome
EICNHL/Europe ALCL 99[32] < 22 yrs	Median 11.0 yrs, range 4 mths–19.5 yrs	352 (100%)	2-yr OS 92.5%	<3 3–16 >16	19 (5%) 308 (88%) 25 (7%)	n.d. n.d. n.d.
SFOP/France HM89 and HM91[33] < 18 yrs	Median age 10 yrs, range 17 mths to 17 yrs	82 (100%)	3-yr OS of 83% (72–90%) 3-yr EFS 66% (54–76%)	≥10	38 (46%)	3-yr EFS 69% (51–82%)
UKCCSG/UK Protocols 9001, 9002/9602, 9003[40] < 18 yrs	Median 11.8 yrs, range of 1.1–16.4 yrs	72 (100%)	5-yr OS 65% (53–76%) 5-yr EFS 59% (47–70%)	< 10	47 (65%)	5-yr EFS 64% (49–77%)
NHL-BFM/Germany, Austria, Switzerland NHL-BFM 90[35] < 18 yrs	Median 10.5 yrs, range 0.8–17.3 yrs	89 (100%)	5-yr EFS 76 ± 5%			
AIEOP/Italy LNH-92[39] < 15 yrs	Median age 11.6 yrs, range 4.2–14.9 yrs	34 (100%)	10-yr OS 85 ± 6% 10-yr EFS 65 ± 8%	≥ 10	23 (68%)	10-yr EFS 65 ± 9%
CCG/US CCG-5941[38] < 21 yrs	n.d.	86 (100%)	5-yr OS 80% (69–87%) 5-yr EFS 68% (57–78%)	< 5 5–9 10–14 ≥14	6 (7%) 29 (34%) 33 (38%) 18 (21%)	n.d. n.d. n.d. n.d.
POG/US APO-POG[37] Stage III/IV < 21 yrs	n.d.	86 (100%)	4-yr OS 88 ± 4% 4-yr EFS 72 ± 6%			

n.d.: no data.

courses and weekly afterwards for a total of 12 months duration of treatment. This trial reported a 2-year survival rate of 92.5% (95% CI 89–95%) for the whole group of 352 ALCL patients. A total of 25 patients (7% of the study population) were 17–21 years of age at diagnosis. Unfortunately, the characteristics and outcomes for this subgroup were not analyzed separately.

Three recent publications on ALCL in pediatric and adolescent patients specified outcome according to age (Table 17.2):

For the French Society of Pediatric Oncology, Brugieres and colleagues reported the outcome of 82 pediatric patients enrolled in the subsequent pediatric French trials HM89 and 91. The overall 3-year EFS for the whole group was 66%. The EFS for the subgroup of patients ≥ 10 years (n = 38) was 69%.[33]

Williams *et al.* reported the results of the UKCCSG trials 9001, 9002/9602 and 9003,[40] with a 5-year EFS of 59% for 72 pediatric and adolescent ALCL patients treated according to protocols 9001, 9002/9602, and 9003. Again, age < 10 years or ≥ 10 years was of no prognostic significance. The 5-year EFS for the pediatric patients < 10 years was 64%.[40]

Rosolen *et al.* reported results of the Italian trial LNH-92.[39] The patient enrollment was restricted to patients < 15 years of age at diagnosis and treatment was based on a modified LSA2-L2 protocol. LSA2-L2 had originally been designed for the treatment of pediatric acute lymphoblastic leukemia. Adapting this regimen for pediatric ALCL patients resulted in a 10-year EFS of 65 ± 8% for the whole population of 34 ALCL patients and 65 ± 9% for the 23 ALCL patients ≥ 10 years at diagnosis.

In all of these reports, outcome for patients age ≥ 10 years was similar to that of pediatric ALCL patients treated according to the same protocol. Interestingly, the French and UK trials were based on the treatment strategy for mature B-NHL lymphoma, while the Italian study used an ALL-type treatment strategy. Therefore, the observation that similar outcome can be achieved with short pulses of intensive chemotherapy, as well as with continuous ALL-type treatment, seemingly holds true not only for pediatric but also for ≥ 10 year aged ALCL patients.

The largest series of adolescents with ALCL treated according to pediatric protocols was reported by the NHL-BFM group.[5,24] The recent analyses included all patients registered in NHL-BFM studies between 1986 and 2007 and reported the outcome for 74 adolescent ALCL patients who were 15–18 years of age at diagnosis. The NHL-BFM protocols used pulse-type treatment as a common backbone strategy for ALCL patients. For the trials NHL-BFM 90 and 95, treatment was stratified by disease stage according to the St. Jude staging system,[36] and the presence of risk factors, including multifocal bone lesions, and for the trial NHL-BFM 95, skin or lung manifestations, the lymphohistiocytic or uncommon morphological variant ALCL or secondary ALCL. The allocation of newly diagnosed ALCL patients into the three risk groups K1, K2, and K3 was 8%, 50%, and 43% for pediatric patients respectively, compared to 0%, 68%, and 32% for the 25 evaluable adolescents with ALCL. These data indicate that the distribution into risk groups is similar for pediatric and adolescents with ALCL. Outcome analysis of the respective populations revealed that in ALCL patients — contrary to other NHL-subtypes — adolescent age was of no prognostic relevance. Outcome for adolescents compared to 290 children with ALCL enrolled during the same period showed no differences between the two age groups (5-year EFS 70 ± 3% vs. 70 ± 6%, Fig. 17.2). The types and rates of events were also comparable for pediatric and adolescent ALCL; in both age groups, there were no deaths due to initial complications of treatment such as fatal tumor lysis syndrome etc. Treatment-related mortality was rare as well, occurring in 2% of the pediatric population and 1% of the adolescents. Lymphoma progression during or after the end of treatment occurred in 28% of pediatric ALCL and 26% of adolescents with ALCL. Secondary malignancies were documented for 1% of children and 3% of adolescents treated according to NHL-BFM protocols which did not include local radiotherapy.

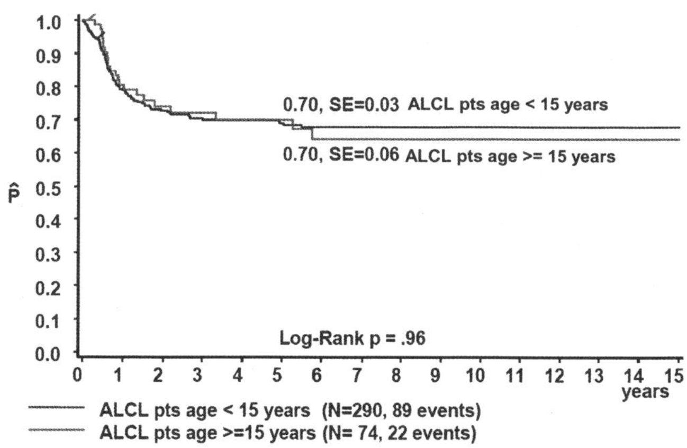

Fig. 17.2. Five-year event-free survival (EFS) analyses for adolescent ALCL patients compared to pediatric ALCL patients treated according to the NHL-BFM based treatment regimen.

Again, contrary to other NHL subtypes in adolescents, there is no significant difference in outcome within the adolescent age group when comparing male and female patients. The 5-year EFS for 45 male patients and 29 female patients treated on pediatric NHL-BFM protocols for ALCL was 73 ± 7% and 64 ± 10%, respectively.

Prognostic factors other than age in pediatric ALCL trials

Within the pediatric multicenter trials, several parameters have been tested for prognostic impact on outcome.

For the French trials HM89 and HM91, which included 82 children and adolescents, visceral involvement (including splenomegaly, hepatomegaly, lung involvement, pleural effusion and other visceral involvement), mediastinal involvement and LDH ≥ 800 U/L were associated with poor prognosis in univariate and multivariate analyses.[33] Age ≥ 10 years at diagnosis and gender were of no prognostic relevance.

In the combined analyses of the UKCCSG trials 9001, 9002/9602, and 9003, visceral involvement and mediastinal involvement were again associated with inferior outcome, and these parameters maintained statistical significance in multivariate analyses.[40] Age ≥ 10 years and gender did not correlate with outcome in that study.

For 34 Italian patients treated according to the ALL-based treatment regimen LNH-92, neither age, gender, stage, site of involvement, histology nor LDH were of prognostic relevance.[39] In the BFM trial NHL-BFM 90, lung involvement, splenomegaly and B symptoms at diagnosis were associated with inferior outcome in univariate analyses, and B symptoms remained prognostic in multivariate analyses. The prognostic relevance of age was not tested.[35]

Finally, for the trial CCG 5941, only bone marrow involvement was found to correlate with lower EFS. Age, gender, race, elevated LDH, and mediastinal involvement were not shown to be suitable prognostic factors for EFS.[38]

In a cooperative analysis of prognostic parameters in pediatric and adolescent ALCL, the available clinical data from the German NHL-BFM, the French SFOP, and the UKCCSG were pooled and analyzed together.[41] The whole series comprised 225 ALCL patients, including 117 patients ≥ 10 years of age at diagnosis. In univariate analysis, age ≥ 10 years was not associated with outcome (RR 0.81 (0.50–1.3, $p = 0.41$)). In multivariate analysis, the risk of progression or relapse was associated with involvement of lung, liver, or spleen, skin lesions, and mediastinal tumor. An advanced stage of disease according to St. Jude or Ann Arbor classification had no additional prognostic value when the three risk factors were taken into account. The risk of progression or relapse increased with the number of risk factors.

Concerning molecular markers, qualitative and quantitative detection of circulating tumor cells in bone marrow or blood by PCR were reported to be strongly associated with poorer outcome, but the analysis was not provided specifically for adolescents with ALCL (see Chapter 10).[42]

ALCL in adults

There are no specific protocols for ALCL in adults. Patients with ALCL are treated with multiagent chemotherapy regimen commonly used for mature B-NHL, mostly CHOP (cyclophosphamide, hydroxydaunorubicine, Oncovin [vincristine], and prednisone) or CHOP-like regimens.

Gascoyne *et al.* analyzed 70 patients with systemic ALCL, including three adolescent patients 15–19 years at diagnosis.[43] The median age was 49 years for the entire population. Within the 70 ALCL patients, ALK-positive patients represented 51% of the cases. Patients were treated with CHOP-like therapy with or without local radiotherapy. However, details of treatment were not reported. The 5-year overall survival was 65% for the whole population. Analysis according to ALK-status yielded an overall survival rate of 79% for the group of 36 ALK-positive ALCL patients (median age: 30 years; range: 15–64 years) and an overall survival rate of 46% ($p = 0.0003$) for the 34 ALK-negative ALCL cases (median age: 61 years; range: 27–75 years). Even though ALK-positivity correlated with younger age, only normal LDH level, International Prognostic Index score ≤ 3 (IPI, based on age, Ann Arbor stage of disease, serum LDH level, ECOG performance status, extranodal site) and ALK-positivity remained prognostic parameters in multivariate analyses for adult patients with ALCL treated with CHOP-like regimen.

Similar results were reported by Falini *et al.* who reviewed 96 ALCL cases and found ALK-positivity in 58 (60%), mostly in children and young adults (mean age 22 ± 11 years) with a male predominance (male/female ratio 3.0). ALK-negative ALCL occurred primarily in older individuals (mean age 43 ± 16 years) and showed a lower M/F ratio (0.9). The overall survival of patients with ALK-positive lymphoma was far better than that of patients with ALK-negative ALCL (71 ± 6% vs. 15 ± 11%, respectively). Outcome analysis of patients with ALK-positive ALCL split according to age revealed no statistically significant difference, with 36 patients alive out of 47 patients, 35 years of age or younger, compared to four patients alive out of six ALK-positive cases older than 35 years of age.[30] However, within the good prognostic category of ALK-positive lymphoma, survival was 94 ± 5% for the low/low intermediate risk group (age-adjusted International Prognostic Index, 0 to 1) and only 41 ± 12% for the high/high intermediate-risk group. Multivariate analysis identified ALK expression and the International Prognostic Index as independent variables and prognostic factors for survival among patients with primary systemic anaplastic large-cell lymphoma.

A recent report of the International Peripheral T-Cell Lymphoma Project including 22 institutions in North America, Europe and Asia reported 87 patients with ALK-positive ALCL and 72 cases with ALK-negative ALCL.[44] For the patients with ALK-positive ALCL, the median age was 34 years, and 74 patients (86%) were less than 60 years at diagnosis. Among ALK-negative patients, median age was 58 years, with 42 patients (58%) being less than 60 years of age. The treatment was a largely anthracycline-based regimen not further specified in the respective publication. The 5-year survival was 70% for the ALK-positive and 49% for the ALK-negative ALCL patients. In line with prior studies, survival rates were superior amongst patients with ALK-positive ALCL compared to patients with ALK-negative ALCL. Patients with ALK-positive ALCL were generally younger than those with ALK-negative ALCL. It is interesting to note that there was no difference in overall survival when the comparison of ALK-negative and ALK-positive patients was limited to those 40 years of age and older (n = 64 and n = 30, respectively) or younger than 40 years (n = 7 and n = 55, respectively). This led to the suggestion that age features as a prominent factor behind outcome differences. Available data on outcome for adolescent and adult patients with ALCL are summarized in Table 17.3.

In conclusion, the available data for ALCL in adolescents indicate that, in contrast to other histological subtypes of NHL, the outcome for ALCL patients treated according to pediatric protocols is similar for adolescents and younger children. In fact, the combined analyses of pediatric and adult patient series indicates that within ALCL, the ALK status might be more important than age, with ALK-positive children, adolescents and young adults representing a distinct subgroup. In these patients, the LDH levels are often within the normal range, although two-thirds or more present with advanced stage III/IV disease according to St. Jude. With pulse-type chemotherapy these patients have an EFS of about 75%. As learned from the pediatric studies, increased intensity of treatment (e.g. the dose of methotrexate) does not necessarily result in increased cure rates. Especially for ALK-positive ALCL, interdisciplinary trials enrolling children, adolescents and young adults might be the approach suited best for the underlying biology of the disease. The use of uniform treatment approaches should add to the elucidation of the prognostic impact of patient age in ALCL.

Table 17.3. Summary of treatment outcome for adolescent and adult patients with anaplastic large cell lymphoma.

Reference	No. of pts	Outcome
Adolescent ALCL patients		
Brugieres *et al.*[33]	38 ALCL pts 10–18 yrs of age	3-yr EFS 69% (51–82%)
Rosolen *et al.*[39]	23 ALCL pts 10–15 yrs of age	10-yr EFS 65 ± 9%
Burkhardt *et al.*[24]	74 ALCL pts 15–18 yrs of age	5-yr EFS 74 ± 6%
Adult ALCL patients		
Gascoyne *et al.*[43]	All 70 ALCL pts	5-yr OS 65%
	36 ALK-positive ALCL pts	5-yr OS 79%
	34 ALK-negative ALCL pts	5-yr OS 46%
Falini *et al.*[30]	53 ALK-positive ALCL pts	OS 71 ± 6%
	23 ALK-negative ALCL pts	OS 15 ± 11%
Savage *et al.*[44]	87 ALK-positive ALCL pts	5-yr OS 70%
	72 ALK-negative ALCL pts	5-yr OS 49%

Lymphoblastic Lymphoma (LBL)

Lymphoblastic lymphoma (LBL) accounts for approximately 20% of pediatric non-Hodgkin lymphoma.[5] LBL can be subdivided in LBL of T-lineage (T-LBL) and precursor B-cell lineage (pB-LBL), comprising 75–80% and 15–20% of cases respectively. Along with mature B-NHL and ALCL, lymphoblastic lymphoma, represents one of the three major subgroups of non-Hodgkin lymphoma in children and adolescents; however, available data on LBL in adolescents is sparse in both the pediatric and adult literature. In the German, Austrian, and Swiss NHL-BFM studies, the frequency of LBL in adolescent NHL patients was 12% for T-LBL and 3% for pB-LBL. This is slightly less than for all pediatric NHL patients, in which T-LBL accounts for 16% and pB-LBL for 5% of all newly diagnosed NHL.[24] Median age at diagnosis was 8.8 years for 335 T-LBL patients and 8.0 years for 97 pB-LBL patients.[5] The NHL-BFM studies were population-based trials in which >95% of all newly diagnosed pediatric NHL patients were enrolled. However, adolescent patients have only recently been registered in the German Childhood Cancer Registry, so the possibility exists that the NHL-BFM data on adolescent NHL patients might not include all newly diagnosed patients. Concerning the absolute incidence of lymphoblastic lymphoma in the pediatric and adolescent population, there is no clear evidence for a change in recent years (see Chapter 16).[2,45]

Although the WHO classification has unified both acute lymphoblastic leukemia (ALL) and lymphoblastic lymphoma (LBL) as precursor lymphoblastic leukemia/lymphoma[46–48] in clinical practice ALL and LBL are usually regarded and treated as separate diseases. Several study groups distinguish between leukemia and lymphoma based on the primary site of involvement. Patients with less than 25% lymphoblasts in the bone marrow and no peripheral blasts are classified as having lymphoblastic lymphoma; patients with 25% or more blasts in the bone marrow patients are classified as having leukemia. Both ALL and LBL are neoplasms of lymphoblasts committed to the lymphoid lineage. The postulated cell of origin is the precursor cell lymphoblast whose differentiation is arrested at discrete stages of maturation. Thus, the malignant clones in patients with ALL or LBL are thought to originate from normal lymphoid progenitor cells arrested at early stages of maturation.

The histopathological and immunophenotypic features of lymphoblastic lymphoma are distinctive, so that diagnosis, if properly approached, is not usually problematic (see Chapter 4). The differential diagnosis includes other NHL subtypes which can be distinguished from ALL and LBL by immunophenotypic characterization of the cells. Further differential diagnostic considerations include other small round-cell tumors. CD99, which is characteristically present on Ewing's sarcoma and peripheral neuroectodermal tumor, is also expressed in lymphoblastic malignancies.[49] Distinction of T-LBL from thymoma is a bit more complicated because both tumors have a thymic T-cell phenotype, but the morphology of the cells is generally different and the characteristic epithelial distribution of thymoma is not present in lymphoma. In addition, cases of thymoma are rare in childhood and adolescence. Morphologically, LBL show diffuse patterns of tissue involvement by a uniform population of small to medium-sized blastic cells. The nuclear cytoplasmic ratio is high. The classically described morphologic findings of LBL correspond to L1 (or L2) acute lymphoblastic leukemia in the French–American–British (FAB) classification of acute lymphoblastic leukemia.[50] LBL is usually TdT-positive, a marker that distinguishes them from all other types of lymphoma. In addition to TdT, CD34 and/or CD99 (MIC2) are also expressed by the majority of LBL and have proved useful in distinguishing this malignancy from other NHL. The immunophenotype of LBL committed to the T-lineage (T-LBL) corresponds to defined stages of intrathymic T-cell differentiation.[51,52] For precursor B-cell lymphoblastic lymphoma, the stage of maturation is differentiated by the expression of surface proteins.

Due to the scarcity of adequate tumor tissue, reported cytogenetic or molecular genetic studies of LBL are rare and include only small numbers of patients. Furthermore, many reports that describe molecular and cytogenetic findings of LBL include cases of ALL and vice versa. An accurate summary of cytogenetic abnormalities in LBL that is devoid of the influence of ALL is still lacking. This lack of cytogenetic and molecular genetic data on LBL hampers the understanding of the pathogenesis and molecular basis of LBL. The principal mechanisms are thought to be analogous to the pathogenic mechanisms in ALL. However, this hypothesis has not yet been proven with experimental data, and recent reports point out that there are a number of distinct molecular differences between ALL and LBL.[24,53–56] In addition to the molecular differences between LBL and ALL, recent data even indicated that there might also be molecular differences between pediatric and adult T-LBL (see below and Chapter 6).[53]

Lymphoblastic leukemia/lymphoma in adolescents

Retrospective analyses of adolescents and young adults (AYA) with newly diagnosed acute lymphoblastic leukemia (ALL) treated either according to pediatric or adult protocols revealed a statistically significant superior outcome for patients treated according to pediatric regimens.[57–61] In the US, the results of such analyses with a clearly inferior outcome for adolescents treated according to adult regimen led to the initiation of a prospective study for AYAs with ALL that uses the more successful pediatric approach (see Chapter 12).[62] Similar analyses of adolescent LBL patients, i.e. comparison of treatment and outcome between pediatric and adult protocols, are lacking so far. Today, the treatment of adolescents with LBL often simply depends on whether the patient is referred to a pediatric or an adult medical department. No clinical trial is open which is focused on adolescents with LBL. However, the lessons learned in adolescents with ALL cannot simply be transferred to LBL. Prior to interdisciplinary discussions regarding improvement of therapy, the clinical and biological characteristics of adolescents with LBL need to be characterized.

Clinical features of lymphoblastic lymphoma in adolescents

Within LBL, the clinical presentation is influenced by the immunophenotype of the cells. T-lineage lymphoblastic lymphoma commonly presents in the mediastinum or as pleural effusions causing respiratory impairment. Pericardial effusion with resulting cardiac tamponade may also occur in individual cases. In addition, signs and symptoms of superior vena cava obstruction may be present. Other potentially involved sites are lymph nodes, liver, spleen, skin, bone, testis, and soft tissue. T-LBL cells have the potential for dissemination to the central nervous system (CNS) which occurs in about 5% of pediatric patient series. Bone marrow (BM) infiltration (> 5% but less than 25% blasts in the BM) is seen in almost 20% of pediatric cases. In the largest series of adolescents (15–18 years) with newly diagnosed T-LBL, the male to female ratio was 3:1, elevated LDH > 500 U/L was reported for 45% of patients, and almost all patients were diagnosed with advanced stage III/IV disease according to the St. Jude staging system[36] due to the mediastinal mass. BM involvement was reported for 16% of adolescent T-LBL patients and CNS involvement for 8%. B symptoms and a poor performance status according to the Karnofsky scale were documented for 35% and 31%, respectively. Compared with the clinical characteristics of 395 pediatric T-LBL patients < 15 years enrolled during the same period into the NHL-BFM trials, there were no differences in the clinical characteristics between adolescent and pediatric T-LBL patients.[24]

In pB-LBL, disease manifestations are frequently localized to the head and neck region, often involving soft tissue, bone or skin.[63,64] The general condition of patients is often normal and symptoms are mild. About one third of patients are diagnosed with BM involvement with > 5% but less than 25% bone marrow blasts. CNS involvement is observed in less than 5% of patients. According to the St. Jude staging system, about one third of patients are diagnosed with limited stage I or II disease. The NHL-BFM studies reported 13 adolescents with pB-LBL vs. 126 pediatric pB-LBL. Of the 13 adolescent patients, six presented with stage I/II disease, elevated LDH was diagnosed in none of the cases, one patient was diagnosed with BM involvement and three with CNS involvement. Compared to the 126 pediatric pB-LBL, CNS involvement was more frequent in adolescents. However, the absolute numbers are clearly too small to draw any conclusion from that aspect.[24]

Treatment and outcome of adolescent LBL patients in pediatric trials

The outcome of pediatric and adolescent patients with lymphoblastic lymphoma improved significantly when combination chemotherapy regimens were introduced, such as the LSA2-L2 protocol[65] and the "Berliner Induktionsprotokoll".[66] Another milestone for the treatment of NHL patients was the therapeutic differentiation to treat lymphoblastic lymphoma with ALL-type treatment regimen and mature B-cell lymphoma with short and intense pulse-type regimen.[67–69] With current treatment approaches, event-free survival rates of 65–90% are reached in pediatric clinical trials (for details see Chapter 16).[70–77] Concerning CNS prophylaxis, intrathecal chemotherapy is part of current regimens for patients without overt CNS disease. Prophylactic cranial irradiation was omitted in recent trials with sufficient CNS-directed therapy using intrathecal MTX and intravenous high-dose MTX.[71,75,77] However, patients with overt CNS disease are usually treated with intrathecal chemotherapy and cranial radiotherapy.

Concerning the outcome of adolescent LBL patients treated with pediatric protocols, the little data that can be collected from recent publications is summarized in Table 17.4. The trial CCG-502 included 281 LBL patients less than 22 years of age at diagnosis who were randomized to receive either a modified LSA2-L2 ALL-type treatment or ADCOMP

Table 17.4. Treatment outcome for lymphoblastic lymphoma patients enrolled in pediatric trials.

	Whole study including children and adolescents					Data according to age groups		
Trial	**Age**	**Stage**	**Treatment**	**Pts**	**pEFS**	**Age (years)**	**Pts**	**pEFS**
SFOP/France LMT81[72]	Median 9 yrs, range 10 mths–16 yrs	I–IV	Modified LSA2-L2	84	75 ± 3%			
CCG/US CCG502[76] ≤ 21 yrs	Median 8.9 yrs, range 5 mths–19.5 yrs	I–IV	Modified LSA2-L2 vs. ADCOMP	143 138	74% 64% (5 yrs)	≤ 10 yrs 10–14 yrs > 14 yrs	156 (56%) 87 (31%) 38 (14%)	RR failure 1.0 RR 1.3 RR 2.7
POG/US POG 8704[70] advanced stage T-LBL ≤ 21 yrs	Median 10–11 yrs, quartiles range 5.7–15.0 yrs	III/IV	L-Asp no vs. L-Asp yes	83 84	64 ± 6% 78 ± 5% (4 yrs)			
NHL-BFM/Germany, Austria, Switzerland NHL-BFM 90[74] T-LBL ≤ 17 yrs	Median 8.8 yrs, range 1.1–16.4 yrs	I–IV (T-LBL)	ALL-BFM	105	90% (5 yrs)	< 10 yrs ≥ 10 yrs	57 (54%) 48 (46%)	89 ± 4% (5 yrs) 94 ± 3% (5 yrs)
NHL-BFM NHL-BFM 95[71] ≤ 18 yrs	Median age 8.6 yrs; range 0.2–19.5 yrs	III/IV	ALL-BFM	169	78 ± 3% (5 yrs)			
EORTC/France, Belgium EORTC 58881[77] ≤ 18 yrs	Median age 8 yrs; range 0–16 yrs	I–IV (T-LBL)	ALL-BFM	119	78 ± 4% (6 yrs)	< 1 yrs 1–9 yrs 10–16 yrs	2 (2%) 68 (57%) 49 (41%)	0% (6 yrs) 82 ± 5% (6 yrs) 74 ± 7% (6 yrs)
COG/US COG pilot[78] < 21 yrs	n.d.	III/IV		85	78 ± 5% (5 yrs)	0–4 yrs 5–9 yrs ≥ 10 yrs	14 (17%) 23 (27%) 48 (56%)	77 ± 12% (5 yrs) 91 ± 6% (5 yrs) 72 ± 7% (5 yrs)
St. Jude/US St. Jude 13[75]	n.d.	III/IV	T-ALL	41	83% (5 yrs)	< 3 yrs ≥ 3 yrs < 10 yrs ≥ 10 yrs	2 (5%) 39 (95%) 17 (42%) 24 (59%)	n.d. n.d. n.d. n.d.

n.d.: no data.

courses. The 5-year EFS rate for the treatment regimens was 74% for LSA2-L2 and 64% for ADCOMP, respectively ($p = 0.17$, adjusted for extent and site of disease). Interestingly, 18 of the 38 adolescent patients enrolled suffered from progression or relapse. The relative risk (RR) of treatment failure was 2.7 for adolescents and 1.3 for patients the 87 patients 10–14 years of age compared to 1.0 for 156 pediatric patients < 10 years of age ($p = 0.0082$). Unfortunately, the adolescent age group was not further analyzed in the paper. The analyses of prognostic parameters revealed only localized vs. disseminated disease vs. BM involvement to be correlated with outcome.[76]

The POG 8704 (T-3) trial was open for patients < 22 years of age. The report by Amylon *et al.* included 195 T-LBL patients with advanced stage disease (167 randomized patients). The median age was 10–11 years with 25% and 75% quartiles of 5.2 and 15.0 years, resulting in a quota of about 25% of patients with adolescent age. Patients received a rotating combination of chemotherapeutic agents and were randomized to receive or not to receive high-dose asparaginase consolidation. The 4-year EFS was 64 ± 6% without and 78 ± 5% with asparaginase. The study reported no correlation with outcome for patient age at diagnosis. In addition, there was no prognostic impact of stage III vs. stage IV disease, sex, presence of mediastinal mass, cytogenetic abnormalities, and ethnicity.[70]

The NHL-BFM 90 trial was based on pediatric ALL-BFM treatment and enrolled 105 evaluable T-LBL patients. The 5-year EFS was 90% for the whole group, and there was no statistically significant difference in EFS according to age, with 89% EFS for patients < 10 years and 94% for the 46% of patients ≥ 10 years. Furthermore, neither gender nor stage of disease, LDH level, immunophenotype, response at day 33 of induction or residual tumor at the end of induction were of prognostic relevance for the risk of relapse.[74] In the subsequent NHL-BFM 95 trial, the ALL-BFM chemotherapy backbone was again used. The study objective was to test against the historical control whether prophylactic CNS radiotherapy can be omitted without an unacceptable increase of relapses. The 5-year EFS was 78% for 169 LBL patients with advanced stage III/IV disease. Outcome according to age was not specified.[71]

The EORTC enrolled 119 evaluable T-LBL patients into the trial EORTC CLG 58881, with modified ALL-BFM treatment without prophylactic cranial radiotherapy. 6-year EFS was 78% for the whole population and 0% for two infants, 82% for 68 children less than 10 years of age and 74% for patients 10–16 years of age at diagnosis. This trend towards inferior outcome for older patients was not statistically significant. The only prognostic parameter with statistical significance for the relapse risk was the response at day 8. None of the 16 patients with complete remission at day eight later suffered from any event, while EFS was only 14% in seven patients with resistant disease at day 8.[77]

In the COG pilot study, 85 patients with advanced stage LBL were enrolled and treated with induction, consolidation and six cycles of maintenance for a total therapy duration of 12 months. 5-Year EFS for the whole group was 78 ± 5%. Interestingly, 5-year EFS appeared to be better for children between 5 and 9 years of age (91 ± 6%) compared to patients 10 years of age or older (72 ± 7%); however, this trend was not statistically significant.[78]

The St. Jude NHL13 trial enrolled 41 evaluable patients with advanced stage III/IV lymphoblastic lymphoma, including 5 pB-LBL, 33 T-LBL, and 3 patients with unknown immunophenotype. The 5-year EFS was 83 ± 6% for the whole patient series. Twenty-four patients (59%) were ≥ 10 years of age or older; however, no outcome analyses were provided for this specific subgroup.[75]

The NHL-BFM group recently reported a detailed review of analyses of adolescent NHL patients treated according to pediatric NHL-BFM protocols. The analyses included all evaluable patients diagnosed between October 1986 and December 2007. A total of 2537 pediatric and 378 adolescents NHL patients were registered, including 395 pediatric and 45 adolescent T-LBL patients. In outcome analyses, 5-year EFS was similar in pediatric and adolescent T-LBL (82 ± 2% vs. 83 ± 7%, respectively, $p = 0.41$, Fig. 17.3A). However, within the adolescent group itself, 5-year EFS was significantly inferior for female T-LBL patients compared to adolescent male T-LBL patients (57 ± 17% vs. 92 ± 6%, respectively; $p = 0.0036$, Fig. 17.3B). Interestingly, clinical characteristics were similar in adolescent male and female patients. This difference in outcome according to gender was not observed in younger patients. 5-Year EFS according to gender in pediatric T-LBL patients < 15 years enrolled during the same time period was 80 ± 4% for 105 girls vs. 83 ± 2% for 290 boys ($p = 0.40$). The available clinical data on pediatric and adolescent T-LBL patients provide no explanation for the inferior outcome for adolescent female T-LBL patients treated according to ALL-BFM based NHL-BFM protocols.[24] Unfortunately, available data on adolescents with

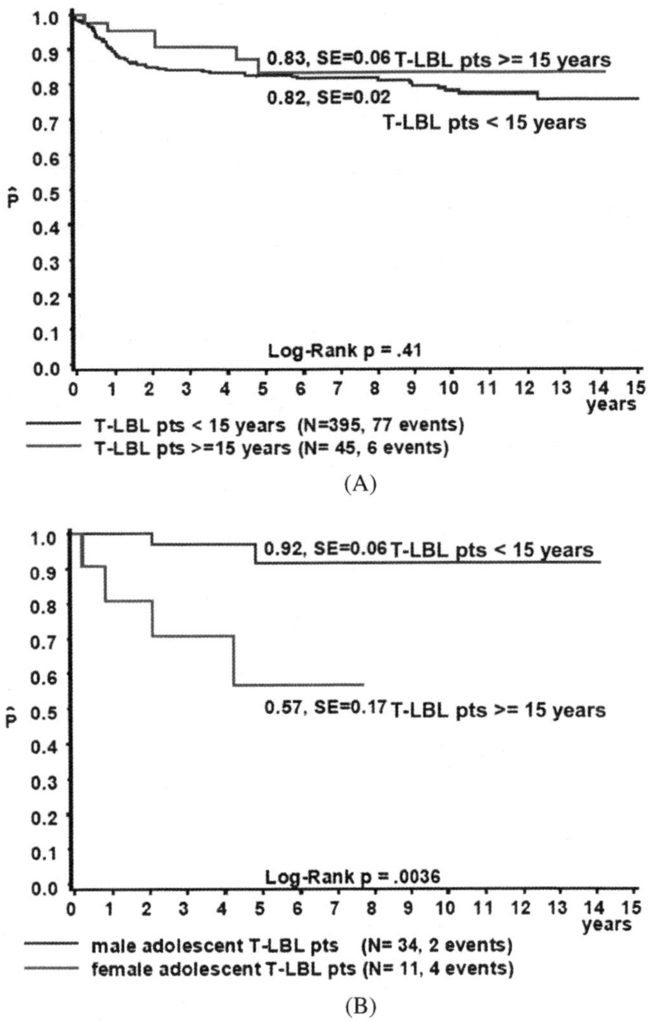

Fig. 17.3. Five year event-free survival (EFS) analyses according to gender for (A) pediatric and (B) adolescent T-LBL patients according to the NHL–BFM-based treated regimen.

T-LBL are extremely limited. Most reports on pediatric clinical trials do not provide characteristic and outcome specifically focused on adolescents and further differentiated according to gender; and even if they did, the numbers would be very small. Combined analyses of data obtained in systematic pediatric trials of pediatric oncology groups may be necessary in order to elucidate the prognostic relevance of adolescent age and female gender in T-LBL patients.

The analyses of the NHL-BFM group reported also on adolescents with pB-LBL, but the absolute number of this specific patient population was limited to only 13 adolescent pB-LBL patients, six boys and seven girls. 5-year EFS was 85 ± 10% for those 13 patients. As mentioned above, overt CNS disease was observed in a quarter of adolescent pB-LBL patients, but this "trend" might have been accidental and caused by the small numbers.[24]

Lymphoblastic lymphoma in adults

Concerning the outcome of LBL patients treated according to adult protocols, variable prognostic impact of patient age at diagnosis was reported for response and survival. Coleman *et al.* analyzed 44 adult patients >16 years of age treated according to two protocols, both of which included induction with cyclophosphamide, doxorubicin, vincristine, prednisone, and asparaginase, CNS prophylaxis, and maintenance therapy with MTX and 6-mercaptopurine. For the whole group of 44 patients, 3-year disease-free survival rate was 56%. In multivariate analyses, Ann Arbor stage I-III and LDH < 300 U/L were favorable prognostic factors, while age below or above 35 years was not a significant prognostic parameter.[79]

Hoelzer *et al.* reported on 45 adult patients with T-LBL (age range 15–61 years) treated according to protocols designed for adult ALL. The 7-year overall survival was 51 ± 10%. Survival according to age was not significantly different, 55% for 12 patients 15–20 years, 46% for 29 patients 21–50 years and 75% for 4 patients >50 years (p>0.5).[80]

Thirty-three adults with lymphoblastic lymphoma were treated with intensive chemotherapy regimens hyper-CVAD with fractionated cyclophosphamide, vincristine, adriamycin, and dexamethasone or modified hyper-CVAD used for ALL. Involved field radiotherapy with 30–39 Gy was given to patients with mediastinal disease at diagnosis. Estimates for 3-year PFS and overall survival were 66% and 70%, respectively. 3-year PFS and overall survival was 72% and 77%, respectively, in 19 patients younger than 30 years vs. 66% and 64%, respectively, in 14 patients 30 years of age or older. The difference in outcome according to age was not statistically significant.[81]

In contrast to these studies with no statistical impact of age, Morel *et al.* reported a study on 80 adult LBL patients. The median age was 34 years (range: 15–76 years) and the distribution according to age groups was: 40 patients age 15–29 years, 22 patients age 30–39 years, 7 patients age 40–49 years and 11 patients above 50 years of age at diagnosis. Patients were treated on two NHL protocols (CHOP or LNH-84) and two French multicenter ALL protocols (FRALLE or LALA). The complete remission duration rate at 30 months was 46%. Parameters associated with poor response were age > 40 years, presence of lumbo-aortic adenopathy, high LDH level, two or more extranodal sites of disease. Age > 40 years retained similar prognostic value when the analysis was restricted to the 59 patients treated with the FRALLE, LALA, or LNH-84 protocol ($p < 0.05$).[82] Available data on outcome for adolescent and adult patients with lymphoblastic lymphoma are summarized in Table 17.5.

Prognostic parameters in lymphoblastic lymphoma

The identification of clinical and/or biological prognostic factors is essential for individual risk-adapted treatment. This is even more true for lymphoblastic lymphoma patients, who face a poor prognosis in case of relapse[24] on the one hand while suffering disproportionately from secondary malignancies and treatment-related toxicity on the other (see Chapter 24). The rate of secondary malignancies is higher for lymphoblastic lymphoma patients when compared with ALCL or mature B-cell lymphoma.[83,84] Also osteonecrosis, a well-known complication of current ALL-type treatment approaches, is diagnosed predominantly in LBL and less frequently in ALCL or B-NHL patients. In addition, numerous ALL studies have shown that osteonecrosis occurs significantly more frequently in adolescents compared to children.[85–87] Due to the higher median age in lymphoma compared to leukemia patients, it is not surprising that osteonecrosis turned out to be a relevant late effect in adolescents with lymphoblastic lymphoma.[88] Taking into account these aspects, prognostic parameters for adequate treatment stratification are essential for LBL patients and especially for adolescents with LBL. Concerning clinical parameters besides age and the above discussed parameters, a handful of small retrospective series of adult patients with lymphoblastic lymphoma identified adverse clinical prognostic factors such as advanced age, Ann Arbor stage of disease, bone marrow or CNS involvement, LDH level, B symptoms, time to attainment of complete response, or International Prognostic Index (IPI).[82,89,90] In pediatric LBL, Riopel *et al.* showed the adverse prognostic effect of advanced Ann Arbor stage of disease, bone marrow involvement, CNS involvement, elevated LDH level and B symptoms.[49] However, in a series of the BFM group including 290 uniformly treated pediatric T-LBL patients, the only parameters with prognostic impact were B symptoms and critically ill condition at diagnosis.[91] Regarding biological parameters, the available data in LBL are too few to prove the possible prognostic impact of a specific genetic alteration or immunophenotypic marker. However, molecular characterization of LBL is advancing, and only recently Baleydier *et al.* performed a detailed molecular characterization of 41 T-LBL patients including nine pediatric cases. Interestingly, none of the nine pediatric cases showed an immature immunogenotype, which was associated with poor prognosis in the corresponding adult cases.[53] In the NHL-BFM series, deletions of chromosome 6q, detected by loss of heterozygosity analyses, were associated with an increased risk of relapse.[54,92] First data on the prognostic impact of minimal disseminated disease (MDD) evaluation in 99 pediatric T-LBL cases using flow cytometry was reported by Coustan-Smith *et al.*,[93] who were able to show that 72% of patients presented with submicroscopic BM involvement at diagnosis. MDD with ≥1% or with ≥5% lymphoblasts, detected by flow cytometry, was associated with unfavorable outcome. In addition, the study showed that monitoring of disease clearance by minimal residual disease (MRD) follow-up samples is feasible. Notably, in that study, stage IV disease with BM

Table 17.5. Summary of treatment outcome for adolescent and adult lymphoblastic lymphoma patients.

Reference	No. of pts	Outcome
Adolescent LBL patients		
Uyttebroeck *et al.*[77]	49 LBL pts 10–16 yrs of age	6 yrs EFS 74 ± 7%
Reiter *et al.*[74]	48 LBL pts 10–17 yrs of age	5 yrs EFS 94 ± 3%
Burkhardt *et al.*[94]	45 LBL pts 15–18 yrs of age	5 yrs EFS 83 ± 6%
Abromowitch *et al.*[78]	48 LBL pts 10–20 yrs of age	5 yrs EFS 72 ± 7%
Adult LBL patients		
Coleman *et al.*[79]	44 LBL pts	3 yrs DFS 56%
Hoelzer *et al.*[80]	all 45 T-LBL pts	7 yrs OS 51 ± 10%
	12 LBL pts 15–20 yrs of age	7 yrs OS 55%
	29 LBL pts 21–50 yrs of age	7 yrs OS 46%
	4 LBL pts > 50 yrs of age	7 yrs OS 75%
Thomas *et al.*[81]	all 33 LBL pts	3 yrs OS 70%
	19 LBL pts < 30 yrs of age	3 yrs OS 77%
	14 LBL pts ≥ 30 yrs of age	3 yrs OS 64%
Morel *et al.*[82]	80 LBL pts	2.5 yrs OS 51%

involvement and/or CNS disease defined according to classical morphological criteria was associated with inferior EFS compared to patients with stage I–III disease (2-year EFS 60 ± 14% for stage IV vs. 90 ± 4%, p = 0.005).[93] The prognostic impact of microscopic and submicroscopic bone marrow involvement might be influenced by the treatment given. In the EORTC and NHL-BFM trials, which used a modified ALL-BFM treatment strategy, the outcome of patients with stage IV disease was not significantly inferior to that of patients with lower stages.[74,77] The prognostic value of minimal disseminated and minimal residual disease examination therefore needs to be elucidated in larger series and within the context of varying treatment strategies (see Chapter 10). In summary, one can safely say that there are presently no consistent prognostic parameters for LBL except for limited stage I/II vs. advanced stage III/IV disease, which is probably the only stratification criterion in use in ongoing clinical trials. Hence, no clear rationale exists for the stratification of the majority of LBL patients with advanced stage disease (80–90% of patients) into risk groups with differences in the treatment intensity.

On the whole, it remains difficult to draw decisive conclusions concerning the relevance of adolescent age in patients with lymphoblastic lymphoma. Treating these patients according to current pediatric regimens might offer event-free survival rates of about 80%. However, there are hints that the outcome of adolescents with LBL might be influenced by gender, with a more favorable outcome in male adolescents T-LBL patients compared females. Pooled analyses, including several trials with similar treatment regimens, accompanied by molecular characterization of disease, are required to assess the risks of LBL in adolescent patients.

Conclusion on Adolescents with NHL

Up to the present time, NHL in adolescent patients is not fully understood in terms of epidemiology, disease biology, adequate treatment, or opportunities to prevent and monitor late effects. One major aspect that contributes to the current situation is the fact that adolescents are underrepresented both in pediatric and in adult clinical trials. To overcome this fact, it is necessary to register all adolescent patients in cancer registries and to enroll as many of them as possible in clinical trials. Only the infrastructure of clinical trials offers the opportunity to adequately address such highly relevant topics as the biological characterization of NHL in adolescents, the analyses of gender-specific differences, the identification of patient subgroups with features resembling that of adult NHL, or the identification of markers which indicate molecular and biologic lymphoma properties that are typically associated with specific prognostic lymphoma subsets. Interdisciplinary efforts and clinical trials will one day offer the chance to adapt treatment strategies specifically to the needs of adolescent patients with newly diagnosed non-Hodgkin lymphoma.

References

1. Bleyer WA, O'Leary M, Barr R, Ries LAG (eds.). (2006) Cancer Epidemiology in Older Adolescents and Young Adults 15–29 Years of Age, Including SEER Incidence and Survival, 1975–2000. *Bethesda, MD. National Cancer Institute.*
5. Burkhardt B, Zimmermann M, Oschlies I, Niggli F, Mann G, Parwaresch R, Riehm H, Schrappe M, Reiter A. (2005) The impact of age and gender on biology, clinical features and treatment outcome of non-Hodgkin lymphoma in childhood and adolescence. *Br J Haematol* **131**: 39–49.
14. Rosenwald A, Wright G, Leroy K, Yu X, Gaulard P, Gascoyne RD, Chan WC, Zhao T, Haioun C, Greiner TC, Weisenburger DD, Lynch JC, Vose J, Armitage JO, Smeland EB, Kvaloy S, Holte H, Delabie J, Campo E, Montserrat E, Lopez-Guillermo A, Ott G, Muller-Hermelink HK, Connors JM, Braziel R, Grogan TM, Fisher RI, Miller TP, LeBlanc M, Chiorazzi M, Zhao H, Yang L, Powell J, Wilson WH, Jaffe ES, Simon R, Klausner RD, Staudt LM. (2003) Molecular diagnosis of primary mediastinal B cell lymphoma identifies a clinically favorable subgroup of diffuse large B cell lymphoma related to Hodgkin lymphoma. *J Exp Med* **198**: 851–862.
18. Patte C, Auperin A, Gerrard M, Michon J, Pinkerton R, Sposto R, Weston C, Raphael M, Perkins SL, McCarthy K, Cairo MS. (2007) Results of the randomized international FAB/LMB96 trial for intermediate risk B-cell non-Hodgkin lymphoma in children and adolescents: It is possible to reduce treatment for the early responding patients. *Blood* **109**: 2773–2780.
23. Cairo MS, Gerrard M, Sposto R, Auperin A, Pinkerton CR, Michon J, Weston C, Perkins SL, Raphael M, McCarthy K, Patte C. (2007) Results of a randomized international study of high-risk central nervous system B non-Hodgkin lymphoma and B acute lymphoblastic leukemia in children and adolescents. *Blood* **109**: 2736–2743.

24. Burkhardt B, Oschlies I, Klapper W, Zimmermann M, Woessmann W, Meinhardt A, Landmann E, Attarbaschi A, Niggli F, Schrappe M, Reiter A. (2011) Non-Hodgkin's lymphoma in adolescents: Experiences in 378 adolescent NHL patients treated according to pediatric NHL-BFM protocols. *Leukemia* **25**: 153–160.
30. Falini B, Pileri S, Zinzani PL, Carbone A, Zagonel V, Wolf-Peeters C, Verhoef G, Menestrina F, Todeschini G, Paulli M, Lazzarino M, Giardini R, Aiello A, Foss HD, Araujo I, Fizzotti M, Pelicci PG, Flenghi L, Martelli MF, Santucci A. (1999) ALK+ lymphoma: Clinico-pathological findings and outcome. *Blood* **93**: 2697–2706.
32. Brugieres L, le Deley MC, Rosolen A, Williams D, Horibe K, Wrobel G, Mann G, Zsiros J, Uyttebroeck A, Marky I, Lamant L, Reiter A. (2009) Impact of the methotrexate administration dose on the need for intrathecal treatment in children and adolescents with anaplastic large-cell lymphoma: Results of a randomized trial of the EICNHL Group. *J Clin Oncol* **27**: 897–903.
33. Brugieres L, Deley MC, Pacquement H, Meguerian-Bedoyan Z, Terrier-Lacombe MJ, Robert A, Pondarre C, Leverger G, Devalck C, Rodary C, Delsol G, Hartmann O. (1998) CD30(+) anaplastic large-cell lymphoma in children: Analysis of 82 patients enrolled in two consecutive studies of the French Society of Pediatric Oncology. *Blood* **92**: 3591–3598.
34. Reiter A, Schrappe M, Tiemann M, Parwaresch R, Zimmermann M, Yakisan E, Dopfer R, Bucsky P, Mann G, Gadner H. (1994) Successful treatment strategy for Ki-1 anaplastic large-cell lymphoma of childhood: A prospective analysis of 62 patients enrolled in three consecutive Berlin-Frankfurt-Munster group studies. *J Clin Oncol* **12**: 899–908.
35. Seidemann K, Tiemann M, Schrappe M, Yakisan E, Simonitsch I, Janka-Schaub G, Dorffel W, Zimmermann M, Mann G, Gadner H, Parwaresch R, Riehm H, Reiter A. (2001) Short-pulse B-non-Hodgkin lymphoma-type chemotherapy is efficacious treatment for pediatric anaplastic large cell lymphoma: A report of the Berlin-Frankfurt-Munster Group Trial NHL-BFM 90. *Blood* **97**: 3699–3706.
37. Laver JH, Kraveka JM, Hutchison RE, Chang M, Kepner J, Schwenn M, Tarbell N, Desai S, Weitzman S, Weinstein HJ, Murphy SB. (2005) Advanced-stage large-cell lymphoma in children and adolescents: Results of a randomized trial incorporating intermediate-dose methotrexate and high-dose cytarabine in the maintenance phase of the APO regimen: A Pediatric Oncology Group phase III trial. *J Clin Oncol* **23**: 541–547.
38. Lowe EJ, Sposto R, Perkins SL, Gross TG, Finlay J, Zwick D, Abromowitch M. (2009) Intensive chemotherapy for systemic anaplastic large cell lymphoma in children and adolescents: Final results of Children's Cancer Group Study 5941. *Pediatr Blood Cancer* **52**: 335–339.
39. Rosolen A, Pillon M, Garaventa A, Burnelli R, d'Amore ES, Giuliano M, Comis M, Cesaro S, Tettoni K, Moleti ML, Tamaro P, Visintin G, Zanesco L. (2005) Anaplastic large cell lymphoma treated with a leukemia-like therapy: Report of the Italian Association of Pediatric Hematology and Oncology (AIEOP) LNH-92 protocol. *Cancer* **104**: 2133–2140.
40. Williams DM, Hobson R, Imeson J, Gerrard M, McCarthy K, Pinkerton CR. (2002) Anaplastic large cell lymphoma in childhood: Analysis of 72 patients treated on The United Kingdom Children's Cancer Study Group chemotherapy regimens. *Br J Haematol* **117**: 812–820.
41. le Deley MC, Reiter A, Williams D, Delsol G, Oschlies I, McCarthy K, Zimmermann M, Brugieres L. (2008) Prognostic factors in childhood anaplastic large cell lymphoma: Results of a large European intergroup study. *Blood* **111**: 1560–1566.
42. Damm-Welk C, Busch K, Burkhardt B, Schieferstein J, Viehmann S, Oschlies I, Klapper W, Zimmermann M, Harbott J, Reiter A, Woessmann W. (2007) Prognostic significance of circulating tumor cells in bone marrow or peripheral blood as detected by qualitative and quantitative PCR in pediatric NPM-ALK-positive anaplastic large-cell lymphoma. *Blood* **110**: 670–677.
43. Gascoyne RD, Aoun P, Wu D, Chhanabhai M, Skinnider BF, Greiner TC, Morris SW, Connors JM, Vose JM, Viswanatha DS, Coldman A, Weisenburger DD. (1999) Prognostic significance of anaplastic lymphoma kinase (ALK) protein expression in adults with anaplastic large cell lymphoma. *Blood* **93**: 3913–3921.
44. Savage KJ, Harris NL, Vose JM, Ullrich F, Jaffe ES, Connors JM, Rimsza L, Pileri SA, Chhanabhai M, Gascoyne RD, Armitage JO, Weisenburger DD. (2008) ALK-anaplastic large-cell lymphoma is clinically and immunophenotypically different from both ALK+ ALCL and peripheral T-cell lymphoma, not otherwise specified: Report from the International Peripheral T-Cell Lymphoma Project. *Blood* **111**: 5496–5504.
45. Kaatsch P, Spix C. (2007) *Annual Report 2006/07 German Childhood Cancer Registry*. Mainz, Germany: German Childhood Cancer Registry.
49. Riopel M, Dickman PS, Link MP, Perlman EJ. (1994) MIC2 analysis in pediatric lymphomas and leukemias. *Hum Pathol* **25**: 396–399.

53. Baleydier F, Decouvelaere AV, Bergeron J, Gaulard P, Canioni D, Bertrand Y, Lepretre S, Petit B, Dombret H, Beldjord K, Molina T, Asnafi V, Macintyre E. (2008) T cell receptor genotyping and HOXA/TLX1 expression define three T lymphoblastic lymphoma subsets which might affect clinical outcome. *Clin Cancer Res* **14**: 692–700.
54. Burkhardt B, Moericke A, Klapper W, Greene F, Salzburg J, Damm-Welk C, Zimmermann M, Strauch K, Ludwig WD, Schrappe M, Reiter A. (2008) Pediatric precursor T lymphoblastic leukemia and lymphoblastic lymphoma: Differences in the common regions with loss of heterozygosity at chromosome 6q and their prognostic impact. *Leuk Lymphoma* **49**: 451–461.
55. Raetz EA, Perkins SL, Bhojwani D, Smock K, Philip M, Carroll WL, Min DJ. (2006) Gene expression profiling reveals intrinsic differences between T-cell acute lymphoblastic leukemia and T-cell lymphoblastic lymphoma. *Pediatr Blood Cancer* **47**: 130–140.
56. Uyttebroeck A, Vanhentenrijk V, Hagemeijer A, Boeckx N, Renard M, Wlodarska I, Vandenberghe P, Depaepe P, de Wolf-Peeters C. (2007) Is there a difference in childhood T-cell acute lymphoblastic leukaemia and T-cell lymphoblastic lymphoma? *Leuk Lymphoma* **48**: 1745–1754.
57. Boissel N, Auclerc MF, Lheritier V, Perel Y, Thomas X, Leblanc T, Rousselot P, Cayuela JM, Gabert J, Fegueux N, Piguet C, Huguet-Rigal F, Berthou C, Boiron JM, Pautas C, Michel G, Fiere D, Leverger G, Dombret H, Baruchel A. (2003) Should adolescents with acute lymphoblastic leukemia be treated as old children or young adults? Comparison of the French FRALLE-93 and LALA-94 trials. *J Clin Oncol* **21**: 774–780.
58. de Bont JM, Holt B, Dekker AW, van der Does-van den Berg A, Sonneveld P, Pieters R. (2004) Significant difference in outcome for adolescents with acute lymphoblastic leukemia treated on pediatric vs adult protocols in the Netherlands. *Leukemia* **18**: 2032–2035.
59. Hallbook H, Gustafsson G, Smedmyr B, Soderhall S, Heyman M. (2006) Treatment outcome in young adults and children >10 years of age with acute lymphoblastic leukemia in Sweden: A comparison between a pediatric protocol and an adult protocol. *Cancer* **107**: 1551–1561.
60. Ramanujachar R, Richards S, Hann I, Goldstone A, Mitchell C, Vora A, Rowe J, Webb D. (2007) Adolescents with acute lymphoblastic leukaemia: Outcome on UK national paediatric (ALL97) and adult (UKALLXII/E2993) trials. *Pediatr Blood Cancer* **48**: 254–261.
61. Schroder H, Kjeldahl M, Boesen AM, Nielsen OJ, Schmidt K, Johnsen HE, Gregersen H, Heyman M, Gustafsson G. (2006) Acute lymphoblastic leukemia in adolescents between 10 and 19 years of age in Denmark — secondary publication. *Dan Med Bull* **53**: 76–79.
62. Stock W, La M, Sanford B, Bloomfield CD, Vardiman JW, Gaynon P, Larson RA, Nachman J. (2008) What determines the outcomes for adolescents and young adults with acute lymphoblastic leukemia treated on cooperative group protocols? A comparison of Children's Cancer Group and Cancer and Leukemia Group B studies. *Blood* **112**: 1646–1654.
63. Lin P, Jones D, Dorfman DM, Medeiros LJ. (2000) Precursor B-cell lymphoblastic lymphoma: A predominantly extranodal tumor with low propensity for leukemic involvement. *Am J Surg Pathol* **24**: 1480–1490.
64. Neth O, Seidemann K, Jansen P, Mann G, Tiemann M, Ludwig WD, Riehm H, Reiter A. (2000) Precursor B-cell lymphoblastic lymphoma in childhood and adolescence: Clinical features, treatment, and results in trials NHL-BFM 86 and 90. *Med Pediatr Oncol* **35**: 20–27.
70. Amylon MD, Shuster J, Pullen J, Berard C, Link MP, Wharam M, Katz J, Yu A, Laver J, Ravindranath Y, Kurtzberg J, Desai S, Camitta B, Murphy SB. (1999) Intensive high-dose asparaginase consolidation improves survival for pediatric patients with T cell acute lymphoblastic leukemia and advanced stage lymphoblastic lymphoma: A Pediatric Oncology Group study. *Leukemia* **13**: 335–342.
71. Burkhardt B, Woessmann W, Zimmermann M, Kontny U, Vormoor J, Doerffel W, Mann G, Henze G, Niggli F, Ludwig WD, Janssen D, Riehm H, Schrappe M, Reiter A. (2006) Impact of cranial radiotherapy on central nervous system prophylaxis in children and adolescents with central nervous system-negative stage III or IV lymphoblastic lymphoma. *J Clin Oncol* **24**: 491–499.
72. Patte C, Kalifa C, Flamant F, Hartmann O, Brugieres L, Valteau-Couanet D, Bayle C, Caillaud JM, Lemerle J. (1992) Results of the LMT81 protocol, a modified LSA2L2 protocol with high dose methotrexate, on 84 children with non-B-cell (lymphoblastic) lymphoma. *Med Pediatr Oncol* **20**: 105–113.
75. Sandlund JT, Pui CH, Zhou Y, Behm FG, Onciu M, Razzouk BI, Hijiya N, Campana D, Hudson MM, Ribeiro RC. (2009) Effective treatment of advanced-stage childhood lymphoblastic lymphoma without prophylactic cranial irradiation: Results of St Jude NHL13 study. *Leukemia* **23**: 1127–1130.
76. Tubergen DG, Krailo MD, Meadows AT, Rosenstock J, Kadin M, Morse M, King D, Steinherz PG, Kersey JH. (1995) Comparison of treatment regimens for pediatric

lymphoblastic non-Hodgkin's lymphoma: A Childrens Cancer Group study. *J Clin Oncol* **13**: 1368–1376.

77. Uyttebroeck A, Suciu S, Laureys G, Robert A, Pacquement H, Ferster A, Marguerite G, Mazingue F, Renard M, Lutz P, Rialland X, Mechinaud F, Cave H, Baila L, Bertrand Y. (2008) Treatment of childhood T-cell lymphoblastic lymphoma according to the strategy for acute lymphoblastic leukaemia, without radiotherapy: Long term results of the EORTC CLG 58881 trial. *Eur J Cancer* **44**: 840–846.
78. Abromowitch M, Sposto R, Perkins S, Zwick D, Siegel S, Finlay J, Cairo MS. (2008) Shortened intensified multiagent chemotherapy and non-cross resistant maintenance therapy for advanced lymphoblastic lymphoma in children and adolescents: Report from the Children's Oncology Group. *Br J Haematol* **143**: 261–267.
79. Coleman CN, Picozzi VJ, Jr., Cox RS, McWhirter K, Weiss LM, Cohen JR, Yu KP, Rosenberg SA. (1986) Treatment of lymphoblastic lymphoma in adults. *J Clin Oncol* **4**: 1628–1637.
80. Hoelzer D, Gokbuget N, Digel W, Faak T, Kneba M, Reutzel R, Romejko-Jarosinska J, Zwolinski J, Walewski J. (2002) Outcome of adult patients with T-lymphoblastic lymphoma treated according to protocols for acute lymphoblastic leukemia. *Blood* **99**: 4379–4385.
81. Thomas DA, O'Brien S, Cortes J, Giles FJ, Faderl S, Verstovsek S, Ferrajoli A, Koller C, Beran M, Pierce S, Ha CS, Cabanillas F, Keating MJ, Kantarjian H. (2004) Outcome with the hyper-CVAD regimens in lymphoblastic lymphoma. *Blood* **104**: 1624–1630.
82. Morel P, Lepage E, Brice P, Dupriez B, D'Agay MF, Fenaux P, Gosselin B, Bauters F, Gisselbrecht C. (1992) Prognosis and treatment of lymphoblastic lymphoma in adults: A report on 80 patients. *J Clin Oncol* **10**: 1078–1085.
83. Leung W, Sandlund JT, Hudson MM, Zhou Y, Hancock ML, Zhu Y, Ribeiro RC, Rubnitz JE, Kun LE, Razzouk B, Evans WE, Pui CH. (2001) Second malignancy after treatment of childhood non-Hodgkin lymphoma. *Cancer* **92**: 1959–1966.
84. Wachowski O, Zimmermann M, Burkhardt B, Determann O, Meyer U, Kaatsch P, Mann G, Parwaresch R, Riehm H, Schrappe M, Reiter A. (2005) Secondary neoplasms subsequent to Berlin-Frankfurt-Muenster (BFM) Therapy of Non-Hodgkin lymphoma of childhood: Significantly higher risk for patients with lymphoblastic lymphoma compared to other NHL-subtypes. *Blood* **106**: 232.
88. Landmann E, Burkhardt B, Zimmermann M, Niggli F, Mann G, Reiter A. (2009) Osteonecrosis in children with non-Hodgkin lymphoma (NHL). *Hematol Meeting Reports* **3**: 87.
91. Pusill-Waschtsmuth B, Oschilies I, Zimmermann M, Ludwig WD, Parwaresch R, Mann G, Schrappe M, Riehm H, Reiter A. (2003) Prognostic factors in childhood T-cell lymphoblastic lymphoma treated in three consecutive NHL-BFM studies. *J Pediatr Hematol Oncol* **25**: S3–S4.
92. Burkhardt B, Bruch J, Zimmermann M, Strauch K, Parwaresch R, Ludwig WD, Harder L, Schlegelberger B, Mueller F, Harbott J, Reiter A. (2006) Loss of heterozygosity on chromosome 6q14-q24 is associated with poor outcome in children and adolescents with T-cell lymphoblastic lymphoma. *Leukemia* **20**: 1422–1429.
93. Coustan-Smith E, Sandlund JT, Perkins SL, Chen H, Chang M, Abromowitch M, Campana D. (2009) Minimal disseminated disease in childhood T-cell lymphoblastic lymphoma: A report from the children's oncology group. *J Clin Oncol* **27**: 3533–3539.

18

Hodgkin Lymphoma in Children, Adolescents and Young Adults

Debra L. Friedman and Anas Younes

Introduction

In 1832, Thomas Hodgkin described seven patients with enlarged lymph glands and spleen. At the turn of the 20th century, histological descriptions of multinucleated giant cells, were described by Sternberg in 1898[1] and Reed in 1902.[2] In the 1960s, the clonality of Reed–Sternberg cell was established[3] and recently, work has been done on the molecular biology of the disease, including the role of immunoglobulin genes, transcription factors, apoptotic pathways and Epstein–Barr virus (EBV) incorporation.[4–7]

Therapeutic advances in HL began in 1902 when Pusey reported on the use of radiotherapy,[8] followed by the use of mechlorethamine (nitrogen mustard) in 1946,[9] then combination chemotherapy with MOPP in 1964[10] and ABVD in the 1970s.[11] Donaldson *et al.* at Stanford introduced the concept of combined modality therapy for pediatric patients using the MOPP backbone and low-dose radiation therapy.[12] (See Table 18.1 for acronyms of treatment protocols.) Multimodality, risk-adapted therapies, designed to balance efficacy with toxicity, as well as the study of adverse long-term outcomes related to the disease and its treatment, are now the standard of care for Hodgkin lymphoma.

Epidemiology

Incidence

Using data from United States Surveillance, Epidemiology End Results (SEER) data,[13] it is clear that Hodgkin lymphoma is a disease that particularly affects adolescents and young adults, and indeed is the most common malignancy in those between the ages of 16 and 19 years (see Chapter 1). Hodgkin lymphoma makes up 8.8% of all childhood cancer under the age of 20 years, but 17.7% of cancer in children between ages 15 and 17 years. The overall annual incidence rate in the United States is 12.1 per million for children under 20 years and increases to 32 per million when limiting the analysis to adolescents between 15 and 19 years. Overall, there is a slight female predominance when considering all children less than 20 years (M:F = 0.9. The Caucasian: African American ratio is 1.3:1.[13]

Adolescent and young adults are most likely to have disease with the nodular sclerosing subtype. While among children < 20 years of age, the nodular sclerosing subtype accounts for 70% of cases, this subtype accounts for 74% of cases in those 15–19 years of age.[13]

Risk factors

There are several factors that are known to increase risk of HL, including family history of HL, EBV infections,

Table 18.1. Common chemotherapy protocols and acronyms.

Acronym	Chemotherapy agents
ABV	Doxorubicin, bleomycin, vinblastine
ABVD	Doxorubicin, bleomycin, vinblastine, dacarbazine (DTIC)
BEACOPP	Bleomycin, etoposide, doxorubicin, cyclophosphamide, vincristine, procarbazine, prednisone
CHOP	Cyclophosphamide, doxorubicin, vincristine, prednisone
COP (P)	Cyclophosphamide, vincristine, procarbazine, (prednisone)
D(A)BVE (PC)	Doxorubicin, bleomycin, vincristine, etoposide, (prednisone, cyclophosphamide)
MOPP	Mechlorethamine (nitrogen mustard), vincristine, procarbazine, prednisone
VAMP	Vincristine, doxorubicin, methotrexate, prednisone
VEPA	Vinblastine, etoposide, prednisone, doxorubicin
OEPA	Vincristine, etoposide, prednisone, doxorubicin
OPPA	Vincristine, procarbazine, prednisone, doxorubicin
ICE	Ifosfamide, carboplatin, etoposide
IV	Ifosfamide, vinorelbine
BEAM	Carmustine, etoposide, cytarabine, melphalan

socioeconomic status and social contacts. For young adult disease (ages 16–44 years), there is a 99-fold increased risk among monozygotic twins and a sevenfold increased risk among other siblings.[14–16] EBV-associated HL, with incorporation of the EBV in the genome, is most commonly reported with the mixed cellularity histologic subtype, in children from underdeveloped and developing nations, and in young adult males. However, a history of infectious mononucleosis and high-titer antibodies to EBV are associated with young adult HL, where incorporation of the EBV genome in the tumor is rare.[7,17–20] The association between HL and socioeconomic status, interestingly also differs by age. In children under 10 years, the disease is associated with lower socioeconomic status and large sibship.[21,22] In contrast, the risk in young adult patients increases with socioeconomic status and with the related characteristics of small nuclear family, single family housing, and fewer siblings or childhood playmates. These findings may be related to an association with infections, where increased infections in early childhood may reduce risk of young adult HL.[23,24] There is inconsistent data regarding clustering of young adult cases.[25,26]

Biology

Reed–Sternberg (RS) cells are embedded within a reactive infiltrate of lymphocytes, macrophages, granulocytes, and eosinophils.[27] The RS cell is the hallmark of classical HL and is a binucleated or multinucleated giant cell that is often characterized with a bilobed nucleus, with two large nucleoli, giving the classically described owl's eye appearance (see Chapter 4).[28] The RS cell and its variants most commonly derive from a neoplastic clone originating from B-lymphocytes in lymph node germinal centers. Molecular sequence analyses of RS cell clones reveal rearrangements of immunoglobulin variable-region genes that result in the lack of immunoglobulin production. Such cells should die from apoptosis, but it is thought that RS cells evade the apoptotic pathway, leading to the genesis of HL.[4,5] The B lymphoid cells from which RS arise have high levels of constitutive nuclear NF-κB, a transcription factor known to mediate gene expression related to inflammatory and immune responses and deregulation of NF-κB has been postulated as a mechanism by which RS cells evade apoptosis.[6,29] NF-κB dimers are held in an inactive cytoplasmic complex with inhibitory proteins, the IkBs.[29] B-cell stimulation by diverse signals results in rapid activation of the IkB kinase (IKK). The IKK complex phosphorylates two critical serine residues of IkBs,[30–32] thereby targeting them for rapid ubiquitin-mediated proteasomal degradation. Active NF-κB dimers are then released and translocated to the nucleus, where they activate gene transcription. Activation of NF-κB appears to be a final common effect of costimulatory interactions, genetic aberrations, or viral proteins that operate in HL.[33]

RS cells express CD40 and CD40 ligand (CD40L) is expressed on inflammatory T and dendritic cells that surround them. CD40/CD40L interactions normally provide a second signal from activated helper T cells to normal B cells, resulting in activation of NF-κB. NF-κB in turn causes proliferation and induces expression of Bcl-x_L, which protects B cells from apoptosis.[34] Tumor necrosis factor receptor-associated factor 1 (TRAF1) is overexpressed in EBV-transformed lymphoid cells and RS cells[35] and is associated with activation of NF-κB and protection of lymphoid cells from antigen-induced apoptosis. Activation of NF-κB, in turn, leads to expression of TRAF1, thereby establishing a positive feedback loop that maximizes NF-κB-dependent gene expression.[36] EBV latent membrane protein 1 (LMP1) interacts with TRAF1, and tumors with TRAF1-LMP1 aggregates exhibit high NF-κB activity.[37,38] LMP1 activates NF-κB by promoting IkBa turnover.[39] RS cells express CD30 and CD30 ligation promotes proliferation of HL-derived cells with constitutive activation of NF-κB.[40]

EBV may play a role in the rescue and repair of RS cells, further aiding in their evasion of apoptosis. Genome fragments can be found in approximately 30–50% of HL specimens[7,41–43] Three latent viral antigens are expressed in EBV-positive HL in RS cells: Epstein–Barr nuclear antigen-1 (EBNA1), required for viral episome maintenance, LMP1 with transforming properties and LMP2, which is non-transforming.[44,45]

Histology

Hodgkin lymphoma can broadly be divided into two pathologic classes: classical Hodgkin lymphoma (CHL) and nodular lymphocyte predominant Hodgkin lymphoma (NLPHL) (see Chapter 4).[46,47] In turn, CHL can be further divided into four subtypes: lymphocyte-rich (LRCHL), nodular sclerosis (NSHL), mixed cellularity (MCHL), and lymphocyte-depleted (LDHL).

Tumor cells (RS cells) in CHL do not express B-cell antigens such as CD45, CD19 and CD79A, but virtually all express CD30 and approximately 70% express CD15, while only 20–30% express CD20.[48] In comparison, the tumor cells of NLPHL do express B-cell antigens such as CD19, CD20, CD22 and CD79A, may or may not express CD30 and do not express CD15.[49] In addition, the OCT.2 and BOB.1 oncogenes are downregulated in CHL but not in NLPHL, correlating with immunoglobulin transcription.[50]

Clinical Considerations

Presentation and staging

The presentation of HL does not differ by age at diagnosis with painless adenopathy as the most common presentation. However, mediastinal involvement is present in approximately 76% of adolescents. A large mediastinal mass with a maximum diameter that is greater than one third of the chest diameter and/or a node or nodal aggregate greater than 10 cm occurs in about 20% of patients.[51,52] Approximately 20% of patients may also have associated "B" symptoms. B symptoms are defined as (1) unexplained loss of > 10% of body weight in the 6 months preceding the diagnosis; (2) unexplained fever with temperatures > 38°C for more than 3 days; or (3) drenching night sweats.[52–54] Staging is now performed clinically, based on the Ann Arbor staging system,[55] as revised in 1989.[53] Approximately 80–85% of children and adolescents with HL have involvement limited to or with direct extension from the lymph nodes and/or the spleen (Stages I–III), whereas 15–20% of patients have involvement of the lung, bone marrow, bone or liver.[55] Staging guidelines are summarized in Table 18.2.

Diagnostic evaluation

History should include elicitation of B symptoms, as that is important in risk stratification. A thorough physical evaluation should be performed and an excisional lymph node biopsy should be performed for tissue confirmation. Computed tomography (CT) scans of the neck, thorax, abdomen, and pelvis should be performed. In addition, an upright chest radiograph (CXR) with posteroanterior (PA) and lateral views are required for documentation of a large mediastinal mass (bulk mediastinal disease), defined as tumor diameter > 1/3 the thoracic diameter (measured transversely at the level of the dome of the diaphragm on a 6-foot upright PA CXR).[56] With changes in the quality of CT and functional imaging, it is likely that this will no longer be standard of care moving forward. FDG-PET imaging is standard of care in Hodgkin lymphoma and response to disease is now judged by FDG-PET alone or in combination with CT. With the advent of combined CT-PET scans, areas of disease can be evaluated simultaneously with both modalities in an overlapping fashion.[57–60] Technicium-99 bone scintigraphy should be considered in patients with bone pain or elevated alkaline phosphatase, although PET may soon obviate the need for this.

Bone marrow biopsy is recommended for all Stage III and IV patients or patients with B symptoms. There are less consistent recommendations for lower stage patients without B symptoms.[61,62] Laboratory studies include a complete blood count, blood chemistries to evaluate hepatic and renal function and acute phase

Table 18.2. Clinical and staging criteria for Hodgkin lymphoma.

A. Stage grouping

Stage I: Involvement of single lymph node region (I) or localized involvement of a single extralymphatic organ or site (IE).

Stage II: Involvement of two or more lymph node regions on the same side of the diaphragm (II) or localized contiguous involvement of a single extralymphatic organ or site and its regional lymph node(s) with involvement of one or more lymph node regions on the same side of the diaphragm (IIE).

Stage III: Involvement of lymph node regions on both sides of the diaphragm (III), which may also be accompanied by localized contiguous involvement of an extralymphatic organ or site (IIIE), by involvement of the spleen (IIIS), or both (IIIE + S).

Stage IV: Disseminated (multifocal) involvement of one or more extralymphatic organs or tissues, with or without associated lymph node involvement, or isolated extralymphatic organ involvement with distant (nonregional) nodal involvement.

B. Symptoms and presentations

"A" Symptoms: Lack of "B" symptoms.

"B" Symptoms: At least one of the following:
- Unexplained weight loss > 10% in the preceding 6 months
- Unexplained recurrent fever > 38°C
- Drenching night sweats.

X Bulk disease (see C below)

E Involvement of a single extranodal site that is contiguous or proximal to the known nodal site

C. Bulk disease

One or both of the following presentations are considered "bulk" disease:

- **Large mediastinal mass:** Tumor diameter > 1/3 the thoracic diameter (measured transversely at the level of the dome of the diaphragm on a 6-foot upright PA CXR). In the presence of hilar nodal disease, the maximal mediastinal tumor measurement may be taken at the level of the hilus. This should be measured as the maximum mediastinal width (at a level containing tumor and any normal mediastinal structures at the level) over the maximum thoracic ratio.
- **Large extra-mediastinal nodal aggregate:** A continuous aggregate of nodal tissue that measures > 6[a] cm in the longest transverse diameter in any nodal area

[a]Some studies use 10 cm for definition of extramediastinal bulk disease.

reactants such as ferritin, erythrocyte sedimentation rate and serum copper, which may be seen as nonspecific markers of tumor activity.

Prognostic factors

Pretreatment factors that have been shown to be associated with adverse outcome include advanced stage, B symptoms, bulk disease, extranodal extension, male sex and elevated erythrocyte sedimentation rate. In some studies, hemoglobin < 11.0 g/dl or white blood cell count > 11,500/mm^3, age 5–10 years, and increased numbers of sites of disease.[63–69] Patients with NLPHL appear to have an overall better prognosis than those with CHL, and amongst those with CHL, histologic subtype is not consistently associated with prognosis.[67,70] Serum markers that may confer adverse prognostic risk, such as soluble vascular adhesion molecule-1, tumor necrosis factor, soluble CD-30, β2 microglobulin, transferin, serum IL-10 and serum CD8 antigen.[71–76] High RS cell levels of caspase 3 may be associated with a more favorable outcome.[77] Early response to treatment, which may be a correlate for biology, may also be an important prognostic factor, allowing titration of therapy to the individual.[68,78–80] Some of these data are summarized in Table 18.3.

Initial Treatment for Hodgkin Lymphoma

Contemporary standard approaches to adolescent and young adult HL include multiagent chemotherapy with or without low-dose involved field radiotherapy. The overriding principles of these treatment regimens are to balance efficacy with both acute and, perhaps, more importantly, long-term toxicities.[81–83] A summary of common protocols for upfront therapy is found in Table 18.4.

Chemotherapy regimens have largely built upon the MOPP and ABVD backbones, and over time have resulted in improved survival.[84,85] To decrease alkylator therapy and potential cardiotoxicity, and provide dose-intensive treatment, the Pediatric Oncology Group (POG) developed a series of studies built upon the ABVD backbone, substituting dacarbazine with etoposide.

Table 18.3. Adverse pretreatment prognostic factors for Hodgkin lymphoma.[a]

Host
Male sex
Age: 5–10 years
Disease
Advanced stage
Increased numbers of sites of disease
Bulk disease
Extranodal extension
Laboratory markers
Elevated erythrocyte sedimentation rate
Hemoglobin < 11.0 g/dl
White blood cell count > 11,500/mm^3
Soluble vascular adhesion molecule-1
Tumor necrosis factor
Soluble CD-30
Beta-2 microglobulin
Transferin, serum IL-10
Serum CD 8 antigen
Clinical presentation
B symptoms

[a]Not consistent across all studies: Therapeutic interventions have been shown to abrograte significance in some studies.

The use of vincristine instead of vinblastine allowed for escalation of doxorubicin and etoposide. POG 9226 piloted therapy with four cycles of DBVE followed by low dose IFRT in patients with Stages I, IIA and IIIA. Five-year EFS was 89%.[86] POG 9426 evaluated the same chemotherapy in a nonrandomized response-based manner. Those with a rapid response (60% tumor reduction, gallium negative) after two cycles proceeded to consolidative IFRT without further chemotherapy; slow responders continued to receive four cycles plus IFRT. In POG 9425 (for patients with advanced stage disease), prednisone and cyclophosphamide were added to the ABVE-PC backbone, with more rapid delivery of therapy to intensify the weekly therapeutic intensity. Response was assessed after three cycles (9 weeks). Those with rapid response did not receive the additional two cycles of chemotherapy. Overall 3-year EFS was 87% and OS 96%, with no difference in EFS between slow and rapid responders and a progressive disease rate of only 1%. All patients received consolidative regional low dose (20Gy) RT.[79,83] Both studies evaluated the efficacy of dexrazoxane in reducing cardiac and pulmonary toxicity. While it is still too early to know whether there was a significant benefit, dexrazoxane was associated with an increased risk of acute (hematologic/infectious) toxicities and development of second malignancies, mostly treatment-related leukemia.[87] In young adults and adults with early favorable classical HL, the current standard of care is two cycles of ABVD plus involved field radiation therapy.[88]

With the goal of continued excellent long-term survival and decreasing long-term effects of treatment, POG and the Children's Cancer Group (CCG) have conducted trials to evaluate elimination of radiation therapy. In the Children's Cancer Group (CCG) 521 study, patients were randomized between 12 cycles of alternating MOPP/AVBD vs. six cycles of AVBD + low-dose regional chemotherapy. Event-free survival was only 77% for Stage III and IV patients and there was excess pulmonary toxicity with ABVD.[84] POG 8725 compared eight cycles of MOPP/AVBD with and without IFRT in Stage IIB, III and IV patients. There was no significant benefit for radiation therapy,[85] but the study used a large amount of chemotherapy, which is associated with potential significant long-term adverse outcomes including gonadal toxicity, cardiac toxicity and secondary leukemia (see long-term outcomes of therapy below). Response post three cycles was a strong prognostic factor, with a 94% EFS in the rapid early responders as opposed to a 78% EFS in those who did not respond quickly.[85] CCG 5942 studied the elimination of radiation therapy in a randomized fashion in all patients who had a complete response following chemotherapy. Patients were treated with four cycles of COPP/ABV, six cycles of COPP/ABV or two cycles each of COPP/ABV, cytarabine/etoposide, and CHOP, depending on stage of disease and presence of bulk disease. Of the 829 eligible patients, complete response was achieved in 83% and 501 were randomized to receive IFRT or no further therapy. Event-free survival for all Stage II, III and IV patients was 84.4%, 76% and 81% at 4 years, respectively. In all groups, the difference in EFS post-randomization was highly significant and overall EFS was 91% for the group who received IFRT and 86% for those who did not receive IFRT. Despite the differences in EFS, early evaluation of overall survival is not affected by the inclusion of IFRT.[63] A pilot study CCG 59704, utilized the German Hodgkin Disease Group's BEACOPP backbone for patients with B symptoms or advanced stage disease. Overall, the 3-year EFS was 95% with patients receiving 6–8 cycles of chemotherapy with or without radiotherapy on the basis of a gender-stratified, response-based therapeutic algorithm.[89]

Studies in the Children's Oncology Group (COG) evaluate the principles of risk-adapted therapy, where therapy is decreased for those at lowest risk and with

Table 18.4. Recommendations for standard therapy in pediatric Hodgkin lymphoma.

Risk group	Stage and presentation	Recommended therapy	Commonly accepted chemotherapy regimens
Low	IA, IIA < 4 nodal regions without B symptoms, bulk disease or extranodal extension	2–4 cycles of non-cross-resistant chemotherapy +/–LD-IFRT	VAMP × 4 COPP/ABV hybrid × 4 DBVE × 4 OEPA or OPPA × 2 CHOP × 3–4 +/– Rituximab ABVD × 2–4
Intermediate	IA, IIA with bulk disease, ≥ 3 nodal regions, or extranodal extension IIB,[a] IIIA, IVA[a]	4–6 cycles of non-cross-resistant chemotherapy +/– LD-IFRT	COPP/ABV × 6 DBVE-PC × 3–5 OPPA/OEPA × 2 + COPP × 2 ANVD × 4–6
High	IIB,[a] IIIB, IVB[a]	4–8 cycles of non-cross-resistant chemotherapy +/– LD-IFRT	DBVE-PC × 3–5 BEACOPP × 8 (or BEACOPP × 4 + ABVD × 2 or + COPP/ABV × 4) OPPA/OEPA × 2 + COPP × 4 Stanford V ABVD × 6

[a]It remains unclear whether IIB disease, particularly with bulk disease is intermediate or high risk. Similarly, some regimens treat all Stage IV patients as high risk, although most studies show that patients with IVA disease have better outcomes than those with IVB.

LD-IFRT: low-dose involved field radiotherapy (15–25 Gy).

favorable early responses to chemotherapy and augmented for those with more advanced disease or a slow response to initial chemotherapy.

The Dana Farber–Stanford–St. Jude pediatric Hodgkin lymphoma consortium studies have focused efforts on reduction in alkylating agent, anthracycline and radiotherapy doses. Low-risk patients have been treated with four cycles of an alkylator-free chemotherapy protocol, VAMP, with radiotherapy doses of 15 Gy or 25.5 Gy based upon response to the first two cycles of chemotherapy. This approach resulted in a 5-year EFS of 93%.[90] For patients with higher risk disease, two protocols have been evaluated, VAMP/COP and VEPA, both with IFRT. Results have been less acceptable with 5-year EFS of 74% and 68%, respectively.[91,92] The group is now evaluating the Stanford V regimen[93] that has been successfully employed in adult patients.

In the same era, the German cooperative groups have built upon COPP chemotherapy in both pediatric and adult Hodgkin lymphoma. The DAL-HL-90 study used OEPA/COPP for males and OPPA/COPP for females, both followed by IFRT. EFS for Stages II, III, and IV were 92, 86 and 90%, respectively.[94] The GPOH-95 study was designed to assess elimination of radiotherapy for those with a complete response. It built on the OPPA/OEPA backbones by adding cycles of COPP for patients with more advanced disease. Radiotherapy dose was determined by the post-chemotherapy disease reduction. Complete response was defined as complete resolution of all disease (as opposed to 70% reduction in CCG 5942 and 59704). Only 22% achieved a complete response. Fifty percent achieved between 75% and 95% disease reduction and were treated with 20 Gy radiotherapy, while 4% had less than a 75% reduction and were treated with 30 Gy. Twenty percent of patients had residual masses treated with boost doses to 35 Gy. Overall, the EFS was 92% for those receiving radiotherapy compared with 88% in those treated with chemotherapy alone. This difference was largely influenced by patients with more advanced stage disease or B symptoms. For patients with IA, IB, and IIA disease, EFS was not different among those with a CR to chemotherapy and no other therapy (97%) and those with a partial response, subsequently treated with radiotherapy (94%). However, for all other patients, the EFS was 79% for those treated with chemotherapy alone compared with 91% for those treated with combined modality therapy.[95]

For low-risk patients, NLPHL some patients may be treated with surgery alone. There are multiple small reports in both adult and pediatric HL of patients of successful treatment of completely resected Stage I disease. For those who did relapse, salvage rates were encouraging and death from disease very low.[96–99] This has prompted a study in the COG to formally evaluate surgery only in patients with involvement of a single completely resected lymph node with NLPHL. The optimal treatment of patients with advanced stage NLPHL remains undetermined. These patients are traditionally treated with regimens that are used for patients with advanced stage classical HL, such as ABVD (doxorubicin, bleomycin, vinblastine, dacarbazine). However, given the similarities between NLPHL and indolent CD20+ B-cell non-Hodgkin lymphoma (NHL), a question remains whether low-grade lymphoma regimens, such as R-CHOP, are more effective. To address this issue, Fanale *et al.* conducted a retrospective analysis of treatment outcomes in patients who received R-CHOP vs. other regimens treated at UT MDACC from 1995 to 2010.[100] Patients treated with R-CHOP were found to have a better 5-year progression-free survival and overall survival compared with those who were treated with HL-directed regimens.[100] However, such a question can only be answered in prospective randomized studies.

Radiotherapy for Hodgkin lymphoma

It has been recognized since the 1950s that HL is an extremely radiosensitive disease. Initially, this therapy was delivered using orthovoltage where limited fields that could safely be treated to high doses. With the advent of the linear accelerator, Kaplan *et al.* at Stanford University developed techniques to safely and effectively treat large fields with high doses.[52] At the present time, for children and adolescents with HL, radiotherapy is exclusively delivered in the context of multimodality therapy. Doses of 15–25 Gy are commonly used, and some experimental protocols are attempting to identify groups of patients for whom the exclusion of radiotherapy is possible, without affecting disease-free survival.[101]

Megavoltage energies are now treatment of choice for pediatric HL. A 4- to 6-MV linear accelerator should be used to treat supradiaphragmatic fields, whereas 8–15-MV machines may be appropriate for treating paraaortic nodes. Distances of less than 80 cm are to be avoided as they will result in suboptimal depth dosage. Although there are differences in treatment techniques among radiation oncologists and specific institutions, the general technical principles remain constant across centers. [102–104] Proton beam radiotherapy is currently under investigation at several centers across the United States.

Table 18.5. Guidelines for involved field radiation.

Involved nodes	Radiotherapy field
Cervical	Neck, supraclavicular/infraclavicular
Supraclavicular	Supraclavicular/infraclavicular, lower neck
Axillary	Axilla ± supraclavicular/infraclavicular
Mediastinum	Mediastinum, hila and infraclavicular/ supraclavicular
Hila	Hila, mediastinum
Spleen	Spleen ± para-aortic
Para-aortic	Para-aortic ± spleen
Iliac	Iliac, inguinal, femoral
Inguinal	External iliac, inguinal, femoral
Femoral	External iliac, inguinal, femoral

The fields of radiotherapy treatment must be meticulously and judiciously designed with the goal to deliver the optimum volume of radiotherapy for disease control, while avoiding normal tissue damage. Similarly, dosage calculations should take into account lack of homogeneity of tissues within a field.[101] Customized shielding blocks should be utilized as appropriate to protect normal tissue. These may include posterior cervical spine, humeral head, laryngeal, occipital, lung, and cardiac blocks. Blocking the genitalia is of specific importance, when pelvic fields are included. In females, while scattered and transmitted dose to the ovaries will be inevitable, medial or lateral transposition of the ovaries (oophoropexy) results in doses of 8–10% and 4–5%, respectively of the pelvic dose, [105,106] which will be compatible with the preservation of fertility. For males, the greatest shielding to the testes is affording by use of a frog leg position together with an individually fitted shield, which will reduce the scatter to approximately 0.75% of the pelvic lymph node dose.[107] Daily radiotherapy is delivered using equally weighted anterior and posterior fields, with fractional doses of 1.5–1.8 Gy daily, five times per week. It is imperative to design fields to minimize re-treatment match line problems if additional radiotherapy is needed to treat recurrence.[101] Radiotherapy information for treatment of HL is found in Table 18.5.

Treatment for Relapsed Hodgkin

Hodgkin lymphoma may be cured even if it has recurred after initial treatment. Potentially curative options include conventional chemoradiotherapy protocols for those with lower risk relapses, radiotherapy alone for those relapsing in a limited nodal pattern, reinduction chemotherapy followed by autologous hematopoietic stem cell transplantation (HSCT) (see Chapter 20), and experimental

Table 18.6. Common treatment options for recurrent Hodgkin lymphoma.

ICE (Ifosfamide, carboplatin, and etoposide)
DECA (Dexamethasone, etoposide, cisplatin, and cytarabine)
IV (Ifosfamide and vinorelbine)
GV (gemcitabine and vinorelbine)
IEP–ABVD–COPP (Ifosfamide, etoposide, prednisone–doxorubicin, bleomycin, vinblastine, dacarbazine–cyclophosphamide, vincristine, procarbazine, and prednisone)
APE (Cytosine arabinoside, cisplatin, and etoposide)
SGN-35 (brentuximab vedotin) antibody–drug conjugate targeting CD30A

therapies such as immunotherapy (see Chapter 21).[108–115] Palliative care should always be considered for patients with refractory or recurrent disease, when curative intent is not likely,[116] but care should be taken not to miss a potential curative opportunity.[117] Some common retrieval regimens are shown in Table 18.6. Much of the data on relapsed HL comes from studies that include both adult and pediatric patients. It remains unclear whether outcomes vary according to age. Chemotherapy agents are chosen, in part dependent upon previous chemotherapy and radiotherapy exposures, as well as planned additional therapy, such as the need for mobilization of stem cells and HSCT. When HSCT is being considered, disease response to cytoreductive therapy prior to HSCT predicts overall survival. HSCT is most effective for patients who enter with minimal or chemosensitive disease.[115,118,119] Two Ifosfamide-based regimens have been used with good response rates, ICE[110,118] and IV.[120] In addition ICE has been used in the preparative regimen in a recently reported tandem transplant regimen.[121] In a recent study comparing ICE to DHAP for patients with relapsed HL and non-Hodgkin lymphoma, ICE had a superior outcome with an overall response rate of 68%.[121] When ICE is used prior to planned stem cell transplant, it has recently been shown that pre-ASCT functional imaging predicted outcome with 4-year EFS rates of 75% for patients transplanted with negative functional imaging, with negative imaging being the only independent prognostic factor in multivariable analysis.[121] In another study of transplant-eligible patients with relapsed or refractory lymphoma using ICE for both salvage and stem cell mobilization, the overall response rate to ICE was 89%.[121] In addition, ICE has been used in the preparative regimen in a recently reported tandem transplant regimen.[121] Ifosfamide has also successfully been paired with Vinorelbine the treatment of recurrent HL with an overall response rate as high as 83%.[121] Gemcitabine has also been used in combination with Vinorelbine with excellent overall response rates in recurrent HL with or without ifosfamide and other cytotoxic agents.[122] In a recently closed trial from the Children's Oncology Group, of 25 evaluable patients overall response was 76% and furthermore, early response to FDG-PET was more prognostic of overall response than CT.[123,124]

Patients with low stage disease (I, II), no B symptoms and no bulk disease who were initially treated with non-dose-intensive chemotherapy and no radiotherapy, may be salvaged with conventional chemotherapy and low-dose involved field radiotherapy, or sometimes standard dose radiotherapy alone[111,125,126] However, B symptoms and extranodal disease at the time of relapse are poor prognostic factors,[127] as is shorter duration of initial remission.[128,129] For those who have previously been treated with chemoradiotherapy, particularly with standard radiotherapy or, with newer dose-intensive regimens, recurrence within 12 months of completion of therapy results in overall survival rates of 10–30% with conventional chemotherapy regimens.[109,114,128,129] Relapses occurring 12 months or greater are more responsive to salvage chemotherapy, but overall survival rates remain low — 20–50% with conventional chemotherapy.[128–130] Thus for patients with advanced stage disease, B symptoms, bulk disease, those previously treated with combined modality regimens that included dose-intensive chemotherapy or standard dose radiotherapy, or those with a short period of remission, reinduction chemotherapy followed by HSCT and radiotherapy remain the treatment of choice, although survival rates range broadly from 25–80%.[108,115,117,131–139] An advantage of transplant has been reported in two randomized trials, from the British National Lymphoma Investigation and the German Hodgkin's Lymphoma Study Group together with the European Group for Blood and Marrow Transplantation, where EFS was superior in the transplant arm compared to the conventional therapy arm, using a backbone of BEAM.[140,141]

Autologous HSCT is most commonly used for recurrent or refractory HD. However, an allogeneic effect has been observed, albeit offset by transplant-related morbidity and mortality.[135–137,142] This has led to research investigating reduced intensity allogeneic approaches, as well as immune modulation and induction of autologous graft vs. host disease, in order to benefit from the allogeneic effect.[143–147]

The treatment of HL patients whose disease relapses after autologous stem cell transplantation, remains challenging, with an estimated median survival of less than 3 years.[148] Drug development in this area represents a significant unmet medical need.[149] Several new compounds have recently demonstrated promising clinical activity in patients with relapsed HL after failing ASCT, including brentuximab vedotin (SGN35), panobinostat (LBH589) and everolimus (RAD001) (see Chapter 22). Although the safety and efficacy of these agents have been examined in young adults, experience with these drug in pediatric patients is currently not available.[150] In a recent multinational, open-label, phase 2 study, the efficacy and safety of brentuximab vedotin was evaluated in 102 patients with relapsed or refractory HL after ASCT.[151] Patients were treated with 1.8-mg/kg brentuximab vedotin by intravenous infusion every 3 weeks. In the absence of disease progression or prohibitive toxicity, patients received a maximum of 16 cycles. Reductions in tumor size were observed in 94% of patients. The ORR was 75%, with a best response of complete remission (CR) achieved by 34% of patients and PR in 40%. The median duration of response was 29 weeks, with 60% of the CR patients remaining in CR after 12 months. The most common treatment-related adverse events were peripheral sensory neuropathy, nausea, fatigue, neutropenia, and diarrhea.[151] In a separate large phase II study, the safety and efficacy of panobinostat, an oral histone deacetylase inhibitor, was evaluated in 129 patients with relapsed HL.[152] Patients were treated with 40 mg three times per week, every week, in 21-day cycles. A reduction in tumor measurements was observed in 99 (77%) patients. Responses were observed in 35 (27%) patients (5 complete responses and 30 partial responses). The median duration of response was 6.9+ months, and the median progression-free survival was 5.7+ months. Common related grades 3 and 4 adverse events included thrombocytopenia, anemia, and neutropenia.[152] Finally, the safety and efficacy of everolimus, an oral mTOR inhibitor, were evaluated in 15 patients with relapsed HL.[153] Patients were treated with daily doses of 10-mg everolimus for up to one year, and seven patients (47%) achieved partial responses. Grade 3 adverse events included thrombocytopenia and anemia. Based on these encouraging data, a phase I/II study combining panobinostat with everolimus is currently being conducted in patients with relapsed HL.[154,155]

Monitoring for adverse long-term outcomes of therapy

The common potential long-term effects of radiotherapy and chemotherapy for HL are summarized together with general monitoring recommendations in Tables 18.7 and 18.8, respectively (see also Chapter 24). To date, there do not exist uniformly effective long-term follow up plans for survivors of childhood HL, as evidenced by published research over the past decade that documents a significant lost-to-follow up rate, lack of knowledge on the part of HL and other childhood cancer survivors about their past treatment and potential for adverse health sequelae, inadequate provision of follow up care and poor utilization of available health services.[147,150,156–163] Various pediatric cooperative groups have addressed the problem

Table 18.7. General guidelines for radiation late effects assessment and management.

System	Potential effects	Monitoring recommendations[a]
Cardiac	Cardiomyopathy Pericarditis Coronary artery disease Valvular disease	Electrocardiogram and echocardiogram
Pulmonary	Pulmonary fibrosis	Pulmonary function tests (PFTs) (including DLCO and spirometry)
Thyroid	Overt or compensated hypothyroidism Thyroid nodules or cancer Hyperthyroidism	Free T4; TSH
Gonadal (female)	Delayed/arrested puberty Early menopause Ovarian failure	FSH, LH, estradiol
Gonadal (male)	Germ cell failure Infertility/azoospermia Leydig cell dysfunction Hypogonadism Delayed/arrested puberty	FSH, LH, testosterone Semen analysis

(*Continued*)

Table 18.7. (*Continued*)

System	Potential effects	Monitoring recommendations[a]
Bone	**Osteopenia** Bone mineral density ≥ 1 and < 2.5 SD below mean **Osteoporosis** Bone mineral density ≥ 2.5 SD below mean **Osteonecrosis** (Avascular necrosis – AVN)	Bone density evaluation (DEXA or quantitative CT) MRI as clinically indicated by signs or symptoms suggestive of AVN
Second malignancies	Sarcomas CNS tumors Breast cancer Melanoma Non-melanoma skin cancer Thyroid cancer Other solid tumors	Routine cancer screening per general population guidelines Mammography to screen for female breast cancer at age 25 years or 10 years post-RT exposure, whichever is later

[a]Monitoring recommendations all include a risk-adapted health history and physical examination. The frequency with which diagnostic studies and laboratories should be performed is dependent on many factors including dose of radiotherapy, chemotherapy exposures, age at exposure and other clinical parameters.

Table 18.8. General guidelines for chemotherapy late effects assessment and management.

System	Agents	Potential effects	Monitoring guidelines[a]
Cardiac	Anthracyclines	Cardiomyopathy, arrhythmias	Electrocardiogram and echocardiogram
Pulmonary	Bleomycin	Restrictive lung disease	PFTs (including DLCO and spirometry)
Gonadal (female)	Alkylating agents	Delayed/arrested puberty, early menopause, ovarian failure	FSH, LH, estradiol
Gonadal (male)	Alkylating agents	Germ cell failure, infertility/ Azoospermia, leydig cell dysfunction, hypogonadism, delayed/arrested puberty	FSH, LH, testosterone
Bone	Corticosteroids[±] Methotrexate Alkylating agents (due to hypogonadism) Corticosteroids	Osteopenia, bone mineral density ≥ 1 and < 2.5 SD below mean, osteoporosis, bone mineral density ≥ 2.5 SD below mean, Osteonecrosis (AVN)	Bone density evaluation (DEXA or quantitative CT). MRI as clinically indicated by signs or symptoms suggestive of AVN
Second malignancies	Alkylating agents: Topoisomerase II inhibitors	Leukemia	CBC/differential
	Cyclophosphamide	Transitional bladder carcinoma	Urinalysis

[a]Monitoring recommendations all include a risk-adapted health history and physical examination. The frequency with which diagnostic studies and laboratories should be performed is dependent on many factors including dose of chemotherapy, radiotherapy exposures, age at exposure and other clinical parameters. AVN: avascular necrosis.

with the development of long-term follow up guidelines, which provide a foundation for what follow up care should be delivered.[164,165] However, the recommendations are not completely consistent with one another and there are, at present, a lack of sufficient resources committed to ensure their implementation.[164–166] Therefore, ongoing research is required to develop a uniform set of "best practice" guidelines that can be utilized as an integral part clinical care for survivors of childhood and adolescent HL.

Conclusions

Hodgkin lymphoma is characterized by complex biology and epidemiology that require additional study to better understand how they interface with one another, affect disease presentation, response to therapy and long-term outcomes. Cure rates remain one of the highest in pediatric oncology, but adverse long-term outcomes are similarly quite frequent in occurrence. Ongoing clinical trials thus seek to balance efficacy with both short and long-term toxicity. For higher risk initial disease, refractory and recurrent disease, the challenge remains increasing the cure rate and incorporating novel agents that may better target the underlying biology and pathophysiology.

References

11. Santoro A, Bonadonna G, Valagussa P, Zucali R, Viviani S, Villani F, Pagnoni AM, Bonfante V, Musumeci R, Crippa F, *et al.* (1987) Long-term results of combined chemotherapy-radiotherapy approach in Hodgkin's disease: Superiority of ABVD plus radiotherapy versus MOPP plus radiotherapy. *J Clin Oncol* 5: 27–37.
12. Donaldson SS, Link MP. (1987) Combined modality treatment with low-dose radiation and MOPP chemotherapy for children with Hodgkin's disease. *J Clin Oncol* 5: 742–749.
20. Sleckman BG, Mauch PM, Ambinder RF, Mann R, Pinkus GS, Kadin ME, Sherburne B, Perez-Atayde A, Thior I, Mueller N. (1998) Epstein-Barr virus in Hodgkin's disease: Correlation of risk factors and disease characteristics with molecular evidence of viral infection. *Cancer Epidemiol Biomarkers Prev* 7: 1117–1121.
21. Grufferman S, Delzell E. (1984) Epidemiology of Hodgkin's disease. *Epidemiol Rev* 6: 76–106.
28. Brauninger A, Schmitz R, Bechtel D, Renne C, Hansmann ML, Kuppers R. (2005) Molecular biology of Hodgkin's and Reed/Sternberg cells in Hodgkin's lymphoma. *Int J Cancer.*
39. Sylla BS, Hung SC, Davidson DM, Hatzivassiliou E, Malinin NL, Wallach D, Gilmore TD, Kieff E, Mosialos G. (1998) Epstein-Barr virus-transforming protein latent infection membrane protein 1 activates transcription factor NF-kappaB through a pathway that includes the NF-kappaB-inducing kinase and the IkappaB kinases IKKalpha and IKKbeta. *Proc Natl Acad Sci U S A* **95**: 10106–10111.
40. Mir SS, Richter BW, Duckett CS. (2000) Differential effects of CD30 activation in anaplastic large cell lymphoma and Hodgkin disease cells. *Blood* **96**: 4307–4312.
48. Tzankov A, Zimpfer A, Pehrs AC, Lugli A, Went P, Maurer R, Pileri S, Dirnhofer S. (2003) Expression of B-cell markers in classical Hodgkin lymphoma: A tissue microarray analysis of 330 cases. *Mod Pathol* **16**: 1141–1147.
51. Mauch PM, Kalish LA, Kadin M, Coleman CN, Osteen R, Hellman S. (1993) Patterns of presentation of Hodgkin disease. Implications for etiology and pathogenesis. *Cancer* **71**: 2062–2071.
57. Friedberg JW, Fischman A, Neuberg D, Kim H, Takvorian T, Ng AK, Mauch PM, Canellos GP, van den Abbeele AD. (2004) FDG-PET is superior to gallium scintigraphy in staging and more sensitive in the follow-up of patients with *de novo* Hodgkin lymphoma: A blinded comparison. *Leuk Lymphoma* **45**: 85–92.
59. Hueltenschmidt B, Sautter-Bihl ML, Lang O, Maul FD, Fischer J, Mergenthaler HG, Bihl H. (2001) Whole body positron emission tomography in the treatment of Hodgkin disease. *Cancer* **91**: 302–310.
63. Nachman JB, Sposto R, Herzog P, Gilchrist GS, Wolden SL, Thomson J, Kadin ME, Pattengale P, Davis PC, Hutchinson RJ, White K. (2002) Randomized comparison of low-dose involved-field radiotherapy and no radiotherapy for children with Hodgkin's disease who achieve a complete response to chemotherapy. *J Clin Oncol* **20**: 3765–3771.
64. Ruhl U, Albrecht M, Dieckmann K, Luders H, Marciniak H, Schellenberg D, Wickmann L, Dorffel W. (2001) Response-adapted radiotherapy in the treatment of pediatric Hodgkin's disease: An interim report at 5 years of the German GPOH-HD 95 trial. *Int J Radiat Oncol Biol Phys* **51**: 1209–1218.
65. Krasin MJ, Rai SN, Kun LE, Merchant TE, Metzger ML, Kaste SC, Howard SC, Hudson MM. (2005) Patterns of treatment failure in pediatric and young adult patients with Hodgkin's disease: Local disease control with combined-modality therapy. *J Clin Oncol* **23**: 8406–8413.
66. Smith RS, Chen Q, Hudson MM, Link MP, Kun L, Weinstein H, Billett A, Marcus KJ, Tarbell NJ, Donaldson SS. (2003) Prognostic factors for children with Hodgkin's disease treated with combined-modality therapy. *J Clin Oncol* **21**: 2026–2033.
68. Landman-Parker J, Pacquement H, Leblanc T, Habrand JL, Terrier-Lacombe MJ, Bertrand Y, Perel Y, Robert A, Coze C, Thuret I, Donadieu J, Schaison G, Leverger G, Lemerle J, Oberlin O. (2000) Localized childhood Hodgkin's disease: Response-adapted chemotherapy with etoposide, bleomycin, vinblastine, and prednisone before low-dose radiation therapy-results of the French Society of Pediatric Oncology study MDH90. *J Clin Oncol* **18**: 1500–1507.
69. Schwartz CL. (2003) Prognostic factors in pediatric Hodgkin disease. *Curr Oncol Rep* **5**: 498–504.
79. Schwartz C, Constine L, London W, Kamps W, Marcus R, Chauvenet A. (2001) Intensive response-based therapy with or without dexrazoxane for intermediate/ high-stage (I/HS) pediatric Hodgkin's disease (HD): A Pediatric Oncology Group (POG) study. *Fifth International Symposium on Hodgkin's Lymphoma.* Koln, Germany.

80. Weiner MA, Leventhal BG, Marcus R, Brecher M, Ternberg J, Behm FG, Cantor A, Wharam M, Chauvenet A. (1991) Intensive chemotherapy and low-dose radiotherapy for the treatment of advanced-stage Hodgkin's disease in pediatric patients: A Pediatric Oncology Group study. *J Clin Oncol* **9**: 1591–1598.
83. Schwartz CL. (2005) Special issues in pediatric Hodgkin's disease. *Eur J Haematol Suppl*: 55–62.
85. Weiner MA, Leventhal B, Brecher ML, Marcus RB, Cantor A, Gieser PW, Ternberg JL, Behm FG, Wharam MD Jr., Chauvenet AR. (1997) Randomized study of intensive MOPP-ABVD with or without low-dose total-nodal radiation therapy in the treatment of stages IIB, IIIA2, IIIB, and IV Hodgkin's disease in pediatric patients: A Pediatric Oncology Group study. *J Clin Oncol* **15**: 2769–2779.
86. Tebbi CK, Mendenhall N, London WB, Williams JL, de Alarcon PA, Chauvenet AR. (2006) Treatment of stage I, IIA, IIIA(1) pediatric Hodgkin disease with doxorubicin, bleomycin, vincristine and etoposide (DBVE) and radiation: A Pediatric Oncology Group (POG) study. *Pediatr Blood Cancer* **46**: 198–202.
88. Engert A, Plutschow A, Eich HT, Lohri A, Dorken B, Borchmann P, Berger B, Greil R, Willborn KC, Wilhelm M, Debus J, Eble MJ, Sokler M, Ho A, Rank A, Ganser A, Trumper L, Bokemeyer C, Kirchner H, Schubert J, Kral Z, Fuchs M, Muller-Hermelink HK, Muller RP, Diehl V. Reduced treatment intensity in patients with early-stage Hodgkin's lymphoma. *N Engl J Med* **363**: 640–652.
89. Kelly KM, Hutchinson RJ, Sposto R, Weiner MA, Lones MA, Perkins SL, Massey V. (2002) Feasibility of upfront dose-intensive chemotherapy in children with advanced-stage Hodgkin's lymphoma: Preliminary results from the Children's Cancer Group study CCG-59704. *Ann Oncol* **13**(1): 107–111.
90. Donaldson SS, Hudson MM, Lamborn KR, Link MP, Kun L, Billett AL, Marcus KC, Hurwitz CA, Young JA, Tarbell NJ, Weinstein HJ. (2002) VAMP and low-dose, involved-field radiation for children and adolescents with favorable, early-stage Hodgkin's disease: Results of a prospective clinical trial. *J Clin Oncol* **20**: 3081–3087.
91. Hudson MM, Krasin M, Link MP, Donaldson SS, Billups C, Merchant TE, Kun L, Billet AL, Kaste S, Tarbell NJ, Howard S, Friedmann AM, Hurwitz CA, Young JA, Marcus KC, Rai S, Cowan T, Weinstein HJ. (2004) Risk-adapted, combined-modality therapy with VAMP/COP and response-based, involved-field radiation for unfavorable pediatric Hodgkin's disease. *J Clin Oncol* **22**: 4541–4550.
92. Friedmann AM, Hudson MM, Weinstein HJ, Donaldson SS, Kun L, Tarbell NJ, Link MP. (2002) Treatment of unfavorable childhood Hodgkin's disease with VEPA and low-dose, involved-field radiation. *J Clin Oncol* **20**: 3088–3094.
93. Horning SJ, Hoppe RT, Breslin S, Bartlett NL, Brown BW, Rosenberg SA. (2002) Stanford V and radiotherapy for locally extensive and advanced Hodgkin's disease: Mature results of a prospective clinical trial. *J Clin Oncol* **20**: 630–637.
94. Schellong G, Potter R, Bramswig J, Wagner W, Prott FJ, Dorffel W, Korholz D, Mann G, Rath B, Reiter A, Weissbach G, Riepenhausen M, Thiemann M, Schwarze EW. (1999) High cure rates and reduced long-term toxicity in pediatric Hodgkin's disease: The German-Austrian multicenter trial DAL-HD-90. The German-Austrian Pediatric Hodgkin's Disease Study Group. *J Clin Oncol* **17**: 3736–3744.
95. Dorffel W, Luders H, Ruhl U, Albrecht M, Marciniak H, Parwaresch R, Potter R, Schellong G, Schwarze EW, Wickmann L. (2003) Preliminary results of the multicenter trial GPOH-HD 95 for the treatment of Hodgkin's disease in children and adolescents: Analysis and outlook. *Klin Padiatr* **215**: 139–145.
99. Murphy SB, Morgan ER, Katzenstein HM, Kletzel M. (2003) Results of little or no treatment for lymphocyte-predominant Hodgkin disease in children and adolescents. *J Pediatr Hematol/Oncol* **25**: 684–687.
100. Fanale MA, Lai C-M, McLaughlin P, Romaguera J, Fayad L, Hagemeister F, Samaniego F, Rodriguez MA, Neelapu SS, Shah JJ, Kwak L, Dong W, Reed V, Dabaja BS, Popat U, Younes A. (2010) Outcomes of Nodular Lymphocyte Predominant Hodgkin's Lymphoma (NLPHL) patients treated with R-CHOP. *Blood (ASH Annual Meeting Abstracts)* **116**: 2812.
108. Glossmann JP, Staak JO, Nogova L, Diehl V, Scheid C, Kisro J, Reis HE, Peter N, Engert A, Josting A. (2005) Autologous tandem transplantation in patients with primary progressive or relapsed/refractory lymphoma. *Ann Hematol* **84**: 517–525.
110. Hertzberg MS, Crombie C, Benson W, Taper J, Gottlieb D, Bradstock KF. (2003) Outpatient-based ifosfamide, carboplatin and etoposide (ICE) chemotherapy in transplant-eligible patients with non-Hodgkin's lymphoma and Hodgkin's disease. *Ann Oncol* **14**(Suppl 1): i11–16.
111. Josting A, Nogova L, Franklin J, Glossmann JP, Eich HT, Sieber M, Schober T, Boettcher HD, Schulz U, Muller RP, Diehl V, Engert A. (2005) Salvage radiotherapy in patients with relapsed and refractory Hodgkin's

lymphoma: A retrospective analysis from the German Hodgkin Lymphoma Study Group. *J Clin Oncol* **23**: 1522–1529.

113. Ruffer JU, Ballova V, Glossmann J, Sieber M, Franklin J, Nogova L, Diehl V, Josting A. (2005) BEACOPP and COPP/ABVD as salvage treatment after primary extended field radiation therapy of early stage Hodgkins disease — results of the German Hodgkin Study Group. *Leuk Lymphoma* **46**: 1561–1567.

115. Yuen AR, Rosenberg SA, Hoppe RT, Halpern JD, Horning SJ. (1997) Comparison between conventional salvage therapy and high-dose therapy with autografting for recurrent or refractory Hodgkin's disease. *Blood* **89**: 814–822.

122. Chen JH, Chang PY, Yao NS. (2009) Gemcitabine plus vinorelbine as an effective salvage chemotherapeutic regimen in advanced Hodgkin lymphoma. *Hematol Oncol Stem Cell Ther* **2**: 371–372.

124. Cole PD, Schwartz CL, Drachtman RA, de Alarcon PA, Chen L, Trippett TM. (2009) Phase II study of weekly gemcitabine and vinorelbine for children with recurrent or refractory Hodgkin's disease: A Children's Oncology Group report. *J Clin Oncol* **27**: 1456–1461.

133. Josting A, Sieniawski M, Glossmann JP, Staak O, Nogova L, Peters N, Mapara M, Dorken B, Ko Y, Metzner B, Kisro J, Diehl V, Engert A. (2005) High-dose sequential chemotherapy followed by autologous stem cell transplantation in relapsed and refractory aggressive non-Hodgkin's lymphoma: Results of a multicenter phase II study. *Ann Oncol* **16**: 1359–1365.

137. Cooney JP, Stiff PJ, Toor AA, Parthasarathy M. (2003) BEAM allogeneic transplantation for patients with Hodgkin's disease who relapse after autologous transplantation is safe and effective. *Biol Blood Marrow Transplant* **9**: 177–182.

138. Lieskovsky YE, Donaldson SS, Torres MA, Wong RM, Amylon MD, Link MP, Agarwal R. (2004) High-dose therapy and autologous hematopoietic stem-cell transplantation for recurrent or refractory pediatric Hodgkin's disease: Results and prognostic indices. *J Clin Oncol* **22**: 4532–4540.

143. Peggs KS, Hunter A, Chopra R, Parker A, Mahendra P, Milligan D, Craddock C, Pettengell R, Dogan A, Thomson KJ, Morris EC, Hale G, Waldmann H, Goldstone AH, Linch DC, Mackinnon S. (2005) Clinical evidence of a graft-versus-Hodgkin's-lymphoma effect after reduced-intensity allogeneic transplantation. *Lancet* **365**: 1934–1941.

150. Chen R, Gopal AK, Smith SE, Ansell SM, Rosenblatt JD, Klasa R, Connors JM, Engert A, Larsen EK, Kennedy DA, Sievers EL, Younes A. (2010) Results of a pivotal phase 2 study of brentuximab vedotin (SGN-35) in patients with relapsed or refractory Hodgkin lymphoma. *Blood (ASH Annual Meeting Abstracts)* **116**: 283.

151. Sureda A, Younes A, Ben-Yehuda D, Ong T-C, Kaufman JL, Corre CL, Gallagher J, Shen A, Engert A. (2010) Final analysis: Phase II study of oral panobinostat in relapsed/refractory Hodgkin lymphoma patients following autologous hematopoietic stem cell transplant. *Blood (ASH Annual Meeting Abstracts)* **116**: 419.

152. Johnston PB, Ansell SM, Colgan JP, Habermann TM, Inwards DJ, Micallef INM, Porrata LF, Reeder CB, Roy V, LaPlant BR, Witzig TE. (2007) mTOR inhibition for relapsed or refractory Hodgkin lymphoma: Promising single agent activity with everolimus (RAD001). *Blood (ASH Annual Meeting Abstracts)* **110**: 2555.

153. Younes A, Copeland A, Fanale MA, Hagemeister F, Fayad L, Pro B, Faria SC, Ji Y, Medeiros LJ, Berry DA, Buglio D. (2010) Phase I/II study of the novel combination of panobinostat (LBH589) and everolimus (RAD001) in relapsed/refractory Hodgkin and non-Hodgkin lymphoma. *Blood (ASH Annual Meeting Abstracts)* **116**: 3964.

154. Lemoine M, Buglio D, Jona A, Derenzini E, Medeiros LJ, Berry DA, Younes A. (2010) The pan-deacetylase inhibitor panobinostat downregulates HIF-1{alpha} and VEGF and, synergizes with everolimus in Hodgkin lymphoma cell lines. *Blood (ASH Annual Meeting Abstracts)* **116**: 2851.

19

Immunodeficiency-Associated Hematological Malignancies

Nader Kim El-Mallawany, Michael R. Bishop and Bruce Shiramizu

Introduction

The immune system's role in the pathophysiology of cancer has been under investigation for well over a century. Early scientific observations from the late 1800s have established important principles that are still applicable today.[1,2] Malignancies, especially hematological, occur with heightened frequency in patients with immune deficiencies. However, the rare occurrence of immune deficiency disorders and the refractory nature of the cancers that occur in their wake render each case a formidable challenge. Furthermore, much remains to be understood about the complex dynamics that exist between the immune system, neoplastic pathways, and viral pathophysiology. This chapter will highlight advancements and an up-to-date understanding of cancer immunology, the role of viruses in relation to malignancies as well as childhood and adolescent primary and acquired immunodeficiency-associated hematological malignancies.

Immunology, Virology and Malignancy

Cancer immunology

Current theories characterizing the interaction between the immune system and cancer biology are built upon the concepts of immune surveillance and immune tolerance.[3–5] Recently, a model described as immunoediting connects these two principles along a dynamic continuum.[6] The theory of cancer immunoediting is based on three processes — elimination, equilibrium, and escape. In this model, malignant cells may thrive due to the inability of immune surveillance to eliminate them or due to their resilience in escaping immune recognition through induction of immune tolerance or otherwise due to a combination of processes falling anywhere along that spectrum (Fig. 19.1). Alas, the vast multitude of interactions between the host immune system and the development of malignancies is at once delicate, intricate, and complex.

A wide diversity of observations in both animal and human subjects has further highlighted the connection between the immune system and cancer biology. After many years of struggling to establish proof of principle, it was shown that immunodeficient mice have a greater propensity to develop malignancy than their healthy counterparts.[7] Meanwhile, in establishing patient registries for children with primary immunodeficiency, it was well documented that these children experience a much higher incidence of cancer compared to the general population.[8] Follow-up studies for patients undergoing organ transplantation,[9] as well as patients infected with human immunodeficiency virus (HIV),[10] also show a significantly increased relative risk of developing cancer.

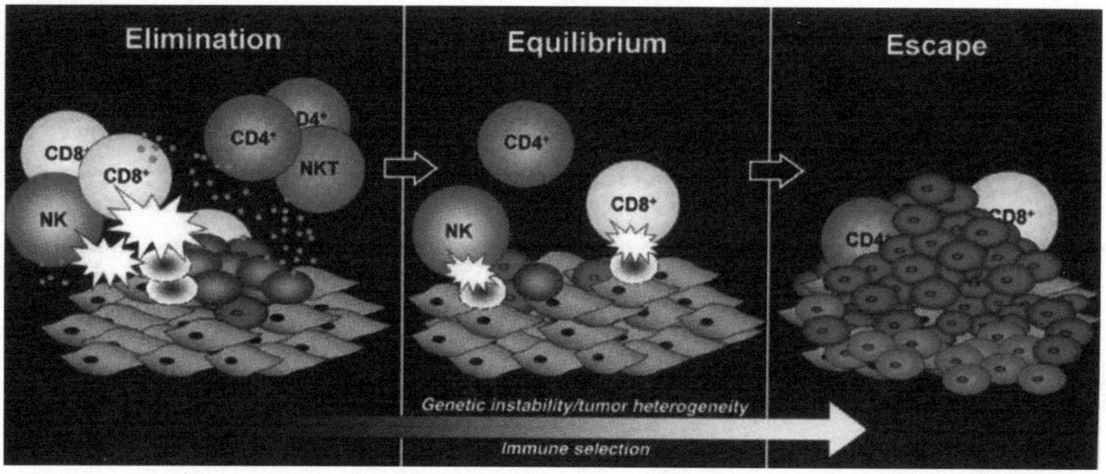

Fig. 19.1. The three Es of cancer immunoediting. Cancer immunoediting encompasses three processes. (A) Elimination corresponds to immunosurveillance. (B) Equilibrium represents the process by which the immune system iteratively selects and/or promotes the generation of tumor cell variants with increasing capacities to survive immune attack. (C) Escape is the process wherein the immunologically sculpted tumor expands in an uncontrolled manner in the immunocompetent host. In Panels (A) and (B), developing tumor cells (blue), tumor cell variants (red), underlying stroma and nontransformed cells (gray) are shown; in Panel (C), additional tumor variants (orange) that have formed as a result of the equilibrium process are shown. Different lymphocyte populations are as marked. The small orange circles represent cytokines and the white flashes represent cytotoxic activity of lymphocytes against tumor cells.

Dunn GP, Bruce AT, Ikeda H, Old LJ, Schreiber RD. (2003) Cancer immunoediting: From immunosurveillance to tumor escape. *Nat Immunol* **3**(11): 991–998.

Further evidence for the link between immunology and cancer lies in unraveling the mechanisms of tumorigenesis associated with the immune response. Histopathologic evaluation of several different types of malignancies illustrates the importance of tumor infiltrating lymphocytes (TIL) in the tumor microenvironment.[11] On the other hand, the presence of regulatory T cells (Tregs) within the tumor microenvironment has been shown to directly suppress the tumor-specific effects of T cells.[12,13] Characterized by CD4 and CD25 antigen expression, Tregs represent tumor-induced immune suppression and serve as a potential target for immunotherapy.[14] In as much, the development of anticancer treatment strategies targeting immunological mechanisms of oncogenesis has offered some of the strongest evidence for the role of the immune system in fighting malignancy.

The diversity and specificity of the human immune system is vast and has inspired the development of a wide array of immunotherapeutic approaches. Anti-cancer therapy has advanced significantly with the advent of monoclonal antibodies targeting antigens expressed on various types of malignant cells. Examples include rituximab against the CD20 antigen expressed on B-cell non-Hodgkin lymphomas, trastuzumab against HER-2/Neu expressed on breast cancer, and gemtuzumab, which targets CD33 expressed on acute myeloid leukemia, amongst many others (see Chapter 21).[15] Meanwhile, targeted immunotherapies utilizing cytotoxic T lymphocytes (CTL) have shown promise in the treatment of melanoma[16] and Epstein–Barr virus (EBV)-positive lymphomas.[17] Adoptive immunotherapies utilizing chimeric antigen receptors have also shown early promise, combining the honing properties of monoclonal antibodies with the cytotoxic potential of T and NK cells.[18] Dendritic cells are an attractive target for anti-tumor vaccine development because they are potent antigen-presenting cells (APC) that stimulate both CD8+ and CD4+ T-cell activation and additionally, can be cultured *ex vivo*.[19,20] Other methods of therapeutic immune activation include manipulation of tumor antigens via conjugation, driving costimulatory pathways to enhance antigen presentation, and the exogenous use of cytokines.[4] In summary, the expanding arsenal of anti-cancer immunotherapeutic options highlights the integral connection between the immune response and cancer biology.

Viral pathophysiology and oncogenesis

The association between viruses and human cancer was first illustrated in the mid 1960s when EBV was discovered in tissue samples of Ugandan patients with

Table 19.1. Expression of EBV latent genes in disease.[a]

Pattern of latency	EBNA-1	EBNA-2	EBNA-3	LMP-1	LMP-2	EBER	Disease
Type 1	+	–	–	–	–	+	Burkitt's lymphoma
Type 2	+	–	–	+	+	+	Nasopharyngeal carcinoma, Hodgkin's disease, peripheral T-cell lymphoma
Type 3	+	+	+	+	+	+	Lymphoproliferative disease, X-linked lymphoproliferative disease, infectious mononucleosis
Other	±	–	–	–	+	+	Healthy carrier

EBV: Epstein–Barr virus; EBNA: Epstein–Barr virus nuclear antigen; LMP: latent membrane protein; EBER: Epstein–Barr virus-encoded RNA.
[a] A plus sign indicates that the gene is expressed in the disease, a minus sign that is not expressed, and the two together that the gene may or may not be expressed.
Cohen JI. (2000) Epstein–Barr virus infection. *N Engl J Med* **343**(7):481–492.

endemic Burkitt lymphoma. This was a hallmark moment for both fields of virology and oncology, as it marked not only the eventual discovery of an entire viral genome, but an etiologic agent for cancer as well. Since that point in history, the connection between viruses and cancer has been magnified greatly. We now know that approximately 15% of human cancers are associated with a number of different viruses including EBV, human herpesvirus-8 (HHV-8), human T-cell lymphotropic virus-1 (HTLV-1), hepatitis B and C viruses, and human papillomavirus (HPV) (Table 19.1).[21] Furthermore, it is well established that the majority of malignancies arising in the setting of a known immunodeficiency disorder are associated with viral infection.[8] The connection between viruses and human cancer is diverse in a variety of ways, ranging in its role in pathophysiology (from a direct causative agent to a contributing cofactor), in the types of cancer that arise (from hematological malignancies to solid tumors), and in its propensity to develop in both patients with and without established immunodeficiency. Further advances in understanding the associations between virology, immunology, and malignancy will continue to foster progress in elucidating mechanisms of oncogenesis as well as developing novel therapeutic approaches.

Epstein–Barr virus

Since the oncogenic potential of EBV was described nearly half a century ago, it has been used as a model for viral oncogenesis through its known characteristics.[22] The viral pathogenesis of EBV, as well as the host immune response to EBV infection, are well established. EBV is associated with a wide variety of human malignancies — both hematological malignancies and carcinomas — under a diverse array of clinical scenarios including patients with known immunodeficiencies as well as in otherwise healthy individuals. Furthermore, the establishment of EBV-immortalized cell lines have provided the basis for subsequent investigations of the transformation potential of the virus within infected B lymphocytes.[23]

The mechanisms of EBV viral pathogenesis are well characterized. A member of the human herpesvirus family, EBV, was the first herpesvirus to have its genome completely cloned and sequenced.[24] The virus is transmitted via salivary secretions, and initial infection occurs in the epithelial cells of the oropharynx. Through binding of a major membrane glycoprotein to the CD21 antigen, the virus infects B lymphocytes within the lymphoid tissue of Waldeyer's ring.[25] After the initial infection and immune response, EBV remains latent within resting B cells. Although the EBV genome encodes for nearly 100 proteins, only 10 viral genes are expressed in latently infected resting B cells. These genes are represented by six nuclear proteins (EBNA-1, EBNA-2, EBNA-3A, EBNA-3B, EBNA-3C, and EBNA-LP), two membrane proteins (LMP-1 and LMP-2), and two types of nontranslated RNA (EBER-1 and EBER-2).[26] In downregulating the expression of viral proteins in latency, EBV is able to evade immune recognition and maintain viral persistence. Additional EBV genes, e.g. BZLF1, are associated with the processes of viral reactivation and lytic replication. Each protein has well described cellular interactions related to important functional pathways including B cell proliferation, apoptosis, and cytokine production, amongst many others. Different combinations of latent viral protein expressions were identified in both healthy carriers and patients with EBV malignancies (Table 19.2), which showed that the profile of latent antigens expressed by the B cells within which EBV persists, played an important role in driving abnormal cellular pathway progression.[22]

Table 19.2. Immunodeficiency cancer registry cases: Distribution of tumors and immunodeficiencies.

Immunodeficiency	Adenocarcinoma	Lymphoma	Hodgkin's disease	Leukemia	Other tumors	Total
Severe combined immunodeficiency	1 (2.4%)	31 (73.8%)	4 (9.5%)	5 (11.9%)	1 (2.4%)	42 (8.4%)
X-linked agammaglobulimemia	3 (14.3%)	7 (33.3%)	3 (14.3%)	7 (33.3%)	1 (4.8%)	21 (4.2%)
Common variable immunodeficiency	20 (16.7%)	55 (45.8%)	8 (6.7%)	8 (6.7%)	29 (24.2%)	120 (24%)
IgA deficiency	8 (21.1%)	6 (15.8%)	3 (7.9%)	0 (0%)	21 (55.3%)	38 (7.6%)
Hyper-IgM syndrome	0 (0%)	9 (56.3%)	4 (25.0%)	0 (0%)	3 (18.8%)	16 (3.2%)
Wiskott–Aldrich syndrome	0 (0%)	59 (75.6%)	3 (3.8%)	7 (9.0%)	9 (11.5%)	78 (15.6%)
Ataxia telangiectasia	13 (8.7%)	69 (46.0%)	16 (10.7%)	32 (21.3%)	20 (13.3%)	150 (30.0%)
Other immunodeficiencies	1 (4.0%)	12 (48.0%)	1 (4.0%)	4 (16.0%)	7 (28.0%)	25 (5.0%)
Total immunodeficiency categories	46 (9.2%)	252 (50.4%)	43 (8.6%)	63 (12.6%)	96 (19.2%)	500 (100%)

Gross TG and Shiramizu B. (2006) Lymphoproliferative Disorders and Malignancies Related to Immunodeficiencies. In Pizzo PA and Poplack DG, eds. *Principles and Practice of Pediatric Oncology,* 5th edition. pp. 748–767, Lippincott, Williams & Wilkins, Philadelphia.

Understanding the immune response to EBV illuminates the mechanisms of pathogenesis in EBV-related disease. EBV infection activates both the humoral and cellular arms of the immune system. Initially, EBV infection of B lymphocytes stimulates B cell production of both EBV-specific and nonspecific antibodies. This is followed by the critically important cell-mediated response which results in CD8+ CTL that are both EBV-specific and nonspecific. A deficient CTL response to EBV could potentially offset the host/virus symbiosis and lead to EBV-driven disruption of the immune response resulting in either uncontrolled B-cell proliferation or a toxic nonspecific T-cell and histiocytic reaction. Ultimately, the CD8+ T cells play the primary role in controlling EBV infection and maintaining a controlled latency stage. In latent disease, a healthy individual will have approximately 10^{-5} to 10^{-6} of the circulating B cells that are latently infected, contrasted to the presence of 1–5% of all circulating CD8+ CTL maintaining the capacity to react to EBV.[26] NK cells and CD4+ T cells play a supporting role for the CTL, while neutralizing antibodies may play a role in thwarting the spread of virus to additional B cells.[27,28]

The spectrum of disease from EBV has enormous range — from asymptomatic infection to mild viral syndrome to infectious mononucleosis to frank malignancy. The vast majority of people are exposed to EBV at a young age and suffer minimal or no complications from infection. Older children who are exposed to EBV for the first time may develop infectious mononucleosis, in which the nonspecific immune reaction described above accounts for the symptomatology. The initial nonspecific humoral response is appreciated by the monospot evaluation, a nonspecific test targeting the heterophil antibody produced in response to infection.[29] The overwhelming nonspecific CTL response that occurs thereafter accounts for the prolonged hyperinflammatory state that characterizes the associated symptoms of mononucleosis.[30] These lymphocytes account for the atypical lymphocytosis classically appreciated on the peripheral blood smear.[27] Eventually though, a specific anti-EBV CTL response assumes control and induces viral latency. Lymphoproliferative consequences of EBV infection are characterized by a heterogeneity of immune responses. Many of the EBV-associated cancers, including Burkitt lymphoma and Hodgkin lymphoma, occur several years after initial EBV infection. Latently infected EBV+ B cells have undergone malignant transformation from additional pathogenetic factors, resulting in the lymphomatous transformation. On the other hand, in immunodeficient patients, primary or reactivated EBV infection can result in a lymphoproliferative disease secondary to the immune system's inability to induce or maintain viral latency. Indeed, the spectrum of potential consequences from EBV infection is broad and is based on the immune system's capacity to respond to the presence of virus.

The importance of the CTL response to EBV infection is emphasized by the high risk for EBV+ B-cell lymphoproliferative disease (LPD) in patients with cell-mediated immune deficiency. This includes patients with both primary immunodeficiency disorders as well as those with secondary immunodeficiency from treatment-related immune suppression (in solid organ and hematopoietic stem cell transplantation) or human immunodeficiency virus (HIV) infection. These patients are at risk for a variety of EBV+ B-cell lymphomas as well as Hodgkin lymphoma. HIV+ pediatric patients are also uniquely at risk for developing EBV+ leiomyomas and leiomyosarcomas, which are otherwise extremely rare smooth muscle tumors. There also exists an entity of EBV+ T-cell LPD that arises both *de novo* and in the setting of patients with chronic active EBV (CAEBV) infection. It is theorized that these patients lack an element of cell-mediated immune function that permits the development of this highly fatal form of EBV-driven T-cell lymphoproliferation, yet the specific immunologic abnormality has yet to be elucidated.[31] Similarly, this theory applies to the closely related EBV+ Hydroa vacciniforme-like T-cell lymphoma.

In contrast, a number of EBV-associated malignancies occur in patients without any evidence of immune dysfunction. These include nasopharyngeal carcinoma, gastric carcinoma, B-cell non-Hodgkin lymphomas (NHL) including Burkitt lymphoma (BL), Hodgkin lymphoma, and also a subset of peripheral T-cell lymphomas including the extranodal nasal type NK/T-cell lymphoma. While EBV+ B-cell NHL and Hodgkin lymphoma can occur in patients with immunodeficiency, they most often occur in otherwise healthy subjects. The diverse propensity to induce oncogenic changes in both healthy and immune-deficient patients underlines the complexity of EBV pathogenesis and its inextricable link to human cancers.

The relationship between EBV and malignancy is unique in many ways. For example, there are distinct demographic characteristics of many EBV-associated malignancies. The endemic subtype of BL that occurs primarily in Sub-Saharan Africa is always EBV+, while only 30% of the sporadic form of BL that occurs in the rest of the world is positive for EBV.[32] EBV-associated T-cell and NK-cell lymphomas, on the other hand, tend to occur in Eastern Asia with much greater frequency than the rest of the world.[33] Another distinct feature of EBV-associated malignancies is that while some diseases occur exclusively in the setting of EBV infection, others exist both secondary to and independent of EBV infection. Malignancies that are nearly always EBV+ include endemic BL, post-transplant lymphoproliferative disease (PTLD), nasopharyngeal carcinoma, and EBV+ T-cell LPD. In contrast, those that are only occasionally EBV+ include Hodgkin lymphoma, gastric carcinoma, and other B-cell lymphomas including sporadic BL. The precise mechanisms of oncogenesis that distinguish between diseases with varied levels of association with EBV are incompletely understood. However, continued progress in shedding light on EBV's diverse manner of involvement in malignancy will foster an improved understanding of the mechanisms of disease pathogenesis and approaches for treatment as well.

EBV infection presents a very unique association with human cancer, especially in the childhood, adolescent, and young adult patient population. Confounded by the fact that more than 90% of the human population are infected by EBV without suffering subsequent oncologic complications, the complex link between EBV infection and malignancy in a relatively minute subset of the human population represents a scientific conundrum that has yet to be fully explained. EBV-associated malignancies are driven by a multitude of different factors including disruption in immune function, epigenetic and genetic changes at the molecular level, and epidemiologic associations with co-morbid diseases. The extensive study of EBV's role in the development of human cancer has fostered immense progress in the understanding and treatment of a wide variety of malignancies. Nonetheless, there remains much to be learned about the subtle complexities of disease pathogenesis in EBV+ cancer and continued growth in the scientific understanding of this unique virus will offer hope for further advances in the fields of immunology, virology, and oncology alike.

Human T-cell lymphotropic virus

The human T-cell lymphotropic virus-1 (HTLV-1) is a retrovirus that is also associated with hematological malignancy. HTLV-1 infects an estimated 10–20 million people worldwide[34] and is endemic in clusters of geographical locations including Japan, the Caribbean, parts of South America, West and Central Africa, and some of the Oceanic Islands.[35] It is primarily transmitted via breast feeding, however spread can occur via sharing of bodily fluids as well.[36] HTLV-1 infection is asymptomatic in the vast majority of patients, however, similar to EBV, a minor subset of patients develop very severe complications. The two major diseases associated with HTLV-1 are adult T-cell leukemia/lymphoma (ATLL)[37] and an inflammatory disease of the central nervous system (CNS) called HTLV-1-associated myelopathy (also known as tropical spastic paraparesis).[38] In endemic areas, HTLV-1 infection occurs early in life, but the progression to ATLL usually occurs in advanced age and in a relative paucity of infected patients.

The viral pathogenesis of HTLV-1 and its progression to malignancy involves a variety of factors. The virus is tropic for CD4+ T cells, but can also utilize CD8+ T cells as a reservoir of infection.[39] Infection is characterized by a slow rate of viral replication and high genetic stability of the virus.[40] Unlike the other human retrovirus HIV, HTLV-1 infection does not result in cytopathic destruction of the CD4+ T cells. Rather, HTLV-1 regulates its own transcription via its regulatory protein Tax. Tax has been shown to have numerous important cellular interactions with host proteins that may promote tumorigenesis including affecting the NF-κB cell proliferation pathway,[41] transactivation of genes favoring T cell proliferation and apoptosis inhibition, repression of cell cycle control and DNA repair, as well as inhibition of several tumor suppressor genes.[42] Another HTLV-1-encoded protein HBZ has also been implicated in disease pathogenesis, affecting both the NF-κB[43] and T cell proliferation pathways.[44] These epigenetic changes are important contributors to the development of HTLV-1 disease pathogenesis, and in as much the virus itself is not a direct oncogenic factor. Infection with HTLV-1 induces both humoral and cellular immune responses, and similar to EBV-induced malignancies, an impaired CTL response to HTLV-1 is associated with the development of ATLL.[45–47]

The association between HTLV-1 and ATLL was established in 1980 when the virus was isolated from tissue samples of a patient with T-cell lymphoma.[48] Infection with HTLV-1 carries an approximate 5% lifetime risk of developing ATLL.[49] There are four clinical variants of the disease — acute, lymphomatous, chronic, and smoldering. The most common variant is the acute type, in which patients often present with disseminated disease and systemic symptoms, organomegaly, and circulating malignant cells. The lymphomatous variant is characterized by prominent lymphadenopathy without involvement of the peripheral blood, while the chronic and smoldering subtypes represent more indolent disease with frequent involvement of the skin — the distinction is that the chronic subtype is marked by peripheral blood lymphocytosis. The immunophenotype of ATLL cells is usually represented by the expression of the CD4, CD2, CD5, and CD25 antigens, with downregulation of CD7. That being said, there exist variants that are CD8+ as well.[50] Patients with ATLL are known to be immunocompromised with an increased risk for opportunistic infections. The prognosis for the acute and lymphomatous subtypes of ATLL is dismal with median survival ranging between 5–13 months using standard chemotherapy treatment protocols.[51] Evidence for the immunological linkage between HTLV-1 and ATLL is substantiated by the improved prognosis (up to 30–40% survival) in treating patients with allogeneic hematopoietic stem cell transplantation (alloHSCT) (see Chapter 20).[52] Both clearance of HTLV-1 proviral loads and suggestion of a graft-vs.-lymphoma effect have been documented in multiple clinical trials, showing promise for this immunotherapeutic approach.[53]

Human herpesvirus-8/Kaposi sarcoma-associated herpesvirus

The other virus known to be associated with hematological malignancies is the human herpesvirus-8 (HHV-8), also known as the Kaposi sarcoma-associated herpesvirus (KSHV). Better known for its association with Kaposi sarcoma (KS) in the setting of HIV infection, HHV-8 is also associated with the primary effusion lymphoma (PEL), multicentric Castleman's disease (MCD, a rare form of lymphoproliferative disease), and a variant of diffuse large B-cell lymphoma (DLBCL) that arises in 15–20% of patients with MCD.[54] HHV-8 viral pathogenesis involves a number of virally encoded genes that drive cellular pathways resulting in tumorigenesis. vFLIP is a potent activator of the NF-κB pathway,[55] while vcyc is a viral D-type cyclin homolog that drives cell proliferation.[56] The latency-associated nuclear antigen (LANA) protein has been linked to tumorigenesis through multiple pathways including disruption of the p53 and Rb tumor suppressor networks.[57,58] HHV-8 also encodes a number of microRNAs that are involved in the disruption of programmed cell death pathways including the Bcl-2 apoptosis network.[59] In addition, a viral homolog for IL-6 is expressed by HHV-8 that has been shown to promote hematopoiesis, plasmacytosis, and angiogenesis and has been implicated in the pathogenesis of PEL.[60] Similar to HTLV-1, HHV-8 pathogenesis is multi-factorial and involves a complex network of cellular pathways moderated by virally encoded proteins.

Although malignancies associated with HHV-8 have been diagnosed in non-immunodeficient patients, it most often occurs in the setting of immune suppression secondary to HIV infection. The HIV epidemic paralleled a drastic increase in the incidence not only of KS, but in lymphoproliferative diseases associated with HHV-8 as well. Further evidence accrued supporting a relationship between immune function and HHV-8-associated malignancies. The cell-mediated immune response is the primary defense mechanism against HHV-8 infection; however, the virus has developed mechanisms to evade the host immune response.[61] A number of viral proteins promote immune evasion by disrupting T-lymphocyte interaction/activation,[62,63] downregulating cytokine activity,[64] and impairing antigen presentation.[65] Evidence of insufficient T-cell response to HHV-8 also correlated with development of cancer in patients vs. those with asymptomatic viral infection.[66,67] Moreover, compromise of both NK cell activity[68] and humoral immune function[69] was implicated in the development of KS. Finally, reports of partial tumor regression with immune reconstitution in HIV+ patients starting highly active anti-retroviral therapy (HAART) without chemotherapy further substantiates the importance of the immune system's role in combating disease.[70,71]

HHV-8 and EBV both fall under the subfamily of gamma herpesviruses, a group of viruses known to play a role in cell proliferation and the development of malignancies. HHV-8 infects a wide variety of cells — B lymphocytes, endothelial cells, macrophages, and epithelial cells. It is endemic in the Mediterranean region as well as sub-Saharan Africa, with low estimated prevalence in most of the rest of the world.[72] Other areas with significant incidence include Thailand, Taiwan, and Brazil.[73–75] HHV-8 transmission can occur through sexual interaction and via blood product exchange, however, virus has also been isolated in saliva and is thought to pass through salivary secretions as well.[76]

The lymphoproliferative diseases associated with HHV-8 are extremely rare. PEL accounts for approximately 4% of all HIV-associated lymphomas. It has a predilection to occur in the large body cavities — within the pleural, pericardial, and peritoneal spaces. It is characterized by lymphomatous serous collections of fluid that are not associated with solid tumor masses.[77] HHV-8 is always present in malignant PEL cells, and a majority of cases are also EBV-positive. However, HHV-8 is thought to be the oncogenic virus driving the disease.[54] There also exists an extra-cavitary variant of the disease that can present as nodal or extranodal masses with or without associated effusion. Genomic studies have identified the cellular origin as a B cell. Overall, survival outcomes for PEL are poor.[78]

MCD is also quite rare and reliable epidemiologic studies of its incidence are not available. Castleman's disease is a lymphoproliferative disorder characterized by angiofollicular lymph node hyperplasia. The two clinical variants include unicentric and multicentric disease. MCD is almost always associated with HHV-8 and carries a much more aggressive clinical course. It is associated with a diagnosis of KS or NHL (usually a variant of DLBCL) in a significant number of patients as well.[79,80] KS is a non-hematological malignancy also associated with HHV-8 infection and will be discussed again later in the chapter.

Hepatitis B, hepatitis C, and human papillomavirus

Viral etiologies for other non-hematological malignancies stem from some of the most common viral infections in the world. Hepatitis B and C viruses (HBV and HCV) are associated with hepatocellular carcinoma (HCC), while the human papillomavirus (HPV), which is mainly associated with cervical carcinoma, is also a causative factor for vaginal, vulval, penile, and anal carcinomas as well. HCC is one of the most common human cancers with nearly 75% of the cases arising from HBV or HCV infection.[21] The precise method of tumorigenesis in hepatitis viruses is still unclear. An indirect mechanism proposes that chronic damage to hepatocytes and the resultant presence of cytokines and inflammation in the microenvironment render the hepatic cells vulnerable to dysplastic changes.[81] This theory is sound for HCV infection, as HCC occurs almost exclusively in the setting of advanced liver cirrhosis in patients with hepatitis C.[82] The onset of HCC in patients with HBV infection, on the other hand, does not necessarily develop in patients with extensive liver damage. In that scenario, an alternate theory implicates a mechanism whereby integration of the HBV viral genome into the host disrupts genes that are important in hepatocellular growth and differentiation.[83] Evidence for a direct oncogenic role for HCV has also been explored focusing on the interaction between the hepatitis C core protein and the RAS, STAT, and MAPK molecular pathways.[84–86] In cervical cancer, integration of the cellular genome by HPV is a critical step in viral oncogenesis as well. Upregulation of the E6 and E7 viral genes encodes for proteins that interact with important tumor suppressor pathways (p53 and Rb networks) playing a critical role in cell proliferation.[87] Considering the extensive worldwide prevalence of cancers caused by all three of these viruses, it follows that immune suppression is not a necessary portal of opportunity for disease. Nonetheless, the incidence of virally induced HCC, cervical carcinoma, and HPV-associated anal carcinoma is greater in HIV-infected patients compared to the HIV-negative population, again suggesting an interplay between immunology and cancer in viral pathogenesis.

One of the most compelling relationships between immunology and cancer is the role of anti-viral vaccines in preventing cancer. This is best illustrated in the case of HBV infection. Highly effective vaccines for HBV have been available in over 100 countries since the turn of the 21st century. In turn, the incidence of HBV infection has declined markedly since implementation of the vaccine, as much as 7.5-fold in Taiwan, and 10-fold in The Gambia. This has fortunately coincided with a decrease in the frequency of HCC compared to historical controls as well as to non-vaccinated populations from the same era, with up to 20 years of follow up.[88,89] Similarly, the recent FDA-approved HPV vaccine in 2006 anticipates efficacy in preventing HPV infection and cervical neoplasia.[90] The prospect of preventing one of the most common cancers in the world offers exciting encouragement in utilizing the immunological aspects of oncology to improve outcomes on a global scale.

Malignancies and Primary Immunodeficiencies

In the contemporary era of advances in diagnosing and treating severe opportunistic infections, the survival curves for patients with primary immunodeficiency disorders have improved considerably and the diagnosis of malignancy in these patients has become more prominent.[91] After infectious mortality, malignancies are the second most common cause of death in this patient population. Since instituting patient registries in the early 1970s, much light has been shed on this unique set of disorders. The overall risk for developing cancer in primary immunodeficiencies is nearly 10,000 times higher than expected for healthy counterparts.[92] The incidence of cancer in these children varies depending on the underlying disorder. It can be as high as 10–25% in the three immunodeficiency disorders associated with the highest prevalence of cancers on the registry — ataxia telangiectasia (AT), Wiskott–Aldrich syndrome (WAS), and common variable immunodeficiency (CVID).[93–95] Overall, the pattern of malignancies in patients with primary immunodeficiency is different than that of otherwise healthy children, adolescents, and young adults with the majority of patients developing non-Hodgkin lymphoma rather than acute leukemia (Table 19.3). While many cases of lymphoma in this setting are associated with EBV infection, non-infectious etiologies for cancer also occur. The primary immunodeficiency disorders associated with malignancy are numerous and include defects of cell-mediated and/or humoral immunity as well as impairment of DNA repair mechanisms.

Treatment of malignancy in patients with primary immunodeficiency is challenging. Despite the aforementioned improvements in the diagnosis and treatment of opportunistic infections, the infectious mortality associated with conventional chemotherapy regimens in this group of patients is high. In addition, patients suffering from end-organ damage prior to the onset of anti-neoplastic therapy also have a lower threshold for treatment-related complications (see Chapter 30).[96] Nonetheless, with diligent supportive care measures in the current era, treatment with standard doses of chemotherapy achieves superior results compared to utilizing reduced doses. Achieving remission is a realistic goal in this group of patients, however relapses are common.[97] Ultimately, treating the underlying immunologic disorder in addition to the malignancy will offer the optimal chance for long-term cure. The use of alloHSCT has the potential to cure the underling immunodeficiency and is recommended when suitable donor options are available. Early intervention with transplantation could potentially avoid the infectious and oncologic complications that patients with primary immunodeficiencies often experience.

Primary combined humoral and cellular immunodeficiencies

Severe combined immunodeficiency

Severe impairment of both cellular and humoral immunity is the common thread between the genetically distinct disorders that result in the syndrome of severe combined immunodeficiency (SCID). A heterogeneous group of disorders, SCID is characterized by the impairment of both T and B lymphocyte function, resulting in a severe level of immune compromise. Universal absence of T cells is the rule, while the presence of B and NK cells is variable. However, the presence of B lymphocytes does not necessarily translate into adequate function, as B cells are highly dependent on T cells to properly execute their role in host defense. SCID is classified according to the level of B and NK cell impairment that corresponds with the defects affecting T lymphocytes. An example of a specific disorder includes X-linked SCID, a disease characterized by a mutation in the interleukin 2 receptor gamma (IL2RG) gene which codes for the common gamma chain protein, leading to a derangement of multiple cytokine pathways. These patients exhibit adequate and sometimes elevated quantitative B cell production compared to patients with adenosine deaminase deficiency in whom B cell and NK cell production is absent.[98] As the majority of SCID patients (approximately 75%) with cancer develop lymphomas of B cell origin, it follows that patients with loss of B cell production are less likely to be affected.[99,100] While EBV is usually implicated in lymphomagenesis, EBV-negative lymphomas can occur as well.[101] Curative therapy in the majority of subtypes of SCID is achieved through alloHSCT as reconstitution of T cell immunity is the ultimate goal. Without alloHSCT, most patients die before they reach their second birthday. Children with adenosine deaminase deficiency can be treated with enzyme replacement instead of alloHSCT. However, while

Table 19.3. Treatment of immunodeficiency-associated hematological malignancies in children, adolescents, and young adults.

Immunodeficiency	Defect	Commonly associated malignancies	Infectious link	Treatment approach
PRIMARY				
Combined deficiencies				
SCID	Impaired T & B cells	B-cell NHL	Often EBV	AlloHSCT (enzyme replacement in ADA def.)
WAS	WASP mutations	B-cell NHL	Often EBV	AlloHSCT
XHIM	CD40L mutations	NHL and HL	Often EBV	IVIG infusions (supportive), AlloHSCT
XLP	SAP defects and BIRC4 mutations	B-cell NHL and EBV-HLH	EBV	AlloHSCT
Humoral deficiency				
CVID	Immunoglobulin (Ig) def.	NHL, esp. MALT lymphomas	H. pylori	IVIG infusions (supportive), chemotherapy
Selective IgA Deficiency	IgA deficiency	Gastric carcinomas	H. pylori	Chemotherapy and supportive care
XLA	Def. of Ig and B cells	Leukemia and NHL	None	IVIG infusions (supportive), chemotherapy AlloHSCT
DNA repair disorders				
Ataxia telangiectasia	ATM mutations	ALL, HL, and NHL	None	Poor tolerance of conventional chemotherapy regimens
Nijmegen breakage syndrome	NBS mutations	NHL and HL	None	Poor tolerance of conventional chemotherapy regimens
Bloom syndrome	BLM mutations	AML, HL, and NHL	None	Poor tolerance of conventional chemotherapy regimens
Other disorders				
Chediak–Higashi syndrome	Lysosomal storage defect	EBV-HLH	EBV	AlloHSCT
Griscelli syndrome type 2	RAB27A mutations	EBV-HLH	EBV	AlloHSCT
ALPS	FAS & caspase mutations	HL and NHL	None	Chemotherapy
SECONDARY				
HIV/AIDS	Destruction of $CD4^+$ cells	NHL, Kaposi's sarcoma, and HL	EBV, HHV-8	HAART plus chemotherapy
Post-AlloHSCT and post-SOT	Medically induced immune suppression	PTLD	EBV	Reduction in immune suppression, chemotherapy with rituximab, EBV-CTL immunotherapy

ADA: adenosine deaminase; AIDS: acquired immunodeficiency syndrome; ALL: acute lymphoblastic leukemia; ALPS: autoimmune lymphoproliferative syndrome; AML: acute myeloid leukemia; AlloHSCT: allogeneic hematopoietic stem cell transplantation; CVID: combined variable immunodeficiency; Def: deficiency; EBV-CTL: EBV-cytotoxic T lymphocyte; EBV: Epstein–Barr virus; HAART: highly active anti-retroviral therapy; HIV: human immunodeficiency virus; HL: Hodgkin lymphoma; HLH: hemophagocytic lymphohistiocytosis; H. Pylori: *Helicobacter pylori*; HHV-8: human herpesvirus-8; IVIG: intravenous immunoglobulin; MALT: mucosal-associated lymphoid tissue; NHL: non-Hodgkin lymphoma; PTLD: post-transplant lymphoproliferative disease; SCID: severe combined immunodeficiency; SOT: solid organ transplantation; WAS: Wiskott–Aldrich syndrome; XHIM: X-linked hyper IgM syndrome; XLP: X-linked lymphoproliferative disease; XLA: X-linked agammaglobulinemia.

this prevents the onset of many life-threatening opportunistic infections, it is insufficient to fully restore cellular immunity as evidenced by the occurrence of lymphomas in patients receiving enzyme replacement for greater than 10 years.[102,103]

Wiskott–Aldrich syndrome

An X-linked disorder characterized by the clinical triad of eczema, micro-thrombocytopenia, and immune deficiency, WAS results from mutations of the Wiskott-

Aldrich syndrome protein (WASP). WASP is expressed predominantly in hematopoietic cells and plays an important role in signal transduction and maintaining cytoskeletal integrity. The immunologic impairment in WAS affects the cell-mediated and humoral systems, involving B and T cells as well as monocyte chemotaxis activity.[104] Lymphopenia after infancy is common and is thought to arise from accelerated cell death and/or abnormal lymphocyte maturation in the thymus and bone marrow.[105] The incidence of cancer in patients with WAS is relatively high in comparison with the other primary immunodeficiency disorders. Similar to SCID, lymphoma is the most common malignancy (approximately 75%) diagnosed in patients with WAS.[91] The vast majority of these lymphomas are EBV-positive with extranodal presentation and a predilection for CNS involvement, similar to cases of NHL presenting in patients with other primary immunodeficiencies.[106,107] Leukemia has also been noted on rare occasion. Two cases of nonmalignant self-limited lymphoproliferation that underwent spontaneous self-resolution have been also reported. However, one of those patients eventually developed a B-cell lymphoma, implicating a role for chronic lymphoid proliferation in the pathogenesis of lymphoma development in these patients.[108,109] Curative therapy and a reduction in the risk for malignancy are achieved through alloHSCT.

X-linked hyper IgM syndrome

X-linked hyper immunoglobulin (Ig) M syndrome (XHIM) is another immunodeficiency disorder characterized by impairment of both cellular and humoral immunity. The molecular defect in XHIM stems from mutations encoding the gene for the CD40 ligand (CD40L), a critical component of T-cell interaction with B cells. CD40L is expressed on CD4+ T cells and its interaction with the CD40 antigen expressed on B cells is important for complete T cell and mononuclear cell activation and Ig class switching.[110] Consequently, only IgM antibody production remains intact (or even elevated) and patients are deficient in IgG, IgA, and IgE. Lymphoma accounted for approximately 80% of the malignant diagnoses in patients with XHIM on the primary immunodeficiency cancer registry, exhibiting a particular predilection for Hodgkin lymphoma (25%) associated with EBV infection.[91] Due to the rare prevalence of XHIM in general, the study of its malignant complications is extremely challenging. Nonetheless, cases have recently been reported in boys with NHL and Hodgkin lymphoma.[111,112] The predisposition for lymphoma in patients with XHIM has also been modeled in transgenic mice with deregulated CD40L expression. One-third of mice with the CD40L mutations developed atypical lymphoid proliferation, many of which progressed into frank lymphomas.[113] Supportive care for patients with XHIM consists of monthly infusions of intravenous immunoglobulin, however the only curative options lies in alloHSCT. Of note, patients with XHIM carry a risk for biliary carcinoma due to a relatively high rate of sclerosing cholangitis secondary to chronic cryptosporidiosis infection.[114]

X-linked lymphoproliferative disease

Another combined cellular and humoral immunodeficiency, X-linked lymphoproliferative disease (XLP) is associated with fatal complications from EBV infection. Two distinct molecular defects have been identified; the more common one involves defects of the SLAM (signaling lymphocyte activation molecule)-associated protein (SAP),[115] while the other is characterized by mutations of the BIRC4 gene.[116] The SAP protein carries out multiple important immunologic functions and its deficiency results in impaired signal transduction between T cells and both APC and B cells.[117] This effectively leads to deficient T and B cell function, while additionally, inhibition of lymphocyte apoptosis renders individuals at risk for uncontrolled expansion of the cellular response to infection.[118] Clinical features of XLP are marked by an extreme incapacity to tolerate EBV infection, resulting in a hemophagocytic syndrome that has been termed fatal infectious mononucleosis (FIM) or EBV-associated hemophagocytic lymphohistiocytosis (HLH). Although these entities are seen on rare occasion in patients without XLP, the severe hyper-inflammatory response characteristic of such an immune reaction has been reported to occur in over 50% of males with XLP.[119] Other clinical complications of XLP include hypogammaglobulinemia (secondary to impaired T and B-cell dynamics), hematologic cytopenias, and in one-fourth of all patients, progression to malignant lymphomas.[120]

In patients with XLP, FIM arises from a massive, toxic immune response to EBV infection. An uncontrolled nonspecific reaction from the cellular immune system primarily results in extensive infiltration of parenchymal organs by lymphoid cells, mostly CD8 cytotoxic T cells, and histiocytes. This eventually culminates in systemic hemophagocytosis and tissue destruction, often leading to multisystem organ failure. Prognosis is guarded as the disease itself carries high mortality rates, and an attempt at treatment with etoposide and immune suppression renders patients further immune compromised.[121] Care must be taken to differentiate a new diagnosis of XLP presenting with FIM from the fulminant form of EBV+ T-cell LPD, which can present with an identical clinical picture marked by a severe systemic inflammatory response to *de novo* EBV infection. Distinction lies in isolating a clonal expansion of EBV+ T cells in the latter.[122]

Lymphomas are a potential serious complication of XLP.[123,124] With onset at a median age of 4 years, most lymphomas diagnosed in patients with XLP are NHL of B cell origin — represented predominantly as BL and DLBCL.[125] However, cases of Hodgkin lymphoma and T-cell NHL have also been described.[126] Based on the extreme sensitivity of patients with XLP to EBV, one would expect the majority of lymphoma cases in XLP to be EBV-positive. Peculiarly though, there have been patients documented with definite XLP genetic mutations and EBV-negative lymphomas, even in the current era of sensitive molecular tests for EBV detection.[127,128] This suggests that general immune dysfunction in XLP renders patients susceptible to not only EBV-induced malignancies, but malignancies in general. As with other cases of primary immunodeficiency, remission from lymphomas can be achieved with conventional dose chemotherapy regimens; however relapse is common, and ultimately alloHSCT with optimized donor sources offers the best option for long-term cure.

Primary humoral immunodeficiencies

Common variable immunodeficiency

Common variable immunodeficiency (CVID) is characterized by impaired B cell differentiation and consequently poor immunoglobulin production. As the name implies, CVID is a relatively common disorder. It is defined by a quantitative deficiency of IgG (plus low levels of IgA and/or IgM), poor response to vaccination, and absence of another defined immunodeficiency state. Some patients experience a mild dysfunction of T lymphocytes as well. CVID presents with a variable range of clinical symptoms including recurrent infections, chronic lung disease, autoimmune disorders, gastrointestinal disease, and a heightened susceptibility to cancer — especially lymphoma and gastric carcinoma.[129,130] Onset of disease in CVID occurs at a median age between 23–28 years. Patients with onset prior to age 16 years have an estimated incidence of cancer to be 2.5%, while those with later onset have an increased incidence to 8.5%. NHL accounts for half of cancers in CVID,[131] with EBV negative B-cell disease being most common. B-cell mucosal-associated lymphoid tissue (MALT) lymphomas show a particular predilection for patients with CVID.[132] Contrasting with the majority of B-cell lymphomas in children, MALT lymphomas are low grade and arise from marginal zone-associated lymphoid cells. And unlike the gastric MALT lymphomas that most frequently occur in non-immunodeficient patients, the lungs are the most common site of presentation in patients with CVID.[133] Cases of T-cell NHL and Hodgkin lymphoma have also been reported.[134,135] It is important to note that there exists a granulomatous variant of CVID notable for lymphoproliferative manifestations including lymphadenopathy, splenomegaly, and interstitial lung disease (including lymphocytic interstitial pneumonitis). It occurs in about 10% of CVID patients and has been noted to progress to frank lymphoma in patients.[136] The complex interplay between immune dysregulation, chronic infection (with *Helicobacter pylori* in addition to viruses), genetic defects, and chronic mucosal antigen stimulation in the setting of hypogammaglobulinemia is theorized to render patients with CVID more susceptible to developing lymphoma.

Selective IgA deficiency

IgA deficiency is the most common inherited immunodeficiency. Fortunately though, it is asymptomatic in 90% of patients. It is characterized by an isolated deficiency of IgA in patients greater than 4 years of age. Those patients that suffer from symptoms will present with recurrent sinopulmonary infections, autoimmune disorders, gastrointestinal disease, and anaphylactic transfusion reactions.[137] Immunodeficiency cancer registry data revealed that 25% of tumors associated with IgA deficiency were lymphomas.[131] Although gastric carcinomas are the most common malignancy in patients with IgA deficiency, there have been rare but recent reports documenting the occurrence of lymphomas in this group of patients as well.[138] Theoretically, loss of mucosal immunity through IgA deficiency renders patients vulnerable to malignant changes of mucosal cell surfaces, however this has yet to be substantiated.

X-linked agammaglobulinemia

X-linked agammaglobulinemia (XLA) is an inherited humoral immunodeficiency characterized by markedly low or absent quantities of immunoglobulins and

B cells. Patients present clinically between 6–18 months of age with recurrent bacterial sinopulmonary tract infections. Due to the importance of humoral immune defense against enteroviral infections, patients are also susceptible to coxsackievirus and echovirus. Immunodeficiency cancer registry data reveals a unique distribution of hematological malignancies and carcinomas in patients with XLA with one-third of patients having leukemia, another third with NHL, and approximately 15% with carcinoma.[91] Other reports have confirmed the occurrence of lymphoid malignancies[139,140] as well as gastric[141] and colorectal carcinoma in young adults with XLA.[142] However, conflicting data exists on cohorts of patients in which no malignancies were found.[143,144] Further epidemiologic analyses, as well as molecular evaluations for oncologic associations with the Bruton tyrosine kinase mutation associated with XLA, may serve to clarify the relationship between this immunodeficiency and cancer.

Other disorders with impaired immunologic function

Chediak-Higashi syndrome and Griscelli syndrome type 2

Chediak-Higashi syndrome (CHS) is a lysosomal storage disorder that is associated with the impairment of both phagocytic and cellular immune function. The molecular abnormality affects the lysosomal trafficking regulator (LYST) gene resulting in abnormalities of cells dependent on lysosomal/granular function. Lysosomes are the key storage compartment for cytolitic proteins including perforin and granzyme B. Consequently, mutation of the LYST gene in CHS results in impaired function of the cytotoxic function of T and NK cells. Other cells impaired by the LYST mutation include neutrophils, melanocytes, platelet dense bodies, and plasma membrane repair mechanisms.[145] The appearance of giant cytoplasmic granules in leukocytes is characteristic. A rare autosomal recessive disorder, CHS is characterized by recurrent pyogenic infections, partial oculocutaneous albinism, platelet storage pool deficiency with associated mild coagulopathy, varied levels of neurologic dysfunction, and a 90% probability prior to the age 20 of developing a lethal hemophagocytic complication associated with EBV infection.[146] Although patients do not develop a malignancy *per se*, progression to what is termed the accelerated phase of disease is marked by a massive lymphohistiocytic infiltration of multiple organs that is clinically indistinguishable from any hemophagocytic syndrome. Impaired cellular response to EBV infection is usually what triggers progression to the accelerated phase and outcomes are dismal. The only curative treatment option is alloHSCT.[147]

Griscelli syndrome (GS) type 2 is clinically very similar to CHS. Also characterized by partial albinism and immunodeficiency, patients present with frequent pyogenic infections, hypopigmented hair and skin, and the majority of patients have primary neurologic manifestations. They also suffer from early death due to complications from HLH. GS is a rare autosomal recessive disorder associated with mutations of the RAB27A gene. RAB27A encodes proteins essential for both perforin-dependent lymphocyte cytotoxicity and melanosome function. The immunologic abnormalities in GS are marked by impaired NK cell function and an absence of delayed-type hypersensitivity. Unlike CHS, morphologic analysis of leukocytes does not reveal giant cytoplasmic granules. However similar to CHS, HLH can be triggered by EBV infection.[148] Again, alloHSCT is the only curative option. Ideally, patients are identified and undergo alloHSCT before the onset of a hemophagocytic syndrome, however patients have been salvaged after developing HLH with HLH-directed therapy followed by alloHSCT.[149]

Autoimmune lymphoproliferative syndrome

Autoimmune lymphoproliferative syndrome (ALPS) represents a constellation of genetic apoptosis defects associated with mutations in the FAS, Fas ligand, and caspase 8 and 10 genes.[150] Ineffective apoptosis disrupts the normal life cycle homeostasis of lymphocytes and patients develop an increased proportion of circulating senescent T lymphocytes (CD4–, CD8–, CD3+).[151] Clinical features usually develop at a young age and include chronic multifocal lymphadenopathy, hepatosplenomegaly, and autoimmune cytopenias. Besides autoimmune irregularities, the immune dysfunction in ALPS is also associated with abnormal programmed cell death pathways, but is not associated with a defect in cell-mediated or humoral immune function. The development of lymphomas in patients with ALPS appears to be tied to the dysregulation of lymphocyte apoptotic pathways.[152] The risk of developing Hodgkin lymphoma in patients with ALPS is 51 times the expected incidence, while the risk of having NHL is 14 times the expected incidence.[153] Further investigations are needed to determine the precise role played by apoptosis pathways in eliminating proliferating lymphocytes with oncogenic potential.[154]

Primary disorders of DNA repair

Ataxia telangiectasia

An autosomal recessive disorder with a predisposition for cancer, ataxia-telangiectasia (AT) has variable and profound manifestations, notably immune deficiency and cerebellar degeneration.[155] The affected gene in AT (also known as ATM) normally plays an important role in DNA repair, serving as a sensor of double-stranded DNA breakage.[156] In response to cellular stress, ATM activates numerous damage repair pathways including cell cycle checkpoint control and the p53 tumor suppressor pathway.[157] ATM is also involved in maintaining the immunologic diversity amongst both B and T cells through productive, purposeful gene rearrangements of the B and T cell receptor molecules.[158]

The gene mutation in AT leads to multiple dysfunctional processes. AT cells fail to normally activate cell cycle checkpoints in response to cellular damage from γ-irradiation or radiomimetic agents. They are characterized by defective DNA repair mechanisms and accelerated telomere loss. Moreover, patients suffer from impaired thymic function resulting in a restriction of both helper and cytotoxic T-cell development. Immunoglobulin deficiencies of IgA, IgG, or IgE — potentially secondary to a failure of immunoglobulin class switching from IgM — are also seen in some patients. Progressive cerebellar degeneration is prominent and represents the first appreciable clinical symptom of AT. Patients usually experience neurologic symptoms including progressive cerebellar ataxia presenting in infancy, abnormal eye movements, and dysarthria.

The development of malignancy is also a prominent feature of AT. Patients with AT accounted for the greatest number of cases on the immunodeficiency cancer registry, in which lymphomas and leukemias represented approximately three-quarters of the cases.[91] Hematological malignancies in AT are distinctly of lymphoid origin.[159] In children and young adults they include Hodgkin and non-Hodgkin lymphomas as well as B and T-cell acute lymphoblastic leukemias.[138,160] Overall, approximately 10% of homozygotes with AT will develop lymphoid malignancies in their lifetimes.[161] Meanwhile, it is important to note that mutations of the ATM gene are also associated with sporadic cases of lymphomas and leukemias in patients unaffected by AT. Well documented in T-cell prolymphocytic leukemia, B-cell chronic lymphocytic leukemia, and mantle cell lymphoma, mutations of the ATM gene have also been reported in a minority of patients with follicular lymphoma, DLBCL, and Hodgkin lymphoma.[162]

Other important aspects of AT include the susceptibility to non-hematological malignancies and unique treatment considerations. Patients with AT also experience significant rates of epithelial cancers involving the skin, gastrointestinal tract, genitourinary tract, and CNS. And an important aspect of management in patients with AT is monitoring for poor tolerance of conventional treatment protocols. Administration of chemotherapy and certainly radiation can be challenging in these patients. In addition, their underlying immune deficiency often results in recurrent sinopulmonary tract infections. Both chronic lung disease and the occurrence of acute pulmonary infections can further complicate the treatment course and adjustments of chemotherapy should be tailored to the individual patient.[163]

Nijmegen breakage syndrome

Nijmegen breakage syndrome (NBS) is another disorder of DNA repair and shares many overlapping features with AT. It is a rare autosomal recessive syndrome that is characterized by combined immunodeficiency, chromosomal instability, predisposition to lymphoid and epithelial cancers, and clinical radiosensitivity. Unique physical features distinguish NBS; most patients have severe microcephaly from birth, short stature, and "birdlike" facies. Mutation of the NBS gene results in dysfunction of the protein Nibrin which plays a critical role in the process of DNA repair.

The onset of cancer in NBS patients is early with a median age for cancer-related death of 9.2 years. The majority of cancers reported were lymphomas, but there have been case reports of glioma, rhabdomyosarcoma, and medulloblastoma.[164] In a cohort of over 100 patients with NBS in Poland, approximately 53% developed cancer with greater than 90% of those cases being lymphoid malignancies. The most common lymphoma subtypes in NBS are DLBCL and T-cell lymphoblastic lymphoma (T-LBL),[165] although others including Hodgkin lymphoma[166] and the rare T-cell-rich DLBCL variant, have been reported as well.[167] Cytogenetic analysis of these lymphomas with fluorescent *in situ* hybridization (FISH) revealed chromosomal breaks in the immunoglobulin or T-cell receptor loci in a majority of patients, reaffirming the theory that impaired DNA repair mechanisms likely lead to lymphomagenesis in patients with NBS.[168]

Similar to patients with AT, children with NBS also develop recurrent sinopulmonary infections and after cancer, chronic lung disease with bronchiectasis is the second leading cause of death. The underlying immunologic deficiency is characterized by hypogammaglobulinemia, lymphopenia, thymic dysplasia, and aberrations at the sites of the T cell and immunoglobulin receptor rearrangement (as is seen in AT as well).[169] Careful precaution must be taken in the administration of chemotherapy in each individual patient as dose adjustments are often needed based upon the patient's ability to tolerate therapy.[163]

Bloom syndrome

Bloom syndrome also shares overlapping features with the other disorders of DNA repair. Patients suffer from immune deficiency, a predisposition to cancer, and physical abnormalities. Unique characteristics of Bloom's syndrome are progeria, sun-sensitive erythema of the face, impaired fertility, and immunodeficiency primarily being associated with defects of humoral immunity. These patients also have short stature and chronic lung disease secondary to recurrent infection. Mutations of the BLM gene cause the syndrome resulting from deficient DNA mismatch repair.[170] These patients have a propensity for cancer, and half of the patients will have developed malignancy by the age of 25. Younger patients tend to develop lymphomas and acute myeloid leukemia (AML), while in older age carcinomas such as colon, skin, and breast predominate.[171] The rare occurrence of Bloom syndrome prohibits extensive investigation of the patterns of hematological malignancies associated with the disease, yet cases of NHL, Hodgkin lymphoma, and AML have recently been reported.[138] The occurrence of myeloid malignancies is rare in patients with DNA repair disorders, thus the association of AML with a total or partial loss of chromosome 7 in Bloom syndrome patients is a quite unique.[172]

Malignancy and Acquired Immunodeficiency

HIV-associated malignancies

The association between HIV and malignancy was first established in a patient diagnosed with Kaposi sarcoma (KS) in the United States in 1981.[173] Since that time, multiple malignancies have been identified as occurring with increased frequency in HIV-positive patients in comparison to persons unaffected by HIV.[174] In addition to determining the relative risk of cancer in the setting of HIV infection, risk factors for developing malignancies have also been established.[175] Causal associations have been unraveled, linking the multi-factorial interplay of HIV infection, host immune suppression, and extrinsic factors such as viral infection with EBV, HHV-8, HPV, and hepatitis B and C viruses.[176] With the advent of highly active anti-retroviral therapy (HAART) in the mid-1990s, improvements in caring for patients infected with HIV have advanced treatment and prevention of HIV-associated malignancies in the western world.[177] However, in the HAART era, disparities in access to healthcare between resource-limited and resource-rich regions have led to increased prevalence of HIV-associated complications including the wide spectrum of malignancies that may occur.

In the pre-HAART era, KS was established as the first AIDS-defining malignancy and subsequently followed by NHL and cervical carcinoma. In the current HAART era, a decrease in incidence of both KS and NHL in the areas of the world where HAART is widely accessible has been reported.[178] In sub-Saharan Africa, on the other hand, cases of KS continue to be widespread and the prevalence of HIV-associated NHL is also increased.[179] The incidence of cervical cancer, on the other hand, has not decreased in the current HAART era in any part of the world. Amongst the non-AIDS defining malignancies, which include Hodgkin lymphoma, leiomyoma, leioymyosarcoma, anal carcinoma, hepatocellular carcinoma, skin cancer, and lung cancer, changing trends have been reported as well. The incidence of non-AIDS defining malignancies has actually increased in the current HAART era, the reasons for which are not completely understood.[180] Linked to chronic immune suppression, non-AIDS–defining cancers have increased in prevalence in both areas where HAART is and is not available, dismissing prior theories that the increase in incidence was secondary to individuals living longer with HIV.[181] Multiple factors probably contribute to this finding including interruptions in HAART, lifestyle habits, coinfection with oncogenic viruses, familial history of cancer, exposure to other carcinogens (e.g. tobacco), and increased genomic instability (from microsatellite alterations for example).[182]

In the most extensive evaluation of risk factors for malignancy in HIV-infected pediatric patients, specific risk factors were not easily identified. EBV viral burden was associated with higher rates of cancer, however the effect was modified by CD4 count. Other risk factors such as route of HIV infection, use of zidovudine, and demographic characteristics were not associated with an increased risk of cancer either.[175] Theoretically, the risk of malignancy in HIV-positive patients ties back to the multiple associations discussed in the preceding sections of this chapter. As HIV infection is tropic to CD4+ cells, one must consider that T-helper cells are not the only ones to express the CD4 antigen. Additionally, macrophages, monocytes, dendritic cells, fetal thymocytes, microglial cells, and placental trophoblasts all express the CD4 antigen and are affected by HIV infection and subsequent cytopathic destruction. With impairment of CD4+ cells, the host immunity loses not only the intricate command that the T-helper cells maintain over all aspects of the immune response, but in addition, suffer the loss of adequate antigen presenting cell and phagocytic function as well. The resultant cellular immunodeficiency renders the host immune system deficient in its capacity for tumor surveillance and for host defense against coinfection. Meanwhile, the ubiquitous presence of oncogenic viruses amidst the multiple pathogenetic co-factors (e.g. cellular transformations, immune dysregulation, and chromosomal abnormalities) potentially drives cellular pathways within tumor microenvironments and possibly facilitates the malignant transformation of cells.[183]

The heightened prevalence of hematological malignancies in patients infected with HIV can also be linked to the increased state of lymphoid proliferation. Lymphoid proliferation is manifested by some of the most common clinical findings in HIV patients — localized or generalized lymphadenopathy, bilateral parotid gland enlargement, and lymphocytic interstitial pneumonitis (LIP). Ultimately, immune stimulation by infectious agents as well as aberrant cytokine patterns drive lymphoid proliferation in HIV-infected patients, leading to an increased incidence of lymphoproliferative disease and lymphoma.[183] The remainder of this section will focus on the specific subtypes of hematological malignancies that occur in children, adolescents, and young adults infected with HIV.

Non-Hodgkin lymphomas

NHL comprises the most common group of malignant diagnoses associated with HIV. A heterogeneous group of disorders, HIV-associated NHL is comprised of several distinct disease entities. The vast majority of cases diagnosed in HIV-infected patients are B cell in origin, although peripheral T-cell lymphomas also occur. Nearly 90% of HIV-associated NHL diagnoses are accounted for by BL, DLBCL, and immunoblastic lymphoma (IL). Other subtypes are quite uncommon and include primary CNS lymphoma (PCNSL), primary effusion lymphoma (PEL), and the plasmablastic lymphoma of the oral cavity (PBL). Most cases are high-grade aggressive lymphomas and are more likely to occur with lower CD4 counts. The advent of HAART has diminished the incidence of NHL in people living with HIV infection. The association with viral infection is variable and depends on the subtype of disease.[176]

There are multiple ways to classify HIV-associated NHL. One stratification system distinguishes between the anatomic site of the disease — systemic NHL vs. CNS NHL (i.e. PCNSL) vs. body cavity NHL (i.e. PEL). Within this classification system, the systemic subtype accounts for all diagnoses except PCNSL and PEL. Another classification system distinguishes between subtypes of NHL that are also seen in immuno competent patients vs. those that are rarely seen outside of the context of HIV infection. BL and DLBCL are two of the most common forms of NHL occurring in non-immunocompromised children and are both seen with increased frequency in HIV-positive children and adolescents. Meanwhile, PCNSL, PEL, and plasmablastic lymphoma of the oral cavity are extremely rare in the absence of HIV infection.

Amongst the more common subtypes of NHL, DLBCL is closely linked to IL. Of note, in HIV-negative patients, IL is considered a variant of DLBCL. However, in the setting of HIV infection, IL exhibits unique properties and morphologically appears similar to anaplastic or plasmacytoid large-cell histology rendering it unique in comparison to DLBCL.[184] Another distinction is highlighted by DLBCL being associated with EBV in approximately 40% of cases, contrasted with EBV-positive disease occurring in 90% of those with IL. DLBCL is also characterized by expression of the germinal center cell marker BCL-6, with a number of cases exhibiting rearrangements of the BCL-6 proto-oncogene. In cases of IL, BCL-6 is not expressed as those cells have progressed beyond the germinal center towards plasmayctoid differentiation.[176] Both DLBCL and IL occur in the setting of advanced immune suppression with the absolute CD4 cell counts usually less than 100 cells/microliter.[185]

BL on the other hand, tends to occur within a wide range of CD4 cell counts and is not necessarily associated with severe immune suppression. While the endemic form of BL that occurs in sub-Saharan Africa is uniformly positive for EBV, both the sporadic and immunodeficiency-associated forms are only EBV+ in 30–40% of cases. BL is characterized by translocation of the c-MYC oncogene with sequences from one of three immunoglobulin genes. c-MYC is a transcription factor with an enormous array of interactions with a vast multitude of different cellular processes. c-MYC deregulation is the quintessential factor driving disease pathogenesis in BL. Both c-MYC and EBV are closely associated with a number of apoptotic pathway mechanisms whose disruption has been shown to contribute to Burkitt lymphoma progression in multiple studies. These epigenetic changes serve as potential mechanisms of lymphomagenesis both in the presence and absence of EBV infection.[186]

PCNSL is an extranodal variant of DLBCL occurring in the CNS. As mentioned above, it is extremely rare except in the setting of HIV infection, where it represents approximately 15% of HIV-associated NHL. It occurs in the setting of HIV at a rate of 1000-fold greater than in uninfected individuals. PCNSL is virtually always EBV-positive. It is associated with severe immune suppression with CD4 cell counts usually less than 50 cells/microliter; patients with a longer duration of HIV infection are at greater risk. Patients with higher CD4 cell counts have been reported who lack EBV-specific CD4+ T-lymphocyte function.[187] Prognosis is very poor for PCNSL and radiation therapy in addition to HAART is the mainstay of therapy.[188]

PEL accounts for approximately 4% of HIV-associated lymphomas. It is discussed in greater detail in the preceding section on the virology of HHV-8. Characterized by HHV-8 infection, PEL is also positive for EBV in the majority of cases. However, it is HHV-8 that is thought to drive viral pathogenesis. Classic PEL presents as serous effusions in the pleural, pericardial, or peritoneal cavities, while the solid extracavitary subtype of PEL presents in extraserous sites such as large bowel, skin, lung, and lymph nodes. Patients diagnosed with PEL have a poor prognosis.

Another extremely rare malignancy, PBL of the oral cavity occurs mostly in the setting of HIV infection. Considered a subtype of DLBCL with plasmablastic features, PBL is defined by histological findings of plasmablastic cells with no or minimal plasmacytoid differentiation, rearrangement of the Ig heavy chain gene, and expression of plasma cell antigens (CD138, MUM1, and CD38). Cases of PBL rarely express the mature B-cell CD20 surface antigen. It was first discovered to exhibit preferential involvement of the jaw and oral cavity in HIV-infected patients.[189] More recently though, plasmablastic lymphomas have been described in HIV-infected individuals occurring in non-oral locations as well — the gastrointestinal tract, lymph nodes, skin and soft tissues, and nasopharyngeal cavity. Subsequently, it has been proposed that the terminology be adjusted to describe PBL as a general entity, and cases involving the jaw and oral cavity to be a unique subset. Two cases of PBL have been reported to occur in children. The largest analysis of PBL in the literature examined 112 cases; EBV was found in 74% of tumors.[190] Representing 2–3% of cases of HIV-associated NHL, it usually occurs in the setting of severe immune suppression. Prognosis is quite guarded in this group of patients as well.

With the heterogeneity of subtypes of NHL that exists, it is postulated that the lymphomagenesis that leads to malignant transformation of the B lymphocytes is likely multifactorial. As indicated above, the rates of EBV infection are variable for the different diseases and thus EBV is not likely the overarching etiologic factor. Chronic B cell stimulation though, could act as a potential unifying mechanism because it can lead to a variety of different cellular changes. In the HIV+ patient, there are multiple factors that could drive overstimulation of B-cell differentiation including coinfection with other viruses such as EBV or HHV-8. Additionally, with the deregulation of cytokines in HIV infection from progressive dendritic cell impairment, IL-6 and IL-10 may play roles in driving lymphoid cell proliferation.[191] Other contributing factors to B cell stimulation include direct effect from HIV pathogenesis. It has been shown that the HIV protein Tat is taken up by B lymphocytes, resulting in dysregulation of the tumor suppressor protein pRb2/p130.[192] Tat has also been implicated in tumorigenesis by augmenting the angiogenic properties of the VEG-F and bFGF pathways.[193] Ultimately, chronic B cell stimulation may result in deleterious cellular transformations induced by rearrangements or mutations of prominent genes such as BCL-6, p53, and c-MYC. In the backdrop of an immune system impaired in its capacity for tumor surveillance, it is logical to understand how a variety of aggregated cellular changes can lead to eventual malignant transformation that proliferates unchecked.

Hodgkin lymphoma

Hodgkin lymphoma (HL) is a non-AIDS–defining malignancy that has actually increased in incidence despite implementation of HAART. The risk of developing Hodgkin lymphoma is increased in HIV-infected patients with a range of 5–20-fold greater than that of the general population.[194] This risk peaks when the CD4 cell counts range from 150–199 cells/mL.[195] The rise in incidence of HL with improvement in CD4 cell counts seems paradoxical. However, the increase in CD4+ T lymphocytes theoretically provides anti-apoptotic pathway mechanisms for HL cells to evade self-destruction — a model well described in non-HIV patients with classical HL.[196]

HIV-infected patients who develop HL are more likely than HIV-negative patients to present with high-risk features. An extensive retrospective review of HL occurring in HIV-positive patients exhibited a significantly higher predilection for histological subtypes that carry a worse prognosis — mixed cellularity and lymphocyte depleted.[197] These patients also tend to present with "B" symptoms, advanced stage disease, or with extranodal presentation. Although HL that occurs in non-HIV infected patients is only EBV+ in 20–50% of cases, HIV-associated HL is virtually always EBV+.[198] The theoretical mechanism for disease pathogenesis suggests that Reed–Sternberg (RS) cells produce growth factors in the local tumor microenvironment, thereby recruiting CD4 and inflammatory cells. This in turn provides proliferation signals for RS cells. In that scenario, EBV infection theoretically can predispose lymphocytes to the proliferative changes that are driven by the inflammatory milieu resulting in tumor formation.[199]

Other hematological malignancies that have been reported in patients infected with HIV do not necessarily occur with greater frequency in HIV+ patients in comparison with the general population and therefore the link between those diseases and immunodeficiency is not clear. They include plasma cell disorders, myeloma, and leukemia.[199]

HIV-associated solid tumors

Solid tumors also occur with increased frequency in HIV+ patients. In children living in HHV-8 endemic regions of the world, Kaposi sarcoma (KS) is one of the most prevalent HIV-associated malignancies. KS is an AIDS-defining malignancy and is associated with infection by HHV-8 as discussed in greater detail in the section on viral oncogenesis. KS is one of three AIDS-defining malignancies — the other two are NHL and cervical carcinoma. Cervical cancer, like KS, is strongly associated with viral infection. The viral culprit for cervical carcinoma is HPV. In the largest assessment of the prevalence of HIV-associated cancers in children in the United States, leiomyosarcoma was found to be the 3rd most common malignancy after NHL and KS.[10] Other solid tumors known to occur with greater frequency in HIV-infected patients include hepatocellular carcinoma, anal carcinoma, and lung cancer. Again, viral associations are important in the etiology of these specific malignancies, with hepatitis B and C viruses playing a prominent role in the onset of hepatocellular carcinoma and HPV being involved in anal carcinoma pathogenesis. Lung cancer is extremely rare in children and young adults with HIV; the etiologic agent tied to its occurrence is cigarette smoking.[199]

Post-transplant acquired immunodeficiency

Another form of acquired immunodeficiency in children, adolescents, and young adults occurs in the post-organ transplantation setting. Organ transplantation provides curative treatment options for diseases that were once considered incurable. However, to successfully perform hematopoietic alloHSCT or solid organ transplantation (SOT), a significant amount of immune suppression must be established in the organ recipient. In the setting of post-transplant immune suppression, the recipient is at considerable risk for both infectious and malignant complications.

Although this section will focus on the hematological malignancies that arise secondary to post-transplant induced immunodeficiency, it is important to note that there is a wide spectrum of malignancies that occur after transplant. Post-transplant lymphoproliferative disease (PTLD) is the most common neoplasm that occurs in children, adolescents, and young adults after both SOT and alloHSCT. Other malignancies that occur in the post-transplantation setting include squamous cell cancers (skin, oral cavity, and genitourinary tract), melanoma, sarcomas, brain tumors, carcinomas (kidney, liver, thyroid, and breast), and leukemia/myelodysplastic syndrome (MDS). Leukemia/MDS is rare post-allogeneic transplant, and similar to many other cancers seen post-alloHSCT, is more likely due to the carcinogenic insult from chemotherapy and/or irradiation than from immunodeficiency *per se*. It is also associated with chronic immune suppression from the anti-metabolite azathioprine post-SOT, which demonstrates both carcinogenic and immune suppressive properties.[200] Ultimately though, immunodeficiency is still implicated in the increased susceptibility to several of the aforementioned malignancies due to either viral associations or the immunogenic nature of specific malignancies.

Pediatric organ transplant recipients are at even higher risk for developing malignancies than their adult counterparts. Reports vary from alloHSCT to SOT, and even within solid organ cohorts based upon the transplanted organ, but the overall incidence of a new malignancy following transplantation in children is approximately 5–12%.[201,202] Generally speaking, the cumulative risk of developing secondary cancers increases with each subsequent year post-transplant. Overall, transplant recipients are at 5–10-fold increased risk of developing cancer compared to the general population. Considering important variables such as a higher incidence of primary EBV infection and an increasing cumulative incidence with time, younger children are at even greater risk with reports of up to 30–50-fold increased risk of developing specific malignancies.[183] As more patients are surviving and living longer post-transplant, awareness of the complications of cancer has heightened in importance as it is now a more frequent cause of death in this population of patients.[203]

Post-transplant lymphoproliferative disease (PTLD)

With the increasing number of both alloHSCT and SOT occurring in children, adolescents, and young adults, PTLD is fast becoming one of the prominent subtypes of NHL in pediatric oncology. PTLD represents a heterogeneous group of lymphoproliferative diseases that occur in the post-transplant setting. PTLD is divided into three groups: early lesions, polymorphic PTLD, and monomorphic PTLD.[204] Early lesions are characterized by reactive plasmacytic hyperplasia and represent an infectious mononucleosis-like illness. It is the most common subtype of PTLD and occurs in about 55% of cases. There are neither cytogenetic abnormalities nor clonal Ig gene rearrangements associated with early lesions. Polymorphic PTLD is marked by evidence of early malignant transformation with cytogenetic abnormalities or Ig gene rearrangements. These cellular proliferations appear polymorphic on histology and are often identified by the presence of infiltrating T cells and a lack of necrosis. Polymorphic PTLD occurs in about 30% of cases. Finally, in monomorphic PTLD (around 15% of cases), clonal transformation has distinctly occurred (Fig. 19.2).[205] On histology, the cells appear as a monomorphic collection of malignant lymphocytes and can represent any of the subtypes of NHL in the World Health Organization (WHO) classification system. B-cell lymphomas represent greater than 90% of PTLD cases, with the most common histology being DLBCL, followed by BL.[206] Less common forms of B-cell NHL have also been reported, including PCNSL[207] and PBL,[208] subtypes that are more commonly seen in HIV-infected patients. Other subtypes of lymphoma that have been reported in PTLD include Hodgkin lymphoma, mature T-cell, and rarely NK-cell lymphomas.[209–211]

The vast majority (approximately 80%) of PTLD are associated with EBV infection. EBV drives lymphocyte proliferation in patients lacking cellular immune function, and if unchecked, can result in lymphomatous transformation. The majority of B-cell and Hodgkin lymphoma cases are EBV-positive, while T-cell or NK-cell PTLD tend to be EBV-negative. In general, EBV-negative and non-B-cell PTLD are often late onset (occurring greater than 1 year after transplant) and are associated with significantly poorer outcomes.[212] Younger children who are EBV-naïve prior to transplant are at risk for EBV-seroconversion post-transplant from primary EBV infection. This group of patients is at highest risk for PTLD, and primary EBV infection usually occurs in the 6 months prior to disease presentation.

There is ample evidence for the direct role of EBV in the pathogenesis of PTLD. EBV latent gene expression in PTLD involves all of the EBNA, EBER, and LMP viral proteins.[213] For this reason, EBV+ PTLD B lymphocytes are highly immunogenic. Furthermore, the presence of clonal EBV within cases of monomorphic PTLD provides evidence for the early role of EBV infection in lymphomagenesis. In addition, there is evidence that other epigenetic changes affecting either oncogenes or tumor suppressor genes contribute to the complex interplay between EBV and malignant transformation of lymphocytes.[205]

Clinical presentations vary depending on the site of PTLD infiltration. Often there are high unremitting fevers with systemic symptoms. Nodal disease can present as a rapidly enlarging lymphatic mass. Extranodal presentation occurs in more than half of patients with PTLD. The gastrointestinal tract, lungs, skin, liver, and CNS are the most common sites of extranodal disease. Up to one-quarter of patients have CNS involvement and in SOT recipients, the allograft itself is involved in another 20–25% of patients. PTLD in the allograft can lead to dysfunction of the given organ and may initially present in failure of the transplanted organ itself.

PTLD treatment can be challenging because it requires careful adjustment of the immune-modulating therapies required for a successful transplant. A delicate balance is required to navigate the interplay between immune suppression and host acceptance of the transplanted organ. The onset of organ rejection in SOT and

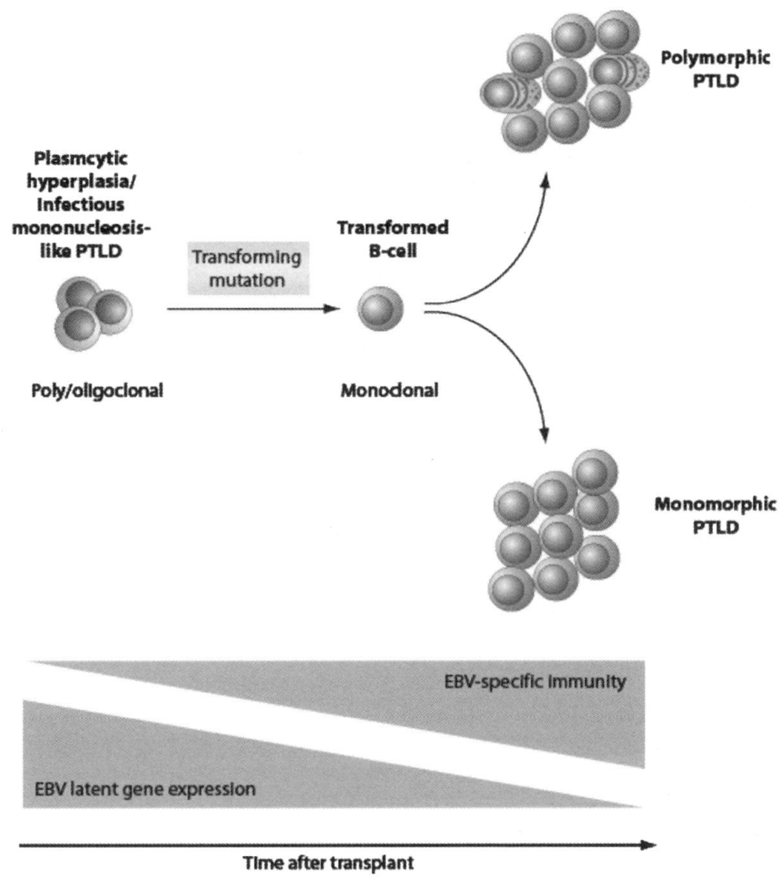

Fig. 19.2. Relationship between EBV latency gene expression, histological subtype of PTLD and recovery of EBV-specific immunity. After transplant, EBV-specific immunity is ablated but gradually returns. In PTLD, a spectrum of EBV latent gene expression is observed, with a broad range of genes tending to be expressed in early onset PTLD, whereas in late onset cases expression is restricted.

Tran H, Nourse J, Hall S, Green M, Griffiths L, Gandhi MK. (2008) Immunodeficiency-associated lymphomas. *Blood Rev* **22**(5): 261–281.

either graft rejection or graft-vs.-host disease (GVHD) in alloHSCT presents a heightened increase in the morbidity and mortality associated with organ transplantation. Although PTLD can spontaneously remit with an initial reduction of immune suppression, in most cases, further therapeutic interventions are required. Established treatments for PTLD include cyclophosphamide plus prednisone, with current regimens adding the anti-CD20 monoclonal antibody rituximab.[214] Adoptive cellular immunotherapy also presents an effective option in the treatment of PTLD. In both SOT and alloHSCT, the use of EBV-specific cytotoxic T-lymphocytes (CTL) has offered hope for the successful implementation of safe and effective immunotherapeutic strategies.[215–217] However, due to the technical difficulty in establishing CTL in the laboratory, this therapy is currently only offered at few select centers throughout the world. Characterized by a mild adverse effect profile with minimal risk for GVHD, CTL offers a highly potent, targeted treatment option without the complications associated with chemotherapy.[218] Prior to the advent of CTL, donor lymphocyte infusions (DLI) were the only form of adoptive cellular immunotherapy available; however, they are associated with significantly high rates of GVHD and its associated complications.

EBV PCR technology has broadened the strategic approach to PTLD. The ability to detect EBV viral DNA in the peripheral blood prior to the presentation of overt PTLD has beckoned the development of pre-emptive interventions in patients post-transplantation. It has been shown that frequent EBV PCR monitoring post-transplant is able to identify patients at risk for both early and late-onset PTLD.[219–221] Based on this information, therapeutic interventions were established utilizing single-agent rituximab as preemptive therapy.[222]

Although preemptive rituximab is unable to completely prevent the onset of PTLD, its use has been shown to decrease the overall incidence of PTLD as well as in one study, abrogate PTLD-related mortality in comparison to historical controls.[223] However, it is important to keep in mind that cases of PTLD have developed despite the use of preemptive rituximab, even in patients with complete initial response documented by clearance of the EBV viral load. The emergence of CD20-negative B cells coinciding with the recrudescence of elevated EBV viral loads has been reported in patients receiving preemptive rituximab. It is worrisome that these patients developed potent immune-evasion properties capable of overcoming targeted monoclonal antibody therapy.[224] An important nuance in EBV PCR technology is the variation in sensitivity that occurs depending on test technique. Different assays may have different levels of sensitivity with regards to detection of virus. In addition, because plasma measurements only capture EBV during its lytic stage, PCR measurements of whole blood or peripheral mononuclear blood cell (PMBC) layer offer a more sensitive technique in analyzing the viral load of EBV. The explanation for this lies in the tropism of EBV for lymphocytes; certainly viral DNA measurements of plasma will be unable to capture virus present within cells.[225] This may be important to remember in patients with borderline plasma EBV PCR values for whom there is a very high index of suspicion for PTLD.

PTLD following blood or marrow transplantation

The immune suppression associated with alloHSCT is uniquely different and slightly more complex than that associated with SOT. For one, alloHSCT recipients are often patients suffering from malignant diseases and have received a considerable amount of chemotherapy and immunosuppressive treatment regimens prior to transplant (see Chapter 20). Beyond that, patients undergoing alloHSCT must not only receive up front immune-modulating therapy to avoid graft rejection, but in addition, they continue to receive immune suppression post-alloHSCT in order to prevent GVHD. To further complicate issues, those that do develop GVHD will require even more intensified immune suppression. In as much, there are multiple significant variables that affect the element of acquired immunodeficiency in alloHSCT recipients.

The onset of PTLD in these patients is distinctly linked with the impaired recovery of cytotoxic T-cell function.[226] Human leukocyte antigen (HLA) disparity,[227] T cell depletion of stem cell grafts,[228] and the use of anti-thymocyte globulin (ATG)[229] are three specific variables that are associated with delayed T-cell immune reconstitution and a heightened risk for PTLD.[230] Meanwhile, chronic GVHD is a distinct risk factor for late onset PTLD.[228] The majority of PTLD cases (82%) occur in the first year post-alloHSCT. Interestingly, although the use of alemtuzumab often parallels the use of ATG in conditioning regimens for immune modulation prior to alloHSCT, alemtuzumab is not associated with an increased risk for PTLD. A monoclonal antibody targeting the pan-lymphocyte CD52 antigen, alemtuzumab effectively depletes both T and B lymphocytes (see Chapter 21). So although the element of T-cell dysfunction in recipients of ATG and alemtuzumab is similar, the paucity of B cells in patients receiving alemtuzumab exerts a protective effect against EBV infection. In alloHSCT recipients, EBV infection is thought to arise in donor lymphocytes. As discussed above, in this group of patients, particularly in SOT recipients, carefully monitoring for EBV by PCR post-transplant is an important aspect of anticipating and preventing the onset of PTLD. While preemptive rituximab is certainly an option for disease prophylaxis, patients at high risk for EBV+ PTLD have been shown to benefit from prophylactic infusions of donor-derived CTL as well.[231] Ultimately, identifying those patients at highest risk for delayed T-cell immune reconstitution as well as those who develop EBV infection post-transplant will enable improved outcomes for the treatment and prevention of PTLD post alloHSCT.

PTLD following solid organ transplantation

Risk factors for PTLD in SOT are also unique and well established. As in alloHSCT, an important variable is the extent of immune suppression incurred by the patient post-transplant. The immune suppression post-SOT is relatively straightforward as patients remain on life-long therapies to prevent graft rejection. However, the extent of immune suppression required varies based upon the individual patient, as well as based on the type of organ transplanted. Lung and small bowel transplant recipients are at higher risk (10–30%) for developing PTLD than their counterparts receiving liver, kidney, or heart transplantation (1–5%). Those receiving prolonged high doses of tacrolimus were at an especially high risk, however careful monitoring of drug levels can offset this risk.[232] Another well-established risk factor is recipients who are EBV seronegative prior to transplant. These tend to be younger patients that have yet to be exposed to EBV. Upon primary exposure post-transplant, they are at considerable risk for developing PTLD. Fortunately though, patients with PTLD associated with primary EBV infection experience better outcomes.[183]

In contrast to PTLD in alloHSCT, EBV tends to arise in host lymphocytes in SOT recipients. Early-onset PTLD (< 1 year post-transplant) typically presents after graft rejection, perhaps due to an element of chronic antigen stimulation incurred from graft rejection. Late-onset PTLD in SOT patients often presents as extranodal disease manifested by organ dysfunction. Poor prognosis is established in patients with multiple sites of disease and CNS involvement, in addition to those with EBV-negative and non-B cell disease. Unlike in PTLD associated with alloHSCT, the use of EBV viral load monitoring is not as well defined in the post-transplant management of SOT recipients. Treatment options are similar as in alloHSCT recipients, however the utility of autologous CTL is a unique option for SOT patients. All in all, the continuous improvements in SOT techniques renders organ transplant an option available to greater numbers of patients than ever before. Therefore, the incidence of PTLD in this population of patients will continue to be an important issue, especially in pediatric transplantation.

Treatment of Immunodeficiency-Associated Hematological Malignancies

Treatment approaches for hematological malignancies associated with immunodeficiency depend on a multitude of variables including the type of malignancy, the nature of the underlying immunodeficiency, the risk for complications from therapy, the utility of hematopoietic alloHSCT as a treatment option, and the availability of immunotherapeutic strategies. Nonetheless, there are a few important principles that can be applied generally. First and foremost, children, adolescents, and young adults with immunodeficiency fare worse than the general population with similar malignancies. This is due to multiple factors, including the aggressive nature of the neoplastic disease, higher rates of treatment-related complications, and the nature of the immunodeficiency rendering the patient at a disadvantage in terms of eradicating the malignancy. Another important general principle centers on boosting the individual's immune system. Any restoration of immunity will enhance efforts to overcome the malignant disease. This boost can occur in the form of HAART implementation in HIV patients, reducing immune suppression in patients post-transplant, or performing alloHSCT in an effort to reverse the underlying immune defect in those with primary immunodeficiency disorders.

The spectrum of hematological malignancies that occurs in immunodeficient children, adolescents, and young adults includes a diverse array of diseases. In general, patients tend to present with advanced stage disease and this alone renders the disease higher risk. However, the more notorious histological subtypes of disease often occur in immunodeficient patients. For example HIV-positive patients more often present with mixed cellularity and lymphocyte depleted Hodgkin lymphoma — subsets of disease with worse prognoses. Treatment must be tailored not only to the specific type of disease, but also focusing on the risk stratification principles that may require a more intensified treatment approach based upon the unique subset of disease classification. Unique diseases, such as PCNSL, require specific treatment strategies like radiation therapy. Others, such as T-cell hematological malignancies, Hodgkin lymphoma, and aggressive B-cell NHL each require very distinct therapeutic approaches in comparison with one another. Careful consideration of the unique pathological characteristics of the malignancy will play a critical role in determining the appropriate therapy for a given patient.

The nature of the underlying immunodeficiency is also crucially important in directing treatment strategies (Table 19.3). Patients with primary immunodeficiencies affecting cell-mediated immunity — including SCID, WAS, XHIM, and XLP — can only be cured of their underlying disorder through alloHSCT. Correction of the underlying immunodeficiency prior to the development of malignancy can successfully serve to prevent malignant complications. However, if cancer develops before a transplant is performed, alloHSCT can then be utilized as a consolidation regimen if able to successfully induce remission with conventional chemotherapy. Other primary immunodeficiency disorders that can be cured successfully through alloHSCT include CHS and Griscelli syndrome type 2.[233]

Risks for complications from therapy are another extremely important consideration. Patients with immunodeficiency may have a higher incidence of treatment-related complications (see Chapter 30). Two particular challenges surround the tolerability of treatment regimens: one is the heightened risk for opportunistic infections in patients with underlying immunodeficiency disorders receiving chemotherapy. The second is marked by the risk for enhanced toxicity from therapeutic agents in patients that are more vulnerable to adverse effects. Patients with DNA repair defects are at particularly high risk for both opportunistic infections and direct treatment-related toxicity secondary to cellular damage. Another important group of patients to consider are those with underlying disorders of cell-mediated immune function because of their heightened risk for viral and fungal complications from standard treatment protocols. Special considerations must be taken with regards to infectious prophylaxis and dose adjustments on an individual basis. One must keep in mind that some patients will be able to tolerate standard therapies despite their immunodeficiency disorder. In that setting, those patients should proceed with standard doses for they will in fact have worse outcomes if downward dose-adjustments are implemented. Ultimately, each individual's risks should be examined closely when tailoring treatment regimens.

HIV-associated malignancies are a perfect example for the need to carefully design treatment strategies based upon the individual patient. The initial treatment regimens for HIV-associated cancers in the pre-HAART era utilized significant decreases in doses of standard chemotherapy; outcomes were generally quite poor with these regimens. After the advent of HAART, patients with immune reconstitution began to tolerate anti-neoplastic therapy better and thereby achieved superior outcomes.[234] Thereafter it became apparent that HIV-infected patients with adequate immune function experienced better outcomes when treated with the same standard dose treatment protocols given to patients without HIV infection.[235] And as the screening, diagnosis, prophylaxis, and treatment of opportunistic infections in HIV have improved, so have the outcomes for patients receiving chemotherapy for HIV-associated malignancies. At this point, even HIV-infected patients with relapsed and refractory lymphoma might benefit from auto- or alloHSCT as long as they are carefully assessed for the risk of potential infectious complications.[236,237]

Another important issue pertains to the utility of hematopoietic alloHSCT as a treatment option (see Chapter 20). While most immunodeficiency-associated hematological malignancies will achieve remission with conventional chemotherapy regimens, the incidence of relapse and refractory disease is considerably high. AlloHSCT serves as a transformative option through reconstitution of the impaired immune system that can thereby prevent the malignant relapse. This applies not only to patients with the aforementioned primary immunodeficiency disorders, but also to patients with EBV+ T-cell lymphoproliferative disease of childhood and HTLV-1+ ATLL. Those patients are quite refractory to conventional treatment regimens and alloHSCT offers them the only hope for long-term cure.[53,238] However, in many of the earlier studies, the reduction in relapse risk was offset by high treatment-related mortality rates. Continued advancements in the field of alloHSCT — in both supportive care and development of unique non-myeloablative conditioning regimens — provide optimism that alloHSCT may provide improved outcomes with decreased treatment–mortality rates.

The immense potential in development of new immunotherapeutic approaches to treating immunodeficiency-associated diseases offers an element of excitement in establishing treatment regimens with enhanced efficacy and fewer complications (see Chapter 21). The outcomes of many B-cell lymphomas have improved significantly with the introduction of the monoclonal antibody rituximab. Radiation-conjugated forms of the anti-CD20 monoclonal antibody have been utilized with modest efficacy against some B-cell lymphomas including PCNSL.[239] Adoptive cell-mediated immunotherapies also offer much hope in the improved outcomes of patients. EBV-specific CTL infusions have shown efficacy in *de novo* EBV lymphomas as well as patients with EBV+ PTLD.[240] In addition, the use of donor-derived EBV-specific CTL infusions are being used post-alloHSCT for enhancement of treatment against primary EBV+ lymphoproliferative disease in addition to its role in prevention of EBV+ PTLD in high-risk recipients. And finally, the role of vaccines may offer another avenue for therapeutic development. While the role of dendritic cell-based vaccines is still being explored, success of the hepatitis B vaccine in decreasing the incidence of hepatocellular carcinoma offers a potential model for decreasing the onset of viral-associated lymphomas. The relationships of EBV to the highly prevalent endemic Burkitt lymphoma in sub-Saharan Africa and that of HTLV-1 to ATLL in endemic regions of the world may serve as a potential platform to investigate the utility of EBV or HTLV-1 vaccines in preventing lymphoma in these high risk endemic populations. Ultimately, continued progress in understanding the delicate interplay between immunodeficiency and the development of malignancy will foster advances in the overall treatment of this unique population of children, adolescents, and young adults.

Conclusion

Discovery of the principle linking the immune system with malignancies has established a foundation upon which a vast amount of knowledge has been built over the past century. It has given rise to understanding the direct etiology and pathogenesis of numerous oncologic diseases while at the same time serving as a model for a general understanding of the mechanistic pathways that drive the formation of malignant cells. In addition, it has shed light upon new horizons for the development of novel therapeutic strategies to improve outcomes for patients with cancer.

A wide variety of hematological malignancies occur with increased frequency in patients suffering from immunodeficiency. Some are driven by viral pathophysiology with EBV, HHV-8, and HTLV-1 being the prominent viral culprits. Primary immunodeficiency disorders impairing the cell-mediated and humoral arms of the immune system, as well as those with DNA repair dysfunction, are at significantly increased risk of developing cancer. Similarly, patients with secondary immunodeficiency from HIV infection or post-transplant immune suppression also develop cancer at greater frequency than the general population. The vast majority of neoplastic diseases associated with immunodeficiency are hematological malignancies with the many subtypes of non-Hodgkin lymphoma representing the greatest proportion of these cases. Although the relatively low overall incidence of immunodeficiency disorders in pediatric patients prohibits large-scale study of the associated malignant complications, the past couple decades have witnessed an improved capacity to identify the unique characteristics of the specific conditions and how treatment options can be tailored to the individual patient.

The outcomes for children, adolescents, and young adults with immunodeficiency-associated hematological malignancies are generally worse than those for their healthy counterparts. However, advances in improving the underlying immunodeficiency as well as in treating opportunistic infections provide improved optimism for better outcomes for this unique population of patients. Continued advances in understanding the principles connecting immune function with cancer pathogenesis has fostered great progress in developing targeted therapeutic regimens. The success of monoclonal antibody therapies and the burgeoning progress achieved through EBV-specific cytotoxic T-lymphocyte infusions serve to pioneer new frontiers for further advances in immunotherapeutic strategies. Ultimately, the goal of enhancing treatment efficacy while diminishing the toxicity associated with conventional chemotherapy regimens may be realized. As the intricate and powerful dynamic between the immune system and hematological malignancies is better defined, exciting developments may offer novel approaches to achieving cures for cancer in both immunodeficient and non-immunodeficient patients alike.

References

4. Pardoll D. (2004) Immunology and cancer. In: MD AJ Abeloff, JE Niederhuber, MB Kastan, WG MCKenna (eds). *Clinical Oncology* (3rd ed). Philadelphia, PA: Elsevier, pp. 113–138.
6. Dunn GP, Bruce AT, Ikeda H, Old LJ, Schreiber RD. (2002) Cancer immunoediting: From immunosurveillance to tumor escape. *Nat Immunol* **3**: 991–998.
10. Biggar RJ, Frisch M, Goedert JJ. (2000) Risk of cancer in children with AIDS. AIDS-Cancer Match Registry Study Group. *JAMA J Am Med Assoc* **284**: 205–209.
17. Heslop HE, Slobod KS, Pule MA, Hale GA, Rousseau A, Smith CA, Bollard CM, Liu H, Wu MF, Rochester RJ, Amrolia PJ, Hurwitz JL, Brenner MK, Rooney CM. (2010) Long-term outcome of EBV-specific T-cell infusions to prevent or treat EBV-related lymphoproliferative disease in transplant recipients. *Blood* **115**: 925–935.
21. Lambert PS B. (2004) Viruses and human cancer. In: MD AJ Abeloff, JE Niederhuber, MB Kastan, WG MCKenna (eds). *Clinical Oncology* (3rd ed). Philadelphia, PA: Elsevier, pp. 207–226.
22. Cohen JI. (2000) Epstein-Barr virus infection. *N Engl J Med* **343**: 481–492.
31. Cohen JI, Kimura H, Nakamura S, Ko YH, Jaffe ES. (2009) Epstein-Barr virus-associated lymphoproliferative disease in non-immunocompromised hosts: A status report and summary of an international meeting, 8–9 September 2008. *Ann Oncol* **20**: 1472–1482.
42. Yoshida M. (2001) Multiple viral strategies of HTLV-1 for dysregulation of cell growth control. *Annu Rev Immunol* **19**: 475–496.
46. Kozako T, Arima N, Toji S, Masamoto I, Akimoto M, Hamada H, Che XF, Fujiwara H, Matsushita K, Tokunaga M, Haraguchi K, Uozumi K, Suzuki S, Takezaki T, Sonoda S. (2006) Reduced frequency, diversity, and function of human T cell leukemia virus type 1-specific CD8+ T cell in adult T cell leukemia patients. *J Immunol* **177**: 5718–5726.

49. Matsuoka M. (2003) Human T-cell leukemia virus type I and adult T-cell leukemia. *Oncogene* **22**: 5131–5140.
53. Shiratori S, Yasumoto A, Tanaka J, Shigematsu A, Yamamoto S, Nishio M, Hashino S, Morita R, Takahata M, Onozawa M, Kahata K, Kondo T, Ota S, Wakasa K, Sugita J, Koike T, Asaka M, Kasai M, Imamura M. (2008) A retrospective analysis of allogeneic hematopoietic stem cell transplantation for adult T cell leukemia/lymphoma (ATL): Clinical impact of graft-versus-leukemia/lymphoma effect. *Biol Blood Marrow Transplant* **14**: 817–823.
54. Carbone A, Cesarman E, Spina M, Gloghini A, Schulz TF. (2009) HIV-associated lymphomas and gamma-herpesviruses. *Blood* **113**: 1213–1224.
71. Wilkinson J, Cope A, Gill J, Bourboulia D, Hayes P, Imami N, Kubo T, Marcelin A, Calvez V, Weiss R, Gazzard B, Boshoff C, Gotch F. (2002) Identification of Kaposi's sarcoma-associated herpesvirus (KSHV)-specific cytotoxic T-lymphocyte epitopes and evaluation of reconstitution of KSHV-specific responses in human immunodeficiency virus type 1-Infected patients receiving highly active antiretroviral therapy. *J Virol* **76**: 2634–2640.
77. Chen YB, Rahemtullah A, Hochberg E. (2007) Primary effusion lymphoma. *Oncologist* **12**: 569–576.
79. Mylona EE, Baraboutis IG, Lekakis LJ, Georgiou O, Papastamopoulos V, Skoutelis A. (2008) Multicentric Castleman's disease in HIV infection: A systematic review of the literature. *AIDS Rev* **10**: 25–35.
80. Stebbing J, Pantanowitz L, Dayyani F, Sullivan RJ, Bower M, Dezube BJ. (2008) HIV-associated multicentric Castleman's disease. *Am J Hematol* **83**: 498–503.
91. Filipovich AH, Heinitz KJ, Robison LL, Frizzera G. (1987) The Immunodeficiency Cancer Registry. A research resource. *Am J Pediatr Hematol/Oncol* **9**: 183–184.
100. Moshous D, Pannetier C, Chasseval Rd R, Deist Fl F, Cavazzana-Calvo M, Romana S, Macintyre E, Canioni D, Brousse N, Fischer A, Casanova JL, Villartay JP. (2003) Partial T and B lymphocyte immunodeficiency and predisposition to lymphoma in patients with hypomorphic mutations in Artemis. *J Clin Invest* **111**: 381–387.
101. Mustillo P, Bajwa RP, Termuhlen AM, Nicol K, Scherzer R, Jaffe R, Filipovich AH, Gross TG. (2008) Tumor immune surveillance defect of X-linked severe combined immunodeficiency is not Epstein-Barr virus specific. *Pediatr Blood Cancer* **51**: 706–709.
102. Husain M, Grunebaum E, Naqvi A, Atkinson A, Ngan BY, Aiuti A, Roifman CM. (2007) Burkitt's lymphoma in a patient with adenosine deaminase deficiency-severe combined immunodeficiency treated with polyethylene glycol-adenosine deaminase. *J Pediatr* **151**: 93–95.
107. Pasic S, Vujic D, Djuricic S, Jevtic D, Grujic B. (2006) Burkitt lymphoma-induced ileocolic intussusception in Wiskott-Aldrich syndrome. *J Pediatr Hematol/Oncol* **28**: 48–49.
108. Rampisela D, Donner LR. (2010) An unusual self-limited clonal Mott cell proliferation with lymphoplasmacytic lymphoma-like features in a child with the Wiskott-Aldrich syndrome and Von Recklinghausen's neurofibromatosis. *Pathol Res Pract* **206**: 467–471.
111. Isam H, Al-Wahadneh A. (2004) Successful bone marrow transplantation in a child with X-linked hyper-IgM syndrome. *Saudi J Kidney Dis Transpl* **15**: 489–493.
112. Bejaoui M, Mellouli F, Chouanine R, Dellagi K, Barbouche MR. (2003) The hyper-IgM syndrome: 13 observations. *Presse Med* **32**: 544–549.
122. Quintanilla-Martinez L, Kumar S, Fend F, Reyes E, Teruya-Feldstein J, Kingma DW, Sorbara L, Raffeld M, Straus SE, Jaffe ES. (2000) Fulminant EBV(+) T-cell lymphoproliferative disorder following acute/chronic EBV infection: A distinct clinicopathologic syndrome. *Blood* **96**: 443–451.
124. Hervier B, Latour S, Loussouarn D, Rimbert M, De-Saint-Basile G, Picard C, Hamidou M. (2010) An atypical case of X-linked lymphoproliferative disease revealed as a late cerebral lymphoma. *J Neuroimmunol* **218**: 125–128.
125. Harrington DS, Weisenburger DD, Purtilo DT. (1987) Malignant lymphoma in the X-linked lymphoproliferative syndrome. *Cancer* **59**: 1419–1429.
126. Gaspar HB, Sharifi R, Gilmour KC, Thrasher AJ. (2002) X-linked lymphoproliferative disease: Clinical, diagnostic and molecular perspective. *Br J Haematol* **119**: 585–595.
127. Strahm B, Rittweiler K, Duffner U, Brandau O, Orlowska-Volk M, Karajannis MA, Stadt U, Tiemann M, Reiter A, Brandis M, Meindl A, Niemeyer CM. (2000) Recurrent B-cell non-Hodgkin's lymphoma in two brothers with X-linked lymphoproliferative disease without evidence for Epstein-Barr virus infection. *Br J Haematol* **108**: 377–382.
131. Mueller BU, Pizzo PA. (1995) Cancer in children with primary or secondary immunodeficiencies. *J Pediatr* **126**: 1–10.
133. Aghamohammadi A, Parvaneh N, Tirgari F, Mahjoob F, Movahedi M, Gharagozlou M, Mansouri M, Kouhi A, Rezaei N, Webster D. (2006) Lymphoma of mucosa-associated lymphoid tissue in common variable immunodeficiency. *Leuk Lymphoma* **47**: 343–346.
134. Gottesman SR, Haas D, Ladanyi M, Amorosi EL. (1999) Peripheral T cell lymphoma in a patient with common

variable immunodeficiency disease: Case report and literature review. *Leuk Lymphoma* **32**: 589–595.

135. Aghamohammadi A, Rezaei N, Gharagozlou M, Ramyar A, Mahjoub F, Rezaei-Kalantari K, Moin M. (2007) Hodgkin lymphoma in two siblings with common variable immunodeficiency. *Pediatr Hematol Oncol* **24**: 337–342.
136. Le Guern V, Le Roux G, Martin A, Feuillard J, Cohen P, Poirel H, Raphael M, Guillevin L, Mouthon L. (2003) Lymphoma complicating common variable immunodeficiency with granulomatous disease: Report of two cases. *Eur J Haematol* **71**: 459–463.
138. Varan A, Buyukpamukcu M, Ersoy F, Sanal O, Akyuz C, Kutluk T, Yalcin B. (2004) Malignant solid tumors associated with congenital immunodeficiency disorders. *Pediatr Hematol Oncol* **21**: 441–451.
139. Gompels MM, Hodges E, Lock RJ, Angus B, White H, Larkin A, Chapel HM, Spickett GP, Misbah SA, Smith JL. (2003) Lymphoproliferative disease in antibody deficiency: A multi-centre study. *Clin Exp Immunol* **134**: 314–320.
140. Winkelstein JA, Marino MC, Lederman HM, Jones SM, Sullivan K, Burks AW, Conley ME, Cunningham-Rundles C, Ochs HD. (2006) X-linked agammaglobulinemia: Report on a United States registry of 201 patients. *Medicine (Baltimore)* **85**: 193–202.
147. Trottestam H, Beutel K, Meeths M, Carlsen N, Heilmann C, Pasic S, Webb D, Hasle H, Henter JI. (2009) Treatment of the X-linked lymphoproliferative, Griscelli and Chediak-Higashi syndromes by HLH directed therapy. *Pediatr Blood Cancer* **52**: 268–272.
148. Meeths M, Bryceson YT, Rudd E, Zheng C, Wood SM, Ramme K, Beutel K, Hasle H, Heilmann C, Hultenby K, Ljunggren HG, Fadeel B, Nordenskjold M, Henter JI. (2010) Clinical presentation of Griscelli syndrome type 2 and spectrum of RAB27A mutations. *Pediatr Blood Cancer* **54**: 563–572.
152. Poppema S, Maggio E, van den Berg A. (2004) Development of lymphoma in autoimmune lymphoproliferative syndrome (ALPS) and its relationship to Fas gene mutations. *Leuk Lymphoma* **45**: 423–431.
159. Taylor AM, Metcalfe JA, Thick J, Mak YF. (1996) Leukemia and lymphoma in ataxia telangiectasia. *Blood* **87**: 423–438.
161. Ziino O, Rondelli R, Micalizzi C, Luciani M, Conter V, Arico M. (2006) Acute lymphoblastic leukemia in children with associated genetic conditions other than Down's syndrome. The AIEOP experience. *Haematologica* **91**: 139–140.
163. Seidemann K, Henze G, Beck JD, Sauerbrey A, Kuhl J, Mann G, Reiter A. (2000) Non-Hodgkin's lymphoma in pediatric patients with chromosomal breakage syndromes (AT and NBS): Experience from the BFM trials. *Ann Oncol* **11**(Suppl 1): 141–145.
165. Dembowska-Baginska B, Perek D, Brozyna A, Wakulinska A, Olczak-Kowalczyk D, Gladkowska-Dura M, Grajkowska W, Chrzanowska KH. (2009) Non-Hodgkin lymphoma (NHL) in children with Nijmegen breakage syndrome (NBS). *Pediatr Blood Cancer* **52**: 186–190.
166. Jovanovic A, Minic P, Scekic-Guc M, Djuricic S, Cirkovic S, Weemaes C, Pasic S. (2009) Successful treatment of Hodgkin lymphoma in Nijmegen breakage syndrome. *J Pediatr Hematol/Oncol* **31**: 49–52.
167. Paulli M, Viglio A, Boveri E, Pitino A, Lucioni M, Franco C, Riboni R, Rosso R, Magrini U, Marseglia GL, Marchi A. (2000) Nijmegen breakage syndrome-associated T-cell-rich B-cell lymphoma: Case report. *Pediatr Dev Pathol* **3**: 264–270.
171. German J. (1997) Bloom's syndrome. XX. The first 100 cancers. *Cancer Genet Cytogenet* **93**: 100–106.
172. Poppe B, van Limbergen H, van Roy N, Vandecruys E, de Paepe A, Benoit Y, Speleman F. (2001) Chromosomal aberrations in Bloom syndrome patients with myeloid malignancies. *Cancer Genet Cytogenet* **128**: 39–42.
175. Pollock BH, Jenson HB, Leach CT, McClain KL, Hutchison RE, Garzarella L, Joshi VV, Parmley RT, Murphy SB. (2003) Risk factors for pediatric human immunodeficiency virus-related malignancy. *JAMA J Am Med Assoc* **289**: 2393–2399.
176. Carbone A, Gloghini A. (2005) AIDS-related lymphomas: From pathogenesis to pathology. *Br J Haematol* **130**: 662–670.
183. Gross T, Shiramizu, B. (2006) Lymphoproliferative disorders and malignancies related to immunodeficiencies. In: PA Pizzo, DG Poplack (ed). *Principles and Practice of Pediatric Oncology* (5th ed). Philadelphia, PA: Lippincott, Williams & Wilkins, pp. 748–767.
187. Gasser O, Bihl FK, Wolbers M, Loggi E, Steffen I, Hirsch HH, Gunthard HF, Walker BD, Brander C, Battegay M, Hess C. (2007) HIV patients developing primary CNS lymphoma lack EBV-specific CD4+ T cell function irrespective of absolute CD4+ T cell counts. *PLoS Med* **4**: e96.
188. Newell ME, Hoy JF, Cooper SG, DeGraaff B, Grulich AE, Bryant M, Millar JL, Brew BJ, Quinn DI. (2004) Human immunodeficiency virus-related primary central nervous system lymphoma: Factors influencing survival in 111 patients. *Cancer* **100**: 2627–2636.
190. Castillo J, Pantanowitz L, Dezube BJ. (2008) HIV-associated plasmablastic lymphoma: Lessons learned from 112 published cases. *Am J Hematol* **83**: 804–809.

191. Biancotto A, Grivel JC, Iglehart SJ, Vanpouille C, Lisco A, Sieg SF, Debernardo R, Garate K, Rodriguez B, Margolis LB, Lederman MM. (2007) Abnormal activation and cytokine spectra in lymph nodes of people chronically infected with HIV-1. *Blood* **109**: 4272–4279.
195. Biggar RJ, Jaffe ES, Goedert JJ, Chaturvedi A, Pfeiffer R, Engels EA. (2006) Hodgkin lymphoma and immunodeficiency in persons with HIV/AIDS. *Blood* **108**: 3786–3791.
196. Carbone A, Gloghini A, Serraino D, Spina M. (2009) HIV-associated Hodgkin lymphoma. *Curr Opin HIV AIDS* **4**: 3–10.
199. Spano JP, Costagliola D, Katlama C, Mounier N, Oksenhendler E, Khayat D. (2008) AIDS-related malignancies: State of the art and therapeutic challenges. *J Clin Oncol* **26**: 4834–4842.
205. Tran H, Nourse J, Hall S, Green M, Griffiths L, Gandhi MK. (2008) Immunodeficiency-associated lymphomas. *Blood Rev* **22**: 261–281.
213. Tanner JE, Alfieri C. (2001) The Epstein-Barr virus and post-transplant lymphoproliferative disease: Interplay of immunosuppression, EBV, and the immune system in disease pathogenesis. *Transpl Infect Dis* **3**: 60–69.
214. Orjuela M, Gross TG, Cheung YK, Alobeid B, Morris E, Cairo MS. (2003) A pilot study of chemoimmunotherapy (cyclophosphamide, prednisone, and rituximab) in patients with post-transplant lymphoproliferative disorder following solid organ transplantation. *Clin Cancer Res* **9**: 3945S–3952S.
230. Landgren O, Gilbert ES, Rizzo JD, Socie G, Banks PM, Sobocinski KA, Horowitz MM, Jaffe ES, Kingma DW, Travis LB, Flowers ME, Martin PJ, Deeg HJ, Curtis RE. (2009) Risk factors for lymphoproliferative disorders after allogeneic hematopoietic cell transplantation. *Blood* **113**: 4992–5001.
233. Dvorak CC, Cowan MJ. (2008) Hematopoietic stem cell transplantation for primary immunodeficiency disease. *Bone Marrow Transplant* **41**: 119–126.
234. Lim ST, Karim R, Nathwani BN, Tulpule A, Espina B, Levine AM. (2005) AIDS-related Burkitt's lymphoma versus diffuse large-cell lymphoma in the pre-highly active antiretroviral therapy (HAART) and HAART eras: Significant differences in survival with standard chemotherapy. *J Clin Oncol* **23**: 4430–4438.
238. Sato E, Ohga S, Kuroda H, Yoshiba F, Nishimura M, Nagasawa M, Inoue M, Kawa K. (2008) Allogeneic hematopoietic stem cell transplantation for Epstein-Barr virus-associated T/natural killer-cell lymphoproliferative disease in Japan. *Am J Hematol* **83**: 721–727.
239. Maza S, Kiewe P, Munz DL, Korfel A, Hamm B, Jahnke K, Thiel E. (2009) First report on a prospective trial with yttrium-90-labeled ibritumomab tiuxetan (Zevalin) in primary CNS lymphoma. *Neuro Oncol* **11**: 423–429.

20

Hematopoietic Stem Cell Transplantation for Children, Adolescents and Young Adults with Hematological Malignancies

Mary Eapen and Vanderson Rocha

Introduction

Hematopoietic stem cell transplantation (HSCT) is a procedure whereby hematopoietic stem cells of any donor type or graft source are given to a recipient with the intention of repopulating and replacing the recipient's hematopoietic system in total or in part. Donor type may be autologous, syngeneic, HLA-matched sibling, other relative or unrelated donor. Graft source may be bone marrow (BM), peripheral blood (PB), or umbilical cord blood (UCB). The role of HSCT for hematological malignancies has evolved concomitantly with nontransplant management such that intensification of front-line therapies for hematological malignancies has led to use of HSCT for salvage rather than front-line treatment. Choice of donor type is dependent on donor availability and an HLA-matched sibling, the donor of choice when available. In the absence of an HLA-matched sibling, alternative donor types including a mismatched relative or an unrelated donor is an acceptable option. Approximately, 50% of allogeneic HSCT now use allografts from a volunteer adult unrelated donor or unrelated cord blood. The use of a syngeneic donor for allogeneic HSCT is obsolete nowadays due to an inadequate graft-vs.-tumor effect, a desirable consequence of allogeneic HSCT for tumor control. Despite the absence of graft-vs.-tumor effects with autologous HSCT, transplantation of autologous graft is the standard of care for relapsed Hodgkin lymphoma and a clinical option (i.e. after careful consideration of the risk vs. benefits for this procedure to nontransplant therapies) for non-Hodgkin lymphoma in second complete remission (CR). Recipients of HSCT receive conditioning regimens prior to infusion of graft. The intensity of the regimen may vary with most pediatric and young adult transplant recipients receiving standard intensity regimens and a minority, reduced intensity regimens. In general, reduced intensity conditioning regimens are reserved for older patients or those with comorbidities or other contraindications that are considered prohibitive for use of standard intensity regimens. Table 20.1 shows the indications for HSCT for children and young adults with hematological malignancies recently revised by the European Blood and Marrow Transplant group (EBMT) according to disease, disease status, and donor source.[1]

Table 20.1. HSCT for children and adolescents with hematological malignancies according to the European Group of Blood and Marrow Transplant.

Disease	Disease status	Allogeneic			Autologous
		Sibling donor	Well-matched unrelated	Mm unrelated > 1 ag mm related	
AML	CR1 (low risk)	GNR/II	GNR/II	GNR/III	GNR/II
	CR1 (high risk)	S/II	CO/II	GNR/III	S/II
	CR1 (very high risk)	S/II	S/II	CO	GNR
	CR2	S/II	S/II	S/II	S/II
	> CR2	CO/II	D/II	D/II	GNR/II
ALL	CR1 (low risk)	GNR/II	GNR/II	GNR/III	GNR/II
	CR1 (high risk)	S/II	CO/II	CO/II	GNR/II
	CR2	S/II	S/II	CO/II	CO/II
	> CR2	S/II	S/II	CO/II	CO/II
CML	Chronic phase	S/II	S/II	D/II	GNR/III
	Advanced phase	S/II	S/II	D/II	GNR/III
NHL	CR1 (low risk)	GNR/II	GNR/II	GNR/II	GNR/II
	CR2 (high risk)	CO/II	CO/II	GNR/II	CO/II
	CR2	S/II	S/II	CO/II	CO/II
Hodgkin's disease	CR1	GNR/II	GNR/II	GNR/II	GNR/II
	1st relapse, CR2	CO/II	D/III	GNR/III	S/II
Myelodysplastic syndromes		S/II	S/II	D/III	GNR/III

S = standard of care; generally indicated in suitable patients. The results of such transplants are reasonably well defined and compare favorably (or are superior to) results of non-transplant treatment approaches.
CO = clinical option; HSCT is a valuable option for individual patients after careful discussions of risks and benefits with the patient but that for groups of patients the value of HSCT for patients included in this category needs further evaluation.
D = developmental; if there is little experience with this particular type of transplant and when additional research is needed to define the role of HSCT. These transplants should be done within the framework of a clinical trial.
GNR = not recommended. It includes early disease stages when results of conventional treatment do not normally justify the additional risk of transplantation-related mortality, or when the disease is so advanced that the chance of success is so small that the risk of the harvest procedure for the normal donor is difficult to justify.
NA = not applicable.
CR1, 2, = first, second complete remission.
I = evidence from at least one well-executed randomized trial;
II = evidence from at least one well-designed clinical trial without randomization; cohort or case-controlled analytic studies (preferably form more than one centre); multiple time series studies; or dramatic results from uncontrolled experiments;
III = evidence from opinions of respected authorities based on clinical experience, descriptive studies or reports from expert committees;
This classification does not cover patients for whom a syngeneic donor is available.

AML: acute myeloid leukemia; ALL: acute lymphoblastic leukemia; CML: chronic myeloid leukemia; NHL: non-Hodgkin lymphoma.

Indications

Acute lymphoblastic leukemia

Allogeneic HSCT, as front-line therapy for acute lymphoblastic leukemia (ALL), is reserved for children with high-risk features such as adverse cytogenetics or molecular biological markers, poor response to prednisone and resistance to initial chemotherapy including persistence of minimal residual disease (see Chapters 11 and 12).[2] Most study groups define these patients as having estimated event-free survival (EFS) of less than 50%. For these patients, HSCT from an human leukocyte antigen (HLA)-matched sibling or suitably matched unrelated donor is an option.[3] As in children, HSCT from an HLA-matched sibling or suitably matched unrelated donor is an acceptable treatment option in young adults with adverse cytogenetics, high white blood cell count, poor response to initial chemotherapy and minimal residual disease.[4,5] ALL patients who experience an early marrow relapse, still have a dismal prognosis when treated with conventional chemotherapy. Although nearly 90% achieve a second remission, most of them subsequently develop progressive disease. For these patients, both matched sibling donor and unrelated donor HSCT are clearly indicated since the outcomes are similar.[6–8] Unrelated donor HSCT appears to be an acceptable option for children and adolescents with ALL in third CR resulting in modest 5-year leukemia-free survival (LFS) of approximately 30%.[9]

Non-Hodgkin lymphoma

More than 95% of pediatric non-Hodgkin lymphoma (NHL) is high-grade disease with excellent results using intensive chemotherapy, including patients with stage III/IV disease (see Chapters 16 and 17). Long-term EFS is between 60–90%, depending on histologic subtype even in those with stage III/IV disease.[10] Consequently, HSCT is reserved for salvage of patients with recurrent NHL and both autologous and allogeneic HSCT are employed. Though allogeneic HSCT are being performed for recurrent NHL, the data thus far have failed to show significant differences in EFS for Burkitt lymphoma, diffuse large B-cell lymphoma and anaplastic large cell lymphoma between allogeneic and autologous HSCT.[10] However, the data support allogeneic HSCT for patients with lymphoblastic lymphoma; EFS rates are higher after allogeneic HSCT compared to autologous HSCT (40% vs. 4%, $p < 0.01$, respectively).

Acute myeloid leukemia

Allogeneic HSCT, as a post-remission strategy for acute myeloid leukemia (AML), is associated with the lowest risk of relapse (see Chapter 13). However, the lower relapse risk after HSCT is limited by the high treatment-related mortality associated with this treatment option. In North America, for children who achieve first CR and have a matched sibling donor, HSCT as post-remission therapy is standard of care with survival rates of 60–70%.[11] This trial failed to show a survival advantage with autologous HSCT compared to intensive chemotherapy. On the other hand, in Europe, the role of HSCT in first CR is declining because of the better outcomes with intensive front-line therapies for good-risk AML and HSCT reserved for high-risk AML.[12] In parallel with interest in limiting the role of allogeneic and autologous HSCT for children and young adults with AML in first CR, there is increased interest in investigating whether unrelated donor HSCT is superior to intensive chemotherapy for those not in first CR or based on risk stratification. In a recent report that examined outcomes after unrelated donor bone marrow transplantation (BMT) in children and adolescents in second CR, in relapse or primary induction failure, disease status at HSCT was the most important predictor for a successful outcome.[13] The 5-year probabilities of LFS were 45%, 20%, and 12% for patients transplanted on second CR, in relapse and primary induction failure, respectively.[13] While it is challenging to examine the importance of adverse cytogenetics and French-American-British (FAB) subtypes in patients with recurrent leukemia, the data suggest unrelated donor HSCT is an effective treatment option for patients with high risk disease. Allogeneic HSCT is often considered for infant AML especially when a matched sibling is available. LFS after matched related and unrelated donor HSCT are similar, with disease status at transplantation being the most important predictor for a successful outcome.[14] The pattern of treatment failure differed by donor type; while relapse was the most common cause of failure after HLA matched sibling HSCT, treatment-related mortality was the most frequent cause of failure after unrelated donor transplantation.

Myelodysplastic syndrome (MDS)

Allogeneic HSCT from a sibling donor is the treatment of choice for children with primary MDS including juvenile myelomonocytic leukemia (JMML) (see Chapters 14 and 15).[15,16] Since the possibility of cure is extremely poor with conventional chemotherapy, allogeneic HSCT from an unrelated donor can also be recommended. The role of autologous HSCT in children with MDS remains controversial and is generally not recommended.

Chronic myeloid leukemia (CML)

CML is a rare disease in children with an incidence 3–5% of all pediatric leukemias (see Chapters 15 and 22). Since the introduction of tyrosine kinase inhibitors (TKIs), which are approved for children and adolescents, HSCT is no longer the first treatment for patients with early phase CML. However, TKIs do not provide cure; life-long medication is necessary, there are treatment failures and continuous contraception is mandatory. Depending on geographic regions, as well as physician and patient preference, HSCT still remains an important treatment option especially for younger patients. HSCT might be postponed for patients who achieve a hematological response at 3 months, followed by a minor cytogenetic response at 6 months and a complete cytogenetic response at 12 months after initiation of TKI (imatinib) at 300 mg/m^2. Once imatinib refractoriness develops, patients should undergo HSCT.

However, prospective studies are needed to address this complex issue and elaborate the best treatment options especially considering the needs of young patients with CML.

Donor Selection

Availability of an appropriately matched donor for HSCT and patient disease status at transplantation are important determinants of success. The optimal donor is an HLA-matched sibling, but less than a third of patients who may benefit from HSCT have a matched sibling.[17] The risk of graft failure and the risk and severity of GVHD after matched sibling donor HSCT is low, resulting in fewer transplant-related morbidities and mortality. The lack of a matched sibling donor for most who may benefit from HSCT led to exploratory transplantation of grafts from alternative donors — mismatched family member or an unrelated donor, usually an adult recruited through the international donor registries that together now list over 14 million donors. Methods of gene definition and HLA-matching have evolved and now involve DNA typing to identify HLA alleles and the most suitably matched donor, since the use of a suitably matched donor reduces the risk of graft failure and GVHD.[18] In general, the recipient's tolerance to mismatching is dependent on the particular epitopes present and younger recipients tolerate mismatching better than older recipients.

Family donors other than matched siblings could be mismatched at a single HLA locus in about 3–5% of cases or more commonly mismatched at two HLA loci (haploidentical). One or more haploidentical family donors can be identified for almost all patients; thus, a the donor will be readily available if transplantation is needed urgently. However, modulation of the graft to overcome the risks of graft failure and GVHD known to occur with the increased donor–recipient mismatching leads to delayed immune reconstitution and consequently infectious complications and death. For most children, parents are the donors of choice and transplantation of the graft from mother to child have better outcomes compared to transplantation of the graft from father to child.[19] The better results observed after maternal–child HSCT may be explained by the mother and child acquiring a life-long partial tolerance to each other because during pregnancy a two-way exchange of cells between mother and child occurs. There are also reports that have shown lower risks of leukemia relapse and higher LFS for patients with AML when the haploidentical donor and recipient are killer immunoglobulin-like receptor (KIR) ligand mismatched in the GVHD direction.[20] Center experience and CD34 cell dose are important factors associated with LFS and should be taken into account when a haplo HSCT is indicated.[21] Importantly, children with ALL in more advanced phases of the disease should not be transplanted with a family HLA mismatched donor.

The other alternative, a volunteer unrelated adult donor, requires stringent donor–recipient matching criteria for optimal survival and identifying an optimally matched donor and recipient often challenging. For example, in a recent analysis of the National Marrow Donor Program's donor registry in the United States, the probabilities of finding an optimally matched volunteer unrelated adult donor were 51% for Caucasians, 30% for Hispanics, 20% for Asians, and 17% for African Americans (M. Maiers, personal communication, August 2008). In countries and regions where the population is less diverse, the probabilities of finding an optimally matched volunteer unrelated donor is easier.[22] In a recent analysis of over 4000 unrelated donor BMT facilitated by the National Marrow Donor Program, United States, HLA matching at HLA-A, -B, -C and -DRB1 (8/8 match) between the donor and recipient was associated with best survival.[18] In that report, a single mismatch at the HLA-DQ locus when donor and recipient were matched at HLA-A, -B, -C, -DRB1 was not associated with adverse outcomes. Further, donor–recipient mismatches at HLA-B or -C appear to be better tolerated than were mismatches at HLA-A or -DRB1 for BMT.[18] As with BMT, an 8/8 match between unrelated adult donors and recipients is associated with best survival after unrelated adult donor peripheral blood progenitor cell (PBPC) transplants, and mismatches at HLA-A, -B or -DRB1 were better tolerated than at HLA-C.[23] In both reports, mortality risks were similar comparing low-resolution (antigen) vs. high-resolution (allele) mismatches, except for HLA-C, where allele-level mismatches were not associated with mortality. Further, the effect of donor–recipient HLA-mismatch on mortality was most evident when transplantation occurred in first CR with an absolute difference of 9–10% in overall survival (OS) after matched and single mismatched transplants.[18] For patients with a more advanced disease, this difference was considerably lower at 3–5%, implying disease status at transplantation is also an important determinant of survival after HSCT.[18] Using unrelated adult donors who are not suitably matched to recipients (i.e. 8/8 match) substantially increases the risk of transplant-related complications, particularly the immunological risk of GVHD, which in turn increases risks of opportunistic infections and consequently mortality. Therefore, novel immunoprophylactic regimens and methods of T-cell depletion were explored to overcome the barrier of GVHD.[24] While GVHD prevention was possible with T-cell depletion, the removal of lymphocytes increased the risks of graft failure, leukemia recurrence and infections which ultimately did not result in the desired survival advantage.[25]

The often futile attempts to identify a HLA-matched sibling or a suitably matched volunteer unrelated adult donor (i.e. an 8/8 matched adult donor) and the complications associated with mismatched related or unrelated donor HSCT led to the search for an alternative source of hematopoietic stem cells namely, umbilical cord blood (UCB). There are several benefits to using UCB including banked UCB, which is immediately available for use, low risk of transmitting infections by latent viruses such as cytomegalovirus (CMV), minimal risk to the donor, and importantly, the less stringent donor–recipient HLA-matching which allows wider access to HSCT to persons with rare haplotypes and ethnic minorities. The less stringent matching requirements can be explained by the immunological naivety of placental T lymphocytes, resulting in lower risks and severity of GVHD. Major disadvantages to using UCB include the low absolute numbers of hematopoietic stem cells and progenitors, the risk of graft failure and inability to contact the donor for additional hematopoietic stem cells for additional infusion and/or cellular therapy.

Graft source

BM obtained by repeated aspiration of the posterior iliac crests of the donor was the first source of hematopoietic stem cells. The donor receives general or local anesthesia during donation and may experience discomfort from the harvesting procedure for a few days after the procedure. Serious side effects are rare and two deaths occurred in 8000 collections.[26] As hematopoietic stem cells continuously detach from the marrow enter the circulation and reenter the marrow, these cells can be collected easily from peripheral blood. Hematopoietic stem cells are collected via a peripheral vein after stimulating the donor's BM with granulocyte colony-stimulating growth factor (G-CSF). In addition to the ease of collection, this avoids exposing the donor to any risks of general anesthesia. However, PBPC transplants have higher GVHD risks compared to BMT and chronic GVHD after PBPC transplants require longer duration of treatment compared to BM.[27] As mentioned above, UCB either from an HLA-matched sibling[28] or a matched or mismatched unrelated donor[29–31] may be used as the graft for children and young adults with hematological malignancies.

Outcomes of HSCT in Children with Acute Leukemia

All published reports comparing transplant outcomes by graft source are retrospective and generally registry based. The logistics of randomizing various graft sources has proven to be challenging; retrospective reports have required careful statistical considerations to enable comparison of grafts and interpretation of results.

Outcomes after PBPC vs. BM from HLA matched sibling donors

There have been several clinical trials that have compared PBPC and BM in adults with leukemias. Briefly, the results of those studies have shown faster hematopoietic recovery, higher incidence of chronic GVHD and a survival advantage for patients transplanted in advanced phase disease after PBPC compared to BM transplants.[32] However, in children and adolescents, only one study has evaluated the impact of PBPC compared to BM from HLA-matched siblings and the outcome differs from that observed in adults.[33] The Center for International Blood and Marrow Transplant Research (CIBMTR) compared the results of 143 PBPC and 630 BMTs from HLA-matched sibling donors in children age 8–20 years, with acute leukemia. PBPC transplant recipients were slightly older, more likely to have advanced leukemia (i.e. in relapse at transplantation), receive growth factors post-transplant and transplanted more recently. As with transplantations in adults, hematopoietic recovery was faster after PBPC transplantation. Though risks of grades 2–4 acute GVHD were similar, chronic GVHD was significantly higher after PBPC transplantation (hazard ratio [HR] 1.85, $p = 0.001$) compared to BM. In contrast to reports in adults, treatment-related mortality (HR 1.89, $p = 0.001$), treatment failure, inverse of

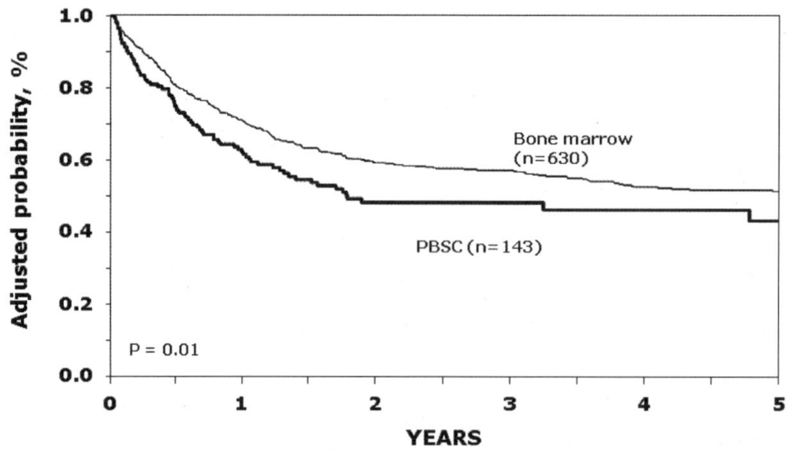

Fig. 20.1. The 3-year probability of overall survival after PBPC and BM transplantation from HLA matched sibling donors, adjusted for disease status at transplantation and use of growth factor for hematopoietic recovery, were 48% and 58%, respectively. Reproduced from the Journal of Clinical Oncology 2004; **22**: 4872–4880. Copyright 2004, with permission from the American Society of Clinical Oncology.

LFS (HR 1.31, $p = 0.03$) and overall mortality (RR 1.38, $p = 0.01$) were higher after PBPC compared to BMT. The risk of relapse was similar in the two treatment groups. After adjusting for other prognostic factors, the 3-year probability of LFS adjusted for disease status and use or non-use of growth factor, were 42% and 51% after PBPC and BMT, respectively. The corresponding 3-year probability of OS was 48% and 58% (Fig. 20.1). The data suggest poorer outcomes after PBPC compared to BMT children and adolescents after adjustment for relevant risk factors and use of PBPC must be discouraged. It is noteworthy that approximately 25% of transplantation for hematological malignancies in children and adolescents continue the use of PBPC grafts.

Outcomes after PBPC vs. BM from adult unrelated donors

PBPC is routinely collected from volunteer unrelated adult donors and account for over 70% of unrelated adult donor transplants. As with matched sibling donor transplants, several reports have compared PBPC and BMT in adults with acute and chronic leukemia.[34] Consistent with the results of sibling donor transplant, risks of GVHD are higher after PBPC transplants compared to BM. However, there were no differences in LFS or OS. A recent report from the CIBMTR and the European Group for Blood and Marrow Transplantation compared transplant outcomes after PBPC and BM unrelated donor transplants in children with acute leukemia.[35] Outcomes of 385 unrelated donor BMTs that were HLA-matched ($n = 186$) or mismatched ($n = 199$) at HLA A, B, C, DRB1 and 110 PBPC transplants that were HLA-matched ($n = 60$) or mismatched ($n = 50$) in patients with acute leukemia younger than 18 years of age were compared. There were no significant differences in patient and disease characteristics, transplant conditioning regimen, GVHD prophylaxis and donor–recipient HLA disparity by graft type. Though the early probability of neutrophil recovery ($\geq 500/\mu l$) was faster after transplantation of PBPC (31% vs. 10% at day 14, $p < 0.001$), the probability of recovery by day 28 was similar after PBPC and BMT (94% and 91%, $p = 0.391$). In contrast, platelet recovery ($\geq 20{,}000/\mu l$) was better after PBPC transplants (86% vs. 76% at day −60, $p = 0.022$). Grade 2–4 acute GVHD was similar (53% vs. 49%) but chronic GVHD higher after PBPC compared to BMT (58% vs. 33%). After adjusting for disease status, donor–recipient HLA disparity and age, transplant-related mortality (20% vs. 24%), relapse (34% vs. 28%), LFS (46% vs. 48%), and OS (49% vs. 49%) were similar after PBPC and BMT (Figs. 20.2 and 20.3). Importantly, these results differ from transplantation of PBPC from HLA-matched siblings where higher chronic GVHD translated into higher transplant-related mortality and lower LFS and OS. The median follow up of surviving patients in this cohort is approximately 2 years and shorter than the 4-year follow up in the HLA-matched sibling report. As the effect of chronic GVHD on survival is a late event, it remains to be seen whether the observed higher chronic GVHD after unrelated donor PBPC transplants will eventually

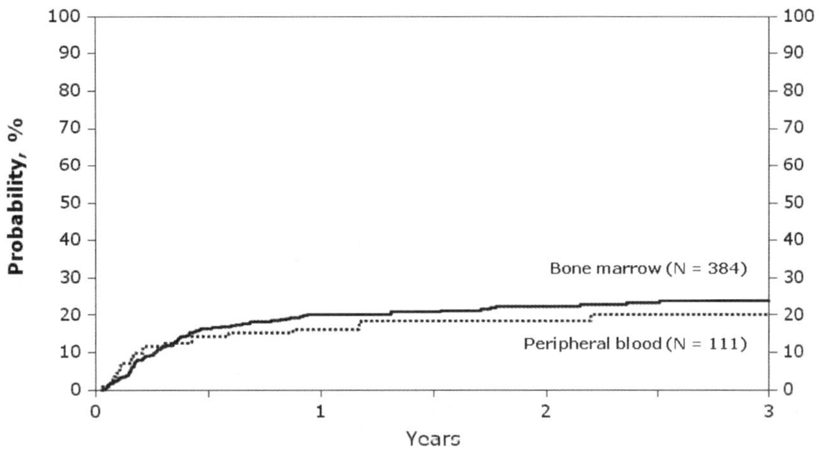

Fig. 20.2. The 3-year probability of transplant-related mortality after PBPC and BM transplantation from adult unrelated donors, were 24% and 20%, respectively.

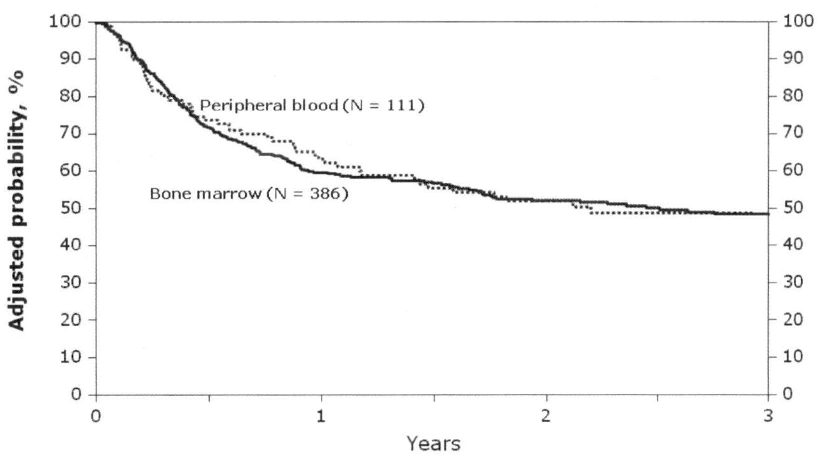

Fig. 20.3. The 3-year probability of overall survival after PBPC and BM transplantation from adult unrelated donors, adjusted for disease status, age and donor-recipient HLA disparity were 49% and 49%, respectively.

lead to the higher mortality or fewer leukemia recurrence in the long-term.

Outcomes after UCB vs. BM from HLA matched sibling donors

In a joint study by the Eurocord and the International Bone Marrow Transplant Registry outcomes of 113 children who received UCB from HLA-matched siblings were compared with those of 2052 children who received BM grafts from HLA-matched siblings.[36] Of the 61 children who were transplanted for a haematological malignancy, 47 had acute leukemia or CML. UCB transplant recipients had slower hematopoietic recovery, and lower risk of acute and chronic GVHD. Among patients receiving transplants for haematological malignancy, 3-year survival was 46% for UCB recipients and 55% for BM recipients ($p = 0.69$). These findings confirm transplantation of an UCB unit with an adequate cell dose from a HLA-matched sibling when available, is comparable to BM. Based on these results, UCB units should be banked when possible for families with a child with hematologic malignancy even when the disease is in remission. To ensure high-quality sibling UCB units, sibling cord blood bank programs must be established and adequately funded.[37]

A recent Eurocord report evaluated the long term outcomes and risk factors influencing outcomes after related HLA-identical UCB transplantation in 147 patients with haematological malignancies.[28] Most patients (74%) had acute leukemia and median follow up approximately 7 years. At transplantation, 40 patients had early disease, 70 intermediate disease, and 37 advanced disease. The median total nucleated cell (TNC) dose was 4.1×10^7/kg after thawing. The cumulative incidence of neutrophil recovery was 90% at day +60 and acute and chronic GVHD, 12% and 10% at 2 years, respectively. At 5 years, the incidence of nonrelapse mortality and relapse were 9% and 47%, respectively; the probability of disease-free survival (DFS) and OS, 44% and 55%, respectively. Among other factors, higher TNC infused was associated with rapid neutrophil recovery and improved DFS. Methotrexate for GVHD prophylaxis lowered the probability of neutrophil recovery. Patients with early and intermediate disease had better DFS and OS. TNC, GVHD prophylaxis and disease status are important prognostic factors that influence outcomes after HLA-matched sibling UCB transplants.

Outcomes after UCB vs. BM from unrelated donors

Comparison of the results of UCB and BM from unrelated donors in children is of paramount relevance because for many patients, the search process will identify both UCB units and an adult unrelated BM donor. Three published studies, two from a single center and one from the Eurocord registry, retrospectively compared outcomes after transplantation of UCB and BM in children with hematological malignancies.[30,38,39] Briefly, in these three reports, recipients of UCB grafts were transplanted sooner compared to recipients of unrelated donor BM grafts, UCB transplants were associated with slower neutrophil and platelet recovery, lower acute GVHD and similar OS after UCB transplant and BMT. In contrast to the single center reports, the report from the Eurocord registry observed higher early transplant-related mortality presumed secondary to infection-related deaths from delayed engraftment or primary graft failure.[28] It is important to note that all patients in the Eurocord report were transplanted before 1998, when UCB was considered as the "last option" for leukemia treatment and the inclusion of heavily pretreated patients as well as those with active disease at transplantation contributed to the higher transplant-related mortality.

All previous comparative studies considered HLA matched for BM grafts using the definition of low resolution typing at HLA-A and -B, and high resolution at HLA-DRB1. A more recent report[29] on behalf of the Centre of the International Bone Marrow Registry and the New York Blood Center, compared outcomes in 503 recipients of UCB with those in 116 recipients of allele-matched BM (HLA-A, -B, -C and DRB1), the current standard when considering an unrelated adult donor. Of the CB recipients, 35 were matched at the HLA-A, -B (antigen-level) and DRB1 (allele-level), 201 were mismatched at 1-locus and 267 were mismatched at 2-loci. All patients were aged < 16 years at transplantation and had acute leukemia. LFS was superior in recipients of HLA-matched CB compared to matched BM and mismatched BM or UCB (60%, p = 0.04). Notably, there were no differences in 5-year LFS after 8/8 HLA matched BM and 1- or 2-loci mismatched UCB (Fig. 20.4). This is in part, explained by differences in risks of transplant-related mortality and relapse between the treatment groups. Compared to HLA-matched BMT, transplant-related mortality was similar in recipients of matched and 1-locus mismatched UCB units with high TNC ($>0.3 \times 10^8$/kg). In UCB recipients who received 1-locus mismatched unit with low TNC ($\leq 0.3 \times 10^8$/kg) and 2-loci mismatched CB (any cell dose), transplant-related mortality was higher (HR 1.88, p = 0.05 and HR 2.31, p = 0.0003, respectively) compared to HLA-matched BM. Approximately 80% of transplant-related deaths in UCB recipients occurred within 3 months after transplantation. Compared to HLA-matched BM, relapse rates were lower in recipients of CB mismatched 2-loci (HR 0.54, p = 0.005). Consistent with other reports, probability of neutrophil recovery (> 500/μl) at day +42 depended on graft type, HLA-match and cell dose (98% with BM; 85% with matched CB; 79% with 1- or 2-loci mismatched CB/high cell dose; 64% with 1- or 2-loci mismatched CB/low cell dose). Compared to HLA matched BM, grades 2–4 and grades 3–4 acute GVHD were lower after matched CB (HR 0.45, p = 0.035, RR 0.51, p = 0.04, respectively) and chronic GVHD was lower after matched or mismatched UCB transplants (HR 0.66, p = 0.04). In a recent analysis that compared outcomes after mismatched UCB and HLA-matched BM or PBPC (matched at HLA-A, -B, -C, -DRB1) in adults, LFS after UCB transplantation was comparable to that observed after 8/8 and 7/8 allele-matched PBPC or BMT.[40] Transplant-related mortality, however, was higher after UCB transplantation compared to 8/8 allele-matched PBPC (HR 1.62, p = 0.003) or BM (HR 1.69, p = 0.003). Grades 2–4 acute and chronic GVHD were lower in UCB recipients compared to allele-matched PBPC (HR 0.57, p = 0.002 and HR 0.38, p = 0.003, respectively),

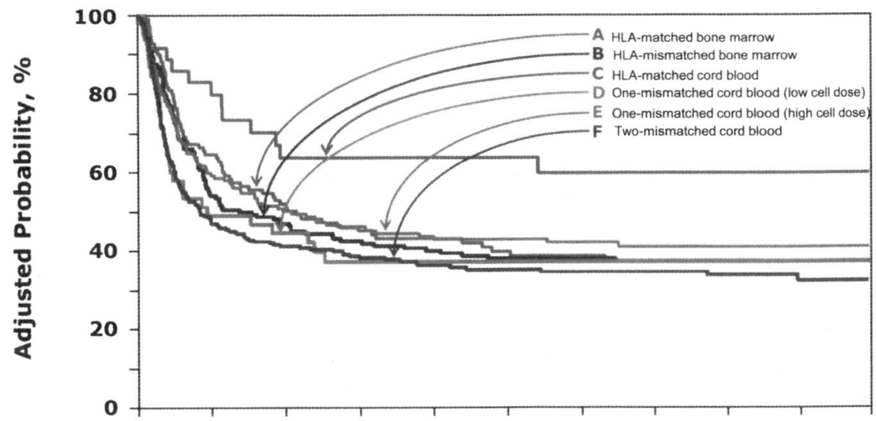

Years:	0	1	2	3	4	5
Line A:	116	62	45	35	29	24
Line B:	166	77	60	53	44	30
Line C:	35	20	17	13	11	8
Line D:	44	19	13	12	10	6
Line E:	157	72	55	44	32	25
Line F:	267	100	67	49	34	21

Fig. 20.4. The 5-year probability of leukemia-free survival adjusted for disease status at transplantation was 38% after HLA matched bone marrow transplant (line A), 37% after mismatched bone marrow transplant (line B), 60% after HLA matched cord blood transplant (line C), 36% after one antigen mismatched cord blood transplant with low cell dose ($\leq 0.3 \times 10^8$/kg total nucleated cells) (line D), 45% after one antigen mismatched cord blood transplant with high cell dose ($> 0.3 \times 10^8$/kg total nucleated cells) (line E) and 33% after two antigen mismatched cord blood transplant (line F). Reproduced from The Lancet 2007; **369**: 1947–1954. Copyright 2007, with permission from Elsevier.

while chronic and not acute GVHD was lower after UCB compared to allele-matched BMT (HR 0.63, p = 0.01). Together, these data support the use of UCB for children or adults with acute leukemia when an HLA-matched unrelated adult donor is lacking and when transplant is urgently needed.

Outcomes after umbilical cord blood vs. full haplotype donor HSCT

The Eurocord group in collaboration with the Acute Leukemia and the Pediatric Diseases Working Parties of the European Group for Blood and Marrow Transplantation retrospectively compared the outcome of patients after unrelated UCB or haplo-transplantation in patients (≤ 16 years) with high risk ALL.[41] Patients received grafts from a haploidentical donor (n = 118) or an unrelated UCB (n = 341). Recipients of haploidentical transplants tended to be older, CMV seropositive and have t(9;22) abnormality. Failure of engraftment was significantly higher after UCB transplant compared to haploidentical transplant (23% vs. 11%, p = 0.007). In multivariate analysis, after adjusting for differences between the two groups and prognostic factors, relapse was higher after haploidentical transplant (HR 1.7, p = 0.01). There were no differences in treatment-related mortality or LFS between the two treatment groups. Therefore, in the absence of an HLA-matched related donor, both strategies are suitable options for children with high risk ALL.

Outcomes after HSCT for Children with MDS

Data on the outcome of children with MDS other than JMML after allogeneic HSCT are scanty; DFS rates are reported to be approximately 60% when the donor is a HLA-matched sibling.[42] However, approximately two-third of patients who may benefit from HSCT lack a matched family donor and a mismatched related or unrelated donor HSCT is considered. Though there are no reports that have compared outcomes after unrelated donor UCB and BMT for MDS, both the Eurocord registry and the CIBMTR have described outcomes after BMT and UCB transplantation separately.

The CIBMTR examined transplant outcomes in 118 patients aged ≤ 18 years with MDS after unrelated BMT in the United States (unpublished data). Disease status and donor–recipient HLA disparity were important prognostic factors; patients with refractory anemia with excess blasts or blasts in transformation were more likely to experience recurrent disease and consequently lower DFS and mismatched transplantations increased the risk of treatment-related mortality. The 8-year DFS for patients with refractory cytopenia after matched and mismatched unrelated donor BMT was 65% and 40%, respectively. Corresponding DFS for patients with refractory anemia with excessive blasts (RAEB) and refractory anemia with excessive blasts in transformation (RAEB-t) was 48% and 28%, respectively.

The Eurocord registry described 70 children with MDS [refractory cytopenia (n = 31) and refractory anemia with excess blasts (n = 30) or blasts in transformation (n = 9)] who received UCB transplantation.[43] As shown for acute leukemia, donor–recipient HLA disparity (mismatched at two HLA loci) and low TNC ($\leq 6 \times 10^7$/kg) had an adverse impact on neutrophil recovery. Of note, the optimal TNC dose is much higher than for acute leukemia. Transplantation period influenced DFS; the 3-year DFS was 50% for transplantations after 2001 compared to 27% for the earlier period ($p = 0.02$). Transplantation period is likely a surrogate for unit TNC and waiting time to transplantation; transplantations after 2001 occurred within 6 months after diagnosis and used UCB units with TNC $> 6 \times 10^7$/kg.

Taken together, these data suggest transplantation with mismatched UCB graft or suitably matched adult unrelated donor is an acceptable alternative for children with MDS who lack a HLA-matched sibling.

Outcomes after HSCT for Children with Lymphoma

With the current upfront chemotherapy regimens, outcome for pediatric NHL is excellent even for those with advanced (stage III or IV) disease. However, the salvaging of patients with refractory or recurrent disease remains very poor. Outcomes after HSCT for patients aged ≤ 18 years with refractory or recurrent Burkitt (n = 41), lymphoblastic (n = 53), diffuse large B cell (n = 52) and anaplastic large cell lymphoma (n = 36), receiving autologous (n = 90) or allogeneic (n = 92 – 43 matched sibling and 49 unrelated donor) were recently reported by the CIBMTR.[10] Patient and disease characteristics of allogeneic and autologous HSCT recipients were similar. There were differences in transplant characteristics; allogeneic donor HSCT was more likely to use irradiation-containing conditioning regimens, marrow stem cells, be performed in more recent years, and for lymphoblastic lymphoma. Disease status at transplantation was important; EFS was lower for patients not in CR at transplantation, regardless of donor type. After adjusting for disease status, 5-year EFS was similar after allogeneic and autologous transplantation for diffuse large B cell (50% vs. 52%), Burkitt (31% vs. 27%), and anaplastic large cell lymphoma (46% vs. 35%). However, EFS was significantly higher for lymphoblastic lymphoma, after allogeneic compared to autologous transplantation (40% vs. 4%, $p < 0.01$). Further, salvage rates were higher for diffuse large B cell and anaplastic large cell lymphoma regardless of donor type. A report from the Berlin-Frankfurt-Munster group on 20 patients with anaplastic large cell lymphoma reported EFS of 75% at 3 years after allogeneic transplantation.[44] These patients received uniform reinduction chemotherapy (NHL BFM 95) and uniform transplant conditioning regimen (total body irradiation, cyclophosphamide and etoposide). In older patients with lymphoblastic leukemia, allogeneic transplantation was associated with higher transplant-related mortality and autologous transplantation with higher disease recurrence, resulting in similar progression-free survival after allogeneic and autologous transplantation.[45] The data support allogeneic transplantation for lymphoblastic lymphoma and anaplastic large cell lymphoma but not for Burkitt or diffuse large B cell lymphoma in children. In young adults, the lower rate of recurrence is offset by higher transplant-related mortality after allogeneic transplantation resulting in comparable progression-free survival after allogeneic and autologous transplantation.[44,46]

As with NHL, children and adolescents with Hodgkin lymphoma have an excellent prognosis even in those with recurrent disease using the various risk adapted treatment strategies that are now available. A recent report from the European Group for Blood and Marrow Transplantation described HSCT outcomes in 91 children and adolescents with recurrent or refractory Hodgkin lymphoma.[47] About half of these patients had failed a prior autologous transplant. OS rates of 45% in a group of patients with aggressive disease and few other salvage treatment options is encouraging and imply this treatment should be considered when a suitably matched donor is available. A limitation of this study is that almost 65% of patients received their allograft from a HLA-matched sibling. Further, relapse was the most common cause of treatment failure. When considering unrelated donor HSCT with its substantially higher risk of treatment-related mortality primarily related to GVHD and in the absence of a demonstrable graft vs. lymphoma effect, the decision to offer this treatment must be considered carefully with other treatment options. Recently, in order to decrease the nonrelapse mortality after allogeneic myeloablative HSCT, some groups have tried to use reduced intensity conditioning (RIC) allogeneic HSCT followed by autologous transplantation. Twelve children, adolescents and young children with relapsed (n = 11) and refractory Hodgkin lymphoma (n = 1) have been transplanted so far in three centers in the U.S.[48] All patients received a myeloablative autograft (carmustine, etoposide and cyclophosphamide) and rituximab (for those with $CD20^+$ Hodgkin lymphoma) prior to a HLA identical sibling-, MUD- or UCBT-RIC (fludarabine + busulfan ± anti-thymocyte globulin. Estimated 2-year OS was 80% (95% confidence interval 41–95%). These interesting results should be further investigated in a larger series of patients and with longer follow up to better evaluate this approach.

Conclusion

HSCT is a curative treatment for selected children who could otherwise not be cured with chemotherapy alone. Advances in treatment of leukemia and molecular diagnosis have helped to select children who may benefit from this approach. While for many years an HLA-matched sibling was the only type of donor routinely employed, more recently, matched unrelated volunteers, full-haplotype mismatched family members, and unrelated cord blood donors are largely utilized to transplant patients lacking an HLA-identical relative. Many significant changes and improvements have occurred over time in the use of HSCT, such as better supportive care and infection prevention and treatment, HLA allelic matching between donor–recipient and therefore better results of unrelated HSCT, strategies of donor choice and patient selection using HLA-mismatched cord blood graft, and new developments in the setting of haploidentical HSCT. Therefore, currently for virtually all patients, a related or unrelated donor can be identified and the decision to perform related or alternative donor HSCT will depend on several patient-, disease-, transplant-, and center-related factors.

References

1. Ljungman P, Bregni M, Brune M, Cornelissen J, de Witte T, Dini G, Einsele H, Gaspar HB, Gratwohl A, Passweg J, Peters C, Rocha V, Saccardi R, Schouten H, Sureda A, Tichelli A, Velardi A, Niederwieser D. (2010) Allogeneic and autologous transplantation for haematological diseases, solid tumours and immune disorders: Current practice in Europe 2009. *Bone Marrow Transplant* **45**: 219–234.
2. Schrauder A, Reiter A, Gadner H, Niethammer D, Klingebiel T, Kremens B, Peters C, Ebell W, Zimmermann M, Niggli F, Ludwig WD, Riehm H, Welte K, Schrappe M. (2006) Superiority of allogeneic hematopoietic stem-cell transplantation compared with chemotherapy alone in high-risk childhood T-cell acute lymphoblastic leukemia: Results from ALL-BFM 90 and 95. *J Clin Oncol* **24**: 5742–5749.
3. Balduzzi A, Valsecchi MG, Uderzo C, de Lorenzo P, Klingebiel T, Peters C, Stary J, Felice MS, Magyarosy E, Conter V, Reiter A, Messina C, Gadner H, Schrappe M. (2005) Chemotherapy versus allogeneic transplantation for very-high-risk childhood acute lymphoblastic leukaemia in first complete remission: Comparison by genetic randomisation in an international prospective study. *Lancet* **366**: 635–642.
4. Marks DI, Perez WS, He W, Zhang MJ, Bishop MR, Bolwell BJ, Bredeson CN, Copelan EA, Gale RP, Gupta V, Hale GA, Isola LM, Jakubowski AA, Keating A, Klumpp TR, Lazarus HM, Liesveld JL, Maziarz RT, McCarthy PL, Sabloff M, Schiller G, Sierra J, Tallman MS, Waller EK, Wiernik PH, Weisdorf DJ. (2008) Unrelated donor transplants in adults with Philadelphia-negative acute lymphoblastic leukemia in first complete remission. *Blood* **112**: 426–434.
5. Moorman AV, Harrison CJ, Buck GA, Richards SM, Secker-Walker LM, Martineau M, Vance GH, Cherry AM, Higgins RR, Fielding AK, Foroni L, Paietta E, Tallman MS, Litzow MR, Wiernik PH, Rowe JM, Goldstone AH, Dewald GW. (2007) Karyotype is an independent prognostic factor in adult acute lymphoblastic leukemia (ALL): Analysis of cytogenetic data from patients treated on the Medical Research Council (MRC) UKALLXII/Eastern Cooperative Oncology Group (ECOG) 2993 trial. *Blood* **109**: 3189–3197.
6. Borgmann A, von Stackelberg A, Hartmann R, Ebell W, Klingebiel T, Peters C, Henze G. (2003) Unrelated donor stem cell transplantation compared with chemotherapy for children with acute lymphoblastic leukemia in a second remission: A matched-pair analysis. *Blood* **101**: 3835–3839.
7. Eapen M, Raetz E, Zhang MJ, Muehlenbein C, Devidas M, Abshire T, Billett A, Homans A, Camitta B, Carroll WL, Davies SM. (2006) Outcomes after HLA-matched sibling transplantation or chemotherapy in children with B-precursor acute lymphoblastic leukemia in a second remission: A collaborative study of the Children's Oncology Group and the Center for International Blood and Marrow Transplant Research. *Blood* **107**: 4961–4967.
8. Locatelli F, Zecca M, Messina C, Rondelli R, Lanino E, Sacchi N, Uderzo C, Fagioli F, Conter V, Bonetti F, Favre C,

Porta F, Giorgiani G, Pession A. (2002) Improvement over time in outcome for children with acute lymphoblastic leukemia in second remission given hematopoietic stem cell transplantation from unrelated donors. *Leukemia* **16**: 2228–2237.

9. Nemecek ER, Carpenter PA, He W, Ellis K, Seber A, Woolfrey A, MacMillan M, Eapen S, Davies HF. (2010) Outcome of unrelated donor blood and marrow transplantation for children with acute lymphoblastic leukemia in third remission. *Biol Blood Marrow Transplant* **16**: S242.
10. Gross TG, Hale GA, He W, Camitta BM, Sanders JE, Cairo MS, Hayashi RJ, Termuhlen AM, Zhang MJ, Davies SM, Eapen M. (2010) Hematopoietic stem cell transplantation for refractory or recurrent non-Hodgkin lymphoma in children and adolescents. *Biol Blood Marrow Transplant* **16**: 223–230.
11. Woods WG, Neudorf S, Gold S, Sanders J, Buckley JD, Barnard DR, Dusenbery K, DeSwarte J, Arthur DC, Lange BJ, Kobrinsky NL. (2001) A comparison of allogeneic bone marrow transplantation, autologous bone marrow transplantation, and aggressive chemotherapy in children with acute myeloid leukemia in remission. *Blood* **97**: 56–62.
12. Gibson BE, Wheatley K, Hann IM, Stevens RF, Webb D, Hills RK, De Graaf SS, Harrison CJ. (2005) Treatment strategy and long-term results in paediatric patients treated in consecutive UK AML trials. *Leukemia* **19**: 2130–2138.
13. Bunin NJ, Davies SM, Aplenc R, Camitta BM, DeSantes KB, Goyal RK, Kapoor N, Kernan NA, Rosenthal J, Smith FO, Eapen M. (2008) Unrelated donor bone marrow transplantation for children with acute myeloid leukemia beyond first remission or refractory to chemotherapy. *J Clin Oncol* **26**: 4326–4332.
14. Eapen M, Rubinstein P, Zhang MJ, Camitta BM, Stevens C, Cairo MS, Davies SM, Doyle JJ, Kurtzberg J, Pulsipher MA, Ortega JJ, Scaradavou A, Horowitz MM, Wagner JE. (2006) Comparable long-term survival after unrelated and HLA-matched sibling donor hematopoietic stem cell transplantations for acute leukemia in children younger than 18 months. *J Clin Oncol* **24**: 145–151.
15. Hasle H. (2007) Myelodysplastic and myeloproliferative disorders in children. *Curr Opin Pediatr* **19**: 1–8.
16. Woods WG, Barnard DR, Alonzo TA, Buckley JD, Kobrinsky N, Arthur DC, Sanders J, Neudorf S, Gold S, Lange BJ. (2002) Prospective study of 90 children requiring treatment for juvenile myelomonocytic leukemia or myelodysplastic syndrome: A report from the Children's Cancer Group. *J Clin Oncol* **20**: 434–440.
17. Rocha V, Locatelli F. (2008) Searching for alternative hematopoietic stem cell donors for pediatric patients. *Bone Marrow Transplant* **41**: 207–214.
18. Lee SJ, Klein J, Haagenson M, Baxter-Lowe LA, Confer DL, Eapen M, Fernandez-Vina M, Flomenberg N, Horowitz M, Hurley CK, Noreen H, Oudshoorn M, Petersdorf E, Setterholm M, Spellman S, Weisdorf D, Williams TM, Anasetti C. (2007) High-resolution donor-recipient HLA matching contributes to the success of unrelated donor marrow transplantation. *Blood* **110**: 4576–4583.
19. Stern M, Ruggeri L, Mancusi A, Bernardo ME, de Angelis C, Bucher C, Locatelli F, Aversa F, Velardi A. (2008) Survival after T cell-depleted haploidentical stem cell transplantation is improved using the mother as donor. *Blood* **112**: 2990–2995.
20. Ruggeri L, Mancusi A, Capanni M, Urbani E, Carotti A, Aloisi T, Stern M, Pende D, Perruccio K, Burchielli E, Topini F, Bianchi E, Aversa F, Martelli MF, Velardi A. (2007) Donor natural killer cell allorecognition of missing self in haploidentical hematopoietic transplantation for acute myeloid leukemia: Challenging its predictive value. *Blood* **110**: 433–440.
21. Klingebiel T, Cornish J, Labopin M, Locatelli F, Darbyshire P, Handgretinger R, Balduzzi A, Owoc-Lempach J, Fagioli F, Or R, Peters C, Aversa F, Polge E, Dini G, Rocha V. (2010) Results and factors influencing outcome after fully haploidentical hematopoietic stem cell transplantation in children with very high-risk acute lymphoblastic leukemia: Impact of center size: An analysis on behalf of the Acute Leukemia and Pediatric Disease Working Parties of the European Blood and Marrow Transplant group. *Blood* **115**: 3437–3446.
22. Tiercy JM, Nicoloso G, Passweg J, Schanz U, Seger R, Chalandon Y, Heim D, Gungor T, Schneider P, Schwabe R, Gratwohl A. (2007) The probability of identifying a 10/10 HLA allele-matched unrelated donor is highly predictable. *Bone Marrow Transplant* **40**: 515–522.
23. Woolfrey AE, Klein J, Haagenson MD, Spellman SR, Battiwalla M, Gajewski JL, Hale GA, Horan J, Hurley CK, Kollman C, Marino S, Oudshoorn M, Petersdorf EW, Ringdén O, Setterholm M, Lee SJ. (2008) Evaluation of human leukocyte antigen (HLA) matching requirements for unrelated peripheral blood stem cell (PBSC) transplantation. *Blood* **112**: 563.
24. Copelan EA. (2006) Hematopoietic stem-cell transplantation. *N Engl J Med* **354**: 1813–1826.
25. Wagner JE, Thompson JS, Carter SL, Kernan NA. (2005) Effect of graft-versus-host disease prophylaxis on 3-year disease-free survival in recipients of unrelated donor

bone marrow (T-cell depletion trial): A multi-centre, randomised phase II-III trial. *Lancet* **366**: 733–741.

26. Anderlini P, Rizzo JD, Nugent ML, Schmitz N, Champlin RE, Horowitz MM. (2001) Peripheral blood stem cell donation: An analysis from the International Bone Marrow Transplant Registry (IBMTR) and European Group for Blood and Marrow Transplant (EBMT) databases. *Bone Marrow Transplant* **27**: 689–692.
27. Flowers ME, Parker PM, Johnston LJ, Matos AV, Storer B, Bensinger WI, Storb R, Appelbaum FR, Forman SJ, Blume KG, Martin PJ. (2002) Comparison of chronic graft-versus-host disease after transplantation of peripheral blood stem cells versus bone marrow in allogeneic recipients: Long-term follow-up of a randomized trial. *Blood* **100**: 415–419.
28. Herr AL, Kabbara N, Bonfim CM, Teira P, Locatelli F, Tiedemann K, Lankester A, Jouet JP, Messina C, Bertrand Y, Diaz de Heredia C, Peters C, Chaves W, Nabhan SK, Ionescu I, Gluckman E, Rocha V. (2010) Long-term follow-up and factors influencing outcomes after related HLA-identical cord blood transplantation for patients with malignancies: An analysis on behalf of Eurocord-EBMT. *Blood* **116**: 1849–1856.
29. Eapen M, Rubinstein P, Zhang MJ, Stevens C, Kurtzberg J, Scaradavou A, Loberiza FR, Champlin RE, Klein JP, Horowitz MM, Wagner JE. (2007) Outcomes of transplantation of unrelated donor umbilical cord blood and bone marrow in children with acute leukaemia: A comparison study. *Lancet* **369**: 1947–1954.
30. Rocha V, Cornish J, Sievers EL, Filipovich A, Locatelli F, Peters C, Remberger M, Michel G, Arcese W, Dallorso S, Tiedemann K, Busca A, Chan KW, Kato S, Ortega J, Vowels M, Zander A, Souillet G, Oakill A, Woolfrey A, Pay AL, Green A, Garnier F, Ionescu I, Wernet P, Sirchia G, Rubinstein P, Chevret S, Gluckman E. (2001) Comparison of outcomes of unrelated bone marrow and umbilical cord blood transplants in children with acute leukemia. *Blood* **97**: 2962–2971.
31. Wagner JE, Barker JN, DeFor TE, Baker KS, Blazar BR, Eide C, Goldman A, Kersey J, Krivit W, MacMillan ML, Orchard PJ, Peters C, Weisdorf DJ, Ramsay NK, Davies SM. (2002) Transplantation of unrelated donor umbilical cord blood in 102 patients with malignant and nonmalignant diseases: Influence of CD34 cell dose and HLA disparity on treatment-related mortality and survival. *Blood* **100**: 1611–1618.
32. Stem Cell Trialist Collaborative Group (2005) Allogeneic peripheral blood stem-cell compared with bone marrow transplantation in the management of hematologic malignancies: An individual patient data meta-analysis of nine randomized trials. *J Clin Oncol* **23**: 5074–5087.
33. Eapen M, Horowitz MM, Klein JP, Champlin RE, Loberiza FR Jr., Ringden O, Wagner JE. (2004) Higher mortality after allogeneic peripheral-blood transplantation compared with bone marrow in children and adolescents: The Histocompatibility and Alternate Stem Cell Source Working Committee of the International Bone Marrow Transplant Registry. *J Clin Oncol* **22**: 4872–4880.
34. Eapen M, Logan BR, Confer DL, Haagenson M, Wagner JE, Weisdorf DJ, Wingard JR, Rowley SD, Stroncek D, Gee AP, Horowitz MM, Anasetti C. (2007) Peripheral blood grafts from unrelated donors are associated with increased acute and chronic graft-versus-host disease without improved survival. *Biol Blood Marrow Transplant* **13**: 1461–1468.
35. Eapen M, Ringden O, Locatelli F, Frangoul H, Remberger M, Laughlin MJ, Rocha V. (2008) Risks and benefits of unrelated donor peripheral blood progenitor cells (PBPC) in children and adolescents with acute leukemia. *Blood* **112**: 977.
36. Rocha V, Wagner JE Jr., Sobocinski KA, Klein JP, Zhang MJ, Horowitz MM, Gluckman E. (2000) Graft-versus-host disease in children who have received a cord-blood or bone marrow transplant from an HLA-identical sibling. Eurocord and International Bone Marrow Transplant Registry Working Committee on alternative donor and stem cell sources. *N Engl J Med* **342**: 1846–1854.
37. Reed W, Smith R, Dekovic F, Lee JY, Saba JD, Trachtenberg E, Epstein J, Haaz S, Walters MC, Lubin BH. (2003) Comprehensive banking of sibling donor cord blood for children with malignant and non-malignant disease. *Blood* **101**: 351–357.
38. Barker JN, Davies SM, DeFor T, Ramsay NK, Weisdorf DJ, Wagner JE. (2001) Survival after transplantation of unrelated donor umbilical cord blood is comparable to that of human leukocyte antigen-matched unrelated donor bone marrow: Results of a matched-pair analysis. *Blood* **97**: 2957–2961.
39. Dalle JH, Duval M, Moghrabi A, Wagner E, Vachon MF, Barrette S, Bernstein M, Champagne J, David M, Demers J, Rousseau P, Winikoff R, Champagne MA. (2004) Results of an unrelated transplant search strategy using partially HLA-mismatched cord blood as an immediate alternative to HLA-matched bone marrow. *Bone Marrow Transplant* **33**: 605–611.
40. Eapen M, Rocha V, Sanz G, Scaradavou A, Zhang MJ, Arcese W, Sirvent A, Champlin RE, Chao N, Gee AP, Isola L, Laughlin MJ, Marks DI, Nabhan S, Ruggeri A,

Soiffer R, Horowitz MM, Gluckman E, Wagner JE. (2010) Effect of graft source on unrelated donor haemopoietic stem-cell transplantation in adults with acute leukaemia: A retrospective analysis. *Lancet Oncol* **11**: 653–660.

41. Hough R, Labopin M, Michel G, Locatelli F, Klingebiel T, Arcese W, Fagioli F, Madero L, Cornish J, Darbyshire PJ, Dini G, Gluckman E, Rocha V. (2007) Outcomes of fully haplo-identical haematopoietic stem cell transplantation compared to unrelated cord blood transplantation in children with acute lymphoblastic leukaemia: A retrospective analysis on behalf of Eurocord, PDWP and ALWP of EBMT. *Bone Marrow Transplant* **39**: S1.
42. Locatelli F, Pession A, Bonetti F, Maserati E, Prete L, Pedrazzoli P, Zecca M, Prete A, Paolucci P, Cazzola M. (1994) Busulfan, cyclophosphamide and melphalan as conditioning regimen for bone marrow transplantation in children with myelodysplastic syndromes. *Leukemia* **8**: 844–849.
43. Moreno-Madureira AB, Eapen M, Locatelli F, Teira P, Zhang MJ, Davies SM, Picardi A, Woolfrey A, Chan K-W, Socie G, Vora A, Bertrand Y, Sales-Bonfim CM, Gluckman E, Niemeyer C, V. R, on behalf of Eurocord-European Blood and Marrow Transplant Group Center for International Blood and Marrow Transplant Registry and the European Working group on childhood MDS. (2010) Analysis of risk factors influencing outcome in children with myelodysplastic syndrome after unrelated cord blood transplantation. *Leukemia* in press.
44. Woessmann W, Peters C, Lenhard M, Burkhardt B, Sykora KW, Dilloo D, Kremens B, Lang P, Fuhrer M, Kuhne T, Parwaresch R, Ebell W, Reiter A. (2006) Allogeneic haematopoietic stem cell transplantation in relapsed or refractory anaplastic large cell lymphoma of children and adolescents — a Berlin-Frankfurt-Munster group report. *Br J Haematol* **133**: 176–182.
45. Levine JE, Harris RE, Loberiza FR Jr., Armitage JO, Vose JM, van Besien K, Lazarus HM, Horowitz MM, Bashey A, Bolwell BJ, Burns LJ, Cairo MS, Champlin RE, Freytes CO, Gibson J, Goldstein SC, Laughlin MJ, Lister J, Marks DI, Maziarz RT, Miller AM, Milone GA, Pavlovsky S, Pecora AL, Rizzo JD, Schiller G, Schouten HC, Zhang MJ. (2003) A comparison of allogeneic and autologous bone marrow transplantation for lymphoblastic lymphoma. *Blood* **101**: 2476–2482.
46. van Besien K, Loberiza FR Jr., Bajorunaite R, Armitage JO, Bashey A, Burns LJ, Freytes CO, Gibson J, Horowitz MM, Inwards DJ, Marks DI, Martino R, Maziarz RT, Molina A, Pavlovsky S, Pecora AL, Schouten HC, Shea TC, Lazarus HM, Rizzo JD, Vose JM. (2003) Comparison of autologous and allogeneic hematopoietic stem cell transplantation for follicular lymphoma. *Blood* **102**: 3521–3529.
47. Claviez A, Canals C, Dierickx D, Stein J, Badell I, Pession A, Mackinnon S, Slavin S, Dalle JH, Chacon MJ, Sarhan M, Wynn RF, Suttorp M, Dini G, Sureda A, Schmitz N. (2009) Allogeneic hematopoietic stem cell transplantation in children and adolescents with recurrent and refractory Hodgkin lymphoma: An analysis of the European Group for Blood and Marrow Transplantation. *Blood* **114**: 2060–2067.
48. Cairo M, Geyer M, Harrison L, Schonfeld T, Bhatia M, Bradley M, Garvin J, George D, Fearon N, Martin P, Kurtzberg J, Schwartz J, Baxter-Lowe L, Satwani P. (2010 (abstract)) Myeloablative (MAC) Autologous Stem Cell Transplantation (AutoSCT) followed by Reduced Intensity (RIC) Allogeneic Stem Cell Transplantation (AlloSCT) in Children, Adolescents and Young Adults (CAYA) with poor risk Hodgkin's lymphoma (HL): Induction of long term GVHL effect. *Biol Blood Marrow Transplant* **16**: S181.

21

Antibody-Targeted Therapy for Children, Adolescents and Young Adults with Hematological Malignancies

Prakash Satwani and Alan S. Wayne

Over the last 4 decades, there have been dramatic improvements in the treatment of children and adolescents with leukemia and lymphoma. Survival rates for pediatric patients diagnosed with acute lymphoblastic leukemia (ALL) and non-Hodgkin lymphoma (NHL) are in the range of 70–90%.[1,2] The intensive chemotherapy regimens, although highly effective, are associated with both short- and long-term morbidities. Furthermore, the outcome of children and adolescents with relapsed ALL and NHL remains poor.[1,3] Thus, novel approaches that can overcome resistance to and decrease nonspecific toxicities associated with chemotherapy regimens are needed to improve the outcome for children and adolescents with ALL and NHL. Targeted monoclonal antibody (MoAb)-based therapies offer potential in that regard.

Introduction

Monoclonal antibodies are the fastest growing class of new therapeutic agents.[4] They hold great promise for the treatment of various malignant and nonmalignant diseases in humans. In 1890, Behring and Kitasato demonstrated that resistance to diphtheria toxin could be transferred from one animal to another by transfer of serum.[5] From this discovery, passive antibody therapy was developed as an effective treatment for infectious diseases and for neutralization of toxins. The concept that antibodies might be effective for the treatment of cancer originated more than a century ago with Paul Ehrlich's hypothesis that it should be feasible to develop a "magic bullet" with affinity for "parasites" but that spares normal tissues.[6] One hundred years elapsed, however, before antibodies were developed as effective agents for the treatment of cancer. In 1975, it become possible to produce identical antibodies specific to a single antigen using the mouse hybridoma technology first developed by Kohler and Milstein[7] for which they received a Nobel prize in 1984. In 1988, Huston *et al.* and Johnson *et al.* reported that antibody variable domains (Fv) could be linked together to make recombinant proteins capable of antigen binding.[8,9] Subsequently, methodologies have been developed to produce MoAbs and their fragments for clinical use and to generate humanized chimeric constructs to reduce immunogenicity. The first MoAb approved for human therapy was the murine monoclonal antibody muromonab-CD3 in 1986. In 1997, rituximab became the first MoAb approved by the US Food and

Drug Administration (FDA) for the treatment of a human cancer (CD20+ NHL). Hematologic malignancies in general are excellent candidates for MoAb-based therapies as they express on their surface normal human differentiation antigens with otherwise limited tissue distribution. In addition, the malignant cells reside predominantly in the vascular and lymphatic compartments and thus are usually accessible to parenterally administered agents.

Antibodies function and structure

Endogenous antibodies are immunoglobulins (Ig) synthesized by B lymphocytes. Each B lymphocyte clone produces a unique and specific immunoglobulin. Antibodies have two separate functions: (i) to bind specific antigen, and (ii) to recruit mediators of the immune stem, including complement and effector cells.

IgG antibodies are large tetrameric molecules composed of two different polypeptide chains: one chain, which weighs approximately 50 kD, is termed the heavy (H) chain; the other chain, which is called the light (L) chain has an approximate weight of 25 kD. Two heavy chains are linked to each other by disulfide bonds, and each heavy chain is linked to a light chain by a disulfide bond to form a three-dimensional "Y"-shaped protein (Fig. 21.1). In any single IgG molecule, the two heavy chains are identical to each another, as are the two light chains.[10] The two outstretched arms of the "Y", known as the "fragment antigen binding" or Fab portion, are responsible for recognizing and binding specific antigens. The Fab comprises constant, variable, and hypervariable regions; the latter of which enable the antibody to bind to the specific cognate antigen epitope. The base of the "Y" is known as the Fc portion, which mediates physiological functions of the antibody such as triggering antibody-dependent cell-mediated cytotoxicity (ADCC) through Fc receptors (FcR) on effector cells as well as providing the site for complement binding.[10]

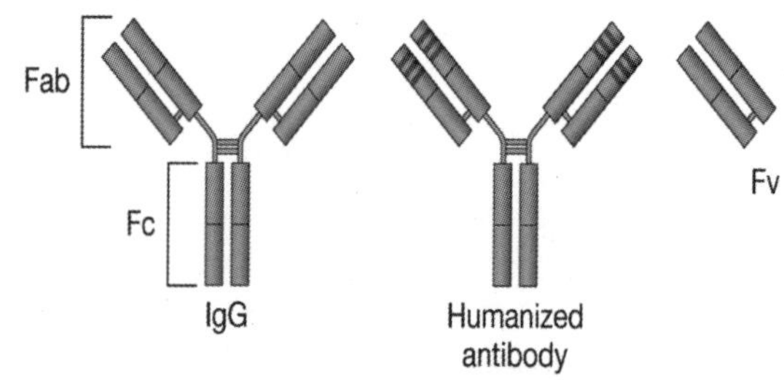

Fig. 21.1. Antibody structure. The IgG molecule is composed of two longer (heavy) chains and two shorter (light) chains that are connected by disulfide bonds. The amino acid sequence of the variable (v) ends of each of the four chains determines the specificity of antigen binding. Humanized MoAb constructs consist predominantly of human amino acid sequences, with the exception of the three hypervariable CDRs, which retain the foreign specie sequences critical for antigen binding. The CDR domains are indicated by the dark bands at the end of the antigen-binding portion of the molecule.

*CDR: complementarity-determining region; Fab: antigen-binding fragment; Fc: crystallizable or complement fixing fragment; Fv: variable fragment; IgG: immunoglobulin G.

Modified and used with permission from Wayne AS, Capitini CM, Mackall CL: Immunotherapy of childhood cancer: From biologic understanding to clinical application. Curr Opin Pediatr 2010; 22(1):2–11.

Nomenclature and classification of MoAbs

Anti-cancer MoAbs are generated by immunization of nonhuman species with tumor-associated antigens (TAA). In chimeric antibodies, the entire variable domain of both heavy and light chains that recognize the TAA represent foreign species-derived amino acids (5–30% of the MoAb composition). This is linked to heavy and light constant regions of human origin. In humanized antibodies, the variable region is modified to contain more of the human amino acid sequence (approximately 90% human homology). Humanized antibodies contain complementary-determining regions (CDR), the antigen-binding sites of nonhuman origin, which recognize the TAA interspersed among variable domain segments of human-derived amino acid sequences. The humanized variable heavy and light domains are linked to heavy and light constant regions of human origin. Such MoAb constructs are less immunogenic in comparison to unmodified MoAbs (Fig. 21.1).

MoAb reagents are named based on their four components according to standards adopted by the US Adoptive Name Council (USANC) (Table 21.1).[11,12] All include a prefix specific to the individual product and end with the suffix "mab". The internal designations specify the disease or target class and the species source. MoAbs can be further classified as unconjugated or conjugated, the names of the latter of which include the specific conjugate compound (e.g. ^{90}Y, ozogamicin, diphtheria toxin).

Mechanism of action of unconjugated MoAbs

Antibodies may mediate anti-tumor effects by a variety of effector mechanisms, including ADCC, complement-dependent cytotoxicity (CDC), cytokine

Table 21.1. Naming system for monoclonal antibody reagents.[a,b]

Prefix	Unique to the reagent
Substem A: Target/Disease class	Bacterial: -b(a)- Cardiovascular: -c(i)- Fungal: -f(u)- Interleukin: -k(i)- Immunomodulatory -l(i)- Neural: -n(e)- Bone: -s(o)- Toxin: -tox(a)- Tumor: -tu(m,z)- Viral: -v(i)-
Substem B: Species source and construct	Rat: a Hamster: e Primate: i Mouse: o Human: u Chimeric: xi Humanized: zu
Suffix	–mab

[a]United States Adoptive Name Council (USANC).
http://www.ama-assn.org/ama/pub/about-ama/our-people/coalitions-consortiums/united-states-adopted-names-council/naming-guidelines/naming-biologics/monoclonal-antibodies.shtml.
[b]The International Nonproprietary Names (INN) Programme of the World Health Organization (WHO).
http://www.who.int/medicines/services/inn/en/index.html.
http://www.who.int/medicines/services/inn/Generalpoliciesformonoclonal antibodies 2009.pdf.

activation, and/or inducing or blocking intracellular signals leading to apoptosis (Table 21.2) (Fig. 21.2). The exact mechanisms of action of many of the clinically active antibodies remain unknown. Understanding these might help to circumvent resistance to MoAbs and to develop therapies to enhance anti-tumor efficacy.

Antibody-dependent cellular cytotoxicity

ADCC is a well-recognized immune effector mechanism in which antigen-specific antibodies direct innate immune effector cells to kill antibody-coated antigen expressing cancer cells.[13] This property is dependent upon interactions between FcRs on immune accessory cells and the Fc portion of an antibody.[14] Fc binding causes cross-linking of FcRs, which leads to effector cell activation. While ADCC can be mediated by natural killer (NK) cells, monocyte-macrophages, and neutrophils, NK cells are the principal ADCC effectors as they express type IIIA FcRs (FcRγIIIa; CD16a) on their surface,[15] which play a dominant role in triggering NK cell-mediated ADCC.[16] The importance of ADCC in the anti-tumor effects of rituximab is demonstrated by the finding that patients with follicular lymphoma who have CD16 polymorphisms associated with high affinity FcRs have improved relapse-free survival after treatment with rituximab.[17]

Complement-dependent cytotoxicity (CDC)

Binding of MoAbs to TAA not only initiates ADCC, but also can result in binding of the antibody Fc to the C1q component of the complement system. This in turn triggers the cascade of complement activation and the formation of the membrane attack complex, which can lead to tumor cell death.

Other mechanisms

Unconjugated MoAbs have a number of additional potential mechanisms of action. Cytotoxicity may result in priming of antigen-specific T cells through the cross presentation of TAAs released by dying cells.[4] Antibodies may induce cell death through the activation of cytokines (e.g. tumor necrosis factor [TNF]α) or signaling pathways (e.g. TNF-related apoptosis-inducing ligand [TRAIL]), or alternatively, through the inhibition of cytokines or signaling pathways necessary for cell survival (e.g. IGF1R). The relative importance of each mechanism varies with the type of malignancy and the specific MoAb agent.[18,19]

Conjugated MoAbs

MoAbs can be rendered highly and directly cytotoxic by conjugation to radioactive isotopes, toxins, or chemotherapeutic agents (Table 21.2). MoAb-based agents armed with such potently cytotoxic moieties do not require active immune response mechanisms for activity, and thus can be effective even in profoundly immunocompromised hosts, such as CAYA with cancer.

Immunotoxins

Bacterial and plant toxins are cytotoxic proteins that induce cell death after internalization through the inhibition of protein synthesis (Fig. 21.3). Plant toxins inhibit protein synthesis by inactivating ribosomes. Examples include ricin A chain (RTA), pokeweed antiviral protein (PAP), and saporin. Bacterial toxins,

Table 21.2. Monoclonal antibody-based reagents for hematologic malignancies in CAYA.

Antigen	Antibody/toxin	Type	Proposed mechanism	Remarks	CAYA clinical trial status
CD19	XmAb5574	Humanized	ADCC, direct cellular cytotoxicity	Enhanced affinity for FcγRIII receptor on effector cells	Pre-clinical studies ongoing
	Anti-B4-bR	Murine	Apoptosis	Ricin toxin conjugate	Pediatric Phase I
CD20	Rituximab	Chimeric	ADCC, CDC, signal inhibition	FDA approved for adult NHL	Pediatric Phase II–II
	Ofatumumab	Human	CDC	Slower off-rate, diminished immunogenicity	Phase I–III adult lymphoma, autoimmune disorders
	Ocrelizumab rhuH27	Humanized	ADCC, CDC, signal inhibition	Binds different epitope than rituximab	Phase I–III adult autoimmune disorders
	PRO131921	Humanized	ADCC	Enhanced affinity for FcγRIII receptor on effector cells	Phase I–II adult CLL, NHL
	Veltuzumab hA20	Humanized	ADCC, CDC, signal inhibition	Slow off-rate, potentially less immunogenic than rituximab	Phase I–II adult NHL
	GA-101	Humanized	ADCC, signal inhibition	Enhanced affinity for FcγRIII receptor on effector cells	Phase I–II adult NHL
	^{90}Y-ibritumomab-tiuxetan	Chimeric	Targeted radiation	β-emitter radioimmunoconjugate composed of the murine parent of rituximab, ibritumomab (Y2B8), an IgG1 antibody, with tiuxetan	Pediatric Phase I
CD22	Epratuzumab	Humanized	ADCC, CDC, signal inhibition	Receptor/antigen complex is rapidly internalized after binding	Pediatric Phase I–II
	90Y-Epratuzumab	Humanized	Targeted radiation	β-emitter radioimmunoconjugate composed of the humanized parent of epratuzumab	Phase II adult follicular NHL
	Inotuzumab ozogamicin	Humanized	Apoptosis	Drug conjugate (calicheamicin)	Phase II adult NHL (with rituximab)
	CAT-3888 (BL22), Moxetumomab pasudotox (CAT-8015, HA22)	Murine	Apoptosis	Pseudomonas exotoxin conjugate	Pediatric Phase I, Phase II adult
	Combotox	Murine	Apoptosis	Mixture of ricin-based immunotoxins targeting both CD22 and CD19	Pediatric Phase I
CD25	Denileukin difititox	Recombinant	Apoptosis	IL-2 conjugated to *diphtheria* exotoxin	FDA approved for adult CTCL
	Daclizumab	Humanized	Apoptosis	Anti-IL-2 receptor α	Phase I–II ATLL
	90Y-Daclizumab	Humanized	Targeted radiation	β-emitter radioimmunoconjugate	Phase II adult hematological malignancies
	LMB-2	Murine	Apoptosis	Pseudomonas exotoxin conjugate	Phase II CLL and CTCL
	CHT-25 ^{131}I	Humanized	Targeted radiation	Chimeric antibody radioconjugate	Phase I HL and NHL
CD30	SGN-30	Chimeric	Growth arrest, apoptosis, ADCC		Phase I–II pediatric and adult HL and ALCL
	XmAb2513	Humanized	ADCC	Enhanced affinity for FcγRIII receptor on effector cells	Phase I adult HL and ALCL

(*Continued*)

Table 21.2. (*Continued*)

Antigen	Antibody/toxin	Type	Proposed mechanism	Remarks	CAYA clinical trial status
	MDX-060	Human	ADCC		Phase I/II ALCL and HL (> 12 yrs)
	MDX-1401	Human	ADCC	Non-fucosylated with enhanced affinity for FcγRIII receptor on effector cells	Phase I HL (> 12 yrs)
	Hefi-1	Murine	Apoptosis		Phase I adults
	Brentuximab vedotin (SGN-35)	Chimeric	Anti-mitotic	Drug conjugate (monomethyl auristatin E, MMAE, a highly potent anti-tubulin agent)	Phase I–III adults, Phase I–II (> 12 yrs)
CD33	Gemtuzumab ozogamicin	Humanized	Apoptosis	Drug conjugate (calicheamicin)	Pediatric Phase I-III, FDA approved for adult AML
	^{131}I-CD33	Humanized	Targeted radiation	β-emitter radioimmunoconjugate	Phase I adult AML
	^{213}Bi-CD33	Humanized	Targeted radiation	α-emitter radioimmunoconjugate	Phase I adult AML
CD52	Alemtuzumab	Humanized	ADCC, CDC, apoptosis	Highly immunosuppressive	AlloSCT conditioning in pediatrics
CD74	Milatuzumab	Humanized	Anti-proliferation, apoptosis		Phase I–II adult CLL and B-NHL
	hLL1-DPOX	Humanized	Apoptosis	Doxorubicin conjugate	Phase I MM
CD80	Galiximab	Primatized	Anti-proliferation, apoptosis, ADCC	Structure indistinguishable from human antibody, less immunogenic in humans	Phase II–III adult NHL
CD2	Siplizumab	Humanized	ADCC	High incidence of EBV-related lymphoproliferative disease	Phase I adults Pediatric Phase I (GVHD)
	Alefacept	Dimeric fusion protein	ADCC	CD2-binding domain of CD58 linked to IgG Fc	Phase I adults
CD3	Muromonab-CD3	Murine	ADCC		Pediatric Phase I–II
	Visilizumab	Humanized	Apoptosis		Phase I adults Pediatric Phase I–II (GVHD)
	A-dmDT390-bisFv (UCHT1)	Murine	Apoptosis	Diphtheria toxin A conjugate	Phase I–II adults
CD4	Zanolimumab	Human	ADCC	Prevents T-cell activation	Phase I–III adult hematologic malignancies

ADCC: antibody dependent cellular cytotoxicity; AlloSCT: allogeneic stem cell transplantation; AML: acute myeloid leukemia; ATLL: adult T-cell leukemia/lymphoma; CDC: complement dependent cytotoxicity; CLL: chronic lymphocytic leukemia; COG: The Children's Oncology Group; CTCL: cutaneous T-cell lymphoma; EBV: Ebstein Barr virus; FDA: Food and Drug Administration; GVHD: graft-vs.-host disease; HL: Hodgkin lymphoma; MM: multiple myeloma; NHL: non-Hodgkin lymphoma; TRAIL: tumor necrosis factor-related apoptosis-inducing ligand.

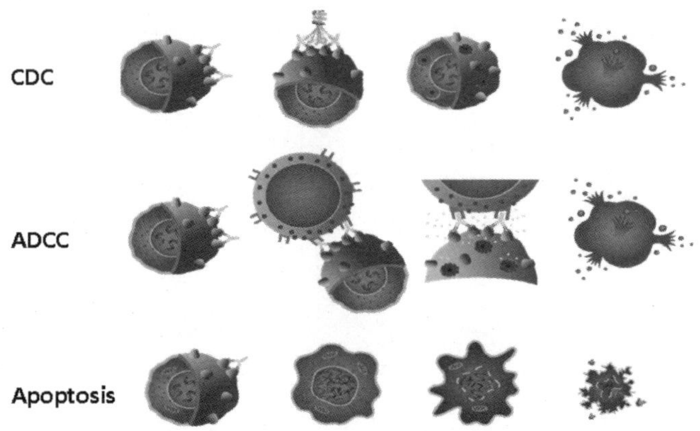

Fig. 21.2. Mechanism of action of monoclonal antibodies.

Complement-Dependent Cytotoxicity (CDC)

MoAbs bind to tumor associated antigens on the cell surface. Subsequently, the Fc portion of the MoAb binds to the C1q component of the complement system. This in turn triggers the cascade of complement activation and the formation of the membrane attack complex, which can lead to tumor cell death.

Antibody-dependent cellular cytotoxicity (ADCC)

Binding of FcRs on immune accessory cells by the Fc portion of MoAbs causes FcR cross-linking, which leads to effector cell activation.

Apoptosis

Binding of MoAb to antigens on the cell surface results in disruption of a cell survival pathway or initiation of a death signal leading to cell death.

including Pseudomonas exotoxin (PE) and Diphtheria toxin (DT), inhibit protein synthesis via inactivation of elongation factor (EF)-2.

Immunotoxins are engineered proteins that consist of two main components: a MoAb or antibody fragment that serves as a binding domain and targets cells that express the cognate antigen, and the toxin moiety. A variety of such agents have been developed for the treatment of hematologic malignancies (Table 21.2). Because small proteins distribute more efficiently through tissues (including tumors), Fv fragments are more commonly employed than larger antibodies in the generation of immunoconjugates for clinical use. In general, clinical development of immunotoxins has been hindered by nonspecific toxicities, immunogenicity, and production difficulties. At the National Cancer Institute (NCI), a 38-kD truncated derivative of Pseudomonas exotoxin A (PE38) has been used in the development of recombinant immunotoxins that target human differentiation antigens.[20] Serial modifications have reduced nonspecific toxicities, increased stability, increased tissue penetration, and improved targeted cytotoxicity.

Radioconjugates

MoAbs that target hematologic malignancy-associated antigens have been linked to radioactive isotopes, most commonly β-emitters (e.g. ^{90}Yttrium, ^{131}Iodine, ^{186}Rhenium) and less frequently α-emitters (e.g. ^{213}Bismuth). Yttrium-90 (^{90}Y) is a pure β-emitting radioisotope. In comparison with iodine-131 (^{131}I), ^{90}Y delivers five times more energy, has a path length of 5 mm vs. 0.8 mm, and has a more favorable half-life of 2.5 days vs. 8 days.[21] Consequently, it is commonly utilized in MoAb-based conjugates. Radioisotopes conjugated to MoAbs offer a number of potential therapeutic advantages. Notably, internalization is not required for activity. Additionally, crossfire from the radioisotope can induce cell death to neighboring cells inaccessible because of tumor bulk, poor vascular supply, and/or low expression of the antigen target. Importantly, radioconjugates that target hematopoietic antigens (e.g. CD45) are concentrated in the marrow and are associated with severe myelosuppression. This is also the case in the treatment of leukemias in general. Consequently, radioimmunotherapy may be employed as part of conditioning prior to stem cell transplant (SCT), although there have been limited studies of this approach in the setting of hematologic malignancies of CAYA. The biophysical properties, advantages and disadvantages of various radioactive isotopes are described in Table 21.3.[22]

Drug conjugates

MoAbs have been conjugated to various cytotoxic drugs. The first of such agent to receive FDA approval was gemtuzumab ozogamicin, which is an anti-CD33 MoAb linked to calicheamicin. The anti-tumor antibiotic calicheamicin binds the minor groove of DNA and induces double-strand breaks leading to cell death. This agent has also been conjugated to anti-CD20 (rituximab)[23] and anti-CD22 (inotuzumab).[24] A number of anthracycline constructs have been developed, including an anti-CD19 conjugate.[25] Anti-CD7 has been conjugated to TRAIL fusion protein.[26]

Possible therapeutic targets of MoAbs in CAYA hematological malignancies

A number of differentiation antigens commonly expressed on the surface of hematologic malignancies encountered in CAYA represent logical targets of MoAb-based therapies (Tables 21.2 and 21.4) (see Chapter 4).

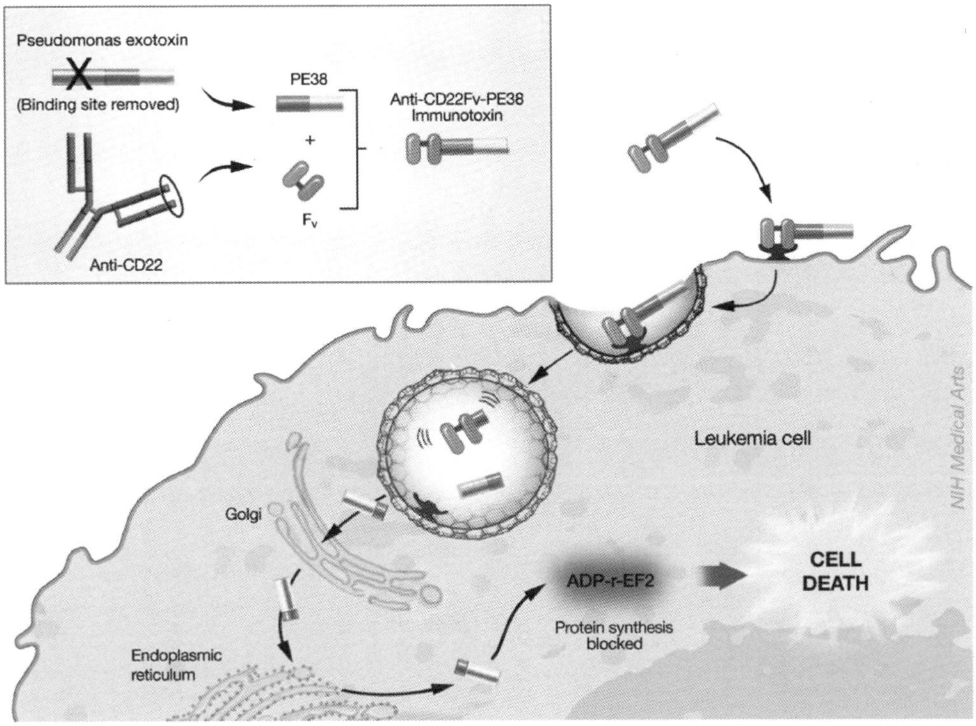

Fig. 21.3. Mechanism of action of immunotoxins. (Inset) Full-length *Pseudomonas* exotoxin A protein contains three functional domains that mediate antigen binding, cytosolic translocation, and cytotoxicity. The recombinant anti-CD22 immunotoxin RFB4(dsFv)–PE38 consists of cloned disulfide-stabilized single-chain Fv from the anti-CD22 MoAb RFB4 and the *Pseudomonas* exotoxin A translocation and killing domains (PE38). Immunotoxin binding to surface CD22 is followed by internalization through endocytosis. Immunotoxin cleavage occurs in the endosome and the C-terminal fragment is transported to the cytosol. ADP-r inactivates EF2, which inhibits protein synthesis causing cell death.

ADP-r: ADP ribosylation; EF2: elongation factor 2; Fv: variable fragment; PE38: 38-kDa truncated derivative of Pseudomonas exotoxin A.

Modified and used with permission from Wayne AS, Capitini CM, Mackall CL: Immunotherapy of childhood cancer: From biologic understanding to clinical application. Curr Opin Pediatr 2010;22(1):2–11.

A Children's Oncology Group (COG) immunohistochemical study of pediatric lymphoma specimens revealed that the majority of B-NHL specimens were positive for CD10, CD19, CD20, CD22, CD52, CD74, and CD80, the majority of T-NHL samples were positive for CD52 and CD25, and anaplastic large cell lymphoma (ALCL) was positive for CD25 (Table 21.4).[27–30] The neoplastic cells in Hodgkin lymphoma commonly express antigens that are targets of available reagents (e.g. CD30). Additionally, infiltrating inflammatory cells that comprise the bulk of Hodgkin lesions can be targeted with MoAbs that target lymphoid antigens. MoAb-based reagents have been developed to target the following antigens relevant to hematologic malignancies of CAYA (Table 21.2).

CD19 is a 95-kD glycoprotein member of the immunoglobulin superfamily expressed throughout the B-cell lineage from the early precursor to the mature B cell, but not on plasma cells. CD19 functions as a costimulatory molecule and a response regulator of B cell signaling. CD19 is internalized after antibody binding, albeit relatively slowly in comparison to other antigens such as CD22.[31] It is expressed in high density on nearly all cases of pre-B, B-cell ALL, Burkitt lymphoma (BL), and diffuse large B-cell lymphoma (DLBCL).

CD20 is a 35-kD glycoprotein expressed on almost all circulating B cells. It is present from the late pre-B cell stage until just prior to terminal differentiation into plasma cells. CD20 mediates intracellular signaling and is believed to play a regulatory role in B-cell proliferation and differentiation. CD20 is not internalized after antibody binding. The majority of children with B-ALL, BL, and DLBCL are positive for CD20. Many patients with nodular lymphocyte predominant Hodgkin lymphoma and a minority of cases of pre-B ALL are CD20 positive as well.

CD22 is a 140-kD glycoprotein member of the immunoglobulin superfamily that functions as a B-cell receptor signal transduction modifier and a cellular

Table 21.3. Radioisotopes used in immunotherapy.

Isotope	$T_{1/2}$ (hrs)	Radiation	Path length (mm)	Advantages	Disadvantages
Iodine-131	193	β, γ	0.8	Simple covalent conjugation Inexpensive Suitable for imaging	Dehalogenation High radiation exposure to others
Yttrium-90	64	β	5.3	Negligible isotope release from chelator High β energy Good tumor penetration Negligible exposure risk	Chelator for labeling Not for imaging Expensive
Copper-67	59	β, γ	0.6	Negligible release from chelator Suitable for imaging	Chelator for labeling Not readily available
Rhenium-186	89	β, γ	1.8	Negligible release from chelator Suitable for imaging	Chelator for labeling Not readily available
Rhenium-188	17	β, γ	4.4	Negligible release from chelator Suitable for imaging Good tumor penetration High β energy	Chelator for labeling $T_{1/2}$ too short for intact IgG monoclonal
Bismuth-212	1	α	0.06–0.1	Excellent cell kill	Short $T_{1/2}$; not useful for imaging
Astatine-211	7	α	0.08	Excellent cell kill	Short $T_{1/2}$; not useful for imaging

Used with permission from Betham Science Publishers: Cheson BD. Radioimmunotherapy of Non-Hodgkin's Lymphomas. Current Drug Targets, 2006, 7, 1293–1300.

Table 21.4. Surface expression of selected differentiation antigens in pediatric leukemia and lymphoma.

Subtype	CD3	CD10	CD19	CD20	CD22	CD25	CD30	CD33	CD52
B-ALL	Rare	50–98%	95–100%	11–40%	96–100%	16–38%	0%	15%	89%
T-ALL	c-100% s-83%	45%	0%	0%	0%	4%	0%	Rare	77–100%
AML	Rare	0%	Rare	0%	Rare	0%	0%	80–100%	36–66%
Burkitt Lymphoma and Leukemia	0%	100%	100%	100%	100%	0%	0%	0%	89%
DLBCL	0%	70–100%	80–90%	100%	98%	0%	0%	0%	98%
T-LBL	c-85% s-46%	57%	Rare	Rare	Rare	8%	6%	14%	100%
ALCL	45%	0%	0%	0%	0%	85%	100%	0%	100%

Data represent percentage of cases that are antigen positive by flow cytometry and/or immunohistochemistry from published series.

ALCL: anaplastic large cell lymphoma; ALL: acute lymphoid leukemia; AML: acute myeloid leukemia; c: cytoplasmic; DLBCL: diffuse large B-cell lymphoma; NA: not applicable; s: surface; T-LBL: T-cell lymphoblastic lymphoma.

adhesion molecule. CD22 appears on the cell surface simultaneously with IgD. Most mature B cells are CD22+ with the exception of plasma cells. CD22 is rapidly internalized after antibody binding. Nearly all children with BL, B-ALL, DLBCL and pre-B ALL have surface expression of CD22.

CD25 The human interleukin-2 receptor (IL-2R) exists in three forms, low (CD25), intermediate (CD122/CD132), and high (CD25/CD122/CD132) affinity. CD25 is a 55-kD inducible receptor that is only expressed on activated T cells, B cells, NK cells, and cells of the monocyte/macrophage system, as well as the regulatory subset of CD4+ cells that express FOXP3 (Treg). CD25 binding dramatically enhances the affinity of the IL-2R, but does not contribute directly to signal transduction. CD25 is internalized upon antigen binding. A soluble form is shed into the circulation serving as a tumor marker. The majority of cases of ALCL in children are CD25+. HTLV-I associated adult T-cell leukemia/lymphoma (ATLL) and certain mature peripheral T-cell lymphomas, although rare in children, are also CD25 positive.

CD30 is a 120-kDa transmembrane glycoprotein of the TNF receptor family that contains six cysteine-rich repeat motifs in its extracellular domain. Like many TNF receptors, CD30 can be shed in a soluble form (sCD30), which can serve as a tumor marker. CD30 is internalized and it is expressed in Hodgkin lymphoma, ALCL, immunoblastic lymphoma and ATLL.

CD33 is a transmembrane receptor expressed on cells of myeloid lineage. It is usually considered myeloid-specific, but it can also be found on some lymphoid cells. It binds sialic acids and is a member of the sialic acid binding Ig-like lectins (SIGLEC) family of lectins. The extracellular portion of this receptor contains two immunoglobulin domains placing CD33 within the immunoglobulin superfamily. The intracellular portion of CD33 contains immunoreceptor tyrosine-based inhibitory motifs (ITIMs) that are implicated in inhibition of cellular activity. CD33 is internalized after binding and this antigen is expressed in AML, JMML, CML and bi-phenotypic leukemia and some cases of infant ALL.

CD52 is a 28-kD glycoprotein expressed on the surface of normal B and T lymphocytes, NK cells, monocytes, macrophages, and granulocytes. CD52 is a non-modulating antigen coupled to the membrane by a glycosylphosphatidylinositol anchor that is neither internalized nor shed. CD52 is expressed by almost all cases of BL, DLBCL, T-cell lymphoblastic leukemia and lymphoma, ALCL, hepatosplenic gamma-delta T-cell lymphoma, and pre-B ALL, and some cases of AML.

CD74 The CD74 antigen represents the non-polymorphic, transmembrane protein invariant chain of the HLA class II molecule.[32] Surface CD74 functions as an accessory signaling molecule and participates in B cell differentiation, maturation, proliferation and survival. This antigen is rapidly internalized and is expressed on a variety of B-cell malignancies including B-NHL.[33]

CD80 or B7.1, is a surface glycoprotein member of the B7-family of costimulatory molecules. It provides critical signals to T cells and is expressed on a subset of normal B cells, antigen presenting cells, subtypes of B-cell lymphomas, and Hodgkin Reed–Sternberg cells.[34]

Additional MoAbs against T-cell malignancies

T-cell malignancies are categorized into two major groups in the current World Health Organization (WHO) classification: (1) immature or pre-thymic T-cell leukemias and lymphomas, and (2) the more mature post-thymic or peripheral T-cell disorders (see Chapters 2 and 4).[35] Mature post-thymic or peripheral T-cell disorders are rare in pediatric populations. T-lineage hematologic malignancies express various surface molecules that can serve as potential targets for MoAbs, immunotoxins or toxin–ligand fusion proteins. These include the pan-T-cell antigen CD2, the T-cell receptor complex CD3, CD4, CD5, various cytokine receptors and their subunits including CD25, CD30, and CD122, and the surface glycoprotein CD52 (Table 21.2). Notably, activity has been observed in adults with T-lineage hematologic malignancies treated with anti-T cell MoAb reagents that have been developed as immunosuppressive agents,[36] and clinical trials in adults with T-cell leukemias and lymphomas have been conducted (Table 21.2).

Clinical trials with MoAbs in CAYA hematological malignancies

Stimulated in part by successes by MoAb-based therapies in adults, trials have recently been conducted in CAYA with hematologic malignancies. The limited number of studies of MoAb-based agents in CAYA populations are reviewed below.

Anti-CD20–targeted therapy

Among the major advances in the treatment of hematologic malignancies over the past decade has been the incorporation of unconjugated anti-CD20 MoAb (rituximab) into the therapy of NHL in adults (see Chapters 16 and 17). Efficacy of rituximab as a single agent and in synergistic combination with chemotherapy has been demonstrated in indolent and high-grade NHL, respectively.[37,38] Trials in adults conducted by the German Multicentre Study Group of Adult ALL[39] and the MD Anderson Cancer Center suggest that rituximab might be safely administered with chemotherapy for B-ALL/Burkitt NHL,[40] and that outcome might be improved in comparison to chemotherapy-treated historical controls. Data on the use of anti-CD20 MoAbs in pediatric lymphoma and leukemia are slowly emerging. The German Berlin-Frankfurt–Munster (BFM) group conducted a Phase II window study to examine the activity of rituximab in children with newly diagnosed B-NHL. Forty-two percent of patients demonstrated histological and/or radiological response to rituximab as a single agent.[41] The most frequent toxicities attributable to rituximab were infusion-related reactions. There were no therapy-related deaths. In a recent COG trial (ANHL01P1), rituximab was added to the induction and consolidation chemotherapy in children with newly diagnosed group B and group C B-NHL (leukemia and lymphoma) treated with the backbone of LMB/FAB-96 therapy. Rituximab infusion appeared to be safe and well tolerated and there was no apparent increase in grade 3–4 toxicities compared to the historical LMB/FAB-96 study. Analysis of event-free survival (EFS) and overall survival in comparison to the LMB/FAB-96 study is in progress. However, a randomized prospective trial is needed in order to evaluate the utility of the addition of rituximab to chemotherapy for children with B-NHL.[42,43] The COG conducted a Phase II pilot study, ANHL0121, to assess the toxicity and efficacy of ifosfamide/carboplatin/etoposide (ICE) chemotherapy in combination with rituximab in children and adolescents with recurrent/refractory B-NHL and mature B-ALL.[44] In this study, a 60% response rate was observed, which appears to be comparable to previous reports of other salvage regimens. Three-year overall survival (OS) for patients who responded was 65% vs. 0% for non-responders ($p = 0.0001$).

^{90}Yttrium-ibritumomab-tiuxetan (^{90}Y-IT) is a radioimmunoconjugate of the murine parent of rituximab, ibritumomab (Y2B8), an IgG1 antibody. In a randomized controlled study comparing ^{90}Y-IT vs. rituximab in adults with relapsed or refractory low-grade follicular or transformed B-NHL, the overall response rate (ORR) and CR rates were significantly improved with radioimmunoconjugate (80% vs. 56%, $P = 0.002$, and 30% vs. 16%, $P < 0.04$ respectively).[21] The COG conducted a phase I study of ^{90}Y-IT in children and adolescents with relapsed/refractory CD20+ NHL. In this study, patients received rituximab on days 0 and 7 and ^{111}Indium ibritumomab–tiuxetan on day 0. Dosimetry studies were done on days 0, 1, 3, and 6. Immediately after rituximab on day 7, patients received ^{90}Y-IT. Five patients were treated and none experienced dose-limiting toxicity (DLT), however, no disease responses were observed.[45] In some studies in adults with aggressive and indolent refractory/relapsed NHL, ^{90}Y-IT and ^{131}I-tositumomab have been integrated in the conditioning regimen for autologous hematopoietic stem cell transplant and reduced intensity conditioning allogeneic stem cell transplant (AlloSCT).[46]

Anti-CD22–targeted therapy

Epratuzumab is a humanized anti-CD22 MoAb. Safety and efficacy of epratuzumab as a single agent and in combination with chemotherapy have been demonstrated in small single center Phase I–II studies in adults with indolent and aggressive B-NHL.[47,48] In recurrent indolent lymphoma, responses were only noted in patients with follicular NHL. Notably, however, a 43% ORR was observed in follicular NHL at doses of 360 mg/m^2/wk.[47] In heavily pretreated adults with aggressive NHL, 10% of patients achieved responses including a few CRs.[48] The combination of rituximab and epratuzumab was associated with ORRs of 60% in recurrent indolent and 67% in aggressive lymphoma.[49] These encouraging results need to be confirmed in larger multicenter Phase II–III studies. To date, no studies of epratuzumab have been conducted in children with B-NHL.

The COG is conducting a pilot study of chemoimmunotherapy reinduction in combination with epratuzumab in children with ALL and marrow relapse (see Chapter 11).[50] This study included an upfront monotherapy phase of epratuzumab that was designed to provide information about single agent activity of epratuzumab in the setting of relapsed pediatric ALL. The single-agent phase consisted of epratuzumab 360 mg/m^2/dose intravenously for four doses. Four weekly doses of epratuzumab were then administered in combination with a three-block reinduction chemotherapy regimen that was previously studied by the COG (AALL01P2 trial).[51] Fifteen patients were enrolled in the first cohort of this study and the response to epratuzumab alone was assessed at the completion of the monotherapy phase.[50] Eleven patients had stable disease, one patient had a PR cytolytic response (defined as complete disappearance of circulating blasts and achievement of at least 50% reduction from baseline in bone marrow blast count), and three had progressive disease. Median absolute blast counts decreased from 384/μL (range: 0–9400/μL) at study entry to 17/μL (range: 0–55,088/μL) at the end of the epratuzumab monotherapy phase. One patient showed a rise in absolute blast count to more than 50,000/μL. Twenty-four hours after the initial dose of epratuzumab 95–98% of the binding sites on leukemic blasts were engaged with epratuzumab as assessed by flow cytometry. At the end of block 1 chemoimmunotherapy, nine patients achieved CR, and seven of these children had no detectable minimal residual disease (MRD). The Phase II portion of this study is currently underway to determine whether remission reinduction rates and MRD responses at the end of block 1 are superior to those achieved with this chemotherapy platform alone based on historical controls.[51]

Anti-CD22 recombinant immunotoxins

The anti-CD22 immunotoxin BL22 or CAT-3888 consists of disulfide-linked Fv portion of the RFB4 MoAb linked to PE38. CAT-3888 was shown to be highly active in a Phase I study in adults with B-lymphoid malignancies with a response rate of 80%.[52,53] CAT-3888 is potently cytotoxic against primary blasts from children with CD22+ ALL.[54] A Phase I trial of CAT-3888 for pediatric CD22+ leukemias and lymphomas was recently conducted at the NCI.[54] This agent was associated with an acceptable safety profile. All adverse events were self-limited, most were Grades 1 and 2, no DLT was observed. There was evidence for clinical activity; pharmacokinetic parameters indicated rapid drug binding by CD22+ blasts.

Moxetumomab pasudotox (HA22 or CAT-8015) is a second-generation anti-CD22 immunotoxin that represents a 3-amino acid Fv mutant of CAT-3888. In comparison to CAT-3888, this agent has an approximately 10-fold increased binding affinity for CD22, which results in an average 10-fold improvement in *in vitro* cytotoxicity in a variety of CD22+ malignancies, including childhood ALL.[55] Phase I clinical trials of moxetumomab pasudotox for adult and pediatric patients with CD22+ hematologic malignancies are in progress and a CR in a child with chemotherapy-refractory ALL has been observed with this agent.[56]

A Phase I trial of a mixture of ricin-based immunotoxins targeting both CD22 (RFB4-dgA) and CD19 (HD37-dgA), also known as Combotox, was recently conducted for pediatric patients with refractory or relapsed ALL.[57] In that trial, clinical activity was observed, including 3 of 17 (18%) CRs. Combotox was associated with severe adverse events and a high incidence of immunogenicity.[57] The maximum tolerated dose (MTD) was determined to be 5 mg/m^2/dose.

Other anti-CD22 targeted agents are in development. For example, a calicheamicin immunoconjugate CMC-544 (inotuzumab ozogamicin) has been shown to be active in preclinical models of ALL and in clinical trials in adults with NHL.[58]

Anti-CD19–targeted therapy

Anti-CD19 PAP was shown to be active against childhood pre-B ALL *in vitro* and in SCID xenografts alone and in combination with chemotherapy.[59,60] Phase I clinical trials of this agent, as well another anti-CD19 immunotoxin, anti-B4-bR, have been conducted in pediatric ALL through the Children's Cancer Group.[61] In the latter study, 19 patients were treated with anti-B4-bR given as two 7-day continuous infusions separated by 7 days. An MTD of 40 μg/kg/day was defined. DLT consisted of capillary leak syndrome. Grade 3 reversible elevation in transaminases was also seen. Human anti-mouse antibodies (HAMA) or human anti-toxin (HATA) antibodies developed in five (26%) patients. No CRs or PRs were observed in that trial.

Anti-CD52–targeted therapy

Alemtuzumab is FDA approved for the treatment of chronic lymphocytic leukemia. A few small studies have been conducted in adults with ALL and AML and rare disease responses using alemtuzumab as a single agent have been reported.[62,63] The COG conducted a Phase II study of single agent alemtuzumab in children with relapsed T-ALL and pre-B ALL. One of 13 (8%) patients achieved a CR.[64] Due to poor accrual, this study was terminated. Alemtuzumab has been used as a part of pretransplant conditioning to promote engraftment after AlloSCT for a variety of conditions including hematologic malignancies in children and young adults.[65]

Anti-CD33–targeted therapy

Gemtuzumab ozogamicin is a recombinant humanized IgG4 antibody directed against CD33 conjugated to a cytotoxic antibiotic, calicheamicin. After gemtuzumab ozogamicin binds to CD33, it is internalized and hydrolyzed, releasing calicheamicin, which intercalates into DNA resulting in cell death.

In a Phase I trial of gemtuzumab ozogamicin in children with relapsed and refractory AML, gemtuzumab ozogamicin was administered at 6–9 mg/m^2 per dose for two doses separated by 2 weeks (see Chapter 13). The MTD of gemtuzumab ozogamicin was determined to be 6 mg/m^2 and disease responses were demonstrated at all dose levels.[66] Notably, 40% of children developed sinusoidal obstruction syndrome (SOS) following AlloSCT. Based on encouraging Phase I results in children, the COG conducted a Phase II trial AAML00P2 to determine the MTD of gemtuzumab ozogamicin in combination with two chemotherapy regimens commonly used in pediatric AML, high-dose cytarabine and mitoxantrone (Arm A), and high-dose cytarabine with L-asparaginase (Arm B).[67] Eligibility included *de novo* AML refractory to initial induction, initial remission duration of less than 1 year, or secondary AML without prior therapy. This study defined the pediatric MTD of gemtuzumab ozogamicin to be 3 mg/m^2 in combination with cytarabine and mitoxantrone and 2 mg/m^2 in combination with cytarabine and L-asparaginase. Approximately 75% of patients in both treatment arms had at least one grade 3 or 4 non-hematologic toxicity reported. Infectious complications were most common, with infection with neutropenia experienced in 40–50% of patients. The incidence of severe SOS (16%) following AlloSCT was comparable to that observed after myeloablative unrelated AlloSCT in general.[67] Approximately 55% of patients in arm A and 40% of patients on arm B achieved either a CR or CR without platelet recovery with 2-year EFS and OS estimates of 31% ± 15% and 45% ± 16%, respectively.[67] The COG is currently conducting a Phase III randomized trial of gemtuzumab ozogamicin combined with conventional chemotherapy for *de novo* AML in children, adolescents, and young adults (AAML0531).

Phase I studies of gemtuzumab ozogamicin as a part of a myeloablative conditioning regimen prior to AlloSCT in high risk AML and another Phase I study of gemtuzumab ozogamicin as a consolidation after reduced intensity conditioning AlloSCT in average risk AML in children are ongoing.[68,69]

Anti-CD30–targeted therapy

Safety and tolerability of the anti-CD30 MoAb SGN-30 were assessed in adults with CD30+ malignancies in a Phase 1 multidose study (2, 4, 8, or 12 mg/kg weekly for 6 weeks).[70] Phase II studies of SGN-30 in adults with recurrent ALCL and Hodgkin lymphoma have been conducted with objective responses observed in ALCL, and stable disease in Hodgkin lymphoma (see Chapter 16 and 18).[71,72] The COG Phase I/II pilot study of ICE chemotherapy and SGN-30 in children with CD30+ recurrent ALCL (ANHL06P1) was closed prior to completion.

The MoAb conjugate SGN-35 (brentuximab vedotin) utilizes the antitubulin agent monomethyl auristatin E. Phase I studies of SGN-35 using 1 or 3 weekly doses have demonstrated modest clinical responses in patients with relapsed or refractory CD30-positive lymphomas.[73,74] SGN-35 is currently undergoing evaluation as monotherapy and in combination with chemotherapy.

Therapeutic combinations

There is rationale for considering various combination regimens. In comparison to chemotherapy, MoAb-based therapies have unique mechanisms of action and resistance, as well as different toxicity profiles. Additive anti-tumor activity is seen when immunotoxins are combined with chemotherapy *in vitro*[75] and synergy has been demonstrated in murine xenograft models.[76] Immunotoxin and/or unconjugated MoAb combinations that target separate antigens have also been shown to result in additive effects.[49, 77]

Gene-modified artificial chimeric receptors

Recently, gene therapy techniques have been utilized to create artificial chimeric T-cell receptors designed to enable immune effector cells to bind to and induce cellular cytotoxicity against malignant cells that express target differentiation antigens (e.g. CD19). Developmental efforts to apply this approach to childhood ALL are underway at a number of centers (see Chapter 23).[78–80]

Bispecific monoclonal antibodies

MoAb constructs with dual specificity for a leukemia-associated antigen and a surface receptor on immune effector cells can serve to direct cell-mediated cytotoxicity. A recombinant anti-CD19/anti-CD3 bispecific antibody (MT103, blinatumomab) has recently been shown to be active in Phase I testing in adults with hematologic malignancies.[81] A Phase II trial in adults with ALL is ongoing and pediatric trials are planned. Importantly, these agents recruit and thus require functional immune effector cells (e.g. T cells) for activity. Consequently, bispecific MoAbs may have increased activity following immune reconstitution after AlloSCT.

Toxicities related to MoAbs

There are a variety of side effects associated with MoAbs and immunotoxins. Acute infusion reactions are relatively common, although rarely treatment limiting. Infusion-related reactions are most likely related to the lysis of normal B and T cells as well malignant cells in circulation followed by release of cytokines, especially TNF.[82] These side effects are often more common with the first dose of therapy and they can usually be managed with antipyretics, antihistamines, and/or corticosteroids.

Depletion of normal hematopoietic cells that express the target antigen (e.g. B cells with rituximab) can be expected. As a result, immunosuppression and increased risk of infection is associated with a number of these agents. Hepatitis B virus reactivation with fulminant hepatic failure has been reported after treatment with rituximab and cytomegalovirus and Epstein–Barr virus reactivation have been observed after alemtuzumab. As noted above, SOS has been associated with gemtuzumab ozogamicin especially in the post-AlloSCT setting. Ibritumomab tiuxetan is associated with myelosuppression due to bone marrow irradiation. Myelosuppression has also been associated with rituximab of unclear etiology and with alemtuzumab presumed due to the expression of CD52 on neutrophils.[83] Post-marketing surveillance of rituximab revealed an association with progressive multifocal leukoencephalopathy, an invariably fatal condition characterized by CNS demyelination caused by reactivation of the JC polyomavirus. Other rare but serious adverse events reported in post-marketing surveillance include severe mucocutaneous reactions and gastrointestinal perforation. In patients receiving B cell-depleting MoAbs, quantitative immunoglobulin levels should be monitored and patients receiving T cell-depleting MoAbs should be monitored for T cell recovery. In general, all patients with hematologic malignancies treated with MoAb-based reagents should have close surveillance for possible infection and empiric antimicrobial therapy should be employed as clinically indicated.

Immunotoxins have been associated with a number of unique toxicities, for example, vascular leak syndrome (VLS) and hemolytic uremic syndrome (HUS). Fluid balance and renal function should be monitored closely. Laboratory abnormalities are relatively common and include hypoalbuminemia and transaminase elevation. Certain toxins have higher rates of toxicity (e.g. ricin). The risk of nonspecific toxin-related toxicity can be decreased through protein modifications.[84]

The impact of MoAb-based therapies on the developing immune system of young children with malignancies has not been well studied. Potential problems would be expected to be target specific and might include thymic damage, lymph node atrophy, reticuloendothelial system dysfunction, hypogammaglobulinemia or agammaglobulinemia, and reduction and slow recovery of B, T, and NK cells. Such effects might result in impaired development of normal immunity, diminished vaccine responses, increased risk of infection, and immune dysregulation (e.g. autoimmunity).

Immunogenicity following administration of MoAbs

Despite the creation of human/murine chimeric ("humanized") antibodies, Fv CDR3 regions are derived from foreign species. Similarly, toxins represent foreign proteins. Thus, antibodies may develop (e.g. HAMA, HATA) that neutralize or diminish drug activity and limit ongoing treatment. Immunogenicity is agent- and disease-specific. In addition, there may be pre-existing antibodies due to prior vaccination (e.g. Diphtheria) or infection (e.g. *Pseudomonas*). A number of approaches have been explored in an effort to reduce the immunogenicity of these agents. Utilization of humanized MoAbs or fragments is the most common employed methodology. Recently, B-cell epitope mapping has been conducted to identify immunogenic amino acids, with the goal to modify immunotoxin sequence in order to generate a less immunogenic protein construct.[85] Finally, combination treatment with immunosuppressive chemotherapy (e.g. fludarabine) is under investigation.

Resistance to MoAb therapy

There are a number of mechanisms that might confer resistance to MoAb therapy (Table 21.5).[86] Primary resistance could be due to (1) low level surface expression of the target on malignant cells or subsets, (2) loss or diminished surface expression due receptor shedding and/or down regulation of TAA, (3) internalization, (4) soluble TAA shed in blood circulation that binds and thus diminishes the efficacy of MoAbs, and (5) FcR polymorphism with impaired ADCC, as reported with rituximab.[86] Secondary resistance could be related to (1) increased catabolism or neutralization by HAMA, human anti-chimeric antibody (HACA), HATA, and human anti-humanized antibody (HAHA), (2) change in cell survival pathways resulting in decreased apoptosis (e.g. activation

Table 21.5. Possible mechanisms of resistance to MoAbs and approaches to overcome.

Mechanism	Example of resistance mechanism	Potential/theoretical mechanism to overcome resistance
TAA binding	Absent expression of TAA	Primary resistance
	Decreased expression of TAA	Frequent dosing of MoAb Administer cytokines to increase expression of TAA
	High soluble TAA concentration in circulation and surrounding tumor cells	Administer cytoreductive therapy with MoAb
	Increase in MoAb metabolism	Frequent dosing of MoAb
	Neutralizing antibodies	Use less immunogenic/antigenic MoAb
	Poor tumor penetration	Alter affinity, charge or size of antibody Use radioconjugated MoAb
Post MoAb binding events	Activation of NF-κB pathway	Use IKK inhibitors Bortezomib + MoAb may circumvent activation of NF-kB pathway
	Decreased apoptosis due to increased bcl-2	Antisense bcl-2 + MoAb MoAb + bcl-2 inhibitor
	Increase in complement inhibitors	Fludarabine can decrease expression of CD55/59 Antibodies to CD55/59
	Decreased ADCC due to FCγRIIIA polymorphism	MoAbs with enhanced affinity for FcγRIII receptor on effector cells (GA-101)
	Decreased effector cells	Autologous infusion of NK cells (collected pre-chemotherapy) Cytokine-mediated expansion of effector cells
	Expression of the multidrug resistance p-glycoprotein (associated with gemtuzumab)	Combination of MoAb and p-glycoprotein modulator

ADCC: antibody-dependent cellular cytotoxicity; IgG: immunoglobulin; IKK: I kappaB kinase; MoAb: monoclonal antibody; NK: natural killer; TAA: tumor-associated antigen.

of NFk-B and increased expression of bcl-2), and (3) expression of drug resistance genes (e.g. p-glycoprotein). Various other mechanisms for resistance and potential ways to overcome these are summarized in Table 21.5.

Conclusions

Efforts to target differentiation antigens expressed on the surface of malignant cells have been facilitated by the development of MoAbs, recombinant immunotoxins, and more recently, artificial chimeric cellular receptors. The optimal agents, dose, schedule, and combination regimens have yet to be defined, but ongoing clinical trials offer promise in that regard. The experience in a number of hematologic malignancies of adulthood suggest that MoAb-based therapies will lead to improvements in disease-free-survival with reduced toxicity in comparison to currently standard treatment regimens for individuals with childhood hematological malignancies.

Acknowledgments

The authors acknowledge Dr. Ira Pastan, Dr. Robert Kreitman, and Dr. David Fitzgerald, colleagues in the Center for Cancer Research, National Cancer Institute. The authors would also like to acknowledge Erin Morris, RN, research nurse at Columbia University Medical Center for editorial assistance.

References

1. Cairo MS, Raetz E, Perkins SL. (2005) Non-Hodgkin's lymphoma in children. In: DW Kufe, RC Bast, WN Hait, WK Hong, R Pollock, RR Weichselbaum, *et al.* (eds). *Cancer Medicine* (7th ed.). Ontario, Canada: BC Decker Inc, pp. 1962–1976.
2. Pui CH, Cheng C, Leung W, Rai SN, Rivera GK, Sandlund JT, *et al.* (2003) Extended follow-up of long-term survivors of childhood acute lymphoblastic leukemia. *N Engl J Med* **349**(7): 640–649.
3. Gaynon PS. (2005) Childhood acute lymphoblastic leukaemia and relapse. *Br J Haematol* **131**(5): 579–587.
4. Cheson BD, Leonard JP. (2008) Monoclonal antibody therapy for B-cell non-Hodgkin's lymphoma. *N Engl J Med* **359**(6): 613–626.
5. Behring E, Kitasato S. (1998) Untersuchungen ueber das Zustandekommen der Diphtherie-Immunitat bei Thieren. In: TD Brock (ed). *Milestones in Microbiology: 1556 to 1940.* ASM Press, p. 141.
6. Ehrlich P. (1900) On immunity with special reference to the cell of life. *Proc R Soc London* **66**: 424–448.
7. Kohler G, Milstein C. (1975) Continuous cultures of fused cells secreting antibody of predefined specificity. *Nature* **256**(5517): 495–497.
8. Huston JS, Levinson D, Mudgett-Hunter M, Tai MS, Novotny J, Margolies MN, *et al.* (1988) Protein engineering of antibody binding sites: Recovery of specific activity in an anti-digoxin single-chain Fv analogue produced in Escherichia coli. *Proc Natl Acad Sci U S A* **85**(16): 5879–5883.
9. Johnson S, Bird RE. (1991) Construction of single-chain Fv derivatives monoclonal antibodies and their production in Escherichia coli. *Methods Enzymol* **203**: 88–98.
10. Janeway CA, Travers P, Walport M, Shlomchik MJ. (2001) *Immunobiology: The Immune System in Health and Disease* (5th ed). New York: Garland Science.
11. AMA (USAN) Monoclonal antibodies. United States Adopted Names. (2007) http://www.ama-assn.org/ama/pub/about-ama/our-people/coalitions-consortiums/united-states-adopted-names-council/naming-guidelines/naming-biologics/monoclonal-antibodies.shtml.
12. International Nonproprietary Names (INN) Programme of the World Health Organization (WHO). (2010) http://www.who.int/medicines/services/inn/en/index.html.
18. Jazirehi AR, Vega MI, Bonavida B. (2007) Development of rituximab-resistant lymphoma clones with altered cell signaling and cross-resistance to chemotherapy. *Cancer Res* **67**(3): 1270–1281.
20. Pastan I, Hassan R, Fitzgerald DJ, Kreitman RJ. (2006) Immunotoxin therapy of cancer. *Nat Rev Cancer* **6**(7): 559–565.
21. Cheson BD. (2003) Radioimmunotherapy of non-Hodgkin lymphomas. *Blood* **101**(2): 391–398.
23. Dijoseph JF, Dougher MM, Armellino DC, Kalyandrug L, Kunz A, Boghaert ER, *et al.* (2007) CD20-specific antibody-targeted chemotherapy of non-Hodgkin's B-cell lymphoma using calicheamicin-conjugated rituximab. *Cancer Immunol Immunother* **56**(7): 1107–1117.
24. Fayad L, Patel H, Verhoef G, Czuczman MS, Foran J, Gine E, *et al.* (2006) Clinical activity of the immunoconjugate CMC-544 in B-cell malignancies: Preliminary report of the expanded maximum tolerated dose cohort of a phase 1 study. *Blood* **108**(11): 766a.
25. Allen TM, Mumbengegwi DR, Charrois GJ. (2005) Anti-CD19-targeted liposomal doxorubicin improves the therapeutic efficacy in murine B-cell lymphoma and ameliorates the toxicity of liposomes with varying drug release rates. *Clin Cancer Res* **11**(9): 3567–3573.

27. Cairo MS, Raetz E, Lim MS, Davenport V, Perkins SL. (2005) Childhood and adolescent non-Hodgkin lymphoma: New insights in biology and critical challenges for the future. *Pediatr Blood Cancer* **45**(6): 753–769.
28. Miles RR, Cairo MS, Satwani P, Zwick DL, Lones MA, Sposto R, *et al.* (2007) Immunophenotypic identification of possible therapeutic targets in paediatric non-Hodgkin lymphomas: A Children's Oncology Group report. *Br J Haematol* **138**(4): 506–512.
29. Miles RR, Raphael M, McCarthy K, Wotherspoon A, Lones MA, Terrier-Lacombe MJ, *et al.* (2008) Pediatric diffuse large B-cell lymphoma demonstrates a high proliferation index, frequent c-Myc protein expression, and a high incidence of germinal center subtype: Report of the French-American-British (FAB) international study group. *Pediatr Blood Cancer* **51**(3): 369–374.
30. Perkins SL, Lones MA, Davenport V, Cairo MS. (2003) B-Cell non-Hodgkin's lymphoma in children and adolescents: Surface antigen expression and clinical implications for future targeted bioimmune therapy: A Children's Cancer Group report. *Clin Adv Hematol Oncol* **1**(5): 314–317.
31. Du X, Nagata S, Ise T, Stetler-Stevenson M, Pastan I. (2008) FCRL1 on chronic lymphocytic leukemia, hairy cell leukemia, and B-cell non-Hodgkin lymphoma as a target of immunotoxins. *Blood* **111**(1): 338–343.
33. Mark T, Martin P, Leonard JP, Niesvizky R. (2009) Milatuzumab: A promising new agent for the treatment of lymphoid malignancies. *Expert Opin Investig Drugs* **18**(1): 99–104.
34. Bhat S, Czuczman MS. (2010) Galiximab: A review. *Expert Opin Biol Ther* **10**(3): 451–458.
37. Coiffier B, Lepage E, Briere J, Herbrecht R, Tilly H, Bouabdallah R, *et al.* (2002) CHOP chemotherapy plus rituximab compared with CHOP alone in elderly patients with diffuse large-B-cell lymphoma. *N Engl J Med* **346**(4): 235–242.
38. Wilson WH, Dunleavy K, Pittaluga S, Hegde U, Grant N, Steinberg SM, *et al.* (2008) Phase II study of dose-adjusted EPOCH and rituximab in untreated diffuse large B-cell lymphoma with analysis of germinal center and post-germinal center biomarkers. *J Clin Oncol* **26**(16): 2717–2724.
39. Gokbuget N, Hoelzer D. (2004) Treatment with monoclonal antibodies in acute lymphoblastic leukemia: Current knowledge and future prospects. *Ann Hematol* **83**(4): 201–205.
44. Griffin TC, Weitzman S, Weinstein H, Chang M, Cairo M, Hutchison R, *et al.* (2009) A study of rituximab and ifosfamide, carboplatin, and etoposide chemotherapy in children with recurrent/refractory B-cell (CD20+) non-Hodgkin lymphoma and mature B-cell acute lymphoblastic leukemia: A report from the Children's Oncology Group. *Pediatr Blood Cancer* **52**(2): 177–181.
47. Leonard JP, Coleman M, Ketas JC, Chadburn A, Ely S, Furman RR, *et al.* (2003) Phase I/II trial of epratuzumab (humanized anti-CD22 antibody) in indolent non-Hodgkin's lymphoma. *J Clin Oncol* **21**(16): 3051–3059.
48. Leonard JP, Coleman M, Ketas JC, Chadburn A, Furman R, Schuster MW, *et al.* (2004) Epratuzumab, a humanized anti-CD22 antibody, in aggressive non-Hodgkin's lymphoma: Phase I/II clinical trial results. *Clin Cancer Res* **10**(16): 5327–5334.
49. Leonard JP, Coleman M, Ketas J, Ashe M, Fiore JM, Furman RR, *et al.* (2005) Combination antibody therapy with epratuzumab and rituximab in relapsed or refractory non-Hodgkin's lymphoma. *J Clin Oncol* **23**(22): 5044–5051.
50. Raetz EA, Cairo MS, Borowitz MJ, Blaney SM, Krailo MD, Leil TA, *et al.* (2008) Chemoimmunotherapy reinduction with epratuzumab in children with acute lymphoblastic leukemia in marrow relapse: A Children's Oncology Group Pilot study. *J Clin Oncol* **26**(22): 3756–3762.
51. Raetz EA, Borowitz MJ, Devidas M, Linda SB, Hunger SP, Winick NJ, *et al.* (2008) Reinduction platform for children with first marrow relapse of acute lymphoblastic leukemia: A Children's Oncology Group study [corrected]. *J Clin Oncol* **26**(24): 3971–3978.
52. Kreitman RJ, Squires DR, Stetler-Stevenson M, Noel P, FitzGerald DJ, Wilson WH, *et al.* (2005) Phase I trial of recombinant immunotoxin RFB4(dsFv)-PE38 (BL22) in patients with B-cell malignancies. *J Clin Oncol* **23**(27): 6719–6729.
53. Kreitman RJ, Wilson WH, Bergeron K, Raggio M, Stetler-Stevenson M, FitzGerald DJ, *et al.* (2001) Efficacy of the anti-CD22 recombinant immunotoxin BL22 in chemotherapy-resistant hairy-cell leukemia. *N Engl J Med* **345**(4): 241–247.
54. Wayne AS, Kreitman RJ, Findley HW, Lew G, Delbrook C, Steinberg SM, *et al.* (2010) Anti-CD22 immunotoxin RFB4(dsFv)-PE38 (BL22) for CD22-positive hematologic malignancies of childhood: Preclinical studies and phase I clinical trial. *Clin Cancer Res* **16**(6): 1894–1903.
55. Salvatore G, Beers R, Margulies I, Kreitman RJ, Pastan I. (2002) Improved cytotoxic activity toward cell lines and fresh leukemia cells of a mutant anti-CD22 immunotoxin obtained by antibody phage display. *Clin Cancer Res* **8**(4): 995–1002.
56. Wayne AS, Bhojwani D, Jeha S, Stetler-Stevenson M, Pui C-H, McDevitt J, *et al.* (2009) Phase I clinical trial of

the Anti-CD22 immunotoxin CAT-8015 (HA22) for pediatric acute lymphoblastic leukemia. *Blood* **114**(22): 345.

57. Herrera L, Bostrom B, Gore L, Sandler E, Lew G, Schlegel PG, *et al.* (2009) A phase 1 study of Combotox in pediatric patients with refractory B-lineage acute lymphoblastic leukemia. *J Pediatr Hematol/Oncol* **31**(12): 936–941.
58. DiJoseph JF, Khandke K, Dougher MM, Evans DY, Armellino DC, Hamann PR, *et al.* (2008) CMC-544 (inotuzumab ozogamicin): A CD22-targeted immunoconjugate of calicheamicin. *Hematol Meeting Reports* **5**(6): 74–77.
59. Jansen B, Uckun FM, Jaszcz WB, Kersey JH. (1992) Establishment of a human t(4;11) leukemia in severe combined immunodeficient mice and successful treatment using anti-CD19 (B43)-pokeweed antiviral protein immunotoxin. *Cancer Res* **52**(2): 406–412.
66. Arceci RJ, Sande J, Lange B, Shannon K, Franklin J, Hutchinson R, *et al.* (2005) Safety and efficacy of gemtuzumab ozogamicin in pediatric patients with advanced CD33+ acute myeloid leukemia. *Blood* **106**(4): 1183–1188.
67. Aplenc R, Alonzo TA, Gerbing RB, Lange BJ, Hurwitz CA, Wells RJ, *et al.* (2008) Safety and efficacy of gemtuzumab ozogamicin in combination with chemotherapy for pediatric acute myeloid leukemia: A report from the Children's Oncology Group. *J Clin Oncol* **26**(14): 2390–3295.
68. Roman E, Cooney E, Harrison L, Militano O, Wolownik K, Hawks R, *et al.* (2005) Preliminary results of the safety of immunotherapy with gemtuzumab ozogamicin following reduced intensity allogeneic stem cell transplant in children with CD33+ acute myeloid leukemia. *Clin Cancer Res* **11**(19 Pt 2): 7164s–7170s.
69. Satwani P, Waxman I, Bhatia M, Jin Z, Kohl V, Baldinger L, *et al.* (2008) Preliminary results of gemtuzumab ozogamicin (GO) during myeloablative conditioning for allogeneic stem cell transplantation (AlloSCT) or following reduced intensity alloSCT (RI-AlloSCT) in children with AML. *J Clin Oncol* **26**(15S): 7038.
77. DiJoseph JF, Dougher MM, Kalyandrug LB, Armellino DC, Boghaert ER, Hamann PR, *et al.* (2006) Antitumor efficacy of a combination of CMC-544 (inotuzumab ozogamicin), a CD22-targeted cytotoxic immunoconjugate of calicheamicin, and rituximab against non-Hodgkin's B-cell lymphoma. *Clin Cancer Res* **12**(1): 242–249.
78. Cooper LJ, Topp MS, Serrano LM, Gonzalez S, Chang WC, Naranjo A, *et al.* (2003) T-cell clones can be rendered specific for CD19: Toward the selective augmentation of the graft-versus-B-lineage leukemia effect. *Blood* **101**(4): 1637–1644.
84. Pastan I. (2003) Immunotoxins containing Pseudomonas exotoxin A: A short history. *Cancer Immunol Immunother* **52**(5): 338–341.
86. Smith MR. (2003) Rituximab (monoclonal anti-CD20 antibody): Mechanisms of action and resistance. *Oncogene* **22**(47): 7359–7368.

22

Novel Therapeutics in Hematologic Malignancies in Children, Adolescents and Young Adults

Nita L. Seibel and Malcolm A. Smith

Introduction

Developing new cancer therapies in children and adolescents presents challenges different from those arising in the adult population. These include the smaller numbers of patients diagnosed with a specific type of cancer as compared to the adult setting and the overall favorable 5-year survival rate for children and adolescents with cancer which is approaching 80%. As a result, there are limited numbers of children and adolescents who are eligible for evaluating experimental therapies. The patients who are available have received multiple therapies and their cancers are highly resistant to therapy. This chapter will focus on the approaches to identify new agents for pediatric oncology and the promising new agents that are being developed to treat hematopoietic malignancies. These agents include inhibitors of BCL-2 family proteins, IAP family proteins, MDM2-p53 interaction, tyrosine kinases [e.g. FLT3, Janus kinases (JAKs), and ALK], mTOR, Notch pathway, mitotic kinases, the ubiquitin–proteasome system, and enzymes involved in epigenetic control of gene expression (Table 22.1).

In order to overcome the limitations in the number of pediatric oncology patients who are available for phases I and II clinical testing and to identify the agents that may have significant benefit for pediatric and adolescent patients, the Pediatric Preclinical Testing Program (PPTP) was implemented by the National Cancer Institute. The PPTP is comprised of a consortium of investigators who integrate *in vivo* and *in vitro* testing with expression and genomic profiling. Standard PPTP testing procedures involve testing novel agents against the 23 cell lines of its *in vitro* panel and against more than 40 solid tumor and ALL xenografts, with most childhood cancer represented by 4–8 xenografts. The objective of the PPTP is to identify agents with significant activity in panels of pediatric preclinical models as a potential mechanism for prioritizing agents for advancement to clinical trials for children with specific cancers, thereby expediting the discovery of more effective therapies for children with cancer. Selected standard agents have been tested in the PPTP, both to calibrate the PPTP tumor panels and to serve as a basis for future combination studies.[1] Testing results for the ALL panel of directly transplanted leukemia xenografts are particularly relevant to prioritizing agents for evaluation in the pediatric leukemia setting.[2]

Pediatric Phase 1 trials of anticancer agents are typically multi-institutional so that accrual is adequate to allow timely completion of the studies. The Children's Oncology Group through their Phase I Consortium conducts many of the pediatric Phase I studies of agents that have relevance to the treatment of hematological

Table 22.1. Summary of the classes of agents, mechanisms of action and targeted malignancies.

Class	Mechanism of action	Disease
BCL-2 family inhibitors	Inhibit prosurvival activity of BCL-2, BCL-X_L, BCL-w, and/or MCL-1	ALL, NHL, AML
Inhibitor of apoptosis proteins (IAP) inhibitors	Inhibit XIAP and induce degradation of cIAP1/cIAP2, thereby promoting apoptosis	ALL, AML
MDM-p53 inhibitors	Inhibit MDM2-mediated degradation of p53; Trigger p53-dependent cell cycle arrest and/or apoptosis	AML, ALL, NHL
Kinases inhibitors		
JAK	Inhibit activating JAK mutations in leukemia cells;	ALL, MDS
ALK	Inhibit constitutively activated ALK in ALK-translocation lymphoma;	Anaplastic large cell lymphoma: Diffuse large B-cell lymphoma
FLT 3	Inhibit FLT 3 signaling	AML (particularly with FLT3 internal tandem duplication with high allelic ratio)
mTOR inhibitors	Inhibit cell growth, protein synthesis, cell-cycle progression induced thru signaling pathways (e.g. PI3K/AKT); In combination with glucocorticosteroids may increase sensitivity of leukemia cells to glucocorticosteroids; may enhance cytotoxicity of existing chemotherapy.	ALL, Ph+ ALL, AML
NOTCH inhibitors	Inhibition of activating NOTCH mutations and induction of G_0/G_1 arrest	T-cell ALL
Mitotic kinase inhibitors	Aurora A and Aurora B kinase inhibit various processes involved in orderly progression through mitosis.	ALL and NHL (Aurora A) AML (Aurora B)
Epigenetic agents		
Histone deacetylase inhibitors	Inhibition of histone deacetylation leading to altered gene expression	NHL, leukemias
Demethylating agents	Incorporation into DNA leading to demethylation and gene reactivation	MDS, AML
Ubiquitin–proteasome system		
Proteasome inhibitors	Inhibition of degradation of key proteins involved in controlling cell cycle progression and cell signaling (e.g. NF-κB pathway)	ALL, AML
NEDD-activating enzyme inhibitor		AML, NHL

ALK: anaplastic lymphoma kinase; ALL: acute lymphoblastic leukemia; AML: acute myelogenous leukemia; Ph+ ALL: Philadelphia chromosome positive acute lymphoblastic leukemia; BCL-2: B cell lymphoma 2 family of proteins; cIAP1: cellular inhibitor of apoptosis 1; FLT 3: Fms-like Tyrosine Kinase-3; JAK: janus kinase; MCL-1: myeloid cell leukemia 1; MDM2: murine double minute 2; MDS: myelodysplastic syndrome; mTOR: mammalian target of rapamycin; NF-kB: nuclear factor kappa-B; NHL: non-Hodgkin lymphoma; PI3K: Phosphoinositide 3-kinase/; XIAP: X-linked inhibitor of apoptosis protein.

malignancies. The Phase I Consortium consists of approximately 20 COG institutions that have expertise in running pediatric Phase I trials and performing pharmacokinetic and pharmacodynamic measurements. Following the completion of the Phase I trial, agents are then tested in the Phase II setting based on the interest and strategic direction of the disease group.

Inhibitors of Pro-Survival Proteins

BCL2 family protein inhibitors

Defects in programmed cell death in cancer cells provide a survival advantage during tumorigenesis as well as resulting in intrinsic resistance to treatment with chemotherapy and radiation therapy. Manipulating the cancer cell's dysregulated apoptosis pathways to favor cell death can enhance treatment effectiveness. In order for this approach to be feasible, the specific apoptosis pathway target of an agent must be one upon which cancer cells are critically dependent and one for which normal cells have much less need. The two primary apoptotic pathways are the extrinsic (death receptor) and intrinsic (mitochondrial) pathway.

BCL-2 family inhibitors

The BCL-2 family of proteins control the key step in the intrinsic apoptotic pathway, permeabilization of the mitochondrial membrane.[3,4] BAX and BAK have been identified as two pro-apoptotic effector proteins in the BCL-2 family that insert after activation into the mitochondrial membrane and allow the efflux of cytochrome c and activation of the caspase cascade. The anti-apoptotic members of the BCL-2 family, including BCL-2, BCL-X_L, and MCL-1, bind to BAX and BAK and block their activation. A set of pro-apoptotic BCL-2 family proteins, the BH3-only proteins including PUMA, NOXA, BIM and BAD, sequester the anti-apoptotic BCL-2 family members, thus promoting BAX and BAK dimerization. The complex balance of these BCL-2 family members determines a cell's susceptibility to apoptosis. The overexpression of anti-apoptotic proteins may confer resistance to chemotherapeutic agents. Inhibitors of the anti-apoptotic/pro-survival BCL-2 family members swing the balance toward apoptosis by neutralizing the effect of these anti-apoptotic proteins. Many ALL leukemia cells are dependent for survival on the apoptotic block provided by BCL-2 family expression.[5,6] ALL cases with MLL gene rearrangement may be particularly responsive to BCL-2 inhibition. Chronic lymphocytic leukemia (CLL) is another lymphoid malignancy that appears to be primed for apoptosis.[6,7]

Small molecule BCL-2 family inhibitors are undergoing clinical evaluation. ABT-263 is an orally bioavailable BH3 mimetic that potently inhibits the pro-survival activity of BCL-2, BCL-X_L and BCL-w. The PPTP studied ABT-263 against its childhood cancer preclinical models, and observed limited single agent activity against solid tumor xenografts, but substantial remission-inducing activity against approximately 50% of the ALL xenografts tested.[7] ABT-263 has entered clinical evaluation in adults, with impressive activity observed in patients with CLL and selected non-Hodgkin lymphomas in the phase 1 setting.[8] ABT-263 has generally been well tolerated, with dose escalation limited by rapid onset, reversible thrombocytopenia. This represents an on-target effect due to the inhibition of BCL-X_L in circulating platelets. The investigation of ABT-263 in ALL is supported by its single agent activity against ALL xenografts, its activity in CLL, and its ability to potentiate the cytotoxic effects of standard anti-leukemia agents.[7,9,10] However, the thrombocytopenia that it induces will be a challenge to overcome in the initial testing of this agent in the relapsed setting. Given the challenges of using the agent when platelet counts are low due to bone marrow infiltration by leukemia, ABT-263 may be most useful in the post-remission setting.

Obatoclax is an intravenous small molecule with pan-BCL-2 family antagonism. It differs from ABT-263 in that it inhibits MCL-1 activity at concentrations similar to those that inhibit Bcl-2 and Bcl-X_L.[11] Dose escalations of obatoclax have been limited by neurotoxicity. It does not induce thrombocytopenia as seen with ABT-263, raising questions about whether *in vivo* levels are adequate to produce robust BCL-X_L inhibition.[12,13] An ALL patient with MLL gene rearrangement achieved a complete response to obatoclax.[12] Subcytotoxic concentrations of obatoclax have been shown to restore the response to dexamethasone in corticosteroid-resistant ALL cells. This could provide a new therapeutic approach to treatment of relapsed, resistant ALL.[14] The Children's Oncology Group is performing a phase I study of obatoclax in combination with standard chemotherapy agents.

IAP family inhibitors

Inhibitor of apoptosis proteins (IAP) are evolutionarily conserved cytoplasmic proteins that directly inhibit caspases resulting in the suppression of apoptosis.[15] There have been eight human IAPs identified and all share a protein domain, the baculovirus IAP repeat (BIR), that is important for their anti-apoptotic activity. The IAPs that have been most studied in cancer are survivin, XIAP, c-IAP1, and cIAP2. XIAP is overexpressed in multiple adult cancers, and elevated XIAP levels appear to be associated with poor prognosis for children with AML.[16,17] XIAP, though its interaction with caspase 9, is able to block apoptosis signaling activated by both the mitochondrial-dependent and the death receptor pathway.

AEG35156 is an XIAP second-generation antisense agent that knocks down the expression of XIAP mRNA and protein in *in vitro* and *in vivo* preclinical models.[18–20] It has been tested in combination with cytarabine and idarubicin in patients with AML. Evidence for significant XIAP knockdown was observed, as was preliminary evidence for enhancement of chemotherapy activity by the agent.[18]

Small molecule inhibitors of IAP family function are also in clinical evaluation.[21] These inhibitors were developed to mimic the interaction between XIAP and SMAC, an inhibitor of XIAP function. Surprisingly, SMAC mimetics were found to induce cell death in sensitive cells independent of caspase 9 and the intrinsic apoptotis pathway.[22,23] Rather, their cytotoxic effect was determined to involve the induction of TNF and subsequent cell death via the extrinsic apoptosis pathway. The initial step in this pathway is the interaction of the SMAC mimetic with cIAP1, which is followed by cIAP1 auto-ubiquitination and degradation, activation of an NF-κB transcriptional program, induction of TNF, caspase activation, and

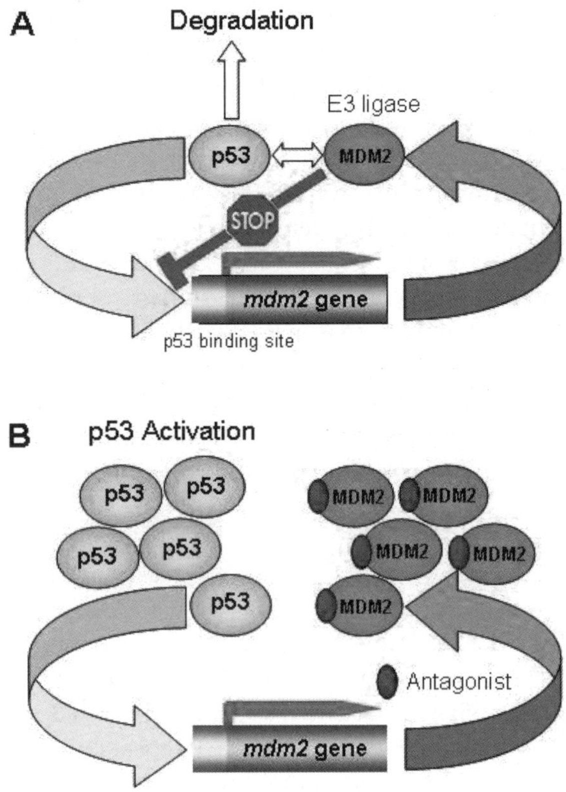

Fig. 22. 1. Small-molecule inhibitors of p53-MDM2 binding interrupt the negative feedback loop by which MDM2 controls p53 level. (A) In unstressed cells, p53 and MDM2 mutually regulate their level through a negative feedback loop. Elevated levels of p53 activate transcription of MDM2. Additionally, MDM2 binds to p53 and inhibits p53 transcriptional activity and facilitates p53 degradation as a specific E3 ubiquitin ligase. (B) Small-molecule inhibitor bind to the p53 pocket which disrupts the p53-MDM2 interaction and frees p53 from MDM2 control. (Adapted and reprinted by permission from Elsevier Ltd.: Vassilev LT, MDM2 inhibitors for cancer therapy, Trends in Molecular Medicine 13(1) 24–33, 2006.).

apoptosis. LCL161 is a SMAC mimetic that shows the predicted pharmacodynamic effects of apoptosis induction associated with cIAP1 degradation and TNF induction in sensitive preclinical models, and it has entered clinical evaluation.[24,25]

MDM2-p53 inhibitors

p53 is the most frequently inactivated protein in human malignancy with more than 50% of all solid tumors carrying mutations in the TP53 gene. The prevalence of TP53 mutations varies according to tumor type and stages of cancer. Many tumors with wild type (WT) TP53 have attenuated p53 function due to negative regulation by other abnormalities. One of these negative regulators is the human homolog of *murine double minute 2* (MDM2), which is located on chromosome 12q15 and encodes a 90-kDa protein that negatively modulates p53 by binding directly to and decreasing p53 stability (Fig. 22.1).[26] A germline single nucleotide polymorphism in the promoter region of MDM2 has been identified and results in an increase in *MDM2* gene expression and is associated with an earlier age of onset of human cancer.[27] In the chronic phase of CML, the incidence of TP53 mutations is 3–5% whereas as the disease progresses to blast crisis, the incidence increases to 25–30%.[28]

Due to the importance of the p53–*MDM2* interaction, restoration of the p53 activity by inhibition of *MDM2* binding represents a novel antineoplastic strategy.[29] Nutlin-3 is a small-molecule antagonist of *MDM2* that binds the p53-binding pocket of *MDM2*, thus inhibiting *MDM2*-mediated degradation of p53 to induce a dramatic increase in its expression and activity.[30] Nutlin-3 has been shown to trigger p53-dependent cell cycle arrest in normal cells and additionally induce apoptosis in tumor cells depending on the tumor cell types. Since the activity of MDM2 inhibitors depends upon p53 activation in cells expressing wild type p53, hematological malignancies are attractive candidates for the MDM2 inhibitor-based therapy because TP53 is infrequently mutated. Studies using cell lines and primary samples from patients with various hematological malignancies, including AML, ALL, CLL, multiple myeloma, and malignant lymphomas, have shown that apoptosis is effectively induced by nutlin-3 in these cells.[31–34] Nutlin-3 synergizes with doxorubicin and cytosine arabinoside in killing myeloblasts in AML. Both the single agent and the combination effect of nutlin-3 are selective for cancer vs. normal cells, as revealed by the lack of toxicity to peripheral blood mononuclear cells or bone marrow-derived hematopoietic progenitors and bone marrow stromal epithelium cells.[32,35,36] A member of the nutlin family of MDM2 antagonists, R7112, is currently undergoing phase I clinical testing in adults with solid and hematological malignancies.[37]

Tyrosine kinases

Janus kinase (JAK) inhibitors

The Janus family of nonreceptor protein kinases include JAK1, JAK2, JAK3 and TYK2. JAK 3 expression is limited to hematopoietic cells whereas JAK1, JAK2 and TYK2 are ubiquitously expressed in mammalian cells. These proteins interact with cytokines and other transmembrane receptors. Various cytokines such as

IL-7 or thymic stromal lymphopoietin activate the JAKs which leads to activation of the STAT pathway.[38] Janus kinase/signal transducer and activator of transcription signaling is important for a wide spectrum of cellular processes, including proliferation, survival or normal functioning of hematopoietic, immune, cardiac, and other cells.

JAK family kinases have gained increasing recognition in the past 5 years as oncology therapeutic targets following the demonstration that most cases of polycythemia vera, essential thrombocythemia, and primary myelofibrosis are associated with a specific JAK2 mutation (V617F) and result in a valine to phenylalanine substitution at codon 617. This mutation is not found in acute lymphoblastic leukemia.[39,40] JAK2 mutations and translocations have been identified in lymphoid malignancies and acute lymphoblastic leukemia in Down syndrome.[41,42]

JAK–STAT activation is relevant in childhood ALL setting. Chromosomal translocations fusing JAK2 and genes encoding various transcription factors lead to the production of constitutively active chimeric proteins which are involved in the pathogenesis of various types of leukemia. In the ALL cases, activation occurs through fusion proteins in which a JAK family member joins with the oligomerization domain of other proteins such as TEL (ETV6) and PCM1.[41,43] Several somatic gain-of-function mutations in JAK1 have been reported in T-cell ALL (adult) where they are present in approximately 20% of the patients. They appear to be less common in children with T-cell ALL and B precursor ALL.[44,45] Activating mutations of JAK1 and JAK2 that occur in a subgroup of pediatric B-cell ALL are associated with IKZF1 deletions and have a poor outcome similar to BCR-ABL 1 pediatric ALL without the fusion protein. These results suggest that inhibition of JAK signaling is a logical target for therapeutic intervention in JAK mutated ALL.

The JAK2 inhibitors are divided into two categories (selective and nonselective) based on their inhibition of JAK2. Both types inhibit other kinases including “off-target” effects against other family members. INCB018424 is the farthest along in clinical development. This is an orally available JAK inhibitor that shows low nanomolar potency against both JAK1 and JAK2.[46] In a large Phase II study of patients with primary myelofibrosis and post-polycythemia vera and essential thrombocythemia myelofibrosis who were treated with INCB018424, durable improvements in constitutional symptoms, reduction in splenomegaly (irrespective of JAK2 mutational status), increased body weight, and reduction of plasma concentrations proinflamatory and angiogenic cytokines and growth factors were observed. The agent was well tolerated and the main toxicity observed was a dose-dependent grade ¾ thrombocytopenia.[47] Other JAK2 inhibitors are TG101348, CYT387, SB1518, and AZD1480. COG is very interested in studying the JAK2 inhibitors in pediatrics and ALL.[48]

Anaplastic lymphoma kinase (ALK)

The ALK receptor tyrosine kinase is a member of the insulin receptor kinase superfamily and is expressed in the developing central and peripheral nervous system. It is activated in anaplastic large cell lymphoma (ALCL) as a result of the t(2;5)(p23;q35) chromosomal translocation which results in the fusion of NPM at 5q35 with ALK at 2p23. The resulting NPM-ALK fusion protein shows constitutive kinase activity. TPM3-ALK, ATIC-ALK, and CLTC-ALK are other fusion proteins involving ALK that have been indentified in ALCL. ALCL cell lines with ALK activation show exquisite sensitivity to small molecule ALK inhibitors (Fig. 22.2). In an *in vivo* model of ALK+, ALCL showed complete tumor regression in response to treatment with the small molecule ALK inhibitor PF-02341066 was observed. PF-02341066 is the first ALK inhibitor to enter clinic trials. The agent was relatively well tolerated by adults, with dose-limiting toxicities being liver enzyme elevations and fatigue. Objective responses were noted in non-small cell lung cancer patients whose tumors had the echinoderm microtubule-associated protein-like 4 (EML4)-ALK translocation.[49] A pediatric Phase I study has been initiated for patients with refractory solid tumors and ALCL.

mTOR inhibitors

The mammalian target of rapamycin (mTOR) is a serine/threonine kinase that functions as a key regulator of cell growth, protein synthesis, and cell cycle progression through interactions with a number of signaling pathways, including PI3K/AKT, ras, TCL1, and BCR/ABL (Fig. 22.3).[50] Rapamycin (sirolimus), a macrocyclic lactone first noted to have significant anticancer activity in preclinical models more than 2 decades ago, was the first mTOR inhibitor to be used in the clinical setting.[51,52] Rapamycin is FDA-approved as an immunosuppressive agent in solid organ transplantation. Most evaluations of mTOR inhibitors for cancer indications involve

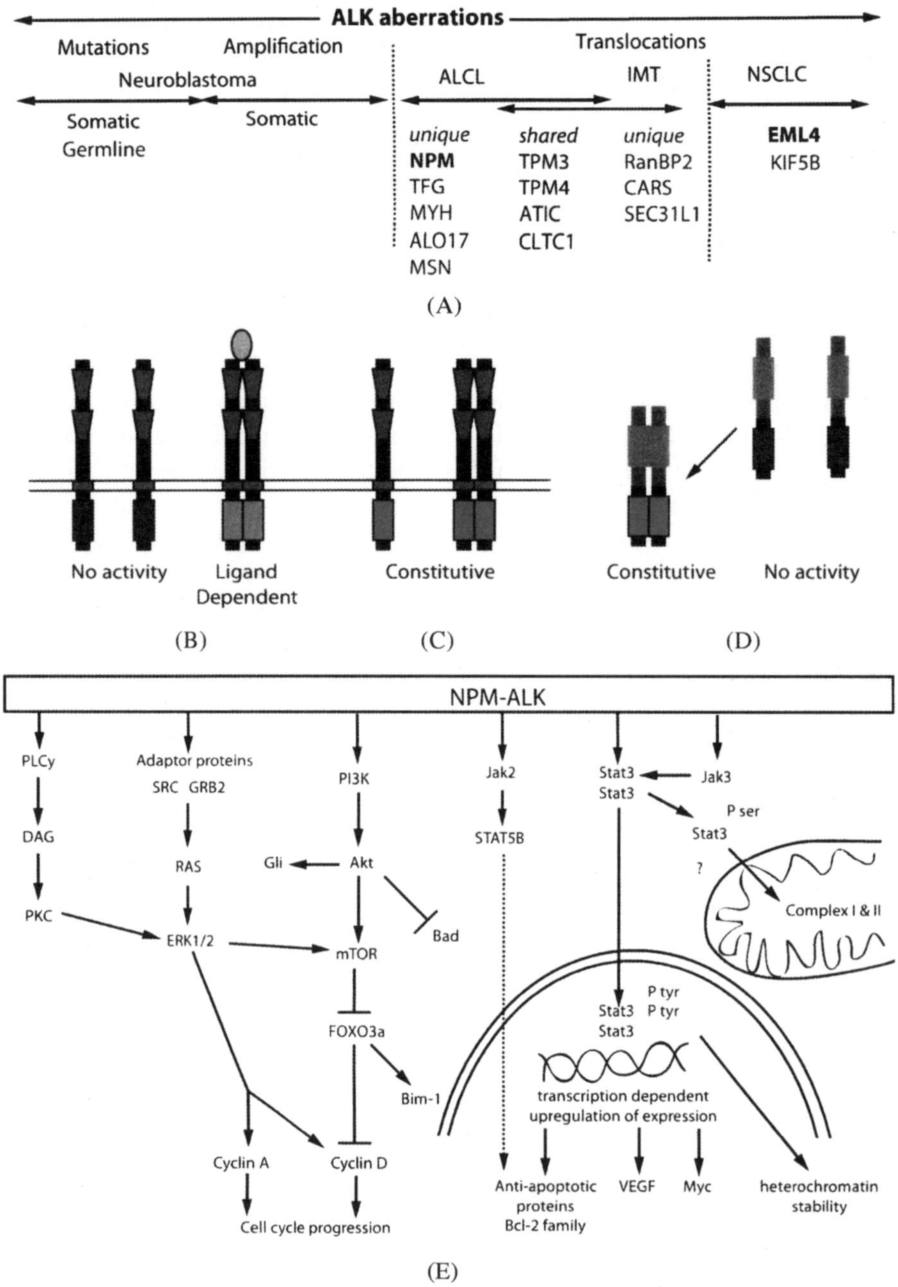

Fig. 22.2. (A) ALK aberrations in human cancer. ALK may be dysregulated by multiple mechanisms in cancer. (B) ALK signaling results from dimerization of the extracellular domain of ALK monomers leading to transphosphorylation of the tyrosine kinase domain. (C) Activating mutations within the tyrosine kinase domain can lead to ligand-independent signaling. (D) Fusion partners approximate the truncated ALK. (E) Constitutive ALK signaling induces transformation through a variety of signaling pathways. (Adapted and reprinted by permission from the American Association for Cancer Research: Mosse YP, Wood A, Maris JM, Inhibition of ALK signaling for cancer therapy, *Clin Cancer Res*, 2009, **15**(18) 5609–5614.).

rapamycin analogs (rapalogs), including temsirolimus (CCI-779), everolimus (RAD001), and ridaforolimus (AP23573, MK-8669). Temsirolimus was the first mTOR inhibitor to gain FDA approval for any malignancy, when it was approved in 2007 for first-line treatment of poor prognosis patients with advanced renal cell carcinoma. Everolimus is approved as second-line therapy for renal cell carcinoma following progression on a VEGF-targeted therapy.[53] When used as monotherapy, mTOR inhibitors are relatively well tolerated with the

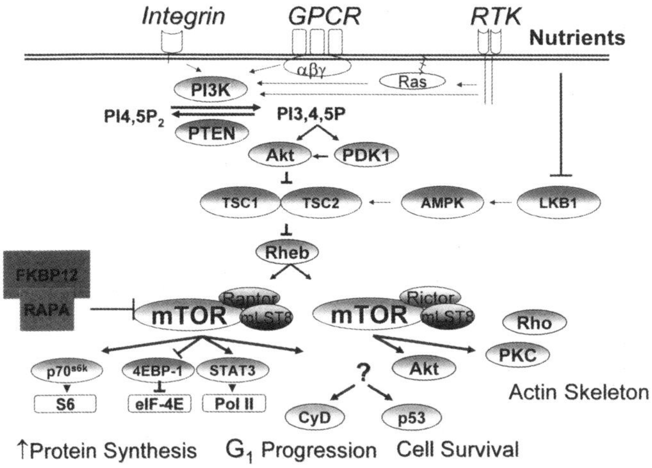

Fig. 22.3. Pathway from growth factor receptor stimulation to mTOR activation (Used with permission and previously published: Dancey JE. Therapeutic targets. *Cancer Biology & Therapy*, 2006, **5**:9, 1065–1073.).

primary toxicities for cancer patients consisting of asthenia, mucositis, thrombocytopenia, hypercholesterolemia, and pneumonitis.[50,54]

Many hematological malignancies have aberrant activation of the mTOR and related signaling pathways. The evaluation of rapamycin by the PPTP showed broad *in vivo* tumor growth inhibition across most of the histologies evaluated, with objective responses (tumor regressions) observed for several diagnoses, including ALL.[55] The activity observed for rapamycin against the ALL PPTP panel is similar to that described in other reports showing *in vivo* activity for rapamycin and rapalogs against ALL xenografts.[56,57] The mTOR inhibitors appear to be active against both B- and T-cell ALL, however they may be more active in T-cell disease.[55] Pediatric Phase I trials of temsirolimus and everolimus have been completed.[58,59] In a Phase I trial of sirolimus in children with relapsed/refractory ALL, all patients tolerated sirolimus and three of seven patients had stable disease.[60]

Because mTOR inhibitors are less likely to be effective in the clinical setting when used as single agents against leukemia, combination treatment is being explored. mTOR inhibitors have been shown to be effective and potentially synergistic in combination with a number of chemotherapeutic agents *in vitro*, such as methotrexate, dexamethasone, etoposide, asparaginases, and doxorubicin.[57,61] The PPTP demonstrated that the combinations of rapamycin with cyclophosphamide or vincristine were well tolerated, with the combinations commonly showing significantly greater antitumor activity than the single agent treatments.[55] Combining corticosteroids with mTOR inhibitors holds promise, as noted by Wei *et al.* based initially on the overlapping gene expression signature of glucocorticoid (GC) sensitivity and the signature induced by rapamycin ALL cells.[62] Other investigators have confirmed the observation that mTOR inhibitors sensitize ALL cells to glucocorticoid-induced cytotoxicity.[63,64] Additionally, since BCR-ABL is upstream of the PI3K/AKT/mTOR signaling pathway, mTOR inhibitors may be effective in Ph+ ALL, including BCR-ABL tyrosine kinase inhibitor resistant disease.[65] However, the PPTP did not show activity for rapamycin against its BCR-ABL-expressing ALL xenograft.[55]

As a result of the potential activity of mTOR inhibitors against ALL, and considering that hematopoietic stem cell transplantation (HSCT) is used as a major salvage for patients with refractory or relapsed ALL and sirolimus has been used as graft-vs.-host disease (GVHD) prophylaxis in a number of transplant trials, the use of sirolimus in the post-HSCT setting is being tested by the Children's Oncology Group. A nationwide Phase III randomized trial, ASCT 0431, is evaluating the addition of sirolimus to GVHD prophylaxis during HSCT for relapsed ALL. The primary hypothesis of this trial is that the addition of sirolimus to GVHD will increase leukemia-free survival compared to a regimen of standard agents, through the novel benefit of using a drug that has the potential to both control GVHD and directly suppress leukemic blasts.

Recent interest has focused on targeting the PI3K/AKT/mTOR pathway in AML, as a majority of patients' blasts have constitutive activation of AKT with subsequent phosphorylation of downstream targets of mTOR.[66] Promising results have been demonstrated using monotherapy with mTOR inhibitors in preclinical models of AML, however these have not translated into substantial clinical benefit in early phase trials.[67,68] Despite these findings, there is interest that targeting the mTOR pathway may enhance the cytotoxicity of existing chemotherapeutic agents and other targeted agents. Sirolimus has been shown to enhance the sensitivity of AML blasts to etoposide *in vitro* and the combination could prevent engraftment of AML cell in NOD/SCID mice better than either single agent alone if cells were treated *in vitro* prior to injection.[69] A cautionary note for combinations of an mTOR inhibitor with cell cycle-specific agents such as etoposide and cytarabine is that mTOR inhibitors potently induce G1 cell cycle arrest, which could limit the effectiveness of cell cycle specific agents during concurrent administration.

Clinical trials testing mTOR inhibitors in combination with standard cytotoxic agents or other molecularly targeted agents are being conducted in adults with AML.

Other inhibitors of the PI3K/AKT/mTOR pathway have been developed and are being tested in clinical trials. These include ATP-competitive inhibitors of mTOR kinase activity (e.g. AZD8055),[70] inhibitors of PI3K (e.g. GDC-0941, NVP-BKM-120, and XL-147), dual inhibitors of PI3K and mTOR (e.g. NVP-BEZ-235 and XL-765), and inhibitors of AKT (e.g. MK-2206).[71,72] The development of these agents is too early to identify specific patient populations in which they offer benefits in comparison to currently available agents that target the PI3K/AKT/mTOR pathway.

Targeting Notch pathway signaling

The Notch signaling pathway regulates cell proliferation and apoptosis and is required for normal embryonic development. Notch1 is a member of a family of highly conserved receptors that normally signal through a series of ligand-induced proteolytic cleavage events. As a result of these events, the intracellular portion of Notch1 (ICN1) gains access to the nucleus where it forms a short-lived transcriptional activation complex resulting in eventual transcription of target genes.[73] The final step of cleavage by γ secretase liberates ICN1. Activating mutations in the Notch1 gene leading to increased levels of ICN1 are present in over 50% of human T-ALL cases as well as many murine T-ALL models.[74] Further studies have shown that ICN1 drives the growth of T-ALL cells by upregulation of MYC expression and enhanced signaling of PI3-kinase/AKT/mTOR pathway. Notch pathway has been shown to be a key regulator of human T-cell acute leukemia-initiating cell activity.[75] Increases in ICN1 levels caused by Notch1 mutations are counteracted by drugs that inhibit γ secretase. Since γ secretase is linked to Alzheimer's disease, it has been a target of interest to pharmaceutical companies. Gamma secretase inhibitors (GSI) can induce G_0/G_1 arrest and decrease cell viability, although the level of apoptosis induced in T-ALL cell lines carrying Notch-activating mutations was modest.[76,77]

The first attempt to treat patients with refractory/relapsed T-ALL with MK-0752, an oral GSI, resulted in treatment failures and significant gastrointestinal toxicity.[78] The toxicity was probably a result of globlet cell metaplasia, as in the absence of Notch signaling the differentiation of epithelial cells lining the small bowel and colon is characterized by a marked increase in goblet cell differentiation and arrested cell proliferation in the intestinal crypts.[79] These failure to observe significant activity could be due to inadequate inhibition of Notch signaling, since dosing was limited by gastrointestinal toxicity, or to the limited levels of apoptosis induced by Notch1-mutant cell lines by GSI.[76,77] Recently, combination therapy using glucocorticoids and GSIs have been shown to improve the antileukemic effects of GSIs, and the glucocorticoids appear to abrogate the development of goblet cell metaplasia associated with GSIs in preclinical models. These results suggest that glucocorticoids plus GSIs may have a role in the treatment of glucocorticoid-resistant T-ALL.[80,81] Altering the schedule of administration of GSIs in mice by using an intermittent, 3-day on/4-day off GSI dosing schedule avoids gut toxicity while maintaining the anti–T-ALL effects, suggesting that alternative scheduling of GSIs may be a useful maneuver in the clinical setting.[82] Rapamycin has been shown to enhance the efficacy of GSIs in mice raising the possibility that combination therapy with GSIs, glucocorticoids, and mTOR inhibitors may have a role in the treatment of T-ALL.[82]

Notch1 mutations are not found in B-ALL and are seen only rarely in AML. The rare human AMLs with Notch1 mutations tend to show minimal myeloid differentiation, frequently express T-cell antigens and fall into a distinct subgroup by expression profiling.[74,83,84] The relationship between the role of the Notch pathway and AML derived stem cells is suggested by overexpression of Jagged-2, one of the Notch ligands, in leukemic stem cells from AML. Incubation of the leukemic stem cells with a GSI-inhibited leukemic stem cell growth in colony formation assays.[85]

Mitotic kinase inhibitors

Kinases play specific roles in the cell cycle, including the itotically active kinases that direct the sequential activation of specific enzymes and transcription factors during progression through the cell cycle, and mitotic kinesins that are motor proteins utilizing energy from ATP hydrolysis to produce directed mechanical force along microtubules of the emerging mitotic spindle. Aurora A and B and Polo-like kinase 1 (PLK1) are examples of mitotic kinases that have been identified as a focus for the development of small molecule inhibitors. Aurora A is a serine–threonine protein kinase that is involved in centrosome duplication and separation, microtubule–kinetochore attachment, spindle checkpoint, and cytokinesis.[86,87] Aurora A kinases are overexpressed or amplified in a number of hematological malignancies and in solid tumors. Aurora B is the kinase component of the chromosomal passenger complex, which additionally includes survivin, inner centromere protein (INCEP), and borealin. Aurora B is required for correct chromosome alignment and segregation as well as for spindle checkpoint function and cytokinesis. Aurora B inhibitors display a distinct molecular mechanism of action in which exposed cells continue to cycle instead of arresting in mitosis, resulting in polyploidy due to DNA replication without cell division. PLKs are a group of highly conserved serine–threonine kinases that play key roles at various stages of mitosis, including centrosome maturation, spindle checkpoint formation, and cytokinesis.

It is unclear whether Aurora A or B will be the better target.[88] In clinical testing of the agents, the common dose-limiting effects are granulocytopenia, nausea, and fatigue. An important question surrounding the use of each of these classes of kinase inhibitors is whether a therapeutic window will exist for them against specific cancers, given that normal proliferating tissues are also susceptible to their effects. The high level of *in vivo* activity of the Aurora A kinase inhibitor MLN8237 observed by the PPTP against neuroblastoma and ALL xenografts at doses producing drug exposures that approximate those tolerable in adults with cancer suggests that clinical benefit against specific cancers maybe achievable for Aurora A inhibitors.[89] As a result of the robust antitumor observed in PPTP, this agent was quickly taken into clinical testing through the COG Phase I Consortium where MLN8237 in a Phase 1/2 trial is being tested in patients with refractory ALL as well as refractory solid tumors such as neuroblastoma.

Inhibitors of Aurora B kinase such as AZD1152 and AT9283 are being evaluated in adults with AML, with single agent activity being observed for each agent.[90] A complicating factor in analyzing responses to these agents in the AML population is that both inhibit FLT3 as well as Aurora B kinase.[90,91] BI 6727 is a PLK1 inhibitor that is being studied in adults with AML.[92] It is a potent, selective inhibitor of PLK1 that was selected for clinical evaluation based on its high and sustained exposure in tumor tissue in preclinical models.[92]

FLT3 inhibitors

Given the poor outcome for children with AML who have FLT3 internal tandem duplication (ITD) with high allelic ratio, therapeutic targeting of FLT3 is a high priority for this subset of patients.[93] A substantial body of data documents that FLT3 inhibition has substantial antileukemia activity in preclinical *in vitro* and *in vivo* models. Many agents with FLT3 inhibitory activity are in clinical evaluation [e.g. AC220, lestaurtinib, tandutinib (MLN-518), lestaurtinib, midostaurin (PKC-412), and sunitinib], with many of these initially being studied because of their effects on other kinases.[94] Among these agents, midostaurin and lestaurtinib appear to be the least selective inhibitors, while sorafenib and AC220 show high specificity for FLT3 in cellular assays.[94,95]

Midostaurin and lestaurtinib have both entered Phase 3 evaluation for FLT3-mutant AML. Lestaurtinib failed to show clinical benefit in its Phase 3 trial for adults with relapsed/refractory FLT3 mutant AML.[96] A likely explanation for this negative result is that maximal FLT3 inhibition was not consistently obtained. Sorafenib has shown single agent activity in patients with FLT3-ITD AML,[97–99] and it has been safely combined with cytarabine and idarubicin in patients with AML.[100] When combined with chemotherapy, it produced a high response rate in newly diagnosed FLT3-mutated patients, with 17 of 18 patients achieving a morphological CR/CRp (94%). For patients with FLT3-mutated AML receiving sorafenib, near complete inhibition of FLT3 signaling was noted in their leukemia cells.[100] Further studies are needed in the pediatric AML population to define the role of FLT3 inhibition for the subset of the overall pediatric AML population that has FLT3-ITD.

Epigenetic Agents

Histone deacetylase inhibitors

One of the critical epigenetic events in oncology is related to aberrant histone modifications.[101] Post-translational modification of histone proteins through acetylation, methylation, and phosphorylation determine how these histone proteins control chromatin remodeling. Histone acetylation is regulated through the opposing actions of histone acetyltransferases (HATs) and histone deacetylases (HDACs), where HATs transfer acetyl moieties to lysine residues and HDACs remove these acetyl moieties. HDAC activity condenses chromatin, preventing access of transcription factors, leading to transcriptional repression. HAT inactivity and HDAC overactivity have been associated with tumorigenesis.[102] HDAC inhibitors have been shown to be effective therapeutic anticancer agents via multiple mechanisms, including inducing cell-cycle arrest, intrinsic and extrinsic apoptotic mechanisms, mitotic cell death, autophagic cell death, reactive oxygen species, inhibiting angiogenesis, and improving NK cell-mediated tumor immunity.[102] These diverse effects on cancer cells make HDAC inhibitors attractive agents not only for monotherapy but also in combination therapy.

The HDAC inhibitor vorinostat has been approved by the US Food and Drug Administration (FDA) as the first HDAC inhibitor for cancer therapy, specifically for relapsed or refractory cutaneous T-cell lymphoma (CTCL). This was based on two successful Phase II trials which demonstrated the effectiveness of vorinostat in relapsed or refractory CTCL.[103]

Many cases of childhood acute leukemia with recurrent chromosomal translocations fuse the DNA-binding domain of a transcriptional activator to a transcriptional repressor, leading to decreased expression of target genes that regulate myeloid differentiation and causing the block in myeloid differentiation that characterizes acute leukemia.[104,105] The processes of histone acetylation and promoter methylation have been shown to contribute to transcriptional repression activity of some of these fusion proteins, including AML1–ETO,[106,107] PML–RARA[108] and TEL–AML1.[109] In addition, the constitutive upregulation of HOX genes essential to leukemogenesis associated with abnormalities in the *MLL* gene at 11q23 has been shown to involve DNA methyltransferase and histone acetylase activity.[110,111]

Pediatric development of HDAC inhibitors has focused on vorinostat and romidepsin. The PPTP evaluated vorinostat and observed *in vitro* activity against all of its cell lines, but observed little *in vivo* activity for vorinostat against either the solid tumor or the ALL xenografts.[112] In the pediatric Phase 1 experience with vorinostat, the dose-limiting toxicities of thrombocytopenia and neutropenia were similar to those reported in adults. Pediatric clinical development of vorinostat centers around combination studies, including vorinostat with the proteasome inhibitor bortezomib, with isotretinoin, and with radiation for children with high grade glioma. One of the challenges with the Phase I studies performed with HDAC inhibitors such as vorinostat is identifying doses and schedules that produce agent blood concentrations comparable to those at which the maximum effective response occurs based on preclinical *in vitro* data. Generally, the drug exposures noted in the clinic for agents like vorinostat have been below the concentrations associated with optimal activity in preclinical studies.

Demethylating agents

5-azacytidine and 5-aza-2-deoxycytidine (decitabine) are nucleoside analogs developed originally as cytotoxic agents, however their hypomethylating properties are being recognized as important in antitumor activity. 5-azacytidine is incorporated into both DNA and RNA whereas decitabine is activated and incorporated only into newly synthesized DNA. Once incorporated in replicating DNA instead of cytosine, they covalently bind and trap DNA methyltransferases, thereby rendering them ineffective and causing passive demethylation of the genomic region. These agents are cell cycle, S-phase specific so they require ongoing cell replication to enable incorporation into the genome with the additional requirement of ongoing cycling to facilitate the demethylation of subsequent "daughter" cells.[113] The therapeutic potential of the now recognized hypomethylation activity of both 5-azacytidine and decitabine at low doses (5-azacytidine 50–75 mg/m^2 decitabine 100–150 mg/m^2) is under evaluation in several types of leukemia, notably myelodysplastic syndromes (MDS) and myeloid leukemias. The Cancer and Leukemia Group B (CALGB) performed a series of clinical trials investigating low dose 5-azacytidine in MDS. The outcome of the Phase II trials (CALGB 8421 and CALGB 8921) and the pivotal randomized Phase III trial (CALGB 9221) that compared low-dose 5-azacytidine to best supportive care confirmed the role for low-dose 5-azacytidine in the management of MDS.[114,115] CALGB 9221 demonstrated 10% complete response rate (CR), 1% partial response rate (PR) and 36% hematological improvement (HI) in the 5-azacytidine arm compared to no CR or PR in the supportive care arm. The cross over design of CALGB 9221 allowing supportive care arm patients to move to the 5-azacytidine arm precluded conclusions on overall survival however, a subsequent randomized trial confirmed that low-dose 5-azacytidine (20 mg/m^2/day × 14 days every 28 days) conferred a survival advantage in high risk MDS compared to conventional treatment regimes (51% vs. 26% at 2 years).[116]

Decitabine, a more potent hypomethylating agent inducing a different profile of gene re-expression compared to 5-azacytidine, is also being explored at low-dose schedules in the treatment of MDS and AML.[117] As with 5-azacytidine, the early phase clinical trials of decitabine demonstrated that low-dose schedules were associated with promising response rates in MDS. This led to a Phase III trial randomizing decitabine against best supportive care.[118] Decitabine was administered at 15 mg/m^2 per dose, 8 hourly, × 3 days every 6 weeks and produced 9% CR, 8% PR, and 13% HI compared to no responses in the supportive care arm. Although the responses were durable (median 41 weeks), they did not translate to a statistically significant overall survival advantage (time to AML or death 12.1 months vs. 7.8 months, $p = 0.16$).[118] On the basis of the results of these Phase III trials, the FDA has approved both 5-azacytidine and decitabine for the treatment of MDS. Studies investigating the therapeutic value of inhibitors of DNA demethylators in pediatric MDS are planned but are compromised by the low patient numbers. Patients with MDS and the chromosomal monosomy 7 abnormality have shown a high rate of cytogenetic responses to low-dose decitabine.[119] Toxicities due to 5-azacytidine and decitabine are mild and include myelosuppression, febrile neutropenia, and gastrointestinal toxicity.[120] Similar to HDAC inhibitors, the optimal dose and duration of treatment with demethylating agents remains unclear. The emphasis on dosing should be based on optimum biological activity rather than maximum tolerated dose.

There is a strong rationale for combining a hypomethylating agent and a HDAC inhibitor in AML and MDS. These combinations are currently in clinical trials in these diseases. In additions combinations with all-trans retinoic acid in acute promyelocytic leukemia are appealing based on the rationale that HDAC inhibition would promote retinoic acid receptor signaling.[121] *In vitro* data with vorinostat, romidepsin, and valproic acid suggest that HDAC inhibitors combination therapy may also prove to be useful in the subgroup of AMLs secondary to core binding factor mutations t(8;21) and inv(16), which also recruit HDACs to silence target genes.[107,122]

Although preclinical evidence supports the importance of epigenetic processes in ALL, including that in the pediatric age group, clinical exploration of epigenetic modifiers in ALL has been limited. There is evidence to suggest that epigenetic modifiers may have specific application in certain subgroups of pediatric acute leukemias. Several recurrent chromosomal translocations characterize subgroups of childhood acute leukemia. Eighty percent of infant ALL harbor MLL gene rearrangements (MLL-r) which is known to harbor domains with epigenetic activity and silencing of several tumor suppressor genes. By examining MLL-r infant leukemia samples, global promoter region CpG island hypermethylation characterized the infant ALL samples in comparison to other ALL samples and normal controls. Additional studies are warranted to determine if this is specific to infants with MLL-r ALL or whether it also applies to older children and adults with MLL-r ALL or to patients of any age with either *de novo* or treatment-related MLL-r AML. The DNA methyltransferase inhibitor decitabine preferentially killed MLL-r ALL lymphoblastic cell lines and this response correlated with the upregulation of several of the identified silenced tumor suppressor genes. Decitabine may represent a novel target treatment for this type of MLL-r infant ALL.[123] In a case report, a 10-year-old girl with multiply relapsed ALL (negative for MLL rearrangement), was treated with decitabine in combination with dexamethasone and attained a complete remission and was able to undergo a second allogeneic stem cell transplant.[124]

Ubiquitin Proteasome System

Proteasome inhibitors

The proteasome is responsible for intracellular protein degradation within the cell. Polyubiquitination marks intracellular proteins destined to undergo degradation at the proteasome. Careful control of the degradation of proteins through the ubiquitin–proteasome pathway is essential for multiple processes in the cell which include orderly progression through cell cycle, p53-mediated responses to cellular stresses and NF-κB activation.[125,126]

The dipeptidyl boronic acid compound bortezomib (PS-341) was the first proteasome inhibitor to proceed into clinical development. Bortezomib induced apoptosis in preclinical studies in leukemic cell lines that were chemotherapy-resistant and radiation-resistant. Based on the multiple signaling pathways affected by proteasome inhibition, there is probably not a single effect of bortezomib that is responsible for all its anticancer activity. One effect of bortezomib is to repress nuclear factor-κB signaling by stabilizing IκB, and allowing IκB to maintain it inhibitory influence over NF-κB. Bortezomib can also stabilize p53, allowing it to function as an apoptotic transcription factor in cells exposed to bortezomib. Proteasome inhibition can induce formation of aggresome formation, endoplasmic reticulum stress, and the unfolded protein response which has special relevance for multiple myeloma cells given their high rates of protein synthesis.[125]

Bortezomib is FDA approved for patients with multiple myeloma and with progressive mantle cell lymphoma. The most common moderate to serious adverse events observed in adults receiving bortezomib have been asthenia, peripheral neuropathy, thrombocytopenia, and neutropenia.[126]

Proteasome inhibition is of interest in AML. Although unstimulated CD34+ stem cells do not express activated NF-κB, NF-κB is constitutively activated in primary AML specimens, and specifically in the CD34+/CD38-leukemic stem cell (LSC) population.[127] The combination of a proteasome inhibitor and idarubicin demonstrates rapid and extensive apoptosis of AML blasts and the LSC population *in vitro* and *in vivo*, while preserving normal hematopoietic stem cells.[128] These data have formed the basis for the hypothesis that by selectively targeting the LSC population in AML, more durable responses will be achieved than with standard therapies alone. A Phase I study of bortezomib in adults with refractory or relapsed acute leukemias established tolerability with twice weekly dosing of 1.25 mg/m^2 for 4 weeks of a 6-week cycle.[129] The combination of bortezomib and pegylated liposomal doxorubicin in adults with advanced hematologic malignancies showed activity in 2 of 5 patients with AML.[130] A Phase I study adding bortezomib to a standard reinduction regimen using idarubicin, and cytarabine demonstrated a good safety profile for the regimen and promising antileukemia activity.[131]

Bortezomib is being investigated in pediatric and adolescent leukemias. The Phase I study of bortezomib in pediatric leukemia identified 1.3 mg/m^2 (given twice weekly for 2 weeks out of 3 weeks) as the recommended Phase 2 dose.[132] Dose-limiting toxicities seen at the 1.7 mg/m^2 dose were altered mental state and grade 4 hypotension followed by grade 5 hypoxia in a patient with fever and neutropenia. The Children's Oncology Group is conducting a Phase II study in patients with relapsed/secondary AML in which bortezomib is combined with two induction regimens (idarubicin/cytarabine or etoposide/cytarabine). Several reports have documented *in vitro* activity against ALL cell lines, although this is a nonspecific observation since many cancer cell lines are sensitive to bortezomib. The PPTP showed that bortezomib had some activity against the ALL xenografts with both of the T-cell ALL xenografts evaluated responding to bortezomib.[133] In the Phase I study of bortezomib for children with recurrent leukemias, there were no responses in nine children with B-cell ALL, all heavily pretreated.[132] Against ALL cell lines, bortezomib was synergistic with dexamethasone and additive with vincristine, asparaginase, cytarabine, and doxorubicin.[134] Bortezomib can be safely administered with standard reinduction therapy in the recurrent ALL setting and 8 of 10 patients treated showed a complete response in the bone marrow.[135] This approach is being piloted by the Children's Oncology Group in COG AALL07P1 which is a Phase II pilot trial of bortezomib in combination with intensive reinduction therapy for children with relapsed ALL and lymphoblastic lymphoma.

Since the proteasome has become a valid target for cancer therapy, development of newer inhibitors that may offer additional benefits continues. Several second-generation proteasome inhibitors have entered Phase I trials in adults, including NPI-0052 (salinosporamide A), carfilzomib (formerly PR-171), and MLN9708. While these agents show potential advantages over bortezomib in preclinical models, further clinical evaluations will be needed to determine whether in the clinical setting they have a broader spectrum of activity and/or less neurotoxicity than bortezomib.[136–140] Another potential interesting target is the immunoproteasome, whose expression may be more tissue restricted than the constitutive proteasome. Currently, all the proteasome inhibitors target both the immunoproteasome and constitutive proteasome. Since the immunoproteasome is expressed predominantly in hematopoietic tissues, less toxicity such as neurotoxicity and gastrointestinal effects may be observed since those tissues express much lower levels of immunoproteasome subunits.[141–143]

NEDD8-Activating Enzyme

While proteasome inhibition is an effective way to modulate the ubiquitin–proteasome system for clinical benefit for some disease, other more focused approaches to blocking activity of this system are in development in hopes that new avenues for clinical benefit will be discovered. The orderly degradation of proteins through the ubiquitin–proteasome system requires the coordinated activity of the ubiquitin-activating enzyme (E1), the ubiquitin-conjugating enzymes (E2s), and ubiquitin ligases (E3). Thus, targeting enzymes in the ubiquitin–proteasome pathway upstream of the proteasome could lead to more specific inhibition of the degradation of one or a few key proteins. The cullin-RING ligases represent the largest subclass of E3 ligases, and they control ubiquitination and turnover of many key substrates with important roles in cell cycle control, NF-κB signaling, DNA replication and repair, oxidative stress response, and hypoxia signaling. Activity of the cullin-RING ligases is controlled by the conjugation of the ubiquitin-like protein NEDD8 to the cullin protein in the multi-subunit cullin-RING ligase complex. The initial step in "neddylation" of the cullin protein is the ATP-dependent activation of NEDD8 by the NEDD8-activating enzyme (NAE), and it is this step that has been targeted for therapeutics development.[144]

MLN4924 is a first-in-class, selective inhibitor of NAE. It potently inhibits the growth of a variety of cancer cell lines and shows *in vivo* activity in xenograft models, inducing regressions in selected AML and NHL models.[145,146] The induction of apoptotic death in cancer cells by MLN4924 involves a novel mechanism of action in which there is deregulation of S phase DNA synthesis.[113,144] Phase I trials in hematological malignancies are currently in progress.

Future Directions

For decades, progress in pediatric oncology has centered around intensifying and refining standard chemotherapy. This is no longer the situation since in some malignancies, the maximum intensity has been reached with standard chemotherapy. As a result, if progress is to continue in treatment outcomes of pediatric cancers, the identification of specific targets within these cancers is essential. This will result in changes in classification of these diagnoses and risk categories for treatment and underlines the important role that these new agents will play in making progress in the future. Never before have we had the tools available to identify potentially active agents to help guide and prioritize studies of new agents. In addition, we are now entering the era in which the recurring genomic and epigenomic alterations present in childhood cancer are being delineated and potentially provide targets for novel agents. The limited numbers of children with any given cancer diagnosis and the even smaller number within any diagnosis that have a specific molecular abnormality demonstrate the importance of international collaboration in order to enroll sufficient number of patients onto clinical trials to define the contribution of novel agents for patient populations whose cancer have specific molecular characteristics. The time is now to be able to take advantage of all of these changes if we hope to attain our goal of curing every child and adolescent diagnosed with cancer.

References

1. Houghton PJ, Morton CL, Tucker C, Payne D, Favours E, Cole C, Gorlick R, Kolb EA, Zhang W, Lock R, Carol H, Tajbakhsh M, Reynolds CP, Maris JM, Courtright J, Keir ST, Friedman HS, Stopford C, Zeidner J, Wu J, Liu T, Billups CA, Khan J, Ansher S, Zhang J, Smith MA. (2007) The pediatric preclinical testing program: Description of models and early testing results. *Pediatr Blood Cancer* **49**: 928–940.
2. Lock RB, Liem NL, Papa RA. (2005) Preclinical testing of antileukemic drugs using an *in vivo* model of systemic disease. *Methods Mol Med* **111**: 323–334.
6. Robinson BW, Behling KC, Gupta M, Zhang AY, Moore JS, Bantly AD, Willman CL, Carroll AJ, Adamson PC, Barrett JS, Felix CA. (2008) Abundant anti-apoptotic BCL-2 is a molecular target in leukaemias with t(4;11) translocation. *Br J Haematol* **141**: 827–839.
7. Lock R, Carol H, Houghton PJ, Morton CL, Kolb EA, Gorlick R, Reynolds CP, Maris JM, Keir ST, Wu J, Smith MA. (2008) Initial testing (stage 1) of the BH3 mimetic ABT-263 by the pediatric preclinical testing program. *Pediatr Blood Cancer* **50**: 1181–1189.
10. Tse C, Shoemaker AR, Adickes J, Anderson MG, Chen J, Jin S, Johnson EF, Marsh KC, Mitten MJ, Nimmer P, Roberts L, Tahir SK, Xiao Y, Yang X, Zhang H, Fesik S, Rosenberg SH, Elmore SW. (2008) ABT-263: A potent and orally bioavailable Bcl-2 family inhibitor. *Cancer Res* **68**: 3421–3428.
11. Nguyen M, Marcellus RC, Roulston A, Watson M, Serfass L, Murthy Madiraju SR, Goulet D, Viallet J, Belec L, Billot X, Acoca S, Purisima E, Wiegmans A, Cluse L, Johnstone RW, Beauparlant P, Shore GC. (2007) Small molecule obatoclax (GX15-070) antagonizes MCL-1 and overcomes MCL-1-mediated resistance to apoptosis. *Proc Natl Acad Sci USA* **104**: 19512–19517.
16. Nachmias B, Ashhab Y, Ben-Yehuda D. (2004) The inhibitor of apoptosis protein Family (IAPs): An emerging therapeutic target in cancer. *Semin Cancer Biol* **14**: 231–243.
17. Tamm I, Richter S, Oltersdorf D, Creutzig U, Harbott J, Scholz F, Karawajew L, Ludwig WD, Wuchter C. (2004) High expression levels of X-linked inhibitor of apoptosis protein and survivin correlate with poor overall survival in childhood *de novo* acute myeloid leukemia. *Clin Cancer Res* **10**: 3737–3744.
30. Vassilev LT. (2004) Small-molecule antagonists of p53-MDM2 binding: Research tools and spotential therapeutics. *Cell Cycle* **3**: 419–421.

32. Kojima K, Konopleva M, Samudio IJ, Shikami M, Cabreira-Hansen M, McQueen T, Ruvolo V, Tsao T, Zeng Z, Vassilev LT, Andreeff M. (2005) MDM2 antagonists induce p53-dependent apoptosis in AML: Implications for leukemia therapy. *Blood* **106**: 3150–3159.
44. Jeong EG, Kim MS, Nam HK, Min CK, Lee S, Chung YJ, Yoo NJ, Lee SH. (2008) Somatic mutations of JAK1 and JAK3 in acute leukemias and solid cancers. *Clin Cancer Res* **14**: 3716–3721.
46. Fridman J, Nussenzveig R, Liu P, Rodgers J, Burn T, Haley P, Scherle P, Newton R, Hollis G, Friedman S, Verstovek S, Vaddi K. (2007) Discovery and preclinical characterization of INCB018424, a selective JAK2 inhibitor for the treatment of myeloproliferative disorders. *Blood* **110**: (abstract 3538).
48. Pardanani A, Gotlib, JR, Jamieson C, *et al.* (2009) A Phase I evaluation of TG101348, a selective JAK2 inhibitor, in myelofibrosis: Clinical response is accompanied by significant reduction in *JAK*2V617F allele burden. *Blood* **114**: 755A.
49. Kwak EL, Camidge DR, Clark J, Shapiro GI, Maki RG, Ratain MJ, Solomon B, Bang Y, Ou S, Salgia R. (2009) Clinical activity observed in a phase I dose escalation trial of an oral c-met and ALK inhibitor, PF-02341066. *J Clin Oncol* **27**: (abstract 3509).
50. Meric-Bernstam F, Gonzalez-Angulo AM. (2009) Targeting the mTOR signaling network for cancer therapy. *J Clin Oncol* **27**: 2278–2287.
54. Baldo P, Cecco S, Giacomin E, Lazzarini R, Ros B, Marastoni S. (2008) mTOR pathway and mTOR inhibitors as agents for cancer therapy. *Curr Cancer Drug Targets* **8**: 647–665.
55. Houghton PJ, Morton CL, Kolb EA, Gorlick R, Lock R, Carol H, Reynolds CP, Maris JM, Keir ST, Billups CA, Smith MA. (2008) Initial testing (stage 1) of the mTOR inhibitor rapamycin by the pediatric preclinical testing program. *Pediatr Blood Cancer* **50**: 799–805.
57. Teachey DT, Sheen C, Hall J, Ryan T, Brown VI, Fish J, Reid GS, Seif AE, Norris R, Chang YJ, Carroll M, Grupp SA. (2008) mTOR inhibitors are synergistic with methotrexate: An effective combination to treat acute lymphoblastic leukemia. *Blood* **112**: 2020–2023.
58. Fouladi M, Laningham F, Wu J, O'Shaughnessy MA, Molina K, Broniscer A, Spunt SL, Luckett I, Stewart CF, Houghton PJ, Gilbertson RJ, Furman WL. (2007) Phase I study of everolimus in pediatric patients with refractory solid tumors. *J Clin Oncol* **25**: 4806–4812.
59. Spunt SL GS, Vik T. (2007) Phase I, safety, pharmacokinetic, exploratory biomarker study of intravenous temsirolimus in children with advanced solid tumors. *Pediatric Blood Cancer.*
60. Rheingold SR SN, Chang YJ *et al.* (2007) A phase I trial of Sirolimus (Rapamycin) in pediatric patients with relapsed/refractory leukemia. *Blood* **110**.
67. Yee KW, Zeng Z, Konopleva M, Verstovsek S, Ravandi F, Ferrajoli A, Thomas D, Wierda W, Apostolidou E, Albitar M, O'Brien S, Andreeff M, Giles FJ. (2006) Phase I/II study of the mammalian target of rapamycin inhibitor everolimus (RAD001) in patients with relapsed or refractory hematologic malignancies. *Clin Cancer Res* **12**: 5165–5173.
68. Rizzieri DA, Feldman E, Dipersio JF, Gabrail N, Stock W, Strair R, Rivera VM, Albitar M, Bedrosian CL, Giles FJ. (2008) A phase 2 clinical trial of deforolimus (AP23573, MK-8669), a novel mammalian target of rapamycin inhibitor, in patients with relapsed or refractory hematologic malignancies. *Clin Cancer Res* **14**: 2756–2762.
72. Courtney KD, Corcoran RB, Engelman JA. The PI3K pathway as drug target in human cancer. *J Clin Oncol* **28**: 1075–1083.
74. Aster JC, Pear WS, Blacklow SC. (2008) Notch signaling in leukemia. *Annu Rev Pathol* **3**: 587–613.
75. Armstrong F, Brunet de la Grange P, Gerby B, Rouyez MC, Calvo J, Fontenay M, Boissel N, Dombret H, Baruchel A, Landman-Parker J, Romeo PH, Ballerini P, Pflumio F. (2009) NOTCH is a key regulator of human T-cell acute leukemia initiating cell activity. *Blood* **113**: 1730–1740.
77. Lewis HD, Leveridge M, Strack PR, Haldon CD, O'Neil J, Kim H, Madin A, Hannam JC, Look AT, Kohl N, Draetta G, Harrison T, Kerby JA, Shearman MS, Beher D. (2007) Apoptosis in T cell acute lymphoblastic leukemia cells after cell cycle arrest induced by pharmacological inhibition of notch signaling. *Chem Biol* **14**: 209–219.
79. Milano J, McKay J, Dagenais C, Foster-Brown L, Pognan F, Gadient R, Jacobs RT, Zacco A, Greenberg B, Ciaccio PJ. (2004) Modulation of notch processing by gamma-secretase inhibitors causes intestinal goblet cell metaplasia and induction of genes known to specify gut secretory lineage differentiation. *Toxicol Sci* **82**: 341–358.
81. Real PJ, Tosello V, Palomero T, Castillo M, Hernando E, de Stanchina E, Sulis ML, Barnes K, Sawai C, Homminga I, Meijerink J, Aifantis I, Basso G, Cordon-Cardo C, Ai W, Ferrando A. (2009) Gamma-secretase inhibitors reverse glucocorticoid resistance in T cell acute lymphoblastic leukemia. *Nat Med* **15**: 50–58.
87. Vader G, Lens SM. (2008) The Aurora kinase family in cell division and cancer. *Biochim Biophys Acta* **1786**: 60–72.

89. Maris JM, Morton CL, Gorlick R, Kolb EA, Lock R, Carol H, Keir ST, Reynolds CP, Kang MH, Wu J, Smith MA, Houghton PJ. Initial testing of the aurora kinase a inhibitor MLN8237 by the Pediatric Preclinical Testing Program (PPTP). *Pediatr Blood Cancer.*
90. Moore AS, Blagg J, Linardopoulos S, Pearson AD. (2010) Aurora kinase inhibitors: Novel small molecules with promising activity in acute myeloid and Philadelphia-positive leukemias. *Leukemia* **24**: 671–678.
92. Rudolph D, Steegmaier M, Hoffmann M, Grauert M, Baum A, Quant J, Haslinger C, Garin-Chesa P, Adolf GR. (2009) BI 6727, a Polo-like kinase inhibitor with improved pharmacokinetic profile and broad antitumor activity. *Clin Cancer Res* **15**: 3094–3102.
93. Meshinchi S, Alonzo TA, Stirewalt DL, Zwaan M, Zimmerman M, Reinhardt D, Kaspers GJ, Heerema NA, Gerbing R, Lange BJ, Radich JP. (2006) Clinical implications of FLT3 mutations in pediatric AML. *Blood* **108**: 3654–3661.
95. Pratz KW, Cortes J, Roboz GJ, Rao N, Arowojolu O, Stine A, Shiotsu Y, Shudo A, Akinaga S, Small D, Karp JE, Levis M. (2009) A pharmacodynamic study of the FLT3 inhibitor KW-2449 yields insight into the basis for clinical response. *Blood* **113**: 3938–3946.
98. Metzelder S, Wang Y, Wollmer E, Wanzel M, Teichler S, Chaturvedi A, Eilers M, Enghofer E, Neubauer A, Burchert A. (2009) Compassionate use of sorafenib in FLT3-ITD-positive acute myeloid leukemia: Sustained regression before and after allogeneic stem cell transplantation. *Blood* **113**: 6567–6571.
100. Ravandi F, Cortes JE, Jones D, Faderl S, Garcia-Manero G, Konopleva MY, O'Brien S, Estrov Z, Borthakur G, Thomas D, Pierce SR, Brandt M, Byrd A, Bekele BN, Pratz K, Luthra R, Levis M, Andreeff M, Kantarjian HM. (2010) Phase I/II study of combination therapy with sorafenib, idarubicin, and cytarabine in younger patients with acute myeloid leukemia. *J Clin Oncol.*
102. Marks PA, Richon VM, Kelly WK, Chiao JH, Miller T. (2004) Histone deacetylase inhibitors: Development as cancer therapy. *Novartis Found Symp* **259**: 269–281; discussion 281–268.
112. Keshelava N, Houghton PJ, Morton CL, Lock RB, Carol H, Keir ST, Maris JM, Reynolds CP, Gorlick R, Kolb EA, Wu J, Smith MA. (2009) Initial testing (stage 1) of vorinostat (SAHA) by the pediatric preclinical testing program. *Pediatr Blood Cancer* **53**: 505–508.
113. Soucy TA, Smith PG, Rolfe M. (2009) Targeting NEDD8-activated cullin-RING ligases for the treatment of cancer. *Clin Cancer Res* **15**: 3912–3916.
118. Kantarjian H, Issa JP, Rosenfeld CS, Bennett JM, Albitar M, DiPersio J, Klimek V, Slack J, de Castro C, Ravandi F, Helmer R, 3rd, Shen L, Nimer SD, Leavitt R, Raza A, Saba H. (2006) Decitabine improves patient outcomes in myelodysplastic syndromes: Results of a phase III randomized study. *Cancer* **106**: 1794–1803.
125. Orlowski RZ, Kuhn DJ. (2008) Proteasome inhibitors in cancer therapy: Lessons from the first decade. *Clin Cancer Res* **14**: 1649–1657.
132. Horton TM, Pati D, Plon SE, Thompson PA, Bomgaars LR, Adamson PC, Ingle AM, Wright J, Brockman AH, Paton M, Blaney SM. (2007) A phase 1 study of the proteasome inhibitor bortezomib in pediatric patients with refractory leukemia: A Children's Oncology Group study. *Clin Cancer Res* **13**: 1516–1522.
133. Houghton PJ, Morton CL, Kolb EA, Lock R, Carol H, Reynolds CP, Keshelava N, Maris JM, Keir ST, Wu J, Smith MA. (2008) Initial testing (stage 1) of the proteasome inhibitor bortezomib by the pediatric preclinical testing program. *Pediatr Blood Cancer* **50**: 37–45.
134. Horton TM, Gannavarapu A, Blaney SM, D'Argenio DZ, Plon SE, Berg SL. (2006) Bortezomib interactions with chemotherapy agents in acute leukemia *in vitro*. *Cancer Chemother Pharmacol* **58**: 13–23.
135. Messenger YH GP, Raetz E *et al.* (2008) Remarkable activity of bortezomib combine with chemotherapy in phase I study of relapsed childhood acute lymphoblastic leukemia (ALL). A report form the Therapeutic Advances in Childhood Leukemia (TACL) Consortium. *Blood* **112**.
144. Soucy TA, Smith PG, Milhollen MA, Berger AJ, Gavin JM, Adhikari S, Brownell JE, Burke KE, Cardin DP, Critchley S, Cullis CA, Doucette A, Garnsey JJ, Gaulin JL, Gershman RE, Lublinsky AR, McDonald A, Mizutani H, Narayanan U, Olhava EJ, Peluso S, Rezaei M, Sintchak MD, Talreja T, Thomas MP, Traore T, Vyskocil S, Weatherhead GS, Yu J, Zhang J, Dick LR, Claiborne CF, Rolfe M, Bolen JB, Langston SP. (2009) An inhibitor of NEDD8-activating enzyme as a new approach to treat cancer. *Nature* **458**: 732–736.

23

Adoptive Cellular and Gene Therapy

Laurence J.N. Cooper and Helen E. Heslop

Introduction

Some, but not all malignancies in children, adolescents, and young adults can be cured by undertaking hemopoietic stem cell transplantation (HSCT) after conventional therapies such as chemotherapy, radiation, and surgery. Allogeneic HSCT provides recipients with an engrafted immune system that can seek and destroy malignant cells (see Chapter 20). To improve the therapeutic potential of immunotherapy to not only increase cure rates, but provide a less toxic therapy, the cellular components of the immune system can be manipulated *ex vivo* for *in vivo* application. In some instances, their function may be further enhanced by gene transfer. Adoptive transfer of immune system effectors targeting antigens expressed on tumor cells may potentially produce long-lived antitumor activity and this approach has already shown activity in selected clinical applications such as donor lymphocyte infusions after HSCT and the use of T cells to treat EBV-associated lymphomas (see Chapter 19). However, broad application of adoptive immunotherapy requires the development of approaches to identify and target less immunodominant antigens and to improve suboptimal persistence of transferred autologous and allogeneic lymphocytes to overcome tumor-evasion strategies.

Allogeneic Donor Lymphocytes Post-HSCT

Allogeneic HSCT is widely used for pediatric patients with high-risk and relapsed hematologic malignancies.[1] Although the chemotherapy and radiotherapy used in conditioning regimens contribute to the therapeutic effect, the role of the immune system in the graft-vs.-leukemia (GVL)-effect has been appreciated in animal models for many years has been and confirmed by clinical observations in recipients who developed graft-vs.-host disease (GVHD) and had a lower incidence of relapse.[2] More recently, the wider use of reduced intensity conditioning regimens has reinforced the role of alloreactivity in eradicating hematologic malignancies with studies showing that antitumor responses post-HSCT correlate with development of a diverse T cell response specific for minor histocompatibility[3] or tumor-associated antigens (TAA) such as WT1.[4]

Donor lymphocyte infusions

The use of donor lymphocyte infusions (DLI) to treat patients with relapse following an allogeneic HSCT has emphasized the role of GVL effects in controlling disease.[5] DLI results in significant clinical responses in relapsed patients, particularly those with chronic myeloid leukemia (CML) and lymphoma.[5] Responses have also been noted in acute myeloid leukemia (AML) and some cases of acute lymphoid leukemia (ALL), but the overall response rate is much lower for acute leukemias.[5] DLI has also been highly effective in treating Epstein–Barr virus (EBV)-associated post-transplant lymphoproliferative disease (PTLD) following allogeneic HSCT.[6] The major drawback of DLI is that the unmanipulated product contains precursors reactive with other host tissues resulting in a significant risk of GVHD and compromised engraftment.[5] As the frequency of TAA-specific T cells is much lower than that of alloreactive T cells within the DLI product, strategies have been developed to either selectively deplete alloreactive cells from a heterogeneous population or to enrich TAA-specific T cells by *ex vivo* expansion.

Allodepletion

One approach to the problem of deleterious alloreactivity is to selectively deplete donor-derived T cells of alloreactive cells which express activation markers including CD69, CD147, and the IL2 receptor CD25, in response to stimulation with alloantigens expressed on recipient cells. Three clinical trials have tested this strategy using a CD25 immunotoxin to deplete alloreactive T cells *ex vivo*.[7–9] Either recipient peripheral blood mononuclear cells (PBMC) or EBV-transformed lymphoblastoid cell lines (LCL) were used as a source of alloantigen for stimulation. In each study, administration of allodepleted T cells promoted the reconstitution of antiviral immunity without inducing GVHD, but the antitumor effects were less convincing.[7–9] Further studies to optimize the process and increase antitumor immunity are underway.[10] Another approach cocultures donor-derived T cells with alloantigens found on recipient PBMC in the presence of costimulatory blockade, for example provided by anti-CD80 and CD86. This leads to desired anergy of the T cells to alloantigens without loss of immune responses to specific viral antigens and TAA; clinical trials are using such anergized T cells to restore immune reconstitution after haploidentical HSCT.[11]

EBV-specific T cells

To overcome the risk of alloreactivity with DLI, investigators developed approaches to generate cytotoxic T cells *ex vivo* for the recipient by repeated stimulation of donor-derived PBMC with antigen-presenting cells (APC) expressing TAAs found on EBV-infected malignant B cells (Fig. 23.1). To translate this approach to the clinic, the EBV-derived antigens expressed by malignant cells were identified and a subset of immunodominant genes were found to be expressed on LCL which could serve as immortalized APC with the necessary costimulation required, thereby triggering an effective T cell response during *in vitro* culture. This approach was initially evaluated in the setting of EBV-associated PTLD which is an excellent model as the outgrowing tumor cells have the same phenotype and pattern of EBV gene expression as EBV-transformed LCL. LCL can be manufactured from the transplant donor by infecting PBMC with a laboratory strain of EBV and used as irradiated stimulator cells to generate autologous EBV-specific cytotoxic T cell lines (CTLs). When EBV-specific CTLs were administered as prophylaxis or therapy for PTLD in high-risk allogeneic HSCT recipients, they have been able to expand and reconstitute immunity to EBV.[12,13] In a long-term follow-up study of four trials, none of the 101 high-risk patients who received CTL prophylaxis developed PTLD compared with 11% of control patients.[12] In addition, 11 of 13 patients treated with CTLs for biopsy-proven or probable PTLD achieved sustained complete remissions.[12]

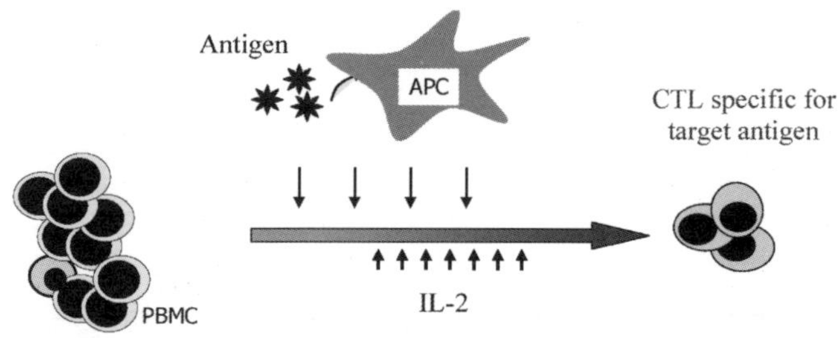

Fig. 23.1. Generating CTLs by repeated *ex vivo* stimulation. Low-frequency virus-specific CTLs in a PBMC population are expanded by primary and secondary stimulation with antigen expressed on APC followed by expansion with IL-2. The resulting population is enriched for T cells specific for the viral antigen.

TAA-specific T cells to treat hematologic malignancies

Most hematologic malignancies do not express viral-derived antigens. Potential TAA are listed in Table 23.1 and include minor histocompatibility antigens, lineage-restricted antigens and novel antigens generated by tumor-specific translocations. Minor histocompatibility antigens are polymorphic genes that differ between donor and recipient. If such antigens are selectively expressed on hemopoietic cells, they may serve as a candidate antigen for targeting by T cells as exemplified by

Table 23.1. Potential tumor antigens.

Target	Examples	Malignancies
Viral antigens	EBV	Non-Hodgkin lymphoma Hodgkin's disease
	SV40	Non-Hodgkin lymphoma
Differentiation antigen	CD19 or CD20	NHL
	CD30	Hodgkin's disease
	PR1	Myeloid malignancies
Cancer testes antigens	MAGE antigens NY-ESO	Testicular and many hematologic malignancies[13]
Minor antigens	HA1, HA2	Hematologic malignancies post transplant
Tumor-specific antigens	Telomerase	Many types of malignancies
	Idiotype	NHL
	WT1	Many hematologic malignancies

a case report that described a patient with relapsed CML who attained complete remission following infusion of minor histocompatibility antigen-specific CTL derived from the donor.[14] A more recent report describes administration of CD8+ CTL-clones specific for tissue-restricted recipient minor histocompatibility antigens.[15] These cells persisted for up to 3 weeks after infusion and induced complete, but transient remissions in 5 of 7 recipients which illustrates the potential of this targeted approach.[15] Unfortunately, pulmonary toxicity was seen in three patients, because of unexpected expression of the targeted minor histocompatibility antigens in normal lung tissue illustrating the difficulty of identifying targets selectively expressed on tumor cells.[15]

Autologous T Cell Infusion

Autologous TAA-specific CTLs

As described above, EBV-PTLD has served as a prototype disease for successful targeting of viral antigens associated with cancer. These results provided the rationale for evaluation of EBV-specific CTLs for treating other EBV-associated malignancies, such as Hodgkin lymphoma, some types of non-Hodgkin lymphoma (NHL), and nasopharyngeal carcinoma. In this setting, autologous EBV-specific CTLs were infused, but initial studies revealed decreased response rates compared to the use of donor-derived CTLs to treat PTLD.[16,17] One explanation is that these tumors, which develop in previously immunocompetent individuals, express a more restricted array of EBV-encoded antigens than EBV-PTLD, which is a highly immunogenic tumor expressing all nine EBV latency antigens including the immunodominant EBNA 3 antigens. In contrast, Hodgkin lymphoma, NHL, and nasopharyngeal carcinoma in the immunocompetent host express only weakly immunogenic EBV antigens (EBNA1, LMP1 and LMP2). Investigators have therefore developed strategies to increase the frequency of CTL clones recognizing these subdominant tumor antigens by stimulating T cells with LMP (latent membrane protein) antigens through enforced expression on APC (dendritic cells or LCLs) using adenoviral vectors.[18] The resulting CTLs are enriched for T cells specific for desired LMP antigens and showed increased activity compared with generic EBV-specific CTLs when administered to patients with EBV+ Hodgkin disease or NHL, either post-HSCT or in the setting of relapsed disease.[18]

T cells non-specifically activated ex vivo

Autologous T cells can be numerically expanded *ex vivo* through polyclonal activation using cross-linked OKT3 (monoclonal (mAb) specific for CD3) or a combination of OKT3 and mAb specific for CD28 antibody and several groups have evaluated whether such propagated T cells might have antitumor activity. Based on reports that correlated faster recovery of lymphocyte counts with improved outcome after autologous HSCT for both NHL and Hodgkin disease, this nonspecific cellular product has mainly been infused after autologous HSCT to augment T-cell function against minimal residual disease.[19,20] Infusion of autologous CD3/CD28-activated T cells is associated with rapid recovery of lymphocyte counts.[21] The strategy has also been combined with vaccination and recipients who received vaccine-primed T cells early after autologous HSCT had better humoral response and better CD4+ proliferative response to the vaccine carrier protein than other treatment groups. These studies provide insights into how vaccination and adoptive cellular therapy can be effectively combined.[22]

Infusion of T Cells Genetically Modified to Redirect Specificity

The engraftment of allogeneic T cells after HSCT provides the pre-eminent example for how donor-derived immune cells can mediate an antitumor effect. However, given the morbidity and mortality of HSCT, investigators have sought approaches to infuse just the T cells themselves, rather than transplanting an entire

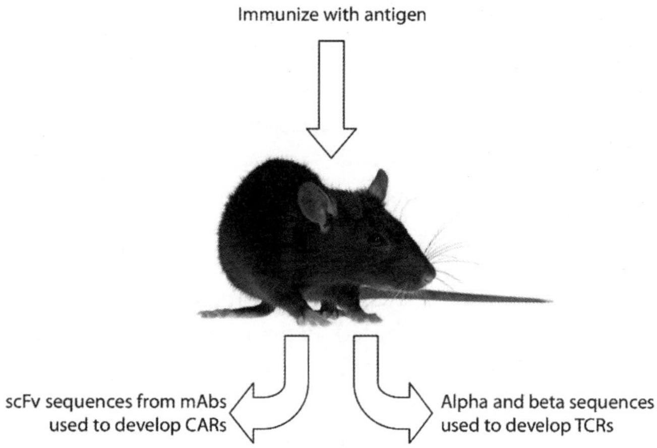

Fig. 23.2. Generating tumor-specific T cells by enforced expression of an immunoreceptor. Immunization of mice with TAA can be used to generate mAbs that recognize tumors. These mAbs can themselves be used as immunotherapy or their antigen-binding domains (scFv region) can be sequenced and used to build CARs. Similarly, immunization with TAA can be used to break T-cell tolerance in mice expressing transgenic human MHC. The murine $\alpha\beta$ TCR genes can be sequenced and used to develop TCRs for expression in MHC-restricted human T cells.

allograft to restore hematopoiesis, in order to produce a potent graft-vs.-tumor (GVT)-effect. One of the obstacles to be overcome with adoptive transfer of T cells is the lack of specificity for TAA. This is especially apparent in the autologous setting, as T cells are tolerized against self-antigens (Table 23.1) which are typically identified as TAA. One approach to overcoming tolerance is through the use of gene therapy to introduce an immunoreceptor to redirect specificity. These immunoreceptors can be derived from mice and the subsequently expressed in human T cells to redirect specificity (Fig. 23.2). There are two pre-eminent examples of using gene therapy to introduce murine sequences that target human TAAs. One approach is based upon the generation of mAbs and cloning of their antigen-binding domains (scFv regions) which are used as a template for the construction of single-chain immunoreceptors termed chimeric antigen receptors (CARs). The CAR when introduced into T cells redirects the specificity independent of major histocompatibility complex (MHC). The other method to break tolerance is to immunize transgenic mice expressing a human MHC molecule, such as HLA A2 and then harvesting the murine $\alpha\beta$ T-cell receptor (TCR) which can be introduced into human T cells to redirect specificity in the context of MHC. Both of these approaches have been used in clinical trials to redirect specificity to desired TAA and both have been associated with imparting an antitumor effect.

Approaches to genetically transfer immunoreceptor genes into T cells

There are two methods to introduce immunoreceptors into T cells which have been used in clinical trials. One uses viral transduction with recombinant retrovirus and the other uses nonviral gene transfer based on electroporation.[23–25] The use of recombinant retrovirus is most common since the gene transfer efficiency has previously been superior to nonviral approaches. Indeed, there are now published clinical data which demonstrate an antitumor effect when T cells are transduced to express a CAR.[26] There are two potential drawbacks to the use of recombinant retrovirus for the genetic modification to T cells. The first involves the economics of preparing and releasing a clinical-grade retrovirus from a limited number of production facilities and the current need for testing of the packaging cells and the patient-specific genetically modified cells for the presence of replication-competent retrovirus. The other issue is that retroviruses have a nonrandom integration pattern into the genome which may lead to insertional mutagenesis. This was apparent in the French gene therapy trial to correct X-linked severe combined immunodeficiency (SCID-X1) when the transduction of autologous CD34+ hematopoietic stem cells resulted in the emergence of a clonal population of T cells with autonomous proliferation mostly due to the integration of retroviral sequences into or near LMO2 proto-oncogene.[27,28] Contrasting viral gene transfer is the use of electroporation to introduce desired transgenes into T cells. This approach has been facilitated by two developments. The first is the availability of the Nucleofector to electrotransfer DNA plasmids into T cells. Investigators now routinely use this device to obtain transient transfection of desired transgenes in greater than 50% of primary T cells from PBMC or umbilical cord blood. One of the problems of electrotransfer of plasmids is the low integration efficiency. This has been overcome by the second major advance surrounding this technology, in which the investigators have used the transposon/transposase systems to improve the integration efficiency. Both the *Sleeping Beauty* (SB) and the *piggyBac* (PB) systems have been adapted for the expression of immunoreceptors in human T cells (Fig. 23.3).[29–32] These transposon/transposase systems can be thought of as similar to retrovirus as the genetic cargo load (transposon) is flanked by internal repeats

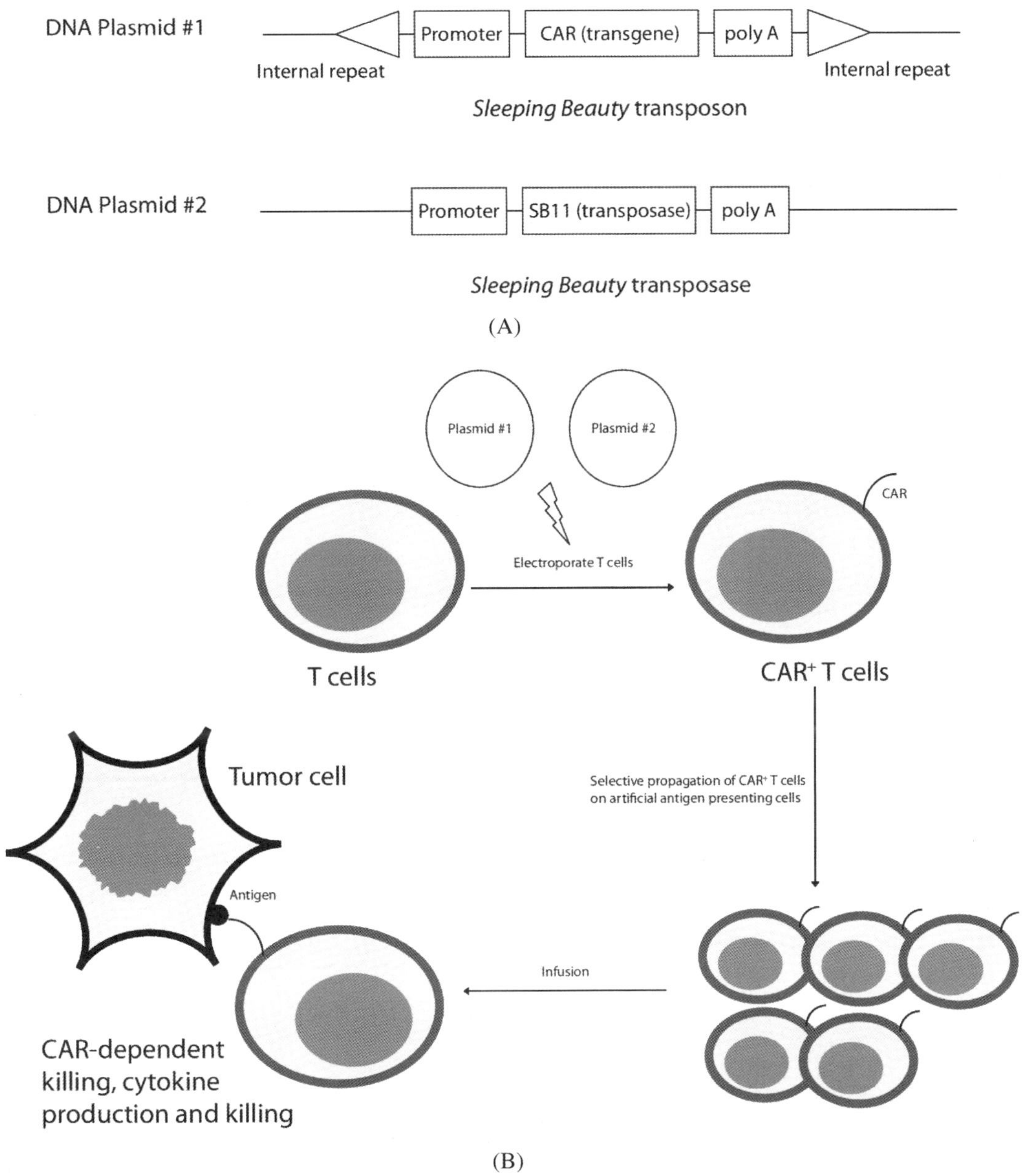

Fig. 23.3. Nonviral gene transfer of *Sleeping Beauty* system to express CAR and numerically expand CAR+ T cells on artificial antigen-presenting cells. (A) The *Sleeping Beauty* (SB) system shown as two DNA plasmids expressing the transposon (in this case a CAR) and transposase (e.g. SB11). The transposase mediates transposition by inserting the transposon, flanked by two internal repeats, into TA dinucleotide repeats in the T-cell genome. (B) Electro-transfer of the SB plasmids into T cells and selective propagation of CAR+ T cells on artificial antigen presenting cells (aAPC). CAR-mediated numeric expansion is achieved by the aAPC expressing antigen recognized by the CAR (e.g. CD19) and desired costimulatory molecules. The CAR+ T cells can recognize tumor cells (e.g. CD19+ malignant B cells) resulting in killing, cytokine release, and proliferation.

(analogous to the long-term repeats in the retroviral expression vector) which is integrated into the T cell genome via a transposase (an enzyme analogous to the integrase found in retrovirus). We have recently been able to adapt the SB system for clinical trials.[33] The advantages of a transposon/transposase system can be considered in reference to the retroviral approaches as the cost for producing clinical grade plasmids is considerably less than that associated with the manufacture of clinical-grade retrovirus. Furthermore, the integration pattern of the SB system into TA dinucleotide repeats appears to be more random than is achieved using retrovirus. Both viral and nonviral gene transfer approaches have their advantages and disadvantages and both are under investigation in clinical trials for the purposes of redirecting T cell specificity.

Introduction to α and β T-cell receptor, two transgenes to redirect T cell specificity

T cells use α and β chains of the TCR to recognize peptide antigens in the context of self-MHC. Engrafted donor-derived T cells are critical for providing and sustaining an antitumor response, whether it be emerging from the bone marrow of patients with leukemia undergoing allogeneic HSCT or intravenously infused in patients with metastatic melanoma.[34] However, investigators have recognized that T cells bearing unmanipulated αβ TCR pairs may not have sufficient functional avidity for desired TAA to produce a sustained or predictable antitumor effect. Thus, investigators have developed genetic approaches to improve TCR avidity, which when introduced into T cells, may increase their therapeutic potential. For example, murine melanoma-specific TCR chains have been expressed in human T cells and used in clinical trials.[35] This approach is complicated by the problems of mispairing between the introduced and endogenous α and β chains resulting in unwanted hybrid molecules which have not be subject thymic deletion and thus may be autoreactive.

Introduction of CAR, a single transgene to redirect T cell specificity

The ability to genetically modify T cells to express TCR chains allows investigators to target the intracellular TAA. The introduction of single chain CARs allows investigators to target self-surfaced TAAs (Fig. 23.4). The former technology uses TCR chains to recognize TAA in the context of MHC whereas the latter approach provides recognition of self-surface TAA independent of MHC. The prototypical CAR uses the scFv region of a mAb, which is held by extracellular scaffolding domains to the T-cell surface and then upon docking with TAA, activates T cells through one or more cytoplasmic signaling domains typically involving CD3-ζ. The CAR-mediated signal is based on recognition of TAA by the scFv and could result in non-physiologic activation. Thus, investigators have extensively modified the structures of CARs, both in terms of the type of scaffolding that as well as the endodomain that activates T cells to recapitulate a fully competent activation signal that accompanies TCR binding to peptide and MHC.[36]

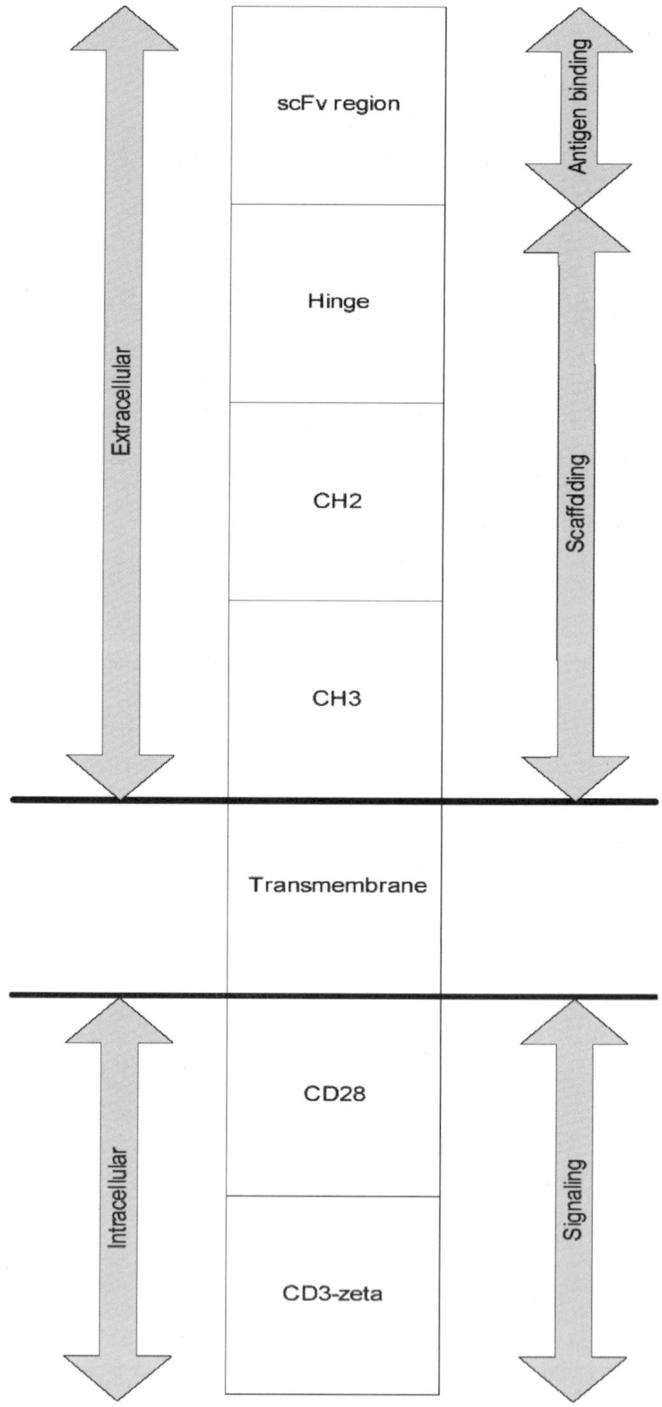

Fig. 23.4. Schematic of a second-generation CAR to target a cell-surface TAA. This prototypical CAR expresses two intracellular signaling domains (CD28 and CD3-ζ) that activate T-cell effector functions upon the extracellular domain docking with antigen via the scFv region. The scFv region is bound to the cell via a scaffold which in this case is derived from human IgG4 hinge, C_H2, and C_H3 regions.

Infusion of T Cells Genetically Modified to Augment Function in the Tumor Microenvironment

While genetically modified T cells may have potent specificity for malignant cells, there are additional obstacles for successful immunotherapy. Tumors possess a number of immune evasion strategies to evade adoptively transferred immune system effectors.[37,38] These include failure to present tumor antigens appropriately to the immune system, loss of targeted TAAs, secretion of cytokines that promote an immunosuppressive environment, and recruitment of regulatory T cells (T_{regs}). These evasion mechanisms can impede *in vivo* persistence, function, and expansion of adoptively transferred T cells. Gene transfer provides a means of modifying infused T cells to confer resistance to these evasion mechanisms. For example, the CD28 chimeric endodomain may help CAR+ T cells avoid T_{reg}-mediated immunosuppression. Many tumor cells or their associated infiltrating cells produce TGF-β which favors the development of immune tolerance and T-cell anergy.[39] If T cells are genetically modified to express a dominant negative (dn) TGF-β receptor however, they can become resistant to the anti-proliferative effects of TGF-β and retain their functionality *in vivo*.[40] An alternative approach is to modify T cells to express cytokine or cytokine receptor genes that reproduce the environment found after lymphodepletion, such as IL-2, IL-7, or IL-15.[41,42] These strategies are promising in preclinical models and will soon be tested in the clinic. Other approaches under evaluation are administration of mAbs to receptors on T cells that have an inhibitory effect on T cell activation such as CTLA4 (cytotoxic T-lymphocyte antigen-4) and PD-1 (programmed death-1).

Infusion of NK Cells

Just as T cells can be genetically modified to improve tumor specificity, immunogenetics can be adapted to improve the antitumor effect of natural killer (NK) cells. This has been exploited to achieve an antitumor effect in two situations.

Example #1

The first example stems from patients with AML who undergo haploidentical HSCT.[43] These patients have been shown to benefit from a NK cell-mediated effect when MHC class I molecules between the donor and recipient are appropriately mismatched so that engrafted NK cells are released from inhibition on account of the killer immunoglobulin receptor (KIR) failing to recognize its MHC ligand on AML blasts.[44,45] The potential for a NK-cell mediated antitumor effect after unrelated HLA-matched HSCT as well as autologous HSCT is being explored to take advantage of the concept of NK-cell licensing.[46] Infusing haploidentical NK cells with KIR-HLA disparity is being undertaken in pilot studies for other hematopoietic tumors such as ALL as well as solid tumors such as neuroblastoma.[47] These clinical trials are supported by the convincing clinical data achieved after the adoptive transfer of NK cells to treat refractory AML. Since persistence of NK cells is correlated with the therapeutic effect, recipients with AML have augmented survival of infused NK cells after receiving lymphodepleting chemotherapy to induce lymphopenia-driven expansion of NK cells when coupled with infusion of the survival cytokine IL-2.

Example #2

In the second example, gene therapy is used to redirect the specificity of NK cell-mediated killing rather than relying on the genetics of KIR and HLA. Genetically modified NK cells can express CAR to redirect specificity.[48,49] The clinical evaluation of these CAR+ cells has lagged behind CAR+ T cells in part because of early difficulties that include (i) propagating NK cells, (ii) genetically modifying NK cells, and (iii) developing CARs with the cytoplasmic domains to provide a fully competent NK cell activation event.[50] These hurdles have now been overcome and it is notable that artificial antigen presenting cells (aAPC) can efficiently numerically expand NK cells to large numbers. One potential clinical scenario that CAR+ NK cell might have a particular roll is infusions after allogeneic HSCT, as donor-derived NK cells are not thought to participate in GVHD.

NKT cell therapy

NKT cells are a subset of T cells that recognize tumor-derived lipids in the context of CD1d, a specialized HLA molecule. NKT cells have several attractive properties for immunotherapy as they have an endogenous ability to kill in response to their TCR recognizing CD1d and lipid thereby, modifying the tumor microenvironment.[51] One lipid that a subset of NKT cells recognizes is the ceramide α-galactosylceramide which can be purified as clinical-grade material. While infusion of this glycolipid antigen by itself failed to provide a significant clinical benefit, this ceramide has been used to propagate NKT cells *in vitro* and infusions of autologous NKT cells has resulted in some clinical responses in patients with recurrent non-small cell lung cancer.[52]

Surival of Infused Lymphocytes

A common theme for all adoptive immunotherapies is that the therapeutic effect is directly dependent on the persistence of the infused cells. Indeed, one limitation of immunotherapy has been the suboptimal persistence of the adoptively transferred cells in many clinical scenarios. The best persistence has been seen when T cells have been administered early post-HSCT into a lympho-depleted environment that promotes T-cell expansion. For example, long-term persistence has also been observed when T cells have been transferred to melanoma patients after intensive lymphodepletion.[34] However, lymphodepletion may not be needed to sustain persistence of infused T cells as a report on long-term follow up of gene-marked, donor-derived, EBV-specific CTLs administered after HSCT (as prophylaxis or therapy for EBV-PTLD) showed survival of marked cells for up to 9 years, implying that transferred cells were able to access the memory pool.[12] In this study, the infused product contained CD4 as well as CD8 cells, which may have promoted long-term persistence and function. However, persistence in other studies has been less optimal[25] and there has been increasing interest in defining the best type of T cell for transfer to ensure robust *in vivo* function. The infused T cells themselves can be manipulated so that they can respond not only to cytokines, but also proliferate in response to anticipated antigen exposure. For example, CARs have been expressed in T cells that recognize viral antigens through defined endogenous $\alpha\beta$ TCR. A recent trial has demonstrated improved antitumor effects in patients with neuroblastoma that received autologous T cells recognizing GD_2 through introduced CAR and EBV through TCR.[26] The biological effect was correlated with improved persistence of the EBV- and GD_2-bispecific T cells, presumably because the TCR recognized latent viral antigens intermittently expressed in the patient. The concept that viral-specific T cells are a preferred cellular substrate for the introduction of CAR fits within a theme that certain T-cell populations may have desired properties for immunotherapy. For example, when targeting tumors for elimination using *ex vivo*-propagated T cells, it is advantageous to prevent the emergence of regulatory T cells (T_{regs}) that may suppress desired T-cell effector functions. This can be accomplished by modifying the tissue culture environment, by including IL-6 and/or IL-21. Other T-cell subsets, such as naïve, memory, and regulatory T cells have been demonstrated to persist when infused in mice and monkeys which raises the possibility that these T cells can be selectively cultured for infusion.[53–55] Manipulation of the T-cell environment *in vitro* and *in vivo* may also promote the improved function of infused immune effectors; this has resulted in a series of studies to manipulate the tissue culture environment to generate cells for infusion with improved proliferative potential and manipulate the recipient to improve engraftment. The pool of lymphocytes within the peripheral blood is maintained by homeostatic levels of cytokines, especially IL-7 and IL-15. Depletion of endogenous lymphocytes, such as with myelosuppressive and myeloablative chemotherapy regimens can therefore be used to induce production of cytokines associated with a favorable milieu for the lymphopenia-induced proliferation and improved persistence of infused lymphocytes.

Combination Immunotherapy

Endogenous and introduced immunoreceptors on T cells can be combined to improve an antitumor effect and T cells and NK cells can be combined with other immunotherapies to strengthen their therapeutic potential. For example, NK cells can be combined with a therapeutic mAb, such as targeting CD20 or GD_2, to improve targeting of tumor cells through antibody-dependent cell-mediated cytotoxicity (ADCC) (see Chapter 21). The ability to conjugate mAb to a survival cytokine (immunocytokine) such as IL-2 has also been used to improve the persistence of T cells.[56] Rather than targeting cytokines to the tumor using immunocytokines, soluble cytokines have been employed to improve the persistence of T cells and NK cells. The most often used is IL-2, but there is concern that high doses lead to unacceptable toxicity and lower doses may lead to stimulation of T_{regs}. Other cytokines, such as IL-7, IL-15, and IL-21, that activate lymphocytes through the common γ receptor chain are now, or about to be, tested in clinical trials. These cytokine are expected to improve the persistence and effector function of infused T cells and NK cells. As previously mentioned, T cells have also been combined with vaccine to improve immune response to a desired antigen. For example, patients can be immunized before and after infusion of *ex vivo* expanded T cells to improve immune response to vaccine following autologous HSCT.[22]

Enhancing Safety

Since genetically modified T cells have the potential to last for many years and perhaps even the lifetime of the host, any adverse effect attributable to gene transfer or gene modified cells may worsen over time. Potential adverse effects of infused T cells include inflammatory reactions, off-target effects mediated through the immunoreceptor, and adverse effects of gene transfer such as insertional mutagenesis. Fortunately, the published data so far suggest the incidence of serious adverse effects is low. We recently reviewed 381 infusions of T-cell products in 180 recipients, who were enrolled on IND studies of T cells targeting malignancies or post-transplant viral infections and found no Grade 3–4 infusion reactions.[57] However, recently, two serious adverse reactions resulting in early and fatal pulmonary toxicity have been reported infusion of T cells genetically modified to express CARs targeting HER2 and CD19[58,59] and in one case, the investigators apparently concluded that the toxicity may have been due to low levels of expression of the target on pulmonary endothelium.[59] Adverse effects, due to on- and off-target effects of infused cells, may also be observed later post-infusion with both native T cells and genetically modified T cells. As mentioned earlier, T cells specific for the minor histocompatibility antigens administered after relapse induced toxicity due to the unexpected presence of the target antigens on lung tissue.[15] Another example is melanoma-specific T cells recognizing melanin-expressing cells in the inner ear and the retina produced by T cells genetically modified with MART-1–specific TCRs, which also induced impressive tumor responses in patients with melanoma.[35] Morbidity can sometimes also be due to on target effects, for example bystander inflammation was reported during therapeutic responses to EBV-specific CTL.[12] In all of these examples, the adverse effects were controlled with short courses of steroids. In the setting of DLI after HSCT, side effects can be minimized if T cells are infused on dose escalation regimens.[5] An alternative strategy is to include a transgene in the construct for conditional ablation to allow the cell to be destroyed on exposure to a specific signal if adverse events occur following infusion. Several suicide genes have been evaluated of which the herpes simplex viral thymidine kinase (TK) gene is the most widely used. The product of TK phosphorylates ganciclovir to the active moiety, allowing ablation of infused T cells if this drug is administered. Several Phase I and II studies have administered TK-transduced DLI products after allogeneic HSCT and the approach has proved effective in allowing the cells to be eliminated if graft vs. host disease occurs.[60] As the TK suicide gene is probably immunogenic, investigators are also developing alternatives such as inducible Caspase9 (icasp9) which is a naturally occurring component of the caspase pathway that can be triggered by administration of a small molecule dimeriser that brings together two nonfunctional icasp9 molecules to form the active enzyme.[10]

Conclusions

One of the benefits of adoptive immunotherapy is that it can be effective irrespective of age of the recipient. Thus, approaches that have been piloted in the adult cancer population can be readily applied in populations of children, adolescent, and young adults. Adoptive cellular immunotherapy has produced definitive benefits in the treatment of relapsed CML, AML, and EBV-associated malignancies after HSCT. However, limitations have been identified including inadequate persistence or expansion. Ongoing research efforts are focused on defining the optimum methodology for generation of T cell and other lymphocyte products, developing gene therapy approaches to enhance the function of adoptively transferred cells, and manipulating the tumor microenvironment to overcome tumor evasion strategies. To broaden the application of these immunotherapy trials, innovation is needed to simplify production so that cellular therapies can be tested in definitive multicenter studies.

References

2. Bleakley M, Riddell SR. (2004) Molecules and mechanisms of the graft-versus-leukaemia effect. *Nat Rev Cancer* **4**: 371–380.
3. Nishida T, Hudecek M, Kostic A, Bleakley M, Warren EH, Maloney D, Storb R, Riddell SR. (2009) Development of tumor-reactive T cells after nonmyeloablative allogeneic hematopoietic stem cell transplant for chronic lymphocytic leukemia. *Clin Cancer Res* **15**: 4759–4768.
4. Rezvani K, Yong AS, Savani BN, Mielke S, Keyvanfar K, Gostick E, Price DA, Douek DC, Barrett AJ. (2007) Graft-versus-leukemia effects associated with detectable Wilms tumor-1 specific T lymphocytes after allogeneic stem-cell

transplantation for acute lymphoblastic leukemia. *Blood* **110**: 1924–1932.

5. Kolb HJ. (2008) Graft-versus-leukemia effects of transplantation and donor lymphocytes. *Blood* **112**: 4371–4383.
6. O'Reilly RJ, Doubrovina E, Trivedi D, Hasan A, Kollen W, Koehne G. (2007) Adoptive transfer of antigen-specific T-cells of donor type for immunotherapy of viral infections following allogeneic hematopoietic cell transplants. *Immunol Res* **38**: 237–250.
7. Amrolia PJ, Muccioli-Casadei G, Huls H, Adams S, Durett A, Gee A, Yvon E, Weiss H, Cobbold M, Gaspar HB, Rooney C, Kuehnle I, Ghetie V, Schindler J, Krance R, Heslop HE, Veys P, Vitetta E, Brenner MK. (2006) Adoptive immunotherapy with allodepleted donor T-cells improves immune reconstitution after haploidentical stem cell transplantation. *Blood* **108**: 1797–1808.
9. Solomon SR, Mielke S, Savani BN, Montero A, Wisch L, Childs R, Hensel N, Schindler J, Ghetie V, Leitman SF, Mai T, Carter CS, Kurlander R, Read EJ, Vitetta ES, Barrett AJ. (2005) Selective depletion of alloreactive donor lymphocytes: A novel method to reduce the severity of graft-versus-host disease in older patients undergoing matched sibling donor stem cell transplantation. *Blood* **106**: 1123–1129.
10. Tey SK, Dotti G, Rooney CM, Heslop HE, Brenner MK. (2007) Inducible caspase 9 suicide gene to improve the safety of allodepleted T cells after haploidentical stem cell transplantation. *Biol Blood Marrow Transplant* **13**: 913–924.
11. Davies JK, Gribben JG, Brennan LL, Yuk D, Nadler LM, Guinan EC. (2008) Outcome of alloanergized haploidentical bone marrow transplantation after *ex vivo* costimulatory blockade: Results of 2 phase 1 studies. *Blood* **112**: 2232–2241.
12. Heslop HE, Slobod KS, Pule MA, Hale GA, Rousseau A, Smith CA, Bollard CM, Liu H, Wu MF, Rochester RJ, Amrolia PJ, Hurwitz JL, Brenner MK, Rooney CM. (2010) Long-term outcome of EBV-specific T-cell infusions to prevent or treat EBV-related lymphoproliferative disease in transplant recipients. *Blood* **115**: 925–935.
14. Falkenburg JH, Wafelman AR, Joosten P, Smit WM, van Bergen CA, Bongaerts R, Lurvink E, van der Hoorn M, Kluck P, Landegent JE, Kluin-Nelemans HC, Fibbe WE, Willemze R. (1999) Complete remission of accelerated phase chronic myeloid leukemia by treatment with leukemia-reactive cytotoxic T lymphocytes. *Blood* **94**: 1201–1208.
15. Warren EH, Fujii N, Akatsuka Y, Chaney CN, Mito JK, Loeb KR, Gooley TA, Brown ML, Koo KK, Rosinski KV, Ogawa S, Matsubara A, Appelbaum FR, Riddell SR. (2010) Therapy of relapsed leukemia after allogeneic hematopoietic cell transplantation with T cells specific for minor histocompatibility antigens. *Blood* **115**: 3869–3878.
16. Bollard CM, Aguilar L, Straathof KC, Gahn B, Huls MH, Rousseau A, Sixbey J, Gresik MV, Carrum G, Hudson M, Dilloo D, Gee A, Brenner MK, Rooney CM, Heslop HE. (2004) Cytotoxic T lymphocyte therapy for Epstein-Barr virus+ Hodgkin's disease. *J Exp Med* **200**: 1623–1633.
17. Straathof KC, Bollard CM, Popat U, Huls MH, Lopez T, Morriss MC, Gresik MV, Gee AP, Russell HV, Brenner MK, Rooney CM, Heslop HE. (2005) Treatment of nasopharyngeal carcinoma with Epstein-Barr virus — specific T lymphocytes. *Blood* **105**: 1898–1904.
18. Bollard CM, Gottschalk S, Leen AM, Weiss H, Straathof KC, Carrum G, Khalil M, Wu MF, Huls MH, Chang CC, Gresik MV, Gee AP, Brenner MK, Rooney CM, Heslop HE. (2007) Complete responses of relapsed lymphoma following genetic modification of tumor-antigen presenting cells and T-lymphocyte transfer. *Blood* **110**: 2838–2845.
21. Laport GG, Levine BL, Stadtmauer EA, Schuster SJ, Luger SM, Grupp S, Bunin N, Strobl FJ, Cotte J, Zheng Z, Gregson B, Rivers P, Vonderheide RH, Liebowitz DN, Porter DL, June CH. (2003) Adoptive transfer of costimulated T cells induces lymphocytosis in patients with relapsed/refractory non-Hodgkin lymphoma following CD34+-selected hematopoietic cell transplantation. *Blood* **102**: 2004–2013.
22. Rapoport AP, Stadtmauer EA, Aqui N, Vogl D, Chew A, Fang HB, Janofsky S, Yager K, Veloso E, Zheng Z, Milliron T, Westphal S, Cotte J, Huynh H, Cannon A, Yanovich S, Akpek G, Tan M, Virts K, Ruehle K, Harris C, Philip S, Vonderheide RH, Levine BL, June CH. (2009) Rapid immune recovery and graft-versus-host disease-like engraftment syndrome following adoptive transfer of Costimulated autologous T cells. *Clin Cancer Res* **15**: 4499–4507.
23. Cooper LJ, Topp MS, Serrano LM, Gonzalez S, Chang WC, Naranjo A, Wright C, Popplewell L, Raubitschek A, Forman SJ, Jensen MC. (2003) T-cell clones can be rendered specific for CD19: Toward the selective augmentation of the graft-versus-B-lineage leukemia effect. *Blood* **101**: 1637–1644.
24. Dotti G, Savoldo B, Brenner M. (2009) Fifteen years of gene therapy based on chimeric antigen receptors: "Are we nearly there yet?" *Hum Gene Ther* **20**: 1229–1239.
25. Till BG, Jensen MC, Wang J, Chen EY, Wood BL, Greisman HA, Qian X, James SE, Raubitschek A, Forman SJ, Gopal AK, Pagel JM, Lindgren CG, Greenberg PD,

Riddell SR, Press OW. (2008) Adoptive immunotherapy for indolent non-Hodgkin lymphoma and mantle cell lymphoma using genetically modified autologous CD20-specific T cells. *Blood* **112**: 2261–2271.
26. Pule MA, Savoldo B, Myers GD, Rossig C, Russell HV, Dotti G, Huls MH, Liu E, Gee AP, Mei Z, Yvon E, Weiss HL, Liu H, Rooney CM, Heslop HE, Brenner MK. (2008) Virus-specific T cells engineered to coexpress tumor-specific receptors: Persistence and antitumor activity in individuals with neuroblastoma. *Nat Med* **14**: 1264–1270.
27. Hacein-Bey-Abina S, Garrigue A, Wang GP, Soulier J, Lim A, Morillon E, Clappier E, Caccavelli L, Delabesse E, Beldjord K, Asnafi V, MacIntyre E, Dal Cortivo L, Radford I, Brousse N, Sigaux F, Moshous D, Hauer J, Borkhardt A, Belohradsky BH, Wintergerst U, Velez MC, Leiva L, Sorensen R, Wulffraat N, Blanche S, Bushman FD, Fischer A, Cavazzana-Calvo M. (2008) Insertional oncogenesis in 4 patients after retrovirus-mediated gene therapy of SCID-X1. *J Clin Invest* **118**: 3132–3142.
28. McCormack MP, Young LF, Vasudevan S, de Graaf CA, Codrington R, Rabbitts TH, Jane SM, Curtis DJ. (2010) The Lmo2 oncogene initiates leukemia in mice by inducing thymocyte self-renewal. *Science* **327**: 879–883.
29. Hackett PB, Largaespada DA, Cooper LJ. (2010) A transposon and transposase system for human application. *Mol Ther* **18**: 674–683.
30. Huang X, Wilber A, McIvor RS, Zhou X. (2009) DNA transposons for modification of human primary T lymphocytes. *Methods Mol Biol* **506**: 115–126.
32. Nakazawa Y, Huye LE, Dotti G, Foster AE, Vera JF, Manuri PR, June CH, Rooney CM, Wilson MH. (2009) Optimization of the PiggyBac transposon system for the sustained genetic modification of human T lymphocytes. *J Immunother* **32**: 826–836.
33. Williams DA. (2008) Sleeping beauty vector system moves toward human trials in the United States. *Mol Ther* **16**: 1515–1516.
35. Johnson LA, Morgan RA, Dudley ME, Cassard L, Yang JC, Hughes MS, Kammula US, Royal RE, Sherry RM, Wunderlich JR, Lee CC, Restifo NP, Schwarz SL, Cogdill AP, Bishop RJ, Kim H, Brewer CC, Rudy SF, VanWaes C, Davis JL, Mathur A, Ripley RT, Nathan DA, Laurencot CM, Rosenberg SA. (2009) Gene therapy with human and mouse T-cell receptors mediates cancer regression and targets normal tissues expressing cognate antigen. *Blood* **114**: 535–546.
36. Kowolik CM, Topp MS, Gonzalez S, Pfeiffer T, Olivares S, Gonzalez N, Smith DD, Forman SJ, Jensen MC, Cooper LJ. (2006) CD28 costimulation provided through a CD19-specific chimeric antigen receptor enhances *in vivo* persistence and antitumor efficacy of adoptively transferred T cells. *Cancer Res* **66**: 10995–11004.
37. Stewart TJ, Abrams SI. (2008) How tumours escape mass destruction. *Oncogene* **27**: 5894–5903.
38. Zou W. (2005) Immunosuppressive networks in the tumour environment and their therapeutic relevance. *Nat Rev Cancer* **5**: 263–274.
39. Petrausch U, Jensen SM, Twitty C, Poehlein CH, Haley DP, Walker EB, Fox BA. (2009) Disruption of TGF-beta signaling prevents the generation of tumor-sensitized regulatory T cells and facilitates therapeutic antitumor immunity. *J Immunol* **183**: 3682–3689.
40. Foster AE, Dotti G, Lu A, Khalil M, Brenner MK, Heslop HE, Rooney CM, Bollard CM. (2008) Antitumor activity of EBV-specific T lymphocytes transduced with a dominant negative TGF-beta receptor. *J Immunother* **31**: 500–505.
42. Vera JF, Hoyos V, Savoldo B, Quintarelli C, Giordano Attianese GM, Leen AM, Liu H, Foster AE, Heslop HE, Rooney CM, Brenner MK, Dotti G. (2009) Genetic manipulation of tumor-specific cytotoxic T lymphocytes to restore responsiveness to IL-7. *Mol Ther* **17**: 880–888.
43. Locatelli F, Pende D, Maccario R, Mingari MC, Moretta A, Moretta L. (2009) Haploidentical hemopoietic stem cell transplantation for the treatment of high-risk leukemias: How NK cells make the difference. *Clin Immunol* **133**: 171–178.
44. Miller JS, Soignier Y, Panoskaltsis-Mortari A, McNearney SA, Yun GH, Fautsch SK, McKenna D, Le C, Defor TE, Burns LJ, Orchard PJ, Blazar BR, Wagner JE, Slungaard A, Weisdorf DJ, Okazaki IJ, McGlave PB. (2005) Successful adoptive transfer and *in vivo* expansion of human haploidentical NK cells in patients with cancer. *Blood* **105**: 3051–3057.
45. Rubnitz JE, Inaba H, Ribeiro RC, Pounds S, Rooney B, Bell T, Pui CH, Leung W. (2010) NKAML: A pilot study to determine the safety and feasibility of haploidentical natural killer cell transplantation in childhood acute myeloid leukemia. *J Clin Oncol* **28**: 955–959.
46. Kim S, Sunwoo JB, Yang L, Choi T, Song YJ, French AR, Vlahiotis A, Piccirillo JF, Cella M, Colonna M, Mohanakumar T, Hsu KC, Dupont B, Yokoyama WM. (2008) HLA alleles determine differences in human natural killer cell responsiveness and potency. *Proc Natl Acad Sci USA* **105**: 3053–3058.
48. Altvater B, Landmeier S, Pscherer S, Temme J, Schweer K, Kailayangiri S, Campana D, Juergens H, Pule M, Rossig C. (2009) 2B4 (CD244) signaling by recombinant antigen-specific chimeric receptors costimulates natural killer cell activation to leukemia and neuroblastoma cells. *Clin Cancer Res* **15**: 4857–4866.

50. Cooper LJ. (2009) Persuading natural killer cells to eliminate bad B cells. *Clin Cancer Res* **15**: 4790–4791.
51. Song L, Asgharzadeh S, Salo J, Engell K, Wu HW, Sposto R, Ara T, Silverman AM, DeClerck YA, Seeger RC, Metelitsa LS. (2009) Valpha24-invariant NKT cells mediate antitumor activity via killing of tumor-associated macrophages. *J Clin Invest* **119**: 1524–1536.
53. Berger C, Jensen MC, Lansdorp PM, Gough M, Elliott C, Riddell SR. (2008) Adoptive transfer of effector CD8+ T cells derived from central memory cells establishes persistent T cell memory in primates. *J Clin Invest* **118**: 294–305.
54. Hinrichs CS, Borman ZA, Cassard L, Gattinoni L, Spolski R, Yu Z, Sanchez-Perez L, Muranski P, Kern SJ, Logun C, Palmer DC, Ji Y, Reger RN, Leonard WJ, Danner RL, Rosenberg SA, Restifo NP. (2009) Adoptively transferred effector cells derived from naive rather than central memory CD8+ T cells mediate superior antitumor immunity. *Proc Natl Acad Sci USA* **106**: 17469–17474.
55. Xie Y, Akpinarli A, Maris C, Hipkiss EL, Lane M, Kwon EK, Muranski P, Restifo NP, Antony PA. (2010) Naive tumor-specific CD4(+) T cells differentiated *in vivo* eradicate established melanoma. *J Exp Med* **207**: 651–667.
56. Singh H, Serrano LM, Pfeiffer T, Olivares S, McNamara G, Smith DD, Al-Kadhimi Z, Forman SJ, Gillies SD, Jensen MC, Colcher D, Raubitschek A, Cooper LJ. (2007) Combining adoptive cellular and immunocytokine therapies to improve treatment of B-lineage malignancy. *Cancer Res* **67**: 2872–2880.
57. Cruz CR, Hanley PJ, Liu H, Torrano V, Lin YF, Arce JA, Gottschalk S, Savoldo B, Dotti G, Louis CU, Leen AM, Gee AP, Rooney CM, Brenner MK, Bollard CM, Heslop HE. (2010) Adverse events following infusion of T cells for adoptive immunotherapy: A 10-year experience. *Cytotherapy* **12**: 743–749.
58. Brentjens R, Yeh R, Bernal Y, Riviere I, Sadelain M. (2010) Treatment of chronic lymphocytic leukemia with genetically targeted autologous T cells: Case report of an unforeseen adverse event in a phase I clinical trial. *Mol Ther* **18**: 666–668.
59. Morgan RA, Yang JC, Kitano M, Dudley ME, Laurencot CM, Rosenberg SA. (2010) Case report of a serious adverse event following the administration of T cells transduced with a chimeric antigen receptor recognizing ERBB2. *Mol Ther* **18**: 843–851.
60. Ciceri F, Bonini C, Stanghellini MT, Bondanza A, Traversari C, Salomoni M, Turchetto L, Colombi S, Bernardi M, Peccatori J, Pescarollo A, Servida P, Magnani Z, Perna SK, Valtolina V, Crippa F, Callegaro L, Spoldi E, Crocchiolo R, Fleischhauer K, Ponzoni M, Vago L, Rossini S, Santoro A, Todisco E, Apperley J, Olavarria E, Slavin S, Weissinger EM, Ganser A, Stadler M, Yannaki E, Fassas A, Anagnostopoulos A, Bregni M, Stampino CG, Bruzzi P, Bordignon C. (2009) Infusion of suicide-gene-engineered donor lymphocytes after family haploidentical haemopoietic stem-cell transplantation for leukaemia (the TK007 trial): A non-randomised phase I-II study. *Lancet Oncol* **10**: 489–500.

24

Late Effects After Treatment for Hematological Malignancies During Childhood, Adolescence or Young Adulthood

Paul C. Nathan, Tara Henderson and Laura Janzen

Introduction

The marked improvement in the survival of many childhood and adolescent cancers over the past several decades has resulted in a growing population of long-term survivors. By 2005, there were almost 330,000 survivors of childhood or adolescent cancers alive in the United States, a third of whom were survivors of a hematological malignancy.[1] ALL, HL, NHL, and AML comprised 15.0%, 9.6%, 5.7%, and 1.9% of all survivors, respectively, with ALL and HL representing the 2nd and 4th most prevalent diagnostic groups among all childhood or adolescent cancer survivors. In addition to this growing population, there are many survivors of hematological malignancies diagnosed and treated during young adulthood. The excellent long-term survival in patients treated on contemporary ALL, HL and NHL protocols will lead to continued growth in the population of survivors of leukemia and lymphoma. Unfortunately, many survivors experience long-term sequelae of their cancer or its therapy. Given the large number of potential life-years impacted by a diagnosis of cancer during childhood, adolescence or young adulthood, efforts have been focused on minimizing toxicity in survivors, either by modifying therapeutic protocols or by intervening to prevent or mitigate the development of late effects after therapy.

There is considerable variation in both the type and severity of late effects observed in survivors of hematological malignancies. In previous treatment eras, cranial radiation therapy (CRT) was an integral component of treatment for ALL. CRT was implicated as a cause of neurocognitive impairment and neuroendocrine dysfunction, and has been eliminated for over 80% of children and adolescents with this disease. Children, adolescents and young adults treated on contemporary ALL protocols who do not receive CRT likely have a lower risk of adverse sequelae, but further monitoring of these survivors will be necessary to determine their long-term outcomes. In contrast, many survivors of HL are at high risk for late sequelae of therapy, including the development of second malignant neoplasms (SMN), thyroid, cardiac, carotid and pulmonary dysfunction, and impaired fertility. Regardless of the primary cancer diagnosis, treatment with hematopoietic stem cell transplantation (HSCT), particularly allogeneic transplantation, is associated with a considerable risk of chronic

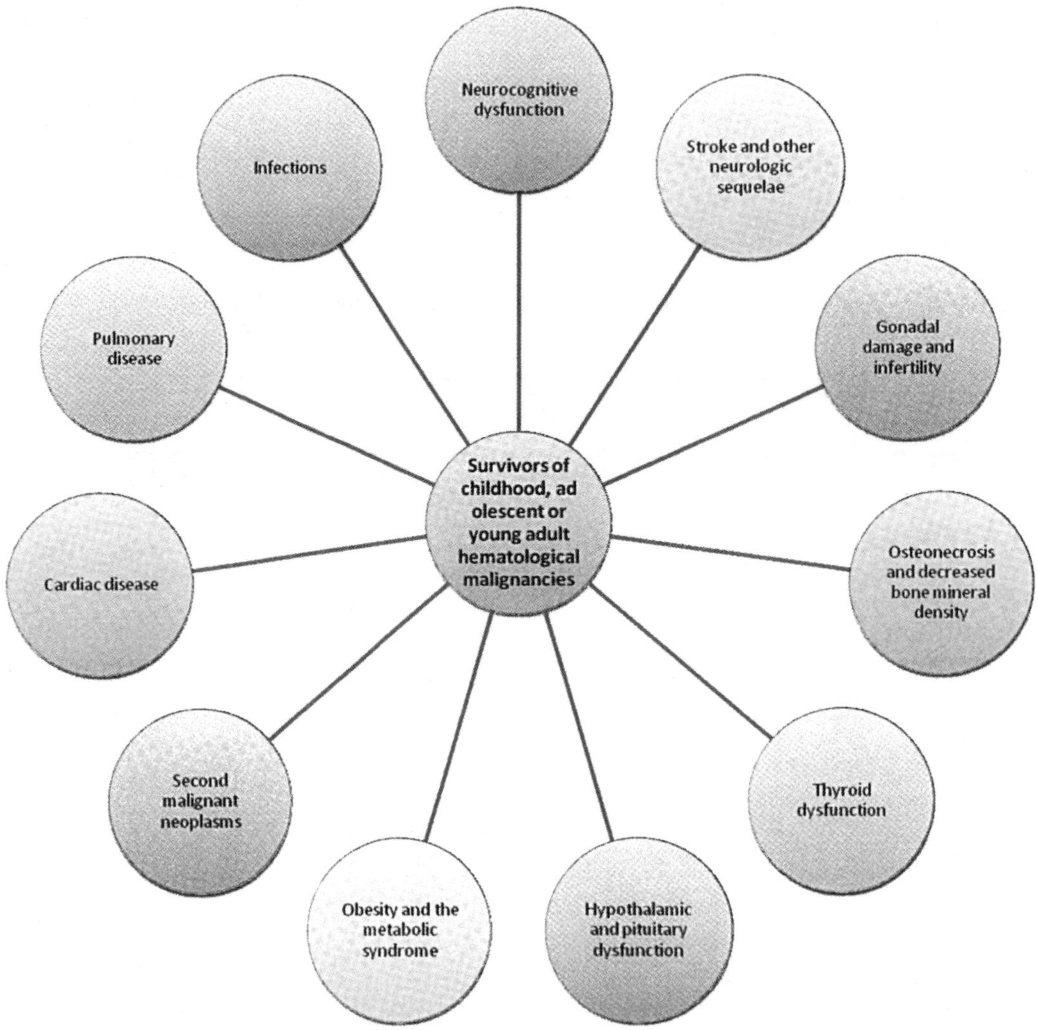

Fig. 24.1. Major physical late effects of therapy seen in survivors of hematological malignancies.

morbidity (see Chapter 20). Since treatment for hematological malignancies varies considerably depending on the treatment era, patient and disease characteristics, the risks of late effects of therapy are more accurately assessed according to specific treatment exposures rather than diagnosis. Radiation therapy, alkylating agents, and anthracycline antibiotics, which are used commonly in the treatment of these malignancies, are associated frequently with long-term sequelae. Recent research has suggested that polymorphisms in genes responsible for chemotherapy metabolism may modify susceptibility to certain late effects of chemotherapy, such as neurocognitive dysfunction after treatment with methotrexate and cardiac toxicity as a result of anthracycline exposure.[2,3]

Health care practitioners that care for long-term survivors of hematological malignancies require knowledge of survivors' treatment histories, understanding of the late effects associated with specific exposures, and access to published guidelines for the long-term care of childhood and adolescent cancer survivors. These data, along with a awareness of survivors' co-morbid health conditions, lifestyle habits and genetic predispositions, will guide decisions about patient counseling and periodic screening and surveillance, with the goal of ensuring life-long health and quality of life (Figs. 24.1–24.2).

Neurocognitive Sequelae

Neurocognitive late effects may occur in survivors whose disease directly involved the CNS, such as CNS-positive ALL and NHL, and those treated with CRT or chemotherapy that crosses the blood–brain barrier following intrathecal or high-dose systemic administration. It is estimated that one-third of survivors of childhood or adolescent ALL and AML

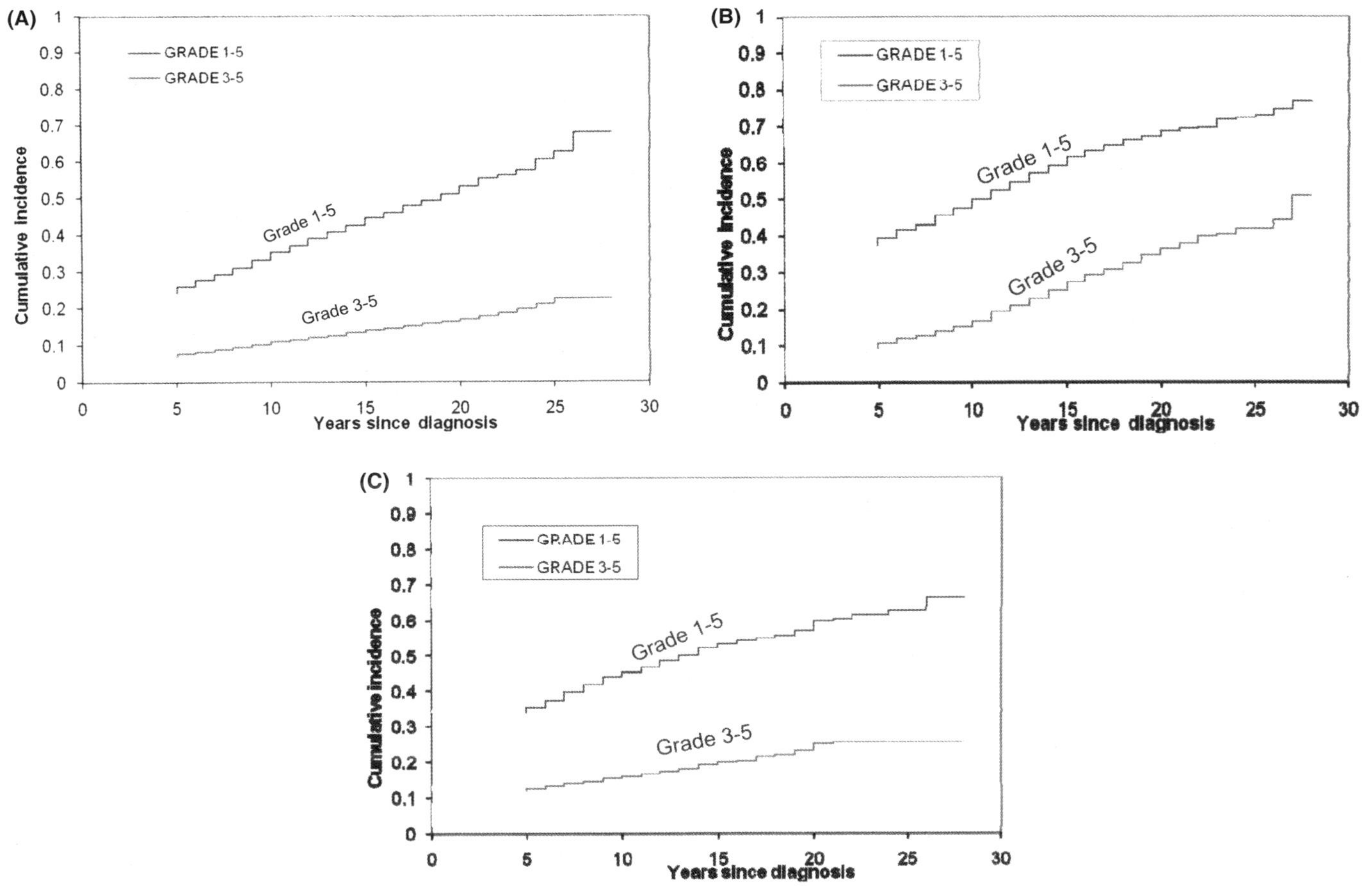

Fig. 24.2 A–C. Cumulative incidence of chronic health conditions in the Childhood Cancer Survivor Study (CCSS) cohort according to the original diagnosis and the severity of the later condition. (A) Leukemia (ALL and AML). The severity of subsequent health conditions was scored according to the Common Terminology Criteria for Adverse Events (version 3) as either mild (grade 1), moderate (grade 2), severe (grade 3), life-threatening or disabling (grade 4), or fatal (grade 5). (B) Hodgkin's lymphoma. (C) C: Non-Hodgkin's Lymphoma.

Kevin C. Oeffinger, M.D., Ann C. Mertens, Ph.D., Charles A. Sklar, M.D., Toana Kawashima, M.S., Melissa M. Hudson, M.D., Anna T. Meadows, M.D., Debra L. Friedman, M.D., Neyssa Marina, M.D., Wendy Hobbie, C.P.N.P., Nina S. Kadan-Lottick, M.D., Cindy L. Schwartz, M.D., Wendy Leisenring, Sc.D., Leslie L. Robison, Ph.D., for the Childhood Cancer Survivor Study Chronic Health Conditions in Adult Survivors of Childhood Cancer. *NEJM* **355**(15): 1572–1582.

experience long-term neurocognitive difficulties. For individual survivors, neurocognitive late effects may limit educational and vocational opportunities and reduce overall quality of life. Further, survivors of childhood or adolescent cancer are at increased risk of adverse social and behavioral outcomes that may limit independence and achievement. At a societal level, long-term leukemia and lymphoma survivors are more likely to require special education services and be underemployed.[4,5]

There is considerable individual variability in neurocognitive outcomes, with myriad disease, treatment and individual factors interacting to contribute to an individual survivor's level of risk. Long-term survivors of ALL, AML and NHL who receive CRT or intrathecal or high-dose systemic methotrexate (MTX) have comparable neurocognitive deficits, while those with HL do not typically require CNS-directed treatment and it is therefore assumed that their cognitive functioning is spared. Disease relapse in ALL, which requires more intensive CNS-directed treatment, is associated with higher rates of neurological complications and greater neurocognitive morbidity.

Of all the treatment modalities, CRT is associated with the poorest neurocognitive outcomes, particularly in females and those treated prior to 5 years of age. There is a dose response relationship; while doses of 24 Gray (Gy) are clearly neurotoxic and are no longer used in ALL treatment, doses less than 15 Gy are thought to have minimal neurotoxic effects, although further investigation of lower dose CRT is required. CRT with 24 Gy is associated with 10–12 point losses in IQ[6,7] along with declines in attention, memory, processing speed, and academics. While outcomes associated with 18 Gy are somewhat better, survivors treated with this dose of CRT and concomitant chemotherapy show IQ declines of approximately 6 points and deficits in other cognitive domains.[8] Current protocols that avoid CRT for the nearly 80% of standard risk ALL patients have significantly reduced neurocognitive morbidity in survivors.

HSCT following ALL relapse or as a first-line or relapse therapy for AML often involves conditioning with total body irradiation (TBI; 12 Gy) or cyclophosphamide. Despite the potential neurotoxicity of these conditioning regimens, minimal late neurocognitive or academic sequelae are evident post-HSCT,[9] consistent with other findings of average neurocognitive functioning for school-aged transplant survivors. However, HSCT may pose greater neurocognitive risks for children under the age of 3 years.

Chemotherapy-only protocols are now the mainstay of ALL treatment, with CNS prophylaxis typically delivered intrathecally (see Chapters 11 and 12). Children or adolescents treated with chemotherapy alone may experience declines in specific neurocognitive functions, albeit to a lesser degree than those treated with CRT. MTX and corticosteroids have received the most attention as contributors to neurocognitive deficits. However, multiple agents are typically used in combination and the timing, dosing, and mode of administration may also be relevant. Intrathecal (IT) MTX alone results in comparable outcomes relative to triple IT treatment consisting of MTX, cytarabine, and hydrocortisone.[10] When MTX is administered intravenously at doses sufficient to cross the blood–brain barrier (high dose to very high dose: 8–33.6 g/m^2), typically followed by leucovorin rescue, there does not appear to be a significant impact on long-term intelligence.[11] However, specific deficits in attention, working memory, and nonverbal functions are related to higher IV MTX dose and rapid infusion rates.[12,13] Corticosteroids are used for a prolonged period of time and at relatively high doses in ALL treatment. Prior research indicated poorer memory in children treated with dexamethasone relative to prednisone.[14] However, new evidence indicates that there are no meaningful differences in long-term ALL survivors who were randomized to receive either dexamethasone or prednisone, except for a slight advantage for the prednisone group in word reading skills.[15]

In addition to disease- and treatment-related factors, there are numerous individual factors that moderate neurocognitive outcomes. Younger age at treatment is a commonly reported risk factor, although a number of individual studies and a meta-analysis failed to demonstrate this relationship.[16,17] Female sex is associated with an increased risk of neurocognitive late effects, although explanations for this sex difference remain elusive.[18] Time since treatment has been variably shown to moderate long-term outcome, supporting the progressive nature of neurocognitive declines which occur rapidly in the first few years post-treatment and more gradually thereafter. Polymorphisms in enzymes responsible for chemotherapy metabolism may modify individual sensitivity to neurotoxic treatments. While this avenue of investigation is relatively new, there is evidence of a relationship between folate pathway polymorphisms and attention difficulties in ALL survivors.[2] Pre-existing developmental vulnerabilities may also increase the risk of poor neurocognitive outcomes following treatment. Finally, socioeconomic status (SES) is a major influence on children's neurocognitive functioning, although it is not consistently analyzed in outcome studies. One study found that SES outweighed all other medical or treatment factors in influencing neurocognitive outcomes in HSCT survivors.[9]

Large group studies indicate that overall intelligence in children and adolescents with ALL treated with chemotherapy alone remains within the average range, despite subtle declines. Specific declines in core cognitive processes such as working memory, processing speed, attention, visual–motor integration, and executive functions are the most commonly reported and are thought to underlie the observed declines in intelligence and academic achievement (Fig. 24.1). Academically, ALL survivors show relative weakness in mathematics and reading achievement, presumably due to a failure to acquire new information or skills at a typical rate.[19] In addition, long-term deficits in gross and fine motor function associated with vincristine may further hinder academic success (Fig. 24.3).[20]

Myelination of the brain occurs in a well-defined sequence which begins prenatally, and continues through childhood and adolescence. Disruption of this protracted process is thought to account for both chemotherapy- and CRT-induced neurocognitive changes. Neuroimaging studies of long-term ALL survivors treated with CRT and chemotherapy reveal cortical and subcortical white matter changes, along with intracerebral calcifications and cortical atrophy.[21] Smaller white matter volumes are associated with greater deficits in intelligence, attention, and academics.[22] Diffusion tensor imaging (DTI), an imaging

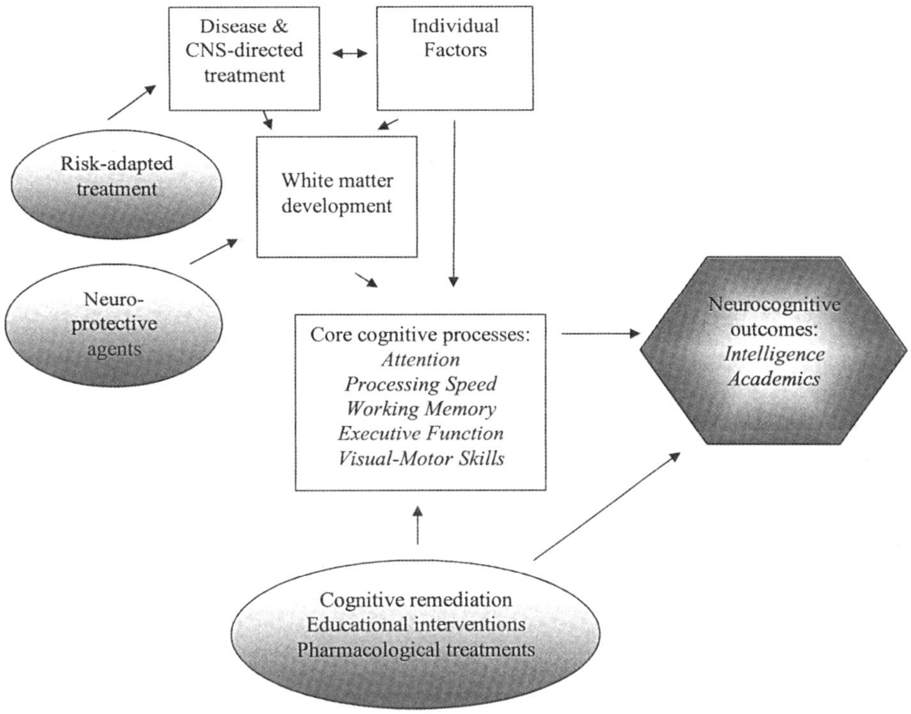

Fig. 24.3. Conceptual Framework: Variables contributing to neurocognitive outcome in survivors of hematological malignancies. Adapted from Palmer SL. Neurodevelopmental impact on children treated for medulloblastoma: a review and proposed conceptual model. Dev Disabil Res Rev. 2008;14(3):203–10 and Askins MA, Moore BD, 3rd. Preventing neurocognitive late effects in childhood cancer survivors. J Child Neurol. 2008 Oct; 23(10):1160–71.

modality that facilitates the study of the integrity of white matter tracts, has revealed white matter structural alterations in adult survivors of childhood ALL and positive correlations between the integrity of white matter tracts and motor and processing speed.[23] Although neuroimaging is essential to understanding the mechanisms of treatment-related neurocognitive changes, it is not recommended as a routine investigation in the clinical care of childhood cancer survivors.

Comprehensive neuropsychological evaluation is highly recommended for all childhood cancer survivors who received CNS-directed therapy or are experiencing new-onset academic difficulties. Neuropsychological assessment is essential to characterize the nature and severity of neurocognitive late effects and to provide developmentally appropriate, individualized recommendations for interventions and accommodations. Butler and Copeland have been at the forefront in developing interventions for childhood cancer survivors aimed at remediating neurocognitive deficits. Their Cognitive Remediation Program (CRP) incorporates attention training, special education strategies and aspects of cognitive–behavioral therapy.[24] Despite the intensity and duration of their intervention, only modest gains have been reported in academic achievement without clear improvement in neurocognitive functioning. Pharmacological interventions that target the attention deficits common in childhood cancer survivors have also been explored. Methylphenidate has been associated with improved attention on standardized tests and parent reports.[25] Educational interventions, including accommodations for unique learning needs and modifications to the curriculum, are required by many survivors. Career and vocational counseling is increasingly available for young adult cancer survivors, providing assistance in the identification of appropriate career options, development of self-advocacy skills and the modification of previously used educational accommodations to facilitate success in post-secondary educational settings and the workplace.

Because the individual and societal costs of neurocognitive late effects in the growing cohort of survivors are substantial, prevention of neurocognitive deficits before they occur has become the ultimate goal. Advances have been made in developing highly individualized treatments based on survival outcomes, and it may be possible to use the same strategies to optimize cognitive outcomes. Exploration of neuroprotective agents also holds promise and may allow for optimal cure rates without compromising neurocognitive function.[26]

Neurologic Outcomes

Stroke is a rare but serious adverse event that has been reported acutely during ALL therapy, and in long-term survivors of ALL and HL. Therapy with L-asparaginase has been associated with both acute hemorrhagic and ischemic stroke with survivors demonstrating variable recovery and long-term deficits. Late-occurring stroke occurs with increased frequency in survivors of ALL or HL treated with radiation to the head or neck. The North American Childhood Cancer Survivor Study (CCSS) demonstrated a 0.73% risk of stroke at 25 years after diagnosis in survivors of leukemia (including both ALL and AML).[27] Survivors with a history of relapse or CRT doses exceeding 30 Gy demonstrated the highest risk, although even those survivors treated with less or no CRT were at increased risk compared to their siblings. Unlike CRT in children with ALL, which causes direct damage to the cranial vasculature, the increased risk of stroke in HL survivors is likely related to thromboembolic disease secondary to radiation-induced cardiac valve damage or premature carotid atherosclerosis. Patients treated with mantle radiation are at particular risk.[28] A Dutch cohort study of 2201 children and adults treated for HL revealed an increased risk of both stroke (standardized incidence ratio 2.2; was 2.2; 95% confidence interval 1.7–2.8) and transient ischemic attacks (standardized incidence ratio 3.1; 95% confidence interval 2.2–4.2) when compared to the general population.[29] The increased risk remained elevated with prolonged follow up, with a cumulative incidence of ischemic stroke or transient ischemic attack at 30 years after HL treatment of 7%. Survivors treated with radiation to the head or neck require an annual neurologic exam, and imaging with carotid ultrasound should be considered in those treated with greater than 40 Gy to the neck.[30] Hyperlipidemia, hypertension or a positive family history should be taken into account when deciding if an individual survivor requires ultrasound surveillance.

Other neurologic abnormalities reported in survivors included peripheral neuropathies, seizures, and headaches. Vincristine can cause peripheral neuropathies during therapy. Although most survivors do not display clinical signs of impaired nerve conduction after the conclusion of therapy, nerve conduction testing often demonstrates residual impairment.[20] Some ALL survivors have persistent fine or gross motor dysfunction which is likely multifactorial in origin since peripheral neuropathy, persistent muscle weakness, and central nervous system damage that affects visual motor integration can all occur in long-term survivors. The CCSS has reported higher rates of seizures and headaches in long-term survivors of ALL,[31] but this awaits confirmation from other studies.

Fertility

For many survivors, alterations in gonadal function and loss of fertility are the most life-altering sequelae of their childhood, adolescent or young adult cancer, impacting their body image, sexuality, dating and marriage relationships, and sense of well-being. Fortunately, most modern ALL protocols and upfront AML chemotherapy regimens that proactively limit gonadotoxic modalities do not impact fertility, and contemporary HL protocols strive to limit the impact of treatment on fertility. However, some treatment plans for relapsed leukemia and lymphoma, including HSCT, can impact fertility. In particular, alkylating agents (such as cyclophosphamide and procarbazine) and radiation that involves the pelvis (e.g. infra-diaphragmatic inverted-Y field and TBI) can cause gonadal damage.

Gonadal damage in males

In males, treatment with alkylating agents is associated with gonadal toxicity and a risk of oligo- or azoospermia. The risk of sterility is proportional to cumulative dose exposure; males who receive < 7.5 g/m^2 of cyclophosphamide (or equitoxic doses of other alkylating agents) are unlikely to suffer decreased spermatogenesis.[32] Such doses are seldom used in contemporary, front-line leukemia protocols, but may be used in HSCT regimens. Treatment of the testes with radiation or TBI can lead to both sterility and impaired production of testosterone. Radiation doses of as low as 4 Gy can damage the germinal epithelium of the testes, while doses of 24 Gy or higher are associated with Leydig cell dysfunction.[32] All prepubertal males treated with 24 Gy of testicular irradiation or higher will require androgen replacement. Most, but not all, boys in puberty at the time of their testicular irradiation will ultimately need testosterone replacement.[33]

Historically, therapy for HL and some NHL utilized high-dose alkylating agents, often including procarbazine and nitrogen mustard, and were associated with irreversible sterility (see Chapters 16, 17 and 18). Six to eight cycles of MOPP chemotherapy causes azoospermia in over 80% of patients.[32] More contemporary ABVD or ABVE-PC–based regimens are associated with transient oligo- or azoospermia in approximately one-third of patients, but most recover spermatogenesis after completing therapy.[34] Thus, the risk of infertility after modern lymphoma therapy is associated with the cumulative dosage of alkylating agents and pelvic radiation. Semen collection and preservation should be considered at the time of cancer diagnosis in all pubertal males whose planned therapy places them at risk for future infertility.

Gonadal damage in females

Exposure to alkylating agents and radiation that involves the ovaries (including cranio-spinal radiation) can destroy primordial follicles, hastening the onset of menopause or, in some cases, causing primary ovarian failure. Fortunately, modern ALL protocols and upfront AML chemotherapy regimens seldom cause ovarian dysfunction. Acute ovarian failure during or shortly after completing cancer therapy is uncommon in children with leukemia or lymphoma,[33] but can occur in girls who receive high-dose pelvic radiation, TBI or very high doses of alkylating agents as a preparative regimen for HSCT. Young girls with primary ovarian failure will require induction of puberty and continued hormonal therapy to allow for normal growth and development. This should be performed by an endocrinologist experienced in the management of pubertal and growth disorders.

Any reduction in the number of primordial follicles places a woman at risk for early menopause (prior to age 40 years).[33] In a case-control study of over 500 female HL survivors treated as adolescents and young adults who were followed for a median of 9.4 years, MOPP chemotherapy was associated with an over fivefold increase in early menopause; MOPP/ABV was also associated with an increased risk of premature menopause, although to a lesser extent (Hazard Ratio [HR] = 2.9). Alkylating agents, especially procarbazine (HR = 8.1) and cyclophosphamide (HR = 3.5), showed the strongest association with premature menopause — a significant dose response was demonstrated.[34,35] In a case-control study of adolescent and young adult survivors of HL treated with ABVD, no significant subfertility was found.[36]

In evaluating a survivor for ovarian dysfunction, it is imperative to take a detailed pubertal and menstrual history. Adult survivors should be asked about symptoms of a low estrogen state (i.e. hot flashes, night sweats, vaginal dryness, altered mood). While it is difficult to predict premature menopause with laboratory testing, a physician can evaluate ovarian potential and reserve by measuring follicle stimulating hormone and estradiol levels in a menstruating woman on day 3 of her cycle. More in-depth investigations should be considered through referral to a reproductive endocrinologist. Further, women at risk of developing premature menopause should be counseled to not delay child-bearing.

Bone Complications

Therapy for hematological malignancies is associated with detrimental effects on the growing skeletal system; these include osteonecrosis (avascular necrosis) and bone mineral density (BMD) loss. These bone problems are predominantly issues following treatment for ALL and T-cell lymphoma because of prolonged exposure to corticosteroids and methotrexate in some patients.

Osteonecrosis

Osteonecrosis is the result of bone death due to inadequate blood supply and bone marrow ischemia. It can lead to an array of symptoms ranging from mild discomfort to debilitating pain and immobility, joint swelling and articular collapse. The overall incidence of osteonecrosis in previous ALL protocols ranged from 1.6–9.3%.[37,38] Higher incidence is associated with older age at cancer treatment (> 10 years).[37] Both genders are affected equally. In one study, the peak incidence was higher in Caucasians and occurred at an older age in boys compared to girls.[39] Treatment-related risk factors include prolonged exposure to corticosteroids, asparaginase, and radiation therapy.[37,40] Corticosteroids are thought to induce osteonecrosis directly by causing apoptosis of osteoblasts and mature osteocytes, and indirectly by increasing the amount of fat content in the bone marrow leading to vascular compression and fat embolization. Dexamethasone therapy, with or without prednisone, appears to confer a higher risk of osteonecrosis than prednisone alone.[37] Asparaginase is associated with a hypercoagulable state that can lead to osteonecrosis in a mechanism similar to that observed in children with thrombophilia.

Symptoms of osteonecrosis usually develop within 2–3 years of treatment.[37,38] Patients most often present with pain, limp, or joint effusions. In over 90% of cases, weight-bearing joints are affected, with hips and knees being most common. Frequently, multiple joints are affected.[37,38] The preferred modality for evaluating osteonecrosis is magnetic resonance imaging (MRI).[41] However, the utility of MRI for surveillance has not been established since not all patients with radiographic evidence of osteonecrosis will develop progressive joint destruction.[42] Depending on the joint location, severity, patient age, and status of cancer treatment, survivors can be treated with physical therapy, limitation of weight-bearing, analgesia, and/or surgery. Of 31 patients who developed osteonecrosis in a cohort of 1951 pediatric patients treated on the ALL-BFM 95 trial, 13 patients required a total of 22 surgical procedures.[43] Surgical interventions for osteonecrosis include core decompression, rotational osteotomy, vascularized bone graft, and joint replacement.

Reduced BMD

Both corticosteroid and methotrexate exposure can lead to loss of BMD. Treatment with CRT or TBI can induce endocrinopathies such as hypogonadism and growth hormone (GH) deficiency that can exacerbate cortical bone loss. Corticosteroids inhibit osteoblast activity, disrupting the bone formation–resorption balance in favor of resorption. Further, corticosteroids interfere with the GH–insulin-like growth factor-1 axis, reduce muscle strength, and disrupt calcium balance, all of which may compound bone loss.[44,45] Methotrexate, often given in conjunction with corticosteroids for ALL therapy, causes osteoblast apoptosis. Studies have shown that ALL survivors have lower BMD than the general population.[46] It is hypothesized (although has not been demonstrated) that survivors who do not reach their optimal peak bone density may be at higher risk of osteoporosis and fractures as older adult. The Children's Oncology Group Long-term Follow-Up Guidelines for Survivors of Childhood, Adolescent and Young Adult Cancers (COG LTFU Guidelines) suggest consideration of a baseline BMD exam upon entry into long-term follow up for all survivors who received corticosteroids, methotrexate or have had evidence of GH deficiency or gonadal failure.[30] Further, survivors should be evaluated for adequate dietary consumption of calcium and Vitamin D. Survivors should be counseled to avoid smoking, alcohol, and excessive caffeine, as these have been shown to exacerbate osteoporosis in adults. Weight-bearing exercise should be encouraged. Survivors with severe BMD loss or multiple bone fractures should be referred to an endocrinologist for consideration of pharmacologic intervention such as calcitonin or bisphosphonates. In survivors referred during childhood or adolescence, the endocrinologist will also assess for the presence of poor growth or gonadal dysfunction that might impact bone health.

Other Endocrinopathies

Most endocrinopathies in childhood, adolescent or young adult cancer survivors are the result of exposure to radiation therapy. Except for the link between alkylating agent chemotherapy and gonadal dysfunction (see Fertility), the chemotherapy agents used in the treatment of leukemia and lymphoma are not associated with endocrine late effects.

Thyroid dysfunction

Survivors of HL and NHL who receive radiation therapy involving the neck, and survivors of leukemia treated with CRT or TBI, are at risk of developing thyroid dysfunction, which presents most commonly as hypothyroidism. The prevalence of hypothyroidism following radiation involving the neck/mediastinum for HL has been estimated to be as high as 47% after 26 years of follow up.[47] The cumulative incidence of hypothyroidism in a cohort of over 3500 ALL survivors (65% of whom were exposed to radiation) was 1.6%.[48] The risk of thyroid dysfunction appears to be dose dependent. In a recent CCSS study of ALL survivors with thyroid dysfunction, increased risk of hypothyroidism was associated with > 20 Gy CRT in addition to any spinal radiotherapy.[48] Hyperthyroidism, benign thyroid nodules, and thyroid malignancies can also occur in radiated survivors. Exposure to any craniospinal radiotherapy has been associated with a threefold risk of hyperthyroidism.[48] The current COG LTFU Guidelines suggest an annual thyroid examination and measurement of TSH and free T4. In patients with palpable nodules, thyroid ultrasound and referral to an endocrinologist should be considered.

Hypothalamic/Pituitary dysfunction

Radiation involving the brain, including CRT and TBI, can cause neuroendocrine dysfunction as a result of hypothalamic or pituitary damage. GH deficiency and precocious puberty are the most common endocrinopathies related to hypothalamic/pituitary dysfunction, while deficiencies of gonadotropin, TSH and ACTH are uncommon in leukemia survivors treated with less than 40 Gy. GH deficiency usually occurs with radiation doses to the hypothalamic–pituitary axis in excess of 18 to 20 Gy but has been reported with lower doses such as those used in TBI. Little is known about the risk after 12 Gy of CRT used in current T-cell ALL protocols. Risk factors include higher doses of radiation, younger age at exposure, and female gender.[49] GH deficiency is associated with diminished linear growth through childhood and adolescence. In adults, GH deficiency is associated with increased rates of dyslipidemia, insulin resistance, osteopenia, cardiovascular mortality and reduced quality of life (see Obesity and Metabolic Complications).

The great majority of leukemia and lymphoma survivors enter puberty at a normal age.[50] Historically, ALL survivors exposed to 18–24 Gy CRT were at increased risk of precocious puberty, with females at greater risk than males.[51] Growth and pubertal development must be monitored closely in all leukemia and lymphoma survivors. They should have yearly physical examinations with special attention to height, weight, and Tanner stage. Children at particular risk should be followed even more closely as the age of puberty approaches. In poorly growing children or early adolescents, an X-ray for evaluation of bone age and thyroid function should be obtained. Those with poor growth or advanced puberty require prompt endocrine evaluation so interventions (such as GH replacement or suppression of precocious puberty) can be implemented with sufficient time to maximize final adult height. Adult survivors at risk for GH deficiency should be referred to an endocrinologist for discussion of the risks and benefits of GH testing and replacement.

Obesity and the Metabolic Syndrome

Obesity

Over the past 25 years, the prevalence of overweight in children and adolescents in the general population has doubled and that of obesity has tripled.[52] The negative consequences of obesity are of particular concern in cancer survivors since being overweight may exacerbate other late effects of therapy, such as cardiovascular and lung disease. Among survivors of hematological malignancies during childhood or adolescence, only those treated for ALL demonstrate an increased risk of being overweight compared to population norms. CRT, particularly at doses above 20 Gy, has been identified as the most important risk factor;[53] however, lower CRT doses have also been associated with weight gain in ALL survivors.[54] Female survivors treated with CRT prior to the age of 4 years old are at particular risk. Potential mechanisms of radiation-induced obesity include GH deficiency and acquired leptin insensitivity. Leptin, an adipose-derived hormone, interacts with receptors in the baso-medial hypothalamus to modulate energy balance by controlling appetite and metabolism. Polymorphisms in the leptin receptor gene (specifically, Gln223Arg) have been demonstrated to significantly increase the risk of developing obesity among female survivors of ALL treated with higher doses of CRT.[55]

Whether ALL therapy, not including CRT, leads to an increased risk of obesity is controversial. While several small studies have shown an increase in BMI while on therapy, longitudinal data to and beyond attainment of final height is still lacking. Corticosteroids increase energy intake and may reduce physical activity through their impact on muscles (myopathy), bones and joints. Risk factors for becoming overweight, common in the general population, including poor dietary choices, increased sedentary behavior, and decreased physical activity may contribute to the risk of overweight in survivors. Children with ALL engage in less habitual physical activity both during and after therapy.[56,57] Young children receiving therapy for ALL demonstrate an earlier adiposity rebound than healthy controls, further potentiating the development of overweight.[58] Since many children or adolescents with ALL become overweight during or shortly after completing therapy, investigators are currently evaluating interventions that focus on combinations of improved diet, increased physical activity and decreased sedentary behavior during therapy. The effectiveness of these interventions remains to be established.

Metabolic syndrome

Beyond obesity, CRT for ALL has been shown to increase survivors' risk of developing the metabolic syndrome. This syndrome, defined by the presence of three or more of central obesity, hypertension, raised fasting glucose, elevated triglycerides, and lowered HDL cholesterol, increases the risk of cardiovascular disease and type 2 diabetes during adulthood. Irradiated survivors are at increased risk of developing both individual components of the syndrome and of meeting its diagnostic criteria.[59] GH deficiency appears to play a central role in CRT-induced metabolic syndrome. CRT has also been demonstrated to promote fat redistribution, particularly the development of visceral adiposity, which is a robust predictor of the development of metabolic abnormalities (such as insulin resistance and hyperlipidemia) and has been linked to premature death in the general population.

Overall, survivors of childhood ALL are more likely to be overweight, sedentary, less physically fit, and demonstrate features of the metabolic syndrome, including visceral adiposity, insulin resistance, and dyslipidemia. Although survivors treated with CRT are at particular risk for early onset of these abnormalities, even those who are not irradiated appear to be at some risk. Regardless of the type of hematological malignancy, and whether or not CRT was used as part of the therapeutic regimen, all survivors need to be counseled about the importance of a healthy lifestyle, including consumption of a healthful diet and engagement in appropriate physical activity. Health care providers should monitor survivors' height, weight and blood pressure annually, and consider evaluation of lipid levels, particularly in overweight survivors.

Second Malignant Neoplasms

Subsequent malignant neoplasms (SMN) are the second leading cause of death in childhood cancer survivors after recurrence of the primary cancer. The reported incidence of SMN after ALL ranges from 1.4% to 5.2%,[60–62] but is lower in non-irradiated survivors (1.2% to 3.1%).[61,63] While the cumulative incidence is relatively low, the risk relative to the general population is high, with ALL survivors five times more likely to develop a new cancer than their age and gender matched peers.[63] In a CCSS study of over 250 AML survivors, the 20-year cumulative incidence of SMN was 1.7%, a 3.5-times increased risk compared to the general population.[64] Similarly, NHL survivors have a 20-year cumulative incidence of 3%, representing a threefold increase in risk.[65] In contrast, survivors of HL have a significantly increased risk of SMN, far higher than that seen after other hematological malignancies. One study of 1300 pediatric HL survivors found a cumulative SMN incidence of 11% at 20 years, increasing to 26% at 30 years, with an over 18-fold risk of subsequent neoplasm as compared to the general population.[66] In the British CCSS, the 20-year cumulative risk of SMN in over 5500 HL survivors was 15%.[67] Lastly, in a Dutch study of SMN in over 1200 HL survivors, the cumulative incidence was 28%, with a relative risk of sevenfold over expected.[68]

Survivors can develop both hematological and solid SMNs. Therapy-related AML (tAML) and myelodysplastic syndrome (MDS) can occur after exposure to epipodophyllotoxins and alkylating agents. Epipodophyllotoxin-related tAML occurs most often within 2–3 years of exposure, has a predominance of monocytic or myelomonocytic features, and frequently is associated with cytogenetic abnormalities involving 11q23. Alkylating agent-related tAML most often occurs 5–10 years following exposure, is characterized by a preceding myelodysplastic phase, and often involves loss or deletions of chromosomes 5 or 7. The risk of these cancers is dose dependent.[69] The relatively low doses of alkylating agents and epipodophyllotoxins used in contemporary leukemia and lymphoma protocols make these SMNs rare. This is fortunate since the outcome is poor, despite the use of HSCT.

Solid tumors are most often the result of radiation exposure. This risk increases with time and in many instances, these neoplasms occur 10–15 years or more following exposure.[70] Excluding non-melanoma skin cancers, the most common solid SMN in irradiated survivors are malignant brain tumors, meningiomas, breast cancer, thyroid cancers, sarcomas, and NHL. The risk of breast cancer and brain tumors is dose dependent,[71,72] while in thyroid cancer, the risk is linear until 20 Gy and then declines.[73] Breast cancer is the most frequent SMN in HL survivors. A systematic review of the literature revealed a 13.3 to 55.5-fold increase in the risk of breast cancer after HL therapy, equivalent to an absolute excess risk of 18.6 to 79.0 per 10,000 person-years. Between 13–30% of female HL survivors treated with radiation will develop a breast malignancy by 40–45 years of age.[74] Increased rates of other solid SMN have been described in large cohorts of HL survivors, including thyroid cancer, bone tumors, colorectal, lung and gastric cancers.[66–68]

Surveillance guidelines have been developed to monitor at-risk survivors for solid tumors. In general, survivors should be educated regarding their risk for solid tumors in the radiation field and should be counseled to report new pain, masses or prolonged fevers. Physicians should order appropriate diagnostic imaging associated with clinical symptoms. In addition, survivors should have yearly exams inspecting the skin, soft tissues and bones in irradiated areas. The *COG LTFU Guidelines* recommend that women exposed to 20 Gy or more of chest radiation begin surveillance mammography and MRI at age 25 or 8 years after completion of radiation therapy, whichever occurs last.[30] In survivors exposed to ≥ 30 Gy abdominal radiation, early surveillance for colorectal cancer is recommended, with colonoscopy every 5 years starting 10 after radiation therapy or age 35 years, whichever occurs last. Surveillance should start sooner in survivors with familial cancer syndromes such as Hereditary Non-Polyposis Colorectal Cancer (HNPCC) or Familial Adenomatous Polyposis (FAP) (Figs. 24.4–24.6).

Cardiac Dysfunction

Cardiac disease is the third most prevalent cause of premature mortality in long-term cancer survivors, after relapse and SMN. The use of anthracycline chemotherapy agents in many leukemia and lymphoma protocols, and the use of mantle radiation in some patients with lymphoma, predisposes many survivors of hematological malignancies to future cardiac dysfunction. Survivors of HL, which is treated often with both anthracyclines and radiation therapy to a field that involves the heart, are as much as 12 times more likely to die from cardiac disease than the general population, while survivors of ALL, AML and NHL have a four- to sixfold increased risk of cardiac death.[75]

Anthracycline cardiomyopathy

Anthracycline antibiotic agents have a high affinity for the mitochondrial membrane phospholipid, cardiolipin,

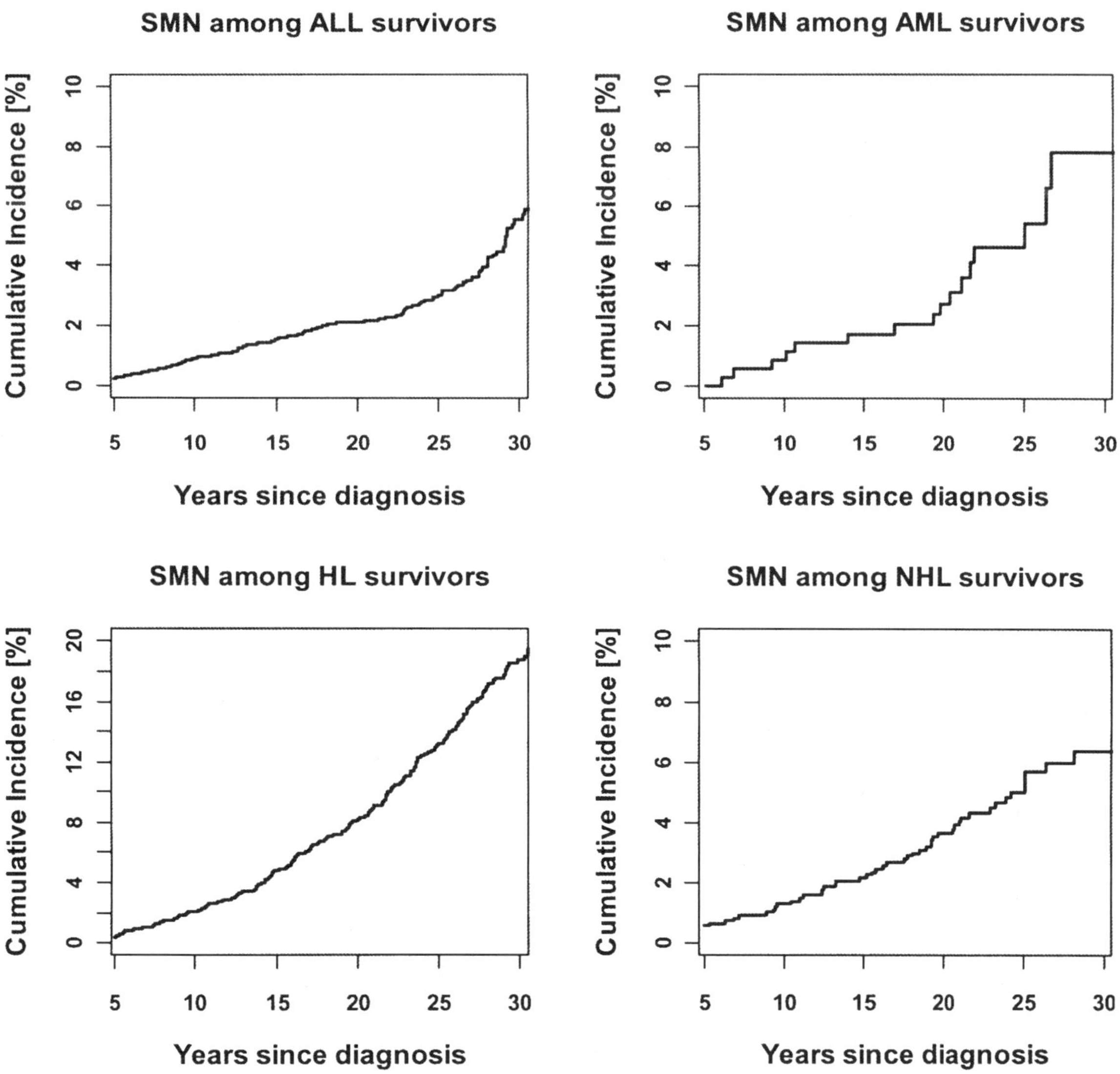

Fig. 24.4. Cumulative incidence of second malignant neoplasms (SMN) in after ALL, AML, NHL, or HL in the CCSS cohort. Unpublished data from CCSS, used with permission.

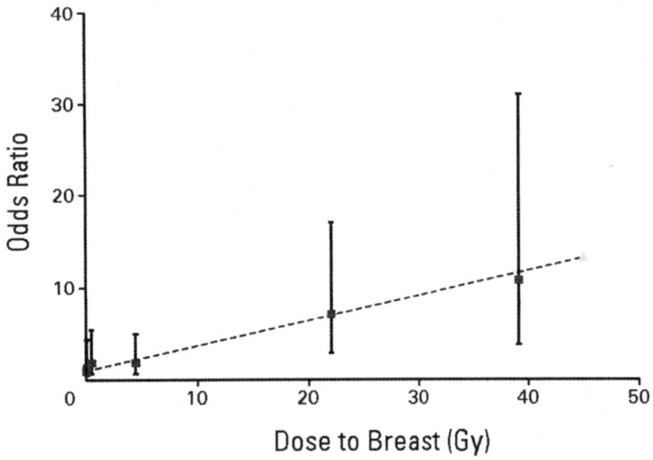

Fig. 24.5. The relationship between radiation dose and the risk of breast cancer in female survivors of all cancers in the CCSS cohort. J Clin Oncol. 2009 Aug 20;27(24):3901–3907. Inskip PD, Robison LL, Stovall M, Smith SA, Hammond S, Mertens AC, Whitton JA, Diller L, Kenney L, Donaldson SS, Meadows AT, Neglia JP. Radiation dose and breast cancer risk in the childhood cancer survivor study.

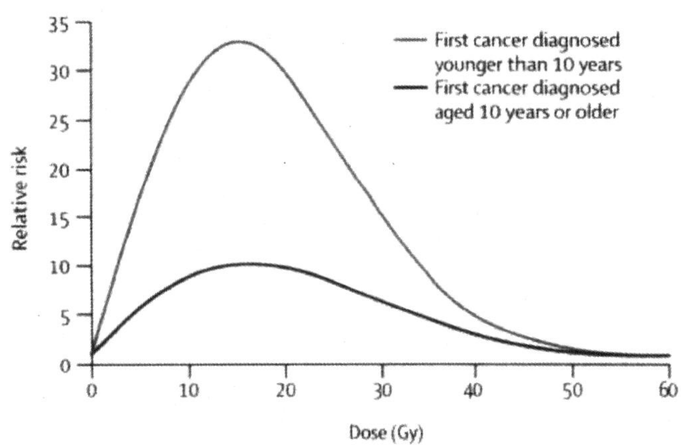

Fig. 24.6. The relationship between radiation dose and the risk of thyroid cancer in survivors of all cancers in the CCSS cohort according to age at diagnosis of their primary cancer. The Lancet. 2005 Jun 11–Jun 17; 365(9476): 2014–2023. Alice J Sigurdson, Cécile M Ronckers, Ann C Mertens, Marilyn Stovall, *et al.* Primary thyroid cancer after a first tumour in childhood (the Childhood Cancer Survivor Study): A nested case-control study.

and consequently accumulate in cardiac myocytes. The mechanisms by which these agents cause myocardial damage are incompletely understood. Through their direct impact on mitochondrial respiration and the formation of anthracycline–iron complexes, they result in the generation of oxygen-derived free radicals which damage lipid, protein and DNA, leading to myocyte death. Cardiac myocytes are particularly susceptible to free radical damage because of their highly oxidative metabolism and relatively poor antioxidant defenses. Myocyte death leads to thinning of the myocardium and dilation of the cardiac chambers. In turn, heart wall thinning leads to increased wall stress, a reduction in ventricular function, and a compensatory increase in renin production. This increases afterload which further increases wall stress, leading to a cycle of cardiac dysfunction that is frequently progressive. The most common manifestation of anthracycline cardiac toxicity is late-onset cardiomyopathy which presents one or more years after the completion of therapy. It can manifest as subclinical abnormalities on cardiac imaging studies such as echocardiography, or with symptoms of congestive heart failure, both related to a reduction in left ventricular function. Risk factors for the development of anthracycline cardiac toxicity include higher cumulative anthracycline dose, younger age at therapy (less than 4–5 years of age), increasing time from therapy, concomitant radiation to a field involving the heart, and possibly female gender. Polymorphisms in genes that regulate anthracycline metabolism may modify toxicity.[3] In patients who receive greater than 300 mg/m^2 of doxorubicin, the risk of congestive heart failure at 20 years approaches 10%.[76] A small number of studies have evaluated the effectiveness of angiotensin-converting enzyme (ACE) inhibition therapy in patients with either clinical or subclinical cardiac toxicity. Although ACE inhibitors demonstrate benefit in some patients, this tends to be transient.[77] Other pharmacologic strategies, such as β blockers require future study (Table 24.1).

Cardiac disease after chest radiation

Mantle field radiation, used in patients with HL and occasionally NHL, delivers radiation to the coronary arteries, most valves, the pericardium, much of the myocardium and the heart's conducting system. Consequently, radiation therapy has been associated with a long-term risk of coronary artery disease (CAD), valvular dysfunction, pericarditis, myocardial dysfunction, and arrhythmias.

The prevalence of CAD has been reported to be between 10% and 20% at 20 years after radiation exposure, although many patients develop atherosclerotic changes as early as 10 years following therapy. The atherosclerotic changes observed in cancer survivors are indistinguishable from those observed in other populations. An increased risk of CAD is associated with higher radiation doses to the coronary arteries. However, myocardial infarction occurs most frequently in survivors with other

Table 24.1. Calculation of doxorubicin isotoxic dose equivalents (30).

Anthracycline agent	Multiply dose by...
Doxorubicin	1
Daunorubicin	0.833
Epirubicin	0.67
Idarubicin	5
Mitoxantrone	4

Long-term follow-up guidelines for survivors of childhood, adolescent, and young adult cancers. In: Hudson M, Landier W, Eshelman D *et al.*, eds: Children's Oncology Group; 2009.

cardiac risk factors. Indeed, traditional risk factors for CAD, such as male sex, hypertension, dyslipidemia, and increasing age impact the risk in lymphoma survivors.

The prevalence of clinically significant valvular disease is as high as 30% in 15-year survivors of chest radiation. Although any of the heart valves can be affected, the aortic valve is the most frequently damaged, with stenosis being the most common manifestation. Radiation dose and time from treatment are the only two identified risk factors.

Radiation is also a risk factor for the development of anthracycline-induced cardiomyopathy, although the interaction between these two modalities in causing cardiac damage is poorly understood. Even those patients treated with chest radiation in the absence of anthracycline chemotherapy are at risk for myocardial dysfunction. This is usually characterized by a restrictive cardiomyopathy due to myocardial fibrosis. Unlike the systolic dysfunction observed after anthracycline therapy, this usually manifests with diastolic abnormalities. Frank congestive heart failure is unusual, but survivors may demonstrate restrictions in exercise capacity.

Surveillance for cardiac dysfunction in survivors of hematological malignancies

COG[30] and other national and international groups[78–80] have published consensus-based guidelines for lifelong surveillance for cardiac dysfunction in survivors. In addition to regular physical examination, COG recommends periodic imaging with echocardiogram or MUGA at frequencies varying from annually to every 5 years depending on age at therapy, cumulative anthracycline dose and radiation exposure (Tables 24.2 and 24.3). In addition, the guidelines highlight the importance of a healthy lifestyle with an emphasis on addressing modifiable risk factors for cardiac disease, such as obesity, dyslipidemia, hypertension, and cigarette smoking.

Pulmonary Disease

Pulmonary disease is the fourth most prevalent cause of premature mortality in long-term survivors. In the CCSS, 2.6% of deaths in 5-year survivors were attributable to diseases of the respiratory system.[75] Patients treated for HL with chest radiation and chemotherapy agents such as bleomycin, and survivors of HSCT are particularly vulnerable to lung disease. Survivors of ALL, AML, NHL and HL are 4.2, 24.9, 10.8, and 9.1 times more likely to die of pulmonary disease than the general population, respectively.[75] The natural history of lung toxicity after cancer therapy is poorly understood due to a paucity of long-term follow up studies, and reliance on survivor self-report in large cohorts such as the CCSS.

Radiation to fields involving the lungs causes direct damage to lung tissue. At higher doses, radiation can also inhibit chest wall growth, particularly when patients are young children at the time of therapy. Acute radiation toxicity is characterized by radiation pneumonitis, which usually occurs within 1 to 3 months after radiation. Symptomatic pneumonitis is usually only observed in patients who receive higher radiation doses (> 30 Gy) to a significant portion of their lungs.[81] However, subclinical radiographic and pulmonary function testing abnormalities have been observed after lower radiation doses. Doses above 15 Gy, or fractionated TBI above 12 Gy, pose the highest risk. In addition to radiation dose and the volume of lung in the radiation field, fractionation and younger age at therapy are also risk factors for toxicity. The acute changes of radiation pneumonitis may evolve to pulmonary fibrosis, which is frequently asymptomatic. PFT abnormalities include evidence of restriction and reduction of diffusing capacity, although obstructive changes have also been observed in some survivors. When symptomatic, pulmonary fibrosis usually presents with exertional dyspnea as well as chronic, nonproductive cough. Changes may be progressive, static or resolve over time.

Bleomycin, an antibiotic chemotherapy agent frequently used in HL protocols, can cause acute pneumonitis as well as chronic lung toxicity. Chronic toxicity presents as pulmonary fibrosis, characterized by impairment of gas diffusion between alveoli and pulmonary capillaries, and evidenced by a reduction in diffusing capacity of the lung for carbon monoxide (DLCO) on PFT. The greatest risk of bleomycin pulmonary toxicity has been observed with doses greater than 400 units/m^2, a dose seldom used in the treatment of pediatric patients. Although less common, pulmonary toxicity has been observed in children treated with 60–100 units/m^2.

Table 24.2. Recommended frequency of cardiac imaging after anthracycline chemotherapy.

Age at treatment	Radiation with potential impact to the heart	Anthracycline dose[a]	Recommended frequency of echocardiogram or MUGA scan
< 1 year old	Yes	Any	Every year
	No	< 200 mg/m^2	Every 2 years
		≥ 200 mg/m^2	Every year
1–4 years old	Yes	Any	Every year
		< 100 mg/m^2	Every 5 years
	No	≥ 100 to < 300 mg/m^2	Every 2 years
		≥ 300 mg/m^2	Every year
≥ 5 years old	Yes	< 300 mg/m^2	Every 2 years
		≥ 300 mg/m^2	Every year
		< 200 mg/m^2	Every 5 years
	No	≥ 200 to < 300 mg/m^2	Every 2 years
		≥ 300 mg/m^2	Every year
Any age with decrease in serial function			Every year

[a]Based on doxorubicin isotoxic equivalent dose (see Table 24.1).

Reproduced from the Children's Oncology Group Long-Term Follow-Up Guidelines for Survivors of Childhood, Adolescent and Young Adult Cancers, Version 3.0, October 2008, used with permission.

Table 24.3. Recommended frequency of cardiac imaging after radiation therapy with potential impact to the heart.

Age at treatment	Radiation dose	Anthracycline dose[a]	Recommended frequency of echocardiogram or MUGA scan
< 5 years old	Any	None	Every 2 years
		Any	Every year
≥ 5 years old	< 30 Gy	None	Every 5 years
	≥ 30 Gy	None	Every 2 years
	Any	< 300 mg/m^2	Every 2 years
		≥ 300 mg/m^2	Every year
Any age with serial decrease in function			Every year

[a]Based on doxorubicin isotoxic equivalent dose (see Table 24.1).

Reproduced from the Children's Oncology Group Long-Term Follow-Up Guidelines for Survivors of Childhood, Adolescent and Young Adult Cancers, Version 3.0, October 2008, used with permission.

Anecdotal reports of progressive pulmonary fibrosis after exposure to high oxygen concentration (e.g. during anesthesia) has prompted the recommendation that survivors treated with bleomycin avoid exposure to concentrated oxygen and wear a MedicAlert bracelet documenting their risk. However, most adverse events have occurred during or shortly after therapy in adults exposed to high doses of bleomycin — thus, the long-term risk in the childhood cancer survivor population is not well defined. Perhaps more important is the recommendation that survivors exposed to bleomycin refrain from smoking and avoid exposure to second-hand smoke.

Busulfan, as well as alkylating agents such as melphalan, has also been established as a pulmonary toxin. Busulfan and melphalan are often used as conditioning agents for HSCT. Their role in causing toxicity after HSCT is difficult to discern as these patients may also be treated with TBI, develop chronic graft vs. host disease or pulmonary infections (viral, bacterial or fungal) which can also lead to chronic lung toxicity. Chronic lung toxicities in transplant survivors include bronchiolitis obliterans, bronchiectasis and chronic bronchitis. Patients who have received prolonged immunosuppression for chronic graft vs. host disease are at particular risk.

Care of survivors at risk for pulmonary toxicity should include an annual history and physical examination. Chest X-ray and pulmonary function testing are recommended at entry into a long-term follow up program and then as clinically indicated in patients with abnormal results or clinical symptoms. Pneumococcal and influenza vaccination should be considered. Finally, an anesthesia consult should be obtained prior to any surgical procedures.

Long-Term Vulnerability to Infection After Therapy

Before the advent of computed tomography (CT) scans, functional imaging and the use of systemic chemotherapy, most patients with HL were evaluated for stage of disease by laparotomy, lymph node biopsy and splenectomy. Thus, many survivors of HL treated in the 1970s–1980s are asplenic. Furthermore, functional asplenia after 40 Gy radiation exposure involving the spleen has been described.[82] Due to poor defenses to encapsulated organisms, these patients have a 2–4% lifetime risk of overwhelming sepsis, with a 1–2% mortality rate.[83,84] To address and reduce the risk of this late effect, health care providers must provide adequate education regarding this risk, appropriate protective immunization, and the need for prompt medical evaluation during febrile episodes.[85,86]

Predicting the Late Effects of New Agents for the Treatment of Leukemia or Lymphoma

Recent therapeutic protocols for leukemia and lymphoma have included novel agents such as monoclonal antibodies and molecular therapeutics (see Chapters 21 and 22). Several such agents are being tested in Phase I or II trials in patients with refractory or recurrent disease who are unlikely to become long-term survivors. However, some of these agents will eventually be incorporated into front-line treatment protocols. Others, such as rituximab, have become core components of some treatment regimens. Although many of these new agents result in less acute toxicity than older, cytotoxic chemotherapy agents, their long-term impact will require further study.

Late-onset cytopenias, particularly neutropenia, have been reported in patients treated with rituximab.[87] However, these tend to occur in the year following therapy and are generally self limiting. Similarly, the drug can cause hypogammaglobulinemia, although this too is transient in nature. Reactivation of hepatitis B and C have been reported after rituximab therapy. Rarely, late pulmonary sequelae have been reported. These may be secondary to acute pulmonary infection during times of decreased immunity, or to an inflammatory reaction resulting in diffuse parenchymal lung disease. This presents most frequently with interstitial pneumonitis. If such complications occur, investigation for infectious etiologies should be undertaken and if negative, a trial of corticosteroids can be considered.[87]

Other novel agents, such gemtuzumab, ozogamicin and imatinib, have not been associated with particular long-term sequelae. However, follow up in survivors treated with these and other agents is short, and there will need to be continued surveillance for late effects in these patients over time.

Risk-Based Care

Since the late effects of cancer and its therapy are associated with decreased quality of life and excess morbidity and early mortality, the Institute of Medicine (IOM) has recommended risk-based long-term follow up care focused on the surveillance, prevention, and treatment of late effects throughout the lifespan.[88] Central to the appropriate care of this complex patient population is the provision of a treatment summary and a survivorship care plan to all childhood, adolescent, or young adult cancer survivors at the conclusion of their therapy (see Chapter 27). These documents are intended to assist both the survivor and their health care providers in assuring appropriate follow up for specific late effects. Individualized care plans should lay out each survivor's required health care visits, surveillance, and the anticipatory guidance needed to minimize their risks of morbidity and premature mortality. In response to the IOM report, guidelines have been developed by numerous national and international organizations, including the COG, Scottish Intercollegiate Guideline Network, and the United Kingdom Children's Cancer Study Group. Given the heterogeneity in treatment protocols for each type of cancer, recommendations are based on treatment exposures rather than primary diagnosis. Thus, it is imperative that both survivors and their physicians have knowledge of their prior therapies, documented in a treatment summary that includes chemotherapy names and cumulative doses (for those agents known to have a relationship between dose and risk), as well as radiation fields and doses.

Despite these recommendations and available practice guidelines, early evidence suggests that only a minority of survivors may be receiving appropriate risk-based health care.[89] One well-described barrier to life-long risk-based care is that childhood cancer survivors are generally poorly informed about their previous therapies, their associated sequelae, and the need for long-term follow up.[90] Further, many survivors have developmental and psychological issues that impact their transition to adult-based care. Recent studies suggest many pediatric oncologists are not aware of the follow up guidelines for childhood or adolescent cancer survivors and are less comfortable caring for survivors once they reach 21 years of age.[91] It has been suggested that given the relatively small size of the childhood, adolescent, and young adult cancer survivor population, many health care providers outside of the oncology specialty are unaware of these patients' long-term risks and their need for risk-based care. Finally, in the United States, inadequate health insurance due to the classification of childhood or adolesecent cancer as a "pre-existing condition" and unemployment are barriers to appropriate care in some survivors.

Conclusion

The optimistic prognosis for many children, adolescents and young adults with newly diagnosed leukemia or lymphoma has allowed oncologists to focus increasingly on preventing or reducing their risk for long-term sequelae of therapy. Avoidance of CRT for most patients with ALL, and elimination or reductions in doses of potentially toxic chemotherapies have been achieved in many treatment protocols without compromising disease survival. Identification of genetic differences between patients that alter their risk for specific toxicities will eventually be used to tailor therapy to individual patients. In addition, future research will focus on ways to prevent or mitigate the natural history of late effects once toxic exposures have occurred. Despite advances in reducing the long-term toxicities of cancer therapy, all survivors of childhood, adolescent or young adult leukemia and lymphoma should continue to receive lifelong medical care and surveillance that focuses on their specific risks in order to maximize both the quantity and quality of their lives.

Patient Vignettes

Here, we present the cases of two patients, each of whom had a history of a hematopoietic malignancy. The table that follows each vignette highlights the risks associated with the cancer in question and the most effective preventive and management strategies for its survivors, based on the COG LTFU guidelines.

Case 1: Acute Lymphoblastic Leukemia

P.G. is a 14-year-old boy in whom high-risk acute lymphoblastic leukemia was diagnosed at the age of 9 years. He was treated with chemotherapy (daunorubicin, 125 mg/m^2; doxorubicin, 150 mg/m^2; high-dose methotrexate; dexamethasone; cyclophosphamide; vincristine; thioguanine; mercaptopurine; cytarabine; PEG-asparaginase; intrathecal methotrexate; and intrathecal cytarabine) and cranial radiation therapy (18 Gy) over the course of 38 months. He has been overweight since completing treatment and has been complaining of right hip pain for the last few months.

Case 2: Hodgkin Lymphoma

J.S. is a 34-year-old woman who just moved to town and presents for a routine physical examination. She had Stage I Hodgkin lymphoma (HL) at age 14; she was treated with 44 Gy mantle radiation following a staging laparotomy and splenectomy. She has not seen an oncologist in over 15 years.

Table 1. Selected treatment-based potential late effects and screening recommendations[a] for asymptomatic survivors of acute lymphoblastic leukemia.

Treatment agent	Potential late effects	Periodic evaluation (timing and frequency)
Any	Psychosocial disorders Social withdrawal Educational problems Fatigue Limitations in healthcare and insurance access	Assessment of educational or vocational progress Psychosocial evaluation
Any blood product (if cancer was diagnosed before 1993)	Chronic hepatitis C	Measurement of hepatitis C antibody (baseline)
Cranial radiation therapy (18–24 Gy)	Neurocognitive deficit	Referral for formal neuropsychological evaluation (baseline and as clinically indicated)
	Growth hormone deficiency	Height, weight, BMI (every 6 months until growth is completed, yearly thereafter)
	Precocious puberty	Tanner stage (yearly)
	Overweight or obesity	Blood pressure (yearly)
	Metabolic syndrome	Measurement of fasting glucose and lipid profile (every 2–5 years)
	Cataracts	Eye examination for visual acuity/lens opacity (yearly) Evaluation by ophthalmologist (every 3 years)
	Dental abnormalities Xerostomia	Dental examination and cleaning (every 6 months)
	Thyroid cancer/nodules	Thyroid examination (yearly)
	Hypothyroidism	Measurements of TSH, free T_4 (yearly)
Methotrexate	Osteopenia and osteoporosis	DEXA or quantitative CT (baseline and as clinically indicated)
	Renal toxicity	Urinalysis (yearly) Measurements of BUN, creatinine, electrolytes, calcium, magnesium, phosphate (baseline and as clinically indicated)
	Hepatic dysfunction	Measurements of AST, ALT, bilirubin (baseline and as clinically indicated)
Daunorubicin and doxorubicin: cumulative dose < 300 mg/m^2	Cardiomyopathy and left ventricular dysfunction	Echocardiogram (every 2 years)
	Arrhythmia	ECG (baseline and as clinically indicated)
Corticosteroids (i.e. dexamethasone)	Osteonecrosis (avascular necrosis)	Musculoskeletal examination (yearly)
Cyclophosphamide	Urinary tract toxicity (e.g. bladder malignancy, hemorrhagic cystitis)	Urinalysis (yearly)
	Acute myeloid leukemia Myelodysplasia	CBC, differential (yearly for 10 years after treatment)
	Hypogonadism Delayed/arrested puberty	Tanner staging (yearly until sexually mature) Measurement of FSH, LH, testosterone (baseline at age 14 and as clinically indicated)
Vincristine	Peripheral sensory or motor neuropathy	Neurological examination (yearly until 2–3 years after therapy)

[a]Although some conditions (e.g. osteoporosis, renal toxicity) are associated with multiple treatment agents, each condition or periodic evaluation is listed only one time.
AST: aspartate aminotransferase; ALT: alanine aminotransferase; BMI: body mass index; BUN: blood urea nitrogen; DEXA: dual X-ray absorptiometry; FSH: follicle stimulating hormone; LH: luteinizing hormone; TSH: thyroid-stimulating hormone.

Table 2. Selected treatment-based potential late effects and screening recommendations* for survivors of Hodgkin lymphoma treated with mantle radiation and a staging laparotomy/splenectomy.

Treatment agent	Potential late effects	Periodic evaluation (timing and frequency)
Any	Psychosocial disorders Social withdrawal Educational problems	Assessment of educational or vocational progress Psychosocial evaluation
Mantle radiation	Breast cancer	Breast self-examination (monthly) Clinical breast examination (yearly until age 25, then every 6 months) Mammogram and breast MRI (yearly, beginning 8 years after radiation or at age 25, whichever occurs last)
	Cardiac toxicity (ischemic coronary artery disease, valvular heart disease, left ventricular dysfunction, arrhythmia)	Measurement of fasting glucose and lipid profile (every 3–5 years) Echocardiogram (every 2 years) ECG (baseline and as clinically indicated)
	Carotid artery disease	Auscultation for carotid bruit (yearly)
	Subclavian artery disease	Evaluate radial and brachial pulses and blood pressure in each arm (yearly)
	Thyroid cancer or nodules	Thyroid examination (yearly)
	Hypothyroidism or hyperthyroidism	Measurement of TSH, free T_4 (yearly)
	Pulmonary toxicity (pulmonary fibrosis, restrictive and/or obstructive lung disease)	Pulmonary function tests with DL_{CO} and chest X-ray (baseline and as clinically indicated)
	Dental abnormalities Xerostomia	Dental examination and cleaning (every 6 months)
	Dermatologic changes in radiation field	Dermatologic examination of irradiated area (yearly)
Splenectomy	Asplenia	When febrile (≥ 38.3°C [101°F]), physical examination and blood culture immunize with *Pneumococcal, Meningococcal,* and *Haemophilus influenzae* vaccines. Pneumovax booster in patients ≥ 10 years old at ≥ 5 years after previous dose

DL_{CO}: diffusing capacity for carbon monoxide; TSH: thyroid-stimulating hormone.
Reproduced, with permission, from The Consultant, May 2008.

References

1. Mariotto AB, Rowland JH, Yabroff KR, Scoppa S, Hachey M, Ries L, *et al.* (2009) Long-term survivors of childhood cancers in the United States. *Cancer Epidemiol Biomarkers Prev* **18**(4): 1033–1040.
4. Mitby PA, Robison LL, Whitton JA, Zevon MA, Gibbs IC, Tersak JM, *et al.* (2003) Utilization of special education services and educational attainment among long-term survivors of childhood cancer: A report from the Childhood Cancer Survivor Study. *Cancer* **97**(4): 1115–1126.
6. Cousens P, Waters B, Said J, Stevens M. (1988) Cognitive effects of cranial irradiation in leukaemia: A survey and meta-analysis. *J Child Psychol Psychiatry* **29**(6): 839–852.
8. Rubenstein CL, Varni JW, Katz ER. (1990) Cognitive functioning in long-term survivors of childhood leukemia: A prospective analysis. *J Dev Behav Pediatr* **11**(6): 301–315.
10. Kadan-Lottick NS, Brouwers P, Breiger D, Kaleita T, Dziura J, Northrup V, *et al.* (2009) Comparison of neurocognitive functioning in children previously randomly assigned to intrathecal methotrexate compared with triple intrathecal therapy for the treatment of childhood acute lymphoblastic leukemia. *J Clin Oncol* **27**(35): 5986–5992.
11. Nathan PC, Whitcomb T, Wolters PL, Steinberg SM, Balis FM, Brouwers P, *et al.* (2006) Very high-dose methotrexate (33.6 g/m(2)) as central nervous system preventive therapy for childhood acute lymphoblastic leukemia: Results of National Cancer Institute/Children's Cancer Group trials CCG-191P, CCG-134P and CCG-144P. *Leuk Lymphoma* **47**(12): 2488–2504.
12. Buizer AI, de Sonneville LM, van den Heuvel-Eibrink MM, Veerman AJ. (2005) Chemotherapy and attentional dysfunction in survivors of childhood acute lymphoblastic

leukemia: Effect of treatment intensity. *Pediatr Blood Cancer* **45**(3): 281–290.
13. Carey ME, Hockenberry MJ, Moore IM, Hutter JJ, Krull KR, Pasvogel A, *et al.* (2007) Brief report: Effect of intravenous methotrexate dose and infusion rate on neuropsychological function one year after diagnosis of acute lymphoblastic leukemia. *J Pediatr Psychol* **32**(2): 189–193.
14. Waber DP, Carpentieri SC, Klar N, Silverman LB, Schwenn M, Hurwitz CA, *et al.* (2000) Cognitive sequelae in children treated for acute lymphoblastic leukemia with dexamethasone or prednisone. *J Pediatr Hematol Oncol* **22**(3): 206–213.
15. Kadan-Lottick NS, Brouwers P, Breiger D, Kaleita T, Dziura J, Liu H, *et al.* (2009) A comparison of neurocognitive functioning in children previously randomized to dexamethasone or prednisone in the treatment of childhood acute lymphoblastic leukemia. *Blood* **114**(9): 1746–1752.
17. Campbell LK, Scaduto M, Sharp W, Dufton L, van Slyke D, Whitlock JA, *et al.* (2007) A meta-analysis of the neurocognitive sequelae of treatment for childhood acute lymphocytic leukemia. *Pediatr Blood Cancer* **49**(1): 65–73.
19. Peterson CC, Johnson CE, Ramirez LY, Huestis S, Pai AL, Demaree HA, *et al.* (2008) A meta-analysis of the neuropsychological sequelae of chemotherapy-only treatment for pediatric acute lymphoblastic leukemia. *Pediatr Blood Cancer* **51**(1): 99–104.
20. Lehtinen SS, Huuskonen UE, Harila-Saari AH, Tolonen U, Vainionpaa LK, Lanning BM. (2002) Motor nervous system impairment persists in long-term survivors of childhood acute lymphoblastic leukemia. *Cancer* **94**(9): 2466–2473.
21. Hertzberg H, Huk WJ, Ueberall MA, Langer T, Meier W, Dopfer R, *et al.* (1997) CNS late effects after ALL therapy in childhood. Part I: Neuroradiological findings in long-term survivors of childhood ALL — an evaluation of the interferences between morphology and neuropsychological performance. The German Late Effects Working Group. *Med Pediatr Oncol* **28**(6): 387–400.
22. Reddick WE, Shan ZY, Glass, JO, Helton S, Xiong X, Wu S, Bonner M, Howard SC, Chistensen R, Khan RB, Pui C-H, Mulhern RK. (2006) Smaller white-matter volumes are associated with larger deficits in attention and learning among long-term survivors of acute lymphoblastic leukemia. *Cancer* **106**: 941–949.
24. Butler RW, Copeland DR, Fairclough DL, Mulhern RK, Katz ER, Kazak AE, *et al.* (2008) A multicenter, randomized clinical trial of a cognitive remediation program for childhood survivors of a pediatric malignancy. *J Consult Clin Psychol* **76**(3): 367–378.
25. Mulhern RK, Khan RB, Kaplan S, Helton S, Christensen R, Bonner M, *et al.* (2004) Short-term efficacy of methylphenidate: A randomized, double-blind, placebo-controlled trial among survivors of childhood cancer. *J Clin Oncol* **22**(23): 4795–4803.
27. Bowers DC, Liu Y, Leisenring W, McNeil E, Stovall M, Gurney JG, *et al.* (2006) Late-occurring stroke among long-term survivors of childhood leukemia and brain tumors: A report from the Childhood Cancer Survivor Study. *J Clin Oncol* **24**(33): 5277–5282.
28. Bowers DC, McNeil DE, Liu Y, Yasui Y, Stovall M, Gurney JG, *et al.* (2005) Stroke as a late treatment effect of Hodgkin's disease: A report from the Childhood Cancer Survivor Study. *J Clin Oncol* **23**(27): 6508–6515.
29. de Bruin ML, Dorresteijn LD, van't Veer MB, Krol AD, van der Pal HJ, Kappelle AC, *et al.* (2009) Increased risk of stroke and transient ischemic attack in 5-year survivors of Hodgkin lymphoma. *J Natl Cancer Inst* **101**(13): 928–937.
30. Hudson M, Landier W, Eshelman D, *et al.* (eds.) (2009) *Long-term Follow-up Guidelines for Survivors of Childhood, Adolescent, and Young Adult Cancers.* Children's Oncology Group.
31. Goldsby RE, Liu Q, Nathan PC, Bowers DC, Yeaton-Massey A, Raber SH, *et al.* (2010) Late-occurring neurologic sequelae in adult survivors of childhood acute lymphoblastic leukemia: A report from the Childhood Cancer Survivor Study. *J Clin Oncol* **28**(2): 324–331.
33. Sklar C. (1999) Reproductive physiology and treatment-related loss of sex hormone production. *Med Pediatr Oncol* **33**(1): 2–8.
34. Anselmo AP, Cartoni C, Bellantuono P, Maurizi-Enrici R, Aboulkair N, Ermini M. (1990) Risk of infertility in patients with Hodgkin's disease treated with ABVD vs MOPP vs ABVD/MOPP. *Haematologica* **75**(2): 155–158.
35. de Bruin ML, Huisbrink J, Hauptmann M, Kuenen MA, Ouwens GM, van't Veer MB, *et al.* (2008) Treatment-related risk factors for premature menopause following Hodgkin lymphoma. *Blood* **111**(1): 101–108.
36. Hodgson DC, Pintilie M, Gitterman L, Dewitt B, Buckley CA, Ahmed S, *et al.* (2007) Fertility among female hodgkin lymphoma survivors attempting pregnancy following ABVD chemotherapy. *Hematol Oncol* **25**(1): 11–15.
39. French D, Hamilton LH, Mattano LA, Jr., Sather HN, Devidas M, Nachman JB, *et al.* (2008) A PAI-1 (SERPINE1) polymorphism predicts osteonecrosis in children with acute lymphoblastic leukemia: A report from the Children's Oncology Group. *Blood* **111**(9): 4496–4499.
42. Ribeiro RC, Fletcher BD, Kennedy W, Harrison PL, Neel MD, Kaste SC, *et al.* (2001) Magnetic resonance

imaging detection of avascular necrosis of the bone in children receiving intensive prednisone therapy for acute lymphoblastic leukemia or non-Hodgkin lymphoma. *Leukemia* **15**(6): 891–897.

43. Burger B, Beier R, Zimmermann M, Beck JD, Reiter A, Schrappe M. (2005) Osteonecrosis: A treatment related toxicity in childhood acute lymphoblastic leukemia (ALL) — experiences from trial ALL-BFM 95. *Pediatr Blood Cancer* **44**(3): 220–225.
44. Atkinson SA, Halton JM, Bradley C, Wu B, Barr RD. (1998) Bone and mineral abnormalities in childhood acute lymphoblastic leukemia: Influence of disease, drugs and nutrition. *Int J Cancer Suppl* **11**: 35–39.
45. Hochberg Z. (2002) Mechanisms of steroid impairment of growth. *Horm Res* **58**(1): 33–38.
47. Hancock SL, McDougall IR, Constine LS. (1995) Thyroid abnormalities after therapeutic external radiation. *Int J Radiat Oncol Biol Phys* **31**(5): 1165–1170.
48. Chow EJ, Friedman DL, Stovall M, Yasui Y, Whitton JA, Robison LL, *et al.* (2009) Risk of thyroid dysfunction and subsequent thyroid cancer among survivors of acute lymphoblastic leukemia: A report from the Childhood Cancer Survivor Study. *Pediatr Blood Cancer* **53**(3): 432–437.
53. Oeffinger KC, Mertens AC, Sklar CA, Yasui Y, Fears T, Stovall M, *et al.* (2003) Obesity in adult survivors of childhood acute lymphoblastic leukemia: A report from the Childhood Cancer Survivor Study. *J Clin Oncol* **21**(7): 1359–1365.
54. Garmey EG, Liu Q, Sklar CA, Meacham LR, Mertens AC, Stovall MA, *et al.* (2008) Longitudinal changes in obesity and body mass index among adult survivors of childhood acute lymphoblastic leukemia: A report from the Childhood Cancer Survivor Study. *J Clin Oncol* **26**(28): 4639–4645.
55. Ross JA, Oeffinger KC, Davies SM, Mertens AC, Langer EK, Kiffmeyer WR, *et al.* (2004) Genetic variation in the leptin receptor gene and obesity in survivors of childhood acute lymphoblastic leukemia: A report from the Childhood Cancer Survivor Study. *J Clin Oncol* **22**(17): 3558–3562.
56. Reilly JJ, Ventham JC, Ralston JM, Donaldson M, Gibson B. (1998) Reduced energy expenditure in preobese children treated for acute lymphoblastic leukemia. *Pediatr Res* **44**(4): 557–562.
57. Warner JT, Bell W, Webb DK, Gregory JW. (1998) Daily energy expenditure and physical activity in survivors of childhood malignancy. *Pediatr Res* **43**(5): 607–613.
58. Reilly JJ, Kelly A, Ness P, Dorosty AR, Wallace WH, Gibson BE, *et al.* (2001) Premature adiposity rebound in children treated for acute lymphoblastic leukemia. *J Clin Endocrinol Metab* **86**(6): 2775–2778.
59. Oeffinger KC, Buchanan GR, Eshelman DA, Denke MA, Andrews TC, Germak JA, *et al.* (2001) Cardiovascular risk factors in young adult survivors of childhood acute lymphoblastic leukemia. *J Pediatr Hematol Oncol* **23**(7): 424–430.
60. Bhatia S, Sather HN, Pabustan OB, Trigg ME, Gaynon PS, Robison LL. (2002) Low incidence of second neoplasms among children diagnosed with acute lymphoblastic leukemia after 1983. *Blood* **99**(12): 4257–4264.
61. Loning L, Zimmermann M, Reiter A, Kaatsch P, Henze G, Riehm H, *et al.* (2000) Secondary neoplasms subsequent to Berlin-Frankfurt-Munster therapy of acute lymphoblastic leukemia in childhood: Significantly lower risk without cranial radiotherapy. *Blood* **95**(9): 2770–2775.
62. Hijiya N, Hudson MM, Lensing S, Zacher M, Onciu M, Behm FG, *et al.* (2007) Cumulative incidence of secondary neoplasms as a first event after childhood acute lymphoblastic leukemia. *JAMA* **297**(11): 1207–1215.
63. Mody R, Li S, Dover DC, Sallan S, Leisenring W, Oeffinger KC, *et al.* (2008) Twenty-five-year follow-up among survivors of childhood acute lymphoblastic leukemia: A report from the Childhood Cancer Survivor Study. *Blood* **111**(12): 5515–5523.
64. Mulrooney DA, Dover DC, Li S, Yasui Y, Ness KK, Mertens AC, *et al.* (2008) Twenty years of follow-up among survivors of childhood and young adult acute myeloid leukemia: A report from the Childhood Cancer Survivor Study. *Cancer* **112**(9): 2071–2079.
65. Bluhm EC, Ronckers C, Hayashi RJ, Neglia JP, Mertens AC, Stovall M, *et al.* (2008) Cause-specific mortality and second cancer incidence after non-Hodgkin lymphoma: A report from the Childhood Cancer Survivor Study. *Blood* **111**(8): 4014–4021.
66. Bhatia S, Yasui Y, Robison LL, Birch JM, Bogue MK, Diller L, *et al.* (2003) High risk of subsequent neoplasms continues with extended follow-up of childhood Hodgkin's disease: Report from the Late Effects Study Group. *J Clin Oncol* **21**(23): 4386–4394.
67. Swerdlow AJ, Barber JA, Hudson GV, Cunningham D, Gupta RK, Hancock BW, *et al.* (2000) Risk of second malignancy after Hodgkin's disease in a collaborative British cohort: The relation to age at treatment. *J Clin Oncol* **18**(3): 498–509.
68. van Leeuwen FE, Klokman WJ, Veer MB, Hagenbeek A, Krol AD, Vetter UA, *et al.* (2000) Long-term risk of second malignancy in survivors of Hodgkin's disease treated during adolescence or young adulthood. *J Clin Oncol* **18**(3): 487–497.
72. Neglia JP, Robison LL, Stovall M, Liu Y, Packer RJ, Hammond S, *et al.* (2006) New primary neoplasms of

the central nervous system in survivors of childhood cancer: A report from the Childhood Cancer Survivor Study. *J Natl Cancer Inst* **98**(21): 1528–1537.

73. Ronckers CM, Sigurdson AJ, Stovall M, Smith SA, Mertens AC, Liu Y, *et al.* (2006) Thyroid cancer in childhood cancer survivors: A detailed evaluation of radiation dose response and its modifiers. *Radiat Res* **166**(4): 618–628.
74. Henderson TO, Amsterdam A, Bhatia S, Hudson M, Meadows AT, Neglia JP, *et al.* (2009) Surveillance for breast cancer in women treated with chest radiation for a childhood, adolescent or young adult cancer: A Report from the Children's Oncology Group. *Ann Intern Med* **152**(7): 444–W154.
75. Armstrong GT, Liu Q, Yasui Y, Neglia JP, Leisenring W, Robison LL, *et al.* (2009) Late Mortality Among 5-Year Survivors of Childhood Cancer: A Summary From The Childhood Cancer Survivor Study. *J Clin Oncol* **27**(14): 2328–2338.
76. van Dalen EC, van der Pal HJ, Kok WE, Caron HN, Kremer LC. (2006) Clinical heart failure in a cohort of children treated with anthracyclines: A long-term follow-up study. *Eur J Cancer* **42**(18): 3191–3198.
77. Lipshultz SE, Lipsitz SR, Sallan SE, Simbre VC II, Shaikh SL, Mone SM, *et al.* (2002) Long-term enalapril therapy for left ventricular dysfunction in doxorubicin-treated survivors of childhood cancer. *J Clin Oncol* **20**(23): 4517–4522.
81. Liles A, Blatt J, Morris D, Wardrop R 3rd, Sharma A, Sznewajs A, *et al.* (2008) Monitoring pulmonary complications in long-term childhood cancer survivors: Guidelines for the primary care physician. *Cleve Clin J Med* **75**(7): 531–539.
82. Coleman CN, McDougall IR, Dailey MO, Ager P, Bush S, Kaplan HS. (1982) Functional hyposplenia after splenic irradiation for Hodgkin's disease. *Ann Intern Med* **96**(1): 44–47.
83. Jockovich M, Mendenhall NP, Sombeck MD, Talbert JL, Copeland EM III, Bland KI. (1994) Long-term complications of laparotomy in Hodgkin's disease. *Ann Surg* **219**(6): 615–621; discussion 21–24.
84. Kaiser CW. (1981) Complications from staging laparotomy for Hodgkin disease. *J Surg Oncol* **16**(4): 319–325.
88. Hewitt M, Weiner SL, Simone JV eds. (2003) *Childhood Cancer Survivorship: Improving Care and Quality of Life.* Washington, D.C.: The National Academies Press.
89. Nathan PC, Greenberg ML, Ness KK, Hudson MM, Mertens AC, Mahoney MC, *et al.* (2008) Medical care in long-term survivors of childhood cancer: A report from the childhood cancer survivor study. *J Clin Oncol* **26**(27): 4401–4409.
91. Henderson TO, Hlubocky FJ, Wroblewski KE, Diller L, Daugherty CK. (2009) Physician preferences and knowledge gaps regarding the care of childhood Cancer Survivors: A Mailed survey of pediatric oncologists. *J Clin Oncol* **28**(5): 878–883.

25

Infectious Complications of Hematological Malignancies in Children, Adolescents and Young Adults

Thomas J. Walsh, Andreas H. Groll and Emmanuel Roilides

Introduction

Infectious diseases are important causes of morbidity and mortality in pediatric patients with hematological malignancies.[1,2] While major advances have been achieved in the management of bacterial, fungal, and viral infections in this most vulnerable population, new pathogens and evolving immunosuppressive modalities present new challenges to practicing physicians. The purpose of this chapter is to review current approaches to the management of infectious complications in children, adolescents, and young adults with hematological malignancies.

Innate Host Defenses and Adaptive Immunity

An understanding of innate host defenses and adaptive immunity is fundamental to assessing the risk, causes, and management of infections in patients with hematological malignancies. Innate host defenses encompass mucocutaneous barriers, phagocytic cells, the toll-like receptor system, other receptors of pathogen-associated molecules, cytokine regulatory networks, natural killer cells, reticuloendothelial system, and colonization resistance by endogenous mucocutaneous microflora. Adaptive immunity encompasses the production of pathogen-specific antibodies and T-lymphocyte cell-mediated immunity (Table 25.1).

Mechanical barriers

A complex set of specialized cells of the skin and the respiratory, gastrointestinal, and genitourinary mucosal function to protect the body from invading pathogens.[3] Mucocutaneous cells express unique proteins, mechanical impediments, and immunological mediators that further confer redundant defenses against microbial invasion. The pseudostratified columnar epithelium of the lower respiratory tract provides a mucociliary "escalator" that propels organisms out of the lungs. Pentraxin and other pulmonary surfactant molecules of the collectin class of molecules opsonize bacterial and fungal pathogens. Alpha-defensins in neutrophils and Paneth cells of the small intestine and β-defensins of the skin and the mucosal surfaces of the respiratory, gastrointestinal, and urinary tracts are antimicrobial peptides against bacteria, fungi and viruses. Apocrine cells of the epidermis elaborate bactericidal fatty acids. Secretory IgA further defends patients against pathogens penetrating mucosal surfaces. Vascular catheters, cytotoxic

Table 25.1. Deficits in innate and acquired host defenses: Associated infections in children with hematological malignancies.

Type of host defense	Immune deficit	Mechanism	Organism	Infections
Innate				
Mucocutaneous barriers	Disruption of mucocutaneous barriers	Cytotoxic chemotherapy, radiation therapy or GVHD of mucosal surfaces Percutaneous vascular catheters	Oral microbes flora, e.g. viridans Streptococci Enteric microbes, e.g. *Escherichia coli* and *Klebsiella* spp. Cutaneous microbes, e.g. *Staphylococcus aureus* and *Staphylococcus epidermidis*	Oral and enteric infections Bacteremia
Neutrophils	Neutropenia	Cytotoxic chemotherapy or total body radiation therapy or aplastic anemia	Enteric microbes, e.g. *Escherichia coli*, *Klebsiella* spp., *Pseudomonas aeruginosa*, and *Candida* spp. Aerosolized fungi, e.g. *Aspergillus* spp., Mucorales, *Fusarium* spp.	Bacteremia, candidemia Pneumonia
Neutrophils	Functional impairment of phagocytosis, oxidative and non-oxidative microbicidal mechanisms	Corticosteroid therapy	*Aspergillus* spp., Mucorales	Pneumonia, sinusitis, disseminated infection
Neutrophils	Mutations in NADPH oxidases	Primary immunodeficiency CGD	*Staphylococcus aureus* *Aspergillus* spp. *Burkholderia cepacia*	Pneumonia, cutaneous infections, disseminated infection
Toll-like receptors, dectin and other receptors of pathogen-associated molecules	Alterations of genes encoding Toll-like receptors, dectin receptors	Absence of functional receptor or decreased affinity of receptor	Infection varies with type of receptor and defect	
Cytokines (e.g. proinflammatory cytokines: TNFα, IL-1β, IL-2, IL-6, IL-12)	TNFα inhibition	Impaired upregulation of phagocytic response against bacteria, mycobacteria, fungi	*Mycobacterium tuberculosis* and *Histoplasma capsulatum*	Lower respiratory tract infection
Spleen and reticuloendothelial system (RES)	Splenectomy	Impaired RES function and antibody synthesis	Encapsulated bacteria: *S. pneumoniae*, *H. influenzae*, and *N. meningitidis*; Fulminant infection: caused by *Capnocytophaga canimorsus* (DF-2), *Babesia microti*, and *Plasmodium falciparum*	Sepsis, pneumonia, sinusitis, and meningitis
Adaptive				
B-cell adaptive immunity	Defective immunoglobulin synthesis or hypogammaglobulinemia	Impaired antibody synthesis	Encapsulated bacteria: *S. pneumoniae*, *H. influenzae*, and *N. meningitidis*	Sepsis, pneumonia, sinusitis, and meningitis

(*Continued*)

Table 25.1. (*Continued*)

Type of host defense	Immune deficit	Mechanism	Organism	Infections
T-cell adaptive immunity	Impaired T-cell function or T-cell number	HIV infection, Hodgkin's and non-Hodgkin's lymphomas, corticosteroids, 6-mercaptopurine (6-MP), fludarabine, daclizumab, and alemtuzumab	Intracellularly replicating bacterial pathogens (e.g. *Mycobacterium tuberculosis, Listeria monocytogenes, Salmonella* species); DNA viruses: HSV, VZV, CMV, HHV-6, HHV-8, EBV, adenovirus, polyoma viruses (BK virus, JC virus) EBV-associated lymphoproliferative disorder Fungi: *Cryptococcus neoformans* *Pneumocystis* Protozoa and helminths: *Toxoplasma gondii* *Cryptosporidium* spp. *Toxoplasma gondii* *Strongyloides stercoralis*	Pneumonia, meningitis, disseminated infection

chemotherapy and graft vs. host disease (GVHD) disrupt these mechanical barriers and afford access of potentially life-threatening pathogens.

Colonization resistance and mucocutaneous microflora

Microbiomic studies are revealing that colonization by normal bacterial flora provides a competitive microbiological barrier that resists colonization by extrinsically acquired bacterial and fungal pathogens. Illness, antimicrobial agents, cytotoxic chemotherapy, and GVHD abrogate this normal bacterial flora.

Phagocytes: Neutrophils, monocytes, and macrophages

These cells assert their antimicrobial effects of phagocytosis, oxidative and non-oxidative mediators, and release of immunoregulatory cytokines. Neutrophils and monocytes are quantitatively depleted during cytotoxic chemotherapy or infiltration of bone marrow by leukemic cells. Pulmonary alveolar macrophages, splenic macrophages, and Kupffer cells constitute an important residual phagocytic barrier during neutropenia, when PMNs and MNCs may be depleted. However, corticosteroids suppress phagocytosis, as well as oxidative and non-oxidative mediators.

Neutropenia increases the risk of infections caused by enteric bacteria (*Escherichia coli* and Klebsiella *pneumoniae*), *Pseudomonas aeruginosa*, and fungi (particularly *Candida* spp., *Aspergillus* spp., *Fusarium* spp., and Zygomycetes (Mucorales)).[4] There are three important determinants of risk of infection associated with neutropenia: (1) the absolute neutrophil count (ANC), (2) the rate of decline of the ANC, and (3) duration of neutropenia. A decline of the ANC to $< 500/\mu l$ increases the risk of bacterial and fungal infections and profound neutropenia ($< 100/\mu l$) markedly increases the risk of infection. The rate of decline of circulating PMNs also is important. For example, patients with rapidly declining ANCs following therapy for acute leukemia appear to be at greater risk for infectious complications than patients with chronic aplastic anemia.[5] The duration of neutropenia is a critical factor in determining risk and outcome of infection. Neutropenia that persists for more than 7–10 days is associated with increased risk for severe, recurrent or new bacterial and deeply invasive fungal infections.

Toll-like receptors, dectin and other receptors of pathogen-associated molecules

Toll-like receptors (TLRs), dectin, and other receptors of pathogen-associated molecules are critical interfaces between invading pathogens and the effector component of innate host defenses. The family of TLRs recognizes pathogen-associated molecular patterns (PAMPs). Different pathogens interact with certain TLRs through distinct repetitive patterns of molecules on their cell surface. Binding of PAMPs to TLRs activates signal transduction molecules, including MYD-88 and NFκ-B–dependent pathways, leading to upregulation of genes encoding cytokines, interferons, and chemokines that in turn may activate effector cells against the infecting pathogen. Allelic polymorphisms in genes encoding TLR2 and TLR4 in the donors of allogeneic HSCT recipients are associated with increased risk of invasive aspergillosis.[6] Similarly, a stop codon in the gene-encoding dectin is associated with increased risk of candidiasis.

Cytokines

Tumor necrosis factor (TNF)-α, interleukin-1 (IL-1), interferon-gamma (INF-γ), interleukin 2 (IL-2), interleukin 6 (IL-6), and interleukin 12 (IL-12) are pro-inflammatory cytokines that upregulate phagocytic response against bacteria, mycobacteria, fungi, and viruses. A T-helper 1 (Th1) type of response increases microbicidal activity against most bacteria, mycobacteria, and fungi and is mediated by IL-1, TNFα, INF-γ, and IL-12. By comparison, a T-helper 2 (Th2) type of response increases antibody production but induces a downregulation of host response against most bacteria, mycobacteria, fungi, and viruses. Th2 responses are mediated by interleukin 4 (IL-4) and interleukin 10 (IL-10). Underscoring the importance of cytokines regulation in innate host defense, the use of infliximab and etanercept, which are used in the management of corticosteroid-refractory GVHD through inhibition of TNF-α, results in increased risk of development of tuberculosis, histoplasmosis, and invasive aspergillosis.

Mechanical obstruction

Narrowing of hollow visci by lymphomas or chloromas in children with hematological malignancies increases the risk for post-obstructive infection in the respiratory, gastrointestinal, and geniturinary tracts. Successful management of these infections usually requires chemotherapy, radiation or surgery, depending upon the neoplasm.

Spleen and reticuloendothelial system (RES)

The spleen functions in both innate host defense through macrophages as immune effector cells and through adaptive immunity as a key site for new antibody synthesis. The spleen contributes to the reticuloendothelial system as a mechanical filter for circulating bacteria and fungi. The spleen also is the principal organ involved in the production of antibodies to polysaccharide antigens, filtering damaged cells and removal of opsonized organisms from the circulation.

Asplenic patients are deficient in antibody production when challenged with particulate antigens and have decreased levels of immunoglobulin M (IgM) and properdin (a component of the alternate complement pathway). Responses to polysaccharide vaccines may be substantially blunted. Asplenic patients carry an increased risk for fulminant and rapidly fatal septicemia caused by encapsulated bacterial pathogens, especially *S. pneumoniae*, *H. influenzae*, and *N. meningitidis*. Asplenic patients are also at risk for severe disseminated infection caused by *Capnocytophaga canimorsus* (DF-2) following a dog bite. Patients in endemic areas may suffer overwhelming infection caused by *Babesia microti*, and *Plasmodium falciparum*.

Adaptive immunity

Adaptive immunity depends upon functional B-cell and T-cell repertoires. Dendritic cells comprise another important component of antigen presenting cells (see Chapter 21). The B cell–plasma cell axis of humoral immunity generates antibodies in response to pathogens. Defective immunoglobulin synthesis or hypogammaglobulinemia particularly leads to increased susceptibility to severe infection caused by encapsulated bacteria, particularly *Streptococcus pneumoniae*, *Hemophilus influenzae* type B (HIB), and *Neisseria meningitidis*. Rituximab therapy may deplete B cells but does not necessarily increase the risk for encapsulated bacterial infections.

Rituximab, which is a chimeric monoclonal antibody against CD-20 on B cells, is used in the treatment of indolent lymphoma and autoimmune diseases.

Although relatively safe as a biological agent, rituximab has been increasingly reported to be associated with reactivation of hepatitis B and with development of progressive multifocal luekoencephalopathy.

By comparison, patients with Hodgkin's and non-Hodgkin's lymphomas, as well as those receiving corticosteroids, 6-mercaptopurine (6-MP), fludarabine, daclizumab, and alemtuzumab have impaired cellular immune response. Patients with deficiencies of cellular immunity have an increased risk of fungal, viral, and intracellularly replicating bacterial pathogens (e.g. *Mycobacterium tuberculosis*, *Listeria monocytogenes*, *Salmonella* species). Patients receiving T cell-depleted HSCT are particularly susceptible infections caused by DNA viruses, especially HSV, VZV, CMV, EBV, and adenovirus.

General Principles in the Evaluation and Treatment of Infections Pediatric Patients with Hematological Malignancies

Fever in neutropenic patients with hematological malignancy is managed as a medical emergency requiring prompt evaluation and therapeutic intervention. Febrile neutropenic patients, who are left untreated, may sustain devastating complications of bacterial sepsis. Localizing signs initially may be muted due to the paucity of inflammatory cells. A meticulous history and physical examination directed toward identifying possible foci of infection is important as a guide to select antimicrobial therapy and any adjunctive supportive measures, such as surgical intervention. Supportive microbiological data and diagnostic imaging procedures will further define the etiology and location of the infection.

Initial Assessment of Infection in Patients with Hematological Malignancies

Care of febrile children with hematological malignancies

General principles

Fever is a common manifestation of infection in children with hematological malignancies. Fever also may be the first and only sign of infection. Thus, fever in a neutropenic patient should be managed as a potential medical emergency. Prompt assessment and initiation of appropriate antimicrobial therapy may be life-saving. Indeed, left untreated, febrile neutropenic patients may sustain devastating complications of bacterial sepsis or invasive fungal infections.

Localizing signs of infection, such as pain, warmth, erythema, and localized swelling, may be muted or delayed due to the quantitative or qualitative defects in inflammatory cells and their regulation in neutropenic children. As patients receiving immunosuppressive dosages of corticosteroids, particularly for GVHD, may have a functional neutropenia, fever in this population also warrants prompt assessment.

Differential diagnosis of fever in children with hematological malignancies

Infections are a common cause of fever in children with hematological malignancies; however, noninfectious causes should also be considered in the differential diagnosis. The initial manifestations of acute lymphoblastic leukemia (ALL) commonly include fever due to the primary neoplastic process; by comparison, fever in patients with acute myelogenous leukemia (AML) is seldom due to the leukemic process and is more likely to be due to a concomitant infection. In addition to the malignant process, pyrogenic medications (particularly cytotoxic agents such as bleomycin and cytosine arabinoside), blood product transfusions, and allergic reactions, also are potential sources of a febrile response. Graft vs. host disease may present with a protean array of clinical features, including fever, rash, diarrhea, and hepatic transaminase elevation.

Evaluation of children with fever and neutropenia

As a guide to the selection of antimicrobial therapy and adjunctive supportive measures, such as surgical intervention, a careful history and meticulous physical examination directed toward identifying possible foci of infection is a critical step in the management febrile children with hematological malignancies. Culture data and diagnostic imaging further define the microbiological etiology and location of the infection, respectively. Continued reevaluation of these patients after this initial assessment is essential to achieve successful outcome from a suspected or documented infection.

Patients should be routinely questioned about the presence of any localizing pain or discomfort. The history and physical examination particularly address possible portals of entry of infectious pathogens. These sites include the oropharynx, sinuses, lower respiratory tract, perianal area, central venous catheter sites, and recent trauma to the skin and soft tissues.

Blood cultures are an essential component of evolution of febrile children with hematological malignancies.[7] Blood cultures are obtained from all lumens of central venous lines, when present. The volume of blood cultures, rather than location, is the most important factor for detection of circulating bacteria and fungi. Pediatric blood collection tubes, vials, or bottles are provided for most automated blood culture detection systems. Given the additional time, discomfort, and increased risk of contamination, peripheral blood cultures are not necessary in patients with a vascular access device when two or more sets of blood cultures have been obtained through the catheter.

Urine cultures should be routinely submitted where feasible. Other cultures of stool, cerebrospinal fluid, central line sites, or wounds should be obtained based on clinical suspicion. Following the completion of cultures, broad-spectrum antibiotics should be started promptly in all febrile neutropenic patients.

A routine complete blood count is obtained to document the presence and extent of myelosuppression and to guide transfusion requirements. A serum chemistry profile is drawn to ensure renal and hepatic function for safe administration of antimicrobials and other needed medications.

A chest radiograph (CXR) is preferably obtained in febrile patients. Although the yield of routine CXRs in asymptomatic neutropenic patients is small, they provide an important baseline for comparison with later films. Suspicious pulmonary infiltrates are further evaluated where feasible with a more definitive CT scan.

Evaluation of afebrile neutropenic patients with localizing signs

The absence of fever does not mitigate a diagnosis of suspected infection in neutropenic or heavily immunocompromised patients. Abdominal pain may signify an evolving intraabdominal infection, such as typhlitis. Neutropenic patients with intra-abdominal infection may be afebrile and complain only of localizing pain despite a perforated bowel. Indeed such patients may present with temperatures less than 37°C.

In other settings, erythema and tenderness along a subcutaneous catheter tunnel track usually indicate the presence of a deep soft tissue infection, despite the absence of fever. Similarly, traumatic skin and soft infection in neutropenic patients may present with only minimal erythema, mild tenderness, and no fever.

Neutropenic or immunosuppressed patients with localizing pain, hemodynamic instability, or altered mental status in the absence of fever, should be considered *a priori* as having infection. Prompt initiation of empirical antibacterial therapy in such patients, pending results of further laboratory studies, may prevent unchecked progression of infection and can be life-saving.

Risk assessment in children with hematological malignancies, fever and neutropenia

The majority of children with hematological malignancies, fever, and neutropenia require hospitalization because of the serious morbidity and potential mortality of life-threatening infection in this setting. However, smaller subsets of patients with fever and neutropenia constitute lower risk groups that may receive oral antibacterial therapy, which may improve quality of life and decrease cost of treatment.

Among the strategies for oral ambulatory antibacterial therapy are (a) initial parenteral therapy followed by oral outpatient management upon recovery from neutropenia for documented infection, (b) initial parenteral therapy without documented infection followed by oral outpatient management for the remainder of neutropenia, and (c) an initial oral antibacterial therapy in the absence of a documented infection.

As the default for febrile neutropenic children should be hospital admission and parenteral therapy, identifying "high-risk" patients is critical. Patients with anticipated long durations (> 7 days) of neutropenia, mucositis, documented infection, relapsed malignancy, and concurrent comorbidities, such as hypotension, tachypnea, hypoxia or chest radiographic changes, warrant hospitalization and initial parenteral therapy, particularly in the setting of AML, high-risk ALL, and Burkitt's lymphoma. Whether such patients can be discharged before recovery from neutropenia on oral therapy should be individualized. Children with no comorbidities, negative blood cultures, no focal signs of infection, and evidence of early recovery from neutropenia would be considered "low risk" for early discharge and ambulatory management.

Careful consideration of infrastructural support is needed before adapting an institutional policy for transferring care of febrile neutropenic children to an outpatient setting of oral therapy. Practitioners should use a validated system to accurately predict a pediatric child's risk of serious complications or death from infection that is relevant to the types of antineoplastic therapy being used in one's center.

The success of an oral outpatient regimen depends upon the adequacy of the supportive care infrastructure: mechanisms for outpatient follow up, assessment of the potential burden on patients and families, level of reimbursement for services and out-of-pocket expenses for patients and their families, availability of reliable telecommunications, proximity to a hospital for emergency transfer, availability of transportation to a medical facility, and a reliable caregiver to assure compliance with oral therapy (see Chapter 27).

Evaluation of febrile non-neutropenic patients

Non-neutropenic children with hematological malignancies may also sustain infections, particularly during the immunosuppressive maintenance phase of pre-B-cell ALL and during treatment of GVHD (see Chapter 20). Increasing use of reduced intensity conditioning regimens for HSCT in pediatric patients with hematological malignancy has led to a new population of patients at risk for infection. Evaluation of febrile non-neutropenic children with hematological malignancy includes a careful history, meticulous physical examination, and blood cultures. Other cultures and microbiological studies are performed depending upon the initial history and physical findings.

Initial empirical therapy is begun depending upon likely pathogens if no focal findings are present. Patients with focal findings should receive appropriate therapy based on the site involved. If blood cultures are negative in such patients, the empirical antibacterial therapy may be discontinued. A broad-spectrum third-generation cephalosporin (e.g. ceftriaxone) offers adequate initial coverage in the absence of an obvious focus unless *P. aeruginosa* is suspected, in which case ceftazidime or cefepime are appropriate. Routine use of vancomycin is discouraged in this setting unless there is a specific focus or a high nosocomial or community risk. Empirical antibacterial therapy may be continued for a 48- to 72-hour trial pending cultures in patients with no focus of infection. If the pre-antibiotic blood cultures are negative and no site of infection is identified, the antibiotics may be discontinued. If the cultures are positive or a site is documented, a full therapeutic course is implemented.

Patients with GVHD receiving corticosteroids constitute an expanding population of children with hematological malignancies. These patients should be considered to have a functional neutropenia that warrants prompt evaluation and intervention similar to that of neutropenic patients. Untreated bacterial infection may be fulminant. As these patients are also at risk for initial presentation of fungal pneumonias, CT imaging may be warranted as an initial diagnostic modality.[8]

Empirical antibacterial treatment of febrile neutropenic patients

General principles

Empirical antibiotic therapy is perhaps the single most important advance in infectious diseases oncology supportive care leading to improved survival in neutropenic children with hematological malignancies. The mortality rate from Gram-negative infections, especially those of *Pseudomonas aeruginosa*, *Escherichia coli*, and *Klebsiella pneumoniae*, approached 80% before this strategy was instituted. By comparison, the overall mortality rate from infections caused by Gram-negative bacteria in neutropenic patients has declined to approximately 10% with current antibacterial therapy.

The rationale for empirical antibacterial therapy in neutropenic patients is to provide emergency initial therapy for the most likely infecting pathogens. In principle, an empirical antibiotic regimen must cover a broad spectrum of bacteria, provide high serum bactericidal drug levels, be stable against the emergence of resistant bacteria, possess minimal toxicity, and be simple to administer. Selection of a specific agent or combination for empirical antibacterial agents by pediatric oncology and HSCT programs should be predicated upon well-conducted clinical trials, specific patterns of bacterial infection in one's own institution, antibiotic susceptibility profiles, cost, and toxicity.

Initial antibacterial combination therapy

The three objectives of combination antibacterial therapy are to (1) provide expanded antibacterial spectrum, (2) enhance synergistic interaction, and (3) prevent the emergence of resistance. These properties were particularly important in treatment of Gram-negative bacterial infections in neutropenic patients approximately 25 to 50 years ago when the most advanced antibacterial agents available were carboxypenicillins (e.g. carbenicillin) and aminoglycosides (e.g. tobramycin) had minimum inhibitory concentrations (MICs) that were often only several times lower than their achievable mean plasma concentrations. A synergistic combination would enhance the efficacy and lower the effective MIC of each compound when used in combination. Spectrum was somewhat expanded and prevention of emergence of resistance for the carboxypenicillin was reduced. The aminoglycoside–penicillin combination, however, also was associated with nephrotoxicity and VIII nerve toxicity. Cumulative aminoglycoside-induced ototoxicity and nephrotoxicity may become debilitating and limit use of immunosuppressive and chemotherapeutic agents.

Initial antibacterial monotherapy

Third- and fourth-generation cephalosporins and carbapenems, by comparison, have significantly lower MICs, broader spectrum and greater resistance to β-lactamase degradation than earlier β-lactam antibiotics. Consequently, addition of an aminoglycoside to third- and fourth-generation cephalosporins or carbapenems contributed no meaningful synergy, did not expand spectrum, or did not prevent emergence of resistance. The use of antibiotic monotherapy for the empirical management of febrile neutropenic patients is preferred because of the reduced toxicity of a single agent vs. an aminoglycoside–β-lactam combination.

Based upon the data from large, well-conducted, randomized controlled trials in adult and/or pediatric patients, the following five antibacterial agents are considered to be effective as empirical monotherapy in febrile neutropenic patients: ceftazidime, cefepime, piperacillin–tazobactam, imipenem, and meropenem. These antimicrobial agents have in common potent activity against the Enterobacteriaciae, such as *E. coli* and *K. pneumoniae*, and *P. aeruginosa*. All have activity against methicillin-susceptible *S. aureus*, while the carbapenems and piperacillin–tazobactam have anti-anaerobic activity. The choice among these agents for monotherapy should be guided by individual institutional variables, including types of organisms, patterns of resistance, safety, and costs.

Role of vancomycin in initial therapy of febrile neutropenic children

Empirical administration of vancomycin is not recommended for routine use in patients with fever and neutropenia. The presence of a vascular catheter *per se* does not warrant the use of empirical vancomycin therapy. However, certain infections and specific neutropenic populations should be treated with or receive vancomycin. Among the infections requiring initial therapy with vancomycin are (1) suspected skin and soft tissue infections, and (2) vascular catheter-related infections of the exit site, tunnel, or entrance site. Specific populations warranting initial therapy with vancomycin include those at risk for infections caused by viridans streptococci (most commonly *Streptococcus mitis*) or methicillin-resistant *S. aureus* (MRSA). Neutropenic patients at risk for *S. mitis* bacteremia include those with severe mucositis and a history of broad-spectrum fluoroquinolone prophylactic antibacterial therapy.[9] Patients with known colonization with organisms treatable only with vancomycin and patients presenting with hypotension should also receive empirical therapy with this antibacterial agent.

If vancomycin is initiated empirically and a Gram-positive organism is identified that is oxacillin-susceptible, then a penicillinase-resistant β-lactam or alternative agent is recommended. If vancomycin is initiated empirically and an infection caused by β-lactam-resistant Gram-positive bacteria is not subsequently documented, it may be discontinued.

Initial management of patients allergic to β-lactam antibiotics

The combination of aztreonam and vancomycin is particularly useful in febrile neutropenic patients with a history of IgE-related reactions to penicillins or cephalosporins. Aztreonam is a monobactam antibiotic that is structurally similar to ceftazidime without the 6-member dihydrothiazine ring. The absence of a dihydrothiazine or thiazolidine component in the monobactam molecule substantially reduces the antigenic cross-reactivity between aztreonam and β-lactam antibiotics. Consequently, aztreonam can be safely used in most patients with IgE-mediated allergic reactions (urticaria or anaphylaxis) to β-lactam antibiotics. As the spectrum of aztreonam is restricted to aerobic Gram-negative bacteria, including most Enterobacteriaciae and *P. aeruginosa*, it should be combined with vancomycin for Gram-positive activity.

Pharmacology of antimicrobial agents

A detailed discussion of the spectrum, pharmacokinetics, and safety of the antibacterial, antifungal, antiparasitic agents used in pediatric hematology is beyond the scope of this chapter. The basic properties of many commonly used agents are summarized in Table 25.2.

Table 25.2. Antimicrobial agents used in children with hematological malignancies.

Class	Agent	Spectrum[a]	Daily dose (maximum)	Comments
Antibacterial agents				
Third-generation cephalosporin	Ceftazidime	Enterobacteriaciae, *Pseudomonas aeruginosa*, some Gram-positive aerobes (MSSA), no anaerobic or enterococcal activity	100 mg/kg divided every 8 hrs (max 6 g/d) IV	Caution in use against *Enterobacter* spp., *Serratia* spp., *Citrobacter* spp., and *Morganella* spp. due to stable derepression of Type I β-lactamases
Fourth-generation cephalosporin	Cefepime	Enterobacteriaciae, *Pseudomonas aeruginosa*, some Gram-positive aerobes (MSSA), no anaerobic or enterococcal activity	100 mg/kg divided every 8 hrs (6 g/d) IV	Caution in use against *Enterobacter* spp., *Serratia* spp., *Citrobacter* spp., and *Morganella* spp. due to stable derepression of Type I β-lactamases
Carbapenem	Imipenem	Most Gram-negative and Gram-positive aerobes, including *P. aeruginosa*; broad anaerobic activity	50 mg/kg divided every 6 hrs (4 g/d) IV	*Stenotrophomonas maltophilia* and *Burkholderia cepacia* not covered
	Meropenem	Similar to imipenem	60–120 mg/kg divided every 8 hrs (3 g/d) IV	Less likely than imipenem to cause seizures
Extended-spectrum penicillin	Piperacillin	Enteric aerobes, including some *P. aeruginosa*, *Enterobacter* spp., *Serratia* spp., anaerobes	300 mg/kg divided every 4 hrs (21 g/d) IV	Must be paired with an aminoglycoside for coverage of *P. aeruginosa*
	Piperacillin-tazobactam	Similar to piperacillin, increased activity vs. some β-lactamase–producing Gram-positive cocci, Gram-negative bacilli, and anaerobes	300 mg/kg divided every 4 hrs (12 g/d) IV	Active against TEM-1 like β-lactamase–producing bacteria but not against ESBL or Type-1–producing β-lactamase–producing bacteria
Monobactam	Aztreonam	Exclusively aerobic Gram-negative aerobes including *P. aeruginosa*	100–150 mg/kg divided every 8–6 hrs (4 g/d) IV	Used in penicillin or cephalosporin allergic patients (not cross-reactive with β-lactam agents) Limited spectrum requires use with vancomycin or other anti–Gram-positive antimicrobial agent
Glycopeptide	Vancomycin	Exclusively Gram-positive bacteria	25–40 mg/kg divided every 6–12 hrs (3 g/d) IV	No need to add vancomycin routinely for empirical coverage for fever and neutropenia
Lipopeptide	Daptomycin	Exclusively Gram-positive, including MRSA and susceptible strains of VRE	4–6 mg/kg/d IV	Adjust for renal insufficiency; monitor CPK enzymes; not for use in pneumonia (inactivated by pulmonary surfactant)
Oxazolidinone	Linezolid	Exclusively Gram-positive, including MRSA, susceptible strains of VRE, and penicillin and cephalosporin-resistant *S. pneumoniae*	10 mg/kg q 12 hrs IV or PO	Excellent oral bioavailability; increased risk of thrombocytopenia, especially after 2 weeks of therapy
Streptogramin	Quinupristin/dalfopristin	Exclusively Gram-positive, similar to linezolid but spectrum does not include *E. faecalis*	7.5 mg/kg q8h IV	Venous irritation, should be given via central venous catheter; increased risk of CPK enzyme elevation and muscle injury
Flouroquinolone	Levofloxacin	Enterobacteriaceae and respiratory pathogens, including *S. pneumoniae*, *H. influenzae*, *Legionella* spp., and *Mycoplasma pneumoniae*	10 mg/kg Q24h in children ≥ 5 yrs 10 mg/kg Q12h in children 6 mths–5 yrs	Levofloxacin may be associated with increased frequency of arthralgias, arthritis, tendinopathy, and gait abnormality in children

(*Continued*)

Table 25.2. (*Continued*)

Class	Agent	Spectrum[a]	Daily dose (maximum)	Comments
Antifungal agents				
Amphotericin B	Deoxycholate amphotericin B	Broad antifungal activity including *Candida* spp., *Aspergillus* spp., Mucorales, *Cryptococcus neoformans, Histoplasma capsulatum*	0.5 mg/kg/d IV once daily for empirical therapy and treatment of candidemia; higher doses (0.75 mg/kg/d-1.0 mg/kg/d IV) may be used for documented infections due to *Aspergillus* spp. and other filamentous fungi	Severe azotemia may be reduced by saline hydration; hypokalemia and hypomagenesemia are not responsive to saline hydration; optimal dosing is not well established
	Lipid formulations [amphotericin B lipid complex (ABLC), amphotericin B colloidal dispersion, and liposomal amphotericin B (LAmB)]	Same spectrum as deoxycholate formulation	3 mg/kg/d IV for empirical therapy; 5 mg/kg/d IV for refractory documented infections due to *Aspergillus* spp. and other filamentous fungi	Significantly less nephrotoxicity with efficacy at least equal to that of DAmB; no significant difference between 3 mg/kg and 10 mg/kg dosages in treatment of invasive aspergillosis by LAmB
Triazole	Fluconazole	*Candida* spp., (not *C. krusei* and not some strains of *C. glabrata*); *C. neoformans, Trichosporon* spp. and *Coccidioides immitis*	Dosage of 12 mg/kg/d IV or PO in children provides comparable plasma exposure of 400 mg/d in adults; lower dosages of 6 mg/kg are used for management of mucocutaneous infections	Excellent bioavailability, independent of gastric acidity
	Itraconazole	*Aspergillus* spp., *Candida* spp. *H. capsulatum, Blastomyces dermatitidis*, and *C. immitis*	3–5 mg/kg/d PO	Absorption erratic but increased with taking drug with meals or by using cyclodextrin formulation (associated with gastrointestinal distress)
	Voriconazole	*Candida* spp., *Aspergillus* spp., *Trichosporon* spp. and some strains of *Scedosporium* spp., and *Fusarium* spp.	6 mg/kg Q12h for empirical therapy and 8 mg/kg Q12h IV for documented infections; higher dosages in pediatric patients are necessary in order to achieve comparable adult drug exposures.	Pediatric suspension is available; bioavailability is reliable and is enhanced with empty stomach
	Posaconazole	*Aspergillus* spp., *Candida* spp. *H. capsulatum, Blastomyces dermatitidis*, and *C. immitis*	Dosages have not been fully characterized in children; pharmaco-kinetic studies are pending	Posacoazole is not indicated as primary therapy for mucormycosis; bioavailability is erratic but increased with taking drug with meals
Echinocandin	Caspofungin	*Candida* spp. and *Aspergillus* spp.	50 mg/m^2/d IV to achieve comparable plasma concentrations in adults receiving 50 mg/d IV	

(*Continued*)

Table 25.2. *(Continued)*

Class	Agent	Spectrum[a]	Daily dose (maximum)	Comments
	Micafungin	*Candida* spp., and *Aspergillus* spp.	1–4 mg/kg/d IV for children > 2 yrs; weight adjusted clearance is approximately 1.35 times in 2–8 yrs	
	Anidulafungin	*Candida* spp., and *Aspergillus* spp.	0.75–1.5 mg/kg/d IV for children > 2 yrs	
Antiviral agents				
Anti-herpetic	Acyclovir	HSV, VZV	HSV: 250 mg/m^2 Q8h or 5 mg/kg Q8h IV VZV: 500 mg/m^2 Q8h or 10 mg/kg Q8h IV	Hydration should be ensured when administering high doses of acyclovir
Anti-CMV	Ganciclovir	CMV, HSV, VZV, HHV-6	For CMV: 5 mg/kg IV every 12 hrs for 14 days induction, then 5 mg/kg/d for maintenance	Neutropenia is the major dose limiting toxicity; not routinely used for HSV, VZV but dose used for CMV is effective for the other herpes viruses
	Foscarnet	HSV, VZV, CMV (including most acyclovir and ganciclovir resistant strains)	CMV: 60 mg/kg/d IV Q8h for 14 d then 90–120 mg/kg/d IV for maintenance VZV, HSV: 40 mg/kg Q8h IV	Nephrotoxicity has a dose-limiting effect, renal function and electrolytes require close monitoring
	Cidofovir	CMV (resistant to acyclovir and ganciclovir) and adenovirus	Low dose: 1 mg/kg IV three times per week (MWF) without probenicid High dose: 5 mg/kg IV once weekly with probenecid	Nephrotoxicity is dose limiting; IV hydration is indicated
Anti-PCP agents				
	Trimethoprim-sulfamethoxazole (TMP/SMX)	*Pneumocystis*	20 mg/kg/d IV in two divided doses for PCP treatment	May cause myelosuppression in high doses; TMP/SMX is active against many Gram-positive and Gram-negative bacteria, including *S. maltophilia* and *B. cepacia*
	Pentamidine	*Pneumocystis*	4 mg/kg/d IV for treatment	Adverse effects include pancreatitis, hypoglycemia, diabetes mellitus, hypocalcemia, and infusional hypotension
	Dapsone	*Pneumocystis*	2 mg/kg/d PO (for prophylaxis) (100 mg max.)	High incidence of hemolytic reactions, can also cause methemoglobinemia
	Atovaquone	*Pneumocystis*	30 mg/kg/d PO (1500 mg/d max.)	Suspension formulation has better bioavailability

[a]Antimicrobial spectrum depicted here is for summary purposes and is not a complete list.

CMV: cytomegalovirus; ESBL: extended spectrum β-lactamases; HHV-6: human herpes virus 6; HSV: herpes simplex virus; MSSA: methicillin susceptible *S. aureus*; MRSA: methicillin-resistant *Staphylococcus aureus*; PCP: pneumocystis pneumonia; VRE: vancomycin-resistant enterococci; VZV: varicella zoster virus.

Antimicrobial resistance, infection control and antibiotic stewardship

The use of any antibacterial regimen may be thwarted by the emergence of resistant bacteria. The advent of aerobic Gram-negative bacteria with powerful resistance mechanisms now threatens the utility of all systemic antibacterial agents. Among these mechanisms are AmpC stably derepressed β-lactamases, extended spectrum β-lactamases, carbapenemases, metallo-β-lactamases, altered porins and increased expression of drug transporters. That Enterobacteriaciae, *P. aeruginosa*, *S. maltophlia*, and *Acinetobacter baumannii* are expressing these resistance mechanisms warrants careful consideration of antibiotic stewardship and infection control measures to preserve the limited antibacterial armamentatrium that we can offer our patients with hematological malignancies.

Modification of Initial Antibacterial Therapy in Persistently Neutropenic Children

Empirical and preemptive antifungal treatment of febrile neutropenic patients

Depending upon the development of new symptoms and signs, the initial empirical antibacterial therapy may require modification. Common modifications of the initial antimicrobial regimen are described in Table 25.3.

For neutropenic patients who remain persistently febrile despite antibiotic therapy, initiation of empirical or preemptive antifungal therapy reduces the frequency of invasive fungal infections by early treatment of mycoses before development of complications and by prophylaxis of subsequent mycoses in high-risk patients.

The empirical use of an antifungal compound in persistently febrile neutropenic patients is based on several lines of reasoning. First, antemortem diagnosis of invasive fungal disease is difficult in an immunocompromised host. Second, withholding antifungal therapy pending a definitive diagnosis may allow local progression or dissemination to occur before the institution of therapy. Third, the outcome of an invasive fungal infection in an immunocompromised patient is improved by early institution of therapy. Fourth, it is possible to identify patients who are at greatest risk for invasive mycoses.

For profoundly neutropenic patients who remain persistently febrile for 5 or more days, despite broad-spectrum antibiotics, the risk of invasive fungal infections increases in direct relation to the duration of neutropenia.[10] Randomized controlled clinical trials

Table 25.3. Common modifications of initial empirical antibacterial therapy for febrile neutropenic children with hematological malignancies.

Symptoms, signs or status	Modifications of primary empirical antibacterial therapy
Persistent or recurrent fever	
Fever for < 5 days and hemodynamically stable with no focal evidence of infections	Continue initial therapy with monitoring closely on at least a daily basis
Persistent for 5 days and hemodynamically stable	Add empirical antifungal therapy
Recurrent fever after 5 days or later in patient with persistent neutropenia	Add empirical antifungal therapy
Hemodynamically unstable: decreased systolic or diastolic blood pressure, diminished urinary output, or tachycardia disproportionate to fever	Initiate salvage antimicrobial therapy with carbapenem, vancomycin, aminoglycoside (or fluoroquinolone), and antifungal agent with consideration of transfer to ICU
Persistent or recurrent fever at time of recovery from neutropenia	Evaluate liver and spleen by abdominal CT, ultrasonography, or MRI, for chronic disseminated (hepatosplenic) candidiasis, and evaluate need for antifungal therapy. If evaluation is negative, consider chest CT for evaluation of untreated or partially treated pneumonia
Infection of chronically indwelling vascular catheter during initial therapy	Emergence of exit site infection: following Gram stain and culture, initiate vancomycin
	Emergence of tunnel infection: remove catheter
Bloodstream	
Cultures drawn before initiation of initial antibiotic therapy	
Gram-positive organism	Add vancomycin pending further identification
Gram-negative organism	Maintain regimen if patient is hemodynamically stable and if isolate is susceptible. If *Enterobacter* spp., *Serratia* spp., or *Citrobacter* spp. or *Morganella* spp., are isolated or if found to be resistant to initial therapy, add a carbapenem to anticipate stably derepressed β-lactamase producers. If ESBL-producing *E. coli* or *Klebsiella* spp. is suspected based upon initial cultures, change to carbapenem, pending definitive MICs. Initiate infection control measures
	If *Pseudomonas aeruginosa* that is not susceptible to initial therapy is recovered, guide treatment according to MICs

(Continued)

Table 25.3. *(Continued)*

Symptoms, signs or status	Modifications of primary empirical antibacterial therapy
Organism isolated during initial antibiotic therapy	
Gram-positive organism	Add vancomycin
Gram-negative organism	Change to combination regimen, such as carbapenem plus aminoglycoside, pending susceptibility
Head and neck infection	
Necrotizing or marginal gingivitis	Add specific anti-anaerobic agent (clindamycin or metronidazole) to empirical therapy
Mucosal vesicular or ulcerative lesions	Suspect HSV infection. Culture and begin acyclovir therapy
Sinus congestion, tenderness or nasal ulcerative lesions	Suspect invasive fungal infection with *Aspergillus*, Mucorales, *Fusarium* or other mould; obtain imaging studies and ENT consultation (request endoscopy if coagulation status permits). Adjust antifungal therapy according to organism recovered
Gastrointestinal tract	
Retrosternal burning pain	Suspect *Candida* or herpetic esophagitis, or both. Add empirical antifungal therapy and acyclovir. Also consider bacterial esophagitis. For patients not responding within 48 hours, endoscopy should be considered
Acute abdominal pain	Suspect typhlitis, as well as appendicitis, if pain in right lower quadrant, even in the absence of fever. If diarrhea is present, consider *C. difficile*-associated diarrhea. Add specific anti-anaerobic coverage (e.g. metronidazole to ceftazidime; or substitution of carbapenem for ceftazidime) to empirical regimen and monitor closely for need for surgical intervention
Perianal tenderness	Evaluate for anal fissures, perianal cellulitis, perianal fistulas, or perirectal abscesses. Add specific anti-anaerobic drug to empirical regimen, as indicated, for perianal cellulitis, fistulas and suspected perirectal abscesses. Monitor need for surgical intervention, especially when patient is recovering from neutropenia. Perianal fissures can be managed with aerobic coverage and topical cleanliness with Sitz baths and gentle wipes
Respiratory tract	
New focal lesion(s) in patient recovering from neutropenia	Observe carefully, as such lesions may be a consequence of inflammatory response to previously occult pneumonic process detected in concert with neutrophil recovery.
New focal lesion(s) in patient with continuing neutropenia	Suspect invasive pulmonary aspergillosis or other cause of fungal pneumonia. Submit serum for galactomannan and (1→3)-β-D-glucan assays. Perform BAL or transthoracic needle aspirate with appropriate direct exams and cultures. Add voriconazole or lipid formulation of amphotericin B, depending upon findings (simultaneous voriconazole and amphotericin B should be avoided as the combination may be antagonistic against *Aspergillus* spp. in neutropenic patients)
New interstitial pneumonitis	Attempt diagnosis by examination of induced sputum or BAL. If patient is symptomatic, begin empirical treatment with trimethoprim-sulfamethoxazole, pending procedure. Evaluate for viral causes, including RSV, CMV, and Metapneumovirus by nasopharyngeal wash or BAL. Consider noninfectious causes, such as bronchiolitis obliterans with organizing pneumonia (BOOP) or drug reaction. Lung biopsy may be warranted in such cases.

of empirical antifungal therapy have been conducted of deoxycholate amphotericin B, liposomal amphotericin B, itraconazole, voriconazole, caspofungin, and fluconazole. With exception of fluconazole, all these agents have activity against *Aspergillus* spp. and other filamentous fungi. Selection of an agent for empirical antifungal therapy will depend upon the patterns of infection in one's institution, use (if any) of prophylactic agents, drug acquisition cost, presence of or risk for end organ toxicity (e.g. renal or hepatic dysfunction), and probability of concomitant invasive aspergillosis, such as the presence of pulmonary infiltrates.

For patients who remain neutropenic, antifungal therapy should be continued until resolution from neutropenia. Persistence or recrudescence of fever should prompt a meticulous investigation for nonfungal infectious causes, such as resistant bacteria or emergent fungal pathogens. These organisms include *Aspergillus* spp., *Trichosporon*, *Fusarium* spp., *Pseudallescheria* spp., *Scedosporium* spp., and Mucorales.

Preemptive antifungal therapy is a logical extension of empirical antifungal therapy. With the advent of assays for detection of circulating fungal cell wall biomarkers (galactomannan and (1→3)-β-D-glucan) and availability of high-resolution CT scanning, more targeted therapy to higher risk patients is possible.

Cordonnier *et al.* recently completed a multicenter, open-label, randomized noninferiority trial that compared an empirical antifungal strategy with a preemptive one using amphotericin B.[11] First-line antifungal treatment was amphotericin B deoxycholate (1 mg/kg/day) or liposomal amphotericin (3 mg/kg/day), depending on daily renal function. The primary efficacy outcome was the proportion of patients alive at 14 days after recovery from neutropenia. By intention-to-treat analysis of 293 enrolled patients, survival was 97.3% with empirical treatment and 95.1% with pre-emptive treatment. However, probable or proven invasive fungal infections were more common among patients who received preemptive treatment than among patients who received empirical treatment (13 of 143 vs. 4 of 150; $P < .05$). Of the 293 patients, 17 (5.8%) developed an IFI. The 12 cases of aspergillosis (2 proven and 10 probable) involved the lungs, and 1 also involved the CNS. The five cases of candidiasis were documented by blood cultures. Thus, empirical antifungal and preemptive AFT were associated with similar survival but greater frequency of invasive fungal infection in the preemptive therapy group.

Evaluation and management of documented infections

Prompt initiation of empirical antibacterial therapy, which is active against the infecting pathogens, at the time of the presentation with fever and neutropenia, is the most important therapeutic intervention for improved outcome. Treatment of documented infections should be based on the antimicrobial susceptibility pattern of the bloodstream isolate while maintaining broad empirical coverage against organisms that may not have been recovered in blood cultures.

Bacteremia

Bacterial infections are documented in approximately 10% to 30% of all febrile neutropenic cancer patients at initial presentation. The causes of bacteremia have changed during the past five decades. Until the late 1970s, aerobic *Gram*-negative bacilli (especially *E. coli*, *K. pneumoniae* and *P. aeruginosa*) were the most frequently isolated pathogens. Subsequently, the pattern of infections shifted toward more *Gram*-positive bacteria. While the majority of these organisms are coagulase-negative staphylococci, patients with mucositis have a higher risk of bacteremia caused by viridans streptococci.[9] Among the factors possibly contributing to this shift are increased used of indwelling central venous catheters, fluoroquinolone prophylaxis, and high-dose chemotherapy-induced oral mucositis. Nonetheless, as the aerobic Gram-negative bacteria cause the greatest infection-related mortality threat to neutropenic patients, the initial antimicrobial regimens are administered with these in mind.

The emergence of multidrug-resistant Gram-negative bacteria is changing patterns of use of initial therapy. Metallo-β-lacatamase–producing *Stenotrophomonas maltophilia*, Amp stably derepressed β-lactamase–producing *Enterobacter species*, extended-spectrum β-lactamase–producing *Escherichia coli* and *K. pneumoniae*, and carbapenemase-producing Enterobacteriaciae are now increasingly emerging as the most frequently isolated aerobic *Gram*-negative bacilli with high level resistance to many front line empirical regimens. These isolates also may carry resistance genes encoding fluoroquinolone and aminoglycoside resistance. While these organisms typically emerge as causes of bacteremias in the course of patient who is already receiving broad-spectrum antibiotics, they may appear as causes of infection at initial presentation. Such patients include those with previous antibiotic exposure, those receiving prophylactic fluoroquinolones, and patients transferred from centers with high endemicity for multidrug-resistant bacteria.[12]

The most common causes of bacteremia due to *Gram-positive* pathogens are coagulase-negative *Staphylococcus* spp, *S. aureus*, viridans *Streptococcus* species (particularly *S. mitis*), and *Enterococcus* species. *Corynebacterium* spp. (e.g. *Corynebacterium jekeium*) and *Bacillus* spp. are less frequently isolated and tend to occur in patients with long episodes of granulocytopenia or those with indwelling vascular access devices, respectively.

Resistant Gram-positive pathogens isolated from febrile neutropenic children and adolescents also have emerged as an increasing challenge. *Enterococcus* species that are resistant to vancomycin, ampicillin, or aminoglycosides, or all of these, have been increasingly reported and are associated with high mortality in immunocompromised patients. Some isolates of *viridans* streptococci are resistant to penicillin and cephalosporins, and therefore require vancomycin for therapy. Isolates of *Streptococcus pneumoniae* with either intermediate or high-level penicillin resistance are now relatively common in many parts of the United States. This is of special concern for those immunocompromised children and adolescents who are at high risk for pneumococcal septicemia; for example, asplenic patients and patients post-HSCT with chronic GVHD are at particularly high risk for pneumococcal sepsis.

The presence of severe (grades 3–4) mucositis in a neutropenic patient is an indication for vancomycin for the empirical treatment of *S. mitis* bacteremia. Bacteremia caused by α-hemolytic or viridans streptococci, most commonly *S. mitis*, may cause rapid onset of hypotension, with progression in approximately one fourth of cases, to a syndrome of shock, diffuse alveolar injury, acute renal failure, and neurologic manifestations. Palmar erythema and subsequent desquamation may also be a feature of this syndrome. Cytotoxic chemotherapy-induced mucosal epithelial disruption is the key risk factor for the *S. mitis* sepsis syndrome. The antecedent administration of high-dose cytosine arabinoside and myeloablative preparative protocols for HSCT facilitates *S. mitis* bacteremia. Administration of antacids or H2-blockers, and prophylactic treatment with TMP/SMX or fluoroquinolone antibiotics, both of which allow for breakthrough growth of α-hemolytic streptococci, are other co-factors contributing to this serious infection.

Vascular catheter-associated bacteremia

Virtually all febrile neutropenic patients with bacteremia have a vascular catheter. Whether the catheter is the source of bacteremia or merely associated with blood stream is difficult to assess. The alimentary tract is an important portal of entry for aerobic Gram-negative, some Gram-positive bacteria and *Candida* spp. in patients receiving cytotoxic chemotherapy and those with GI GVHD. The risk of routine removal of central silastic venous catheters in such patients may substantially outweigh any putative benefits given the pathogenesis in such patients.

Positive blood cultures drawn through a venous catheter can be considered to have arisen from one of three possible sources: (1) infection of the line from external sources (skin, catheter hub); (2) hematogenous seeding of the catheter from an internal source, particularly from the alimentary tract with mucosal disruption; and (3) rarely, contaminated infusate (parenteral nutrition solution or platelets with bacterial contamination).

Peripheral blood cultures in pediatric patients are painful, and are associated with increased contamination from cutaneous flora, and contribute little to increasing the diagnostic yield of bacteremia; thus, their utility is questionable. The volume of blood drawn is the critical determinant for recovery of bacteria from blood stream infections. Thus, two or three blood cultures through the central venous catheter (one set through each lumen) will provide a yield similar to that of central cultures plus peripheral cultures but without the patient discomfort and the potential for increased contamination from cutaneous flora.

Chronic indwelling central venous catheters do not require routine removal for treatment of bacteremias under most conditions provided that the catheter is treated effectively. Removal and replacement of chronic indwelling catheters carries the risk of general anesthesia, pneumothorax, and hemorrhage, particularly in thrombocytopenic patients. Removal of chronic indwelling central venous catheters is best determined by the type of organism recovered, the hemodynamic stability of the patient, and the presence of persistent bacteremia, rather than by differences in colony counts suggesting evidence of direct involvement of the catheter.

Among the relative indications for removal of a chronically indwelling catheter are bacteremias caused by *S. aurous*, *Bacillus* spp., and atypical mycobacteria, such as *Mycobacterium fortuitum* and *Mycobacterium chelonei*. Catheter-related bacteremia due to *S. maltophilia* also may cause refractory bacteremia and warrant catheter removal. Most catheter-associated infections caused by coagulate-negative staphylococci can be controlled without removal of the catheter.

Bacteremias caused by *Gram*-negative bacilli can be treated with intravenously delivered antibiotics without removal of the vascular catheter. For double- or triple-lumen catheters, the antibiotics are infused simultaneously in split doses among the lumens. Rotation of infusions among lumens is less advantageous as the lumens are exposed less frequently to antibiotics. If, despite these measures, blood cultures remain persistently positive 48–72 hours later or there is recurrent bacteremia of the same organism after completion of therapy, catheter should be removed. Oral antibiotics are not able to achieve adequate intralumenal concentrations and are therefore not recommended for managing the vascular catheter.

Vascular catheter-associated candidemia

Depending upon the study, *Candida spp.* are the third to fourth most common causes of healthcare-associated bloodstream isolates nationwide. While *Candida albicans* is the most common species isolated, constituting approximately 50% of isolates among all patients with candidemia, centers report a marked shift toward non-*albicans* species in patients with hematological malignancies. These non-*Candida albicans* spp. consist principally of *C. glabrata*, *C. tropicalis*, *C. parapsilosis*, and *C. krusei*. The shift toward non-C. *albicans* is multifactorial and likely includes the effects of triazole prophylaxis, altered innate host defenses, immunosuppressive agents and antibacterial therapy.

Identification of *Candida* spp. carries important prognostic and therapeutic implications. As antifungal susceptibility profiles are often not available for several days in most centers, an assumption of possible resistance patterns is made based upon species identification. For example, *Candida glabrata* may emerge as a cause of fungemia in patients who are already receiving antifungal triazole prophylaxis. Such isolates are typically resistant to antifungal triazoles and possibly to amphotericin B. *Candida tropicalis* has a more severe clinical course than does *C. albicans* in neutropenic patients and is associated disproportionately with the syndrome of acute disseminated candidiasis (cutaneous dissemination; arthralgias, myalgias, and renal failure). *Candida parapsilosis* is associated with vascular catheters and total parenteral nutrition. *Candida krusei*, an uncommon cause of fungemia and is virtually always resistant to fluconazole. Following exposure to amphotericin B, some isolates of *Candida lusitaniae*, *Candida guilliermondii*, and *Candida lipolytica* isolates are resistant to polyenes.

All episodes of candidemia require therapy, regardless of the clinical and host immune status. Among the therapeutic options for initial treatment of candidacies in children with hematological malignancies, echinocandins provide the most rational strategy in treating triazole resistant isolates, preventing hepatic or renal toxicity, minimizing drug interactions, providing fungicidal activity against *Candida* spp., exerting a antibiofilm property, and affording antifungal spectrum that includes *Aspergillums* spp.

Management of chronically indwelling central venous catheters in patients with candidemia hematological malignancies is controversial. Some experts assert that because the gastrointestinal tract is the principal portal of entry for *Candida* spp. in oncology-HSCT patients, catheter removal may not improve outcome. On the other hand, vascular catheters also may become the target for seeding by organisms hematogenously disseminated from the GI tract. A reasonable approach to management of uncomplicated candidemia is to remove vascular catheters, where feasible, unless there are extenuating circumstances such as limited vascular access or transfusion-refractory thrombocytopenia. For patients whose vascular catheter cannot be readily removed, all lumens of the vascular device should be simultaneously treated with an echinocandin or polygene for the duration of management of candidemia.

Local infections of vascular catheters

Local infections of chronic indwelling vascular catheters of the Hickman or Broviac type may be classified as exit site infections, entrance infections, and tunnel infections. For catheters with subcutaneous ports, the classification further includes pocket space abscesses and pocket space cellulitis. Exit site infections may be managed conservatively with local care with or without systemic antibiotics. Exit site infections usually can be managed without catheter removal; however, if *P. aeruginosa* is cultured from the exit site, catheter removal may be required, particularly for resistant organisms.

By comparison, tunnel infections, entrance infections, and pocket space infections of chronic indwelling catheters usually warrant removal of the vascular device. Tunnel infections are characterized by spreading cellulitis in the subcutaneous tissues along the tunnel tract of long term intravenous catheters. Unlike exit site infections, these infections are often associated with serious local morbidity and bacteremias. The infected tunnel tract may require surgical debridement in advanced infections. Antibacterial therapy is directed at the pathogens observed on Gram stain and recovered from culture.

Respiratory tract infections

Infections of the upper respiratory tract

Acute bacterial sinusitis in immunocompetent children is most commonly caused by *S. pneumoniae, H. influenzae, and Moraxella catarrhalis*, while chronic sinusitis is most commonly caused by *Staphylococcus aureus*, *Gram*-negative bacilli (*including P. aeruginosa*), anaerobic bacterial species, and fungi such as *Aspergillus* spp. As sinusitis in neutropenic or otherwise immunocompromised children may be caused by any of the foregoing pathogens, as well as members of the fungal order Mucorales, a rapid diagnostic assessment by a pediatric otolaryngologist to identify the microbial pathogen is warranted. Patients with obstruction of the sinuses by tumor, such as Burkitt's lymphoma or rhabdomyosarcoma, are especially at risk for bacterial sinusitis.

Until definitive microbiological results are available, broad-spectrum empirical antibacterial therapy is instituted. Empirical antifungal therapy also is warranted in patients who are neutropenic, diabetic, or who are receiving corticosteroids.

Fungal sinusitis in neutropenic patients and HSCT recipients most commonly are caused by *Aspergillus* spp., Mucorales, *and Fusarium* spp. A microbiological diagnosis from direct examination and culture obtained through endoscopy or nasal speculum examination of infected turbinates is needed to guide definitive antifungal therapy of fungal sinusitis. A microbiological diagnosis is important, particularly to distinguish aspergillosis from mucormycosis. Voriconazole is used for primary treatment of *Aspergillus* sinusitis, while amphotericin B is used for mucormycosis. Given the heightened probability of mucormycosis as a cause of sinusitis in immunocompromised patients, the broader spectrum amphotericin B formulation is used initially pending a definitive microbiological diagnosis.

The presence of ethmoidal fungal sinusitis requires urgent otolaryngological and medical intervention in neutropenic patients. Invasion by fungi through the lamina papyrecea causes post-septal periorbital infection, threatens the ocular globe, entraps extraocular muscles, and may result in the orbital apex syndrome with infarction of the optic nerve and central retinal artery. As the cavernous sinuses receive the venous drainage of the ethmoid sinus, fungal ethmoidal sinusitis may result in cavernous sinus thrombosis and invasion of the cranial nerves III, IV, V-1, V-2, and VI, as well as the internal carotid artery.

Ear infections

Otitis media may follow a viral upper respiratory illness, especially when related to respiratory syncytial virus. Otitis media in children with hematological malignancies may be particularly tenacious and refractory to conventional therapy. Children with anatomic alterations (e.g. radiation damage) of the external or middle ear or Eustachian tube are particularly susceptible to recurrent infectious episodes. Broad-spectrum antibacterial therapy is used for treatment of acute otitis media in children with hematological malignancies and HSCT patients unless a specific pathogen has been identified.

Immunosuppressed patients, particularly those with an anatomic abnormality of the middle ear are at increased risk for the development of mastoiditis. Without adequate management, mastoiditis may cause chronic osteomyelitis, subdural empyema, cortical vein thrombosis, septic thrombosis of the transverse venous sinus, and cerebral abscess. In addition to bacterial pathogens associated with mastoiditis, fungi may also cause mastoiditis in patients with prolonged neutropenia or other forms of chronic immunosuppression. Patients should undergo appropriate evaluation, including computed tomography (CT) scans of the mastoids if they have symptoms or signs, such as localized erythema, swelling, tenderness, referable to the mastoid. Surgical drainage of the infected mastoid sinus in immunocompromised patients is often necessary for definitive diagnosis and management of mastoiditis.

Infections of the lower respiratory tract

Diagnosis of pulmonary infiltrates

The relatively large number of infectious and noninfectious causes of pulmonary infiltrates that must be considered in the differential diagnosis, including progression of the underlying malignancy, drug reactions, emboli, hemorrhage, engraftment syndrome, as well as bronchiolitis obliterans and its variants is a formidable challenge in the management of pulmonary infiltrates in the children with hematological malignancies.

Evaluation of immunocompromised children with suspected pneumonia includes a chest radiograph, CT scan, blood cultures, hematological indices, pulse oximetry, and collection and microbiological examination of available respiratory secretions. Nasopharyngeal washes or swabs for viral pathogens, including respiratory RSV, influenza, parainfluenza, and adenovirus, are important in patients with concomitant upper respiratory tract symptoms. Radiographic evaluation with a CT scan is more sensitive than conventional chest radiography and may more provide information regarding the pattern and extent of disease that may not be evident on plain film alone.

Flexible fiberoptic bronchoscopy with bronchoalveolar lavage (BAL) can provide evidence for a specific microbiological diagnosis in immunocompromised patients with pneumonia. The yield of bronchoscopy depends on the clinical situation and the extent of prior therapy. A BAL can yield a specific diagnosis in most cases of newly established bacterial pneumonias and *Pneumocystis* pneumonia (PCP); whereas, it is significantly less sensitive for detection of invasive fungal infections or bacterial infections in patients who have received prior antibiotic therapy.

Transthoracic needle biopsy can be useful for the assessment of disease that is focal and in the periphery of the pulmonary parenchyma. Video-assisted thoracoscopy (VAT)-guided lung biopsy also can provide excellent pathologic samples as well as an ability to visualize superficial lesions; however, this procedure is limited in small children by the size of the instruments required. Although open lung biopsy is time-honored "gold standard" for the diagnosis of pulmonary pathology, it is limited by intraoperative sampling error and postoperative morbidity. At the same time, open lung biopsy may also provide definitive therapy by permitting resection of solitary infectious lesions, such as a focus of invasive fungal infection.

A practical approach for the evaluation of pulmonary infiltrates in immunocompromised patients is to categorize patients according to the anatomic distribution of the infiltrative lesion (i.e. localized or diffuse) and the granulocyte count (i.e. neutropenic or not). This classification permits rapid evaluation, identification of likely pathogens, and prompt institution of appropriate therapy to optimize the probability for a successful therapeutic intervention.

Localized pulmonary infiltrates in non-neutropenic patients

The common causes of localized pulmonary infiltrates in children with hematological malignancies include the common bacterial, viral and mycoplasmal organisms isolated from immunocompetent patients as well as opportunistic pathogens found in immunocompromised hosts.

Non-neutropenic immunocompromised children, such as those receiving maintenance chemotherapy for ALL and HSCT recipients who are receiving immunosuppressive therapy for GVHD are also at risk for less common pathogens that are dependent upon an intact T-cell response. These pathogens include *M. tuberculosis*, atypical mycobacteria, *Nocardia* spp., *Legionella* spp., and fungi, such as *Aspergillus* spp., *C. neoformans*, and certain endemic dimorphic fungi such as *C. posadasii (immitis)* and *H. capsulatum.*

Children with documented drug-susceptible *M. tuberculosis* receive 9 to 12 months of therapy with at least two effective anti-tuberculosis agents (e.g. isoniazid and rifampin). Multidrug-resistant strains of *M. tuberculosis* should be considered in those patients from endemic areas. Those infected with atypical mycobacteria, such as *M. kansasii* or *M. avium-intracellulare* are treated with agents active against these pathogens.

Legionella spp. are commonly found in water sources and may be found in the hospital environment, leading to nosocomial acquisition. Legionella pneumonia in immunosuppressed pediatric patients is heralded by the abrupt onset of nonspecific symptoms such as fever, malaise, anorexia, lethargy, and headache. A nonproductive cough develops in most patients; chest pain, dyspnea, diarrhea, and neurologic symptoms may be prominent features. A lobar, patchy, alveolar infiltrate is most commonly produced by *L. pnuemophila*; although, diffuse infiltrates also may occur. By comparison, *Legionella micdadei* is more commonly associated with nodular infiltrates then is *Legionalla pneumophila.*

As *Legionella* grows optimally on buffered charcoal yeast extract agar, this medium is optimally included in the BAL examination procedure. The combination of culture of respiratory secretions or BAL fluid, urinary antigen assay, and pan-*Legionella* PCR optimize diagnostic sensitivity for detection of *Legionella* pneumonia.

As the urinary antigen test is specific only for *Legionella pneumophila* type 1, *L. micdadei* pneumonia cannot be excluded by a negative assay.

Legionella pneumonia in children is treated with erythromycin or azithromycin for 3 weeks. Rifampin may be added for seriously ill patients. Fluoroquinolones are employed only in pediatric patients who are refractory to or intolerant of the macrolides.

Nocardia spp. present most frequently as a localized or nodular pulmonary infiltrate. Patients with a pulmonary nocardiosis also may have concomitant CNS involvement, particularly brain abscesses. *Nocardia* infections are most frequent in patients with impaired T-cell immunity. Diagnosis depends on positive cultures or histopathologic demonstration of tissue invasion by the organisms. TMP/SMX (15 mg/kg/d trimethoprim component) for 6 months is the most widely employed therapy. A carbapenem with an aminoglycoside is an alternative for patients who are intolerant of or refractory to TMP/SMX for treatment of nocardiosis. Therapy should be guided by antibacterial susceptibility profiles.

With an increasing burden of immunosuppression in HSCT applied to management of GVHD, pulmonary aspergillosis has emerged as the most common cause of infectious pneumonic mortality in HSCT recipients and a common cause of community-acquired pneumonia after patients are discharged. Infiltrates in this setting are often nonspecific bronchopneumonias. Primary treatment consists of voriconazole. Alternative agents include an LFAB or echinocandin.

Localized pulmonary infiltrates in neutropenic patients

Specific findings of a "halo" sign, crescent sign, nodular infiltrate, or wedge shape infiltrate are indicative of a possible angioinvasive filamentous fungus, including, but not limited to, *Aspergillus* spp. *Pseudomonas aeruginosa* and other angioinvasive fungi, such as *Fusarium* spp., *Scedosporium* spp., and the Mucorales, may produces radiologically indistinguishable lesions.

Gram-positive or Gram-negative bacteria, fungi and viruses may all cause localized pulmonary infiltrates in neutropenic patients. Bacterial pathogens predominate in patients with neutropenia lasting less than 10–14 days. *Aspergillus* spp., Mucorales, *Fusarium* spp., and *Scedosporium* spp. emerge in patients with longer periods of neutropenia. Where possible, a BAL, percutaneous needle aspirate, VAT biopsy, or open lung biopsy should be performed. The halo sign in neutropenic patients may distinguish angioinvasive fungi from other pathogens, these findings are not specific for aspergillosis. A definitive diagnosis depends on microbiologic or histopathologic confirmation in specimens obtained from BAL or other procedure. Serum galactomannan and $(1\rightarrow3)$-β-D-glucan are valuable biomarkers in detection of invasive aspergillosis. Galactomannan may also be measured directly in the BAL fluid. Coupled with a CT scan that is radiographically compatible with invasive pulmonary aspergillosis in the appropriate host population, a positive serum galactomannan assay establishes a diagnosis of probable invasive aspergillosis in neutropenic patients and HSCT recipients.

Successful management of invasive pulmonary aspergillosis requires an early diagnosis and prompt therapeutic intervention with voriconazole or lipid formulations of amphotericin B as an alternative if hepatic transaminases are elevated. Surgical resection of pulmonary lesions in invasive pulmonary aspergillosis and other mycoses due to these filamentous fungi may provide definitive and potentially life-saving therapy. Surgical resection should be considered in the following situations: hemoptysis from a single cavitary lesion; progression of a solitary lesion despite antifungal therapy; and infiltration into contiguous structures, including pericardium, great vessels, esophagus, or chest wall while receiving antifungal therapy.

Diffuse pulmonary infiltrates in patients with cancer

Pneumocystis pneumonia (PCP) is an important treatable cause of diffuse pulmonary infiltrates in pediatric oncology patients. In assessing *a priori* risk, the probability of developing PCP is increased in relation to impaired T-cell immunity.[13] Patients with PCP most commonly present with fever, a nonproductive cough, tachypnea, dyspnea, and hypoxemia. The time course of the symptoms ranges from a chronic, indolent course (characteristic of AIDS patients) to an acute, fulminant presentation, more commonly observed in pediatric oncology patients. Although adventitious lung sounds are not usually detectable on auscultation in most cases of PCP, patients receiving corticosteroids may have evidence of rales. Radiographic examination usually reveals bilateral diffuse alveolar-interstitial infiltrates, often originating at the hilum and extending peripherally. Microbiological diagnosis of PCP requires demonstration of cysts or trophozoites on direct exam or DNA by PCR in pulmonary material from patients with a clinically compatible course. TMP-SMX is initiated IV as the preferred first line agent. Acutely ill patients who do not respond to TMP/SMX may receive an alternative regimen, such as IV pentamidine, clindamycin plus primaquine, or dapsone plus pyrimethamine. Orally administered atovaquone is another option for patients who are not acutely ill; however, response rates are lower than those of TMP-SMX and bioavailability may be erratic. Adjunctive administration of corticosteroids may improve outcome in pediatric oncology-HSCT patients with moderate to severe PCP, as defined by a room air arterial partial pressure of oxygen ≤ 70 mm Hg or an alveolar-arterial gradient > 35 mm Hg on presentation. While the optimal dosage and duration of corticosteroid therapy in children have not been defined, an estimated adult equivalent for children is 1 mg/kg twice daily for the first 5 days, 1 mg/kg daily for the next 5 days, and 0.5 mg/kg daily for the remainder of a 14- to 21-day course of therapy.

Mycoplasma pneumoniae and *Chlamydiophila pneumoniae* also can cause diffuse pulmonary infiltrates in immunocompromised children. Considerable advances have been achieved in evaluation of BAL fluid by PCR for detection of *Mycoplasma* and *Chlamydia* DNA, thus enabling more specific pathogen-directed therapy. If reliable diagnostic assays are not available, an empirical course of azithromycin is warranted in immunocompromised children with diffuse pulmonary infiltrates.

RSV may cause severe lower respiratory tract disease with a high mortality rate, especially in patients undergoing therapy for acute myelogenous leukemia or HSCT. RSV usually can be diagnosed rapidly, using a direct immunofluorescent antibody stain performed on a nasopharyngeal wash specimen. Although no randomized controlled studies have addressed the utility of ribavirin in immunocompromised cancer patients, survival appears to be improved particularly if ribavirin is administered early in the course of infection. There is evidence from several small case series reports that RSV pneumonia also may respond favorably to ribavirin aerosol in addition to therapy with intravenous immune globulin or RSV immune globulin.

Children with cancer are at increased risk for influenza. Pattern and extent of symptoms are not different from those in immunocompetent children. However, the course of influenza may be prolonged. While bacterial superinfections of the respiratory tract are frequent, there is no specific propensity for primary influenza pneumonitis. Options for therapeutic intervention include oseltamivir and zanamivir.

CMV pneumonitis most often occurs between days 30 and 100 after allogeneic bone marrow transplantation, coinciding with the period of highest risk for the development of acute GVHD.[14,15] CMV pneumonitis is characterized radiographically by diffuse bilateral linear or nodular infiltrates. However, CMV pneumonitis occasionally may present as a lobar or segmental consolidation or as a solitary nodule. As the result of prospective surveillance for antigenemia or PCR signal in allogeneic HSCT recipients, CMV pneumonia is seldom observed. A diagnosis of CMV pneumonia is established by demonstration of cytopathic effect on a BAL specimen in a patient with a radiologically compatible pneumonic process. Such findings should prompt the institution of a treatment course with ganciclovir.[16] Foscarnet is an appropriate alternative to ganciclovir, particularly in those at risk for myelotoxicity or who are intolerant of or refractory to ganciclovir.

VZV and HSV can also cause diffuse pneumonitis in immunocompromised patients. VZV may reactivate late in the course of HSCT, particularly in those not receiving acyclovir suppressive therapy. These viruses, however seldom cause isolated pulmonary disease, but instead are associated with cutaneous disease and visceral dissemination, including lung, liver and CNS. While parainfluenza, influenza, adenovirus, and HHV-6 have been described as causes of interstitial pneumonitis in pediatric cancer patients, these respiratory viruses more commonly cause tracheobronchitis and bronchopneumonia, rather than a diffuse interstitial process.

For any child presenting with pulmonary infiltrates consistent with a viral process, either a BAL or at minimum a nasopharyngeal wash is performed for detection of influenza, RSV, adenovirus, and parainfluenza. Infections caused by influenza and RSV carry important therapeutic implications, while all of these viruses have important infection control implications to prevent transmission to other immunocompromised patients. Moreover, there is increasing recognition of the role for rhinoviruses, coronaviruses, and metapneumovirus as causes of lower respiratory tract infections in immunocompromised patients with hematological malignancies.

Infections of the oral cavity

Among the common oral infections occurring in children with hematological malignancy are oropharyngeal candidiasis ("thrush"), HSV mucocutaneous lesions, and periodontal disease. Oropharyngeal candidiasis is a superficial infection caused most commonly by *C. albicans*. This infection is usually controlled by topical antifungal agents, such as clotrimazole troches or nystatin suspension or by oral fluconazole.

Perioral and intraoral HSV lesions usually appear as clear painful vesicular eruptions, frequently in clusters or "crops" on an erythematous base. However, intraoral lesions may be nondescript, often ulcerative, and can be confused with the stomatotoxicity usually attributed to chemotherapy. Diagnosis of HSV oral infection may be confirmed by rapid shell vial culture (requiring 24–48 hours) or may be made presumptively by the identification of multinucleated giant cells (positive Tzanck preparation) or by a positive fluorescent antibody reaction. Acyclovir (750 mg/m^2 per day divided every 8 hours or 5 mg/kg every 8 hours) is the preferred treatment because of its infrequent toxicity, ease of administration, and documented efficacy in reducing the duration of viral shedding and shortening the time to healing.

Gingivitis is an inflammation of the superficial structures of the mucosal epithelium, and periodontitis describes an involvement of the supportive structures of the teeth. Cultures of infected sites revealed mixed aerobic and anaerobic flora. *Capnocytophaga ochracea* (formerly DF-1) may cause necrotizing gingivitis and Gram-negative sepsis in patients receiving cytotoxic chemotherapy. The presence of marginal or necrotizing gingivitis, characterized by an erythematous periapical gingiva, is caused by anaerobes and should be treated with specific anti-anaerobic agents such as piperacillin–tazobactam, clindamycin, metronidazole, or carbapenem.

Esophageal infections

Fungal, viral, and bacterial organisms can all cause an infectious esophagitis in the immunocompromised host. Infectious esophagitis most commonly occurs among neutropenic patients. Chemotherapy-induced mucositis, neutropenia, mediastinal radiation, and gastroesophageal reflux are important risk factors. Patients most often present with subacute onset of retrosternal burning chest pain, dysphagia, and odynophagia. HSV, CMV, and bacteria may coincide with or precede esophageal candidiasis. The absence of oral lesions cannot be used to discount the presence of esophageal candidiasis in neutropenic patients. Given the difficulty in performing esophagoscopy in neutropenic children, a reasonable approach to symptomatic esophagitis in such patients is empirical initiation of acyclovir for HSV and fluconazole or an echinocandin for *Candida*. If resolution of symptoms does not occur, endoscopy is warranted.

Intraabdominal pain and selected infections of the gastrointestinal tract

Intraabdominal pain in a neutropenic must be expeditiously evaluated with a thorough physical examination, laboratory screening studies, diagnostic imaging and prompt administration of empirical antibacterial therapy that includes anti-anaerobic activity. Typhlitis (necrotizing infection of the cecum) or neutropenic colitis is a common cause of abdominal pain in persistently neutropenic children. Patients most often present with subacute or acute onset of right lower quadrant abdominal pain and tenderness, which frequently becomes generalized over several hours. As fever may be absent early in the course of neutropenic colitis, the presence of abdominal pain in a neutropenic patient should prompt the administration of empirical antibacterial therapy for aerobic and anaerobic pathogens. As *Clostridium difficile* is recognized increasingly as an important cause of typhlitis, metronidazole with ceftazidime or cefepime is a logical combination. CT scan should be performed where feasible in all neutropenic patients with right lower quadrant pain for staging of extent of infection. CT imaging may reveal localized thickening of the bowel wall, mucosal edema, right lower quadrant inflammatory mass, and pericecal fluid. Most patients with typhlitis can be medically managed without surgical resection of the involved segment of colon.

Clostridium difficile colitis arises in the setting of prolonged administration of broad-spectrum antibacterial antibiotics, including cephalosporins, carbapenems and fluoroquinolones.[17] Symptoms and signs include abdominal pain, fever, and/or diarrhea, which may be watery or mucoid. Evaluation includes routine stool cultures and a *C. difficult* toxin assay or PCR. Metronidazole is administered for primary treatment of mild to moderate *C. difficile*-associated colitis while oral vancomycin is reserved for patients severe or complicated infection. Infection control measures are important adjuncts for prevention of nosocomial transmission.

Hepatic infections

The hepatitis viruses A, B, C, D, and E infect the liver as the primary target, while other viruses, such as HSV,

CMV, EBV, VZV, Coxsackie B virus, and adenovirus, as well as the protozoan *Toxoplasma gondii* and fungi, such as *Candida*, infect the liver during the process of general dissemination. A detailed description of all of these viral processes is beyond the scope of this chapter. Nevertheless, some general principles pertain to these agents. Active viral infection of the liver may alter hepatic metabolism of compounds used for direct antineoplastic therapy or the HSCT preparative regimen. Active viral infection of the liver may increase the risk of additive injury from hepatotoxic agents used in cytotoxic chemotherapy or anti-infective therapy, as evidenced by the rapid rise of hepatic AST and ALT. Such injurious viral infections of the liver may limit the use of potentially life-saving chemotherapy of HSCT. Children with hematological malignancy who also have clinical or biochemical evidence of hepatitis should undergo a serologic and molecular evaluation to attempt to characterize the etiologic agent.

Hepatitis B virus (HBV) may result in acute or chronic infections, including chronic active hepatitis, chronic persistent hepatitis, and asymptomatic carrier states. Immunosuppressive therapy may increase the probability of development of a fulminant hepatic infection or of a chronic carrier state among patients infected with HBV, underscoring the need to know the patient's hepatitis status before initiating antineoplastic therapy. While the presence of circulating hepatitis B surface antigen (HBsAg) is not a contraindication to chemotherapy, an acute hepatic failure syndrome may result from acute HBV infection in an immunosuppressed patient. The pre-transplant HBV DNA viral load is an important risk factor for post-transplant HBV reactivation. Thus, lowering the HBV DNA viral load before chemotherapy or HSCT with lamivudine (3-TC) may improve outcome. Moreover, lamivudine (3-TC) starting 1 week before and continuing until 52 weeks after allogeneic HSCT significantly reduced HBV exacerbation in a small randomized clinical trial.

Some patients with chronic HCV infection can be effectively treated with a combination of interferon-α2b plus ribavirin. The decision to who and when to treat is based on a number of factors, including severity of disease, concurrent comorbidity and pre-existing contraindications to ribavirin or interferon-α2b.

Hepatic candidiasis

Hepatic candidiasis is included within a syndrome, which is also known as hepatosplenic candidiasis or chronic disseminated candidiasis, that occurs in patients following recovery from a period of prolonged (> 7 days) neutropenia during which time they have sustained hematogenous seeding of *Candida* spp. to the liver and other tissue sites. The infection may have been manifest only as an earlier episode of candidemia but may have had no evidence of antecedent candidemia until recovery from neutropenia. Patients characteristically have persistent fever after recovery from an episode of neutropenia, right upper quadrant discomfort, nausea, weight loss, and increased serum alkaline phosphatase. Following recovery from neutropenia, it is characterized by the presence of multiple "bull's eye" lesions in the liver on ultrasound or CT scan. The diagnosis of hepatic candidiasis is based on a high index of suspicion and should be confirmed with an open liver biopsy as percutaneous needle aspirates have not been historically successful. Treatment of hepatic candidiasis requires long courses of treatment with the duration of antifungal therapy ranging from approximately 6 to 12 months until full resolution of symptoms. An initial course of an echinocandin followed by oral fluconazole is a tenable approach.

Anorectal infections

Anorectal infections may be classified anatomically according to their location: perianal fissures, perianal cellulitis, and perirectal infections. Anal fissures in neutropenic patients present as painful linear tears in the mucocutaneous integrity of the anal orifice and are most commonly cause by aerobic Gram-negative bacilli, such as *E. coli*, *Klebsiella* spp. and *P. aeruginosa*. Uncomplicated anal fissures can be successfully treated with an initial antibacterial regimen targeting aerobic Gram-negative bacilli, such as ceftazidime or cefepime.

Perianal cellulitis presents as pain, tenderness, and erythema extending beyond the anal orifice. As extension of tenderness and erythema into the surrounding soft perianal tissue may involve anaerobic flora, the presence of perianal cellulitis warrants the addition of anti-anaerobic coverage, such as metronidazole, to ceftazidime or cefepime or the use of a single agent such as piperacillin–tazobactam. Additional supportive measures include Sitz baths three or four times daily, stool softeners, a low-bulk diet, and avoidance of unnecessary rectal manipulation, especially repetitive digital examinations. Surgical intervention is seldom warranted.

True perirectal infections are uncommon complications in neutropenic patients. Developing as the result of disruption of the rectal mucosa and extension of infection into the pelvic perirectal tissues, the diagnosis is suspected in patients with intractable perianal cellulitis, development of perianal fistulas, suggesting a tract between the skin and deeper pelvic tissues, and the presence of persistent fever. Diagnosis is confirmed by pelvic CT scan or MRI. Therapeutic approaches to perirectal abscesses include anti-anaerobic coverage and timely surgical or percutaneous catheter drainage of collections.

Infections of the central nervous system

Among the infections of the CNS in children with hematological malignancies, are meningitis, encephalitis, brain abscesses, and involvement of shunts and Ommaya reservoirs. Infectious meningitis, albeit uncommon in pediatric oncology patients, is associated with significant morbidity and mortality. As meningitis in cancer patients can be subtle in presentation in imunocompromised children with cancer, patients presenting with fever and signs or symptoms of CNS dysfunction should be promptly evaluated by lumbar puncture and radiographic evaluation through a head CT scan with contrast or an MRI scan with gadolinium. Evaluation of CSF includes aerobic culture and Gram stain, cryptococcal antigen, fungal culture, and cytological analysis in addition to cell count and differential, protein, and glucose.

Children with intraventricular shunts and *Ommaya* reservoirs are at high risk for development of CNS infection. The responsible pathogens are most commonly those colonizing the adjacent skin: coagulase-positive and coagulase-negative staphylococci, *Corynebacterium* species, and *Propionibacterium acnes*; rarely, they are Gram-negative bacilli. Patients may have fever, headache, increased intracranial pressure, and meningismus. Patients also may be asymptomatic, in which case the diagnosis may be made by noting cerebrospinal fluid cultures being repetitively positive for the same organism. Most patients with *Ommaya* reservoir infections can be treated successfully without the need to remove the device; however, this may require a combination of intraventricular and intravenous therapy. Antimicrobial therapy is directed at the organism recovered from CSF and usually consists of vancomycin, which may be administered parenterally and intraventricularly.

Encephalitis

The relative prevalence of the different viral, bacterial, parasitic, fungal, and rickettsial agents associated with encephalitis or encephalomyelitis is altered in different populations of immunodeficient patients. For example, patients with humoral immune abnormalities, especially hypogammaglobulinemia, may have chronic encephalitis caused by poliovirus or echovirus. Patients with abnormalities of cell-mediated immunity may have encephalitis caused by measles. Although HSV reactivation is common during cancer chemotherapy, herpes encephalitis does not appear to be more common in immunosuppressed patients. Encephalitis may be caused by other viral pathogens, such as EBV, CMV, VZV, and HHV-6. Current data indicate that HHV-6 is an increasingly common cause of infectious encephalitis in allogeneic HSCT recipients. Detected by PCR in the cerebrospinal fluid, HHV-6 may cause a fatal encepholapathy.

West Nile virus (WNV) is the most recently recognized cause of mosquito-borne encephalitis in North America that clearly poses a threat particularly to ambulatory pediatric oncology patients. Although most human cases of WNV infection are acquired via bites from an infected mosquito, blood products and transplanted cells and tissues are other potential vehicles of transmission. Allogeneic HSCT increase the risk for severe WNV infection due to prolonged immune impairment. Pediatric oncology patients should adapt the current precautions issued by CDC for avoidance mosquito bites to prevent infection by WNV.

Patients with encephalitis or encephalomyelitis commonly present with signs of meningeal irritation (e.g. fever, headache, nuchal rigidity) and evidence of altered mentation. Confusion may progress to stupor and finally to coma. Focal neurologic signs and seizures are relatively common. Patients with WNV infection may present with flaccid paralysis of the lower extremities. Cerebrospinal fluid examination may demonstrate a pleocytosis (10–2000 cells/mm^3), with a predominance of mononuclear cells. An increased number of erythrocytes has been reported with HSV encephalitis. Protein levels are usually elevated, and the glucose characteristically remains within the normal range except for a decreased level in mumps infection.

For cancer patients with focal neurologic deficits or altered mentation, recognition of other infectious, metabolic, toxic, and neoplastic causes is important. CT scan or MRI of the brain may help in some instances, especially if a focal lesion is visualized, but specific diagnosis of encephalitis in an immunocompromised patient is often difficult.

The application of PCR to CSF is improving diagnostic sensitivity in patients with possible CNS viral infections. The impact of PCR on diagnosis of HSV encephalitis is especially apparent. Previously requiring a brain biopsy, PCR of cerebrospinal fluid now allows for prompt, sensitive, and highly specific diagnostic accuracy for HSV encephalitis with excellent correlation with brain biopsy results. Nevertheless, when PCR is not available, acute and convalescent serum antibody titers against herpesviruses, echoviruses, and the less common arboviruses should be measured. Specific cerebrospinal fluid antibody may be detected in cases of mumps, HSV, or VZV.

Toxoplasmosis of the CNS is a treatable infection that can present as encephalitis in an immunosuppressed oncology patient or HSCT recipient. Caused by the obligate intracellular protozoan, *Toxoplasma gondii*, toxoplasmosis may represent newly acquired or reactivated infection and is rarely limited to the central nervous system, usually occurring in concert with fever, lymphadenopathy, hepatitis, pneumonia, myocarditis, and pericarditis. The cerebrospinal fluid typically manifests a mononuclear pleocytosis, elevated protein, and a normal glucose concentration. A battery of serologic tests is available for the diagnosis of toxoplasmosis, but most of these are limited in their applicability to the immunosuppressed patient because of suboptimal antibody responses. Definitive diagnosis requires demonstration of the parasite within tissue sections. Recent advances in PCR of CSF may detect CNS toxoplasmosis non-invasively.

Pyrimethamine combined with sulfadiazine, with the addition of folinic acid to reduce pyrimethamine-induced myelotoxicity is considered standard treatment of active toxoplasmosis. For immunodeficient patients, therapy should be continued for 4–6 weeks after the resolution of all clinical symptoms and signs. The combination of high-dose intravenous clindamycin with the usual doses of pyrimethamine appears to be a useful alternative for treatment of toxoplasmosis in patients who are unable to tolerate sulfonamide-based drugs. Other agents combined with pyrimethamine, such as atovaquone, dapsone, or the newer macrolides, may also be effective in treatment of toxoplasmosis in immunocompromised hosts.

Brain abscesses

The differential diagnosis in cancer patients with evidence of a focal lesion within the central nervous system is between metastatic or primary malignancy and a brain abscess. Predisposing factors for brain abscess include a contiguous infected site (e.g. otitis, sinusitis, dental abscess), a history of recent neurosurgery, congenital cardiac disease, bacterial endocarditis, and pulmonary infection. The common organisms causing brain abscesses in immunocompetent and immunosuppressed patients are typically aerobic and anaerobic bacteria derived from the oral cavity. However, as pediatric oncology patients are immunosuppressed, nocardiosis and invasive fungal infections also rank highly in the differential diagnosis for brain abscess in this population. Consequently, a definitive microbiological diagnosis of the cause of brain abscess in pediatric oncology patients is necessary.

Early evaluation and specific diagnosis are crucial in the management of brain abscess because effective antimicrobial or neurosurgical therapy is available. Diagnosis is commonly made by radiographic demonstration of a localized mass and followed by an open or closed procedure to aspirate or resect the localized lesion. As CNS nocardiosis and invasive fungal infections are usually associated with preceding pulmonary infiltrates, a less invasive diagnostic approach is to establish a microbiological cause of the lung infection.

Underscoring the importance of CNS fungal infections as a cause of brain abscesses in immunocompromised oncology patients, a review of brain abscesses complicating HSCT found that 53 (92%) of 58 cases of were caused by fungi. *Aspergillus* spp., were the most common pathogen, followed by *Candida* spp. Whereas, only four (7%) had a bacterial brain abscess and one patient had cerebral toxoplasmosis. *Aspergillus* species accounted for ~60% of isolates and one-third were caused by *Candida* species. Mortality associated with these treatable infections was 97%.

Manifestations of CNS aspergillosis include focal seizures, hemiparesis, cranial nerve palsies, and hemorrhagic infarcts due to vascular invasion. CSF cultures are usually negative and most cases are associated with pulmonary lesions. The presence of pulmonary infiltrates and focal neurological deficits in an immunocompromised patient were significantly more predictive of CNS aspergillosis than for CNS candidiasis or cryptococcosis in a multivariate discriminant analysis of autopsy-proven CNS mycoses. Although a specific diagnosis of CNS aspergillosis historically has been difficult to establish, recent case reports illustrate that galactomannan detected by EIA in cerebrospinal fluid may permit a noninvasive means of detecting this frequently lethal infection.

Prevention of Infection

Prophylactic antimicrobial agents

Antibacterial prophylaxis

Fluoroquinolones have been studied in adult patients for oral antibacterial prophylaxis because of their favorable bioavailability, tolerability, and broad spectrum. These agents have been widely used in adult oncology patients with considerable success in reducing bacteremic events during neutropenia; however, they have not been widely used for prophylaxis in children because of concerns of chondrotoxicity associated with long-term exposure. Moreover, none of the studies of antibacterial prophylaxis has demonstrated a reduction in infection-related mortality. The recent development of fluoroquinolone-resistant *C. difficile* and potential for selection of emergence of resistance over time to fluoroquinolines on a pediatric oncology unit is another potential limitation to their use as in-patient prophylactic agents. Nonetheless, thoughtfully designed and carefully implemented studies should be considered in selected pediatric patient populations.

TMP-SMX, which was once used for selective decontamination of the gastrointestinal tract, is now restricted for use as prophylaxis against PCP. Other classes of antibacterial agents, such as β-lactam antibiotics, are seldom used for prophylaxis in neutropenic patients.

Pneumocystis prophylaxis

TMP/SMX is routinely used for prevention of PCP in childhood leukemia, other intensively treated pediatric cancers, as well as HSCT recipients.[18] The recommended prophylactic regimen is TMP/SMX with 150 mg TMP/m^2/day and 750 mg/m^2/day of SMX to a total upper limit dose of 160/800 mg given orally in divided doses twice a day during 3 consecutive days per week. Alternative compounds for patients intolerant of or allergic to TMP/SMX are aerosolized pentamidine (once or twice monthly), pentamidine IV 2 mg/kg once monthly to a total upper limit dose of 100 mg, dapsone PO 2 mg/kg to a total upper limit dose of 100 mg (exclude GCPD deficiency) and atovaquone PO (dosages vary with age) to a total upper limit dose of 1500 mg/d thrice weekly. As sulfones, such as dapsone, have structural similarities to sulfonamides, caution is used in administering this compound to patients with TMP/SMX.

Antiviral prophylaxis

Post-exposure antiviral chemoprophylaxis with oseltamivir or zanamivir are effective in protecting patients developing influenza and from its pneumonic complications. While chemoprophylaxis with antiviral medications is not a substitute for influenza vaccination, such interventions may be especially beneficial in immunocompromised patients in whom the antibody response may not be universally protective.

Acyclovir, given orally or intravenously, is effective prophylaxis against reactivations of HSV in seropositive patients with acute leukemia as well as in HSCT recipients. Prophylactic IV dosages range from 250 mg/m^2 every 8 hours to 5 mg/kg every 12 hours, and oral doses of 10 mg/kg PO given three times daily up to a total oral dose of 400 mg. Such dosages are also effective in reducing the frequency of VZV reactivation.

Guided by CMV PCR on whole blood or by circulating CMV, initiation of ganciclovir for CMV is increasingly used in pre-emptive strategies for prevention of CMV disease. This approach selects for the highest risk patients with molecular evidence of infection but before development of clinically overt CMV disease in tissues.

Immunization

The American Academy of Pediatrics and the CDC regularly publish updated guidelines regarding immunization practices in healthy and immunocompromised pediatric patients. The current website address is http://www.cdc.gov/vaccines/pubs/ACIP-list.htm. Table 25.4 summarizes current recommendations. The website should be reviewed for updates and revisions of current practices. Among the challenges in vaccinating immunocompromised patients, are the potential impairment of immunogenicity of the vaccine, knowing when to reschedule vaccine administration following immunological reconstitution, and whether the vaccine itself in the case of attenuated live organisms may cause disease?

Live or attenuated vaccines

Administration of live attenuated viral vaccines is usually contraindicated in immunocompromised children. Measles–mumps–rubella (MMR) is a live attenuated virus vaccine that is contraindicated in patients undergoing active chemotherapy. If these patients are exposed

Table 25.4. Immunizations in children with hematological malignancies.[a]

Children receiving chemotherapy for leukemia and lymphoma	
DTaP	For children less than 7 years, given 3–6 months after completion of therapy
HiB	Given 3–6 months after completion of therapy
IPV	OPV should not be given to patients or their household contacts, IPV given 3–6 months post completion of therapy
MMR[b]	Given 3–6 months post completion of therapy
VZV[b]	Should be considered in ALL patients after remission for one year, otherwise at 3–6 months post completion of therapy
Influenza	Should be given each autumn, household contacts should also be immunized
Hematopoietic stem cell transplant recipients	
dT	Given at 12, 14 and 24 months post-transplant for those > 7 years of age
DTaP	Given at 12, 14, and 24 months post-transplant for those < 7 years of age
HiB	Given at 12, 14 and 24 months post-transplant
13-VCPP[c]	Given at 12 and 24 months post-transplant
MMR[b]	Given at 24 months post-transplant in those patients without significant GVHD
VZV[b]	Given at 24 months post-transplant
IPV	Given at 12, 14 and 24 months post-transplant, OPV should not be given
Influenza	Given each autumn (greater than 6 months post-transplant), household contacts should also be immunized
Hep B	Given at 12, 14 and 24 months post-transplant

[a]Recommendations are based on limited data. Immunization schedules may need to be individualized based on the patients underlying disease and degree of immunosuppression.
[b]Live attenuated virus vaccines should not be administered during immunosuppression.
[c]13-VCPP: 13-valent conjugated pneumococcal polysaccharide vaccine.

DTaP: Diphtheria, tetanus, and pertussis; HiB: Haemophilus influenzae type B; Hep B: hepatitis B vaccine IPV MMRb: measles, mumps, rubella vaccine; OPV: injectable polio vaccine/oral polio vaccine; VZVb: varicella zoster virus vaccine.

to measles, immunoglobulin should be administered regardless of previous vaccination status. However, MMR immunization is recommended for patients with ALL, but not for Hodgkin's lymphoma, after completion of therapy with a waiting period of 6–12 months to allow for T-cell reconstitution. Household contacts can be safely vaccinated because transmission of the vaccine virus does not occur. For HSCT recipients, administration of MMR vaccine is recommended at 24 months or after discontinuation of immunosuppression, whichever is later.

The oral polio vaccine (OPV), which also is a live virus vaccine, is contraindicated in immunocompromised patients and their household contacts. Instead, inactivated polio vaccine (IPV) should be used after completion of chemotherapy or HSCT.

The current varicella vaccine, which uses the live attenuated Oka strain, has been extensively studied in immunocompromised children. The vaccine is safe in children with ALL with the most common toxicity being a mild rash occurring in approximately 50% of those treated. Although the varicella vaccine is safe and effective in children with leukemia, it is still considered investigational in the United States in immunocompromised patients. Passive immunoprophylaxis either with varicella zoster immune globulin (VZIG) within 96 hours of exposure is indicated in the high risk children with no reliable history of varicella.

Toxoids, inactivated bacteria, inactivated viruses, polysaccharide–protein conjugates

The diphtheria-pertussis-tetanus (DPT) vaccine is immunogenic and protective in infants and children receiving chemotherapy. The diphtheria-tetanus-acellular pertussis (DTaP) vaccine, containing the acellular form of the pertussis component, decreases the risk of seizures and is the currently recommended preparation. While DTaP may be administered at scheduled times during active chemotherapy, an alternative approach to assure greater immunogenicity is to immunize at the end of antineoplastic therapy.

Current guidelines recommend the vaccination of all immunosuppressed individuals with heptavalent conjugated pneumococcal polysaccharide, *Hemophilus influenzae* B conjugated polysaccharide, and, where appropriate, meningococcal vaccines. For HSCT recipients, the current guidelines recommend administration of three doses of DTaP, as well as inactivated polio, HIB, and HBV vaccines as early as 6 months, while some still recommend 12, 14, and 24 months post-HSCT.

Influenza is the most common cause of seasonal excess mortality in the United States. Annual influenza vaccination all immunocompromised children and their household contacts before the onset of influenza season. Similarly, lifelong seasonal administration of influenza vaccine for HSCT recipients is recommended before transplantation and resuming six months after transplantation.

Current challenges and future directions

Among the foremost challenges facing immunocompromised children with hematological malignancies are the inexorable rise of multidrug-resistant bacteria, emergence of invasive fungal infections, and development of refractory viral infections.[19] For many of these infections, there are limited or no effective therapies. Further compounding these challenges are the increasing uncertainties of the impact of new immunosuppressive and other therapies on host defenses. Translational research in infectious diseases supportive care is critical to meeting these formidable challenges and to providing life-saving strategies in our most immunologically vulnerable patients.

References

1. Bailey LC, Reilly AF, Rheingold SR. (2009) Infections in pediatric patients with hematologic malignancies. *Semin Hematol* **46**: 313–324.
2. Castagnola E, Faraci M. (2009) Management of bacteremia in patients undergoing hematopoietic stem cell transplantation. *Expert Rev Anti Infect Ther* **7**: 607–621.
3. Bow EJ. (2009) Neutropenic fever syndromes in patients undergoing cytotoxic therapy for acute leukemia and myelodysplastic syndromes. *Semin Hematol* **46**: 259–268.
4. Wittman B, Horan J, Lyman GH. (2006) Prophylactic colony-stimulating factors in children receiving myelosuppressive chemotherapy: A meta-analysis of randomized controlled trials. *Cancer Treat Rev* **32**: 289–303.
5. Valdez JM, Scheinberg P, Young NS, Walsh TJ. (2009) Infections in patients with aplastic anemia. *Semin Hematol* **46**: 269–276.
6. Zaoutis TE, Heydon K, Chu JH, Walsh TJ, Steinbach WJ. (2006) Epidemiology, outcomes, and costs of invasive aspergillosis in immunocompromised children in the United States, 2000. *Pediatrics* **117**: e711–e716.
7. Bravo LT, Procop GW. (2009) Recent advances in diagnostic microbiology. *Semin Hematol* **46**: 248–258.
8. Dornbusch HJ, Manzoni P, Roilides E, Walsh TJ, Groll AH. (2009) Invasive fungal infections in children. *Pediatr Infect Dis J* **28**: 734–737.
9. Bruckner L, Gigliotti F. (2006) Viridans group streptococcal infections among children with cancer and the importance of emerging antibiotic resistance. *Semin Pediatr Infect Dis* **17**: 153–160.
10. Groll AH, Tragiannidis A. (2009) Recent advances in antifungal prevention and treatment. *Semin Hematol* **46**: 212–229.
11. Cordonnier C, Pautas C, Maury S, Vekhoff A, Farhat H, Suarez F, Dhedin N, Isnard F, Ades L, Kuhnowski F, Foulet F, Kuentz M, Maison P, Bretagne S, Schwarzinger M. (2009) Empirical versus preemptive antifungal therapy for high-risk, febrile, neutropenic patients: A randomized, controlled trial. *Clin Infect Dis* **48**: 1042–1051.
12. Pournaras S, Iosifidis E, Roilides E. (2009) Advances in antibacterial therapy against emerging bacterial pathogens. *Semin Hematol* **46**: 198–211.
13. Pyrgos V, Shoham S, Roilides E, Walsh TJ. (2009) Pneumocystis pneumonia in children. *Paediatr Respir Rev* **10**: 192–198.
14. Hiemenz JW. (2009) Management of infections complicating allogeneic hematopoietic stem cell transplantation. *Semin Hematol* **46**: 289–312.
15. Sullivan KJ, Goodwin SR, Sandler E, Joyce M. (2005) Critical care of the pediatric hematopoietic stem cell recipient in 2005. *Pediatr Transplant* **9**(7): 12–24.
16. Jancel T, Penzak SR. (2009) Antiviral therapy in patients with hematologic malignancies, transplantation, and aplastic anemia. *Semin Hematol* **46**: 230–247.
17. Gray TL, Ooi CY, Tran D, Traubici J, Gerstle JT, Sung L. (2010) Gastrointestinal complications in children with acute myeloid leukemia. *Leuk Lymphoma* **51**: 768–777.
18. (2009) Guidelines for preventing infectious complications among hematopoietic cell transplant recipients: A global perspective. *Bone Marrow Transplant* **44**: 453–558.
19. Walsh TJ. (2009) Advances and challenges in infectious diseases supportive care of patients with hematologic malignancies, hematopoietic stem cell transplantation, and severe aplastic anemia. *Semin Hematol* **46**: 191–197.

26

Integrative Therapies for Children, Adolescents and Young Adults with Hematological Malignancies

Shana S. Jacobs and Kara M. Kelly

Introduction

Integrative therapies (IT), sometimes referred to as complementary and alternative medicine (CAM) is defined as "a group of diverse medical and healthcare systems, practices, and products that are not presently considered to be part of conventional medicine."[1] Integrative therapies include both nonbiological and biological agents (Table 26.1).

Evidence for IT in children and adolescents with hematological malignancies is slowly evolving. The ideal model of integrative pediatric oncology would offer IT modalities that are deemed safe and effective, in conjunction with effective conventional medical treatments. Because of potential interactions, herbs and other dietary supplements should be used with caution, especially during active therapy. Symptom management and wellness should be the emphasis, with IT therapies supporting health promotion and key disease prevention strategies for childhood cancer survivors. All uses, responses, and effects of IT therapies should be carefully documented. A desire to use IT therapies may be an effort to become an active participant in the healing process. Health care providers should encourage, not discourage this partnership.

Integrative Therapy Use in Children

Pediatric use of IT is common and increasing, with usage rates ranging between 20% and 40% in the general pediatric population.[2] In children with chronic illnesses, the rates are often higher as parents seek to maximize the treatment options available for their children.[3,4] IT are widely turned to in children and adolescents with asthma;[5] obesity;[6] and mental and behavioral disorders such as attention-deficit/hyperactivity disorder and autism[7] and depression. A large number of pediatric hospitals now offer IT services; a survey of pediatric pain management services affiliated with major universities found IT offered at 86% of the centers.[8] However, despite the popularity of IT for many of these disorders, there is little research on the effectiveness of most IT for many of these conditions, particularly in children.

Integrative therapy use in children and adolescents with all types of cancer

In pediatric cancer, surveys demonstrate up to 59–84% usage of IT.[9,10] The majority of children and adolescents who turn to IT use these therapies in an "integrated" approach, along with, rather than conventional therapies,

Table 26.1. Integrative therapies.

Whole medical systems	Homeopathic medicine (Europe)	Small doses of diluted substances that in larger doses would produce illness
	Naturopathic medicine (Europe)	Dietary and lifestyle changes with herbs, massage and joint manipulation aiming to support the body's own healing
	Traditional Chinese medicine	Combination of herbs, meditation, massage, and acupuncture that aim to aid healing by restoring the yin-yang balance and the flow of qi
	Ayurveda (India)	Combination of herbs, massage, and yoga aiming to integrate the body, mind, and spirit to prevent and treat disease.
Mind-body medicine	Mental control and meditation	Hypnosis, hypnotherapy, meditation, faith healers, imagery
	Creative outlets	Art, music, or dance
Biologically based therapies	Herbal products	For example: Curcumin, mistletoe, ginseng, mushrooms, milk thistle, echinacea, saw palmetto, essiac, selenium, ginkgo biloba, valerian, green tea
	Dietary supplements	Vitamins, minerals, fatty acids, amino acids, garlic
Manipulative and body-based practices	Osteopathic manipulation	
	Massage	
Energy medicine	Biofield therapies	Acupuncture, acupressure, reiki, qi gong, therapeutic touch
	Bioelectromagnetic-based therapies	Use of electromagnetic fields, such as pulsed fields, magnetic fields, or alternating-current or direct-current fields

Adapted from http://nccam.nih.gov/health/whatiscam/overview.htm.

to help manage the side effects associated with cancer therapy, to augment the efficacy of conventional medications, and to provide psychological support for coping with the diagnosis of cancer (see Chapter 28). Parents pursue IT to ensure that they have left "no stone unturned" and that they are doing all they can to help their child be cured or support them during cancer therapy.

Despite the high prevalence of IT during cancer therapy, many patients and parents do not discuss their use of IT with their physicians,[10] and most pediatric oncologists do not ask about IT use.[11] The discrepancy between patient use and discussions with health care providers is potentially dangerous for patients, especially since up to 20% of children with cancer are using nonvitamin, nonmineral biological IT,[12] which have the highest potential to interact with chemotherapy. Additionally, when physicians ask about and show an interest in patient IT use, patients and families are more likely to share honestly and seek IT in conjunction with the health care team.

An often under-recognized observation is that IT are used frequently among children and adolescents enrolled on clinical trials.[10] Therefore concomitant use of any IT must be recorded, so that any potential interactions can be carefully monitored. The family and healthcare provider's decision to include IT should be based on available evidence and not include those therapies that require a tremendous burden with unproven benefit or that might lead to obstacles for the child to adhere to the conventional therapy.

Integrative therapy use for children and adolescents with hematological malignancies

Specific prevalence data on the use of IT among children and adolescents with hematological malignancies has generally not been reported in the surveys, although IT were used by 53 of 60 children with leukemia in a recent Malaysian study.[13] While as with all pediatric cancers, most parents of children and adolescents with hematological malignancies use IT in conjunction with chemotherapy, a review of court cases involving parents seeking alternative therapies in lieu of conventional chemotherapy revealed that there are some parents who seek alternative therapies instead of chemotherapy for children with favorable outcome hematological malignancies.[13] Although there has been a significant increase in research on IT for cancer, there is still a paucity of data to guide clinical practices incorporating IT for children and adolescents with hematological malignancies.

Research in Integrative Therapy

With the greater use of IT by children and adolescents with hematological malignancies, increasing scientific attention is being directed towards the investigation of these therapies. Research has evolved from testimonials of "miraculous" cures, case series, and single arm outcome studies to underpowered clinical trials and, more recently, to randomized clinical trials investigating efficacy.[14] However, research on IT is complex and usually more difficult than that of conventional anticancer therapies, particularly in children with cancer. Preclinical and Phase I studies are often not done, and this may impact the conduct of Phase III trials. Traditional Chinese medicine (TCM) and other traditional medicine techniques use a very personalized approach that individualizes treatment, using multiple herbs simultaneously, to restore an individual's well-being rather than focusing more generally on a type of disease. The whole concept of disease and wellness is different than in Western medicine, and the herbs used have multiple components. These aspects of TCM make good randomized clinical trials very challenging.[12,15] Investigations of nonpharmacologic therapies such as acupuncture are hampered by the lack of validated assessment tools in children, as well as the challenges of finding appropriate placebos.[16] The rarity of childhood cancer further reduces the incentive for many IT providers to scientifically evaluate therapies in children and adolescents.

Despite these limitations, there is a strong imperative to test IT which are already in widespread use, both to expand the repertoire that Western medicine has available for supportive care and to investigate potential toxicities of combining IT with cancer-directed therapies. Additionally, botanical drug development offers many advantages over the combinatorial chemistry approach currently in use for anticancer agents.[15]

Direct Antileukemia or Lymphoma Effects

There is very limited evidence for IT use for anticancer purposes for hematological malignancies in children or adults. There is limited preclinical evidence of cytotoxic activity of specific biological agents in leukemia cell lines, though clinical trial data is almost nonexistent. For a full discussion of the use of herbs and botanical compounds in pediatric and adult cancers, refer to reviews by Miller[17] and Melnick.[12,15]

Several Ayurvedic herbs have undergone preclinical testing in leukemias and other cancers. Ashwagandha, a traditional Ayurvedic herb, is typically used to improve vitality and normalize bodily functions; its putative active constituent, withaferin A, was found to cause apoptosis in human leukemia HL-60 cells via oxidative stress and mitochondrial dysfunction.[18] *Streblus asper* Lour. (shakhotaka), another Ayurvedic herb, showed cytotoxic effects on mouse lymphocytic leukemia.[19] *Rubia cordifolia* L. demonstrated antitumor activity against P388 leukemia similar to that of deoxybouvardin and vincristine, and has been tested in a Phase I study demonstrating safety.[17] Curcumin, another herb from Ayurvedic tradition, has been evaluated in pediatric acute lymphoblastic leukemia (ALL) cells, with modulation of leukemia cell resistance achieved through a reduction in multiple drug resistance gene mRNA levels.[17]

Preclincal studies showed that an essential oil from a lemongrass variety of *Cymbopogon flexuosus* (CFO) and its major chemical constituent could induce apoptosis by increased expression of mitochondrial cytochrome c and apical death receptors in human leukemia HL-60 cells.[15] In another study, extracts of Annona glabra (pond apple), an herb used in Mexican, Chinese and Japanese traditional health systems, were highly cytotoxic to drug sensitive (CEM) and multidrug-resistant leukemia (CEM/VLB) cell lines.[13] In contrast, *in vitro* investigation of extracts of mistletoe (Viscum album) and two Peruvian herbs, Uncaria tomentosa (Vilcacora) and Croton lechleri (Sangre de drago) in 51 patient leukemia samples and four leukemia cell lines (Jurkat, CCRF-CEM, HL-60, K-562) demonstrated stimulation of cell growth.[19]

Traditional Chinese medicine (TCM) has been used to treat adults with leukemia. There is one report from China of successful treatment of adults with acute myelocytic leukemia (AML) with TCM.[20] Indigo naturalis (2,2′-bisindole) was identified as the active ingredient of the TCM treatment of a number of diseases including chronic myelocyctic leukemia. BIO-112, a synthetic derivative of indirubin, which is a by-product of indigo

Table 26.2. Integrative therapies that have been investigated for use as a supportive care therapy in children with hematological malignancies (See reviews (22,96)).

Symptom	Whole medical systems	Mind–body medicine	Biologically based therapies	Manipulative and body-based practices	Energy medicine
Nausea/vomiting	Acupressure (–)	Cognitive distraction[a] (+) Hypnosis[a] (+) Music[a] (+)		Massage (–)	
Mucositis	Homeopathic mouth rinse[a] (+/–)		Glutamine[a] (+)		
Pain				Massage[a] (–)	
Procedural pain		Music (+) Hypnosis[a] (+) Art			
Fatigue				Massage[a] (–)	
Cachexia			Fish oil[a] (+)		
Anxiety/Insomnia		Hypnosis[a] (+)		Massage[a] (+)	
Weight gain			Creatine (+)		
Constipation					
Hepatotoxicity			Milk thistle[a] (+)		
Mood				Massage[a] (+)	

[a] Randomized controlled trial; (+) Positive results observed; (–) Negative results observed.

naturalis, is undergoing testing in Phase II clinical trials for leukemia in Europe.[17] Triptolide, a diterpine triepoxide derived from the Chinese plant *Tripterygium wilfordii*, is an inhibitor of heat shock transcription factor 1. Omtriptolide, a derivative of triptolide, is in early phase clinical trials for the treatment of acute myelogenous leukemia. In pediatric patients, there is an ongoing trial of β-glucans in combination with rituximab for refractory leukemia and lymphoma.[21] Beta-glucans are derived from medicinal mushrooms, which are used in TCM to treat various types of cancer.

Practicing Integrative Oncology in the Care of Children and Adolescents with Hematological Malignancies

There are many aspects of childhood cancer therapy where IT may have a beneficial role, especially as a component of the multidisciplinary approach often utilized in childhood cancer therapy (see Chapter 27).[22] The aims of the IT interventions are to assist with the minimization of pain and suffering and to provide practical, emotional and physical support. While the existing research on IT in children and adolescents is not specific to hematological malignancies, many of the side effects and symptoms targeted by IT are experienced by patients with leukemias and lymphomas, and the results can often be extrapolated for leukemia and lymphoma patients. Several types of integrative therapies can be considered for symptom control in the care of the child or adolescent with hematological malignancies at this time, and some of these are described below and in Table 26.2.

Massage

In adults with cancer, positive effects have been noted for a range of symptoms including pain, nausea, depression, anger, stress, fatigue, and anxiety.[23–27] Anxiety appears to be the symptom most consistently reported as positively affected by massage, especially immediately after the massage.[28–31] Additionally, physiologic markers of anxiety (heart rate, blood pressure) have been shown to be reduced immediately following massages.[31] Most positive effects are short lived (immediately following the massage to within a half hour after), though some longer term effects have been noted.[32,33]

Of the integrative therapies, massage is one of the more popular in pediatric patients, with about 30% of children in general[9] and 60% of children with cancer[9] reporting use. In a review of massage in pediatric patients, Beider and Moyer reported on 24 randomized controlled trials, accounting for 200 participants, completed between 1992 and 2006. While the authors point out the statistical and design flaws of the studies, they are still able to conclude that evidence is strong for the effect of massage on anxiety in children, particularly after repeated sessions of massage.[34]

Only two studies have been published on massage therapy in pediatric oncology patients. The first involved 23 children and adolescents with cancer, ages 1 to 18 years. Massage had positive effects on reducing heart rate and anxiety, and participants had very positive evaluations of their massage experience.[35] In the second study, 50 children aged 1–19 with cancer undergoing bone marrow transplantation received professional massage, parent massage or were controls. Results indicated statistically significant differences in days to engraftment in the combined (parent and professional) massage group. Results from the professional massage group yielded a significant decrease in immediate anxiety and discomfort.[36]

Sleep disturbances and fatigue are common problems for children and adolescents taking steroids,[37] and massage can be helpful for these symptoms as well as the resultant mood disturbances and anxiety. In addition, corticosteroid and vincristine therapy can cause extreme pain which may be relieved by massage or reflexology.

Acupuncture and acupressure

Acupuncture describes a family of techniques in which small needles, heat, or electrical stimulation are placed at very precise anatomical points. Acupuncture is a key component of TCM. According to TCM, acupuncture points are situated on meridians along which qi (a "life energy") flows. Acupressure applies pressure (by hand or by another device) to the same acupuncture points.

While evidence regarding use of acupuncture in pediatric conditions is somewhat lacking due to a paucity of well-designed clinical trials,[16] there is evidence of efficacy in adult cancer patients with symptoms such as nausea and vomiting,[38,39] pain, fatigue, anxiety and insomnia,[22,40] symptoms that are equally burdensome to pediatric oncology patients. In addition, acupuncture has been shown to be well tolerated in children[41,42] and has been shown to help some children, particularly with pain management.[8,43,44] Acupuncture has been investigated in one pediatric oncology study of chemotherapy-induced nausea and vomiting where it was found to significantly decrease need for rescue nausea medications as well as vomiting episodes.[45] Very few adverse events have been noted. A retrospective safety review of children receiving acupuncture demonstrated no bleeding complications, even when acupuncture was administered with platelet counts less than 20,000/μl.[46]

Acupressure has the advantages of not requiring highly trained practitioners or specialized equipment and avoiding needles for needle phobic children or adolescents. Although its feasibility has been shown among children and adolescents with ALL, it has not yet demonstrated efficacy for chemotherapy-associated nausea.[13] A systematic review of 10 studies of acupressure for CINV in adults found the studies to be inconclusive but promising for an effect of acupressure for this purpose.[47] A study of acupressure to prevent delayed nausea and vomiting in children receiving highly emetogenic chemotherapy is under development.

Mind–body therapies

Mind–body therapies, especially hypnosis, cognitive distraction, art therapy and music therapy, may be effective adjunctive therapies in managing procedural pain, anxiety, and nausea.[13] Hypnosis can be particularly effective in children, especially between the ages of 7 and 14.[48] In a study of 54 children with cancer, Zeltzer *et al.* found hypnosis to be effective (compared with both cognitive distraction/ relaxation and placebo) in reducing anticipatory and chemotherapy-induced nausea and vomiting (CINV).[49] Self-hypnosis and guided imagery have been found to be helpful for management of pain in children, particularly headaches.[50] Hypnosis is often used to reduce procedural pain and anxiety, and several small studies have found positive effects in pediatric oncology patients undergoing bone marrow aspirates and spinal taps.[51–55] Overall, however, the evidence supporting its use, while promising, is inconclusive.[48]

In a small study of children with leukemia, art therapy before and after lumbar punctures was associated with more collaborative behavior and fewer resistive behaviors compared to an historical comparison.[56]

Exercise

In adults with cancer, exercise has been shown in repeated studies to be safe and to improve fatigue, pain, nausea, sleep, and mood.[57,58] In pediatrics, exercise programs have been found to be safe and effective in improving aerobic fitness, strength, and functional mobility in children and adolescents with ALL.[59,60] A review of research related to physical activity during treatment for pediatric cancer found that reduced physical activity is common in patients during and after therapy, including during maintenance therapy for ALL, and that exercise interventions provided promising results in patients on therapy and in survivors.[61]

Select herbs and biological therapies

Many herbs and biologic therapies are in use by patients with cancer and other disorders, and a full review of all potential biologic therapies is beyond the scope of this chapter. Pertinent reviews include those by Miller,[17] Melnick,[12,15] and Ladas.[22] Select agents with evidence of effectiveness in symptoms that affect children and adolescents with hematological malignancies or evidence of potential harm are discussed.

Ginger (Zingiber officinale) is often used as an antiemetic. It has been shown to be effective for nausea and vomiting associated with pregnancy,[62–65] and has shown promising, but inconsistent effects, on post-operative nausea and vomiting.[66–69] Seven studies have assessed ginger for CINV in adults. In the largest study to date, Ryan *et al.* compared nausea severity in 644 adults receiving single-day chemotherapy who received one of three doses of ginger (0.5g, 1.0g, 1.5g) to placebo. All doses of ginger significantly reduced nausea severity on ($p = 0.003$), with the largest reduction in nausea severity at the 0.5 g/d and 1.0 g/d doses.[70] A study of ginger for CINV in children and adolescents is in development.

Probiotics are one of the most frequently used biological IT in children and adolescents. A number of studies have investigated lactobacillus GG in children with viral-induced diarrhea and have reported encouraging findings. Because probiotics contain live active organisms, there has been hesitation in prescribing their use in immunocompromised patients. However, large randomized clinical trials in immunocompetent patients, including newborns, have rarely reported any adverse events.[22] Probiotics may be beneficial in the setting of allogeneic stem cell transplant. In a murine model of acute graft vs. host disease (aGVHD), *Lactobacillus rhamnosus* GG before and after transplantation resulted in improved survival and reduced aGVHD.[71] No studies have been published in children or adolescents with cancer, though a study in children receiving stem cell transplants is in development.

Glutamine is a conditionally essential amino acid during severe catabolic states and has been used for the prevention of mucositis and peripheral neuropathy. In studies of children undergoing SCT, glutamine decreased duration of fever,[72] and decreased TPN and narcotic use.[13] Glutamine has also been found to be helpful in preventing peripheral neuropathy in adults with cancer. A review of oral glutamine for prevention of peripheral neuropathy found a few small studies in patients receiving paclitaxil and oxaliplatin.[73] Though larger studies are needed, glutamine appears promising for this purpose as well, and no toxicities have been reported.

Carnitine deficiency has been noted in children and adolescents receiving chemotherapy, and has been found to correlate with fatigue.[74] In open-label studies in adult cancer patients, supplementation with L-carnitine has been found to reduce cancer-related fatigue,[75] though large randomized controlled trials have not been reported. Carnitine may also have cardioprotective effects with anthracycline chemotherapy, however this has not been investigated in clinical trials.[76]

Valerian (Valeriana officinalis L.) is a popular European herb used for its mild sedative and tranquilizing properties. Multiple studies have shown Valerian to improve sleep without increasing daytime sleepiness. Additionally, it appears to have a wide margin of safety and it is not metabolized via the cytochrome enzymes, suggesting no interaction with chemotherapy agents. However, it has not been well studied in cancer patients or in children, and effects of long-term use are unknown. Another herb often used as a sleep aid is Kava (*Piper methysticum* G. Forst). While Kava also appears to be efficacious and is generally well tolerated, there have been a few reports of hepatic failure associated with kava use, making it not advisable to use concurrently with chemotherapy.[77]

Antioxidants (such as β-carotene, lycopene, vitamins C, E, and A, and other substances) are one of the most common classes of supplements used by patients with cancer; these supplements are used for direct cytotoxic effects, or for synergy with conventional therapy or to mitigate conventional therapy induced toxicity. In a prospective observational study conducted among children with ALL, low plasma and dietary antioxidant levels[13] directly correlated with treatment-related toxicity. However, there is concern that supplements promoted for their antioxidant qualities may diminish the efficacy of anticancer treatments, particularly radiation, that work through the promotion of oxidizing free radicals.[12,78] Studies adequately evaluating the impact of supplementation on toxicity and disease free survival have not been completed.

Immune modulators are another broad category of CAM therapies that are often used by cancer patients.[79] Popular immune-enhancing herbs and dietary supplements include astragalus, echinacea, β-glucans, and mushroom extracts (especially Reishi, Maitake, Shitaki). Agents such as Asian mushrooms[80] and mistletoe[81] have been shown to increase cytotoxic T lymphocytes, natural killer cells, or endogenous production of cytokines. However, these agents have not been shown to be efficacious or safe in cancer patients. Finally, little is known about the potential interactions of immune modulators with chemotherapy or the appropriate dose, toxicities, and length of treatment in children or adolescents with cancer. No clinical trials specifically in children or adolescents have been reported in the English language literature.

Creatine monohydrate may attenuate corticosteroid associated increases in body fat accumulation, a common complication of therapy for childhood ALL and lymphoma.[13]

Milk thistle a hepatoprotective herb, is associated with reductions in serum transaminases in children receiving maintenance chemotherapy for ALL.[13] Its use may reduce the need for dose reductions in chemotherapy for hepatotoxicity. No interactions with chemotherapy were observed in a T-cell ALL cell line.

Risks of Integrative Therapy

Similar to the situation in adults, the integration of complementary therapies in the management of children and adolescents with leukemia and lymphoma is controversial. Most surveys demonstrate that the biologically active herbs and other dietary supplements are the most common type of IT in use with conventional therapies,[10,82] yet there are very few clinical trials in adults or children examining their safety and efficacy. Ernst describes case reports of adverse events related to IT use, often due to heavy metal contamination of botanical products, which can lead to gastric upset, hematologic problems and neurocognitive difficulties.[83] Microbial contamination of herbal products may be associated with even more significant risks in immunocompromised children and adolescents, especially for those children undergoing stem cell transplantation. Direct toxicities of dietary supplements have been observed, but the prevalence is unknown as systematic reporting is not legally mandated.[13] However, it is important to remember that adverse effects and drug interactions are frequently observed with conventional medications as well. The compelling issue with the biologically active ITs is that they remain largely unstudied, particularly in children and adolescents with cancer. Known and theoretical interactions are summarized in Sencer and Kelly.[79]

The non-biologically based therapies are generally considered safe. For example, in a review of adverse events observed among children and adolescents receiving acupuncture, the incidence rate of side effects is estimated to be only 1.55 per 100 treatments, with the most common side effect being redness at the puncture site.[84] Only one serious adverse event was observed among 1865 treatments. Similar safety records have been reported for yoga[85] and massage.[86] Nonetheless, although there is a low risk of interference with conventional therapies, training programs for integrative therapies practitioners often have little to no standards for training with children, let alone children receiving intensive conventional treatment for hematological malignancies. Furthermore, most pediatric hematology/oncology fellowship curricula have not incorporated formal educational opportunities on integrative therapies,[13] so pediatric oncologists have little information to advise patients on how to safely incorporate IT into their treatment.

Decisions about the Choice of Integrative Therapy

The decision to use a particular IT will in part be based on the developmental stage of the child or adolescent. Children with fear of needles and discomfort with the invasiveness of the conventional treatment such as intrathecal chemotherapy injections and bone marrow aspirations may have added anxiety with the use of acupuncture; in this instance acupressure, massage, or hypnosis may be more appropriate options. Young children often have a fear of strangers and may assume that all health care providers may induce unintentional pain. Introduction of the relatively noninvasive IT modalities of reflexology, energy therapies, or aromatherapy may be a more effective strategy. This is particularly true for younger patients who may not have the language skills to articulate their fears, yet have strong imaginations to understand concepts such as energy fields, guided imagery, and meditation. Children and adolescents may be hesitant in using IT because of the fear of what the therapy may feel like, therefore an effective strategy may be to first observe a session on another patient, parent, or sibling.

Integrative Therapies and Survivorship

There are a huge number of adult survivors of childhood leukemia and lymphoma, who are at risk for medical and psychosocial sequelae that may adversely affect their health status.[87] Survivors are challenged with issues not limited to energy balance, fatigue, bone health, pain syndromes, and anxiety, and are at increased risk for many long-term sequelae including cardiac dysfunction, stroke, osteoporosis and osteonecrosis, infertility, and second malignancies.[88] The use of IT extends into survivorship to reduce risk of relapse, cope with late effects from cancer therapy, or reduce their risk of developing a late effect.[89]

The use of IT as a component of a healthy lifestyle may provide support to survivors for coping with many of the late effects of cancer therapy. For example, yoga and meditation may help to reduce the feelings of anxiety associated with cancer recurrence, may lessen the functional impact of disturbances in balance or gait, or assist with maintenance of a healthy weight. Acupuncture may provide relief to patients who are challenged with fatigue, recurrent pain, or infertility. Use of dietary supplements is less complicated as concerns for interactions with conventional chemotherapy or radiation therapy are not issues, and may help patients with physical late effects such as lack of bone density and with psychological well being.[90]

Integrative Therapies and Palliative Care

Pain and suffering at the end of a child's life is often not adequately managed with conventional approaches. The most common symptoms experienced by children and adolescents at this time include fatigue, pain, dyspnea, anorexia, nausea, and vomiting, constipation and diarrhea, with many of these symptoms not adequately treated by conventional means, as 89% of parents in one study reported that children suffered "a lot or a great deal" within the last month of life.[91] Therapies to be considered for their adjunctive role include acupuncture, aromatherapy, massage, energy therapies, and mind-body approaches. Palliative care should include interventions offered to parents and siblings, who often suffer both psychological and physical distress during the child's end of life and consequent phase of bereavement.[92] A recent survey investigating the current practices and resources surrounding palliative and end-of-life care among participating institutions of the Children's Oncology Group demonstrated that integrative services were widely available, with 39% of institutions directly providing services. 95% had services available in the communities that these institutions serve.[93] Of the 50 institutions that offered IT, 76% of the oncology divisions made direct referrals for these therapies, highlighting the acceptance of IT in the palliative care setting.

How can we Best Counsel our Patients about Integrative Therapies?

As more parents of children and adolescents with cancer seek integrative care, pediatric institutions face the need to answer patients' and healthcare providers' questions about integrating these therapies in the care of children and adolescents with hematological malignancies. In a study performed at a pediatric institution with an established IT consultation service, consultations were most frequently requested by oncology patients primarily for assistance with symptom management, and with questions on various therapies, especially herbs and dietary supplements.[94] As healthcare providers, we educate patients and parents about their disease and the various treatment modalities available. Similarly, we need to offer easy-to-understand information about integrative approaches. Table 26.3 lists reputable internet resources for clinicians and patients. We can encourage patients and parents to talk with us when they hear of anecdotal use of unproven modalities, and discourage the use of most biologically based IT until studies are undertaken to prove their safety and efficacy. Most of all, we can remind them that we are their partners in care, that we care about and take seriously their wishes to use IT in the best interests of their child.[95]

Summary

The goal of an integrative approach in the care of children and adolescents with hematological malignancies is to provide IT modalities that are deemed safe and effective in conjunction with effective conventional medical treatments. There is significant need for research evaluating the roles of IT for direct treatment of hematological malignancies and for symptom control of toxicities related to conventional therapies. More formal education opportunities on ITs in the training of pediatric oncologists and other healthcare providers working with children and adolescents with cancer should be implemented. Healthcare providers should consider how IT services may be beneficial to children

Table 26.3. Integrative oncology resources.

Government Resources
National Center for Complementary Alternative Medicine, National Institute of Health: http://nccam.nih.gov
Office of Cancer Complementary Alternative Medicine, National Cancer Institute, National Institute of Health: http://occam.nci.nih.gov
PDQ®. Cancer Information Summaries: Complementary and Alternative Medicine, National Cancer Institute, National Institute of Health: http://www.cancer.gov/cancertopics/pdq/cam
Office of Dietary Supplements, National Institute of Health: http://ods.od.nih.gov/
U.S. Food and Drug Administration, Department of Health and Human Services: http://www.fda.gov/
Academic Institutions
Integrative Therapies Program for Children with Cancer, Columbia University Medical Center: http://integrativetherapies.columbia.edu/
About Herbs, Botanicals and Other Products, Memorial Sloan Kettering Cancer Center: http://www.mskcc.org/mskcc/html/11570.cfm
Complementary/Integrative Medicine, MD Anderson Cancer Center: http://www.mdanderson.org/departments/cimer/
Zakim Center for Integrative Therapies, Dana Farber Cancer Institute: http://www.dana-farber.org/pat/support/zakim/default.html
Databases
Natural Standard http://www.naturalstandard.com/
Cochrane Reviews on Complementary Medicine, The Cochrane Collaboration: http://cochrane.org/reviews/en/topics/22_reviews.html
CAM Clinical Trials from NCI's PDQ® Database: http://www.cancer.gov/cam/clinicaltrials_pdq.html
CAM on PubMed, National Library of Medicine:
http://www.ncbi.nlm.nih.gov/sites/entrez?db=pubmed&orig_db=PubMed&cmd_current=Limits&pmfilter_Subsets=Complementary%20Medicine

and adolescents with leukemia or lymphoma. However, until the evidence for or against an integrative modality is more conclusive, the provider's role is to ask about and document the use of IT, critically evaluate the evidence or lack of evidence, balance the potential risks with possible benefits, and assist the family in their decisions regarding use of integrative approaches for their child.

References

3. Kemper KJ. (2001) Complementary and alternative medicine for children: Does it work? *West J Med* **174**: 272–276.
4. Kemper KJ, Vohra S, Walls R. (2008) American Academy of Pediatrics. The use of complementary and alternative medicine in pediatrics. *Pediatrics* **122**: 1374–1386.
5. Mark JD. (2007) Integrative medicine and asthma. *Pediatr Clin North Am* **54**: 1007–1023; xii.
6. McClafferty HH. (2007) Integrative approach to obesity. *Pediatr Clin North Am* **54**: 969–981; xi.
7. Weber W, Newmark S. (2007) Complementary and alternative medical therapies for attention-deficit/hyperactivity disorder and autism. *Pediatr Clin North Am* **54**: 983–1006; xii.
10. Kelly KM, Jacobson JS, Kennedy DD, Braudt SM, Mallick M, Weiner MA. (2000) Use of unconventional therapies by children with cancer at an urban medical center. *J Pediatr Hematol Oncol* **22**: 412–416.
14. Post-White J, Hawks R, O'Mara A, Ott MJ. (2006) Future directions of CAM research in pediatric oncology. *J Pediatr Oncol Nurs* **23**: 265–268.
18. Malik F, Kumar A, Bhushan S, Khan S, Bhatia A, Suri KA, Qazi GN, Singh J. (2007) Reactive oxygen species generation and mitochondrial dysfunction in the apoptotic cell death of human myeloid leukemia HL-60 cells by a dietary compound withaferin A with concomitant protection by N-acetyl cysteine. *Apoptosis* **12**: 2115–2133.
19. Rastogi S, Kulshreshtha DK, Rawat AK. (2006) Streblus asper Lour. (Shakhotaka): A review of its chemical, pharmacological and ethnomedicinal properties. *Evid Based Complement Alternat Med* **3**: 217–222.

20. Hu XM, Liu F, Zheng CM, Li L, Liu C, Zhang SS, Xiao HY, Yang XH, Wang HZ, Xu YG, Hu NP, Ma R. (2009) Effect and prognostic analysis of treatment for acute myeloid leukemia using Chinese drugs combined with chemotherapy. *Chin J Integr Med* **15**: 193–197.
24. Jane SW, Wilkie DJ, Gallucci BB, Beaton RD. (2008) Systematic review of massage intervention for adult patients with cancer: A methodological perspective. *Cancer Nurs* **31**: E24–E35.
25. Wilkinson S, Barnes K, Storey L. (2008) Massage for symptom relief in patients with cancer: Systematic review. *J Adv Nurs* **63**: 430–439.
26. Myers CD, Walton T, Small BJ. (2008) The value of massage therapy in cancer care. *Hematol Oncol Clin North Am* **22**: 649–660; viii.
27. Russell NC, Sumler SS, Beinhorn CM, Frenkel MA. (2008) Role of massage therapy in cancer care. *J Altern Complement Med* **14**: 209–214.
28. Ahles TA, Tope DM, Pinkson B, Walch S, Hann D, Whedon M, Dain B, Weiss JE, Mills L, Silberfarb PM. (1999) Massage therapy for patients undergoing autologous bone marrow transplantation. *J Pain Symptom Manage* **18**: 157–163.
30. Cassileth BR, Vickers AJ. (2004) Massage therapy for symptom control: Outcome study at a major cancer center. *J Pain Symptom Manage* **28**: 244–249.
33. Listing M, Reisshauer A, Krohn M, Voigt B, Tjahono G, Becker J, Klapp BF, Rauchfuss M. (2009) Massage therapy reduces physical discomfort and improves mood disturbances in women with breast cancer. *Psychooncology* **18**: 1290–1299.
37. Hinds PS, Hockenberry MJ, Gattuso JS, Srivastava DK, Tong X, Jones H, West N, McCarthy KS, Sadeh A, Ash M, Fernandez C, Pui CH. (2007) Dexamethasone alters sleep and fatigue in pediatric patients with acute lymphoblastic leukemia. *Cancer* **110**: 2321–2330.
38. Melchart D, Linde K, Fischer P, Berman B, White A, Vickers A, Allais G. (2001) Acupuncture for idiopathic headache. *Cochrane Database Syst Rev* **1**: CD001218.
39. Ernst E. (2009) Acupuncture: What does the most reliable evidence tell us? *J Pain Symptom Manage* **37**: 709–714.
41. Kemper KJ, Sarah R, Silver-Highfield E, Xiarhos E, Barnes L, Berde C. (2000) On pins and needles? Pediatric pain patients' experience with acupuncture. *Pediatrics* **105**: 941–947.
43. Kundu A, Berman B. (2007) Acupuncture for pediatric pain and symptom management. *Pediatr Clin North Am* **54**: 885–889; x.
44. Tsao JC, Meldrum M, Bursch B, Jacob MC, Kim SC, Zeltzer LK. (2005) Treatment expectations for CAM interventions in pediatric chronic pain patients and their parents. *Evid Based Complement Alternat Med* **2**: 521–527.
46. Taromina K LE, Rooney D, Hughes D, Meyer A, Kelly K. (2007) Acupuncture is feasible in children with cancer with low platelet counts. *J Soc Integr Oncol* **5**: 178–188.
49. Zeltzer LK, Dolgin MJ, LeBaron S, LeBaron C. (1991) A randomized, controlled study of behavioral intervention for chemotherapy distress in children with cancer. *Pediatrics* **88**: 34–42.
50. Tsao JC, Zeltzer LK. (2005) Complementary and alternative medicine approaches for Pediatric Pain: A review of the state-of-the-science. *Evid Based Complement Alternat Med* **2**: 149–159.
51. Wall VJ, Womack W. (1989) Hypnotic versus active cognitive strategies for alleviation of procedural distress in pediatric oncology patients. *Am J Clin Hypn* **31**: 181–191.
52. Liossi C, Hatira P. (1999) Clinical hypnosis versus cognitive behavioral training for pain management with pediatric cancer patients undergoing bone marrow aspirations. *Int J Clin Exp Hypn* **47**: 104–116.
54. Kellerman J, Zeltzer L, Ellenberg L, Dash J. (1983) Adolescents with cancer. Hypnosis for the reduction of the acute pain and anxiety associated with medical procedures. *J Adolesc Health Care* **4**: 85–90.
58. Speed-Andrews AE, Courneya KS. (2009) Effects of exercise on quality of life and prognosis in cancer survivors. *Curr Sports Med Rep* **8**: 176–181.
62. Fischer-Rasmussen W, Kjaer SK, Dahl C, Asping U. (1991) Ginger treatment of hyperemesis gravidarum. *Eur J Obstet Gynecol Reprod Biol* **38**: 19–24.
63. Keating A, Chez RA. (2002) Ginger syrup as an antiemetic in early pregnancy. *Altern Ther Health Med* **8**: 89–91.
67. Bone ME, Wilkinson DJ, Young JR, McNeil J, Charlton S. (1990) Ginger root — a new antiemetic. The effect of ginger root on postoperative nausea and vomiting after major gynaecological surgery. *Anaesthesia* **45**: 669–671.
68. Phillips S, Ruggier R, Hutchinson SE. (1993) Zingiber officinale (ginger) — an antiemetic for day case surgery. *Anaesthesia* **48**: 715–717.
69. Visalyaputra S, Petchpaisit N, Somcharoen K, Choavaratana R. (1998) The efficacy of ginger root in the prevention of postoperative nausea and vomiting after outpatient gynaecological laparoscopy. *Anaesthesia* **53**: 506–510.
74. Hockenberry MJ, Hooke MC, Gregurich M, McCarthy K. (2009) Carnitine plasma levels and fatigue in children/adolescents receiving cisplatin, ifosfamide, or doxorubicin. *J Pediatr Hematol Oncol* **31**: 664–669.

76. McFalls EO, Paulson DJ, Gilbert EF, Shug AL. (1986) Carnitine protection against adriamycin-induced cardiomyopathy in rats. *Life Sci* **38**: 497–505.
80. Borchers AT, Stern JS, Hackman RM, Keen CL, Gershwin ME. (1999) Mushrooms, tumors, and immunity. *Proc Soc Exp Biol Med* **221**: 281–293.
81. Ernst E, Schmidt K, Steuer-Vogt MK. (2003) Mistletoe for cancer? A systematic review of randomised clinical trials. *Int J Cancer* **107**: 262–267.
87. Hudson MM, Mertens AC, Yasui Y, Hobbie W, Chen H, Gurney JG, Yeazel M, Recklitis CJ, Marina N, Robison LR, Oeffinger KC. (2003) Health status of adult long-term survivors of childhood cancer: A report from the childhood cancer survivor study. *JAMA* **290**: 1583–1592.
90. Kemper KJ, Shannon S. (2007) Complementary and alternative medicine therapies to promote healthy moods. *Pediatr Clin North Am* **54**: 901–926; x.
92. Lannen PK, Wolfe J, Prigerson HG, Onelov E, Kreicbergs UC. (2008) Unresolved grief in a national sample of bereaved parents: Impaired mental and physical health 4 to 9 years later. *J Clin Oncol* **26**: 5870–5876.
94. Kemper KJ, Wornham WL. (2001) Consultations for holistic pediatric services for inpatients and outpatient oncology patients at a children's hospital. *Arch Pediatr Adolesc Med* **155**: 449–454.
96. Myers C, Stuber ML, Bonamer-Rheingans JI, Zeltzer LK. (2005) Complementary therapies and childhood cancer. *Cancer Control* **12**: 172–180.

27

Nursing Considerations and Acute Side Effects for Children, Adolescents and Young Adults with Hematological Malignancies

Rita Secola, Lauren Harrison and Diane Altounji

Introduction

As there is great effort in achieving long-term survival of children, adolescents and young adults with hematological malignancies, the demand for nursing excellence has never been so great. Knowledgeable and well-trained nurses are critical in providing safe and effective care. Nurses who care for these patients are challenged with providing outstanding clinical care and maintain the frontline leadership in the multidisciplinary team approach of care required for these patients and their families. Nurses are the consistent professionals who interact with patients and families at diagnosis, throughout treatment and in every patient care setting. Over extended lengths of time, nurses develop rapport with patients and families and thus provide a superior source of trust, support, and information for the team to optimize the plan of care. The trajectory of care for these patients includes nursing roles that encompass bedside clinical care provider, educator, consultant, manager, advocate, researcher, and communicator. Their roles are critical to help manage patients through short- and long-term cancer treatments, life after cancer treatment, and when the end of life is near. Children, adolescents, and young adults with hematological malignancies may undergo a host of treatment-related side effects that will require an immense amount of physical and psychosocial support (see Chapter 28). Nurses are at the forefront of providing that support.

Patients with hematological malignancies may be at greater risk for particular cancer treatment effects. An overview of specialized nursing roles, selected acute and long-term treatment-related effects, health promotion after cancer treatment, special considerations for adolescents and young adults and end-of-life considerations in caring for this patient population are described.

Specialized Nursing Roles

Nursing is a unique profession as there are a variety of roles that nurses can fulfill. The opportunities for advancement are expanding as the need for nurses increase worldwide. An extensive range of nursing professionals is required to meet the diverse needs of children, adolescents and young adults with cancer.

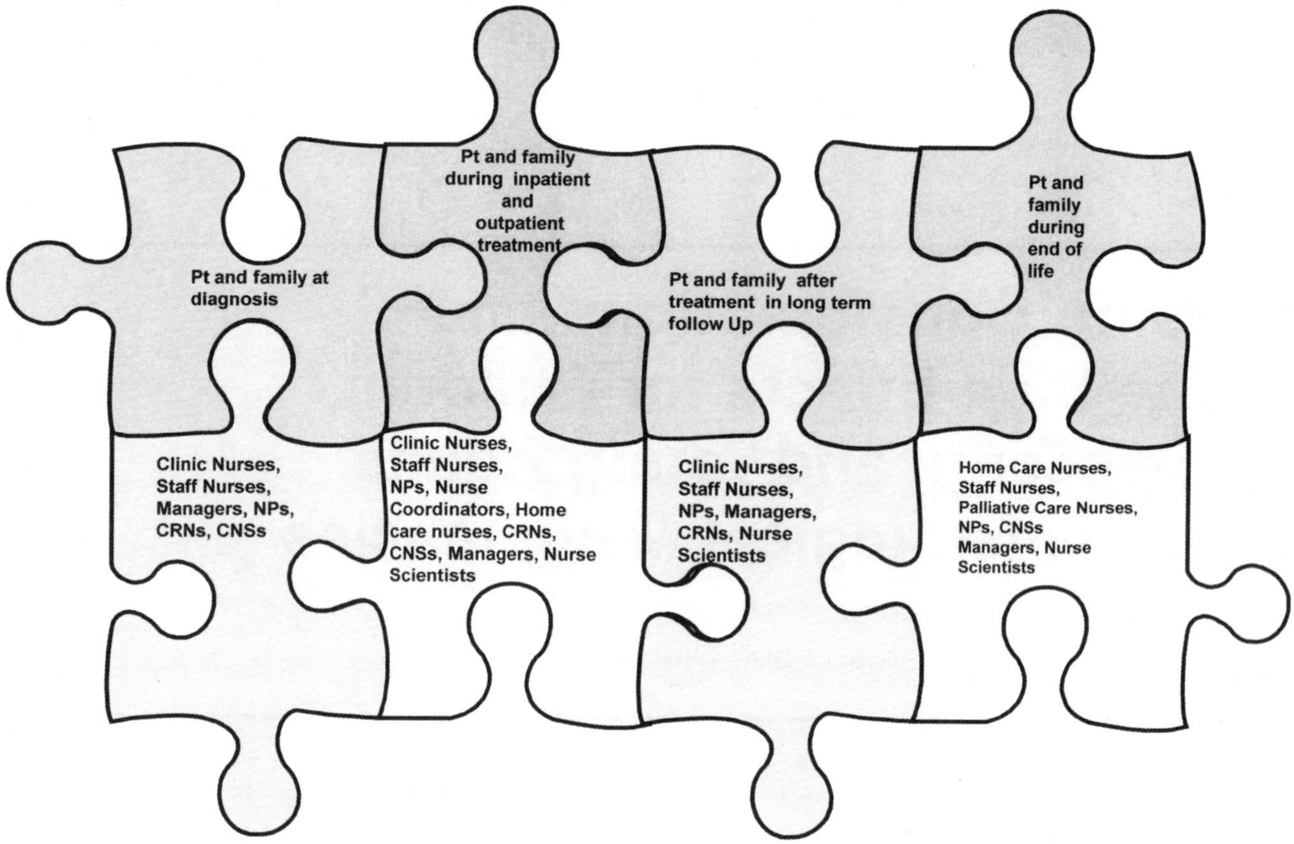

Fig. 27.1. Nursing roles throughout the patient and family cancer experience.
CNSs: clinical nurse specialists; CRNs: clinical research nurses; Pt: patient; NPs: nurse practitioners.

The multidisciplinary team must rely on nurse's various skills and knowledge in partnering toward the long-term survival of these patients. As a specialized nurse, oncology nurses at all levels have a critical role in every step of patient care. Each role brings a focus of caring for this special population of patients. All oncology nurses are committed to providing expert quality clinical care, education and support to patients and families. Selected specialized oncology nursing roles that facilitate the complex care that is required for these patients and families is reviewed. Figure 27.1 depicts various nursing roles that connect the pieces to care for and support patients and families throughout their cancer experience.

Nurse practitioners

Nurse practitioners (NPs) are advanced practice nurses who have completed their masters or doctoral degree and have passed their State board certification in pediatric oncology, pediatrics, or family disciplines. They have been trained in the diagnosis and management of medical conditions. Their responsibilities routinely include performing history and physicals, organizing and monitoring of treatment therapies, interpreting test results, prescribing medications, educating patients and families, and providing patient care. The NP role is widely used in pediatric oncology in various care settings including inpatient, outpatient and private practice settings. NPs usually work in concert with physicians to develop and provide the prescribed plan of care.

Nurse coordinators/navigators

The role of the nurse coordinator is an integral part of the care team. Nurse coordinator responsibilities may vary; however, they remain a designated contact person for patients and families throughout the trajectory of care beginning from the time of diagnosis. Nurse coordinators orchestrate patient referrals, communicate with insurance companies, maintain treatment summaries, coordinate care among multidisciplinary teams, and assist in providing ongoing education to patients and families. NPs often participate in this role, allowing an expanded capacity to perform triage duties and prescribe supportive care when needed. Recently, the term "patient navigator" has been used to describe this role and function appropriately so, as patients are steadily guided and directed to receive their necessary care and support.[1]

Clinical research nurses

Clinical research plays a central role in the advancement of the treatment of childhood cancer. A majority of pediatric oncologists participate in clinical trials either through cooperative groups such as the Children's Oncology Group, the Pediatric Blood and Marrow Transplantation Consortium or through smaller multicenter clinical trials. Patients are strongly encouraged to be treated according to clinical trials as the treatment programs are often the best available therapy or pose opportunity for improved cancer treatment options. The clinical research nurse (CRN) plays an essential role in the research process. The CRN performs an initial patient screening to determine study eligibility and assists the NP or physician in crucial discussions related to the specific treatment plan with patients and families. Providing continuing education to patient and families, clinical care nurses and physicians, and monitoring study patients for any adverse events are definitive aspects of the CRN role. In collaboration with the principal investigating physician, the CRN has responsibility to ensure that the patient receives the correct therapy as outlined in the protocol and has successfully met all pretreatment criteria in a timely manner. Additionally, CRNs maintain regulatory files for all patients on clinical trials and communicates routinely with outside services, groups or industries as appropriate. Nurses who have a background in oncology often find the transition into a research role attractive and feasible and may give them a sense of expanded nursing autonomy. Many clinical research centers also have clinical research associates (CRAs) in place who assist in the data management processes and work closely with CRNs.

Clinical nurse specialists/clinical managers

Clinical nurse specialists (CNSs) or clinical managers are advanced practice nurses who have completed their masters degree and typically work in clinical practice leadership positions. They have received extensive education on the specialized physiological and psychological needs of cancer patients along with nursing leadership and administrative roles. They work closely with nursing staff to ensure ongoing expert clinical care is provided. They also lead and provide patient family and staff education on current and new treatment regimens and modalities. Additionally, they work toward advancing nursing practice through evidence-based research and performance improvement initiatives.

Nurse research scientists/PhDs

Nurse research scientists or nurses with a Doctor of Philosophy (PhD) degree are nurses who have completed a rigorous course of study which is research oriented. The focus of study is on clinical nursing research designed to provide theoretical and scientific knowledge necessary to perform as nursing scholars. The role of these specialized nurses is to build upon and generate new nursing scientific knowledge for the advancement of nursing practice, research, and health care policy. Nurse scientists may practice in academic or clinical practice settings or more recently noted in a combination of both settings. Their expertise and knowledge can assist in bridging the gap between academia and clinical practice to lead nursing research endeavors at the bedside. In relation to caring for children, adolescents and young adults with hematological malignancies, these endeavors may encompass generating new knowledge for improvement of models of care, nursing education, patient outcomes, pain management, and acute side effect management, and quality of life, end-of-life, long-term survivorship and patient family education. These nurses have opportunities to lead a multidisciplinary comprehensive scientifically sound approach in caring for patients with cancer and their families.

Acute Treatment-Related Effects

Despite the successes that have been made in recent years regarding cancer treatment, patient and family untoward experiences related to acute treatment effects remains. Nurses play a vital role in the delivery and administration of cancer treatment protocols. As importantly, nurses are at the forefront in the prevention and management of unpleasant effects that patients may experience. A selection of common acute treatment-related effects in children, adolescents, and young adults with hematological malignancies is reviewed.

Myelosuppression and risk for infection

In general, cancer treatment is myelosuppressive and leaves patients at high risk for infection (see Chapter 25). Patients with hematological malignancies may be at higher risk for infection due to the nature of their illnesses directly involving the bone marrow and a decrease in normal blood cell precursors. Prevention of infection is a significant aspect of providing nursing and supportive care during treatment.[2]

Supportive care medications are used to decrease the risk of infection. Administration of blood growth factors such as granulocyte-colony stimulating factor (G-CSF) and granulocyte macrophage-colony stimulating factor (GM-CSF) may reduce the rate of infection and length of hospitalization in children (0–18 yrs) receiving myelosuppressive chemotherapy.[3] Administration usually begins 24–36 hours following chemotherapy and concludes as per treatment protocol or institutional guidelines. Common practice for the duration of blood growth factors administration is generally 10–14 days or when the absolute neutrophil count (ANC) reaches ≥ 500 mm^3.[4,5] A significant concern when a patient's ANC decreases to suboptimal levels is the risk for opportunistic infections. *Pneumocystis carinii* is an organism that is not usually harmful to those with normal immunity; however it can cause serious complications in an immunocompromised patient. The use of prophylactic trimethoprim-sulfamethoxazole (TPM-SMX) has proven to be effective in the prevention of developing *Pneumocystis carinii* pneumonia (PCP).[2] Guidelines for the administration of TPM-SMX are 150 mg/m^2 twice a day for 3 consecutive days per week.[2] Pentamidine, given aerosolized or intravenously, or an oral medication, dapsone, may be utilized preventatively for patients who cannot tolerate TPM-SMX.[2] Though these alternative prophylactic medications are costly, they are the only option for patients with hypersensitivities to TPM-SMX.[2]

Nurses must be educated on and well prepared to deliver these medications while caring for patients with hematological malignancies throughout their treatment course. Providing patient and family education that includes signs of infection and medication-related side effects such as fever, bone pain, rash, difficulty breathing, uncontrolled diarrhea, or vomiting, is crucial for the well being of these patients and in determining their tolerance of required therapies.

The placement of a central venous catheter (CVC), which provides long-term venous access, is often necessary for the delivery of chemotherapy, blood products, nutrition, and supportive care medications and to obtain frequently required blood specimens in patients with hematological malignancies. Despite the significant advantages of a CVC, this device carries a high risk of morbidity and mortality related to infection as it has direct access into the bloodstream of immunocompromised patients for extended lengths of time. CVC-related infections may be identified by the patient's clinical condition and laboratory-confirmed organisms found in blood samples obtained via the CVC, the catheter tip, and peripheral blood.[6] The source of infectious organisms may be directly related to the port of entry at the exit site of the catheter or from intrinsic immunocompromised patient flora. Skin organisms may easily migrate through subcutaneous tissue and colonize at the tip of the catheter. The catheter hub is also a common site of infection that may harbor organisms to cause CVC bacteremia.[7] It is imperative that nurses provide evidence-based CVC care for the prevention of potentially life-threatening infections. There is ongoing national effort to implement and enforce a collective set of evidence-based CVC care guidelines known as CVC evidence-based bundles. When CVC bundles of care are performed collectively and consistently, there are reports of reduced CVC-related bloodstream infections.[8–10] Nurses are the frontline CVC care providers and are responsible for consistent adherence in performing CVC evidence-based bundle care. Evidence-based CVC bundle care includes appropriate hand hygiene, maximum sterile barrier precautions upon CVC insertion, skin and site care with 2% chlorhexidine (Chloraprep®), applying a chlorhexidine-impregnated patch (biopatch®) directly over catheter exit site, and utilizing an occlusive dressing over the exit site.[11]

Prior to a patient's initial discharge to return home with a CVC in place, the patients and families must be competent in CVC home care. They must be able to perform dressing changes, cap changes, saline and heparin flushes, verbalize recognition of signs and symptoms of infection, and perform CVC emergency care. Nurses are responsible to ensure patients and families are able to verbalize and demonstrate adequate CVC home care techniques. Proper home care is essential in the prevention of CVC-related infections.[6,7] Table 27.1 provides a summary of general CVC home care guidelines.

In the event of a fever-related admission, nurses must assess patients for signs of infection. If a child is hospitalized for fever and neutropenia, they are at great risk for septic shock.[2] Vital signs must be closely monitored. Early signs of septic shock include fever (temperature > 38.5 °C) or hypothermia, delayed capillary refill, and weak peripheral pulses. Delayed signs are hypotension, tachycardia, changes in level of consciousness, and decreased urine output. Early recognition and intervention

Table 27.1. General central venous catheter (CVC) home care guidelines.

Locate and properly utilize CVC clamp	Locate and demonstrate open and closed position, close on thick padded part when not in use.
Recognize signs or symptoms of infection	Notify MD immediately for fever, chills, redness, tenderness, swelling or pain.
Special reminders	Wash hands thoroughly with alcohol-based waterless gel or soap and water prior to all CVC care. Protect from water during bathing or showering. Always have clamp available. Never reuse supplies. No rough play or contact sports. Inform school nurse, staff or new healthcare providers of CVC in place. Coil, tape, and secure CVC. CVC care done in a clean dry room. Seek a helper during CVC care for small children. Always close CVC clamp when injection cap if off and CVC line is open to air.
CVC site care	Change dressing weekly, when wet, soiled or falling off or as directed. Check site for signs of infection with each dressing change. Utilize appropriate skin care to CVC site: > 2 months chloraprep® swab/biopatch®; < 2 months alcohol and betadine Cover with transparent dressing.
CVC flush procedure	Daily flush or as directed. Utilize weight-appropriate heparin flush as directed. Always check expiration date of heparin flush
CVC cap change	Change cap weekly or as directed Prep cap and catheter junction with alcohol or chloraprep® as directed NS and/or heparin flush CVC prior to applying new injection cap Careful not to contaminate new injection cap prior to placing on CVC
Emergency care	Notify MD immediately for any signs of infection. Clamp CVC immediately if torn, cut or leaking. Apply pressure to exit site if CVC has been pulled or falls out. Clamp CVC if injection cap comes off. Secure dressing and notify MD if CVC cuff is exposed out of exit site. If CVC does not flush easily, do not force and notify MD. Call 911 if patient becomes short of breath, complains of chest pain or turns a dusky blue color and lie patient on their left side.

Adapted from Childrens Hospital Los Angeles, CVC Home Care Guidelines, Secola, R. *et al.*, 2009.

is imperative to ensure a positive patient outcome. Nurses should be prompt in assessing for signs of septic shock and aggressive in obtaining orders for rapid interventions, including oxygen and support ventilation, isotonic fluid bolus, administration of antibiotics, or electrolyte correction as needed. If the patient does not respond to initial interventions, vasopressors and close monitoring in the intensive care unit is often warranted.[12]

Teaching patients and families about myelosuppression and the risk of infection is a vital aspect of nursing care for these patients. It is critical for patients and families to be knowledgeable about the risk of immunosuppression in order to most effectively prevent infection.[13]

Proper handwashing is the primary form of prevention against nosocomial infection and limits the spread of antimicrobial resistance.[14] Nurses should wash hands before and after each contact with a patient and, most importantly, prior to CVC care. Patients and families must be properly educated on the importance of handwashing in order to further increase the protection of the patient.[2] Conducting hand washing demonstrations for patients and families and having pictures and signs available are ways in which nurses can assist in patient family understanding and adherence to proper hand hygiene.

Avascular necrosis and osteoporosis

Avascular necrosis (AVN) is classified by decreased bone density and manifests as joint pain, generally caused by slipped capital femoral epiphysis (see Chapter 24)[4,7] AVN is most commonly seen in children less than 4 years of age during the treatment of Hodgkin lymphoma (HL) and non-Hodgkin lymphoma (NHL); however, it can be seen in adolescents and young adults.[4] It is commonly attributed to radiation therapy and corticosteroid administration; however, certain chemotherapeutic agents have been implicated such as methotrexate, cyclophosphamide, and fluorouracil.

AVN is most commonly seen in children with hematological malignancies vs. other pediatric cancers.[4] Nurses must be vigilant in monitoring for any patient complaints of bone or joint pain upon physical assessment.

The use of corticosteroids in the treatment of hematological malignancies in children, adolescents, and young adults increases the risk of osteoporosis, along with the added poor nutrition, weight loss, low body weight, and decrease physical activity often seen in patients with hematological malignancies secondary to chemotherapy and radiation therapy treatment.[15] Thirty to fifty percent of patients develop osteoporosis, with the fastest decrease of bone density experienced within the first 6 months to 1 year of treatment.[15]

Osteopenia and osteoporosis are caused by multiple factors seen throughout cancer treatment. The intake of calcium can aid in bone reabsorption. Its absorption in the gut depends on the presence of vitamin D. Nurses should ensure that their patients are receiving adequate, age-appropriate doses of calcium and vitamin D throughout treatment to help decrease their risk of developing significant bone density loss.[15]

Central nervous system toxicities and cognitive impairment

Though most central nervous system (CNS) toxicities manifest as late effects of treatment, acute CNS toxicities are seen in children, adolescents, and young adults with hematological malignancies (see Chapter 24). Most commonly, the CNS is affected due to chemotherapeutic drugs. Vinca alkyloids are the main class of chemotherapy that causes cranial nerve and CNS deficits.[16] Symptoms attributed to CNS toxicity include jaw pain, ptosis of the eye, vocal cord paralysis, and foot drop. Peripheral neuropathy, numbness, or tingling is linked to cytotoxic agents such as vinca alkyloids and additionally to cisplatin, carboplatin, etoposide, cytarabine, and taxanes.[16,17] L-asparaginase and methotrexate toxicity can lead to encephalopathy. Administration of intrathecal chemotherapy increases the risk of CNS acute effects, such as encephalopathy and seizures.[18]

Acute cognitive and behavioral changes in patients with hematological malignancies are often attributed to their treatment regimen of chemotherapy, corticosteroid administration, and radiation therapy. Altered mental status can be seen as a result of chemotherapy, including L-asparaginase, cisplatin, carboplatin, ifosfamide, and methotrexate.[16,17] Symptoms will manifest as personality changes, mood swings, depression, failure to meet developmental milestones, and loss of short-term memory. Confusion and alteration in level of consciousness may also occur.[16]

Management of acute CNS effects begins with a thorough neurological assessment. The nurse must have a baseline for the patient's neurological status in order to note any significant changes. Assessment should include level of consciousness, alertness of patient, cranial nerve testing, strength and sensation in extremities, deep tendon reflexes, and observations of gait. Once a change in the neurological examination is noted, further assessment and investigation should take place.[16,18] Nurses must provide thorough patient family education on the side effects and monitoring for neurological consequences of chemotherapy agents known to cause CNS toxicities or cognitive impairments. Noted toxicities or impairments may lead to necessary adjustment in treatment regimens to prevent any further injury.

Bleeding and thrombosis

The intense therapy utilized to treat patients with hematological malignancies often causes thrombocytopenia (see Chapter 30). Thrombocytopenia occurs due to the destruction of rapidly dividing blood cells, particularly fragile megakaryocytes which produce platelets. Though there is varying protocol or institutional guidelines regarding prophylactic platelet transfusions, it is important for nurses to assess patients for signs of bleeding. Spontaneous life-threatening hemorrhage can occur if platelet levels fall below 20,000/mm^3 but is rarely seen among children in treatment. However non–life-threatening bleeding may lead to more serious complications if left untreated.[4] Current research is addressing the fact that children may be able to tolerate low platelet levels without incident.[4,19]

When caring for patients who are thrombocytopenic, the nurse should place them on bleeding precautions and educate patients and families. These precautions may include brushing teeth using soft toothettes, eating soft foods, and avoiding contact sports or rough play. The use of medications such as aspirin and ibuprofen are contraindicated due to their anticoagulation effect.[7] Female patients should be placed on oral contraceptives to suppress menstruation. Nurses must observe the patient for significant bruising, gingival bleeding, epistaxis, and bloody stools. Furthermore, the nurse must note any significant drop in hemoglobin. Signs of active bleeding will require blood product transfusion.[2,7]

More serious than thrombocytopenia is the occurrence of disseminated intravascular coagulation (DIC). DIC most commonly occurs during induction therapy.[20] When initial chemotherapy is administered, cancerous cells release procoagulant substances.[20] This process leads to the formation of microthrombi, the consumption of platelets and clotting factors, and ultimately concurrent thrombosis and hemorrhage. The patient will demonstrate signs of DIC with a decreased platelet count, increased prothrombin, decreased fibrinogen, and positive D-dimer.[7,20] DIC is potentially life threatening, thus early detection of DIC is imperative, including close monitoring of the patient's laboratory values. In addition to monitoring laboratory values, nursing interventions include monitoring the patient for signs of bleeding and ensuring adequate oxygenation and tissue perfusion. Medical management of DIC involves blood product transfusion, such as fresh frozen plasma (FFP), platelets, cryoprecipitate and packed red blood cells.[7]

Cerebrovascular accidents (CVA) can occur in patients with cancer due to several factors. Patients with hyperleukocytosis which involves an abnormally excessive number of leukocytes in the blood that may block blood supply to vital organs such as the brain and may be detected in patients with acute myeloid leukemia (AML), acute monoblastic leukemia, or acute lymphocytic leukemia (ALL), are at increased risk.[4] CVAs are generally seen during induction therapy. If a patient is in DIC, the formation of thrombi may lead to a CVA.[4]

Liver and renal dysfunction

Patients undergoing intense chemotherapy and radiation therapy are at risk for chemical hepatitis.[16] Defined as a nonviral inflammation of the liver, chemical hepatitis results when hepatocytes are destroyed and enzymes are released into the bloodstream. The enzymes, alanine transaminase (ALT) and aspartate transaminase (AST), will be elevated in serum laboratory values. Infants are at an increased risk of developing this complication, as their immature organs metabolize chemotherapeutic drugs less efficiently than older children.[16] Nurses must be aware of trends in liver function laboratory values before determining the safety of administering chemotherapy.

The renal system is also at risk for developing complications as a result of treatment. Through the administration of chemotherapy, precipitation of metabolites may occur, causing an obstruction in the renal tubules.[16] Drugs associated with acute renal failure are ifosfamide, methotrexate, carboplatin, and cisplatin.[21] Nurses should monitor for renal dysfunction symptoms including unbalanced input and output, weight gain, hypertension, tachycardia, tachypnea, abnormal urine chemistry, and ascites. Significant changes in laboratory values, such as elevated serum creatinine, BUN, and uric acid, and abnormal electrolyte values, may indicate renal complications.[21] Renal impairment is generally not a chronic issue, however early identification and adequate hydration during chemotherapy administration is necessary for the least long-term effects.[21]

Gastrointestinal effects

Acute gastrointestinal (GI) side effects that patients may experience are the direct result of the chemotherapeutic agents and/or radiation therapy administered. The rapidly dividing cells of the lining of the GI tract are easily damaged by the cytotoxic therapies and subsequently produce a range of mild to severe symptoms.

As the intensity of chemotherapy regimens has increased, so has the incidence of oral mucositis/stomatitis in children, adolescents, and young adults. Stomatitis/mucositis is a known GI side effect of cancer treatment. This condition can range from a localized oral mucosal erythema to a moderate to severe GI tract hemorrhage. During daily oral and GI assessments, nurses are able to identify the presence of symptoms related to mucositis and stomatitis such as mucosal swelling, redness, ulcers, bleeding, oral or GI pain, or bloody emesis or stool. Appropriate nursing management includes enforcement of basic oral hygiene and pain control. Optimal oral hygiene is the first-line defense against developing complications associated with mucositis/stomatitis. Optimal oral care is generally defined by regular tooth brushing two to three times daily with oral rinses of non-abrasive solutions. In the case of thrombocytopenia, a toothette may replace a regular toothbrush.[22]

Pharmacological prevention and treatment regimens for oral mucositis may vary among institutions, as there has been little research to prove that one agent is superior to another. However, medications commonly used are chlorhexidine gluconate mouthwash, nystatin swish and swallow solution, and clotrimazole troches.[7] Pain control may include basic analgesics, such as acetaminophen. For more intense complaints of pain or the progression of mucositis/stomatitis, the patient may require intravenous opioids. Since oral mucosal cells and leukocytes have similar renewal rates, there has been a positive correlation made between myelosuppression and mucositis.[23]

Children, adolescents, and young adults undergoing cancer treatment are at high risk of developing malnutrition due to the effects of aggressive treatment, such as nausea, vomiting, diarrhea, taste changes, mucositis, and anorexia. A patient's nutritional status should be assessed within 24 to 48 hours upon every admission. Changes in weight and oral intake should be noted. Generally, a nutritional screening is conducted by a registered dietician; however, it is a nursing responsibility to note any changes in weight, oral intake, or any significant changes in laboratory values, such as hypoglycemia and decrease high-density lipoprotein (HDL) levels — both signs of malnutrition.[24] Providing patients and families with suggestions on foods and fluids high in protein and calories or high caloric food additives are key nursing interventions.

Nausea and vomiting are among the most common side effects of chemotherapy treatment. Nausea is a subjective symptom described as the need to vomit, while vomiting is the actual contraction of abdominal muscles and expulsion of gastric contents.[7,25] Nausea and vomiting can occur acutely, during or shortly after a chemotherapy infusion, or delayed, meaning 24 hours or more after chemotherapy is administered. Vomiting is one of the most "dreaded" side effects of treatment, thus it is the nurse's responsibility to try to manage this symptom as effectively as possible.[25] Furthermore, vomiting can lead to additional complications, such as dehydration, electrolyte imbalances, weight loss, and potential aspiration, especially in the case of infants undergoing treatment.

Effective antiemetics include ondansetron, lorazepam, metoclopramide with diphenhydramine, promethazine, hydroxyzine, and dronabinol. Dexamethasone may be administered if the patient is not on a steroid regimen.[7] Table 27.2 lists commonly used pharmacologic regimens for chemotherapy-induced nausea and vomiting. The nurse should continuously assess the effectiveness of antiemetic therapy and seek alterative or adjunct regimens or interventions including for patients who experience anticipatory nausea or vomiting. Table 27.3 describes nursing management for anticipatory nausea and vomiting.

Allergic and hypersensitivity reactions

Allergic reactions and hypersensitivity reactions may occur when a patient is exposed to certain chemotherapy or biological agents, and often manifests as bronchospasm, airway edema, or sudden drop in blood pressure.[16] Less severe reactions include rash, chills, fever, pruritis, hives, redness or swelling at injection site. Allergic reactions are normally graded based on the severity of the patient's symptoms. Chemotherapeutic agents most commonly associated with allergic reactions are etoposide and L-asparaginase.[16] Noncytotoxic therapies that patients may receive throughout their treatment course such as blood products and antibiotics, specifically vancomycin or amphotericin B, may also elicit allergic or hypersensitivity reactions.[16]

Nursing management involves immediate interruption of intravenous infusions, administration of medications such as diphenhydramine or hydrocortisone, and the possible use of epinephrine in severe cases.[16] Documentation of patient allergies or previous allergic type reactions and patient and family teaching regarding allergic reactions is necessary to prevent future reactions. Preventative interventions may include premedications prior to future administrations or a change in the route or duration of administration of the identified drug.[16]

Table 27.2. Commonly used pharmacologic regimens for chemotherapy-induced nausea and vomiting.

Agents with low emetic potential (e.g. vincristine, L-asparginase, etoposide)	**Agents with moderate emetic potential (e.g. doxorubicin, cyclophosphamide, ifosfamide, methotrexate)**	**Agents with high emetic potential (e.g. cisplatin, high-dose cyclophosphamide and cytarabine)**
1st Line: Ondansetron prior to chemotherapy	**1st Line:** Ondansetron prior to chemotherapy and at 4–6 hrs post (max: 2–3 doses daily)	**1st Line:** Ondansetron prior to chemotherapy and every 4–6 hrs ATC
2nd Line: Ondansetron prior to chemotherapy and at 4–6 hrs post (max: 2 doses daily)	**2nd Line:** Add dexamethasone, unless contraindicated due to diagnosis or medication regimen	**2nd Line:** Add dexamethasone, unless contraindicated due to diagnosis or medication regimen
	3rd Line: **Additional alternatives:** • Promethazine • Hydroxyzine • Metoclopramide with diphenhydramine • Aprepitant • Palonosetron	**3rd Line:** Add dronabinol
		4th Line: Stop ondansetron and start granisetron every 12 hrs.
		5th Line: **Additional alternatives:** • Promethazine • Hydroxyzine • Metoclopramide with diphenhydramine • Aprepitant • Palonosetron

ATC: Around the clock.
Adapted from Nursing Care of Children and Adolescents with Cancer, Baggot, C.R., *et al.*, W.B. Saunders Co., 2002.

Table 27.3. Nursing management for anticipatory nausea and vomiting.

Distraction	**Chemotherapy infusion accommodations**	**Pharmacological interventions**
• Television • Music • Favorite movies • Card games • Board games • Video/electronic games • Arts and crafts • Books	• Begin while patient is sleeping, nighttime delivery options • Keep medication or infusions out of patient's direct view • Cover or disguise bottle/bag of chemotherapy out of patient's direct view	• Premedication for patient with lorazepam or other anti-anxiolytic or sedative agents.

Pain

Pain is experienced by patients undergoing treatment due to several factors, such as the disease itself, effects of treatment, painful procedures, or issues unrelated to the hematological malignancy, such as preexisting problems or acute trauma.[7] It is the responsibility of the nurse to assess the location, quality, and intensity of pain. The nurse must "listen", "support", and record the patient's self report as pain is subjective and always what the patient states it is.[26] It is important that the nurse utilizes an age-appropriate pain assessment tool to establish the intensity of the patient's pain, and thus determine what class of analgesic is the most appropriate.[5] Non-steroidal anti-inflammatory drugs (NSAIDS), such as acetaminophen, are useful for mild chronic or acute pain. However, the uses of opioids are the most effective intervention for pain management for moderate to severe pain.[7]

In addition to using medication for pain management, there are appropriate nonpharmacological nursing interventions that can be employed. Applying heat or cold to the affected area is a common practice, though contraindicated where there is any tissue breakdown, as extreme temperatures may cause further damage and pain.[7] Distractions, such as toys, games, books, television, or movies, can divert the patient's focus from their pain to an enjoyable activity. Guided imagery helps the patient imagine being in a pleasant and safe place. It involves breathing exercises, leading to muscle relaxation, and subsequent pain relief.[7]

Tumor lysis syndrome

A significant metabolic complication associated with initial chemotherapy administration for various subtypes of hematological malignancies is known as tumor lysis syndrome (TLS) (see Chapter 30). TLS is defined as the development of severe metabolic abnormalities that include hyperuricemia, hyperphosphatemia, hypocalcemia, and hyperkalemia.[27] These abnormalities can lead to acute renal failure and more significantly life-threatening complications. Due to the high growth fraction, high proliferative rate and the hypersensitivity to cytotoxic therapy of these diseases, there is abrupt release of intracellular ions, nucleic acids, proteins and their metabolites which may overwhelm the patient's normal homeostatic mechanisms and cause severe metabolic disorders.[28] Therefore, these patients are at great risk for TLS. Vigorous measures should be taken to minimize the risk of patients developing severe TLS, renal failure or life-threatening metabolic complications.

Nursing responsibilities include working collaboratively with the team to, first and foremost, identify patient risk factors for TLS. Furthermore, nursing interventions should include completing a thorough patient history, physical assessment, obtaining and evaluating initial laboratory findings, initiating adequate intravenous hydration, and administering anti-hyperuricemic agents prior to the initiation of cytotoxic therapy. Once the patient begins treatment, nursing care includes astute monitoring of laboratory values, intake and output, vital signs and any signs and symptoms of potential metabolic abnormalities. Ongoing cares entails administration of supportive medications, intravenous fluids, and prompt communication to the team for the management of any metabolic abnormalities that may arise. It may be necessary to collaborate with critical care teams to ensure that a higher level of monitoring or interventions is readily available if needed. Table 27.4 reviews nursing guidelines for the prevention and management of TLS.

Long-Term Treatment-Related Effects

Over the past 20 years, advancements for the treatment of childhood cancer has led to an 80% overall survival rate.[29,30] It is estimated that there are currently 270,000 survivors of childhood cancer, and that 1 in 570 of them are ages 20 to 40 years.[30,31] However, survivors of childhood cancer may face additional complications stemming from the cancer itself, the chemotherapy and/or radiation, and the supportive care that they received (see Chapter 24). It is estimated that approximately 50% of all survivors will experience some dysfunction as a result of their cancer treatment.[29] Many studies have shown that two out of three survivors of childhood cancer experience at least one long-term effect.[30] Nursing plays a vital role in the management of long-term effects through monitoring, providing education to increase awareness, providing recommendations and resources for screening of long-term effects, as well as providing support and management as conditions occur. Offering these resources, nurses can empower patients to be vigilant about continuing to seek follow up care related to known long-term effects. For example, nurses can provide education to patients who have received mediastinal or testicular radiation on the importance of and how to conduct breast or testicular self-examinations. Nurses can direct discussions on risk factors and signs and symptoms related to long-term effects. Additionally, nurses should review the patient's current health problems and medication use, reproductive status, health behaviors, quality of life, and psychosocial functioning.[32]

Childhood, adolescent and young adult cancer survivors may face physical, developmental, and psychological problems following their therapy. These problems may include anxiety, hearing loss, cataracts, obesity, thyroid problems, as well as major organ toxicities. The following is a selection of the most common late effects that have been described in the literature.

Cardiac dysfunction

The effects of certain chemotherapeutic agents, notably anthracyclines and high-dose cyclophosphamide, as well as mediastinal radiation therapy, may lead to a number of cardiac complications. These complications may appear months and years following completion of therapy.

Table 27.4. Nursing management for tumor lysis syndrome (TLS).

TLS pretreatment measures and prevention	▶ Maintain intravenous hydration-3L/m^2/day D5 ¼ **NO Potassium** ▶ Maintain urine output > 100cc/m^2/hr ▶ Maintain urine specific gravity < 1.010 ▶ If required, maintain $NaHCO_3$ alkalinization with urine pH 6.5–7.5 ▶ Obtain weight BID ▶ Administer antihyperuricemic agent as ordered ▶ Administer diuretic(s) as indicated ▶ Obtain baseline hematology and chemistry blood specimens ▶ Monitor VS, lab values ▶ Place on cardiac monitor as indicated ▶ Minimize additional potassium or phosphorous intake ▶ Ensure metabolic stability **PRIOR** to the start of cytotoxic therapy
Treatment plan and medication delivery	▶ Administer cytotoxic therapy as ordered ▶ Administer antihyperuricemic agent as ordered → Allopurinol (Alloprim™) PO divided BID or TID → Allopurinol (Alloprim™) IV divided in 1–3 doses → Rasburicase (Fasturtec®/Elitek®) IV Q day for 1–3 days ▶ Maintain $NaHCO_3$ alkalinization if required ▶ Obtain and frequent monitoring of laboratory specimens as ordered ▶ Ongoing assessment and monitoring for signs or symptoms of metabolic abnormalities
Management of metabolic abnormalities	▶ Hyperkalemia ≥ 6.0 mEq/L → As indicated: sodium polystyrene sulfonate; furosemide, glucose/insulin, sodium bicarbonate, hemofiltration/dialysis, calcium gluconate ▶ Hyperphosphatemia ≥ 6.5 mg/dL → As indicated: aluminum hydroxide, dietary and medication phosphate restriction, glucose/insulin, furosemide, hemofiltration/dialysis ▶ Hypocalcemia ≤ 7.0 mg/dL → As indicated: control hyperphosphatemia, seizure precautions, calcium gluconate

BID: twice a day; PO: by mouth; TID: three times a day; VS: vital signs; IV: intravenous.
Adapted from: The Childrens Oncology Group (COG) Tumor Lysis Nursing Guidelines. Secola, R. *et al.*, COG Nursing Discipline, 2006.

The therapy may cause permanent damage to the myocytes, which has been known to lead to cardiomyopathy, congestive heart failure, coronary artery disease or arrhythmias.[29] Cerebrovascular disease is another complication in patients with ALL or HL who have received radiation therapy. In particular, leukemia survivors reported a stroke rate of 58 per 100,000 person years, with a relative risk of 5.9 compared to their healthy siblings.[31] HL survivors had a 5.6-fold increased risk for stroke compared to their health siblings if they were treated with mantle radiation therapy.[31]

Nursing care for patients at risk for cardiac complications focuses on maintaining a healthy lifestyle by eating a well-balanced heart healthy diet, maintaining a healthy weight, and incorporating exercise into their daily routines. Nurses continually need to educate patients and families on the risks, signs and symptoms of cardiac problems, and encourage them to receive routine follow up care.

Pulmonary dysfunction

Chronic dysfunction of the respiratory system, especially in those patients who have received radiation therapy to their lungs, or treatment with known pulmonary toxic agents such as bleomycin, busulfan, or carmustine, has been widely reported in childhood cancer survivors.[33] It is common that patients report symptoms indicative of pulmonary fibrosis including, dyspnea on exertion, fatigue, and cough. Younger children are susceptible to these complications as the therapy impairs normal growth and development of their anatomy.[29] A Childhood Cancer Survivor study reported that survivors had an increased relative risk compared to healthy siblings of pulmonary dysfunction, including respiratory distress, diminished lung capacity, collapsed lung and lung calcification.[33] Of significance, this study reported that lung transplantation had occurred at least 5 years into survivorship. The rate of lung fibrosis was higher for patients diagnosed at age 15 years or more compared to those diagnosed at less than 5 years of age. However, for those who received both pulmonary toxic chemotherapy alone or in combination with chest radiation had an increased incidence of lung fibrosis up to 15 years after diagnosis. The incidence for patients who received chest radiation continued to increase up to 25 years after diagnosis.[33]

The risks of pulmonary complications are often discussed with patients and families before, during, and after the completion of cancer treatment. However, ongoing nursing education with patients and families includes the potential risks, and monitoring for symptoms, as well as providing support and resources for long-term pulmonary complications.

Neurological complications

Neurocognitive complications can be devastating for patients and families. Patients who received whole-brain irradiation, or treatment with certain chemotherapeutic agents, such as methotrexate, are at risk for developing neurocognitive problems following completion of therapy.[34] Subtle changes may be observed such as a decline in their academic achievements, delay in motor function and memory, or overt symptoms such as seizures and leukoenchephalopathy.[29] Recently, treatments for certain childhood cancers are decreasing or eliminating radiation therapy in hopes to mitigate this long-term sequelae.[35]

The literature reveals that the most common neurocognitive complications with chemotherapy alone for treatment of ALL include problems with visual processing, visual-motor functioning, attention and executive functioning.[35] Nurses play an essential role in monitoring patients for neurocognitive changes, as well as providing support and educational resources for patients and families as needed. Such resources may include: referrals for neurocognitive testing, and information on federal laws regarding The Americans with Disability Act and the Individuals with Disabilities Education Act. Additionally, nurses can work with the patient's school administrators, staff and teachers, on a plan for the patient's transition back to school, and provide education on and monitoring for potential neurocognitive long-term effects that may develop.[36]

Fertility issues

The effects of chemotherapy and/or radiation therapy on reproductive organs in both males and females have been widely reported, suggesting that these patients have a higher risk of fertility issues. It is estimated that 15–30% of pediatric cancer survivors are sterile.[37] The Children's Oncology Group (COG) performed a retrospective review of 6000 women childhood cancer survivors. The results reported that overall female survivors were less likely to become pregnant compared to healthy siblings.[38] A detailed analysis revealed that survivors who were young (0–4 years) at diagnosis had the highest risk of becoming pregnant.[38] Risk factors for an increased incidence of ovarian failure included hypothalamic/pituitary radiation at doses greater than 30 Gy, ovarian/uterine radiation at doses greater than 5 Gy, and treatment with alkylating chemotherapeutic agents.[38]

Upon completion of therapy and during yearly follow up visits, ongoing nursing assessment of the patients' sexual function and development will aid in detecting long-term fertility issues. Nurses may also provide education and resources regarding fertility options for developmentally and age-appropriate patients both prior to initiation of therapy as well as post-therapy.[36] Nurses also play a role in ensuring fertility options such as sperm or egg banking is presented to patients and families at the time of diagnosis.

Secondary malignancies

Over the past 20 years, the advancements in the treatment for children with hematological malignancies have led to the rise in both disease-free and overall survival rates. However, the incidence of these survivors developing treatment-related secondary malignancies is two- to threefold greater than the general population.[39] The highest incidences of secondary primary cancers are divided into two groups: chemotherapy-related myelodysplasia (MDS)/AML and radiation-related solid tumor second malignant neoplasm. The former develops less than 3 years from the original diagnosis.[39] Known chemotherapeutic agents that cause MDS and AML include alkylating agents and topoisomerase II inhibitors.[39,40] The development of a solid tumor after radiotherapy accounts for about 80% of all secondary malignancies, and the most prevalent are lung, breast, and thyroid cancers as well as brain tumors and sarcomas.[39] Historically, these types of secondary malignancies do not present until 5 to 10 years after treatment.[40] Early detection and routine screening is essential in this group of patients.

Nurses are at the forefront in providing education and resources for patients and families as patients transition into adult care settings. Secondary cancers are the leading cause of nonrelapse late mortality and serious morbidity for childhood cancer survivors.[39] With early detection and continued education, there may be a decrease in this high incidence and provision of improved quality of life for these patients.

Health Promotion After Childhood Cancer

As more children become survivors of childhood cancer, there has been a large movement to develop long-term effects clinics and programs. The development of multidisciplinary teams to address long-term physical, as well as psychosocial effects of survivorship, is critical to provide comprehensive and holistic care to this population. Nurses are a primary source of support and information, and play a critical role in ensuring successful transition of patients and families once they leave the oncology setting. Nurses are able to empower patients and families to advocate for themselves by preparing them to navigate the healthcare system to ensure adequate long-term follow up care for monitoring and managing any long-term effects.[30] A multidisciplinary team in the COG developed Long-Term Follow-Up Guidelines for survivors of childhood, adolescent and young adult cancers in 2008.[41] These guidelines include a comprehensive review of and recommendations for the prevention and management of treatment-related long-term effects and survivorship issues. Table 27.5

Table 27.5. Long-term effects of cancer survivors.

System	Known causes	Long-term effects	Symptoms	Special monitoring
Cardiac	Doxorubicin Daunorubicin Idarubicin Mitoxantrone Epirubicin Radiation therapy Chest or thorax Spine Abdomen Total body irradiation	Left ventricular dysfunction Cadiomyopathy Arrhythmias Valvular stenosis/insufficiency Pericardial fibrosis Coronary artery disease	Shortness of breath Fatigue Dizziness Chest pain Lower extremity edema Irregular and/or rapid heartbeat	EKG Echocardiogram/ MUGA scan Cardiac stress test Blood work: lipid profile and fasting glucose
Pulmonary	Bleomycin Carmustine Lomustine Busulfan Chest radiation therapy Total body irradiation Chronic GVHD Surgery to lungs/chest	Pulmonary fibrosis Recurrent lung infection Bronchiolitis obliterans Restrictive/obstructive lung disease	Shortness of breath Frequent coughing/wheezing Chest pain Infection	Chest X-ray Pulmonary function tests
Neurological	Diagnosis at a very young age Cytarabine (high dose) Brain surgery Radiation (brain, TBI) Cisplatin/carboplatin Methotrexate	Difficulties learning	Problems with: Attention span Ability to complete tasks on time Memory Planning/organization Problem solving	Neuropsychological testing

(*Continued*)

Table 27.5. (*Continued*)

System	Known causes	Long-term effects	Symptoms	Special monitoring
Female Health	Cyclophosphamide Carboplatin Cisplatin Nitrogen mustard Busulfan Carmustine Melphalan Thiotepa Ifosfamide Radiation	Failure to enter puberty Cessation of menstrual cycles Lack of estrogen production Infertility pregnancy risks		Yearly check-up Blood tests: FSH, LH, estradiol Possible endocrinologist referral Bone density test
Male Health	Cyclophosphamide Busulfan Carmustine Ifosfamide Melphalan Carboplatin Cisplatin Nitrogen mustard Procarbazines Testicular radiation Brain radiation TBI	Infertility Testoterone deficiency		Yearly check-up including hormone and puberty status Possible endocrinologist referral Blood tests: FSH, LH, testosterone
Secondary Cancers	Cyclophosphamide Nitrogen mustard Etoposide Teniposide Doxorubicin Daunorubicin Hematopoietic cell transplant Radiation therapy	Leukemias Solid tumors	New/persistant symptoms including: easy bruising/ bleeding, paleness of skin, fatigue, bone pain, abdominal pain, blood in stool/urine, lumps, shortness of breath, persistant headaches,	Yearly comprehensive health check-up

EKG: electrocardiogram; FSH: follicle-stimulating hormone; GVHD: graft-vs.-host disease; LH: luteinizing hormone; MUGA: multigated acquisition scan; TBI: total body irradiation.
Adapted from: The CureSearch Children's Oncology Group Long-Term Follow-Up Guidelines, October 2008, Health Links at www.survivorshipguidelines.org.

highlights a sample of some known long-term effects, causes, symptoms and special monitoring that are detailed on the health links related to these survivorship guidelines.

Nurses should also continually assess patients and families for signs of concern regarding the fear of relapse. Triggers for this concern may include frequent questioning about results, or the need for frequent checkups or testing, or specific patient complaints that may indicate a sign of relapse. Open discussions and exploring with them what might happen or ensuring them that there will be assistance if needed may alleviate their levels of fear and anxiety.

Special Nursing Considerations for Adolescents and Young Adults

Adolescent and young adult patients present additional psychosocial and physical issues that require special attention during their diagnosis, treatment and in long-term follow up (see Chapter 3). Their quality of life is influenced by unique issues including sense of mortality, self-image, independence, self-esteem, potential physical, and/or cognitive changes as well as financial issues, family responsibilities and job stability. Each of these areas need to be examined and addressed in hopes to support this population of patients to thrive as independent adults with a desirable quality of life.

The development of independence at this stage of life is dramatically affected by a cancer diagnosis. Rather than strive towards independence, patients tend to become more dependent and angry, and parents may tend to become overprotective.[37] Although they are currently "children", it is imperative to include adolescents and young adults along with their parents or significant others in treatment discussions. These crucial conversations should include potential side effects and their management, to better prepare them physically and emotionally during treatment and post-treatment courses. Physical changes such as losing hair, central venous catheter placement, undergoing surgery and potential remaining limitations or scars, gaining or losing weight, or isolation from peers or coworkers may have negative consequences on their quality of life. These changes may also make it difficult for them to cope with diagnosis and treatment and affect their mood and self-esteem. A change in physical appearance may have a greater impact than the cancer diagnosis and treatment for some adolescents and young adults.[37] Providing resources for physical and emotional support for this vulnerable patient population will greatly impact their ability to cope with their diagnosis and treatment course and future lives. Additionally, nurses must work closely with this subpopulation to educate them on the added risks of participating in unhealthy behaviors, such as smoking, sun exposure, alcohol consumption, unprotected or risky sexual encounters as well as use age-appropriate health promotion strategies to help them maintain a healthy lifestyle.[36] Table 27.6 highlights the unique issues that should be assessed when developing a cancer treatment plan and long-term follow up for adolescents and young adults with hematological malignancies.

Table 27.6. Unique issues to address in caring for adolescents and young adults during and post-cancer treatment.

Assess for non-adherence
Assess mental status and any signs of depression
Assess for signs of low self esteem, body image, social isolation
Assess for family support, status of personal relationships
Assess level of understanding and education
Assess level of autonomy and independence
Assess accessibility to healthcare team and follow up
Assess financial status, responsibilities, burdens, school reintegration, career
Assess for current or future parenthood, fertility concerns

End of Life Issues

Though parents of children with hematological malignancies often receive encouraging statistics of long-term survival at the time of diagnosis, the nature of pediatric cancer, particularly depending on the exact type of hematological malignancy, is that of uncertainty. Unexpected event-free or long-term survival may happen, contrarily, unexpected deterioration or disease progression may occur. For all cancer patients, there may come a time when it is determined that there are no curative solutions. However, according to De Graves and Aranda, it is important to the families of these patients to maintain some level of hope while gradually introducing the idea of palliative care.[42] It is imperative for the treatment team to provide a high level of care and support to reassure patients and families that their well being is still a priority. As nurses, it is important to pay close attention to the new set of needs these patients and families have at such a difficult time.[42]

The main goal of palliative care is to ensure the patient's comfort and to maximize the patient's quality of life. End-of-life can bring about many physiological complications that can be addressed by nurses. The main concerns are pain, dyspnea, and agitation.[43] Common medications used to remedy these concerns are opioids, such as morphine, fentanyl, or hydromorphone that are often administered via continuous intravenous drips. Used as adjunct therapy to decrease dyspnea and agitation, nurses may administer anxiolytics, such as lorazepam or midazolam.[7,44] Nursing interventions should be individualized and based on the patient's needs, the patient's and family's values, culture, spirituality and personal interactions.[44] Table 27.7 exemplifies an end-of-life nursing care plan.

The ongoing evolution of nursing considerations for children, adolescents and young adults with hematological malignancies is inherent. The constant change, growth and development that this dynamic subspecialty will endure are inevitable. These frequent advances in science and treatment protocols will continue to rely on a workforce that is able to collaborate utilizing a wide range of skills for the provision of innovative care for these patients in a variety of care settings. Partnerships with nursing are a priority and at the core of this collaborative workforce. Nurses will continue to be pivotal in ensuring the delivery of safe quality care via their unique and indispensable roles as expert clinician, educator, manager, researcher, communicator, consultant, and advocate.

Table 27.7. Nursing plan of care for end-of-life.

Goals	Interventions
Short-term: • Patient will demonstrate comfort, i.e. report minimal pain scale (FACES/FLACC) scores, decreased agitation, sleeps comfortably, relaxed facial expression, absence of tachycardia and tachypnea. • Parent and patient (if age appropriate) will verbalize understanding of what is medicinally available to decrease discomfort. • End-of-life/Hospice arrangements will be made that are agreeable to patients and their families. **Long-term:** • Patient will verbalize age appropriate understanding of end-of-life. • Parents/Guardians will be able to openly discuss end-of-life with patient. ▪ Patient and family will report a positive end-of-life experience.	**Pain Management:** • Intermittent or continuous administration of opioids in correlation with patient's pain level. • Non-pharmacological intervention, e.g. guided imagery, distraction, relaxation **Nutrition:** • TPN/intralipids • Enteral tube feeds • Withdrawal of enteral/parenteral nutrition • Withdrawal of IV fluids **Cardiorespiratory Monitoring:** • CR monitor on or off depending on family's preference • Reduction of vital signs to Q12H, QDay, or stopped **Psychosocial Needs:** • Anxiety management: Intermittent or continuous administration of anxiolytics drugs • Encourage patient and family to recognize grief • Assess for causative and contributing factors that may delay the grief process • Allow frequent opportunity for questions • Encourage expressions of anger/concern • Provide privacy for patient and family/offer private room • Allow family's support system unlimited visitation **Referrals:** • Palliative care team • Pain team • Social work • Child life • Spiritual care/chaplain • Psychiatry • Home health/hospice

CR, cardiorespiratory; FLACC: face, legs, activity, cry, consolability.
Adapted from: Childrens Hospital Los Angeles (CHLA) End of Life Care Plan. Altounji, D. & Wise, C., 2010.

References

1. Wilcox B, Bruce SD. (2010) Patient navigation: A "win-win" for all involved. *Oncol Nurs Forum* **37**: 21–25.
2. Hockenberry M, Kline N. (2006) *Nursing Support of the Child with Cancer*. Philadelphia: Lippincott, Williams and Wilkins.
3. Sasse EC, Sasse AD, Brandalise S, Clark OA, Richards S. (2005) Colony stimulating factors for prevention of myelosuppressive therapy induced febrile neutropenia in children with acute lymphoblastic leukaemia. *Cochrane Database Syst Rev* **3**: CD004139.
4. Pizzo P, Poplack D (eds). (2006) *Principles and Practices of Pediatric Oncology*. Philadelphia: Lippincott, Williams and Wilkins.
5. Kline N (ed). (2008) *Essentials of Pediatric Hematology/Oncology Nursing: A Core Curriculum*. Glenview: Association of Pediatric Hematology/Oncology Nurses.
6. Flynn PM, Shenep JL, Stokes DC, Barrett FF. (1987) *In situ* management of confirmed central venous catheter-related bacteremia. *Pediatr Infect Dis J* **6**: 729–734.
7. Baggot C, Kelly K, Fochtman D, Foley G (eds). (2002) *Nursing Care of Children and Adolescents with Cancer*. Philadelphia: W.B. Saunders Company.
8. Mermel LA. (2000) Prevention of intravascular catheter-related infections. *Ann Intern Med* **132**: 391–402.
9. Institute for Healthcare Improvement (2005) 100,000 lives campaign. http://www.ihi.org/IHI/Programs/ Campaign/ 100kCampaign Overview Archive.htm.

10. Institute for Healthcare Improvement (2006) Getting started kit: Prevent central line infections. http://www.ihi.org.
11. O'Grady NP, Alexander M, Dellinger EP, Gerberding JL, Heard SO, Maki DG, Masur H, McCormick RD, Mermel LA, Pearson ML, Raad, II, Randolph A, Weinstein RA. (2002) Guidelines for the prevention of intravascular catheter-related infections. The Hospital Infection Control Practices Advisory Committee, Center for Disease Control and Prevention, U.S. *Pediatrics* **110**: e51.
12. Ralston M, Hazinski M, Zaritsky A, Schexnayder S, Kleinman M (eds). (2005) *Pediatric Advanced Life Support Provider Manual.* Dallas: American Heart Association.
13. Kelly KP, Porock D. (2005) A survey of pediatric oncology nurses' perceptions of parent educational needs. *J Pediatr Oncol Nurs* **22**: 58–66.
14. Longtin Y, Sax H, Leape LL, Sheridan SE, Donaldson L, Pittet D. (2010) Patient participation: Current knowledge and applicability to patient safety. *Mayo Clin Proc* **85**: 53–62.
15. Pagano-Therrien J, Santacroce SJ. (2005) Bone mineral density decrements and children diagnosed with cancer. *J Pediatr Oncol Nurs* **22**: 328–338.
16. Kline N (ed). (2004) *The Pediatric Chemotherapy and Biotherapy Curriculum.* Glenview: Association of Pediatric Oncology Nurses.
17. Ruland CM, Hamilton GA, Schjodt-Osmo B. (2009) The complexity of symptoms and problems experienced in children with cancer: A review of the literature. *J Pain Symptom Manage* **37**: 403–418.
18. Ablin A. (1997) *Supportive Care of Children with Cancer: Current Therapy and Guidelines from the Children's Cancer Group.* Baltimore: John Hopkins University Press.
19. Stanworth SJ, Hyde C, Heddle N, Rebulla P, Brunskill S, Murphy MF. (2004) Prophylactic platelet transfusion for haemorrhage after chemotherapy and stem cell transplantation. *Cochrane Database Syst Rev* **4**: CD004269.
20. Dixit A, Chatterjee T, Mishra P, Kannan M, Choudhry DR, Mahapatra M, Choudhry VP, Saxena R. (2007) Disseminated intravascular coagulation in acute leukemia at presentation and during induction therapy. *Clin Appl Thromb/Hemostasis* **13**: 292–298.
21. Krawczuk-Rybak M, Kuzmicz M, Wysocka J. (2005) Renal function during and after treatment for acute lymphoblastic leukemia in children. *Pediatr Nephrol* **20**: 782–785.
22. Hogan R. (2009) Implementation of an oral care protocol and its effects on oral mucositis. *J Pediatr Oncol Nurs* **26**: 125–135.
23. Cheng KK. (2008) Association of plasma methotrexate, neutropenia, hepatic dysfunction, nausea/vomiting and oral mucositis in children with cancer. *Eur J Cancer Care (Engl)* **17**: 306–311.
24. Mosby TT, Barr RD, Pencharz PB. (2009) Nutritional assessment of children with cancer. *J Pediatr Oncol Nurs* **26**: 186–197.
25. Robinson DL, Carr BA. (2007) Delayed vomiting in children with cancer after receiving moderately high or highly emetogenic chemotherapy. *J Pediatr Oncol Nurs* **24**: 70–80.
26. McCaffery M, Pasero C. (1999) *Pain Clinical Manual.* St. Louis, MO: Mosby, Inc.
27. Secola R, Reid D. (2008) Oncologic emergencies: Acute tumor lysis syndrome. In: N Kline (ed). *Essentials of Pediatric Hematology/Oncology Nursing: A Core Curriculum.* Glehview: Association of Pediatric Hematology/Oncology Nurses.
28. Cairo MS, Bishop M. (2004) Tumour lysis syndrome: New therapeutic strategies and classification. *Br J Haematol* **127**: 3–11.
29. Bottomley SJ, Kassner E. (2003) Late effects of childhood cancer therapy. *J Pediatr Nurs* **18**: 126–133.
30. Eshelman D, Landier W, Sweeney T, Hester AL, Forte K, Darling J, Hudson MM. (2004) Facilitating care for childhood cancer survivors: Integrating children's oncology group long-term follow-up guidelines and health links in clinical practice. *J Pediatr Oncol Nurs* **21**: 271–280.
31. Morris B, Partap S, Yeom K, Gibbs IC, Fisher PG, King AA. (2009) Cerebrovascular disease in childhood cancer survivors: A Children's Oncology Group report. *Neurology* **73**: 1906–1913.
32. Hudson MM, Hester A, Sweeney T, Kippenbrock S, Majcina R, Vear S, Wiard S, Kaplan S. (2004) A model of care for childhood cancer survivors that facilitates research. *J Pediatr Oncol Nurs* **21**: 170–174.
33. Mertens AC, Yasui Y, Liu Y, Stovall M, Hutchinson R, Ginsberg J, Sklar C, Robison LL. (2002) Pulmonary complications in survivors of childhood and adolescent cancer. A report from the Childhood Cancer Survivor study. *Cancer* **95**: 2431–2441.
34. Goldsby RE, Liu Q, Nathan PC, Bowers DC, Yeaton-Massey A, Raber SH, Hill D, Armstrong GT, Yasui Y, Zeltzer L, Robison LL, Packer RJ. (2010) Late-occurring neurologic sequelae in adult survivors of childhood acute lymphoblastic leukemia: A report from the Childhood Cancer Survivor Study. *J Clin Oncol* **28**: 324–331.
35. Anderson FS, Kunin-Batson AS. (2009) Neurocognitive late effects of chemotherapy in children: The past 10 years of research on brain structure and function. *Pediatr Blood Cancer* **52**: 159–164.

36. Bronowicki PA, Houlahan KE, Conley SB. (2009) Nursing care of patients with childhood cancer. In: *Oncology of Infancy and Childhood.* Philadelphia, PA: Saunders, an imprint of Elsevier Inc.
37. Grinyer A. (2007) *Young People Living with Cancer.* Bershire: Open University Press.
38. Green DM, Kawashima T, Stovall M, Leisenring W, Sklar CA, Mertens AC, Donaldson SS, Byrne J, Robison LL. (2009) Fertility of female survivors of childhood cancer: A report from the Childhood Cancer Survivor study. *J Clin Oncol* **27**: 2677–2685.
39. Oeffinger KC, Bhatia S. (2009) Second primary cancers in survivors of childhood cancer. *Lancet* **374**: 1484–1485.
40. Bhatia S, Sklar C. (2002) Second cancers in survivors of childhood cancer. *Nat Rev Cancer* **2**: 124–132.
41. CureSearch. (2008) *Long-term Follow-up Guidelines for Survivors of Childhood, Adolescent and Young Adult Cancers (ed version 3.0).* Arcadia: Children's Oncology Group.
42. De Graves S, Aranda S. (2005) When a child cannot be cured — reflections of health professionals. *Eur J Cancer Care (Engl)* **14**: 132–140.
43. Houlahan KE, Branowicki PA, Mack JW, Dinning C, McCabe M. (2006) Can end of life care for the pediatric patient suffering with escalating and intractable symptoms be improved? *J Pediatr Oncol Nurs* **23**: 45–51.
44. Kline N. (2004) Care of the terminally ill child and the family. In: N Kline, J Brace-O'Neill, M Hooke, (eds). *Essentials of Pediatric Oncology Nursing: A Core Curriculum.* Glenview: Association of Pediatric Oncology Nurses, pp. 243–244.

28

Psychosocial and Neurocognitive Late Effects

Stephen A. Sands and Keith Pasichow

Introduction

Most of the original work in psycho-oncology began in the 1960s and 1970s when survivorship for childhood acute lymphoblastic leukemia (ALL), the most common childhood leukemia, was only around 53%[1] and for lymphoma was around 40%.[2] As such, the literature regarding long-term psychological and social-emotional effects from this time is very limited. Given the poor prognosis of the patients in this era, psychosocial research focused mainly on coping with death, communicating disease information to children, and examining how parents dealt with the loss of a child.[3] With the dramatic improvement in the ALL cure rate reaching 89% in the 1990s[1] and as high as 90% in some recent studies,[4] there has been a shift in the focus of psychosocial researchers to long-term survivorship and social-emotional adjustment among childhood and adolescent patients.[3,5]

The literature in the area of psycho-oncology as it relates to pediatric leukemias is somewhat limited with most of the research focusing on the more common ALL, rather than other less frequent diagnoses such as acute myeloblastic leukemia or the chronic leukemias. Additionally, much of the research into long-term effects has focused on neurocognitive sequelae such as effects on IQ and learning disabilities, use of special education services and attention deficits. As such, this review of the psychological sequelae includes information on both the neurocognitive as well as the psychosocial late effects.

As leukemia treatment modalities have evolved over the years, the psychological research has adjusted to take into account the potential treatment risks to patients. As an illustration, when ALL patients were originally treated with radiation to the CNS, researchers looked into the late effects of ionizing radiation on the brain in various stages of development (see Chapters 11 and 12). With the introduction of intrathecal (IT) chemotherapy and clinical trials reducing or omitting CNS radiation, psychological studies compared the efficacy and late effects of IT chemotherapy with and without cranial irradiation. Similarly, researchers have recently begun to examine the psychological and neurocognitive sequelae of IT and high-dose (HD) systemic steroid use in children and adolescents with leukemia.

Unfortunately, there is still little information available on the psychosocial sequelae of childhood lymphoma patients and survivors. As such, we have utilized articles examining the psychosocial functioning and HRQoL of adult lymphoma patients, in the hopes of providing a basis for future research into these same areas in pediatric patients. This chapter sets out the research findings in psychosocial and neurocognitive sequelae among leukemia and lymphoma survivors in the basic order that treatment regimens have progressed, starting with research into effects of CNS radi-

Table 28.1. Neurocognitive sequelae.

Patients who receive CRT	
• Learning disabilities	
• Poor academic achievement	
• Psychological distress	
• Lower scores on intelligence testing	
• Problems related to attention	
Patients who do not receive CRT	
• Problems related to attention (i.e. focus, sustained attention)	

CRT: cranial radiation therapy.

ation among ALL survivors and moving forward from there in order to provide a more complete picture of the progression of knowledge in this area.

Neurocognitive Sequelae

In most early ALL therapeutic trials, curative treatment was achieved with the use of CRT which many studies have found to be a significant risk factor for long-term psychosocial and neuropsychological morbidity[6–9] (Table 28.1). As a result, much of the early research into long-term sequelae in ALL and other leukemias has focused on the risks of CRT in survivors[8–14] including attention deficits,[9,14,15] deficits in intelligence,[6,9,16] a reduced likelihood of attending college[7] and even altered non-dominant hemisphere functioning[12] (see Chapter 24). The majority of studies focused on measuring IQ and reported that most survivors who had been exposed to CNS radiation had IQ deficits when compared to healthy, age matched children,[17] and were significantly more likely to have learning disabilities.[11] Studies linked these deficits to poor academic achievement, especially in math and reading[8] and reported that survivors who had received CRT had lower rates of secondary education as compared to their siblings.[18] One study examined 80 survivors and their healthy siblings for signs of "sluggish cognitive tempo" defined as lethargy, daydreaming, and disorganized thought. They found that the survivors who had received CRT were significantly more likely to present with symptoms of "sluggish cognitive tempo" than their siblings.[19] A finding of great importance to early researchers was that patients treated without cranial radiation therapy (CRT) lacked these same deficits, suggesting that disease and chemotherapy alone were not sufficient to cause significant long-term neurocognitive sequelae,[10] such that a reduction in the use of CRT or elimination of CRT in most patients would likely help to alleviate these neurocognitive findings.

Recent studies in this population of patients have demonstrated a connection between CRT and increased levels of psychological distress, as well as poor body image and depression.[6,7,12] Interestingly, there has been some data to suggest that lower intelligence in patients treated with CRT is correlated with poor use of coping mechanisms, such as one study of 102 adult survivors of childhood ALL and Wilm's tumor compared with age and geographically matched controls.[6] Indeed, in one large retrospective study of 555 adult survivors of ALL, comparing treatment using CRT and chemotherapy with treatment using only chemotherapy, survivors treated with high-dose CRT (>21 Gy) self-reported a significantly higher incidence of mood disturbances, including depression, than those patients treated with low-dose (<21 Gy) or no CRT.[7] Likewise, a study comparing 106 patients aged 3–6.5 years old, treated with IT methotrexate, various regimens of systemic chemotherapy and either CRT or no CRT found that those patients treated with CRT scored significantly lower on all scales of general cognitive and motor abilities than those treated without CRT. This same study found no differences between the different systemic chemotherapy regimens in either the CRT or no CRT subgroups.[20] Additional studies have also demonstrated that groups treated with CRT performed significantly lower than controls (those treated with chemotherapy only) and population norms in areas such as intelligence, academic achievement[9] and problems with attention,[9,14,17] as well as behavioral areas such as adaptability.[21] While the original standard dose of CRT was as high as 24 Gy, results from protocols using 18 Gy[22] and, more recently, 12 Gy[23] have been encouraging, both in their survival rates and the decreased incidence of both neurocognitive and psychosocial sequelae.

As treatment regimens have continually reduced or omitted exposure to CRT, many of the neurocognitive sequelae previously reported have abated. In one study of 99 childhood oncology patients with various malignancies outside the CNS, treated with systemic chemotherapy, no CRT and either IT chemotherapy or no IT chemotherapy, no long-term intelligence or neurocognitive effects were noted in either group.[24] This study, in addition to several other large studies around the same time,[25–28] suggest that treatment of the CNS does not in itself cause long-term neurocognitive sequelae. Rather, they imply that the use of CRT specifically was the cause of many of the detrimental effects reported in the early literature.

Table 28.2. Psychosocial sequelae.

Increased psychological distress
Problems related to attention
Symptom-related distress
Avoidance coping mechanisms
Impaired functioning in close relationships
Lower physical functioning
Overall similar HRQoL to survivors of other cancers

Unlike some of the other neurocognitive sequelae that have abated as the use of CRT diminished, attention problems are still commonly reported in pediatric oncology patients even among those treated with only chemotherapy.[10, 29] Previously, patients treated with CRT were found to have problems in many areas of attention, including the ability to focus and the ability to sustain attention.[9,15] Recent studies examining neuropsychological sequelae in ALL patients treated with chemotherapy only have continued to find that, as compared to healthy controls, attention is significantly more impaired in ALL survivors.[8,16,21,30] This consistent finding suggests that there is a strong relationship between the neurotoxicities of the various ALL treatment regimens and the development and maintenance of attentional processes. Future research will need to examine the differences between patients on various chemotherapy regimens and the neurocognitive development of childhood oncology patients to help determine what factors are significantly associated with these late effects, and consequently how to proactively address them.

Psychosocial Sequelae

As treatment modalities shifted away from the use of CRT in standard risk patients, psychosocial research focused more upon those patients treated with chemotherapy only (Table 28.2). Many studies in this population have found increased psychological distress,[4,6,17,31] continuing problems with attention and focus,[10,15] and a range of social skills deficiencies[4,32] as compared to peers and siblings. In fact, in one review of the Childhood Cancer Survivors Study, it was demonstrated that survivors of childhood lymphoma tend to report higher levels of emotional distress than leukemia survivors.[33] A similar review found that Hodgkin's lymphoma survivors self-reported higher levels of symptom-related distress than survivors of leukemia and even of non-Hodgkin's lymphomas.[34] Despite this, most studies to date have reported that the increased incidence of these deficits is not clinically significant and that survivors tend to compare favorably with both siblings and healthy controls in most areas of psychosocial adjustment.[3,11,12,32,34,35]

Specific problem areas commonly reported in the literature involve the increased use of avoidance as a coping mechanism, especially in interpersonal relationships[6] and depression.[34,36] Despite a lack of increased incidence of psychiatric disorders, survivors of pediatric cancers, such as ALL and lymphoma, demonstrated impaired functioning in close relationships, suggesting that a social-emotional problem, albeit subclinical, exists amongst survivors. In one study, avoidant behaviors were exhibited by survivors in all interpersonal relationships, were more pronounced shortly after finishing treatment, and tended to wane as time from treatment increased.[6] There was no relationship between avoidant behaviors and intelligence, and avoidant behaviors are still reported at an increased rate among survivors treated with chemotherapy only, suggesting that these effects are not related to the neurocognitive effects of CRT.[3,6] One area for future research will be to examine the relationship between coping mechanisms and the use of avoidant behaviors.

It is important to note that there appears to be an overall positive tone to the findings of much pediatric psycho-oncology research; however, some recent studies have cast doubt on the idea that survivors are generally well psychologically, especially when measures of health related quality of life (HRQoL) are used. Health-related quality of life is used to refer to the perception of a person's health and the effects that perception has on the person's life.[37] Trude *et al.* reported in 2007 that survivors demonstrated lower HRQoL when compared with healthy controls[31] while Waters *et al.* reported in 2003 that survivors experienced poorer physical, social and emotional health than population controls.[4] Some of this effect may be explained by the finding that adolescent patients in particular tend to self-rate as having lower HRQoL than age-matched controls, as opposed to younger patients who tend to rate themselves as on par with their peers.[38] Additionally, a German study published in 2007 concluded that patients who rated themselves as having poorer body image and physical functioning than healthy controls were typically those patients with solid tumors,[39] suggesting that there is a subset of pediatric oncology patients who fall into a higher risk category, and may be skewing some of the data looking at all diagnoses in this population. Taking these possible confounding factors into account, it is reasonable to conclude that while there may be some deficits in psychosocial functioning among cancer survivors in general, those with leukemias most likely fall into the group of survivors who self-rate as having similar HRQoL to that of the healthy population.

Similarly, several studies comparing adult lymphoma survivors to those with other cancers, as well as the general population, have found that overall psychological QoL is not generally lower among survivors.[40] These studies often note a significant decrease in the rating of physical functioning among lymphoma survivors, including a higher than expected incidence of chronic fatigue syndrome.[41] One study which compared adult survivors of lymphoma with breast cancer survivors, found that those who had received systemic therapy, as compared to local therapy only, scored significantly lower on measures of physical functioning,[40,42] including decreased libido, limited energy, fatigue, and irritability.[43] However, as we have often seen in studies of pediatric cancer survivors, these physical deficits do not appear to correlate with decreased psychosocial QoL.

Indeed, despite the publication of some studies reporting lower QoL among survivors, the majority of studies indicate that survivors are generally doing well. One large study of 150 children with ALL in Switzerland reported that 84% of survivors had minimal or no late toxicity, with 94% reporting normal schooling and 90% reporting adequate psychosocial integration. The Swiss study did identify several areas where ALL survivors in particular were deficient as compared to the general population, though all were within the neurocognitive category, including IQ and memory deficits, and all were related to cranial irradiation therapy.[11]

Risk Factors

Corticosteroids

Most recently, there has been an increase in the research examining long-term sequelae in patients treated with chemotherapy combined with steroids. The majority of these studies compare the use of prednisone with dexamethasone; two of the most commonly used corticosteroids in pediatric leukemia treatment. It is known from studies of other chronic childhood diseases such as asthma, that long-term use of corticosteroids can negatively affect mood and behavior, as well as neurocognitive functioning.[44] Among pediatric leukemia patients, some studies indicate that those treated with dexamethasone as compared to prednisone demonstrate poorer performance in several areas of academic achievement and memory testing,[44,45] while others suggest that beyond a certain age, while sequelae still exist, there is no difference between the two medications.[46–48] Regardless of the differences between dexamethasone and prednisone, most researchers agree that behavioral problems, such as mood swings, depression, and anxiety, are all increased by the use of corticosteroids.[44–46] There has not been a large volume of research into the long-term effects of steroid use in pediatric leukemia patients, but much of the current research appears to suggest that the majority of these effects are transient[46] and may even be alleviated by switching from dexamethasone to prednisone. As an example, one British study in 2005 found that the negative behavioral effects of dexamethasone use could almost always be alleviated by switching to prednisone, and that these effects did not recur.[45]

Age at diagnosis

In addition to treatment modality, many studies have examined other risk factors for psychosocial sequelae (Table 28.3). Age at diagnosis has been shown to be negatively correlated with psychological and neurocognitive sequelae, though a specific age cutoff has been elusive. One study from 2003 reported that preadolescent age was a strong predictor of mood disturbances, especially among patients treated with CRT. The impact of age was not mediated by educational achievement, suggesting that IQ deficits or learning disabilities, as discussed previously in this chapter, were not a contributing factor to the mood disturbances reported by these patients.[7]

Table 28.3. Risk factors.

Corticosteroids
• Behavioral problems
• Mood disorders
Age at Diagnosis
• Younger age at diagnosis correlated with better psychosocial functioning after treatment
• Positively correlated with physical function deficits, especially among adults
Gender
• Females at higher risk for:
— Lower IQ
— Poorer neurocognitive performance
— Higher incidence of mood disturbances
Length of Follow-up
• Increased incidence of depression

Another study investigating age at diagnosis found that patients diagnosed before 7 years had higher levels of learning disabilities and school performance deficits. Again this study examined patients who were treated with CRT, and found that compared to their siblings, survivors had higher levels of learning disabilities and lower educational achievements. This study also found that emotional functioning was unrelated to educational achievement. They did not measure emotional functioning as a primary end point and so were unable to comment on the differences between emotional functioning in survivors compared to siblings.[18] Still other studies suggest 5 years of age[49] or even 3 years of age[13,17] to be the cutoff for psychological and neurocognitive risk. It appears that while young age is a significant risk factor for psychological sequelae among pediatric leukemia patients, there is no definite age when patients can be considered "safe" from the impact of treatment.

Some studies of adults undergoing treatment for lymphoma have found that age is positively correlated with an increase in the incidence of reported physical functioning problems.[42] While these results were not compared to psychosocial QoL, they do raise the possibility that, like young age among pediatric survivors, older age among adult patients is a risk factor for worsening QoL, a possibility that deserves further scrutiny. Additionally, it is important to examine pediatric lymphoma patients to see if these same findings hold true among a younger population, as the treatment regimens may be the risk factor for lymphoma patients at any age.

Gender

Gender has been demonstrated to be a risk factor for cognitive impairment in survivors of childhood cancers, with most studies indicating that females are at higher risk for lower IQ and poorer performance on various measures of neurocognitive function than males,[8,17,49,50] as well as higher incidence of mood disturbances among girls as compared with boys.[7,51] A large review of the published data concluded that most early studies showed a decrease in IQ in females compared to males, among patients treated with and even without CRT.[50] Similarly, a study in the early 1990s on 51 patients treated with either 18 Gy or 28 Gy CRT found that in both groups, a onetime infusion of high-dose IV MTX was associated with a significantly lower IQ score in girls but not in boys.[52] Interestingly, the 1990s study found no difference among girls based on age at diagnosis,[52] which is consistent with other ALL studies,[53] whereas the review article found a significant difference based on age, with girls who were younger at diagnosis displaying significantly more neurocognitive impairments than girls who were older at diagnosis, though no specific ages were mentioned.[50]

One study comparing lymphoma survivors and patients still undergoing active treatment with healthy controls found a higher incidence of self-reported poor psychological functioning and poor overall outlook in female patients and survivors and compared both to healthy female controls and, perhaps more importantly, to both male patients and male controls.[54] Additionally, female participants in another study were more likely than male participants to have a clinically significant level of somatic distress when compared with males.[34] This finding indicates that there may be an increase in risk for psychosocial sequelae, both on and off treatment, in female patients and suggests an important area for future research among lymphoma patients.

Length of follow up

Length of time from treatment has been examined at as both a positive and negative risk factor for long-term sequelae. Among those patients who experience significant impairment, there appears to be an increased incidence of depression and a more external locus of control as time from treatment increases,[17] suggesting that certain late-effects may develop beyond the scope of many of the published treatment efficacy studies. Therefore, even if many patients are free of sequelae in the relative short-term (5–10 years for most studies), further longitudinal research is warranted to adequately determine if there are emerging late effects as patients progress through life (see Chapter 24).

Conclusion

As we continue to advance in the treatment of childhood leukemia, it is imperative that psychosocial and neurocognitive late effects continue to be studied and risk factors identified, so that early interventions can be developed and tested to minimize late effects for survivors. Treatment options completely avoiding the use of CRT for ALL patients have been reported recently through risk-stratified chemotherapy regimens.[55] Such approaches would provide a means of avoiding many of the devastating effects seen with early treatments involving radiation therapy and may allow survivors to attain a higher quality of life. However, despite these advances, there are still a significant number of questions left unanswered about the psychosocial QoL of pediatric cancer patients. The dearth of information available on survivors of pediatric lymphomas leaves entire populations at risk for long-term sequelae. As demonstrated in this chapter, the only information currently available in any significant quantity on this topic relates only to adult lymphoma patients and survivors, a fact which makes it difficult to accurately assess the risk of younger patients. As psychological research in the field of pediatric oncology and hematology continues to advance and expand, it is critical that researchers include a wider variety of diagnoses among their participants.

Along with advances in the treatment of childhood cancers and a steady increase in the cure rates, the understanding and management of psychosocial and neurocognitive sequelae has progressed from a time when most research was concerned with helping parents manage death, to the current day when most research focuses on the long-term effects to the survivors. While most patients today appear to have minimal late effects when compared with their healthy peers, there is evidence that an underlying level of psychological distress and social-emotional difficulties co-exist for some survivors. Future research into the psychosocial and neurocognitive difficulties in this subset of survivors may help to further elucidate the nature and severity of these problems so that interventions aimed at ameliorating the long-term effects of diagnosis and treatment for all types of childhood cancers can be developed. Additionally, as the majority of research available to date focuses on patients with a limited number of tumor types, it is important that future studies examine these same issues in children with rarer leukemias, lymphomas and other underrepresented morphologies to determine if the same difficulties that are found in survivors of ALL and adult lymphomas, are also found in survivors of other pediatric cancers. The ultimate goal in the treatment of childhood leukemia, lymphoma, and indeed childhood cancer in general, continues to be not only a cure for the physical disease, but also the development of mechanisms that allow patients to progress through life with as few psychological effects as possible.

The authors wish to extend their appreciation to Chloe. A. Greenbaum for all of her help in completing the research necessary for the publication of this chapter.

References

1. Pickard AS, Topfer LA, Feeny DH. (2004) A structured review of studies on health-related quality of life and economic evaluation in pediatric acute lymphoblastic leukemia. *J Natl Cancer Inst Monogr* **33**: 102–125.
2. Hodgkin Lymphoma Facts & Statistics. http://www.leukemia-lymphoma.org/all_page.adp?item_id=8312. (accessed on September 18) (updated on September 2, 2010)
3. Patenaude AF, Kupst MJ, (2005) Psychosocial functioning in pediatric cancer. *J Pediatr Psychol* **30**: 9–27.
4. Waters EB, Wake MA, Hesketh KD, *et al.* (2003) Health-related quality of life of children with acute lymphoblastic leukaemia: Comparisons and correlations between parent and clinician reports. *Int J Cancer* **103**: 514–518.
5. Noll RB, Gartstein MA, Vannatta K, *et al.* (1999) Social, emotional, and behavioral functioning of children with cancer. *Pediatrics* **103**: 71–78.
6. Mackie E, Hill J, Kondryn H, *et al.* (2000) Adult psychosocial outcomes in long-term survivors of acute lymphoblastic leukaemia and Wilms' tumour: A controlled study. *Lancet* **355**: 1310–1314.
7. Glover DA, Byrne J, Mills JL, *et al.* (2003) Impact of CNS treatment on mood in adult survivors of childhood leukemia: A report from the children's cancer group. *J Clin Oncol* **21**: 4395–4401.
8. Catherine CP, Courtney EJ, Lisa YR, *et al.* (2008) A meta-analysis of the neuropsychological sequelae of chemotherapy-only treatment for pediatric acute lymphoblastic leukemia. *Pediatr Blood Cancer* **51**: 99–104.
9. Spiegler BJ, Kennedy K, Maze R, *et al.* (2006) Comparison of long-term neurocognitive outcomes in young children with acute lymphoblastic leukemia treated with cranial radiation or high-dose or very high-dose intravenous methotrexate. *J Clin Oncol* **24**: 3858–3864.
10. Rodgers J, Marckus R, Kearns P, *et al.* (2003) Attentional ability among survivors of leukaemia treated without cranial irradiation. *Arch Dis Child* **88**: 147–150.
12. Hill JM, Kornblith AB, Jones D, *et al.* (1998) A comparative study of the long term psychosocial functioning of childhood acute lymphoblastic leukemia survivors treated by intrathecal methotrexate with or without cranial radiation. *Cancer* **82**: 208–218.
13. Waber DP, Shapiro BL, Carpentieri SC, *et al.* (2001) Excellent therapeutic efficacy and minimal late neurotoxicity in children treated with 18 grays of cranial radiation therapy for high-risk acute lymphoblastic leukemia. *Cancer* **92**: 15–22.

14. Brouwers P, Poplack D. (1990) Memory and learning sequelae in long-term survivors of acute lymphoblastic leukemia: Association with attention deficits. *Am J Pediatr Hematol/Oncol* **12**: 174–181.
15. Rodgers J, Horrocks J, Britton PG, *et al.* (1999) Attentional ability among survivors of leukaemia. *Arch Dis Child* **80**: 318–323.
16. Williams JPD, Berry DHMD, Caldwell DMsCCC, *et al.* (1992) A comparison of neuropsychological and psychosocial functioning after prophylactic treatment for childhood leukemia in monozygotic twins. *Am J Pediatr Hematol/Oncol* **14**: 289–296.
17. Eiser C. (1991) Cognitive deficits in children treated for leukaemia. *Arch Dis Child* **66**: 164–168.
19. Reeves CB, Palmer S, Gross AM, *et al.* (2007) Brief report: Sluggish cognitive tempo among pediatric survivors of acute lymphoblastic leukemia. *J Pediatr Psychol* **32**: 1050–1054.
20. MacLean WE, Jr., Noll RB, Stehbens JA, *et al.* (1995) Neuropsychological effects of cranial irradiation in young children with acute lymphoblastic leukemia 9 months after diagnosis. *Arch Neurol* **52**: 156–160.
21. Waber DP, Turek J, Catania L, *et al.* (2007) Neuropsychological outcomes from a randomized trial of triple intrathecal chemotherapy compared with 18 Gy cranial radiation as CNS treatment in acute lymphoblastic leukemia: Findings from Dana-Farber Cancer Institute ALL Consortium Protocol 95-01. *J Clin Oncol* **25**: 4914–4921.
22. Waber DP. (2002) More good news about neuropsychological late effects in long-term survivors of acute lymphoblastic leukemia. *J Pediatr Hematol Oncol* **24**: 86–87.
23. Pui C-H, Howard SC. (2008) Current management and challenges of malignant disease in the CNS in paediatric leukaemia. *Lancet Oncol* **9**: 257–268.
24. Copeland DR, Moore BD, III, Francis DJ, *et al.* (1996) Neuropsychologic effects of chemotherapy on children with cancer: A longitudinal study. *J Clin Oncol* **14**: 2826–2835.
25. Ochs J, Mulhern R, Fairclough D, *et al.* (1991) Comparison of neuropsychologic functioning and clinical indicators of neurotoxicity in long-term survivors of childhood leukemia given cranial radiation or parenteral methotrexate: A prospective study. *J Clin Oncol* **9**: 145–151.
26. Mulhern R, Fairclough D, Ochs J. (1991) A prospective comparison of neuropsychologic performance of children surviving leukemia who received 18-Gy, or no cranial irradiation. *J Clin Oncol* **9**: 1348–1356.
27. Dowell R, Copeland DR, Judd B. (1989) Neuropsychological effects of chemotherapeutic agents. *Dev Neuropsychol* **5**: 17–24.
29. Jansen NCAJ, Kingma A, Schuitema A, *et al.* (2008) Neuropsychological outcome in chemotherapy-only-treated children with acute lymphoblastic leukemia. *J Clin Oncol* **26**: 3025–3030.
30. Brown RT, Madan-Swain A, Pais R, *et al.* (1992) Chemotherapy for acute lymphocytic leukemia: Cognitive and academic sequelae. *J Pediatr* **121**: 885–889.
32. Mulhern RK, Friedman AG, Stone PA. (1988) Acute lymphoblastic leukemia: Long-term psychological outcome. *Biomed Pharmacother* **42**: 243–246.
33. Zeltzer LK, Buchbinder D, Zebrack B, *et al.* (2009) Psychological status in childhood cancer survivors: A report from the childhood cancer survivor study. *J Clin Oncol* **27**: 2396–2904.
34. Zebrack BJ, Zeltzer LK, Whitton J, *et al.* (2002) Psychological outcomes in long-term survivors of childhood leukemia, Hodgkin's disease, and non-Hodgkin's lymphoma: A report from the childhood cancer survivor study. *Pediatrics* **110**: 42–52.
35. Donna BG, Alice BK, James EH, *et al.* (1997) Quality of life for adult leukemia survivors treated on clinical trials of cancer and leukemia group B during the period 1971–1988. *Cancer* **80**: 1936–1944.
36. von der Weid N. (2008) Adult life after surviving lymphoma in childhood. *Supportive Care Cancer* **16**: 339–345.
37. CDC U. (2009) Health-related quality of life. http://www.cdc.gov/hrqol/. (accessed on April 7) (updated on January 6, 2009).
38. Bauld C, Anderson V, Arnold J. (1998) Psychosocial aspects of adolescent cancer survival. *J Pediatr Child Health* **34**: 120–126.
40. Ahles TA, Saykin AJ, Furstenberg CT, *et al.* (2005) Quality of life of long-term survivors of breast cancer and lymphoma treated with standard dose chemotherapy or local therapy. *J Clin Oncol* **23**: 4399–4405.
41. Oldervoll LM, Loge JH, Kaasa S, *et al.* (2007) Physical activity in Hodgkin's lymphoma survivors with and without chronic fatigue compared with the general population — a cross-sectional study. *BMC Cancer* **7**: 210–221.
42. Johnsen A, Tholstrup D, Petersen M, *et al.* (2009) Health related quality of life in a nationally representative sample of haematological patients. *Eur J Haematol* **83**: 139–148.
43. Devlen J, Maguire P, Philips P, *et al.* (1987) Psychological problems associated with diagnosis and treatment of lymphomas. 1: Retrospective study. *Br Med J (Clin Res Ed)* **295**: 953–954.
44. Waber DP, Carpentieri SC, Klar N, *et al.* (2000) Cognitive sequelae in children treated for acute lymphoblastic

leukemia with dexamethasone or prednisone. *J Pediatr Hematol/Oncol* **22**: 206–213.
45. Stuart FA, Segal TY, Keady S. (2005) Adverse psychological effects of corticosteroids in children and adolescents. *Arch Dis Child* **90**: 500–506.
46. Mrakotsky CM, Silverman LB, Dahlberg SE, *et al.* (2010) Neurobehavioral side effects of corticosteroids during active treatment for acute lymphoblastic leukemia in children are age-dependent: Report from Dana-Farber Cancer Institute All Consortium Protocol 00–01. *Pediatr Blood Cancer.*
47. Kadan-Lottick NS, Brouwers P, Breiger D, *et al.* (2009) A comparison of neurocognitive functioning in children previously randomized to dexamethasone or prednisone in the treatment of childhood acute lymphoblastic leukemia. *Blood* **114**: 1746–1752.
48. Annemieke IB, Leo MJdS, Marry MvdH-E, *et al.* (2005) Chemotherapy and attentional dysfunction in survivors of childhood acute lymphoblastic leukemia: Effect of treatment intensity. *Pediatr Blood Cancer* **45**: 281–290.
49. Haupt R, Fears TR, Robison LL, *et al.* (1994) Educational attainment in long-term survivors of childhood acute lymphoblastic leukemia. *JAMA* **272**: 1427–1432.
50. Armstrong GT, Sklar CA, Hudson MM, *et al.* (2007) Long-term health status among survivors of childhood cancer: Does sex matter? *J Clin Oncol* **25**: 4477–4489.
51. Bitsko MJ, Dillon R, Russell EC, *et al.* (2008) Happiness and time perspective as potential mediators of quality of life and depression in adolescent cancer. *Pediatr Blood Cancer* **50**: 613–619.
52. Waber DP, Tarbell NJ, Kahn CM, *et al.* (1992) The relationship of sex and treatment modality to neuropsychologic outcome in childhood acute lymphoblastic leukemia. *J Clin Oncol* **10**: 810–817.
53. Precourt S, Robaey P, Lamothe I, *et al.* (2002) Verbal cognitive functioning and learning in girls treated for acute lymphoblastic leukemia by chemotherapy with or without cranial irradiation. *Dev Neuropsychol* **21**: 173–195.
54. Wu E, Jenney M, Rockwood T, *et al.* (2007) Assessment of health related quality of life of adolescent cancer patients using the Minneapolis-Manchester quality of life adolescent questionnaire. *Pediatr Blood Cancer* **48**: 678–686.
55. Pui C-H, Campana D, Pei D, *et al.* (2009) Treating childhood acute lymphoblastic leukemia without cranial irradiation. *N Engl J Med* **360**: 2730–2741.

29

Special Considerations in Low and Middle Income Countries

Shripad D. Banavali, Scott C. Howard, Parth S. Mehta, Alessandra Sala, Ronald Barr and Ian Magrath

Introduction

There has been remarkable improvement in increasing survival rates in children and adolescents with hematological malignancies and understanding their pathogenesis in the course of the last 4 decades. However, the bulk of the research and improvements in outcome have occurred in the high income countries while of the more than 250,000 children and adolescents who develop cancer each year, approximately 80% are in the low and middle income (L and MI) countries (Table 29.1). While the children with cancer living in high-income (HI) countries enjoy approximately 80% overall cure rates, those living in L and MI countries tend to have poor cure rates, although available data is limited and in some institutions results can approach those obtained in HI countries. The worse outcome in L and MI countries relates to a broad range of social, economic and cultural barriers limiting access to and delivery of therapy (Fig. 29.1). It is even more unfortunate that this survival gap has widened over the past few decades and advances in treatment have not percolated down to lower income countries, or are not feasible in these settings.[1–3] Often, treatment is dictated by what patients can afford, what drugs are available, or what therapies are feasible in the context of available supportive care, rather than being selected as an optimal treatment regimen for the type and stage of disease. An unknown number of children receive no therapy at all and even palliative care is very limited, such that most children with cancer in the world die in extremely unpleasant circumstances.

Childhood cancer in L and many MI countries is not a health priority for governments due to other much more common competing causes of death such as infections and malnutrition. However, due to the rapidly changing economic and social climate in these countries, cancer is likely to become one of the leading causes of disease-related death in the near future, as is already the case in high income countries.[2,4,5] Furthermore, treatment costs are lower and there is a trend towards single child families. These factors, coupled to the greater potential number of years of life lost in the event that children and adolescents die, result in a greater impact on the economy and a compelling case to invest to a much greater extent than has been the case to date in improving access to care for children with cancer in L and MI countries. Such countries, given the paucity of their resources and the persisting focus, for the most part, on infectious diseases, their predominant health problem to date, have not created an evidence base of their own relating to the care of children with cancer. In contrast, in technologically advanced countries, improvements in outcomes in recent decades have been largely due to a systematic scientific approach involving the conduct of clinical

Table 29.1. Estimates of numbers of children and adolescents with cancer in the world. Based on globocan and cancer on five continents.

	0–14 yrs	15–19 yrs	0–19 yrs
Less developed	133,931	46,538	180,469
More developed	26,964	8907	35,871
World	160,882	55,445	216,327

Estimate for 15–19 yrs is 25–33% of cancer 0–19.

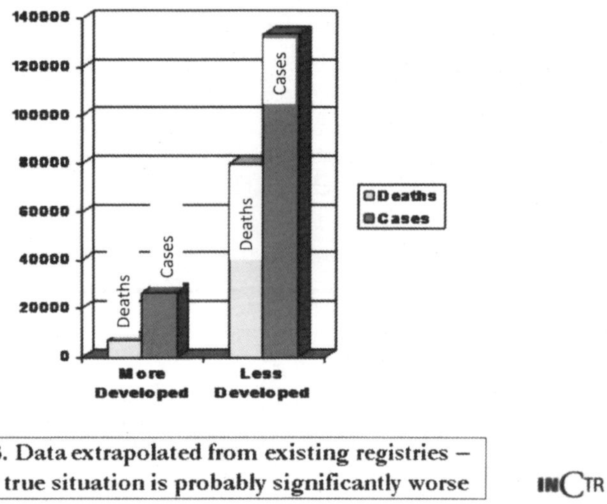

Fig. 29.1. Annual incident cases vs. annual deaths (actual numbers) in children up to 14 years of age in more and less developed countries.

trials in which the majority of children with cancer have participated (although a lesser proportion of adolescents). The use of regimens developed in resource-rich countries, however, is not always possible in L and MI countries because of the challenges brought about by poverty, which affects both the family's ability to obtain prompt treatment and to sustain itself through serious disease and the ability of health providers to deliver appropriate care. Poverty and limited resources lead to advanced disease at the time of presentation and greatly limits either access to, or the ability to use the kinds of intensive chemotherapy regimens, or sophisticated surgical or radiotherapeutic techniques that are widely available in HI countries. Consequently, treatment approaches, with rare exceptions, need to be adapted to the local circumstances, avoiding regimens that are costly or highly toxic and ensuring that family members, who must often travel long distances to reach a center competent to deal with the child's illness, receive the necessary psychosocial, and where necessary, financial support. In its absence, the rates of abandonment of therapy or loss to follow up — and a consequent inability to assess efficacy of the chosen therapy — will be high.

Expanding access to treatment for the large childhood cancer population in L and MI countries is not purely a question of a child's right to the best available therapy, but also has implications for improving pediatric cancer at a global level — currently, only a few countries undertake research in pediatric cancer, and increasing the amount of research performed throughout the world should result in benefits to all; the systematic study of genetic and environmental factors involved in the genesis of childhood cancers in multiple ethnic groups and geographical contexts should greatly increase our understanding of these diseases and provide a more complete picture of their epidemiology and etiology — opening up the possibility of prevention, which, except in rare circumstances (e.g. hepatocellular carcinoma associated with Hepatitis B virus (HBV) is not yet possible. Furthermore, large-scale global trials would provide much needed impetus to ongoing pediatric oncology clinical research, particularly in the less common diseases and would be likely to raise standards of care because of the need to collect highly accurate data, because of the necessary surveillance of clinical practice and because of the increased communication among pediatric oncologists that automatically follows from participation in clinical trials. Finally, the application of novel low-cost strategies obligated by resource-constrained environments could lead to alternative, less toxic therapies in at least some cancers.[6]

In this chapter, we describe the challenges and opportunities of treating hematological childhood cancers in L and MI countries, provide information on results being achieved, where data exists, and discuss future strategies designed to improve access to effective therapy of the 80% of children with cancer who live in L and MI countries.

Epidemiology and Presentation

Incidence

While international patterns of childhood cancer have been relatively well documented, those pertaining to adolescents (15–19 years of age) are much less well described[7] and there is very little information relevant to cancer in young adults (more than 20 years of age), particularly in developing countries. The incidence of cancer in adolescents in Europe varies from 186 per million in the East to 210 per million in the North[8] and rises progressively with age. From age 20 to 60 years, incidence rates in successive 5-year age groups are 362,

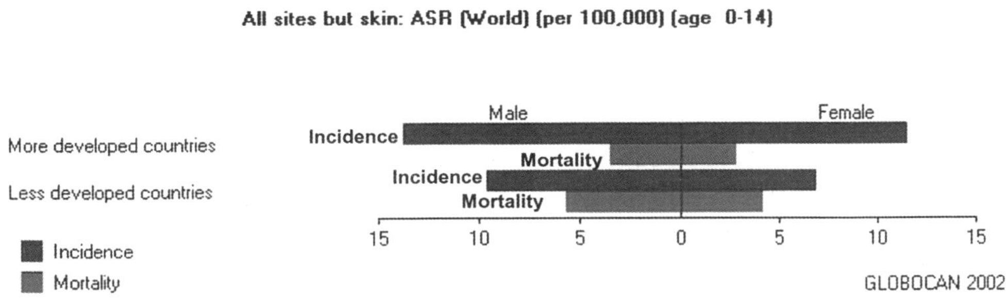

Fig. 29.2. Incidence and mortality rates (age-standardized to a world population) in more and less developed countries.

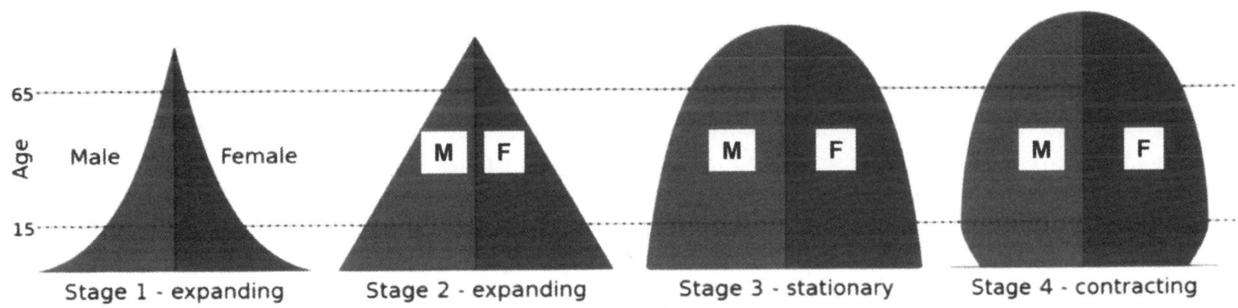

Fig. 29.3. Population pyramids in relationship to the stages of demographic transition. Stage 1 is prior to the industrial revolution. Most L and MI countries are in stages 2 and 3. The wealthiest high income countries are in stage 4. Stage 1: High birth and death rate, short life expectancy. Stage 2: High birth rate, fall in death rate, longer life expectancy, therefore marked population expansion. Stage 3: Declining birth rate, low death rate, more living into old age — population expansion stabilizes. Stage 4: Low birth and death rates — population begins to contract.

554, 827, and 1217 per million.[9] Moreover, the incidence in all age groups has been rising inexorably over time, presumably due to increased exposure to potential environmental carcinogens, although improved detection may have contributed (to an unknown degree) to the increased incidence[8,9] (see Chapter 1).

There is considerable geographic variation in the overall incidence of cancer in young people,[7,10] and on average the incidence of childhood cancer is lower in L and MI countries (Fig. 29.2), but because of the fact that 85% of the world's population lives in L and MI countries, and the age structure of the latter is considerably skewed towards a younger age (Fig. 29.3), more than 80% of the global burden of cancer in childhood, as reflected in incident cases, occurs in developing countries.[11] This is also true when hematological cancers — which account for the bulk of pediatric cancer — are considered separately. Similarly, a high proportion of cancers in adolescents and young adults — it has been estimated that there are 1 million new incident cases per year in the age group 15–39 years[12] — occurs in such countries, if for no other reason, due to their population structures. Interestingly, in low income countries where infectious diseases in childhood are prevalent, the under-5 mortality rate (a good indicator of child health in a population) correlates inversely with the incidence of leukemia but not of solid tumors.[11]

Disease distribution

In industrialized countries, the distribution of malignant diseases varies considerably across the age span,[9] but for the most part, lymphoid neoplasms comprise a third to a half of all pediatric cancers throughout the world. During adolescence, lymphomas predominate in Europe[8] and North America,[9] but in young adults, there is a progressive increase in the proportion of epithelial tumors such as breast cancer with a notable reduction in leukemias and lymphomas, especially the former. Moreover, there are clear gender differences in disease distribution, e.g. a much higher incidence of thyroid cancer in young females, and the distribution of diseases has changed over time in both Europe[8] and North America.[9]

Similar age-related differences exist in less privileged societies, although the proportional representation of individual diseases may vary widely in different settings. As examples, retinoblastoma is more prevalent than acute lymphoblastic leukemia (ALL) in children in some parts of the developing world,[10] while Burkitt lymphoma (BL) is generally the most common tumor in young people in equatorial African countries.[10] Neuroblastoma and the Ewing sarcoma family of tumors are encountered much less frequently in many developing countries than in North America and Western Europe,[13] while the reverse is true of carcinoma of the cervix in young people, albeit, the incidence of this disease, which is caused by human papillomavirus (HPV) and therefore is essentially unknown prior to sexual activity, is rare below the age of 30 years.[14] Furthermore, the age distribution of individual malignant diseases may vary in different parts of the world; for example, Hodgkin lymphoma is seen more often in preschool-aged children in low income than in high income countries.[15]

Such differences are likely to reflect differences in tumor biology caused by environmental and genetic differences in the tumor cells themselves, the latter derived partly from differences in ethnicity and partly from environmental exposures and lifestyles. For example, chronic infections are more important as a cause for cancer in L and MI countries. This is discussed in the next section. In many circumstances, the explanations for differences in incidence are unknown, or is associated with an environmental or lifestyle difference (such as low socioeconomic status) with no knowledge of the specific factor or factors involved. Biological heterogeneity of individual diseases is well described across the age spectrum from childhood to young adult life.[13,16]

Subgroup distributions of AML and ALL also demonstrate geographic variation. APML, which has a high incidence in some populations in Latin America, is a striking example. Within the spectrum of ALL there tends to be a higher proportion of T-cell phenotypes in resource poor countries,[17] particularly in low socioeconomic strata, although this probably reflects a decreased incidence of pre-B ALL than an increase in T-cell ALL status.[18] Likewise, a deficit in cases exhibiting the RUNX1 or TEL-AML1 translocation has been reported from India and Taiwan.[19,20]

Typically, Hodgkin lymphoma (HL) is much less common in adolescents in low income than in high income countries[21] but the proportion of EBV positive cases is higher.[22] Again, there is considerable variation in the proportions of subtypes of non-Hodgkin lymphoma (NHL) in young people in developing countries. Although BL is the most frequent NHL in children across the world, its incidence also varies dramatically, being markedly higher in Sub-Saharan Africa (see below). In older patients, there are marked differences in the pattern of cancer among low income countries, and between low and high income countries.[23] Some of these differences may be attributed to the variations in the prevalences or peak age of infection of HIV, EBV and *Helicobacter pylori* infections (early infection with EBV, for example, could account in part for the high prevalence of BL, HL in children less than 5 years and possibly T-cell lymphomas in the context of hemophagocytic syndromes, as occur particularly in SE Asia[24] (see Chapter 19). Other differences may relate to infections with other agents, some of which may yet to be defined. In general, indolent subtypes of NHL, such as follicular lymphoma, are more common in industrialized countries than in less privileged societies, while the reverse is true for high-grade diseases, although more indolent lymphomas are rare in children and adolescents everywhere, and may be biologically different when they do occur.

The reasons for differences in the spectra of childhood and adolescent cancers in different world regions is clearly due to a combination of genetic make-up and environmental exposures. The relative importance of these is unknown, and they may result in differences of the genetics of the prevalent tumors. Molecular epidemiologic studies of BL, for example, have revealed different genetic profiles in different parts of the world[25] and similar heterogeneity has been described in T-cell ALL.[10]

Apparent differences in disease distribution may sometimes be misleading because of cultural factors and resource constraints. The former are reflected in the disadvantage experienced by females in India and China in accessing healthcare[10] while the latter is exemplified by the probable under-ascertainment of brain tumors in much of Africa, although under-diagnosis is always an inference and may or may not account for apparent differences in incidence of specific diseases.[26] Another reason for differences in incidence and frequency, often ignored in discussions of this type, is the variability and quality of pathological diagnosis in different parts of the world. Some countries or regions of countries may have no pathologists, or no pathologists skilled in the diagnosis of pediatric cancer, while cancer registries, with rare exceptions, are located in urban areas, which may differ markedly from rural areas in a number of respects, including the pattern of cancer and access to care (and hence, therefore, may not be registered).

The International Classification of Childhood Cancer[27] is manifestly appropriate for global use, but a proposed

Table 29.2. Ratio of deaths to cases in children up to 14 years of age in more and less developed countries. This gives an approximate estimate of survival rates.

	Deaths	Cases	Ratio
More developed	6893	26,864	0.256
Less developed	80,116	133,931	0.598

Data extrapolated from the few existing registries — nearly all in urban regions: the true situation is probably significantly worse.

system for cancer in adolescents and young adults[28] has yet to be validated on a worldwide basis. Moreover, the disease distribution profile is subject to changes over time, as reflected in HIV-related malignancies in both resource-rich and resource-poor countries.

Survival and mortality

In high-income countries, the survival rate for adolescents and young adults with cancer may exceed that for children, as has been described recently in Canada.[29] In general, the survival rates[30] are lower in children with cancer in resource-poor than in resource-rich countries as is indicated by incidence/mortality ratios (Table 29.2). There is virtually no comparative information in adolescents and young adults. Important factors contributing to these differences in outcomes, in addition to disparities in human and other resources, are the greater frequency of presentation with advanced disease in low-income countries, higher treatment-related mortality rates (reflective, to a considerable degree, of prevalent comorbidities — especially infection) and abandonment of therapy.[31] Severe malnutrition also makes a contribution,[32] though whether this is a direct causal mechanism or a surrogate for other disadvantages occasioned by low socio-economic status remains unresolved. The quality of care is also, of course, a major factor, as evidenced by the advances made when there is long-term collaboration with partners from high-income countries.[33,34]

Clinical presentation

Although there are examples of clinical manifestations that are especially common in some settings, such as the remarkable prevalence of chloromas in young people with acute leukemia in Turkey,[35] the dominant characteristic of patients with cancer in under-resourced countries is that of advanced disease at diagnosis. It is likely that this represents delayed presentation in most instances, but the particular biological features of tumors — or environmental factors that influence anatomical distribution by creating microenvironments more conducive to tumor cell survival and growth — may play an additional role. A classical example is the markedly higher proportion of jaw tumors in BL in Sub-Saharan African children and children from New Guinea, (some 60% of patients have jaw tumors at the time of presentation, while these are also age-associated, being much more common in young children). Both Sub-Saharan Africa and New Guinea are regions of holoendemic malaria, but also have higher rates of infection and infestation in general. The increased likelihood of infection should also sound a warning note with regard to diagnosis. Tuberculosis, for example, is still a frequent cause of lymphadenopathy in many poor countries and should always be included in the differential diagnosis of persistently enlarged lymph nodes.

Other considerations

In the face of limited resources, the care of such patients is especially challenging. Management of tumor lysis syndrome in patients with BL (see Chapter 30) and of the "ATRA syndrome" in those with APML (see Chapter 13) are obvious examples. The paucity — sometimes complete absence of radiotherapeutic services — in Africa, and in other developing countries, adds to the difficulty of treating patients optimally, although radiation therapy is a relatively minor element of the treatment of most hematological neoplasms. According to the International Atomic Energy Agency, just 15 countries own half of all radiation therapy machines in the world.

Poor socio-economic circumstances significantly compromise the care of young people with cancer in low-income countries. The cost of travel to one of the few facilities where children with cancer are managed, the lack of knowledge of both families and their primary care providers of even the existence of cancer in children and adolescents, and the family difficulties occasioned by the need for long periods away from home (including a dramatic drop in income) are just some of the possible reasons why patients either fail to receive any therapy, or abandon treatment before completion. Poor hygiene may contribute to increased toxicity and cultural barriers, such as preference for traditional practices, also play their part.

Biology: Is It Different?

The differences in incidence of childhood cancer between high income and L and MI countries (Fig. 29.2)

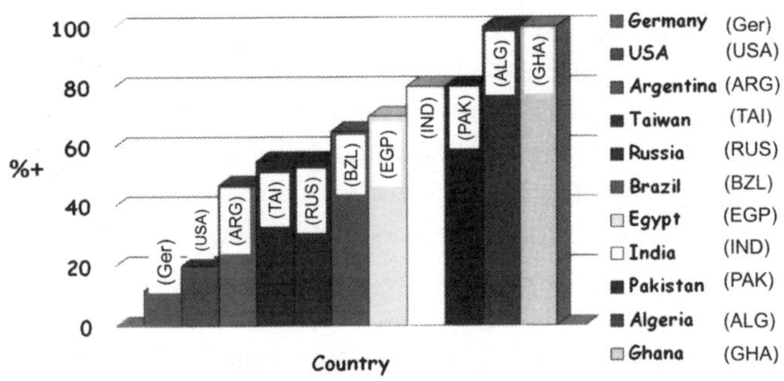

Fig. 29.4. Percentage of cases of Burkitt lymphoma that are EBV positive in various published series.

must be a consequence of differences in the incidence of specific subtypes of cancer. This is verified by the fact that although ALL is the most common childhood cancer at a global level, this is not the case in equatorial Africa, where Burkitt lymphoma (BL) accounts for approximately half of all childhood cancers (except in countries in which Kaposi's sarcoma has increased dramatically as a consequence of the AIDS epidemic in Africa.[36–38] This remarkably high incidence of BL is almost certainly a result of environmental rather than genetic differences, as suggested by the marked difference in EBV association with BL in different world regions[39] (Fig. 29.4) but environmental differences may well influence the biology of childhood cancers — potentially via a direct influence on pre-malignant cells in terms of the genetic changes induced, or, alternatively, through influencing the likelihood that particular biological subtypes will arise (this could result from differences in both the macro and microenvironments). The variability in incidence of ALL in different world regions referred to earlier, for example, appears to be due particularly to variability in the most frequent subtype — CD10+ precursor B-cell ALL.[39,40] There was a progressive increase in incidence/mortality (incidence and mortality were essentially identical in the years before effective therapy was available) of leukemia between the ages of 2–5 years in England and Wales after 1920.[41] This early age peak, now know to be caused by the increased incidence of CD10+ pre-B ALL,[42] which accounts for perhaps 80% of all cases of ALL in this age-group (2–5 years),[42] appeared sequentially throughout the century in various population groups (e.g. American whites before blacks, and is still not present in most under-resourced countries.[43] In such countries, if CD10+ pre-B ALL is considered alone, the early age peak is immediately apparent, consistent with the interpretation that its absence is due to a low proportion of pre-B CD10+ cases,[40] which appears, therefore, to be a disease of higher socioeconomic status — a conjecture supported by the increase of the early age peak throughout the 20th century in parallel with socioeconomic development.[41] Young patients with CD10+ ALL are also frequently associated with TEL-AML1 translocations, although there is evidence that the frequency of different translocations and potentially other genetic abnormalities may also differ geographically[44–46] (see Chapters 5, 6, 7, 8). These differences in the occurrence of ALL subtypes in time and place suggest a close link between the occurrence of specific translocations (some of which are detectable at birth in normal babies) and one or more environmental factors in the genesis of precursor B-cell ALL. The nature of such cofactors remains elusive, although there has been much speculation centered on either "late" infection with a common childhood infectious agent (the delay being incurred by improved hygiene or greater isolation of the infant in higher socioeconomic circumstances), or infection in the neonatal period, resulting in immune dysregulation that predisposes to the later appearance of ALL. To date, the evidence supporting these theories remains indirect.[47–49]

Early infection with malaria and EBV appear to predispose, separately or together, to the likelihood of the development of BL and Hodgkin lymphoma in L and MI countries; both of which are almost invariably associated with the presence of EBV in the tumor cells in children (in the case of Hodgkin lymphoma, particularly prior to the age of 10 years.[39,50] Both malaria and EBV are B-cell mitogens; malaria is known to increase the proportion of circulating B lymphoctyes that contain EBV, albeit in an essentially quiescent state.[39] This gives rise to the possibility that EBV is at least a co-factor in the pathogenesis of some B-cell neoplasms, such as BL and HL, although it clearly plays no role in the development of ALL. The possibility that malaria has a suppressive influence on ALL, whose incidence appears to be low where that of BL is high (namely, in equatorial Africa) cannot be excluded. While geographic differences in genetic polymorphisms in various EBV genes have been well described,[39] whether or not such polymorphisms are relevant to lymphomagenesis remains unknown. The predisposing effect of malaria on BL remains unproven, in so far that a defined mechanism has not been identified, although it's strongly positive effect on B-cell ontogeny and its ability to increase the proportion of circulating EBV-containing cells may be sufficient to increase the likelihood of BL development; although a role for additional infections that influence the cellular composition of the immune system cannot be excluded.[51]

Although definitive evidence of a predisposing role for malaria remains elusive, quite persuasive evidence is provided by the relationship between the likelihood of developing BL and the severity of infection by malaria.[52] The well-described protective effect of sickle cell anemia and (probably) of heterozygotism for the thalassemias, on the severity of malaria[53] might be supposed — if malaria is a co-factor for BL — to have a measurable effect on incidence, but this has never been definitively shown, possibly because numbers are too small to demonstrate a statistically significant difference. The relationship may also have been obscured by failing to take into consideration recent evidence that suggests that heterozygosity for more than one of the monogenetic anemias negatively influences the protective effect of these diseases against malaria.[53]

The possibility that a difference in the relative frequency or type of genetic lesions associated with leukemia/lymphoma influences the response to treatment, and could account for at least a part of the reason for worse results in under-resourced countries is worthy of consideration. Genetic lesions of this type could result in more extensive diseases at presentation, but there can be little doubt that the disease extent is to a large extent determined by a host of socioeconomic factors discussed earlier in this chapter and elsewhere.[54] Differences in the relative proportions of specific chromosomal translocations in ALL known, at least in high-income countries, to be associated with outcome have been reported, those associated with a worse prognosis (e.g. 9;22 translocations) appearing to be more common than in technologically advanced countries, and those associated with a better prognosis (e.g. TEL-AML1) less common than in technologically advanced countries.[45] Again, the influence of such genetic lesions is likely to be obscured by the many other factors that influence outcome, such as delay in initiating treatment, the availability of appropriate treatment and effective supportive care.[54]

Outcomes of Common Childhood Hematological Malignancies in L and MI Countries

The success of developed countries in treating childhood hematological malignancies has not been achieved in L and MI countries. There are several factors contributing to this discrepancy in outcomes, discussed in more detail in the next section, that deserve mention here. These include limited access to care, poverty, poor hygiene, late presentation, limited availability of chemotherapy agents, inadequate supportive care, lack of professional skills and knowledge, and lack of salvage therapy where primary treatment fails. Furthermore, accurate outcome results are hampered by inadequate incidence data and insufficient research to properly delineate treatment outcomes in L and MI countries. Similarly, there is limited information on late effects and quality of life of cancer survivors in L and MI countries, although as survival rates increase, this will become, as it has in HI countries, of increasing importance.[55]

ALL

Acute lymphoblastic leukemia (ALL), the most common childhood cancer worldwide, accounts for approximately a third of childhood malignancy in most world regions; it has an overall 5-year survival rate (OS) as high as 95% in high-income countries for selected subtypes and risk groups and a combined OS rate of approximately 80% (see Chapters 11 and 12). In L and MI countries, the incidence is generally significantly lower for reasons already discussed. In series published from Cuba, Uruguay and Turkey in the 1990s, 5-year OS estimates were 68%, 52% and 40% respectively.[56–58] During a similar time period from 1998–2003, one institution in China reported a 5-year OS rate of 57.7% in children treated on a standard treatment protocol.[59] Improved results have been seen in India and Latin America, particularly where twinning programs and training have been established.[33,34,54] Incidence, treatment, and survival data for the majority of equatorial Africa remains scarce, largely because of the paucity of ALL.

AML

Acute myeloid leukemia (AML) represents a much smaller fraction of leukemia in children in high-income countries, although a rather higher fraction in those countries in which ALL is less common. It has a worse prognosis than ALL everywhere in the world and is particularly difficult to treat in L and MI countries because of the need for intensive supportive care during therapy. In Latin America, patients treated on treatment protocols through the Monza International School of Pediatric Hematology/Oncology (MISPHO) achieved 10–20% lower overall survival as compared to the same regimen used in Italy. This difference was attributed to higher rates of toxic deaths, default, and relapse.[34] The outcome for acute promyelocytic leukemia, however, can be excellent if specific therapy, namely all-trans retinoic acid (ATRA) is available. This has been reported from Iraq[60] and more recently from China. In the latter study, an intensive regimen involving high dose Ara-C and anthracycline gave a 3.5-year EFS of 37.5% with toxic deaths and abandonment of therapy being common. When a less toxic regimen, including ATRA, was introduced, the 3.5-year EFS more than doubled to 79.6%.[61]

NHL

Non-Hodgkin lymphoma (NHL) represents a single term for a group of molecularly and biologically diverse diseases, although in childhood and adolescence the range of common subtypes is much more limited than in adults (see Chapters 16 and 17). Five-year OS for NHL of 62%, 51% and 35% for Cuba, Uruguay and Turkey respectively have been reported.[56–58] In contrast, 5-year OS in high-income countries ranges from 70–90+%, even for patients with stage IV disease.[58,62–64]

HL

HL has four recognized histological subtypes that are variably amenable to therapy in high-income countries (see Chapter 18). Outcomes in L and MI countries continue to be somewhat lower than those from developed countries. This may be because of the relatively lower intensity therapy and broad range of successful chemotherapy regimens such that drug substitution creates less of a difference in outcome. Indeed, despite significantly lower 5-year OS for leukemias and NHL, for HL OS rates values range from 72–87% for Cuba, Uruguay, and Turkey.[56–58] In high-income countries, rates are generally in the region of 90–95%.[58,64]

To improve outcomes, the various barriers to optimal treatment of children with cancer must be recognized and addressed. These barriers are discussed below.

Barriers to Optimal Treatment of Children with Hematological Malignancies in L and MI Countries

Determinants of cancer cure rates

There are many barriers to optimal treatment of children with cancer in L and MI countries (Fig. 29.5). Optimal treatment, and ultimately cure, depends on a series of steps which can be conceptualized as links in the chain of care (Fig. 29.6).[11] The cancer must be suspected, and the patient brought to primary care, referred to tertiary care, diagnosed correctly, treated appropriately, and supported through treatment. These steps can be summarized as three types of access to healthcare services: access to diagnosis, access to treatment, and access to event-free survival (Table 29.3). The cure rate is the product of these three types of access, and the barriers to cure therefore, differ significantly among countries and regions. For example, in Guatemala, only 44% of children with cancer each year receive care in the country's only pediatric cancer center and event-free survival is only 43%. Despite this, 19% of children in the country are cured because 100% of those who reach the center have access to treatment, since the costs of care are covered by a non-profit foundation Ayúdame a Vivir (Help Me to Live, www.ayuvi.org.gt). In contrast, in China about 95% of children have access to diagnosis and event-free survival is excellent, but only about 7% of children are cured because of the lack of access to treatment, which depends on out-of-pocket payment by families.

Access to diagnosis

An accurate and prompt diagnosis for children with cancer in high-income countries is often taken for granted, but if any link in the chain of care is broken, diagnosis will be delayed or missed entirely. Indeed, the most extreme lack of access to diagnosis of acute leukemia is seen in parts of Africa, where the reported incidence is less than 10% of that in high-income countries.[11] This should come as no surprise in regions where endemic malaria affects approximately 200,000 children per million per year, compared to an expected 40, at most, incident cases of acute leukemia; it is noteworthy that the disparity in reported incidence between high- and low-income countries is less marked in patients with solid tumors, in whom the presence of a visible mass or other obvious signs makes confusion with malaria or other endemic infections less likely and in whom clinical manifestations usually only lead to death in advanced stages. Poverty, lack of health insurance, or adequate public health infrastructure delay prevent access to even primary care for many of the world's children, and many L and MI countries have few or no pediatric cancer units so that even patients who receive

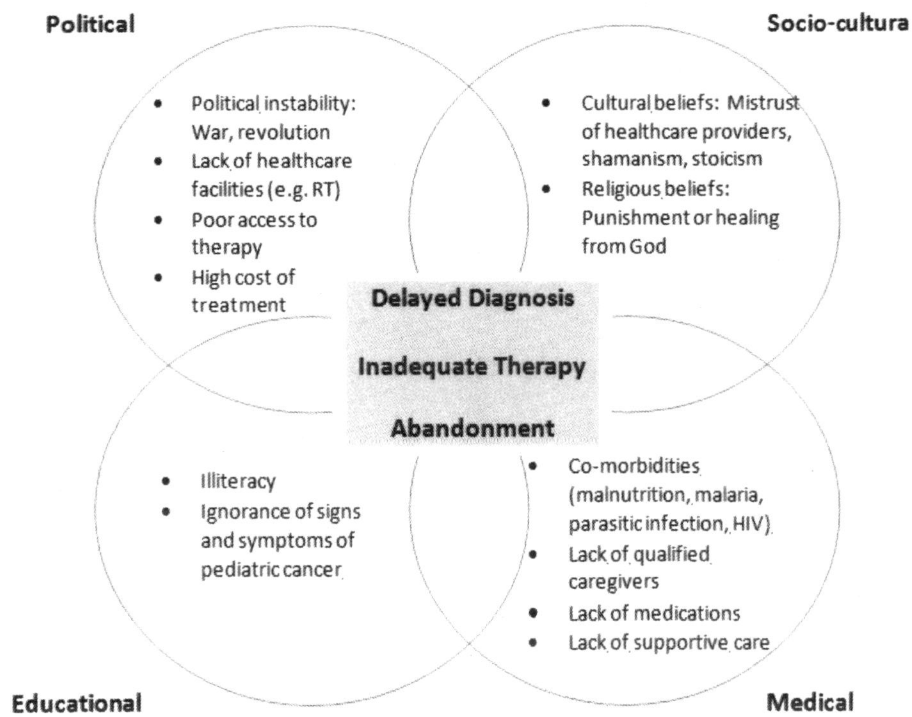

Fig. 29.5. Obstacles to care of children with cancer in low income countries. Published with kind permission of St. Jude Children's Research Hospital (www.Cure4kids.org).

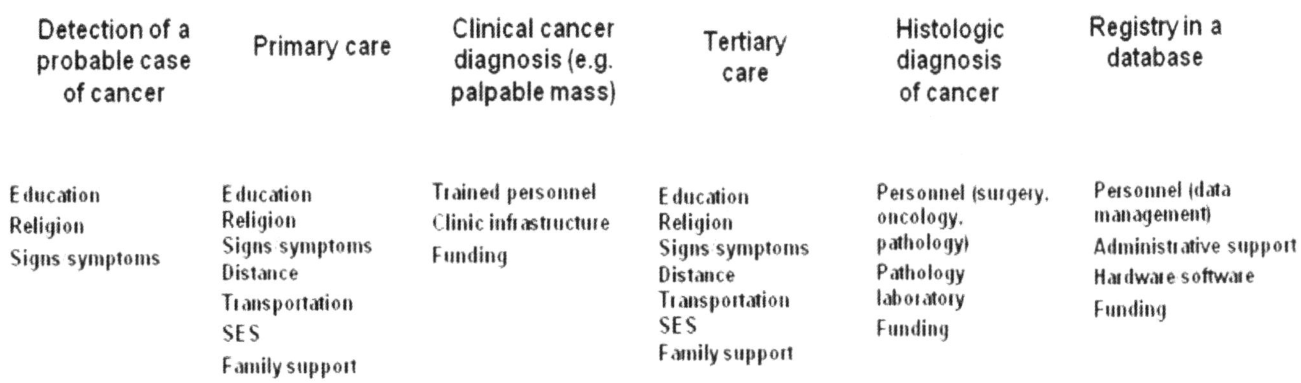

Fig. 29.6. Links in the chain of care for children with cancer. Used with permission from Cancer. Howard SC, Metzger ML, Wilimas JA, Quintana Y, Pui CH, Robison LL, Ribeiro RC. (2008) Childhood cancer epidemiology in low-income countries. *Cancer* **112**: 461–472.

effective primary care and an expeditious referral may not reach a center at which adequate cancer treatment is available. Compounding the economic and health system barriers are low literacy rates, false health beliefs, alternative medicine practitioners, and the inferior position of female children in some societies. The same difficulties that make access to cancer care problematic also make completion of a long cancer treatment regimen very difficult, such that many who have access to diagnosis abandon treatment before cure is achieved.[65,66]

Lack of availability of special diagnostic methods in L and MI countries, such as molecular testing, cytogenetics, and flow cytometry, has often been discussed. However, the effect of these diagnostic tools on cure rates is minimal, and when the patient has to bear the costs of treatment, as long as accurate diagnosis is assured, the top priority must be therapeutic agents, supportive care, and non-medical necessities to prevent abandonment (e.g. transportation, housing near the cancer center, and food). With that in mind,

Table 29.3. Determinants of cure for children with cancer: access to diagnosis, treatment, and event-free survival in selected regions and countries.

Country or region	Approximate rate of access to diagnosis (%)	Approximate rate of access to treatment (%)	Approximate event-free survival of treated patients (%)	Estimated cure rate (%)
High-income countries	100	100	80	80
Upper middle-income countries	95	95	70	63
Guatemala	44	100	43	19
China	95	10	70	7
Malawi	20	30	40	2

Published with kind permission of St. Jude Children's Research Hospital (www.Cure4Kids.org).

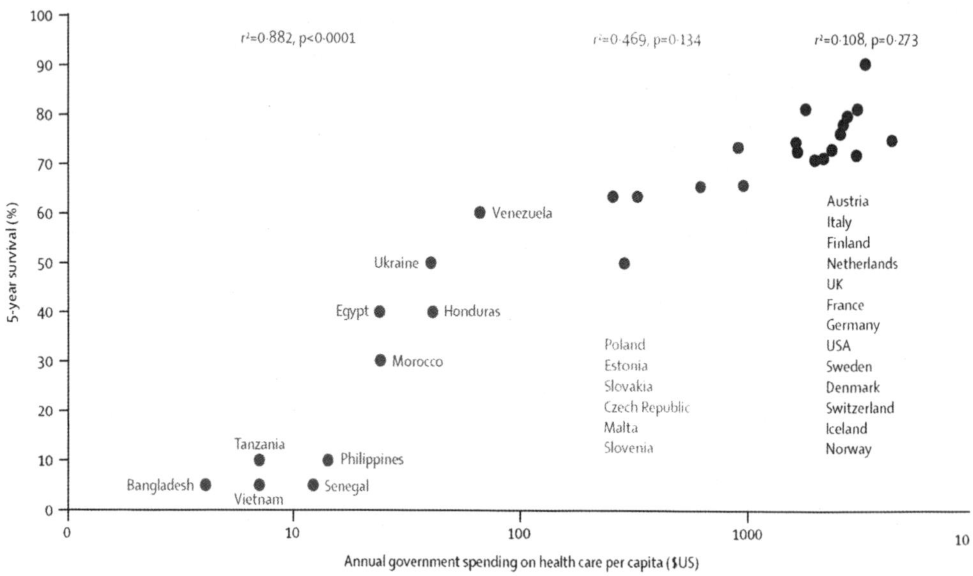

Fig. 29.7. Childhood cancer survival and government annual healthcare spending per capita ($US). Used with permission from Lancet Oncology. Ribeiro RC, Steliarova-Foucher E, Magrath I, Lemerle J, Eden T, Forget C, Mortara I, Tabah-Fisch I, Divino JJ, Miklavec T, Howard SC, Cavalli F. (2008) Baseline status of paediatric oncology care in ten low-income or mid-income countries receiving My Child Matters support: A descriptive study. *Lancet Oncol* **9**: 721–729.

immunohistochemistry should be a top priority for diagnosis of solid tumors and lymphomas and flow cytometry for acute leukemias (see Chapter 4). Indeed, in middle-income countries, the use of flow cytometry for diagnosis and risk-stratification of acute leukemias is cost-saving, since incorrect treatment in even a small percentage of cases is not only morbid, but costly.[67]

Access to treatment

Government spending on healthcare per capita is the strongest predictor of childhood cancer survival, even more so than per capita gross national income (Fig. 29.7). Even modest increases in public healthcare expenditures have a dramatic impact on survival, since they represent improved infrastructure and access at all levels of care. For example, an increase from $10 per person per year to $100 is associated with an increase in pediatric cancer survival from 10% to almost 60%. However, since improving the entire public health infrastructure is not within the purview of most pediatric oncologists, specific strategies are needed to improve pediatric cancer units and access of patients to such units, even when the public health care system is severely under-resourced.

Event-free survival

For patients with access to diagnosis and treatment, EFS poses the final hurdle to achieving cure. Access to surgery,

Table 29.4. Correlation of health and economic indicators with childhood cancer survival in ten low- and lower middle-income countries.

	Pearson's correlation coefficient (*r*)	Pearson's r^2	*P*-value
Government annual health-care expenditure per capita	0.94	0.88	<0.001
Total annual healthcare expenditure per capita	0.87	0.76	0.001
Per capita gross domestic product	0.78	0.60	0.008
Per capita gross national income	0.76	0.57	0.011
Physicians per 1000 population	0.75	0.56	0.013
Nurses per 1000 population	0.71	0.51	0.032
Human development index	0.63	0.40	0.050
Human poverty index	0.59	0.35	0.093
Mortality in people younger than 5 years	−0.58	0.33	0.081

The World Bank divides economies according to their 2009 gross national income per capita into low income ($995 or less), lower middle income ($996–$3945), upper middle income ($3946–$12,195), and high income ($12,196 or more), calculated using the World Bank Atlas method (http://data.worldbank.org/about/country-classifications/world-bank-atlas-method).

indwelling central intravenous line placement (only realistic if effective line-care can be assured), chemotherapy, and radiation therapy are fundamental to oncology treatment regimens (although not necessarily all in the same patient). In some settings chemotherapy supplies are limited by the hospital budget or the family's resources, and in other settings certain agents are not available even to those willing and able to pay. Radiation therapy facilities are lacking or inadequate in many parts of the world, and travel to a neighboring country for care only feasible to a small proportion of patients.

Trained personnel are needed to prescribe, deliver, and monitor these therapies. The number of nurses and physicians per 1000 population correlates strongly with cancer survival (Table 29.4), and the number of health care providers with expertise in pediatric oncology in L and MI countries is usually far less than that in high-income countries. For example, at one center in India, four pediatric oncologists oversee the care of 1500 newly diagnosed children with cancer each year, compared with 20 to 25 per pediatric oncologist per year at many academic centers in the USA and Europe. In addition to the enormous clinical workload, doctors in L and MI countries must also shoulder administrative responsibilities, help patients with social problems, identify the least costly care that will suffice for each patient, and assist with teaching, training, hospital infrastructure improvements, and in many cases with fund-raising. In some cases, no pediatric oncologist is available and pediatricians or medical oncologists with little pediatric experience must do their best to manage children with cancer. In most L and MI countries, nurses are in short supply, and required to rotate among all the hospital services, such that none gain expertise in oncology nursing (see Chapter 27).

Lack of sufficient space in the intensive care unit, blood product shortages and safety issues[68] limited clinical laboratory services, venous access problems, and other aspects of supportive care sometimes limit the intensity of therapy that can be delivered safely. The presence of comorbidities like malnutrition, anemia, infections (e.g. tuberculosis, malaria, parasites, hepatitis) further complicate management (see Chapter 25).

The way forward

Clearly, the interventions needed in, for example, Guatemala differ dramatically from those needed in China, but identification of the type of access lacking, the broken links in the chain of care, is an essential step to make progress. In this regard, the pediatric oncology unit of Guatemala is developing plans to provide national coverage using satellite centers and improving EFS by promoting early diagnosis and locally adapted protocol-based care.[69] Meanwhile, several regions of China have implemented social insurance plans to cover the costs of catastrophic illness and thus in those regions have increased access to treatment to almost 100%.[69] These and other strategies to improve cure rates are discussed in the following section.

Strategies to be Adopted by L and MI Countries to Improve Outcomes for Young People with Hematological Malignancies

Although significant improvements have been made in treatment outcome in some countries, these gains are not evenly distributed, being substantially more limited in L and MI countries. The most striking gains have been accomplished by co-operative programs in which resource-rich and resource-poor partners establish formal linkages, often termed "twinning" programs.[70] This model is discussed below. Whether or not an external partner is available, local initiative accompanied by at least some resources can lead to benefits for children with cancer. The International Society of Pediatric Oncology advocates the establishment of specialized pediatric cancer units.[3] These would normally be located in major urban centers and may start with a single unit in a country with a small population, e.g. fewer than 10 million inhabitants. Such units provide foci of excellence in health service delivery, education and clinical research; and can promote equitable access to care while contributing to national programs in cancer control, including the registration of incident cases.[11,14] Concentration of resources and expertise in this fashion poses challenges for rural populations and families living in smaller conurbations, but these can be offset by assisting with transportation and accommodation while networks of satellite clinics are established to meet components of continuing care closer to home. Such a framework allows optimization of scarce components required for the successful treatment of malignant diseases and provides the best opportunities for gaining experience in the safe and efficacious delivery of chemotherapy while minimizing treatment-related morbidity and mortality.[30] Strategies for progressive intensification of therapy in accordance with the incremental acquisition of expertise have been suggested.[71]

The pursuit of better outcomes through contemporary multi-modality treatment demands that close attention be paid to supportive care. Components of this essential element that require particular attention in the L and MI country setting include nutritional supplementation, given the prevalence of under nutrition in many of these countries,[32] and the provision of blood products that are screened for HIV, hepatitis B and C and syphilis. The latter is no small undertaking, but at the World Blood Donor Day on June 14, 2007, no fewer than 10 low income countries reported that they had reached this goal.

Administration of treatment with curative intent is the cornerstone of cancer control in young people. In L and MI countries, the difficulty in improving outcomes through intensive therapy is compounded by the need to address comorbidities,[14] especially infectious diseases (notably HIV/AIDS, malaria and tuberculosis). Other special considerations include bridging traditional and "modern" health care practices (investment of effort in this area often brings surprising rewards, as exemplified by experience in the most populous countries — India and China);[14,72] and the harsh reality of judging the best use of limited resources in the face of primary disease with a very poor prognosis (such as advanced neuroblastoma) and early relapse of disease in which the attainment of cure is highly unlikely, e.g. Wilms tumor. These circumstances demand substantive, elective discussion of the ethical dilemmas in local situations. Similarly, there is a need to plan for the delivery of palliative and end-of-life care for which imaginative solutions can be achieved.[73] Again, continuing monitoring/surveillance of survivors, for the early detection of "late effects" and other objectives, such as health promotion, demand the development of locally appropriate programs for which, all too often, resources are extremely limited.[74]

Faced with such hurdles, what can the pediatric oncology communities do to perform as agents of change? Since financial constraints are paramount in low-income countries, attention must be paid to the principle of cost effectiveness.[75] Examples of success include the investment in a regional facility for flow cytometry in Guatemala, serving much of Central America;[67] and the treatment of children with BL in Africa with drug costs of $<$ US $50 per child,[76] albeit, results with such regimens are far from optimal. The latter experience highlights the need for a formulary of drugs in L and MI countries, relating to cancer in young people,[77] linking with the thrust by WHO to develop a list of essential medicines for children. Not only will this serve as a useful guide to governments but it could afford opportunities for bulk-purchasing and cost-sharing with respect to both drugs and other medical supplies, although the opportunity is much less than when the same therapy can be given to literally millions of children, e.g. in the case of malaria or even HIV. Moreover, training in pharmacy and procurement is essential if these endeavors are to be successful.

Even the complete absence or non-availability of an entire treatment modality (radiotherapy) does not preclude progress in attaining improvements in outcomes for young people with cancer in L and MI countries (particularly in hematological malignancies). The achievements of colleagues in Nicaragua, with respect to survival rates for children with Wilms tumor[30,78] and HL,[79] are notable in this regard.

Abandonment of therapy, the ultimate expression of non-compliance, has been the commonest cause of treatment failure in L and MI countries.[66] Understanding the basis of this phenomenon,[31] which is decidedly uncommon in resource-rich countries, has allowed the evolution of effective strategies to combat the challenge.[80] This can lead to remarkable progress, as exemplified by the initiative of the government of Mexico in reducing the abandonment rate in children with ALL to less than 1%.[81]

Poor socio-economic status is generally at the root of abandonment — either because of an inability to afford the predominently out-of-pocket expenses of treatment, or to spend time away from the family source of income. Poverty is also linked to basic disease biology (such as immunophenotype in ALL,[18] malnutrition[82] and overall survival.[83]

A key to success is the training of a large enough work force of health professionals, and sometimes reassignment of specific tasks (e.g. giving nurses a more important role). Successful programs have been established for physicians both at the national level, as in India,[84] and regionally, as in Guatemala serving the needs of Central America. Programs in pediatric oncology for nurses have also been developed.[85]

Under-pinning the provision of health services should be a commitment to locally relevant research. This is not a luxury but is essential and must address the "10/90" gap — only 10% of the world's health research funding supports studies of 90% of the diseases affecting the global population.[86] Investment in research can lead to good data management, building knowledge and experience, enhancing health care delivery, and establishing higher standards of clinical practice;[86] all advances that will surely lead to better outcome for young people with cancer in L and MI countries. Building training programs locally and improving professional opportunities is critical to the prevention of migration of health workers to wealthier countries. In this respect, effective partnerships through videoconferencing can be effectively employed; case discussions provide an effective approach to learning.

Contributions of High-Income Countries to Improving Outcome of Children with Hematological Malignancies in L and MI Countries

Institutions and individual in high income countries can contribute significantly to childhood cancer care in L and MI countries. The most effective efforts are those that build local capacity and include education, training, access to experts, twinning programs, clinical research, and development of regional and global networks.

Education and training

The critical importance of well-trained health care professionals is universally recognized. All major medical societies for both adult and pediatric oncology have education programs, support exchange visits among institutions, foster research and clinical collaborations, and provide scholarships for meeting attendance by colleagues from L and MI countries. Many also provide free access to their journal, provide discounted membership to professionals from poorer countries and post educational materials for download on their web sites (e.g. www.siop.nl, www.ASPHO.org, www.inctr.org, www.hematology.org). These efforts over the years have led to a large number of satisfying professional and personal connections across continents that have improved care, research, and morale in the global pediatric oncology community. The use of video- and internet-conferencing (e.g. www.cure4kids.org, made available by St. Jude Children's Research Hospital) complements participation in international meetings and workshops, and has become a routine method of sharing information and experiences, discussing individual patients and reviewing protocol information among colleagues practicing in similar circumstances. Some major centers in L and MI countries (e.g. the Tata Memorial Center and Cancer Institute (WIA) in India have already established extensive web-based networks with peripheral centers for purposes of training, education and patient care.

Educational programs must not be limited to oncology professionals, but must also extend to primary care clinicians, families, and society as a whole. For example, a society-wide education campaign to identify retinoblastoma at an earlier stage in Honduras was associated with a reduction in extra-ocular disease (which is uniformly fatal in Honduras) from 73% to 35%, an intervention that saved the lives of more children with retinoblastoma than any imaginable new chemotherapy regimen.[87] Education of parents whose child already has been diagnosed is also critical to promote adherence to therapy and prevent abandonment, as documented in Indonesian children with ALL[65,88] living.

Access to experts

Although protocol-based care results in standardized treatment regimens for cancer patients, the application of the protocol in the real-world setting often leads to doubts and controversies. Pediatric oncologists practicing in L and MI countries rarely have the luxury of specializing in a subset of childhood or adolescent cancers and often lack access to experts for day-to-day advice and discussion. Furthermore, they are expected to manage large numbers of patients with little time (and sometimes little access) to information resources and may not be in a position to deliver recommended care for a variety of reasons. Cure4Kids and similar educational sites provide access to current online textbooks and seminars at no cost, but do not address the need to discuss specific patients, obtain second opinions about controversial patients or assist in making decisions about protocol modifications dictated by the local situation. Other web-based applications exist in which case-based discussions as well as other forms of distance learning are possible, including iPath[89] and RAFT[90] created by the universities of Basel and Geneva respectively. Many experts in high-income countries routinely provide emailed advice about patients to their colleagues, but may sometimes lack awareness of the conditions in which the patient is being treated, such that advice may not be relevant or practical. Twinning programs and networks of clinicians provide access to experts and a means to develop local expertise, and are further discussed below.

Twinning programs

Twinning programs are defined as long-term partnerships between institutions for the purpose of exchange of information and mutual development. They may be highly focused, or broad-based, bilateral or multilateral, such that a precise definition pediatric oncology twinning programs between centers, high-income countries, and those in L and MI countries have proved to be one of the most successful approaches to improve care in poor resource settings LIC when used to the full and sufficiently well funded, although improvements may take place only in the course of many years. A broad range of educational, and service related programs can be subsumed under this heading. Several twinning programs have been operating for many years, including the partnerships between La Mascota Hospital in Nicaragua and collaborators in Monza, Italy;[70,91,92] among centers in Amsterdam, South Africa, Indonesia and Malawi;[65,88,93–97] between St. Jude Children's Research Hospital's International Outreach Program and centers in Latin America, Africa, and Asia;[33,80,98–101] and many others.[102] Many twinning programs have been partially or entirely supported by non-profit, non-governmental foundations, including the Keira Grace Foundation (www.keiragracefoundation.com), Jiv Daya Foundation (www.jivdayafound.org), World Child Cancer (www.worldchildcancer.org), Fundación Ayúdame a Vivir (www.ayuvi.org.gt), and many others. The International Union Against Cancer (UICC) and Sanofi-Aventis' My Child Matters program has supported more focused projects, each of which has a mentor, in many countries, and performed a comprehensive evaluation of cancer care in 10 of them.[69]

Clinical research as a necessity

In the past, conducting research was considered a luxury for those centers with ample human and financial resources, in which personnel could be assigned exclusively to conduct research activities. However, it is now clear that in L and MI countries, clinical research is obligatory to understand how to use scare resources optimally to cure the maximum number of children possible. Protocols that work well in high-income countries may cause disastrous toxicity in L and MI countries, as occurred when a St. Jude regimen was adopted in El Salvador without modification[99] so very often, adapted regimens are needed.[71] Research in which an external partner is involved is particularly valuable, since it provides an opportunity to evaluate and assist in the improvement of a variety of aspects of patient care (including diagnosis and supportive care)[30] as well as infrastructural issues, such as drug procurement and management. Ideally, centers in which patients are able to receive effective therapy can be used as training centers at national or international levels. Where possible, frequent meetings to compare results among centers and share best practices can be extremely valuable.[33,54,100,103–109]

Conducting clinical research and the process of continuous quality improvement requires a data management program.[110] Funding for the data manager salary often comes from non-governmental agencies until the value of the role can be demonstrated to hospital and government administration. Training of data managers is essential, but equally important is daily supervision, quality monitoring, and collaboration with the pediatric oncologists who will use the data to improve care. It should be made clear that the Principal Investigator bears primary responsibility for the accuracy of the data — all too often, this critically important task is left to junior staff with minimal surveillance. A database of some kind is essential. Many databases are available at no cost to store pediatric oncology information ranging from, at the simplest level, an open access spreadsheet (www.OpenOffice.org) intermediate level databases such as EpiInfo (www.cdc.gov/epiinfo/) or POND (wwww.POND4Kids.org) to sophisticated databases with built in business rules available, for example, from caBIG of the NCI, USA, or developed by cooperative groups or other organizations conducting research (e.g. the International Network for Cancer Treatment and Research, INCTR) for specific studies.

The third component of data management programs, data analysis, is often neglected. The authors have encountered many situations in which data has been collected (sometimes meticulously) but never analyzed with a view of how to improve care. In this regard, identifying preventable toxic deaths, abandonment, and relapse, as well as measuring survival, should be the main goals of any pediatric oncology data management program. Since so few pediatric oncologists in L and MI countries have any formal training in research, clinical studies are best undertaken with the support and encouragement of more expert regional or international colleagues in the context of regional and global networks, as discussed in the next section.

Regional and global networks

Twinning partnerships provide opportunities for rapid progress and mobilize resources on both sides of the partnership to support pediatric oncology, but their impact, at least, in terms of reduced toxicity or improved survival, depending upon dissemination plans via regional or international meetings, is often limited to the participating centers. Regional and global networks can extend their benefits to entire countries or continents, and allow colleagues to learn from colleagues who practice in a similar setting and face similar problems. Furthermore, the research required to adapt treatment regimens and document their efficacy, feasibility and sustainability in the local setting can only be conducted in L and MI countries. Finally, protocol development and implementation, as well as consultation with regional colleagues, and applications for funding are much more successful when several centers combine their efforts.

The formation of national pediatric oncology groups is a good first step, and includes long-standing groups like those in Argentina (www.gatla.org.ar), Brazil (www.sobope.org.br), and Mexico (Agrupación Mexicana de Onco–Hematología Pediátrica en México); as well as relatively new groups, like those in India (Indian Pediatric Oncology Group) and Colombia (Asociación Colombiana de Hematología y Oncología Pediátrica). It is noteworthy that in Colombia, the alliance of oncology centers and several non-governmental organizations (NGO's) has led to effective advocacy for childhood cancer at the governmental level and the passage of legislation similar to that in Mexico, that covers the costs of childhood cancer care and provides some essential healthcare rights.

Regional programs also play a vital role in allowing professionals from neighboring countries to compare healthcare services and share best practices in similar circumstances. Implementing specific projects, such as a shared treatment regimen for a particular disease, can provide a focal point for collaboration. However, saving lives by improving each pediatric cancer unit should remain the primary focus, with use of a specific disease or protocol as the point of departure. This method has been very successful in French-speaking Africa, Sub-Saharan Africa, India, and Latin America.[33,34,54,67,105,106,111,112]

A number of other disease-specific or treatment modality-specific collaborations complement the other activities described above. For example, INCTR (www.inctr.org) provides education, facilitates implementation of protocol-based care, develops cancer prevention programs, and advocates to keep cancer on the global agenda.[113–115] The Program of Action in Cancer Therapy of the International Atomic Energy Agency has been active globally to improve radiation therapy for cancer patients[116] and international collaboration for retinoblastoma education, treatment, and research has been extremely productive.[117–119] The Children's Oncology Group of the USA has actively sought collaborations with other cooperative groups and includes international outreach in its mission.

Frequent communication is the cornerstone of successful collaboration.[120–122] It not only demonstrates the commitment of participants, but increases that commitment through frequent interactions, mutual assistance with patients, sharing of administrative tasks (e.g. development of supportive care guidelines), and building friendships. Online meetings via www.Cure4Kids.org have transformed the twinning programs and regional collaborations of several of the authors. One example is the weekly meeting that has taken place between three centers in Morocco, St. Jude Children's Research Hospital, and many guests from several continents since 2005. Other examples include the neurooncology collaboration between colleagues at the Hospital for Sick Children in Toronto, Canada and the King Hussein Cancer Center in Amman, Jordan.[123]

Optimal Use of Limited Resources

Not all children with cancer receive everything needed for optimal diagnosis and treatment. When parents in L and MI countries, whose resources are often severely constrained, must pay out of pocket for each diagnostic test and therapeutic intervention, the necessity and cost-effectiveness of each potential expense must be considered.[124,125] Some sophisticated diagnostic tests may add little to the diagnosis, but will add to the financial burden — possibily to the level of unsupportability — and leave no funds over for treatment. The reverse may apply, where savings on diagnostic tests lead to inaccurate diagnosis and unnecessary expenditure on incorrect treatment with a potentially bad outcome for the patient. Similar considerations apply to staging studies. Tests for relapse should be carefully considered and it is generally best to continue with current therapy until clear progression indicates relapse rather than undertake costly and even potentially hazardous tests (e.g. surgical procedures) when diagnosing relapse slightly earlier has not been shown to be beneficial. When the cost of treating relapse is high and success highly unlikely, it must be decided, with the family, whether further specific treatment or palliative care represent the best option. The performance of phase I studies is particularly problematic from the ethical perspective in very poor populations, since even if the drugs are paid for, the likelihood of benefit is small and the family may suffer major financial loss from being away from home and their source of income.

The importance of good palliative care cannot be overemphasized. Unfortunately, for various reasons, particularly the frequently limited (or no) access to opioids, few patients receive this essential component of care for patients who never had, or have exhausted all therapeutic options (the term "palliative care" is often now extended to all aspects of symptom control and psychosocial care in patients with potentially fatal diseases). In L and MI countries, where a high fraction of patients present with incurable disease, palliative care should be given a particularly high priority.

Summary and Future Directions

While children in high-income countries presently have 5-year survival rates of 70–80%, such that relatively small increments in survival are likely to occur in the coming years, improved care of the 80% of children and adolescents with cancer in low-and middle-income countries could make an enormous difference to global survival rates. Unfortunately, resources in these countries are very limited, and improvements are unlikely to be rapid, except in those countries presently undergoing rapid economic growth — and assuming that health care expenditure keeps pace with economic development. Paramount in improving survival rates is the building of human capacity for diagnosis, treatment (including palliative care) and supportive care. Children also have special needs, such that many more specialized pediatric oncology units associated with required resources such as pediatric psychosocial workers and teachers will be needed. It is also important to remember that successful treatment of the child with cancer must also be associated with minimizing the long-term or late effects of treatment.

One of the important determinants of improved survival rates in children with cancer in the west was the formation of Cooperative Groups and treating all patients uniformly on clinical studies, thus having outcome data on almost every child with cancer. Eventually, the recognition that the prognosis of children with the same disease varied in a reproducible way (usually relating to the tumor burden or degree of dissemination of disease) led to the recognition of risk groups and the realization that some children required more intensive therapy than others. Treatment could then be tailored to the degree of "risk", generally measured by tumor stage. The concept of risk stratified treatment is particularly important in L and MI countries where cost and supportive care can be prohibitive of many intensive regimens used in technologically advanced countries. In order to extend effective treatment to those with advanced disease — unfortunately, generally a higher fraction in the L and MI countries — it will be important to develop not only specialization within the discipline of pediatric oncology, but cooperative groups in which protocols can be designed and applied uniformly for specific stages of specific diseases and data acquired about their feasibility, effectiveness and cost of treatment in resource poor contexts. Ideally, of course, earlier detection programs (essentially, in pediatric cancer, education of the public and primary care providers) with efficient referral systems should be put in place to ensure that the maximum number of patients have early stage disease at the time of treatment.

In this increasingly globalized world, all stakeholders involved in the care of children with cancer, irrespective of geographical boundaries should advocate for equity and should honor the right of every child to full access to potentially curative treatment of cancer and the highest attainable standard of health as enunciated by United Nations as well as the Ponte De Legno working group.[2,5] However, at the same time, the treatment of childhood cancers in low- and middle-income countries is severely constrained by resource deficiencies (human and otherwise) and the many health problems that are at least equally deserving of attention. Few patients in developing countries have medical insurance, which makes little sense to families whose income is barely sufficient for food and shelter. Decisions have to be taken every day whether to use the limited available funds to treat many children with curable cancers like HL, or to provide care for a few children with a low chance of cure, including children with recurrent disease. At least some of these children may be curable with expensive therapy such as high-dose therapy followed by stem-cell transplantation, but few can afford such treatment, and the number of units able to deliver such care is extremely limited such that access may be unavailable even for those who can afford it — tempting the richest to travel overseas for care, and potentially inhibiting the development of even a small number of such units that can provide focal points from which specialized skills can be developed and disseminated as national economic development occurs.[2,4,125]

Inevitably, the enormous disparities in resources between high-income and low-income countries undermine declarations of the right to effective health care. Unfortunately, the vast majority of wealthy countries do not meet their pledges for official aid of any kind and cancer remains a neglected health problem in L and MI countries, whose health systems remain adapted to infectious diseases. While the millennium goals, which focus on poverty, education and primary health care are critically important, and solving these problems is essential to improving access to care for children (and adults) with cancer at a point in their disease when they retain a significant chance of cure, it is not appropriate to wait until these problems are solved, since this would result in large numbers of deaths, while in fact, there is much that can be done now to improve survival rates in children with cancer, particularly via collaboration among rich and poor — one of the main points that this chapter attempts to make. Childhood cancers are among the most curable of cancers, and children have their entire lives to lead, such that saving the life of a child can lead to significant economic benefits to the country. Moreover, since childhood cancer accounts for a higher proportion of cancer in L and MI countries, and is generally curable, it can serve as an important model to convince policy makers that cancer should be recognized as a health problem everywhere in the world. Fortunately, there are signs that slowly but surely, the world is waking up to this inconvenient truth — inconvenient because of the complexities and cost of developing effective cancer control programs. Many valuable models exist with respect to what can be done to improve capacity for the care of pediatric cancer. The next step is to expand efforts in order to have an impact at national and international levels. While civil society and academia have important roles to play, this will not be achieved in the absence of "buy-in" from governments. It will be essential to work with advocates from other disciplines, to convince policy makers of the importance of cancer, including pediatric cancer, as a global health problem at humanitarian and economic levels. Improving health and education at a global level is not only worthwhile in its own right, but will do much to improve political relations among the worlds nations and to enhance cooperation that is vital to dealing with global problems such as the overuse of fossil fuels at the expense of the environment, the catastrophic impact humans are having on biodiversity and the serious risks posed by nuclear proliferation.

References

7. Stiller CA. (2007) International patterns of cancer incidence in adolescents. *Cancer Treat Rev* **33**: 631–645.
9. Bleyer A, Barr R. (2009) Cancer in young adults 20 to 39 years of age: Overview. *Semin Oncol* **36**: 194–206.
11. Howard SC, Metzger ML, Wilimas JA, Quintana Y, Pui CH, Robison LL, Ribeiro RC. (2008) Childhood cancer epidemiology in low-income countries. *Cancer* **112**: 461–472.
12. Stiller CA. (2006) Personal Communication
17. Paes CA, Viana MB, Freire RV, Martins-Filho OA, Taboada DC, Rocha VG. (2003) Direct association of socio-economic status with T-cell acute lymphoblastic leukaemia in children. *Leuk Res* **27**: 789–794.
18. Sazawal S, Bhatia K, Gutierrez MI, Saxena R, Arya LS, Bhargava M. (2004) Paucity of TEL-AML 1 translocation, by multiplex RT-PCR, in B-lineage acute lymphoblastic leukemia (ALL) in Indian patients. *Am J Hematol* **76**: 80–82.
21. Glaser SL, Lin RJ, Stewart SL, Ambinder RF, Jarrett RF, Brousset P, Pallesen G, Gulley ML, Khan G, O'Grady J, Hummel M, Preciado MV, Knecht H, Chan JK, Claviez A. (1997) Epstein-Barr virus-associated Hodgkin's disease: Epidemiologic characteristics in international data. *Int J Cancer* **70**: 375–382.
22. Naresh KN, Advani S, Adde M, Aziz Z, Banavali S, Bhatia K, Belgaumi A, Ezzat A, Khaled H, Mokhtar N, Norton A, Rohatiner A, Sagar TG, Taciyliz N,

Temmim L, Venkatesh C, Yan Tang J, Magrath I. (2004) Report of an International Network of Cancer Treatment and Research workshop on non-Hodgkin's lymphoma in developing countries. *Blood Cells Mol Dis* **33**: 330–337.

26. Steliarova-Foucher E, Stiller C, Lacour B, Kaatsch P. (2005) International classification of childhood cancer, third edition. *Cancer* **103**: 1457–1467.
27. Barr RD, Holowaty EJ, Birch JM. (2006) Classification schemes for tumors diagnosed in adolescents and young adults. *Cancer* **106**: 1425–1430.
29. Gupta S, Bonilla M, Fuentes SL, Caniza M, Howard SC, Barr R, Greenberg ML, Ribeiro R, Sung L. (2009) Incidence and predictors of treatment-related mortality in paediatric acute leukaemia in El Salvador. *Br J Cancer* **100**: 1026–1031.
30. Bonilla M, Rossell N, Salaverria C, Gupta S, Barr R, Sala A, Metzger ML, Sung L. (2009) Prevalence and predictors of abandonment of therapy among children with cancer in El Salvador. *Int J Cancer* **125**: 2144–2146.
33. Howard SC, Ortiz R, Baez LF, Cabanas R, Barrantes J, Fu L, Pena A, Samudio A, Vizcaino M, Rodriguez-Galindo C, Barr RD, Conter V, Biondi A, Masera G. (2007) Protocol-based treatment for children with cancer in low income countries in Latin America: A report on the recent meetings of the Monza International School of Pediatric Hematology/Oncology (MISPHO) — Part II. *Pediatr Blood Cancer* **48**: 486–490.
34. Ulu EM, Tore HG, Bayrak A, Gungor D, Coskun M. (2009) MRI of central nervous system abnormalities in childhood leukemia. *Diagn Interv Radiol* **15**: 86–92.
37. Sasco AJ, Jaquet A, Boidin E, Ekouevi DK, Thouillot F, Lemabec T, Forstin MA, Renaudier P, N'Dom P, Malvy D, Dabis F. (2010) The challenge of AIDS-related malignancies in sub-Saharan Africa. *PLoS One* **5**: e8621.
38. Magrath IT. (2010) *The Lymphoid Neoplasms.* London: Hodder.
40. Brown WM, Doll R. (1961) Leukaemia in childhood and young adult life. *Br Med J* **1**: 981–988.
41. Hjalgrim LL, Rostgaard K, Schmiegelow K, Soderhall S, Kolmannskog S, Vettenranta K, Kristinsson J, Clausen N, Melbye M, Hjalgrim H, Gustafsson G. (2003) Age- and sex-specific incidence of childhood leukemia by immunophenotype in the Nordic countries. *J Natl Cancer Inst* **95**: 1539–1544.
44. Siraj AK, Kamat S, Gutierrez MI, Banavali S, Timpson G, Sazawal S, Bhargava M, Advani S, Adde M, Magrath I, Bhatia K. (2003) Frequencies of the major subgroups of precursor B-cell acute lymphoblastic leukemia in Indian children differ from the West. *Leukemia* **17**: 1192–1193.
46. Greaves M. (2006) Infection, immune responses and the aetiology of childhood leukaemia. *Nat Rev Cancer* **6**: 193–203.
49. Rao CR, Gutierrez MI, Bhatia K, Fend F, Franklin J, Appaji L, Gallo G, O'Conor G, Lalitha N, Magrath I. (2000) Association of Burkitt's lymphoma with the Epstein-Barr virus in two developing countries. *Leuk Lymphoma* **39**: 329–337.
50. Chene A, Donati D, Orem J, Mbidde ER, Kironde F, Wahlgren M, Bejarano MT. (2009) Endemic Burkitt's lymphoma as a polymicrobial disease: New insights on the interaction between Plasmodium falciparum and Epstein-Barr virus. *Semin Cancer Biol* **19**: 411–420.
53. Magrath I, Shanta V, Advani S, Adde M, Arya LS, Banavali S, Bhargava M, Bhatia K, Gutierrez M, Liewehr D, Pai S, Sagar TG, Venzon D, Raina V. (2005) Treatment of acute lymphoblastic leukaemia in countries with limited resources; lessons from use of a single protocol in India over a twenty year period [corrected]. *Eur J Cancer* **41**: 1570–1583.
55. Boschmonar MG, Alvarez YG, Garcia AM, Soto TN, Roger MC, Garrote LF. (2000) Childhood cancer survival in Cuba. *Eur J Epidemiol* **16**: 763–767.
60. Luo XQ, Ke ZY, Huang LB, Guan XQ, Zhang YC, Zhang XL. (2009) Improved outcome for Chinese children with acute promyelocytic leukemia: A comparison of two protocols. *Pediatr Blood Cancer* **53**: 325–328.
61. Patte C, Auperin A, Gerrard M, Michon J, Pinkerton R, Sposto R, Weston C, Raphael M, Perkins SL, McCarthy K, Cairo MS. (2007) Results of the randomized international FAB/LMB96 trial for intermediate risk B-cell non-Hodgkin lymphoma in children and adolescents: It is possible to reduce treatment for the early responding patients. *Blood* **109**: 2773–2780.
63. Jemal A, Thomas A, Murray T, Thun M. (2002) Cancer statistics, 2002. *CA Cancer J Clin* **52**: 23–47.
65. Arora RS, Eden T, Pizer B. (2007) The problem of treatment abandonment in children from developing countries with cancer. *Pediatr Blood Cancer* **49**: 941–946.
66. Howard SC, Campana D, Coustan-Smith E, Antillon FG, Bonilla M, Fu L, Pui CH, Ribeiro RC, Wilimas JA, Lorenzana R. (2005) Development of a regional flow cytometry center for diagnosis of childhood leukemia in Central America. *Leukemia* **19**: 323–325.
68. Ribeiro RC, Steliarova-Foucher E, Magrath I, Lemerle J, Eden T, Forget C, Mortara I, Tabah-Fisch I, Divino JJ, Miklavec T, Howard SC, Cavalli F. (2008) Baseline status of paediatric oncology care in ten low-income or mid-income countries receiving My Child Matters support: A descriptive study. *Lancet Oncol* **9**: 721–729.

70. Hunger SP, Sung L, Howard SC. (2009) Treatment strategies and regimens of graduated intensity for childhood acute lymphoblastic leukemia in low-income countries: A proposal. *Pediatr Blood Cancer* **52**: 559–565.
71. Kumar S. (2000) India's government promotes traditional healing practices. *Lancet*: 1252.
75. Hesseling PB, Molyneux E, Tchintseme F, Welbeck J, McCormick P, Pritchard-Jones K, Wagner HP. (2008) Treating Burkitt's lymphoma in Malawi, Cameroon, and Ghana. *Lancet Oncol* **9**: 512–513.
76. Barr RD, Sala A, Wiernikowski J, Masera G, Mato G, Antillon F, Castillo L, Petrilli S, Quintana J, Ribeiro R, Agarwal B, Hesseling P. (2005) A formulary for pediatric oncology in developing countries. *Pediatr Blood Cancer* **44**: 433–435.
77. Baez F, Fossati Bellani F, Ocampo E, Conter V, Flores A, Gutierrez T, Malta A, Mendez G, Pacheco C, Palacios R, Sala A, Galimberti S, Cavalli F, Masera G. (2002) Treatment of childhood Wilms' tumor without radiotherapy in Nicaragua. *Ann Oncol* **13**: 944–948.
78. Baez F, Ocampo E, Conter V, Flores A, Gutierrez T, Malta A, Pacheco C, Palacios R, Biondi A, Riva L, Sala A, Silvestri D, Cavalli F, Sessa C, Casanova M, Masera G. (1997) Treatment of childhood Hodgkin's disease with COPP or COPP-ABV (hybrid) without radiotherapy in Nicaragua. *Ann Oncol* **8**: 247–250.
81. Barr RD. (2002) Nutrition, cancer, and children. A "confluence" impacting predominantly on the disadvantaged. *Nutrition* **18**: 434–435.
82. Viana MB, Fernandes RA, de Carvalho RI, Murao M. (1998) Low socioeconomic status is a strong independent predictor of relapse in childhood acute lymphoblastic leukemia. *Int J Cancer Suppl* **11**: 56–61.
84. Wilimas JA, Donahue N, Chammas G, Fouladi M, Bowers LJ, Ribeiro RC. (2003) Training subspecialty nurses in developing countries: Methods, outcome, and cost. *Med Pediatr Oncol* **41**: 136–140.
85. Global Forum for Health Research. (2002) The 10/90 report on health research, 2001. Geneva: Global Forum for Health Research.
86. Leander C, Fu LC, Pena A, Howard SC, Rodriguez-Galindo C, Wilimas JA, Ribeiro RC, Haik B. (2007) Impact of an education program on late diagnosis of retinoblastoma in Honduras. *Pediatr Blood Cancer* **49**: 817–819.
88. Brauchli K, Oberholzer M. (2005) The iPath telemedicine platform. *J Telemed Telecare* **112**: S3–S7.
91. Masera G, Baez F, Biondi A, Cavalli F, Conter V, Flores A, Fontana G, Fossati Bellani F, Lanfranco P, Malta A, Mendez G, Ocampo E, Pacheco C, Riva L, Sala A, Silva F, Sessa C, Tognoni G. (1998) North-South twinning in paediatric haemato-oncology: The La Mascota programme, Nicaragua. *Lancet* **352**: 1923–1926.
96. Israels T, Ribeiro RC, Molyneux EM. (2010) Strategies to improve care for children with cancer in sub-Saharan Africa. *Eur J Cancer* **46**: 1960–1966.
103. Lemerle J, Barsaoui S, Harif M, Hireche K, Ladjadj Y, Moreira C, Andoh J, Doumbe P, Togo B, Kam L, Rafaramino F, Patte C, Tournade MF, Raphael M, Boccon-Gibod L, Mallon B, Raquin MA, Msefer Alaoui F. (2007) Treatment of childhood cancer in Africa. Action of the Franco-African childhood cancer group. *Med Trop (Mars)* **67**: 497–504.
108. Ayoub L, Fu L, Pena A, Sierra JM, Dominguez PC, Pui CH, Quintana Y, Rodriguez A, Barr RD, Ribeiro RC, Metzger ML, Wilimas JA, Howard SC. (2007) Implementation of a data management program in a pediatric cancer unit in a low income country. *Pediatr Blood Cancer* **49**: 23–27.
110. Kruk ME, Wladis A, Mbembati N, Ndao-Brumblay SK, Hsia RY, Galukande M, Luboga S, Matovu A, de Miranda H, Ozgediz D, Quinones AR, Rockers PC, von Schreeb J, Vaz F, Debas HT, Macfarlane SB. (2010) Human resource and funding constraints for essential surgery in district hospitals in Africa: A retrospective cross-sectional survey. *PLoS Med* **7**: e1000242.
112. Magrath I. (2007) Building capacity for cancer control in developing countries: The need for a paradigm shift. *Lancet Oncol* **8**: 562–563.

30

TLS and Other Emergencies

Jessica C. Hochberg and Stanton C. Goldman

Introduction

The majority of children, adolescents and young adults with hematological malignancies have diseases in which the expectation, even in advanced disease, is cure. Early mortality due to emergency complications usually occurs soon after or concomitant with initial diagnosis and is an especially painful and tragic occurrence for families and the medical team. Critical to the success of therapy for rapid proliferating hematopoietic malignancies is timely administration of chemotherapy without delay or dose reduction. We have increasingly better tools to appropriately recognize and manage oncologic emergencies using a patient- and disease-specific approach with an emphasis on prevention. This chapter will concentrate on summarizing several non-infectious causes of morbidity and mortality that can occur in patients with hematological malignancies: tumor lysis syndrome (TLS), hyperleukocytosis (HL), superior mediastinal syndrome (SMS) and coagulopathy/thrombosis (C/T) (Table 30.1). Besides briefly outlining the pathophysiology of these emergencies, we will try to emphasize recent advances in therapy and controversial issues in prophylaxis and management. An overriding theme is that early recognition for all these emergent complications is the most important key to successfully improving outcome.

Tumor Lysis Syndrome

Tumor lysis syndrome (TLS) is a group of metabolic abnormalities resulting from the rapid release of intracellular components from dying malignant cells. The body's homeostatic mechanisms become overwhelmed by such rapid release of intracellular metabolites leading to hyperuricemia, hyperkalemia, and hyperphosphatemia with secondary hypocalcaemia. The severe consequence of this combination can lead to uremia and renal failure, arrhythmias, seizures, and even death.[1–4] Complications resulting from TLS not only compromise the ability to deliver appropriate chemotherapy treatment but can have a significant impact on morbidity, mortality and health economics.[5]

TLS is most frequently associated with aggressive non-Hodgkin lymphoma (NHL) as well as other hematological malignancies, such as acute myeloid leukemia (AML) and acute lymphoblastic leukemia (ALL).[6–8] General risk factors for TLS include the type of malignancy, tumor burden, chemosensitivity and underlying renal dysfunction.[1–3]

Definition

Although the metabolic abnormalities comprising TLS are generally agreed upon, there is no uniform system for classification and grading. The first classification system was proposed in 1993 by Hande and Garrow.[9] This was based upon defining laboratory TLS (LTLS) or clinical TLS (CTLS).[9] While this system helped determine which patients required therapeutic intervention vs. those who did not, there were clear shortcomings which subsequently led to under recognition of patients

Table 30.1. Oncologic emergencies in hematologic malignancies.

Emergency complication	At-risk patient population	Recent advances	Controversies
TLS	Burkitts, ALL with WBC > 100 K	Rasburicase	Continued use of alkaline hydration
HL	ALL (esp. infant and T-ALL), CML and AML with WBC > 100–400 K	Pediatric apheresis technology imatinib (CML)	Chemoreduction vs. exchange/ apheresis procedure
C/T	APML ALL (2nd asparaginase)	ATRA (APML) ATIII?	Monitoring and preemptive therapy for asparginase C/T
SMS	T-ALL, T-NHL	Conformal radiation therapy, Flow cytometric diagnosis	Emergency XRT vs. chemotherapy

C/T: coagulopathy and thrombosis; HL: hyperleukocytosis; SMS: superior mediastinal syndrome; TLS: tumor lysis syndrome.

experiencing life-threatening clinical abnormalities. In order to address these shortcomings, Cairo and Bishop developed a modification to the Hande–Garrow classification system for defining both LTLS and CTLS.[1]

Under this definition, LTLS is considered to be present if two or more serum values of uric acid, potassium or phosphate are above or calcium below normal at presentation, or change by 25% within 3 days before or 7 days after the initiation of treatment (Table 30.2). CTLS requires the presence of LTLS in addition to one or more of the following clinical complications: renal insufficiency, cardiac arrhythmias/sudden death, or seizures (Table 30.3). Using this system, clinical grading of TLS is possible. LTLS is considered to be either present or absent, while the grade of CTLS is defined by the maximal grade of the clinical manifestation (Table 30.4).[1,2]

Table 30.3. Cairo-Bishop definition of clinical tumor lysis syndrome (CTLS).[a]

(1)	Creatinine[a]: $x \geq 1.5$ ULN[b] (age > 12 years or age adjusted)
(2)	Cardiac arrhythmia/sudden death[a]
(3)	Seizure[a]

Modified from Hande and Garrow (Hande and Garrow 1993).

Clinical tumor lysis syndrome (CTLS) assumes the laboratory evidence of metabolic changes and significant clinical toxicity which requires clinical intervention. Clinical TLS is defined as the presence of LTLS and any one or more of the following criteria:

[a]Not directly or probably attributable to a therapeutic agent (e.g. rise in creatinine after amphotericin administration).

[b]Creatinine levels: Patients will be considered to have elevated creatinine if their serum creatinine is 1.5 times greater than the institutional upper limit of normal (ULN) below age/gender defined ULN.

Used with permission from John Wiley and Sons/Blackwell Publishing Ltd. Cairo MS. and Bishop M. Tumour lysis syndrome: New therapeutic strategies and classification. *British J Haematol* 2004; **127:** 3–11.

Pathophysiology

Upon initiation of therapy, there is a rapid release of intracellular anions, cations, and the metabolic products of proteins and nucleic acids into the bloodstream. The increased concentrations of uric acid, phosphates, potassium, and urea can overwhelm the body's ability to process and excrete these materials and result in the clinical spectrum associated with TLS (Fig. 30.1).[3]

Table 30.2. Cairo-Bishop definition of laboratory tumor lysis syndrome (LTLS).

Uric acid	$x \geq 8$ mg/dL or 25% increase from baseline
Potassium	$x \geq 6.0$ mEq/L or 25% increase from baseline
Phosphorous	$x \geq 2.1$ mmol/L children, $x \geq 1.45$ mmol/L (adults) or 25% increase from baseline
Calcium	$x \leq 1.75$ mmol/L or 25% decrease from baseline

Modified from Hande and Garrow (Hande and Garrow 1993).

Laboratory tumor lysis syndrome (LTLS) is defined as either a 25% change or level above or below normal, as defined above, for any two or more serum values of uric acid, potassium, phosphate, and calcium within 3 days before or 7 days after the initiation of chemotherapy. This assessment assumes that a patient has or will receive adequate hydration (± alkalinization) and a hypouricaemic agent(s).

Used with permission from John Wiley and Sons/Blackwell Publishing Ltd. Cairo MS. and Bishop M. Tumour lysis syndrome: New therapeutic strategies and classification. *British J Haematol* 2004; **127:** 3–11.

Hyperuricemia results from the catabolism of intracellular nucleic acids. Complications from hyperuricemia are the most frequently recognized manifestations of TLS and can lead to many of the other clinical derangements. Purine nucleic acids are catabolized to hypoxanthine, then xanthine, and finally to uric acid by xanthine oxidase (Fig. 30.2).[10] Prevention and control of hyperuricemia is critical in the successful management of TLS.

Hyperphosphatemia results from the rapid release of intracellular phosphates from malignant cells, which contain up to four times the amount of organic and inorganic phosphates as normal cells. Phosphate precipitation with calcium in renal tubules can lead to the development of

Table 30.4. Cairo-Bishop grading classification of tumor lysis syndrome.

	Grade 0[a]	Grade I	Grade II	Grade III	Grade IV	Grade V
LTLS	–	+	+	+	+	+
Creatinine[b,c]	≤ 1.5 × ULN	1.5 × ULN	> 1.5–3.0 × ULN	> 3.0–6.0 × ULN	> 6.0 ULN	Death[d]
Cardiac arrhythmia[c]	None	Intervention not indicated	Non-urgent medical intervention indicated	Symptomatic and incompletely controlled medically or controlled with device (e.g. defibrillator)	Life-threatening (e.g. arrhythmia associated with CHF, hypotension, syncope, shock)	Death[d]
Seizure[c]	None		One brief generalized seizure; seizure(s) well controlled by anti-convulsants or infrequent focal motor seizures not interfering with ADL	Seizure in which consciousness is altered; poorly controlled seizure disorder; with breakthrough generalized seizures despite medical intervention	Seizure of any kind which are prolonged, repetitive or difficult to control (e.g. status epilepticus, intractable epilepsy)	Death[d]

Clinical tumor lysis syndrome (CTLS) requires one or more clinical manifestations along with criteria for laboratory tumor lysis syndrome (LTLS).

Maximal CTLS manifestation (renal, cardiac, neuro) defines the grade.

[a]No LTLS.

[b]Creatinine levels: Patients will be considered to have elevated creatinine if their serum creatinine is 1.5 times greater than the institutional upper limit of normal (ULN) below age/gender defined ULN.

[c]Not directly or probably attributable to a therapeutic agent (e.g. rise in creatinine after amphotericin administration).

[d]Attributive probably or definitely to CTLS.

Used with permission from John Wiley and Sons/Blackwell Publishing Ltd. Cairo MS. and Bishop M. Tumour lysis syndrome: New therapeutic strategies and classification. *British J Haematol* 2004; **127**: 3–11.

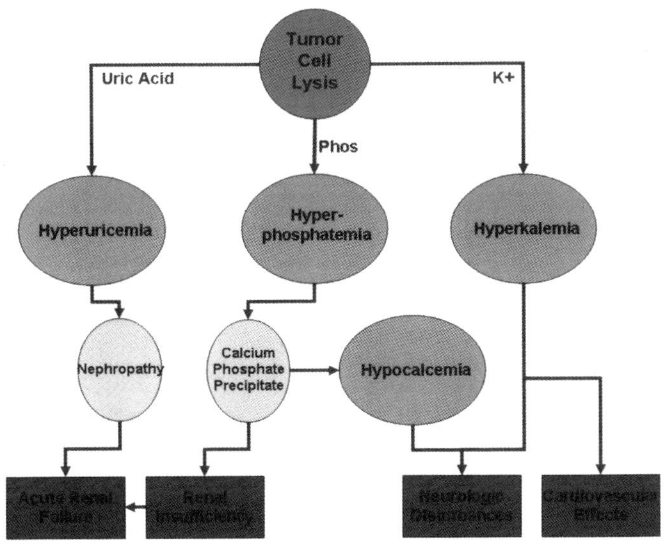

Fig. 30.1. Schematic of the metabolic abnormalities associated with the development of tumor lysis syndrome and the clinical complications stemming from these metabolic derangements.

From Hochberg J, Cairo MS, Coccia PF. Tumor lysis syndrome. Clinical Oncology 4th Edition, Abeloff MD, Armitage JO (ed.). (2008) Elsevier Churchill Livingston, Philadelphia.

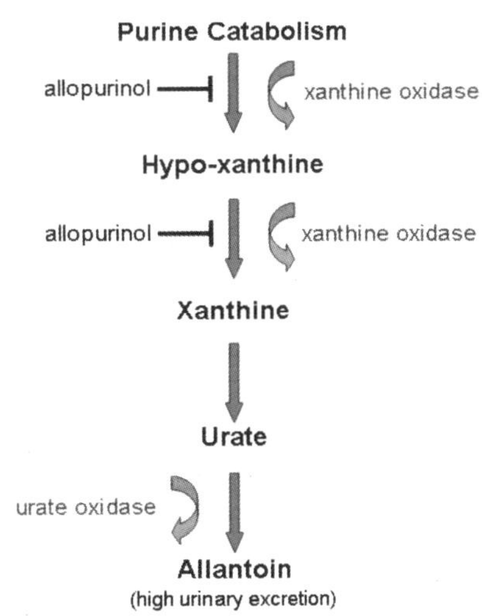

Fig. 30.2. Purine catabolism pathway.

acute renal failure (ARF), often requiring dialysis. The serum concentration of calcium rapidly decreases as precipitation with phosphate occurs. Hypocalcaemia is one of the most serious clinical manifestations of TLS and has been associated with the development of severe muscle cramping, tetany, and cardiac arrhythmias.

Hyperkalemia may also be a life-threatening consequence of TLS. Hyperkalemia results from the inability to clear the significant increase of intracellular potassium released by lysed tumor cells. This can lead to neuromuscular symptoms such as muscle weakness, cramps, and paresthesias as well as severe cardiac manifestations including ventricular tachycardia or fibrillation, syncope, and asystole.

Finally, increases in blood urea nitrogen and creatinine levels occur with worsening renal impairment associated with acute uric acid crystal nephropathy, calcium-phosphate crystals, or a combination of both. This leads to an acute obstructive uropathy syndrome with clinical manifestations of uremia, edema, hypertension, congestive heart failure, and further exacerbations of metabolic disturbances.

Incidence of TLS

The exact incidence of TLS is not well established. Overall, there appears to be an increased risk for tumor lysis in the pediatric population compared to adults. This likely reflects differences in the subtypes of hematologic malignancies found between the two groups as well as the more aggressive nature of pediatric hematologic malignancies and the difference in intensity of treatment protocols. Consequently, many of the clinical trials looking at management of tumor lysis were performed in the pediatric and young adult population, prior to being trialed in adults. An observational study of patients with AML observed LTLS in 17% (130 of 772) of patients and was considered the major cause of death in 2% of patients.[6] ALL patients are also at high risk of developing TLS with an overall incidence of hyperuricemia reported to be up to 21.4%. In a retrospective study of 102 patients with high-grade NHL, the incidence of TLS was reported to be as high as 42% as determined by serial laboratory testing although clinically significant TLS was only 6%.[9] More recent multicenter studies of 1791 children and adolescents with NHL showed that clinically significant TLS occurred in 8.4% (66 out of 790) of patients with Burkitt lymphoma.[11] The development of TLS has been observed with the administration of chemotherapy, corticosteroids, radiation, hormonal agents, and biologic response modifiers, as well as spontaneously prior to the initiation of therapy.[7,12–14]

Certain intrinsic tumor-related factors have been shown to increase the risk for development of TLS. These include high tumor cell proliferation rate, large tumor burden, tumor chemosensitivity, and increased lactate dehydrogenase (LDH) levels.[1,9,15] Thus, the risk of TLS is influenced by a number of characteristics including the type of malignancy, as well as the intensity of cytotoxic treatment. The acute leukemias, AML and ALL, have the potential to be high risk depending on WBC count, significant adenopathy or hepatosplenomegaly or significant elevations in LDH. The highest risk for TLS, and subsequently the most studied, are the high grade lymphomas such as Burkitt's and lymphoblastic lymphomas which are almost always considered high risk.[16]

Treatment

The identfication of patients at risk for the development of TLS is the most important aspect of management so that prophylactic measures may be initiated prior to or concomitantly with beginning chemotherapy. Delay in treatment of TLS can be life-threatening and costly. Recently, an international panel of TLS and hematological malignancy experts was assembled to develop a comprehensive TLS classification system based on type of malignancy and known risk factors.[16,17] This tool can be used to identify cancer patients at risk of developing TLS. (Figs. 30.3, 30.4A–B).[17] Further characterization of risk is determined by the presence of renal risk factors such that those with low or medium risk disease may necessitate upstaging to higher risk of TLS based on poor renal function. In addition, the group provided uniform, risk based TLS management guidelines that may be utilized in practice as well as future TLS studies (Table 30.5).[10,16]

Cytotoxic therapy should be delayed if possible in patients at high risk for development of tumor lysis syndrome until prophylactic measures can be initiated. The patient's vital signs, weight, urinary output, and fluid intake need to be carefully monitored. Serum creatinine, blood urea nitrogen, sodium, potassium, calcium, phosphorous, LDH and uric acid levels should be determined at baseline and every 4–6 hours for the first 48–72 hours after the initiation of tumor therapy. Patients with hyperkalemia and/or hypocalcemia should have a baseline electrocardiogram and continuous cardiac monitoring until normalization of metabolic parameters. Attempts should be made to correct fluid overload, dehydration, electrolyte and acid–base abnormalities, and to establish adequate urinary output before the initiation of therapy.

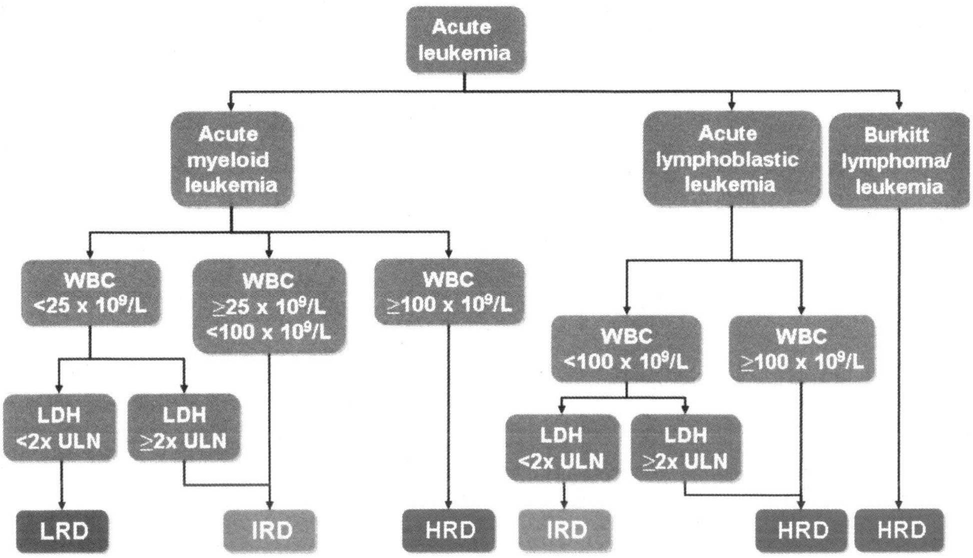

Fig. 30.3. TLS risk assessment for acute leukaemia. Adapted post-medical decision tree for risk assessment of TLS.

This research was originally published in British Journal of Hematology. Mitchell S. Cairo, Bertrand Coiffier, Alfred Reiter, Anas Younes, on behalf of the TLS Expert Panel. Recommendations for the evaluation of risk and prophylaxis of tumor lysis syndrome (TLS) in adults and children with malignant diseases: An expert TLS panel consensus. British Journal of Haematology, 149, 578–586.

HRD: high-risk disease; LRD: low-risk disease; MRD: medium-risk disease; WBC: white blood cell count.

Hydration

Intravenous hydration at 2500–3000 mL/m^2/24 hours, should ideally begin 24–48 hours before the initiation of therapy and continue for 48–72 hours after completion of chemotherapy.[16,18] Recent use of rasburicase for TLS prophylaxis and treatment can reduce the prehydration to a little as 4 hours prior to the initiation of chemotherapy. Administration of lasix or mannitol may be considered to aid in diuresis as needed but overuse of diuretics should be avoided as this can lead to dehydration and worsening of kidney perfusion. The practice of alkalinizing the urine with intravenous sodium bicarbonate has traditionally been recommended as part of TLS prevention and management strategies. However, while alkaline urine promotes the excretion of uric acid, it has the opposite effect on the solubility of xanthine.[15] Particularly after allopurinol treatment, levels of this metabolite are increased, which can lead to the precipitation of xanthine crystals in renal tubules, resulting in an obstructive uropathy similar to the more common uric acid nephropathy. Furthermore, alkalinization increases the risk of calcium phosphate precipitation which can lead to further renal dysfunction. Currently, due to the risks involved and the lack of clear benefit over aggressive hydration alone, the use of sodium bicarbonate for the prevention and treatment of TLS is not necessary when utilizing rasburicase for anti-hyperuremic therapy. Because allopurinol does not decrease the preexisting uric acid load, high-risk patients receiving allopurinol prophylaxis should receive alkalinization to a target urine pH 6.5–7.5 at least during the first 24–48 hours of chemotherapy.

Electrolyte imbalances

Hyperkalemia should be treated expediently with standard measures such as the administration of a potassium-binding resin, sodium polystyrene sulfonate 1 gm/kg/dose (max 15 g) every 6 hours. Patients with elevated potassium > 6.5 meq/kl should be monitored with continuous EKG for peaked T waves with early consideration of dialysis to avoid arrhythmias. Temporizing measures for extreme elevation of potassium could include calcium gluconate intravenous infusion (reduce cardiac excitation) and/or glucose/insulin administration (drives potassium into cells).

Aluminum hydroxide, given orally or through a nasogastric tube at a dose of 50–150 mg/kg/day divided every 4–6 hours, should be used to treat hyperphosphatemia. Treatment of asymptomatic hypocalcemia is generally not recommended as this may increase the

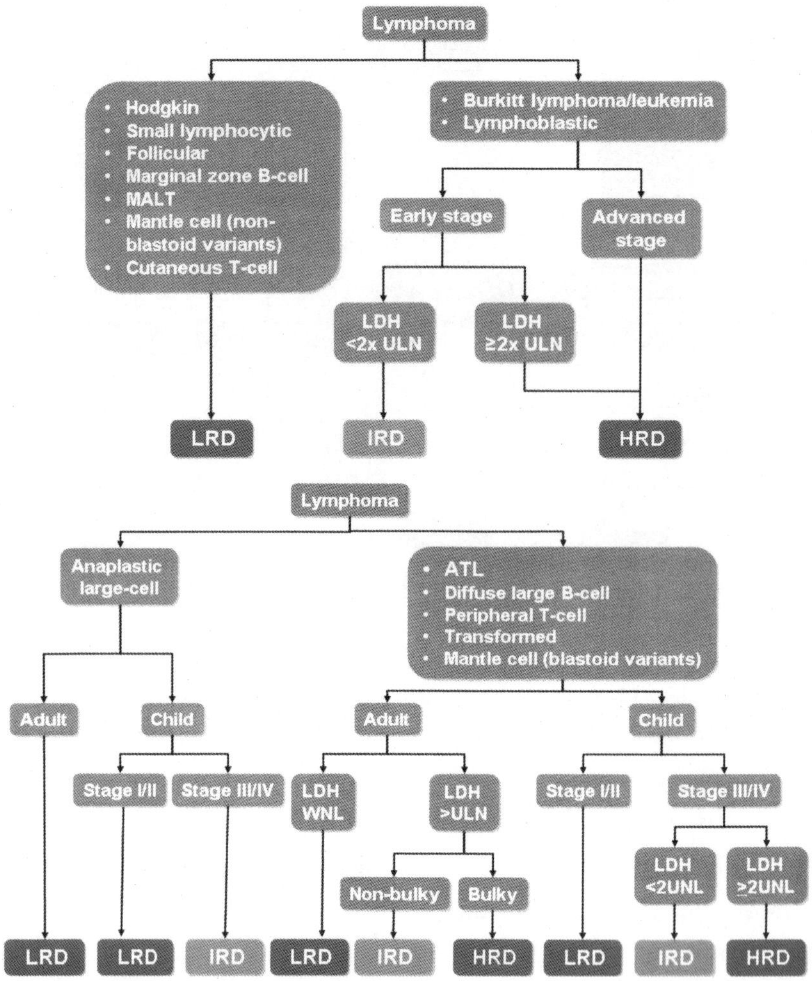

Fig. 30.4. TLS risk assessment for pediatric lymphomas. Adapted post-medical decision tree for risk assessment of TLS.

This research was originally published in British Journal of Hematology. Mitchell S. Cairo, Bertrand Coiffier, Alfred Reiter, Anas Younes, on behalf of the TLS Expert Panel. Recommendations for the evaluation of risk and prophylaxis of tumor lysis syndrome (TLS) in adults and children with malignant diseases: an expert TLS panel consensus. British Journal of Haematology, 149, 578–586.

ALCL: anaplastic large cell lymphoma; B-cell lymphoma; DLBCL: diffuse large; HRD: high-risk disease; LRD: low-risk disease; LDH: lactate dehydrogenase; MALT: mucosa-associated lymphoid tissue; MRD: medium-risk disease; PTCL: peripheral T-cell lymphoma.

risk for calcium phosphorus deposition in the renal tubules. In patients with symptomatic hypocalcemia, intravenous calcium gluconate (50–100 mg/kg per dose) may be administered to correct clinical symptoms.

For patients who have acute renal failure, significant uremia, or severe electrolyte abnormalities hemodialysis should be initiated as soon as possible. Continuous hemofiltration has been used to correct fluid overload and electrolyte abnormalities associated with tumor lysis syndrome in children.[19] The failure to promptly initiate hemodialysis for acute renal failure may turn a potentially reversible clinical situation into an irreversible one.

Hyperuricemia

In addition to hydration, the most important management strategy for TLS is the administration of a hypouricaemic agent, either allopurinol or rasburicase, prior to the initiation of chemotherapy. Allopurinol is a potent inhibitor of xanthine oxidase and blocks the conversion of hypoxanthine and xanthine to uric acid.[20] Allopurinol is used as prevention of new uric acid formation and does not reduce the amount of uric acid already present. Thus, it should be initiated 2–3 days before starting cytotoxic therapy when used in patients with elevated uric acid at baseline. Allopurinol

Table 30.5. TLS prophylaxis recommendations based on TLS risk.

Low-risk disease (LRD)	Intermediate-risk disease (IRD)	High-risk disease (HRD)
ST[a]	N/A	N/A
MM	N/A	N/A
CML	N/A	N/A
Indolent NHL	N/A	N/A
HL	N/A	N/A
CLL[b]	N/A	N/A
AML and WBC < 25 K/mm^3 and LDH < 2 × ULN	AML with WBC 25–100 K/mm^3 AML and WBC < 25 K/mm^3 and LDH ≥ 2 × ULN	AML and WBC ≥ 100 K/mm^3
Adult intermediate grade NHL and LDH < 2 × ULN	Adult intermediate grade NHL and LDH ≥ 2 × ULN	N/A
Adult ALCL	Childhood ALCL stage III/IV	N/A
N/A	Childhood intermediate-grade NHL stage III/IV with LDH < 2 × ULN	N/A
N/A	ALL and WBC < 100 K/mm^3 and LDH < 2 × ULN	ALL and WBC ≥ 100 K/mm^3 and/or LDH ≥ 2 × ULN
N/A	BL and LDH < 2 × ULN	BL stage III/IV and/or LDH ≥ 2 × ULN
N/A	LL stage I/II and LDH < 2 × ULN	LL stage III/IV and/or LDH ≥ 2 × ULN
N/A	N/A	IRD with renal dysfunction and/or renal involvement
		IRD with uric acid, potassium and/or phosphate > ULN
Prophylaxis recommendations		
Monitoring	Monitoring	Monitoring
Hydration	Hydration	Hydration
± Allopurinol	Allopurinol	Rasburicase[c]

[a]Rare solid tumors such as neuroblastoma, germ cell tumors and small cell lung cancer or others with bulky or advanced stage disease may be classified as IRD.
[b]CLL treated with fludarabine, rituximab and/or those with high WBC (≥ 50 K/mm^3), should be classified as IRD.
[c]Contraindicated in patients with a history consistent with G-6PD. In these patients, rasburicase should be substituted with allopurinol.

ALCL: anaplastic large cell lymphoma, ALL: acute lymphoblastic leukaemia, AML: acute myelogenous leukaemia, BL: Burkitt lymphoma/leukaemia, CLL: chronic lymphoid leukaemia, CML: chronic myeloid leukaemia, HL: Hodgkin lymphoma, LDH: lactate dehydrogenase; LL: lymphoblastic lymphoma; MM: multiple myeloma; NHL: non-Hodgkin lymphoma, N/A: not applicable; ST: solid tumors; ULN: upper limit of normal; WBC: white blood cell count.

is generally given as an oral dose of at least 300 mg/m^2/day and continued through the start of therapy until the patient no longer shows evidence of TLS. Allopurinol via its known mechanism of action will interfere with the clearance of 6-mercaptopurine, 6-thioguanine, and azathioprine. To avoid severe mucositis and marrow toxicity, dosing adjustments of 50–75% should be made in patients receiving these agents.

Rasburicase is used either as an alternative to or in conjunction with allopurinol to control hyperuricemia. Rasburicase is a recombinant form of urate oxidase that works by promoting the catabolism of uric acid to allantoin (Fig. 30.2). Allantoin is 5 to 10 times more soluble in urine than uric acid. The gene encoding urate oxidase is absent in humans but has been cloned from *Aspergillus flavus*, allowing production and purification of a recombinant enzyme.[21] Although initial studies were performed using rasburicase daily for 5–7 days, subsequent clinical experience has demonstrated that much less frequent dosing is sufficient.

The safety and efficacy of rasburicase in children has been widely studied in the United States and Europe. A phase I/II multicenter trial conducted by Pui *et al.* in the United States, Canada and France enrolled 131 pediatric patients, aged 9 months to 20 years at high risk of developing TLS.[22] The majority of the patients had pre-B-cell ALL, T-cell ALL or advanced-stage NHL (stage III/IV) and approximately 50% had hyperuricemia at presentation. The first phase of the study established an effective dose of 0.2 mg/kg of rasburicase. This was effective at decreasing uric acid levels to undetectable levels within 48 hours of rasburicase initiation. In the subset of patients with hyperuricemia at the time of presentation, the median uric acid level decreased from 577 μmol/l

(9.7 mg/dl) to 60 μmol/l (1.0 mg/dl) ($p = 0.0001$). In addition, phosphorus and potassium levels remained stable throughout treatment duration and the median serum creatinine levels decreased significantly after only 1 day of treatment. Pharmacokinetic analysis revealed a half-life of rasburicase between 16–20 hours. Rasburicase treatment was well tolerated and no patients developed severe TLS or renal failure. Although antibodies to rasburicase did develop in approximately 15% of patients, they did not appear to be neutralizing or cause subsequent adverse events upon rechallenge of rasburicase.

Goldman *et al.* conducted the first randomized comparison of rasburicase to allopurinol in 52 pediatric patients with hematologic malignancies at high risk of TLS.[23] This multicenter, randomized trial compared 0.2 mg/kg/day of rasburicase given intravenously to oral allopurinol, 300 mg/m^2/day in three divided doses. Study subjects were stratified according to disease type and presenting uric acid levels. They were then randomized to receive rasburicase or allopurinol treatment for a total of 5–7 days. Four hours after drug administration uric acid levels decreased by 86% with rasburicase as compared to only 12% with allopurinol ($p < 0.0001$). The mean area-under-the-curve (uric acid plasma concentration vs. time) was significantly lower for patients treated with rasburicase (128 mg/dl/hour ± 70) compared to those receiving allopurinol (329 mg/dl/hour ± 129) ($p < 0.0001$). This represented a 2.6-fold decrease in uric acid exposure in the rasburicase vs. allopurinol treatment (Fig. 30.5).[23] Patients with hyperuricemia in the rasburicase arm experienced a decline from baseline serum creatinine levels while the patients with hyperuricemia assigned to allopurinol demonstrated a rise in serum creatinine levels. In this study, no patients developed allergic-type reactions, antibodies to rasburicase or grades III to IV toxicity attributed to rasburicase.

Pui *et al.* reported results of a multicenter compassionate use trial of rasburicase for the prophylaxis and treatment of hyperuricemia in 245 pediatric and adult patients with cancer at high risk of TLS.[24] Rasburicase was administered intravenously at a dose of 0.2 mg/kg for up to 7 days (median of three doses). Children receiving rasburicase for the treatment of hyperuricemia had a median decline of uric acid levels from 577 μmol/l (9.7 mg/dl) to 36 μmol/l (0.6 mg/dl) ($p < 0.001$). Ten pediatric patients (total of 4.1%) required hemodialysis for management of electrolyte disturbances. Eight of these patients had ARF on presentation and progressed to dialysis despite low uric acid levels post rasburicase. Overall rasburicase was well tolerated with only nine patients

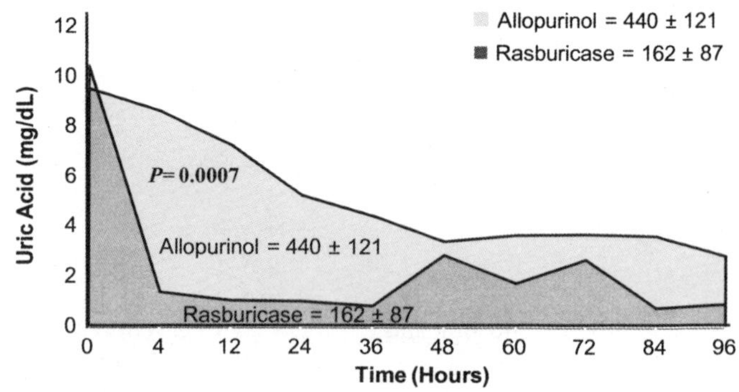

Fig. 30.5. Uric acid AUC 0–96 h mg/(dl h) by treatment.

This research was originally published in Blood. Goldman SC, Cairo MS, *et al.* A randomized comparison between rasburicase and allopurinol in children with lymphoma or leukemia at high risk for tumor lysis. Blood 2001; **97**: 2998–3003. © The American Society of Hematology.

experiencing mild adverse events. Bosly *et al.* also reported on a multicenter, international, compassionate use study using rasburicase in 278 adult and pediatric oncology patients.[25] Twenty-four percent of pediatric patients had elevated plasma uric acid levels at presentation. Median plasma uric acid levels decreased dramatically in children (672–12 μmol/l [11.3–0.2 mg/dl]) after rasburicase administration at 0.2 mg/kg for 1–7 days. Drug-related adverse events were observed in < 2% of patients and included headache, fever, rigors and mild allergic reaction (0.7%).

Recently, the Children's Oncology Group reported their results from the ANHL01P1 study on the assessment of toxicity from the addition of rasburicase in combination with cyclophosphamide, vincristine and prednisone (COP-R) during reduction therapy in children with advanced stage (St. Jude's Stages III, IV and Burkitt leukemia) B-cell NHL.[26] Part of the objectives of this study was to determine the safety of rasburicase administration, the incidence of both LTLS and CTLS during COP-R in children with B-NHL, and to estimate the percentage of children developing renal failure as well as those requiring renal support during reduction therapy. Standard intravenous fluid hydration was given to all patients without alkalinization and rasburicase was administered at a dose of 0.2 mg/kg intravenously on day 0 (4 hours prior to COP chemotherapy). Optionally dosing at days −3 to −1 and on days +1 to + 4 was permitted. Patients with French–American–British (FAB) group B disease (intermediate risk; $n = 48$) had no reported serious adverse events to single dose of rasburicase and no incidence of assisted renal support (dialysis or continuous veno-venous hemofiltration).

Patients with FAB group C disease (bone marrow ≥ 25% L3 blasts and/or central nervous system disease) are at greatest risk of metabolic complications during the COP reduction therapy. In ANHL01P1, data is available on 35 group C patients treated with reduction therapy, recombinant urate oxidase (Rasburicase) and non-alkaline hydration. Eighty-six percent of patients had an elevated LDH (> 2 times upper limit of normal) with the mean LDH ~ 6.5-fold greater than the upper limit of normal. Forty-four percent of patients had hyperuricemia at baseline with a mean uric acid of 714 µmol/l (12 mg/dl) in hyperuricemic patients. About half of FAB group C patients received optional doses of rasburicase prior to day 0 with the median number of total doses being two. There were no serious adverse events attributed to rasburicase administration. Ninety-four percent of patients had an improved estimated glomerular filtration rate at Day 7 of COP reduction. The initial mean glomerular filtration rate ± SD vs. end of COP reduction were 108 ± 42 and 173 ± 64 ml/min/1.73m^2, respectively (p, 0.05). Four patients required assisted renal support but all did so prior to initiating rasburicase. Three of four of these patients were successfully weaned from renal support by the end of COP reduction. Of the remaining patients, there was a 19% and 0% incidence of LTLS and CTLS after rasburicase, respectively. The addition of rasburicase to FAB COP reduction was well tolerated and demonstrated excellent control of tumor lysis and prevention of renal failure.[27]

Cost analysis

The results of a randomized international study of high-risk children and adolescents compared the overall incidence of renal insufficiency, TLS and dialysis during initial chemotherapy.[28] Patients treated in France (SFOP [Societe Francaise d'Oncologie Pediatrique]) had access to non-recombinant urate oxidase but those patients enrolled in Children's Cancer Group (CCG) did not and thus were treated with standard allopurinol instead. The overall incidence of renal insufficiency, TLS, and dialysis was significantly less in SFOP vs. CCG (renal insufficiency 11% vs. 27%, p < .005; TLS 9% vs. 26%, p < .002; and dialysis 3% vs. 15%, p < .004) (Table 30.6).[28] More specifically, total costs of care in both pediatrics and adults have been demonstrated to increase three- to fivefold with the development of renal failure and the need for dialysis.[5,29] Data from the Healthcare Cost and Utilization Project 2004 showed that among

Table 30.6. Incidence of TLS, renal failure and dialysis during radiation therapy (COP) for children with group C B-ALL ± CNS B-NHL FAB/LMB 96.

	All patients	SFOP non-recombinant urate oxidase	CCG allopurinol	*P*-Value
TLS	16%	11%	27%	0.005
Renal failure	20%	9%	26%	0.002
Dialysis	10%	3%	15%	0.004

B-ALL: B-cell acute lymphoblastic leukaemia; B-cell non-Hodgkin lymphoma; CCG: Children's Cancer Group; CNS: central nervous system; COP: cyclophosphamide; vincristine: prednisone; TLS: tumor lysis syndrome; B-NHL: FAB/LMB 96: French–American–British/mature lymphoma B; SFOP: Societe Francaise d'Oncologie Pediatrique.

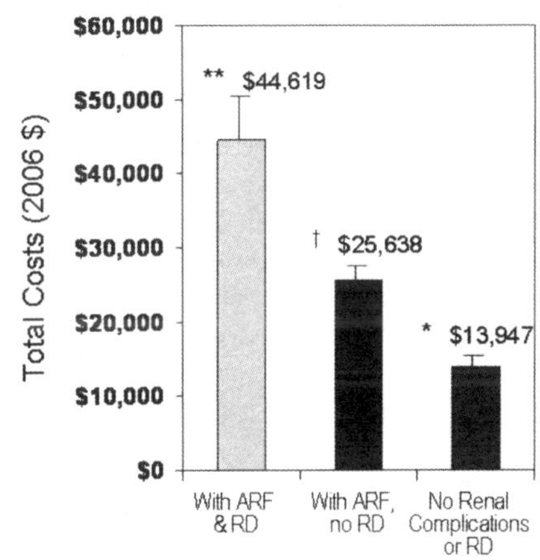

Fig. 30.6. (A) Mean total cost among patients with a hematologic malignancy with and without acute renal failure with or without renal dialysis.

Results represent the mean and 95% confidence interval limits of the total cost (in 2006 dollars).

**P* < .05; patients with acute renal failure with renal dialysis vs. patients with no renal complications or renal dialysis.

†*P* < .05; patients with acute renal failure with renal dialysis vs. patients with acute renal failure without renal dialysis.

‡*P* < .05; patients with acute renal failure without renal dialysis vs. patients with no renal complications or renal dialysis.

ARF: acute renal failure; RD: renal dialysis.

patients with hematologic malignancies undergoing induction chemotherapy who developed ARF, the mean length of stay and costs for patients with ARF with dialysis vs. without renal dialysis were 17.6 vs. 12.2 days, and $44,619 USD vs. $25,638 USD, respectively (Figs. 30.6A–B).[29] Clearly, reducing the incidence of ARF and the requirement for renal dialysis in patients with hematologic malignancies can alleviate some of the economic burden that accompanies these cases.

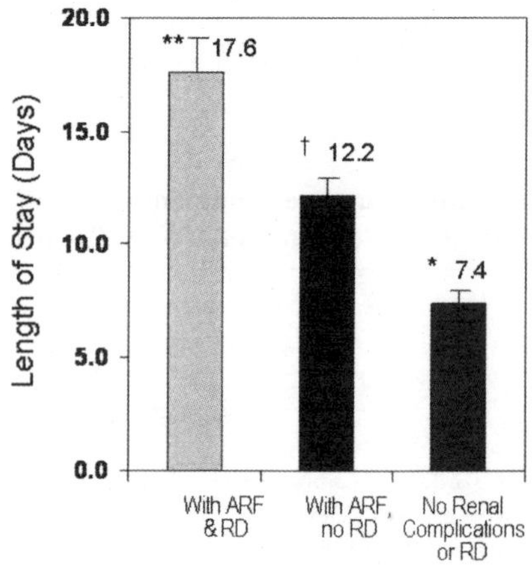

Fig. 30.6. (B) Mean length of stay among patients with a hematologic malignancy with and without acute renal failure with or without renal dialysis.
Results represent the mean and 95% confidence interval limits of the length of stay (in days).
*$P < .05$; patients with acute renal failure with renal dialysis vs. patients with no renal complications or renal dialysis.
†$P < .05$; patients with acute renal failure with renal dialysis vs. patients with acute renal failure without renal dialysis.
‡$P < .05$; patients with acute renal failure without renal dialysis vs. patients with no renal complications or renal dialysis.
ARF: acute renal failure; RD: renal dialysis.
Candrilli S., Bell T., Irish W., Morris., Goldman S., and Cairo M.S A comparison of inpatient length of stay and costs among patients with hematologic malignancies (excluding Hodgkin disease) associated with and without acute renal failure. Clinical Lymphoma and Myeloma 2008; 8(1):44–51.

Hyperleukocytosis

Definition and pathophysiology

Hyperleukocytosis denotes extreme elevation in the circulating WBC due to acute (AML, ALL) or chronic (CML) leukemias. The most widely reported definitional value is WBC > 100K but children can often tolerate much higher WBC before the clinical manifestations of hyperleukocytosis occur (Table 30.7). While complications of hyperleukocytosis such as coagulopathy and tumor lysis syndrome are discussed separately, the main clinical manifestation is leukostasis, a process of vascular obstruction leading to end organ damage and possible early death. The lungs and brain are the most commonly affected organs.[30]

The process of leukostasis has traditionally thought to be due to physical obstruction of the massive leukemic blasts (leukocrit) in the microcirculation. Because myeloblasts are ~ 2-fold larger than lymphoblasts, increased risk of leukostasis has been reported in both adult and pediatric AML patients.[31] Although extreme elevations in the WBC may increase blood viscosity, the usual severe anemia associated with newly diagnosed leukemia may have a compensatory role in reducing viscosity.[31] Recent elegant *in vitro* data points to the role of leukemic blast interaction with vascular endothelium as a key to the molecular pathology of leukostasis. Multiple adhesion receptors (L-selectin, E-selectin, VCAM-1 and CD11/CD18) are involved in blast cell adhesion to cytokine primed endothelium. For example, cytokine (TNF-alpha, IL-1 beta) secretion by myeloblasts in combination with upregulation of adhesion receptors (ICAM-1, and E-selectin) promotes a cascade of adhesion of leukemic blasts to vascular endothelium.[32]

Table 30.7. Key features of hyperleukocytosis.

- Definition is WBC > 100K but symptoms occur generally when:
  - AML (FAB M5) > 100K
  - AML > 200K
  - CML > 300K
  - ALL > 400K
- Symptoms related to upregulation of multiple adhesion receptors as well as cytokine secretion by myeloblasts promoting adhesion of leukemic blasts to vascular endothelium.
- Respiratory and CNS symptoms predominate including severe dyspnea and hypoxia, evidence of pulmonary vascular congestion on CXR, pulmonary hemorrhage and a range of mental status changes from subtle to seizure and obtundation.
- Therapy involves supportive care to promote tissue oxygenation and hemodynamic stability followed by early leukapheresis (or exchange transfusion) for significant clinical symptoms. Prompt initiation of disease specific therapy is crucial.

Evaluation and therapy

A WBC > 100 K at diagnosis should alert the clinician to look for the clinical signs and symptoms of hyperleukocytosis. Children with Philadelphia-chromosome positive CML more often present with higher WBC and clinical symptoms than adults. In one retrospective series, symptoms of leukostasis developed in 60% of pediatric CML (vs. 10% of adults) with a mean initial WBC count of 510 K in childhood cases with clinical symptoms (CNS and/or respiratory).[33] The recent addition of tyrosine kinase inhibitors (imatinab) to the treatment of CML in addition to early use of hydroxyurea for cytoreduction may decrease the need for early leukapheresis. In acute leukemia, pediatric AML has a four- to fivefold risk of mortality over ALL with elevated initial WBC > 100 K. In one large series of hyperleukocytosis in pediatric leukemia only 2 (1.2%) of ALL patients developed CNS manifestations (cerebral hemorrhage) as a result of leukostasis and both presented with WBC > 400 K.[34] In a review of treatment-related mortality in German trials of childhood AML, low performance status, hyperleukocytosis and FAB M5 phenotype were the main risk factors in death during the first 2 weeks of therapy.[35] In a large recent retrospective review at St. Jude's hospital of pediatric AML patients with initial WBC > 100 K ($n = 106$), investigators found that M5 and M4 phenotypes and higher initial WBC were strongly correlated with early deaths.[36]

The clinical evaluation of patients with suspected hyperleukocytosis should focus on the lungs and CNS.[31,37] Pulmonary symptoms may include severe dyspnea and hypoxia with "whited-out" chest radiographs and pulmonary vascular congestion. Pulmonary hemorrhage with hemoptysis and need for mechanical ventilation are ominous signs. Chest radiographs, pulse oximetry, and arterial blood gas analysis should be monitored serially in severely affected patients. CNS manifestations can range from asymptomatic to subtle mental status changes with progression to severe irritability/headache and eventually seizures/obtundation. A thorough view of the optic disks for signs of papilledema is helpful to diagnosis increased intracranial pressure. Early neuroimaging (preferably gadolinium-enhanced MRI) for patients with hyperleukocytosis and CNS symptoms is warranted prior to diagnostic/therapeutic lumbar puncture. MRI findings include cerebral vascular occlusion as well as parenchymal infarcts/hemorrhage.

Therapy for hyperleukocytosis begins with supportive therapy to promote tissue oxygenation and vascular volume in the critically ill patient. Platelet transfusions should be administered for bleeding and/or thrombocytopenia (< 20–30 K) but red cell administration should be done cautiously because of increased blood viscosity associated with red cells. The chief decision of the treating oncologist is whether to initiate specific oncological therapy or first initiate leukapheresis or exchange transfusion.[38] Unfortunately, there are no controlled studies to address this question but practical guidelines suggest that leukapheresis should be considered in those patients with clinical symptoms of leukostasis rather than an absolute white cell threshold. Both leukapheresis and exchange procedures are expected to reduce the WBC by approximate half per procedure. A recent single center experience in children reports an incidence of hyperleukocytosis of 14% in newly diagnosed leukemia patients over a 10-year period and reports successful therapeutic leukopheresis or exchange in 6 out of 11 patients with no procedural complications.[39] Patients with APML should not undergo leukapheresis as it may trigger worsening coagulopathy upon lysis of the leukemic blasts. Mechanical removal of malignant blasts is a temporizing measure that should be followed by disease specific chemotherapy as soon as possible. Cranial radiation therapy for CNS leukostasis is no longer recommended.[40,41] Although we are unlikely to ever have future multicenter trials, it would be helpful to establish clinical registries to investigate, prospectively, the benefits and complications of leukapheresis as well as short and long-term survival of pediatric patients requiring hyperleukocytosis intervention. One area of future research may be the use of pharmacological inhibitors of the interaction of the vascular endothelium and leukemic blast. Discouragingly, despite the improvement in supportive care and decreased early deaths in the more modern era in AML patients with hyperleukocytosis, the ultimate survival remains ~ half that of patients without hyperleukocytosis.[36]

Superior Mediastinal Syndrome

Definition and pathophysiology

Superior mediastinal syndrome (SMS) is an inclusive term that refers to clinically significant compression by a mediastinal mass of the superior vena cava (often referred to as SVC syndrome) and/or airway. In pediatric hematopoietic malignancies, SMS may present as the first manifestation of a new diagnosis and may even lead to cardiorespiratory arrest prior to diagnosis and initiation of therapy.[42] Unlike adults, pediatric patients most often present with external compression of their airway. Younger children are especially vulnerable due to the smaller diameter of the airway and increased developmental compliance of the trachea and main-stem bronchi. Although Hodgkin lymphoma, mediastinal B-cell lymphoma, and anaplastic large cell lymphoma frequently present with mediastinal masses and may have respiratory symptoms, the most notable pediatric malignancy to cause acute airway compromise is T-ALL/T lymphoblastic lymphoma with reports of up to 90% of patients with SVC obstruction subsequently found to have one of these two diseases.[43] The clinical diagnosis of SMS rests on carefully evaluating the patient for airway and cardiovascular compromise. Patients may present with cough, dyspnea, orthopnea and signs of positional distress. Depending on the level of compression, upper airway (stridor) and/or lower airway (wheezing/decreased

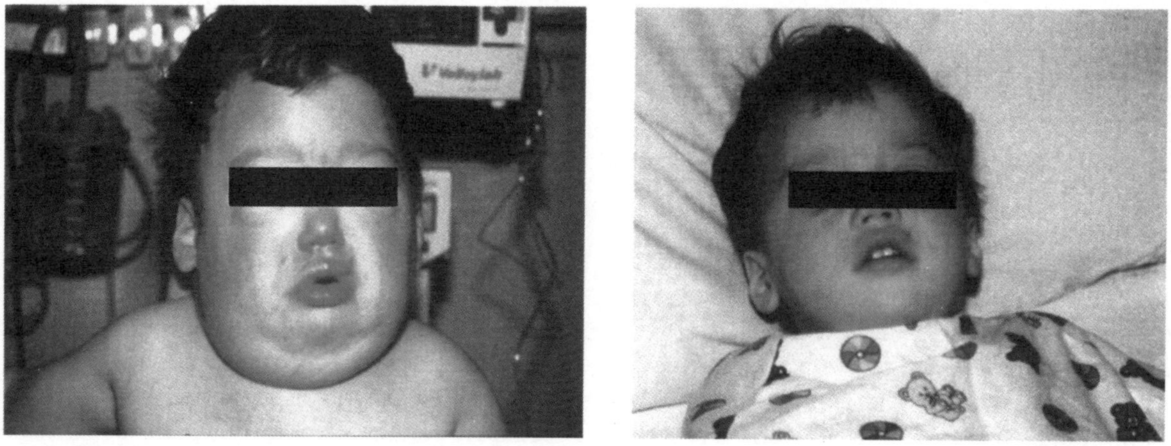

Fig. 30.7. Clinical appearance of superior mediastinal syndrome. A 5-year-old boy with massive facial and periorbital edema secondary to superior mediastinal syndrome both pre- and post-initiation of treatment.

breath sounds) findings may predominate. When upper venous return to the heart is compromised patients may complain of facial swelling that can be mistaken for acute anaphylaxis by families and caregivers. Figure 30.7 shows a 5-year-old boy with new onset T-ALL presenting with massive facial/periorbital edema. Not uncommonly, patients may have received several steroid pulses for clinical diagnosis of asthma or allergic reaction prior to their correct diagnosis.

Diagnosis and management

The diagnosis of SMS rests on careful history and physical exam. In younger anxious children (much like croup), the ideal location for exam is on their parent's lap. A two-view chest radiograph is essential to define the level of tracheal compression and/or deviation. An echocardiogram is extremely useful to define the compromise to venous return and any associated pericardial effusions. Computerized tomography of the chest is also very useful to define the size of the mass and accurately demonstrate airway narrowing (Fig. 30.8) but may be difficult due to sedation concerns in younger children and worsening airway compromise associated with supine position. The chief management balance is to rapidly make a diagnosis of the underlying malignancy (and start appropriate therapy) in the least invasive manner possible. For example, for the patient shown in Fig. 30.7, conscious sedation was performed by an experienced pediatric anesthesiologist in the sitting upright position and a lumbar puncture and anterior crest bone marrow aspirate demonstrated T-ALL. The patient was managed with several days of intravenous steroids prior to general anesthesia and placement of central venous catheter for multiagent chemotherapy. When peripheral studies are negative, CT or ultrasound guided mediastinal biopsies may be accomplished. A recent report demonstrates the utility of flow cytometry in the diagnosis of mediastinal tumors with rapid turnaround time and high accuracy.[44] Children with anterior mediastinal lymphoma and leukemia may experience significant risks with general anesthesia including death. General anesthesia relaxes bronchial and respiratory smooth muscle tones and diminishes lung volumes which can lead to cardiovascular failure. Ricketts suggests that when baseline peak expiratory flow rate and the tracheal cross-sectional area are both less than 50% of predicted values that general anesthesia should not be undertaken.[45] A more recent single center review found that perioperative respiratory complications were confined to patients with an isolated tracheal cross-sectional area less than 30% normal or less than 70% with associated bronchial compression.[46] In the largest series reported to date, investigators at St. Jude's found that 9.4% of patients with mediastinal masses developed anesthesia related complications and that the preoperative features associated with complications included upper body edema (OR 8), orthopnea, main-stem bronchus compression and great vessel compression (OR ~ 5).[47] Finally, it is the rare patient who requires emergent empiric therapy prior to histological diagnosis. Both low-dose steroids and emergent low-dose radiation[48] have been successfully used in this setting.

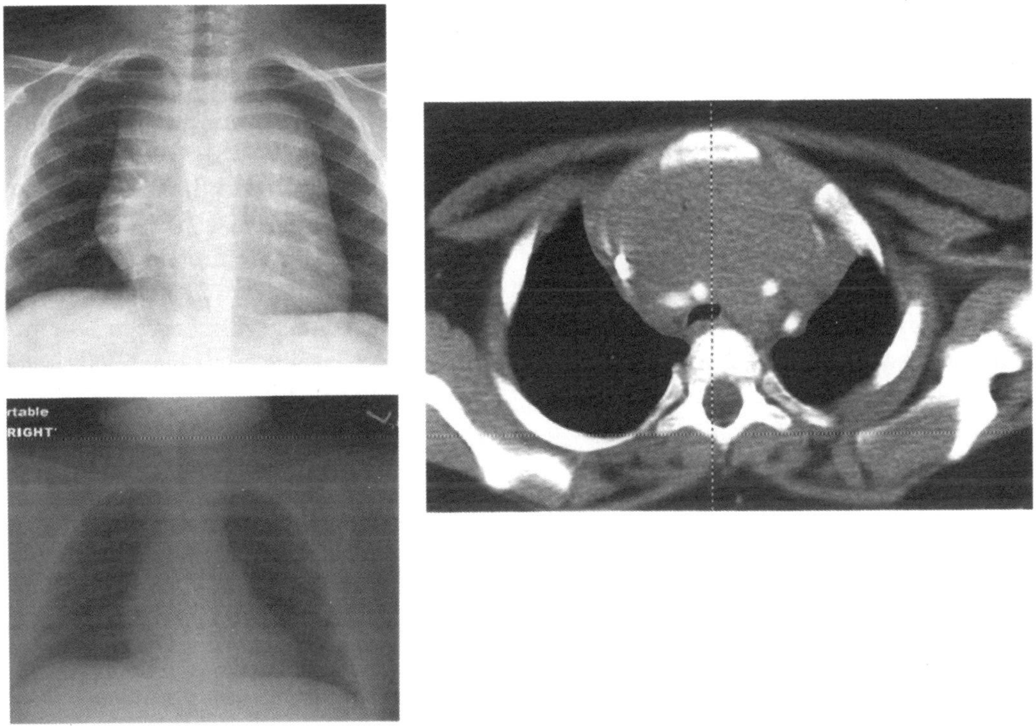

Fig. 30.8. Computerized tomography of a patient with superior mediastinal syndrome. CXR and CT scan of the chest showing a large mediastinal mass causing displacement and compression of the trachea.

Coagulopathy and Thrombosis

Thrombocytopenia

Thrombocytopenia is a commonly encountered presenting symptom in patients with hematologic malignancies and can result from either underproduction or consumption. Often, this has led to bleeding symptoms ranging from mild to severe that have prompted further evaluation thus leading to a diagnosis. Many patients present with mild bleeding symptoms such as bruising, petechiae or controlled epistaxis. However, a subset of patients may present with life-threatening hemorrhage. The definition of thrombocytopenia is a platelet count < 150,000. However, risk for life threatening bleeds is usually not increased until severe thrombocytopenia develops (platelets < 50,000). Aggressive transfusion support to maintain platelet counts above this range is critical, especially in the bleeding patient. Although there is no definitive data to suggest an absolute threshold to maintain platelets, most oncologists choose prophylactic platelet transfusions to keep platelet counts at least above 10,000 which has led to a decrease in bleeding complications allowing for improved survival. However, confirmatory studies in support of this practice are still needed. In addition to this, correction of abnormal-associated coagulopathy with FFP, cryoprecipitate or recombinant FVIIa is beneficial in the management of hemorrhage in patients with concurrent thrombocytopenia.

Coagulopathy associated with pediatric acute promyelocytic leukemia (APL)

APL is a subtype of AML with an excellent long-term prognosis when treated with combination chemotherapy and differentiation therapy such as all-trans retinoic acid (ATRA) (see Chapter 13). Coagulopathy, with both hemorrhagic and thrombotic complications, remains an early source of mortality with CNS hemorrhage an especially devastating early treatment event. Evidence of disseminated intravascular coagulation, fibrinolysis and proteolysis often occur simultaneously. Increased annexin II expression in the APL cell, circulating tumor-derived microparticles, and cerebral microvasculature with resultant fibrinolysis has been recently suggested to play a key role in the pathogenesis of the bleeding diathesis.[49,50] Because of the relative rarity in pediatrics there are few reports of incidence. A large Spanish pediatric (< 18 years) cohort reported three fatal CNS hemorrhages during induction among 66 patients treated with combination ATRA and idarubicin.[51] Likewise, Chinese investigators reported two fatal CNS bleeds among 19 newly diagnosed APL patients treated with arsenic trioxide monotherapy.[52] Spanish investigators have found increased peripheral blast counts and presence of coagulopathy as risk factors for development of fatal hemorrhage during induction.[53] Both prophylactic anticoagulation therapy (heparin, LMWH) and/or antifibrinolytic therapy have not been demonstrated to prevent bleeding or thrombosis in children and adults with APL.[53] All patients should be serially monitored with coagulation studies (including PT, aPTT, fibrinogen and fibrin split products) and complete blood counts with early administration of platelet transfusions, FFP and cryoprecipitate. The most important management is rapid initiation of ATRA which can begin to correct the coagulopathy within 24–48 hours and has been demonstrated to decrease the need for blood product replacement.[54,55]

Asparaginase-associated thrombosis

Pathogenesis and epidemiology

Unlike many adult protocols, asparaginase is an integral component of most induction and consolidation treatments of pediatric acute lymphoblastic leukemia including T and pre B-cell phenotypes. The inhibition of protein synthesis induced by asparaginase has long been known to have profound effects on the procoagulant (e.g. fibrinogen) and anticoagulant proteins (e.g. AT III) which can lead to both hemorrhagic and thrombotic complications.[56] Although children and adolescents in general have less thrombotic complications than their adult counterparts, clinicians should have a heightened awareness for signs and symptoms of venous thromboembolism (VTE) in children treated with asparaginase chemotherapy. This could include central venous catheter obstruction, extremity swelling and/or pain and most importantly CNS symptoms which can vary from headache to rapid onset seizures or obtundation. The cerebral sinovenous system should be imaged with MRI including magnetic resonance venography in children with neurological deterioration receiving asparaginase. The reported prevalence of VTE in pediatric ALL patients receiving asparaginase varies widely based on the intensity of screening methods used. For example, Canadian investigators found a venous thromboembolic incidence of $>1/3$ when screening all patients with bilateral venograms, ultrasound, MRI and echocardiography.[57] A large meta-analysis in >1700 pediatric ALL patients from 17 prospective studies found an overall symptomatic VTE incidence and cerebral sinus thrombosis incidence of 5% and 3%, respectively.[58] Additional risk factors for VTE include age >10 years, CVL-dysfunction and intrathoacic tumor.[59] Concomitant of use steroid therapy, inherited prothrombotic states and the presence of antiphospholipid antibodies have all been reported to increase the risk of symptomatic VTE.[57,60]

Monitoring and therapy

Unfortunately, there is a lack of evidence-based recommendations for monitoring the coagulation system in children with ALL receiving asparaginase during the early phases of therapy. There is also no randomized study in children proving prophylactic therapies actually prevent thrombotic complications in children treated with asparaginase. Thus, monitoring and therapy seems to be institutionally and historically based. A prospective study of fibrinogen monitoring and replacement with fresh frozen plasma (FFP) failed to show even a benefit in biochemical parameters such as ATIII and plasminogen.[61] A recent study examined historical cohorts of patients treated with BFM-based therapy. All patients received antithrombin supplementation to maintain plasma AT III levels $>50\%$ but the more recent cohort of patients received concomitant low molecular weight heparin (LMWH) prophylaxis. Nine out of seventy-one (including three CNS) symptomatic thrombotic events occurred in the AT III only group and 0 out of 41 in the AT III/LMWH group.[62] Investigators in two Canadian institutions with different monitoring and prophylaxis strategies investigated their institutional incidence of CNS thrombosis. At the "prophylactic" institution prospective fibrinogen and AT III monitoring with supplementation with cryoprecipitate and FFP, respectively were employed with an incidence of 0 out of 240 ALL patients experiencing CNS thrombosis vs. 7 out of 479 in the other institution.[63] With the recent approval of oral direct thrombin inhibitors and recombinant antithrombin, one hopes that a prospective study could be undertaken to guide clinicians as to what (if any) is the appropriate preemptive monitoring and prophylactic strategy. Once a clinically recognized VTE occurs, the treatment should include restoration of normal anticoagulation proteins with supplemental FFP, cryoprecipitate and AT III as appropriate followed by anticoagulation therapy. Unique challenges in the pediatric ALL patients include concomitant thrombocytopenia and frequent need of invasive procedures such as lumbar punctures. LMWHs (e.g. enoxaparin) are attractive because of their short half lives and less need for frequent monitoring. Once clinical and radiographic improvement is seen future asparaginase is probably warranted. For the rare child with CNS or other life-threatening hemorrhages associated with asparaginase, rapid correction of thrombocytopenia and coagulopathy is necessary. A recent report details the successful use of recombinant factor VIIa as additional therapy.[64]

Conclusion

Current advances in the treatment of hematologic malignancies in children, adolescents and young adults have provided an expectation of cure. Life-threatening complications from oncologic emergencies in the initial diagnostic and treatment phases can be devastating and can often be avoided or successfully managed if vigilant monitoring and aggressive treatment is initiated. This chapter detailed several of these complications, including tumor lysis syndrome (TLS), hyperleukocytosis (HL), superior mediastinal syndrome (SMS), and coagulopathy/thrombosis (C/T). Recent guidelines in the recognition of at risk patient groups for development of TLS have led to earlier interventions and aggressive control of hyperuricemia and its resulting complications using hydration, allopurinol and newer agents such as rasburicase. This will not only lead to reductions in prolonged hospital stays, but more importantly, ability to give full dose cytoxic therapy without delay. Similarly, early recognition of hyperleukocytosis with CNS and pulmonary symptoms as well as significant coagulopathies and evidence of superior mediastinal syndrome also requires identification of at risk patients and careful clinical evaluation. Once identified, appropriate supportive care should be initiated promptly so that treatment can begin and catastrophic events avoided. Even with improved tools to manage oncologic emergencies, knowledge and prevention remain key to improving outcomes in all patients with hematologic malignancies.

References

1. Cairo MS, Bishop M. (2004) Tumour lysis syndrome: New therapeutic strategies and classification. *Br J Haematol* **127**(1): 3–11.
2. Del Toro G, Morris E, Cairo MS. (2005) Tumor lysis syndrome: Pathophysiology, definition, and alternative treatment approaches. *Clin Adv Hematol Oncol* **3**(1): 54–61.
3. Hochberg J, Cairo MS. (2008) Tumor lysis syndrome: Current perspective. *Haematologica* **93**(1): 9–13.
4. Jeha S. (2001) Tumor lysis syndrome. *Semin Hematol* **38**(4 Suppl 10): 4–8.
5. Annemans L, *et al.* (2003) Incidence, medical resource utilisation and costs of hyperuricemia and tumour lysis syndrome in patients with acute leukaemia and non-Hodgkin's lymphoma in four European countries. *Leuk Lymphoma* **44**(1): 77–83.
6. Montesinos P, *et al.* (2008) Tumor lysis syndrome in patients with acute myeloid leukemia: Identification of risk factors and development of a predictive model. *Haematologica* **93**: 67–74.
9. Hande KR, Garrow GC. (1993) Acute tumor lysis syndrome in patients with high-grade non-Hodgkin's lymphoma. *Am J Med* **94**(2): 133–139.
10. Hochberg J, Cairo MS. (2008) Rasburicase: Future directions in tumor lysis management. *Expert Opin Biol Ther* **8**(10): 1595–1604.
11. Wossmann W, *et al.* (2003) Incidence of tumor lysis syndrome in children with advanced stage Burkitt's lymphoma/leukemia before and after introduction of prophylactic use of urate oxidase. *Ann Hematol* **82**(3): 160–165.
15. Bessmertny O, Robitaille LM, Cairo MS. (2005) Rasburicase: A new approach for preventing and/or treating tumor lysis syndrome. *Curr Pharm Des* **11**(32): 4177–4185.
16. Coiffier B, *et al.* (2008) Guidelines for the management of pediatric and adult tumor lysis syndrome: An evidence-based review. *J Clin Oncol* **26**(16): 2767–2778.
17. Goldman S, *et al.* (2009) A medical decision tree for the prophylaxis (P) and treatment (T) of tumor lysis syndrome (TLS): An international TLS consensus panel. *J Clin Oncol* **27**: (abstract e17575a).
18. Rampello E, Fricia T, Malaguarnera M. (2006) The management of tumor lysis syndrome. *Nat Clin Pract Oncol* **3**(8): 438–447.
20. Klinenberg JR, Goldfinger SE, Seegmiller JE. (1965) The effectiveness of the xanthine oxidase inhibitor Allopurinol in the treatment of Gout. *Ann Intern Med* **62**: 639647.
21. Legoux R, *et al.* (1992) Cloning and expression in Escherichia coli of the gene encoding Aspergillus flavus urate oxidase. *J Biol Chem* **267**(12): 8565–8570.
22. Pui CH, *et al.* (2001) Recombinant urate oxidase for the prophylaxis or treatment of hyperuricemia in

patients with leukemia or lymphoma. *J Clin Oncol* **19**(3): 697–704.
23. Goldman SC, *et al.* (2001) A randomized comparison between rasburicase and allopurinol in children with lymphoma or leukemia at high risk for tumor lysis. *Blood* **97**(10): 2998–3003.
24. Pui CH, *et al.* (2001) Recombinant urate oxidase (rasburicase) in the prevention and treatment of malignancy-associated hyperuricemia in pediatric and adult patients: Results of a compassionate-use trial. *Leukemia* **15**(10): 1505–1509.
25. Bosly A, *et al.* (2003) Rasburicase (recombinant urate oxidase) for the management of hyperuricemia in patients with cancer: Report of an international compassionate use study. *Cancer* **98**(5): 1048–1054.
26. Goldman S, *et al.* (2009) Effective and safe acute tumor lysis syndrome (ATLS) prophylaxis with Rasburicase and non-alkaline hydration in children and adolescents with advanced stage III/IV intermediate risk B-cell non-Hodgkin lymphoma (B-NHL): A Children's Oncology Group Report. *Pediatr Blood Cancer* **52**(6): 145.
27. Goldman S, *et al.* (2009) Preliminary results of the addition of Rasburicase to the reduction cycle and Rituximab to the induction and consolidation cycles of FAB group C chemotherapy in children and adolescents with advanced stage (bone marrow ± CNS) mature B-cell non-Hodgkin lymphoma (B-NHL): A Children's Oncology Group Report in *American Society of Hematology* (abstract). New Orleans, LA.
28. Cairo MS, *et al.* (2007) Results of a randomized international study of high-risk central nervous system B non-Hodgkin lymphoma and B acute lymphoblastic leukemia in children and adolescents. *Blood* **109**(7): 2736–2743.
29. Candrilli S, *et al.* (2008) A comparison of inpatient length of stay and costs among patients with hematologic malignancies (excluding hodgkin disease) associated with and without acute renal failure. *Clin Lymphoma Myeloma* **8**(1): 44–51.
31. Porcu P, *et al.* (2000) Hyperleukocytic leukemias and leukostasis: A review of pathophysiology, clinical presentation and management. *Leuk Lymphoma* **39**(1–2): 1–18.
32. Stucki A, *et al.* (2001) Endothelial cell activation by myeloblasts: Molecular mechanisms of leukostasis and leukemic cell dissemination. *Blood* **97**(7): 2121–2129.
34. Bunin NJ, Pui CH. (1985) Differing complications of hyperleukocytosis in children with acute lymphoblastic or acute nonlymphoblastic leukemia. *J Clin Oncol* **3**(12): 1590–1595.
35. Creutzig U, *et al.* (2004) Early deaths and treatment-related mortality in children undergoing therapy for acute myeloid leukemia: Analysis of the multicenter clinical trials AML-BFM 93 and AML-BFM 98. *J Clin Oncol* **22**(21): 4384–4393.
36. Inaba H, *et al.* (2008) Clinical and biologic features and treatment outcome of children with newly diagnosed acute myeloid leukemia and hyperleukocytosis. *Cancer* **113**(3): 522–529.
38. Blum W, Porcu P. (2007) Therapeutic apheresis in hyperleukocytosis and hyperviscosity syndrome. *Semin Thromb Hemostasis* **33**(4): 350–354.
39. Haase R, *et al.* (2009) Leukapheresis and exchange transfusion in children with acute leukemia and hyperleukocytosis. A single center experience. *Klin Padiatr* **221**(6): 374–378.
42. Hon KL, *et al.* (2005) Critical airway obstruction, superior vena cava syndrome, and spontaneous cardiac arrest in a child with acute leukemia. *Pediatr Emerg Care* **21**(12): 844–846.
43. Arya LS, *et al.* (2002) Superior vena cava syndrome. *Indian J Pediatr* **69**(4): 293–297.
45. Ricketts RR. (2001) Clinical management of anterior mediastinal tumors in children. *Semin Pediatr Surg* **10**(3): 161–168.
46. Hack HA, Wright NB, Wynn RF. (2008) The anaesthetic management of children with anterior mediastinal masses. *Anaesthesia* **63**(8): 837–846.
47. Anghelescu DL, *et al.* (2007) Clinical and diagnostic imaging findings predict anesthetic complications in children presenting with malignant mediastinal masses. *Paediatr Anaesth* **17**(11): 1090–1098.
48. Bertsch H, *et al.* (1998) Emergent/urgent therapeutic irradiation in pediatric oncology: Patterns of presentation, treatment, and outcome. *Med Pediatr Oncol* **30**(2): 101–105.
49. Tallman MS, Abutalib SA, Altman JK. (2007) The double hazard of thrombophilia and bleeding in acute promyelocytic leukemia. *Semin Thromb Hemostasis* **33**(4): 330–338.
50. Stein E, *et al.* (2009) The coagulopathy of acute promyelocytic leukaemia revisited. *Best Pract Res Clin Haematol* **22**(1): 153–163.
52. Zhou J, *et al.* (2009) Single-agent arsenic trioxide in the treatment of children with newly diagnosed acute promyelocytic leukemia. *Blood* **115**(9): 1697–1702.
53. de la Serna J, *et al.* (2008) Causes and prognostic factors of remission induction failure in patients with acute promyelocytic leukemia treated with all-trans retinoic acid and idarubicin. *Blood* **111**(7): 3395–3402.
54. Tallman MS, *et al.* (2004) Effects of all-trans retinoic acid or chemotherapy on the molecular regulation of systemic blood coagulation and fibrinolysis in patients with

acute promyelocytic leukemia. *J Thromb Haemostasis* **2**(8): 1341–1350.

55. di Bona E, *et al.* (2000) Early haemorrhagic morbidity and mortality during remission induction with or without all-trans retinoic acid in acute promyelocytic leukaemia. *Br J Haematol* **108**(4): 689–695.
56. Earl M. (2009) Incidence and management of asparaginase-associated adverse events in patients with acute lymphoblastic leukemia. *Clin Adv Hematol Oncol* **7**(9): 600–606.
57. Mitchell LG, *et al.* (2003) A prospective cohort study determining the prevalence of thrombotic events in children with acute lymphoblastic leukemia and a central venous line who are treated with L-asparaginase: Results of the Prophylactic Antithrombin Replacement in Kids with Acute Lymphoblastic Leukemia Treated with Asparaginase (PARKAA) study. *Cancer* **97**(2): 508–516.
58. Caruso V, *et al.* (2006) Thrombotic complications in childhood acute lymphoblastic leukemia: A meta-analysis of 17 prospective studies comprising 1752 pediatric patients. *Blood* **108**(7): 2216–2222.
59. Athale U, *et al.* (2008) Epidemiology and clinical risk factors predisposing to thromboembolism in children with cancer. *Pediatr Blood Cancer* **51**(6): 792–797.
60. Athale UH, Chan AK. (2007) Thromboembolic complications in pediatric hematologic malignancies. *Semin Thromb Hemostasis* **33**(4): 416–426.
62. Meister B, *et al.* (2008) Comparison of low-molecular-weight heparin and antithrombin versus antithrombin alone for the prevention of symptomatic venous thromboembolism in children with acute lymphoblastic leukemia. *Pediatr Blood Cancer* **50**(2): 298–303.
63. Abbott LS, *et al.* (2009) The impact of prophylactic fresh-frozen plasma and cryoprecipitate on the incidence of central nervous system thrombosis and hemorrhage in children with acute lymphoblastic leukemia receiving asparaginase. *Blood* **114**(25): 5146–5151.
64. Ucar C, Caliskan U. (2006) Successful treatment of acute lymphoblastic leukemia with L-asparaginase-induced intracranial hemorrhage to activated recombinant factor VIIa in a child. *Pediatr Hematol Oncol* **23**(4): 339–345.

Index